THIRD EDITION

THERAPEUTIC EXERCISE

for

MUSCULOSKELETAL INJURIES

ATHLETIC TRAINING EDUCATION SERIES

Peggy A. Houglum, PhD, ATC, PT

Duquesne University

• • •

David H. Perrin, PhD, ATC
Series Editor
University of North Carolina at Greensboro

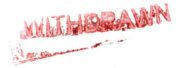

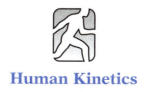

Human Kinetics

Library of Congress Cataloging-in-Publication Data

Houglum, Peggy A., 1948-
   Therapeutic exercise for musculoskeletal injuries / Peggy A. Houglum. -- 3rd ed.
      p. ; cm. -- (Athletic training education series)
   Includes bibliographical references and index.
   ISBN-13: 978-0-7360-7595-4 (print)
   ISBN-10: 0-7360-7595-X (print)
   1. Sports injuries--Exercise therapy. 2. Musculoskeletal system--Wounds and injuries--Exercise therapy. I. Title. II. Series: Athletic training education series.
   [DNLM: 1. Athletic Injuries--therapy. 2. Exercise Therapy--methods. 3. Musculoskeletal System--injuries. 4. Sports Medicine--methods. QT 261 H838t 2010]
   RD97.H6843 2010
   615.8'2--dc22
                                2009024390

ISBN-10: 0-7360-7595-X (print)
ISBN-13: 978-0-7360-7595-4 (print)

The Web addresses cited in this text were current as of June, 2009, unless otherwise noted.

Acquisitions Editor: Loarn D. Robertson, PhD; **Series Developmental Editor:** Amanda S. Ewing; **Developmental Editor:** Jillian Evans; **Managing Editor:** Katherine Maurer; **Assistant Editor:** Steven Calderwood; **Copyeditor:** Joyce Sexton; **Proofreader:** Red Inc.; **Indexer:** Andrea J. Hepner; **Permission Manager:** Dalene Reeder; **Graphic Designer:** Bob Reuther; **Graphic Artist:** Dawn Sills; **Cover Designer:** Keith Blomberg; **Photographer (cover):** © Human Kinetics; **Photographer (interior):** © Human Kinetics unless otherwise noted. Photos on pages 136, 329, 332, 422, 434, 473, 507, 513, 634, 639, 719, 721, 722 by Neil Bernstein; photos on pages 330, 510, 777 courtesy of Peggy Houglum. **Visual Production Assistant:** Joyce Brumfield; **Photo Production Manager:** Jason Allen; **Art Manager:** Kelly Hendren; **Associate Art Manager:** Alan L. Wilborn; **Illustrators:** Argosy, Angela K. Snyder, Dawn Sills, and Mike Meyer; **Printer:** Courier Companies, Inc.

We thank the Palumbo Center at Duquesne University in Pittsburgh, Pennsylvania, for assistance in providing the location for the photo shoot for this book.

Printed in the United States of America   10   9   8   7   6

The paper in this book was manufactured using responsible forestry methods.

Human Kinetics
Web site: www.HumanKinetics.com

United States: Human Kinetics
P.O. Box 5076
Champaign, IL 61825-5076
800-747-4457
e-mail: humank@hkusa.com

Canada: Human Kinetics
475 Devonshire Road Unit 100
Windsor, ON N8Y 2L5
800-465-7301 (in Canada only)
e-mail: info@hkcanada.com

Europe: Human Kinetics
107 Bradford Road
Stanningley
Leeds LS28 6AT, United Kingdom
+44 (0) 113 255 5665
e-mail: hk@hkeurope.com

Australia: Human Kinetics
57A Price Avenue
Lower Mitcham, South Australia 5062
08 8372 0999
e-mail: info@hkaustralia.com

New Zealand: Human Kinetics
P.O. Box 80
Torrens Park, South Australia 5062
0800 222 062
e-mail: info@hknewzealand.com

E4585

For Dan. I am so very pleased with your willingness to carry on for the next generation of athletic trainers in health care.

CONTENTS

CHAPTER 8   The ABCs of Proprioception 255

CHAPTER 9   Plyometrics 271

CHAPTER 10   Functional and Activity-Specific Exercise 295

| PART III | General Therapeutic Exercise Applications | 319 |

INTRODUCTION TO THE ATHLETIC TRAINING EDUCATION SERIES

The six titles of the Athletic Training Education Series—*Core Concepts in Athletic Training and Therapy, Examination of Musculoskeletal Injuries, Therapeutic Exercise for Musculoskeletal Injuries, Therapeutic Modalities for Musculoskeletal Injuries, Management Strategies in Athletic Training,* and *Developing Clinical Proficiency in Athletic Training*—are textbooks for students of athletic training and references for practicing certified athletic trainers. Other allied health care professionals, such as physical therapists, physician's assistants, and occupational therapists, will also find these texts to be invaluable resources in the prevention, examination, treatment, and rehabilitation of injuries to physically active people.

The rapidly evolving profession of athletic training necessitates a continual updating of the educational resources available to educators, students, and practitioners. The authors of the six books in the series have made key improvements and have added information based on the most recent version of the NATA *Athletic Training Educational Competencies* before publication.

- *Core Concepts in Athletic Training and Therapy,* which replaces *Introduction to Athletic Training,* is suitable for introductory athletic training courses. Part I of the text introduces students to the idea of prevention. It also addresses the preparticipation exam (PPE), introduces aspects of fitness testing and conditioning in athletes, looks at the nutrition aspects of health and performance, examines how the environment affects athletic participation, looks at the protective devices used in various sports, and introduces methods of taping and bracing. Part II covers clinical examination and diagnosis, including injury mechanism and classification; the principles of primary and secondary surveys; injuries and conditions that affect the upper and lower extremities, spine, head, neck, thorax, and abdomen; and general medical conditions. Part III covers acute and emergency care, including planning for emergency situations, immediate care for emergency situations, moving and transporting injured athletes, creating an emergency care plan, and obtaining consent for emergency care. Part IV covers therapeutic interventions, including rehabilitation and healing, therapeutic treatment modalities used in athletics, therapeutic exercise parameters and techniques, and pharmacology in athletic training. Part V introduces topics related to health care administration, including information on management functions and insurance. Part VI covers advanced concepts, such as pathophysiology of tissue injury, psychology of sport injury, and evidence-based practice in athletic training. *Core Concepts in Athletic Training and Therapy* fills the need for a text that covers myriad topics at an introductory level. It sets the stage for the other books in the series, which delve much deeper into specific topics.

- In *Examination of Musculoskeletal Injuries,* new information about sensitivity and specificity strengthens the evidence-based selection of special tests, and an increased emphasis on clinical decision making and problem solving and the integration of skill application in the end-of-chapter activities are now included.

- Two new chapters have been added to *Therapeutic Exercise for Musculoskeletal Injuries.* Chapter 16 focuses on arthroplasty, and chapter 17 contains information regarding various age considerations in rehabilitation. This text also provides more support of evidence-based care resulting from a blend of research results and the author's 40 years of experience as a clinician.

- The new edition of *Developing Clinical Proficiency in Athletic Training* contains 26 new modules, and embedded within it is the NATA *Athletic Training Educational Competencies.* The concepts of progressive clinical skill development, clinical supervision and autonomy, and clinical decision making are introduced and explained. The nature of critical thinking and why it is essential to clinical practice are also discussed.

- The third edition of *Therapeutic Modalities for Musculoskeletal Injuries* continues to provide readers with information on evidence-based practice and includes recent developments in the areas of inflammation and laser therapy.

- The fourth edition of *Management Strategies in Athletic Training* continues to help undergraduate and graduate students master entry-level concepts related to administration in athletic training. Each of the 10 chapters is thoroughly updated, and new material is presented on topics such as evidence-based medicine, professionalism in athletic training, health care financial management, cultural competence, injury surveillance systems, legal updates, and compensation for athletic trainers.

The Athletic Training Education Series offers a coordinated approach to the process of preparing students for the Board of Certification examination. If you are a student of athletic training, you must master the material in each of the content areas delineated in the NATA *Athletic Training Educational Competencies.* The Athletic Training Education Series addresses each of the competencies sequentially and thoroughly. The series covers the content areas developed by the NATA Executive Committee for Education of the National Athletic Trainers' Association for accredited curriculum development. The content areas and the texts that address each content area are as follows:

- Risk management and injury prevention *(Core Concepts* and *Management Strategies)*

- Pathology of injury and illnesses *(Core Concepts, Examination, Therapeutic Exercise,* and *Therapeutic Modalities)*

- Orthopedic assessment and diagnosis *(Examination* and *Therapeutic Exercise)*

- Acute care *(Core Concepts, Examination,* and *Management Strategies)*

- Pharmacology *(Core Concepts* and *Therapeutic Modalities)*

- Conditioning and rehabilitative exercise *(Therapeutic Exercise)*

- Therapeutic modalities *(Core Concepts* and *Therapeutic Modalities)*

- Medical conditions and disabilities *(Core Concepts* and *Examination)*

- Nutrition aspects of injury and illness *(Core Concepts)*

- Psychosocial intervention and referral *(Therapeutic Modalities* and *Therapeutic Exercise)*

- Administration *(Core Concepts* and *Management Strategies)*

- Professional development and responsibilities *(Core Concepts* and *Management Strategies)*

The authors for this series—Craig Denegar, Peggy Houglum, Richard Ray, Jeff Konin, Ethan Saliba, Susan Saliba, Sandra Shultz, Ken Knight, Kirk Brumels, Susan Hillman, and I—are certified athletic trainers with well over a century of collective experience as clinicians, educators, and leaders in the athletic training profession. The clinical experience of the authors spans virtually every setting in which athletic trainers practice: high schools, sports medicine clinics, universities, professional sports, hospitals, and industrial settings. The professional positions of the authors include undergraduate and graduate curriculum director, head athletic trainer, professor, clinic director, and researcher. The authors have chaired or served on the NATA's most prominent committees, including Professional Education Committee, Education Task Force, Education Council, Research Committee of the Research and Education Foundation, Journal Committee, Appropriate Medical Coverage for Intercollegiate Athletics Task Force, and Continuing Education Committee.

This series is the most progressive collection of texts and instructional materials currently available to athletic training students and educators. Several elements are present in most of the books in the series:

- Chapter objectives and summaries are tied to one another so that students will know and achieve their learning goals.

- Chapter-opening scenarios illustrate the relevance of the chapter content.

- Thorough reference lists allow for further reading and research.

To enhance instruction, various ancillaries are included:

- All of the texts (except for *Developing Clinical Proficiency in Athletic Training)* include instructor guides and test banks.
- *Therapeutic Exercise for Musculoskeletal Injuries* includes a presentation package plus image bank.
- *Core Concepts in Athletic Training and Therapy, Therapeutic Modalities for Musculoskeletal Injuries,* and *Examination of Musculoskeletal Injuries* all include image banks.
- *Examination of Musculoskeletal Injuries* includes an online student resource.
- *Core Concepts in Athletic Training and Therapy* includes a web resource.

Presentation packages include text slides plus select images from the text. Image banks include most of the figures, tables, and content photos from the book. Instructors can use these images to create their own presentations and to enhance lectures and demonstration sessions. Other features vary from book to book, depending on the subject matter; but all include various aids for assimilation and review of information, extensive illustrations, and material to help students apply the facts in the text to real-world situations.

The order in which the books should be used is determined by the philosophy of each curriculum director. In any case, each book can stand alone so that a curriculum director does not need to revamp an entire curriculum in order to use one or more parts of the series.

When I entered the profession of athletic training over 30 years ago, one text—*Prevention and Care of Athletic Injuries* by Klafs and Arnheim—covered nearly all the subject matter required for passing the Board of Certification examination and practicing as an entry-level athletic trainer. Since that time, we have witnessed an amazing expansion of the information and skills one must master in order to practice athletic training, along with an equally impressive growth of practice settings in which athletic trainers work. You will find these updated editions of the Athletic Training Education Series textbooks to be invaluable resources as you prepare for a career as a certified athletic trainer, and you will find them to be useful references in your professional practice.

David H. Perrin, PhD, ATC, FNATA
Series Editor

PREFACE

When Dave Perrin invited me to write the first edition of this textbook, it wasn't the first time someone had broached the topic with me. It was, however, the first time I took the task to heart and decided to pursue the idea. Several years before Dave made his invitation, Pete Koehneke had approached me with the idea. At that time there was no textbook on rehabilitation of athletic injuries. By the time I began writing the first edition, textbooks on the subject had been written or edited. Why, then, did I decide to write the book?

The answer is complex. Although several textbooks are now in print on the topic of athletic rehabilitation, prior to the publication of the first edition of *Therapeutic Exercise for Musculoskeletal Injuries* (formerly *Therapeutic Exercise for Athletic Injuries*), none satisfied the needs of the clinician beyond the technical level. Instructors across the country had repeatedly told me that they did not use a textbook because those available were either incomplete or did not meet their needs. Others told me that they used more than one text because there was no single textbook that addressed all of the content of their courses. In addition to these textbook shortcomings, the past few years have seen a number of advances and revolutionary changes in the rehabilitation of musculoskeletal injuries. Additionally, advancements in surgical techniques have demanded a concomitant advancement of rehabilitation techniques. The rehabilitation process must constantly evolve and become more sophisticated with surgical technique enhancement, equipment development, and newly acquired knowledge in health care.

Overall, available textbooks did not satisfy instructional needs. They addressed how to perform rehabilitation techniques, but they did not discuss what occurs physiologically, why applications are important, and how treatments are effective. As clinicians who rehabilitate musculoskeletal injuries, athletic trainers are health care professionals who are obligated to understand the therapeutic exercise and rehabilitation techniques they use to treat their patients. This textbook differs significantly from other rehabilitation textbooks because it deals with information vital to these concepts. The reader is guided through a progression of information designed to reveal the whys, hows, whens, and whats of rehabilitation—the essential building blocks that will provide the clinician with the skills to safely and successfully rehabilitate injured individuals.

Instructors using this text in their courses will find an instructor guide, test bank, and presentation package plus image bank available to them at www.HumanKinetics.com/TherapeuticExerciseforMusculoskeletalInjuries. The instructor guide includes chapter and suggested lecture outlines, as well as student activities for the classroom, and the test bank includes numerous questions that can be used to create or supplement tests and quizzes. The presentation package plus image bank offers instructors detailed lecture notes and also includes most of the art, figures, and tables from the text, which can be used to create custom presentations.

STRUCTURE AND ORGANIZATION

This text is divided into four parts. Each part builds on the information presented in previous parts. Part I deals with the basic concepts: what is important in a therapeutic exercise program, what factors affect a program, the team members involved, and the components involved. It also addresses what happens physiologically to the injury site and emotionally to the individual following an injury, as well as principles of physics, assessment techniques, and record keeping.

Part II presents specific techniques and concepts—including manual therapy and concepts involving range of motion, strength, proprioception, and functional activities—to serve as a foundation for parts III and IV. Reporting tools for findings and progressions are also discussed. These techniques are the cornerstone of the establishment, progression, and conclusion of a therapeutic exercise program for musculoskeletal injuries.

Part III contains information on general therapeutic exercise application. These chapters cover topics such as posture evaluation, gait analysis, aquatic exercises, Swiss ball and foam roller exercises, and tendinopathy treatment strategies. These techniques are all used

eBook
available at
HumanKinetics.com

throughout a treatment program and can be applied to many different body segments. This material becomes a set of building blocks for the last section of the book, part IV, which deals with specific application to each body segment of the techniques discussed in parts I, II, and III. Specific rehabilitation techniques and progressions are presented for each area of the body, with special attention to common problems or unique programs that a body segment requires.

TERMINOLOGY

As health care professionals, we should be familiar with terms commonly used in the context of identifying, treating, and managing musculoskeletal injuries. Though our patients may be athletes, industrial workers, or computer programmers, as long as a person is under medical care, that individual is considered a patient first. Therefore, individuals needing rehabilitation are referred to as *patients*. Some health care professionals refer to patients as *clients*. I personally have a difficult time with this term since, to me, it implies someone who is obtaining a service for a fee. We should be concerned primarily with the individual's health care, not what we may be paid, so *patient* better reflects what should be our priority—improving that individual's health status. As health care professionals, athletic trainers provide myriad services. Athletic trainers are well-rounded clinicians with education and skills in all aspects of patient care from prevention to immediate care to rehabilitation. Since this textbook deals with the topics of rehabilitation generally and therapeutic exercises specifically, the athletic trainer who offers this treatment is referred to as a *rehabilitation clinician* or *clinician*.

Treatment is offered in a *clinic*. The clinic can be an athletic training room, an outpatient clinic, a conditioning facility, or an industrial clinic; as long as the individual offering therapeutic exercise rehabilitation is a health care professional and the individual receiving that service is a patient, the facility is a clinic.

NEW TO THIS EDITION

This third edition of *Therapeutic Exercise for Musculoskeletal Injuries* contains much of the information that appeared in the former editions, but it also is substantially different from the previous editions. Two new chapters in part III are among the most substantial additions to this edition. Chapter 16 focuses on arthroplasty, and chapter 17 provides information regarding different age considerations in rehabilitation. Both of

these chapters are included because approximately 50% of graduating athletic training students will end up working in orthopedic or sport clinics. This means that they will treat patients older and younger than those seen in high school and university settings. Clinicians must be aware of the issues relevant to young and old patients and of the need to treat them differently from the "average" 18- to 25-year-old. Additionally, we are already seeing athletes undergo joint replacement and return to sport and recreation; this trend will only increase as technological improvements continue and more individuals remain active as they age. Clinicians must also know and appreciate the surgical procedures, precautions, and rehabilitation needs of one of the most frequently performed orthopedic procedures, arthroplasty.

In addition, there is more information in several of the other chapters, in the form of either new information or expansion of existing information. The chapters that address new topics include chapter 2, which presents a more detailed description of articular cartilage healing; this was important to add since so many new surgical techniques are being developed to treat articular surface injuries. Along with this is more detail on the rehabilitation of knee articular resurfacing in chapter 23. Chapter 18 on the spine has an added section on stabilization and another section on McKenzie and Williams' exercises. Since core stabilization is being recognized as important for many other body segments besides the trunk, this topic needed to be expanded in the current edition. It was not long ago that a physician would ask the clinician to instruct a patient in Williams' flexion exercises, but we do not see McKenzie and Williams' flexion exercises prescribed as a group as they were in the past. However, individual exercises from these two groups remain relevant, and since we do use the exercises individually, I thought it was necessary to recognize the foundation of these exercise programs by identifying them with reference to their original authors and the theories they proposed at the time.

Two chapters, 10 and 15, have had name changes. Chapter 10 is now "Functional and Activity-Specific Exercise." *Functional* exercise is not *specific* exercise, and I feel that it is important to make this distinction. The difference between functional and activity-specific is discussed in this chapter. One of the important and unique aspects of athletic trainers' education that distinguishes athletic trainers from other health care professionals is that their rehabilitation education includes the terminal aspects of rehabilitation. This terminal aspect is the specific activities that the patient will be required to perform once he or she returns to full and normal function. Since athletic trainers rehabilitate more types of people than just athletes, the specific exercises may be sport-related activities or job tasks. Both "sport-specific" and "activity-specific" are used to refer to that final phase of rehabilitation where the athletic trainer's role is to prepare patients to return to whatever demands and skills they must perform. Chapter 15 received a significant upgrade. Its title, "Therapeutic Exercise for Tendinopathy," refers to the terminology changes in the chapter. "Tendinitis" is no longer the common term for common tendon pathology since it is now recognized that the tendon is usually not inflamed. The title, however, is only one small part of the changes in this chapter. As with all the chapters, the information is updated to reflect the most current knowledge and trends in care.

In an effort to facilitate quicker reading of some of the chapters as well as easier location of information, I have described many of the manual techniques and exercises within brief, specially formatted sections. Accompanying photos are easily referred to, but these descriptions are also easy to locate and read. I have divided the techniques and exercises into their various categories for easy distinction among the different types of techniques and exercise groups. I have added at least one other kind of figure to each chapter in part IV. These figures provide a timeline of goals and suggestions for some exercises and identify procedures that may be used within each timeline. Each figure is divided into four segments, based on the healing timeline. Specific days from injury are not the guideline, as would be the case in a cookbook; since each person's response to injury varies, the timeline is determined by a combination of when the patient reaches established goals and the patient's evidence of healing. These figures may assist the visual learner in identifying progressions in therapeutic exercise programs.

Finally, this text provides more evidence for treatment programs than in the past. One of the terms frequently used today in health care is "evidence-based" care. We must remember that evidence-based care is an accumulation of knowledge and information gleaned from research as well as from clinical experience. To that end, I have incorporated into this third edition many evidence-based treatment techniques that are a blend of research results and my own experiences as a clinician over almost 40 years of practice. As I continue to read professional journals to grasp current knowledge in the field, I also use my own clinical techniques to discover what works and what does not work as I provide patient care. Clinical practice must include a routine merger of scholarly literature and clinical treatment with persistent assessment of this amalgamation to identify what is best for the patient; this textbook provides you with the beneficial results of this professional blend.

PURPOSE

This text is a compilation of nearly 40 years of experience in the field of athletic training, as well as in orthopedic, physical therapy, and sports medicine clinics and hospitals; and it provides what I believe is comprehensive information on therapeutic exercise for musculoskeletal injuries. It is meant to be an educational tool for the entry-level student as well as a reference text for the practicing rehabilitation clinician. It is meant to offer established and new information and to challenge both the neophyte and experienced rehabilitation clinician to provide a new level of insight and information about therapeutic exercise and our health care professions.

This text does *not* take a cookbook approach to therapeutic exercise. Instead it provides the knowledge and tools you will need in order to develop the skills for determining what to use for each patient you encounter. It provides the instruments you will need to decide the best course of action, as well as the knowledge about why you are using them; it tells you what to expect when you use a technique and explains the dangers and advantages of various applications, proper progressions, and ways to apply the knowledge and techniques to specific injuries. As each patient is different and responds differently to injury and treatment, it is neither fair to the patient nor realistic for you to believe that a cookbook approach would be helpful to either the patient or to you. The best course of action for you as a rehabilitation clinician is to provide the best therapeutic exercise program you can with your knowledge, skills, understanding, and appreciation of the whats, whys, and hows of therapeutic exercise. If you possess these attributes, you won't need or want a cookbook. This text offers you the tools to develop your own therapeutic exercise programs for your patients. It is your responsibility to use those tools and your own imagination to provide a sound therapeutic exercise program that is fun for you and your patient.

ACKNOWLEDGMENTS

As with any huge project, this text was completed only with the contributions of many people. These special people are intertwined within three categories: My family, my friends, and my Duquesne University family are at the top of the list of people I must acknowledge. I am fortunate that my siblings are my friends, that my friends seem as close as brothers and sisters, and that the people with whom I work at Duquesne University are more friends than colleagues. Without question, these people have provided me with support and assistance. With sometimes painful frankness, they have told me when I was off base. And most of all, with their own stellar performances they have inspired me to make my own actions worthy of their esteem. They may not feel that they have assisted with this text, but without them, there would have been no first edition, let alone a second or third.

Students and instructors who contact me are a consistent and necessary force that keeps me on my toes. They have noticed items in the text and interpreted segments in a way that provided me with an entirely new perspective on what I have written. Their comments and suggestions gave me a desire to present a better edition, an improved outlook, and another way of translating information to make it more relevant, more interesting, and more understandable. This is especially true of my students at Duquesne University, who provide me with a daily dose of inspiration and perception. Thanks to each of you who have provided your input into this new edition. You have made a difference.

I would be remiss not to mention the outstanding team of personnel at Human Kinetics. Without them, I would still not be finished rewriting this edition! They tried their best to keep me on task, and they helped me to make this edition the best one yet. A special thank-you goes to Loarn Robertson, whose enthusiasm for this project has never failed. Another special thank-you must go to Amanda Ewing, Developmental Editor for the Athletic Training Education Series, and Jillian Evans and Kate Maurer, Developmental Editors for this text. They each have put up with a lot from me to make this edition a reality. They showed saintly persistence even though I imagined them pulling their hair out because of my incomplete submissions and late deadlines. In spite of a probable urge to wring my neck over e-mail, they were always courteous and showed more patience than I deserved.

PART

I

Basic Concepts

I keep six honest serving men
(They taught me all I knew)
Their names are What and Why and When
And How and Where and Who.

RUDYARD KIPLING, *The Elephant Child*

What, why, when, how, where, and *who* are questions that are continually asked in medicine. Knowing the answers to them is not always easy or even possible. Understanding them can be even more difficult. Attempting to know and understand the answers, however, is the goal of health care professionals. Knowing and understanding these whats, whys, whens, hows, wheres, and whos of health care define the differences between technicians and professionals.

It is one thing to merely do something, and another to understand why something is done. To be a true health care professional, you must not only know how to perform the techniques and skills that are a part of the profession, but even more important, you must have the knowledge to appreciate why a technique or skill is used and understand the impact of its application. The challenge does not lie in applying a weight to an ankle but in knowing *why* it is done, *when* it should be done, and *what* impact this action has on the body. In a speech delivered in 1985, Diane Ravitch said, "The person who knows 'how' will always have a job. The person who knows 'why' will always be his boss." The technician knows how; the health care professional knows why. A technician can apply the technique, but a professional knows, appreciates, and understands the technique.

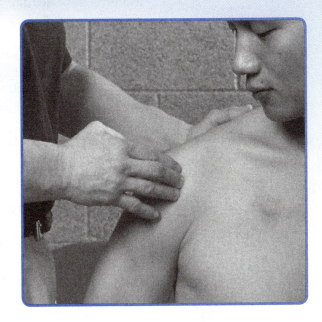

To develop as a professional and gain this knowledge, appreciation, and understanding of therapeutic exercise, you must first establish a foundation. Once this foundation is established, the larger concepts of therapeutic exercise can be addressed.

The fundamentals on which therapeutic exercise is formulated include factors such as interpersonal relationships; ethical, moral, and legal considerations; principles, goals, and objectives of rehabilitation; psychological factors affecting the program progression and success; and the basic components necessary to a successful program. These factors are building blocks for therapeutic exercise and are covered in chapter 1. Unfortunately, they are often omitted from therapeutic exercise programs but nevertheless play important roles in the overall rehabilitation process.

In chapter 2 you are introduced to what happens within the body when an injury occurs. Initiating an activity before healing tissue is able to tolerate the stress can be very detrimental, so understanding the healing process is vital to appreciating the impact of therapeutic exercise during healing. You must be continually aware of the timing of the healing progression during your administration of the rehabilitation program if the program is to be successful.

There are many different ways therapeutic exercises can be applied to the body. Simply changing a patient's position from sidelying to supine can significantly change the stress of an exercise and therefore the effect of that exercise. In chapter 3 you are introduced to forces that are applied to the body and how they can be changed. Understanding basic physics principles that directly apply to a therapeutic exercise program is fundamental to establishing a sound, beneficial program for the physically active.

How do you know whether what you are doing is working? How do you judge whether your efforts are producing the desired effect? One of the most important ways to answer these questions is to assess the results of your treatments. Even before you can determine what treatment techniques you should use, you must examine the patient. In chapter 4 the aspects and techniques of evaluation and examination that will guide your decisions for a treatment program are presented. Recording these findings is a part of the evaluation and examination process and is also addressed.

Once these foundations have been established, we can move on to other factors that are critical to a total rehabilitation program. Specifically, we explore in detail techniques and applications for therapeutic exercise. First, however, as you read through part I, think of individuals you have observed or in whose rehabilitation process you have been involved. You will begin to realize that these foundational concepts do indeed play a vital role on a daily basis for any rehabilitation clinician. An understanding and appreciation of these basic concepts is imperative if you are to create and administer a successful rehabilitation program.

Concepts of Rehabilitation

OBJECTIVES

After reading this chapter, you should be able to do the following:

1. Identify rehabilitation team members and their roles.
2. Discuss the qualities of professionalism in rehabilitation.
3. Discuss the principles, goals, and objectives of rehabilitation.
4. Describe the relationship among goals, progression, and examination.
5. Outline the importance of outcomes-based rehabilitation.
6. Outline the basic components of a therapeutic exercise program and their interrelationship.
7. Identify the stages of grief and the rehabilitation clinician's role in assisting the patient through these stages.

▶ Pam Lee had been in her first athletic training position for three weeks. She felt good about her position as assistant athletic trainer at the Division I university and was excited about being the athletic department's first rehabilitation coordinator. Until now, the athletic trainers had delivered rehabilitation to patients in a haphazard, inconsistent manner, but it was Pam's task to organize and ensure consistent, efficient, and cooperative rehabilitation programs for all the patients.

Coincidentally, the athletic department also hired a new orthopedic surgeon, Dr. Roberts, as the team physician. Dr. Roberts came to the university with extensive experience at another school where there was good communication and cooperation between the doctor's office and the athletic training staff. Pam looked forward to establishing a good relationship with Dr. Roberts.

Pam's first real challenge came early in the football season when the first-string quarterback, Bob "Fastgun" Gullaver, underwent a surgical reconstruction of his anterior cruciate ligament (ACL). Bob was a promising athlete whose football future depended on good rehabilitation of the knee. Pam felt a lot of pressure and mistrust from the coaching staff, Bob's parents, and Bob himself. Pam wasn't sure whether these anxious feelings were because of the injury, the history of the department's care of these types of injuries, or her own limited experience. Pam felt the best way to gain their trust was to handle Bob's case well. Pam knew she must do a good job not only of rehabilitating Bob's knee, but also of communicating with all the people involved.

Teamwork is the ability to work together toward a common vision.

ANDREW CARNEGIE

The preceding quote by Mr. Carnegie reminds us of the importance of working together to achieve a common goal. In therapeutic exercise, that common goal is successful rehabilitation of the patient. This chapter will provide you with an understanding of the basics of rehabilitation: professional interaction with others, the goals and objectives of rehabilitation, and the components of a good rehabilitation program. Although this chapter includes varied topics, they all form the foundation for the therapeutic exercise program that a clinician as part of a team provides for a patient. To provide a program that works and is successful, you must understand who affects the process and how team members work together to see their common vision become reality.

THE REHABILITATION TEAM

Physicians and health care personnel, including rehabilitation clinicians, use common medical terminology to communicate. An individual who receives medical care is referred to as a patient. The term *patient* is used in this text when referring to the person receiving treatment and care from a clinician, physician, or other rehabilitation team member. The injured individual is part of the rehabilitation team. Without the patient, there would be no need for the team. The clinician, physician, parents, and additional medical and health care personnel are the rest of the members of the primary team. If the patient is an athlete—as often those with musculoskeletal injuries are—then the athletic training student and coach will also be part of the team. In addition, there can be other team members who play an indirect, or secondary, role. These people do not usually affect the rehabilitation process directly but may have some impact on its ultimate result. These members may include athletic administrators, sport team members, equipment managers, orthotists, pharmacists, nutritionists, teachers, and attorneys.

■ Primary and Secondary Rehabilitation Team Members

Primary Team Members

Athletic trainer (athletic therapist in Canada) as rehabilitation clinician

Physician

Patient

Orthopedist

Podiatrist

Ophthalmologist

Psychologist or counselor

Physical therapist

Additional Primary Team Members for Athletes

Athletic training student (athletic therapy student in Canada) or other health care student

Parents or spouse

Coach

School nurse

Secondary Team Members

Emergency medical technicians

Orthotist

Pharmacist

Kinesiologist

Exercise physiologist

Nutritionist

Attorney

Supervisor

Peers

Secondary Team Members for Athletes

Sport team members

Equipment manager

Teachers

Athletic administrator

Athletic Trainer as Rehabilitation Clinician

The athletic trainer is the clinician most often responsible for rehabilitation of musculoskeletal injuries in the athletic environment. Often, this clinician is the health care professional relegated to rehabilitate musculoskeletal injuries in other environments as well.

The athletic trainer wears several different hats as a health care professional. When dealing with patients who require rehabilitation before returning to full participation in physical activity or sports, the athletic trainer (Canadian athletic therapist) wears the hat of a rehabilitation clinician. This role is different from the role played during the immediate care and treatment of musculoskeletal injuries at the time of their occurrence. As we will discuss, the clinician's role requires many professional and interpersonal skills.

At the center of the rehabilitation team, regardless of which or how many people make up the team, is the rehabilitation clinician. As the person who has daily contact with the patient and often the only one who has contact with all the other involved parties, the athletic trainer as clinician is the coordinator and leader of the rehabilitation team.

Interpersonal Skills

As a vital rehabilitation team member, the rehabilitation clinician must possess good interpersonal skills. Besides being dedicated to the rehabilitation process, the clinician must be competent and energetic, for the rehabilitation process can be very challenging and lengthy. The rehabilitation clinician's interest in the program and empathy for what the patient is enduring has a profound impact on the patient. The rehabilitation clinician must act professionally toward all rehabilitation team members. Your consideration, respect for others, confidence, honesty, and sincerity inspire the patient to comply with the rehabilitation program you provide and reassure parents, physicians, and other team members that you possess the knowledge, ability, and skill required to be the coordinator for their rehabilitation team.

The rehabilitation clinician also needs good active listening skills. Being an active listener means being involved in the conversation, participating appropriately, and understanding what the other person is saying. These qualities can be reflected by simply paraphrasing to the other person what he or she has just said. This technique imparts to the other person that you are listening and also helps you to understand clearly what is being said.

Record Keeping

One role of the rehabilitation clinician is to keep accurate records regarding the injury, evaluation, rehabilitation treatment, and response to treatment. Summaries, written or verbal, are communicated to the physician. Record keeping is a part of the process until the patient returns to competition or normal activity. Record keeping is discussed in more detail in chapter 4.

Educating Others

As rehab team coordinator, educating the patient, family members, and coach or employer is an important task of the rehabilitation clinician. Understanding the injury, the healing process, and the expected rehabilitation response is important to these individuals. Education prepares the patient for the rehabilitation procedure and prevents surprises. If the patient knows what to expect, he or she has less fear and will be more compliant with the rehabilitation program. Family members' fears are calmed with education. If family members are informed, they are also more willing and able to assist the clinician in helping the patient achieve a successful rehabilitation outcome. Finally, educating the coach provides the coach with a better understanding of what the patient is going through and an appreciation of the time it may take to complete the rehabilitation process.

Health Care Students

Health care students are in the unique position of acting as the rehabilitation clinician for a patient but not having the independence of a credentialed clinician. They operate under the supervision of their approved clinical instructor (ACI). They must be aware of their own limitations and not hesitate to consult the clinician whenever they feel they need advice or assistance.

Physician

As the medical chief of the team, the physician diagnoses the patient's injury, determines the course of treatment, oversees the rehabilitation program, and determines when the patient is ready to resume sports participation or normal activity. The physician and rehabilitation clinician must cooperate and have respect for and confidence in one another. Each should understand the other's role and appreciate the importance of good communication for a successful rehabilitation outcome.

Efforts to plan, communicate, and work together to establish protocols and systems of rehabilitation treatment help to minimize conflicts. It is important for physicians and rehabilitation clinicians to know and understand each other's rehabilitation philosophies and preferred methods of treatment before a rehab program begins. It is not unusual for rehabilitation clinicians and physicians to differ in their perspectives, but it is important for them to reach an understanding and develop a common ground so that they can respect their differences and work with each other in achieving what they both ultimately want: the successful rehabilitation of a patient's injuries.

It is the responsibility of the physician to educate the rehabilitation staff, patient, and family members as the need arises. Communication is the key for everyone to have a good understanding of the injury and the recovery course to be taken.

Family

Family members are important rehabilitation team members. When a patient lives at home, the family members play a vital role because they can assist the patient in complying with the home rehabilitation program. If you are dealing with an individual at the collegiate level, the patient may not live at home, so family members have a less significant role in assisting with compliance, but they are frequently involved with more serious injuries. More often than not, the rehabilitation clinician maintains the most frequent contact with the family.

Coach/Supervisor

Dealing with a coach obviously only applies if the patient is an athlete. If the patient is an employee, the supervisor takes on the role of "coach." But as a coworker with the clinician, the coach relies on the clinician for information on the current status of the patient. The coach plays an important role on the rehabilitation team regarding the injured athlete's restrictions on participation in practice and competition, through communication with the rehabilitation clinician. If participation is restricted, the coach can help the injured individual continue to feel he or she is part of the team by including the patient in practices, team meetings, and strategy sessions and having the patient assist with sideline activities.

Patient

The patient should inform the athletic trainer of any injury he or she sustains and seek treatment as soon as possible following injury. Delay in treatment can often mean needless prolongation of an injury and can retard or prevent the patient's return to full function.

When an injury occurs, it is important that the patient maintain good nutrition to enhance the healing process. Patients must take responsibility for their rehabilitation program's success by adhering to the recommendations of the physician and rehabilitation clinician. Performing the home treatment regimen provided by the clinician is crucial to the overall success of the rehabilitation program.

Other Team Members

Occasionally, other medical and paramedical professionals are included on the rehabilitation team. They are often called on as consultants by the primary or team physician when their special expertise is indicated to enhance the rehabilitation process. Examples of some ancillary team members include podiatrists, orthopedists, ophthalmologists, psychologists, physical therapists, and emergency medical technicians. Rehabilitation techniques that have been used to treat the patient, peers, the plan for care, and the response to treatment may be among the information that is conveyed by the rehabilitation clinician to the consulting medical professional.

Other peripheral team members may include attorneys, school administrators, sports teammates, and other non–medical team members. Which of these team members is involved varies according to the specific situation and circumstances. Attorneys may be involved in cases of negligence; school administrators may be active in a variety of situations, such as when rules and regulations require reassessment or when there is a conflict among involved parties; sports teammates or peers can play an important support role for the patient. The level of involvement of these team members varies greatly. When these team members do play a role, the rehabilitation clinician should be aware of this and interact with them appropriately.

INTERACTING WITH TEAM MEMBERS

Now that you have an awareness of the roles of each of the rehabilitation team members, the importance of good interaction among these members becomes apparent. Also apparent is why the rehabilitation clinician is the coordinator for this team. The rehabilitation clinician is easily accessed by the other team members, has daily contact with the patient, has a good understanding of the injury and the healing process, guides the patient along in the rehabilitation program, sees the response to treatment, and knows the expected progression of rehabilitation.

The primary rehabilitation team members are the patient, athletic trainer as rehabilitation clinician, rehabilitation student, physician, patient's family, coach (if the patient is an athlete), and additional medical and health care personnel. Secondary members include others who play a less significant or less direct part in the patient's rehabilitation. The rehabilitation clinician plays a central role as coordinator of the rehabilitation team.

The athletic trainer or athletic therapist is the center of the communication process. The clinician communicates with the patient, the parents or spouse, the coach or supervisor, the physician, the ancillary medical personnel, and the specialists. Each of these rehabilitation team members may speak with another, but the clinician is in contact with all of them.

With this key position comes responsibility. The rehabilitation clinician must be sure any information conveyed is accurate and not a guess. Saying "I don't know" generates more respect than guessing the correct response. "I don't know" accompanied by "but I'll find out and get back to you" is even more appreciated.

Communicating With the Patient

Being responsible in communication also means knowing when to say something, when to withhold information, and how to communicate effectively and appropriately. When a patient has just been injured and feels distraught, then is not the time to explain in detail the process that will occur during rehabilitation. Using big words and complicated medical terminology is not practical when speaking with most patients or family members, especially if they are upset. Even in a good situation, a person normally has difficulty recalling more than five instructions at one time (Rastall et al., 1999). In a stressful situation the ability to understand or retain unfamiliar information is impaired. It is recommended that patients receive as few instructions at one time as possible and that those instructions be reinforced with a handout or some method of recall (Rastall et al., 1999). I have found from clinical practice that keeping the number of home exercises given in one session to three assures better compliance by the patient.

Using good judgment about what to say and when to say it is a skill. The skill develops with practice and observing others who are good at it. Be patient with yourself as you develop this skill. Contemplate what you will say before you say it, and put yourself in the place of the patient or family member with whom you are talking. Ask yourself how you would like to be addressed at that time, what information you would want or be able to comprehend without any medical knowledge, and then proceed to listen to and observe that person's responses as carefully as you listen to your own words to him or her.

You should communicate with the patient with sincere compassion, understanding of the individual situation, and confidence in your own knowledge of injuries and rehabilitation. It is important to instill in the patient confidence in your ability to treat the injury. This is done by providing the patient with the information he or she seeks about the extent of the injury, the time it will take to heal, and the treatment plan. As mentioned, not all of this information should be provided at once or at the time of injury. Your best judgment about when to provide this information is important in establishing confidence and trust.

Communicating With the Physician

You should not hesitate to contact the physician regarding the patient's injury or response to treatment. Communication between the rehabilitation clinician and the physician is important to the outcome of rehabilitation. Both must be aware of the seriousness and extent of the injury, the patient's response to the injury and treatment, and his or her compliance with the rehabilitation program. Both must also agree with the treatment course and appreciate and respect each other's contributions to the rehabilitation process. This is accomplished by communicating and establishing a rapport with each other. Rehabilitation clinicians communicate with physicians by telephone, through e-mail, in person, and through written reports. Telephone and face-to-face, informal conversations are ways to understand general philosophies and develop rapport. Written and verbal patient reports are also vital to an ongoing professional relationship between the physician and the rehabilitation clinician.

Communicating With Family Members

Depending on the situation, communication with the patient's family varies considerably. At the high school level, parents commonly are intimately involved with the injured youth's recovery process from the start. Communicating with family members at the time of injury is important because it is an opportunity for the rehabilitation clinician to establish a rapport with the family if one has not been established already. It also will reassure parents and calm their fears about serious or lasting results of their son's or daughter's injury. When a patient lives at home, you can inform his or her parents or spouse of home activities that can expedite the rehabilitation program.

When the patient does not live at home, family members do not play as important a role in the rehabilitation program. Occasionally, however, when the patient's injury is more serious and the rehabilitation process is longer and more complicated, family involvement may be more direct. For example, if the patient is to have surgery, he or she may choose to go home for the surgery or following surgery. In other situations—with an injured collegiate athlete, for example—patients may return home at the end of the school year when their rehab program is not yet concluded. In these situations the family may be requested to assist with the rehabilitation program or consult with a local facility to continue the rehabilitation process you have started.

Communicating With the Coach/Supervisor

When a coach or supervisor has confidence and trust in the rehabilitation clinician, cooperation in restricting the patient's workouts is more likely. Impressing upon the coach or supervisor the extent of the patient's injury, the limitations placed on the injured part, and the importance of his or her involvement in the rehabilitation process helps to ensure the success of the rehabilitation program.

Communicating With Secondary Team Members

When a patient is referred to other medical specialists, input from the rehabilitation clinician is appreciated. It provides the specialist with information regarding the patient's injury in the event that the rehabilitation clinician has witnessed the injury. It also provides the specialist with insight regarding the rehabilitation program thus far and the patient's responses to it. The rehabilitation clinician can also assist in and complement the specialist's course of treatment.

Like all primary rehabilitation team members, secondary team members' communication with other team members should be honest, constructive, and professional. The ultimate goal of all team members should be to assist in whatever way appropriate for their position within the team to provide the patient with satisfactory and successful rehabilitation. Acting responsibly by performing their roles unselfishly, appropriately, and cooperatively ensures that this goal is achieved.

Cautions on Communication

With the recent advance of the Health Insurance Portability Accountability Act (HIPAA), the rehabilitation clinician is under legal obligation when it comes to what information regarding a patient's injury can be provided to whom. An initial segment of HIPAA requirements was instituted in 2003. The regulation affects several aspects of health care, including the right to privacy regarding health, illness, and injury. Not all rehabilitation clinicians are directly affected by this law; the extent to which it affects communication depends on the type of health care environment of the facility and whether billing is involved. The government Web site regarding HIPAA is www.hhs.gov/ocr/hipaa/. Specific information, requirements, and regulations can be found at that Web site.

Courteous, professional, accurate, and appropriate communication among all rehabilitation team members is essential for a successful rehabilitation program.

QUALITIES OF PROFESSIONALISM

Being a professional means looking and acting like one. A true professional gives something back to the profession by being an active member of professional associations and organizations (for example, the National Athletic Trainers' Association or NATA), and making a positive contribution.

Being a professional also means adhering to the legal standards determined by the state's regulating body and complying with the ethical standards established by your professional organization. Awareness of these professional standards is the responsibility of every individual who considers himself or herself a professional.

Using your knowledge to provide the patient with the best care possible is an undisputed precept of the profession. This means taking the responsibility to learn current information and practices in the profession and delivering only the care you feel confident in providing.

The years you spend in college to attain a degree and become a clinician provide you with a base upon which you will mold your career within the profession. There are more specialized techniques, more complicated information, and more sophisticated treatment application methods that will become available to you as you continue beyond your entry-level education in rehabilitation. Attending postgraduate seminars, participating in professional meetings, and reading professional publications to learn current information regarding rehabilitation and other topics within the profession are means by which professionals keep up to date.

It is your responsibility to yourself and to the patients you treat to be aware of the new and ever-evolving methods of treatment and rehabilitation. Medical science is continually advancing, and research is continually being conducted around the world to lead us to better understanding of treatment methods. As a professional, you have an ethical and moral responsibility to provide the best care you can to a patient. Participating in different types of continuing education to optimize your health care knowledge, techniques, and skills is an important aspect of fulfilling that responsibility.

Treating the patient with concern, respect, and a consistently professional attitude is vital. This attitude establishes the patient's confidence in your ability to give quality care and guide the patient to a successful rehabilitation outcome.

Looking Like a Professional

Dressing appropriately and being neatly groomed when working as a rehabilitation clinician reflect not only your attitude toward yourself, but also your pride in being a health care professional. If you dress professionally and are neat, clean, and well groomed, you present an appearance that encourages confidence and respect from others. If you are to be taken seriously, you should look like a professional.

Acting Like a Professional

Showing respect and consideration for others, colleagues or patients, is part of acting like a professional. Acting professionally also involves being sensitive to the privacy of the patients you treat. Privacy is important when taking a patient's medical history or exposing a body part in the clinic. Acting professionally means being morally and legally responsible and conducting yourself in a manner that reflects well on your medical profession.

Being a Professional

Being a professional goes beyond looking and acting like one. A true professional also attends professional meetings and becomes active in professional associations. The needs of professionals are met through the profession's association. The association's needs are met through the active participation of its members. It should be the professional responsibility of each clinician to contribute at the local, state, regional, district, or national level to make the association effective and provide vitality to the profession. A professional cannot stand alone, and a profession needs the energy and dedication of its members to play a viable and convincing role in the medical arena today.

The athletic trainers' professional association is NATA. If you plan to work with athletes and are not yet a member, I encourage you to ask your athletic training curriculum program director for information regarding student membership in NATA or to contact the NATA office directly to obtain a student membership application.

> ### ■ NATA National Contact Information
>
> Phone: 214-637-6282
> Fax: 214-637-2206
> Membership e-mail: membership@nata.org
> Web site: www.nata.org

Ethical and Legal Standards

As health care professionals, rehabilitation clinicians have a responsibility to themselves, to their profession, to their employers, and to the patients they rehabilitate to act in a consistently professional manner, including following ethical and legal guidelines.

In today's medical environment the legal aspects of athletic training have become more important than in years past. Ethics, however, has always been an important part of this profession. NATA scripted its *Code of Ethics* in its very early days. The founders of NATA realized the importance of providing guidelines for standards of behavior and ensuring high-quality, principled care for patients by athletic trainers. The NATA *Code of Ethics* has since been revised to keep in stride with current issues, but the primary precepts have remained the same. Even if you do not work with or do not plan to work with patients, I suggest that you obtain a copy of this document and familiarize yourself with it. The NATA *Code of Ethics* can be found online here: www.nata.org/codeofethics/code_of_ethics.pdf.

Some of the topics presented here lie in the legal arena, some in the ethical arena, and some in both. These subjects are important enough in the rehabilitation of patients that you should spend a little time understanding them.

State Regulations

Each state has different legal guidelines. The majority of states now have some type of regulation in the form of licensure, certification, registration, or exemption that determines the legal parameters within which a rehabilitation clinician must operate. It is your responsibility to know and operate within the regulations of the state in which you practice.

Consent

Rehabilitation clinicians use their professional skills, knowledge, and best judgment to decide the course of rehabilitation for a patient. Sometimes the patient may not wish to follow the course of treatment that the clinician has proposed. The patient may refuse to perform a specific activity. Although you may attempt to convince the patient that the activity is appropriate for a variety of reasons, you must remember that if the patient refuses to perform the activity you request, you cannot force the patient to do it. For example, if a gymnast who suffered an ankle sprain refuses to do the non-weight-bearing pool therapy that you recommend, you would probably attempt to make her understand why you want her to go into the water. Regardless of the reasons, if she continues to refuse, you cannot force her into the pool. It is up to you to find an alternative program for her. Likewise, if you want a basketball player with a subluxating shoulder to start doing medicine-ball work, but he refuses because he lacks confidence that his shoulder could tolerate the exercise, the same policy would apply. You would attempt to explain why this is an important activity and reassure him that you would not have him do it unless you thought the shoulder was ready. If he still refuses, you must use a different type of exercise that would be less threatening to him yet still accomplish the same goal. You can attempt to reintroduce the activity later in the program, once the patient's confidence has improved and he is less likely to object.

Rehabilitation clinicians demonstrate their professionalism by maintaining a professional appearance and demeanor, continuing their education within the profession, contributing to the profession by being active in professional associations and organizations, and adhering to legal and ethical standards.

In other words, the patient always has the last say on what is or is not done with his or her body. The patient gives consent for treatment by performing what is requested during the rehabilitation program, but the patient always has the right to say no. The patient's consent is assumed to be given in the treatment process until it is taken away. As a rehabilitation clinician, you must always respect the patient's right to consent to or refuse treatment. Generally, your knowledge, skill, and past experiences with the patient give the patient the confidence and trust in you to ultimately comply with your rehabilitation procedures. Occasionally, however, perhaps because the patient lacks confidence in him or herself, has too much pain, or does not feel comfortable with the activity, he or she refuses to perform it. In those cases, you must respect the patient's refusal and remember that, even though you may disagree, it is the patient who has the final control. Your best defense against this situation is to possess the knowledge to create an appropriate rehabilitation program, self-confidence in your knowledge and mastery as a health care professional, and an ability to create the same confidence in your patients.

Touch

Athletic training is a touching profession. We palpate injuries on a daily basis, feel for spasm and temperature, and touch painful and swollen areas routinely. For this reason, touch becomes something we often do not think about, but we must be continually sensitive to the patient's perception of our touch.

Touching a patient should always be purposeful, with a specific reason and goal in mind. For example, if you touch the thigh of a patient who has received a contusion to the quadriceps, the pressure applied and area palpated should be appropriate.

Touching is an integral and necessary part of a rehabilitation clinician's duties, but you must be acutely aware that a patient may not be accustomed to the intimacy of touch in this context. Presenting yourself in a professional manner, being deliberate in how you touch, demonstrating respect for the patient, and having sensitivity for the patient's situation help to reassure the patient and permit you to perform your tasks appropriately.

If you are unsure of how a patient will respond to your touch, it is best to have another professional present. In today's litigious environment, touch—even when it is purely professional and necessary—can be questioned. If you work with athletes, you will find that most injured athletes are treated in an athletic training clinic where other people are around. However, if you find yourself in an isolated situation or when you feel that questions may potentially arise later, you should take precautions, such as having another professional or someone else present, keeping the treatment room door open, or providing the treatment in a common room where others are present. It is often wise to listen to your instincts; if you have an uneasy feeling about a situation, be cautious.

COMPONENTS OF A REHABILITATION PROGRAM

This section deals with the general principles, objectives, and goals of a musculoskeletal rehabilitation program. An overview of the components of a rehabilitation program is presented. We also take a brief look at assessing the patient's status, evaluating program progression, and measuring the outcomes of the program.

Rehabilitation Principles, Objectives, and Goals

The principles of rehabilitation are used to achieve the goals and objectives of a therapeutic exercise program. The ultimate design of each therapeutic exercise program is based on these principles, goals, and objectives of rehabilitation. The principles and objectives are constants in a therapeutic exercise program. The goals are established for each individual patient in each situation.

Principles

There are seven principles of rehabilitation. Principles are the foundation upon which rehabilitation is based. This mnemonic may assist you in remembering the principles of rehabilitation: ATC IS IT.

Avoid aggravation

Timing

Compliance

Individualization

Specific sequencing

Intensity

Total patient

A: Avoid Aggravation   It is important not to aggravate the injury during the rehabilitation process. Therapeutic exercise, if administered incorrectly or without good judgment, has the potential to make the injury worse. A prime rule was put forth by Hippocrates when he said, "As to diseases, make a habit of two things: to help, or at least to do no harm." This precaution serves rehabilitation clinicians as well.

Rehabilitating the injured individual in a continually progressive manner without aggravating the injury is a primary concern throughout the therapeutic exercise program. Knowledge of how the body responds to injury, aptitude in determining which exercises to use, good judgment in deciding when the program should progress, and skill in observing the patient's response are needed to recognize when and how far to advance the therapeutic exercise program without aggravating the injury.

T: Timing   The therapeutic exercise portion of the rehabilitation program should begin as soon as possible without aggravating the injury. The sooner the patient can begin the exercise portion of the rehabilitation program, the sooner he or she can return to full activity. Following injury, rest is sometimes necessary. Studies have demonstrated, however, that too much rest is actually detrimental to recovery. Appell (Appell, 1990) reported the significance of inactivity when he estimated that during the first week of immobilization, 3% to 4% of an individual's strength is lost each day. This strength is not recovered in the equivalent amount of time, but takes much longer (Staron et al., 1991). In chapter 2 we investigate the deleterious effects of prolonged rest and immobilization.

Some studies indicate that the rate of recovery is much slower than the rate at which strength is lost. This finding emphasizes the importance of beginning a therapeutic exercise program as soon as is safely possible. The longer the initiation of therapeutic exercises is delayed, the longer the recovery process will take. For example, if a patient is inactive for two days with an injury, it may take a week for full recovery to occur. If a patient is put on rest for four days, it may take perhaps as long as three weeks to return to normal activity or competition.

C: Compliance   Without a compliant patient, the rehabilitation program will not be successful. To ensure compliance, it is important to inform the patient of the content of the program and the expected course of rehabilitation. The patient will be more compliant when he or she is better aware of the program to be followed, the work he or she will have to do, and what the whole rehabilitation process entails.

Often an injured individual feels powerless after suffering an injury. That feeling of powerlessness can prevent a successful return to sport participation or normal activity. Knowledge empowers the patient. Empowerment engenders compliance. Compliance leads to success.

Compliance includes several elements. Compliance means that the program is carried out consistently, allowing progressive recovery and improvement. Compliance means that the patient performs whatever exercises or tasks the rehabilitation clinician has instructed the patient to perform outside of the clinic. Compliance means that the patient attends treatment sessions consistently and during those sessions performs whatever activities are included in the program to the best of his or her ability.

I: Individualization   Each person responds differently to an injury and to the subsequent rehabilitation program. Expecting a patient to progress in a program the same way as the last patient you had with a similar injury will prove to be frustrating for both you and the patient. It is no more realistic to compare one patient to another than it is for a parent to compare one child to its sibling. It is first necessary to recognize that each person is different. It is also important to realize that even though an injury may seem the same in type and severity as another, undetectable differences can change an individual's response to the injury. Individual physiological and chemical differences profoundly affect a patient's specific responses to an injury. Several other nonphysical variables can influence the recovery of the patient, including the outside support the patient has from friends, teammates, and family; the patient's psychological makeup and response to the injury; the degree and types of outside pressures the patient may feel to return to competition; and the goals and rewards the patient may want to achieve.

It is your responsibility to understand that these differences exist, be aware of the patient's responses to the injury and rehabilitation program, and design the therapeutic exercise program accordingly to guide the patient through the rehabilitation program as effectively, safely, and efficiently as you can.

S: Specific Sequencing   A specific sequence of events should be followed in a therapeutic exercise program. This specific sequence is determined by the body's physiological healing response. This topic is covered later in this chapter in the section "Basic Components of Therapeutic Exercise."

I: Intensity   The intensity level of the therapeutic exercise program must challenge the patient and the injured area, but at the same time the intensity must not aggravate the injury. Knowing when to increase intensity without overtaxing the injury requires observation of the patient's response and knowledge of the healing process. The healing process is covered in chapter 2.

For you to use the correct exercise intensity in the therapeutic exercise program, knowledge of the progression of exercises and the amount of stress that each exercise imposes is also important. Along with this knowledge, you should have an imagination. This is important because if an exercise is too severe or too easy for the patient to perform, modifying it can permit the right intensity for the patient to progress appropriately. Sometimes all it takes is a slight modification, and other times the modification is more complex. For example, if a patient finds it easy to balance on one leg, having the patient perform the same activity on an unstable surface such as a mini-trampoline makes it more difficult. If doing this exercise on the floor is too easy but doing it on the trampoline is too difficult, you can have the patient perform the exercise on the floor but with eyes closed. Using your imagination and resourcefulness is especially vital if you have a limited equipment budget.

If you combine your knowledge and imagination, you can design a therapeutic exercise program that is challenging and provides the correct intensity level for achieving the goals that have been established. Being imaginative also makes the therapeutic exercise program more interesting for both you and the patient. Making the program interesting enhances the patient's desire to comply and therefore increases the likelihood of a successful outcome.

T: Total Patient   You must consider the total patient in the rehabilitation process. It is important for the injured person to stay finely tuned in the unaffected areas of his or her body. This means keeping the cardiovascular system at a pre-injury level and maintaining range of motion, strength, coordination, and muscle endurance of the uninjured limbs and joints. When a patient is injured, the whole body must be the focus of the rehabilitation program, not just the injured area. Remembering that the total patient must be ready for return to normal activity or competition and providing the patient with a program to keep the uninvolved areas in peak condition, not just rehabilitating the injured area, better prepares the patient physically and psychologically when the injured area is completely rehabilitated.

Objectives

There are two basic objectives for any therapeutic exercise program. The first is related directly to the principle just discussed of treating the total patient. This objective is to prevent deconditioning of uninjured areas. The second objective is to rehabilitate the injured part in a safe, efficient, and effective manner.

Prevent Deconditioning   Preventing deconditioning includes providing exercises for the cardiovascular system, the uninvolved areas of the injured extremity or segment, and the uninvolved extremities. For example, if the patient has a knee injury preventing weight bearing on that leg, the patient can maintain cardiovascular conditioning by performing pool exercises or working out on an upper-body ergometer. The patient can also maintain good strength and range of motion of the trunk, upper body, and uninvolved lower extremity by using weights and other exercises for these segments. Exercises for the involved extremity's hip and ankle can also be used to prevent deconditioning of those areas without applying undue stress to the injured knee.

Similarly, another patient who has suffered a left shoulder injury can exercise the left elbow, wrist, and hand. Even after surgery and immobilization a patient may be able to perform some wrist and hand exercises to help maintain that part's strength and range of motion.

Because of the nature of the injury or the medical restrictions involved, it may sometimes take some imagination on your part to develop exercises that challenge the uninjured parts while not harming the injured area, but it is important for you to design programs with the objective of maintaining current conditioning levels as much as possible.

Rehabilitate the Injured Part   Good knowledge of the injury, healing process, and methods of rehabilitation is paramount in achieving the objective of rehabilitating the injured part. You must use good judgment along with this knowledge to enable the patient to progress safely and effectively through the therapeutic exercise program.

Therapeutic exercise can be used effectively to enhance and promote recovery, but it can also be harmful and ineffective if used incorrectly. It is your responsibility to know the appropriate use of this highly effective yet potentially dangerous therapy.

Goals

Goals are results one strives to achieve. In therapeutic exercise the ultimate goal is the return of the patient to his or her former activity. That return, however, should be safe yet quick, effective yet efficient, and pursued in an aggressive yet guarded manner. This means that you must work diligently with all the tools available to you to enhance the healing of the injury, restore the deficient parameters that have been lost because of the injury, and regain the patient's self-confidence to permit him or her to return with at least the same level of competence as before the injury. This is done in the minimum amount of time that allows the healing process to occur and also provides enough time to rehabilitate the injured area without undue time lost away from the sport or activity.

There is often a fine line between going too slowly and advancing too quickly. The program should stress the patient just enough to provide gains, not losses, with regular progression. The following image might help you to grasp this concept: Each treatment session, it is your responsibility to push the patient up a hill to its peak, applying enough stress to gain as much as possible in an exercise session. At the same time, it is very important to avoid pushing so far that the patient goes over the top and down the other side (applying so much stress that it causes deleterious effects).

Objective and Measurable Goals   Goals should be objective and measurable whenever possible. Goals are occasionally subjective; for example, pain is subjective. However, some objectivity is possible in measuring pain by asking the patient to rate his or her pain on a 10-point scale. Other parameters such as girth, range of motion, and strength can be measured as objective and more concrete goals.

■ Sample Goals

These are examples of long- and short-term goals that could be set for a patient with a shoulder injury.

Long-term goal

The patient will have full strength in all rotator cuff muscles at the conclusion of the rehabilitation program.

Short-term goal

Two weeks from today's treatment session, the patient will have 4/5 strength in the sub-scapularis, 3+/5 strength in the teres minor and infraspinatus, and 3/5 strength in the supraspinatus (using the scoring system discussed in chapter 7 in which 5 = full strength and 0 = complete loss of voluntary contraction).

An alternate short-term goal

Two weeks from today's treatment session, the patient will increase strength in each rotator cuff muscle by 1/2 grade from today's evaluation scores.

It is necessary to record these measurements at various stages in the therapeutic exercise program, most obviously at the beginning and conclusion of the program. Throughout the program, the patient is reassessed routinely as well. Any changes should be recorded. This is important in assisting you and the patient to identify improvements. This record can also help you more easily notice when changes do not occur as frequently as expected and decide what specific modifications are needed in the program.

Short- and Long-Term Goals When an injury is severe enough to restrict sport participation or normal activity for at least a month, both long-term and short-term goals should be set. A long-term goal is the final, desired outcome of a therapeutic exercise program. For example, returning the patient to a former level of athletic competition would be a long-term goal. Specifically, this involves returning the patient to normal levels of all parameters that allow full return to sport participation, including flexibility, strength, endurance, coordination, and skill execution. Definitive levels of these parameters are different for each patient and depend on the patient's sport, specific position, age, skill level, and level of participation. These parameters are discussed in more detail later in this chapter in the section "Basic Components of Therapeutic Exercise."

Short-term goals provide both you and the patient with objective aims to guide you toward the long-term goals. Both short-term and long-term goals are specific as to objective measures of what is to be accomplished by the patient within what time frame, and under what conditions. Short-term goals are established weekly or biweekly and depend on the patient's response to the injury and ability to progress, the stage of the rehabilitation process, and the severity of the injury. A short-term goal may be to reduce edema by 1 cm and increase range of motion by 15° in one week. Other short-term goals may be to increase strength by half a grade (the scoring system for muscle strength is discussed in chapter 7), reduce pain to 3 on a scale of 0 to 10, and ambulate with one crutch in 5 days.

Short-term goals are important because they give the patient something concrete to work toward and the psychological boost to achieve them. Looking at long-term goals can be overwhelming, but focusing on short-term goals gives the patient direction and establishes a logical progression for the rehabilitation process.

Short-term goals should be reasonable and attainable yet challenging for the patient. They should be realistic to allow the patient to achieve them within the time established without irritating the injury or frustrating the patient. Establishing realistic goals takes skill, knowledge, practice, and judgment on your part. You must also be aware of additional factors that may affect the patient's ability to achieve these goals, such as the patient's personality and how he or she responds to injury, challenges, and discipline; outside pressures such as from income or scholarships, family, supervisor or coach, and friends; the patient's other activities, including recreational activities, work, and school; the severity, type, and healing process of the injury; and the level of dysfunction involved.

All injuries involve precautions and contraindications. Complications can occur regardless of the quality of care provided. You must establish goals and place demands on the patient with these factors in mind.

Examination and Assessment

Rehabilitation clinicians continually examine and assess injuries, from the time the injury occurs to the time the patient is ready to return to sport participation or normal activity. Therapeutic exercise programs are one area in which clinicians make frequent assessments.

The only way to establish goals is to examine the patient and make an assessment of the patient's current condition. How much swelling is present? How much range of motion is lost? What is the status of the injured area's strength? These and other questions are assessed on the first day of rehabilitation. They are also reexamined regularly throughout the rehabilitation treatment.

To create short- and long-term goals, you must first establish the current status of the deficient parameters. Then you decide what realistic short-term goals the patient can achieve in a specific amount of time. Once those goals are achieved, you once again perform an examination and make an assessment to decide new and appropriate short-term goals.

You must continually examine and assess the patient's condition to provide the patient with an accurate therapeutic exercise program with appropriate goals. Since examination is performed frequently and throughout the rehab process, it will be covered in more depth in chapter 4.

Progression

A good therapeutic exercise program progresses in a challenging yet safe manner. Accurate examination and assessment of the patient's response to the exercises and treatment is necessary for this to occur. The progression should be in accordance with the severity of the injury, the type of injury, and the patient's response to the injury and treatment. A good progression challenges the patient without causing deleterious effects such as increased pain or swelling or decreased ability to perform.

Exercise Progression

One aspect of progression is the type of exercise. For example, a strength progression may advance from **isometrics** to **isotonics** to **isokinetics** to **plyometrics.** The patient begins with a level that is challenging but not irritating to the injury, which is determined, in part, by the severity of the injury and the rehabilitation clinician's assessment of the patient's current ability. A patient with a mild ankle sprain who is ambulating without crutches may be able to forgo isometrics and begin isotonic and weight-bearing resistive exercises. However, a patient with profound swelling who is on crutches may be able to tolerate only non-weight-bearing range-of-motion and isometric exercises.

Program Progression

Another level of progression involves the program itself: A program should be designed to emphasize different types of goals as it progresses. Keep in mind that you cannot expect a patient to perform advanced skill drills before flexibility and strength have been achieved, and that full strength cannot be achieved until flexibility is restored. This is discussed in the section "Basic Components of Therapeutic Exercise" later in this chapter.

Outcomes-Based Rehabilitation

Today's buzzword in medicine is *outcomes.* Outcomes are important to the understanding, use, and justification of programs used to treat patients. The outcome of a treatment program is often assessed using a tool that has been devised for measuring the patient's response and satisfaction following a treatment that is given for a specific injury or condition. The outcome tool is most often a questionnaire that is given before the start of the program, sometime during its course, and at its conclusion. Questions often relate to the patient's condition before and after treatment and to the patient's perception of different aspects of the treatment, including quality of care, professional attitudes, and effectiveness of the program in achieving goals. Input from the clinician providing the treatment program is also obtained. Final results are then compiled and statistically analyzed to provide a variety of information to today's medical providers, patients, and payers. Figure 1.1 shows the Lower Extremity Functional Scale (LEFS), an example of a specific outcomes questionnaire.

Outcomes tools are divided into two categories—a general health status measurement tool and a region-specific measurement tool. A generic status measurement tool is used to assess a patient's physical, social, and emotional health and is used for a variety of illnesses and treatment environments. The gold standard for the generic health status tool is the SF-36, originally advanced by John E. Ware, Jr. (Ware et al., 1995; Ware & Sherbourne, 1992). Although it has been demonstrated to be a reliable and valid tool, it is time consuming to administer and was not designed as a tool with which to make treatment decisions for individual patients (Brinkley, Stratford, Lott, & Riddle, 1999). A variety of condition-specific outcomes tools have been developed in an attempt to more accurately examine and assess items that are related to the specific injury or illness and will reveal changes with treatment applications. For example, a commonly used condition-specific outcomes tool that examines changes in back pain is the Roland-Morris Questionnaire (Stratford, Binkley, Riddle, & Guyatt, 1998).

Some of the problems that are recognized in selecting an assessment tool that restricts the reliability of one tool to assess treatment effects for different conditions include the difficulty in using a tool's scale for different injuries, the shortcomings a tool has in its application to specific individuals, and the clinician's lack of confidence in the meaningfulness of the scores (Brinkley et al., 1999). For example, a condition-specific tool that is designed to measure patellofemoral injury treatment outcomes may not be considered a reliable tool to measure outcomes of treatment for a shoulder dislocation, and a tool designed to measure treatment outcomes on a high school athlete may not be applicable to measuring treatment outcomes on a middle-aged laborer.

Outcomes are important in many fields of medicine. They are used in physicians' offices, outpatient clinics, and hospitals. They are used to modify treatment, justify treatment, evaluate the effectiveness of protocols, judge the appropriateness of treatment responses, and assist in authorization of payment. An outcomes assessment tool can be provided by an outside agency, which analyzes the results from many different treatment providers around the country, or it can be devised and analyzed by a single facility.

A couple of the more commonly used outcome research tools used today in rehabilitation are the Functional Independence Measure (FIM) (Keith, Granter, Hamilton, & Sherwin, 1987), a tool used primarily for inpatient rehabilitation facilities, and Focus on Therapeutic Outcomes (FOTO), a tool for outpatient rehabilitation facilities.

Different users of an assessment tool evaluate outcomes differently, depending on their perspective. For example, an insurance company may use outcomes research results to decide what is usual and customary for expected duration and treatment cost of a specific injury. A patient may use them to see whether the treatment program met his or her needs. Health care providers may look at the outcomes study results to assess whether the programs being used to treat specific injuries and individual patients in their facility are effective, cost efficient, and achieve the goals of the professional administering the treatment. There are occasions, however, when outcomes assessments are used incorrectly to generalize results to a larger

LOWER-EXTREMITY FUNCTION

It will be useful in your rehabilitation program to know if you are having difficulty with any specific activities at this time. Please indicate your ability for each activity by circling the appropriate number. Your selected number should reflect what you feel you are able to do today.

Activity	Unable to perform	I can perform but with great difficulty	I can perform with moderate difficulty	I can perform with a little difficulty	I can perform without difficulty	This is something I do not do regularly
Any of your usual work, housework, or school activities	0	1	2	3	4	5
Your usual recreational activities	0	1	2	3	4	5
Your usual hobbies	0	1	2	3	4	5
Getting into the bath	0	1	2	3	4	5
Getting out of the bath	0	1	2	3	4	5
Walking in the house	0	1	2	3	4	5
Putting on shoes and socks	0	1	2	3	4	5
Lifting objects such as a grocery bag	0	1	2	3	4	5
Performing light activities at home	0	1	2	3	4	5
Performing heavy activities at home	0	1	2	3	4	5
Getting in and out of the car	0	1	2	3	4	5
Walking more than 15 minutes	0	1	2	3	4	5
Walking less than 15 minutes	0	1	2	3	4	5
Going up or down 1 flight of stairs	0	1	2	3	4	5
Standing more than 15 minutes	0	1	2	3	4	5
Standing more than 1 hour	0	1	2	3	4	5
Running on flat ground	0	1	2	3	4	5
Running on hills	0	1	2	3	4	5
Hopping/jumping	0	1	2	3	4	5
Getting out of bed	0	1	2	3	4	5

▶ **Figure 1.1** Sample outcomes assessment tool.

Data from J.M. Binkley et al., 1999, "The lower extremity functional scale (LEFS): Scale development, measurement properties, and clinical application," *Physical Therapy* 79(4): 383.

A rehabilitation program should be designed with seven essential principles, two main objectives, and specific long- and short-term goals in mind. The overall program and individual exercises should progress safely and effectively. Rehabilitation clinicians should know how to assess the patient's status and evaluate the program's outcomes.

■ Outcomes Resources

- *Guide for the Uniform Data Set for Medical Rehabilitation (Adult FIM), version 4.0.* 1993. Buffalo, NY: University of New York at Buffalo/UB Foundation Activities.
- Lewis, C., and T. McNerney. 1994. *The functional tool box.* Washington, DC: Learn.
- McDowell, I., and C. Newell. 1996. *Measuring health.* 2nd ed. New York: Oxford University Press.
- Medical Outcomes Trust approved instruments. 1996. *Medical Outcomes Trust Bulletin* 4(1).
- Scientific advisory committee instrument review criteria. 1995. *Medical Outcomes Trust Bulletin* 3(Sept.).

---

population or different situation. Inappropriate inferences should be avoided, for they are misleading, unfair, and erroneous.

Because it is imperative for a rehabilitation clinician to be as effective and efficient as possible in treating patients and returning them to sport participation or normal activity, clinicians are inherently concerned with outcomes. Outcomes assessments may not be as critical, however, for clinicians who practice in an athletic training clinic or industrial setting as for those who practice in other settings, such as orthopedic clinics or hospitals. However, as systems of health care and payment continue to change, all rehabilitation clinicians will eventually be compelled to deal with outcomes assessments more formally than is currently typical.

BASIC COMPONENTS OF THERAPEUTIC EXERCISE

In the total rehabilitation program, there are two basic elements, therapeutic modalities and therapeutic exercise. Modalities are used to treat and resolve those effects first seen in injury: spasm, pain, and edema. Although modalities are an essential component of a rehabilitation program, they will not be presented in detail in this text. Therapeutic exercise (therex) is an essential and critical factor in returning the patient to sport participation or normal activity. If the therapeutic exercise program is to be effective, however, specific parameters must be addressed sequentially. Each of these parameters must be restored to at least pre-injury levels if the patient is to safely resume full sports participation or normal activity. These parameters in their proper sequence are

1. flexibility and range of motion,
2. strength and muscle endurance, and
3. proprioception, coordination, and agility.

Each of these parameters is based on the previous ones, much like a pyramid, stones placed one on the other, layer by layer until the structure is complete. This concept will become clearer as we discuss each parameter.

Flexibility and Range of Motion

There is a technical difference between flexibility and range of motion, but in functional terms the difference is nominal. The term **flexibility** is often used when referring to the mobility of muscles and the length to which they can extend. If a muscle is immobilized for a period of time, it tends to lose its flexibility, or degree of mobility. If stretching exercises are incorporated as part of a routine conditioning program, the muscle tends to maintain its flexibility or length. Inflexibility usually means that a muscle, not a joint, has limited mobility.

Range of motion, however, refers to the amount of movement possible at a joint. For example, the normal range of motion for shoulder **abduction** is 170°. Range of motion is affected by the flexibility of the muscles and muscle groups surrounding the joint. If a muscle lacks flexibility, the joint may not have full range of motion. Range of motion is also affected by other factors such as mobility of the joint capsule and ligaments, fascial restraints, and regional scar tissue.

Range of motion is also affected by strength. For example, if a patient does not have the strength to lift the arm fully against gravity, active shoulder range of motion will not reach 170°. This is one reason why active and passive range-of-motion measurements are usually different from each other, passive range of motion being greater than active. Active and passive ranges of motion are discussed in chapter 5.

Because of their close clinical relationship, the terms *range of motion* and *flexibility* are often used interchangeably. We will treat these terms as synonyms throughout the text, but keep in mind that technical differences do exist between them.

A properly designed therapeutic exercise portion of a rehabilitation program places a priority on regaining lost range of motion and flexibility first. Achieving flexibility early in the therapeutic exercise program is necessary for two important reasons. First, the other parameters are based on the flexibility of the affected area. To make this point clear, consider how handicapped a hurdler would be if the hamstrings were inflexible. The patient's strength and timing would be of little importance if the flexibility necessary to extend the leg over the hurdle was lacking. Using an upper extremity example, a baseball pitcher with less than full shoulder range of motion is at a distinct disadvantage. Lacking full shoulder motion, the pitcher lacks power and is at risk for injury, regardless of strength, endurance, or timing.

The second reason to emphasize regaining range of motion first in the therapeutic exercise program is the impact of the healing process (discussed in chapter 2). As injured tissue heals, scar tissue is laid down. As scar tissue matures, it contracts. This is important in eventually minimizing the size of the scar, but it also can be detrimental because as the tissue contracts, it pulls on surrounding tissue, causing loss of motion, especially if the scar crosses a joint.

During healing there is a window of opportunity during which scar tissue mobility can be influenced and changed. Once that time frame has passed, the likelihood of successfully achieving full range of motion is diminished considerably. If efforts are not made during the remodeling phase, when the newly formed scar tissue is most easily influenced, attempts to improve range of motion will be very difficult and frustrating at best and futile at worst. Although restoration of other parameters is also sought during the first stage of therapy, flexibility must be the primary emphasis.

Strength and Muscular Endurance

As the patient progresses, achieving normal strength and muscular endurance becomes the priority. With any injury some strength is lost. The amount of strength and muscular endurance lost depends on the area injured, the extent of the injury, and the amount of time the patient has been disabled by the injury.

Muscular strength refers to the maximum force that a muscle or a muscle group can exert. It is most often measured by determining the amount of weight that the muscle or group can lift in one repetition. **Muscular endurance** is the muscle's ability to sustain a sub-maximal force in either a static activity or a repetitive activity over time. An example of muscular endurance in a static activity is the length of time a gymnast can maintain an iron-cross position on the rings. A runner in a marathon and a starting pitcher are examples of athletes who perform repetitive activities that require muscular endurance.

Of all the parameters achieved during therapeutic exercise, strength is probably the most obvious and most frequently sought following an injury. It is obvious because it is easily understood that a weightlifter cannot return to competition following a sprain until full knee strength is achieved. It is just as obvious that a wrestler must have normal shoulder strength to return to competition after suffering a dislocation.

The need for muscular endurance and the relationship between muscular strength and endurance are sometimes not considered, however. If a baseball pitcher has good rotator cuff strength but no endurance beyond 10 repetitions, how is he going to manage pitching more than a couple of innings in a game? If a basketball center can leg press 225 kg (496 lb) but can last only five repetitions, will she be able to recover rebounds for an entire game?

Muscular strength and endurance are two dimensions within a continuum of muscle resistance. They also affect each other. When strength improves, there are also gains in endurance, and vice versa. This is an important factor to remember in establishing a therapeutic exercise program for patients. For example, if a patient is attempting to recover from patellofemoral pain syndrome, the patient may not be able to tolerate heavy weights to achieve the strength you would like to see. Exercises for endurance may be more tolerable and will still produce gains in strength until the patient becomes strong enough to tolerate higher resistance. Essential concepts of muscle strength and endurance are presented in chapter 7.

Proprioception, Coordination, and Agility

Proprioception, coordination, and agility are often omitted in a therex program. It is too often assumed that because range of motion and strength are restored, the patient is ready to resume full sport participation or normal activity. This is not the case at all. Impaired balance, proprioception, or coordination—either from injury to the structures controlling these parameters or from lack of practice in a specific skill—increases risk of injury.

A variety of factors affect a patient's proprioception, coordination, and agility. A number of factors in turn are affected by these elements, including muscular power, skill execution, and performance. (The factors that affect and are affected by proprioception, coordination, and agility are discussed later in chapter 8.) To develop appropriate proprioception and coordination skills, enough flexibility and strength must first be achieved. Coordination and agility are based on the patient's having enough flexibility to perform the skill through an appropriate range of motion and enough strength, endurance, and power to perform it repeatedly, rapidly, and correctly. This is the reason that proprioception, coordination, and agility are the last parameters to focus on: they need the foundations of good flexibility, strength, and endurance to be optimal.

Although not all health care professionals emphasize this parameter, a total rehabilitation program must include the recovery of proprioception, coordination, and agility. Consider a tennis player who has suffered a back injury that has kept him out of competition for two months. The timing of his serve, the coordination of his response to his opponent's serve, and the agility of his feet in sudden lateral movements on the court may all be impaired. Simple exercises for proprioception are introduced early in the therapeutic exercise program, but proprioception, coordination, and agility are not emphasized until after strength and range of motion are achieved. Development of execution skills is the last step before a patient's return to full sport participation. Accurate execution of functional and sport-specific skills requires attainment of all parameters.

The final stage of emphasis on coordination and proprioception evolves into the execution of normal drills that mimic the patient's actual activities. The final step before returning to competition involves execution of these sport-specific activities. In this final stage the patient regains the confidence necessary to perform at his or her prior activity level. When the patient can perform well and with confidence, the rehabilitation clinician can be assured that the goal of fully rehabilitating the patient has been achieved.

RETURN-TO-COMPETITION CRITERIA

If you work with athletes, returning to competition is nearly always the goal of the therapeutic exercise program. By the time the patient is ready to return to full sport participation, you have fully examined and assessed the injured area, the patient's ability to withstand the

Therapeutic exercise must address the following physiological parameters in proper order: first, flexibility and range of motion, then muscular strength and endurance, and finally, proprioception and coordination.

demands of the sport, and the patient's readiness to return to competition. Full readiness to resume sport participation means that the injured area has no pain, swelling, or atrophy and has full range of motion, flexibility, strength, and endurance and that the patient can perform the sport skills and coordination tasks at an appropriate functional level.

You and the patient must remember that the physician has the final word on when the patient is able to return to competition. It is through your communication with the physician regarding the patient's response to treatment, the patient's ability to perform activities required in the sport, and the injured area's status that the physician can make that determination.

> The physician determines when a patient is ready to return to competition based on an examination of the patient and the information provided by the rehabilitation clinician about the patient's status.

PSYCHOLOGICAL CONSIDERATIONS

Many psychological factors have a direct and sometimes profound influence on the overall results of the rehabilitation program. The rehabilitation clinician must be aware of these factors not only to be able to promote optimal results of the therapeutic exercise program but also to encourage and provide needed support to the patient.

Stages of Grief

Kubler-Ross (Kubler-Ross, 1969) outlined stages of grief that people go through when confronted by the knowledge of their own death or that of a loved one. Although it has never been measured or conclusively proven, others (Peterson, 1986; Rotella, 1985) have suggested that patients who have experienced a disabling injury that keeps them out of competition also go through this process. Since anecdotal reports indicate injured athletes go through this process, it will be explained here. Kubler-Ross's stages of grief are denial, anger, depression, and acceptance.

1. **Denial.** At first, the patient doesn't believe that the injury is severe and feels that he or she will return to competition in a day or two.

2. **Anger.** As the reality of the severity and consequences of the injury sets in and the patient is forced to see the difficulty he or she is having in recovery, the patient expresses anger as a release of the genuine feelings of frustration and helplessness. This anger is often directed at whomever is present. It is helpful to remember that during this phase the patient is angry because of the injury and the situation he or she is in, not because of any action or words of those who are around. Attempts to calm, rationalize with, or help the patient see what is really happening are often futile at this point. The patient wants only to express this anger and does not want to be told why he or she should not be angry or that things will get better.

During this stage, you should attempt to prevent the injury from becoming aggravated by any harmful activities the patient may attempt. You should also be a sounding board for the patient, letting the patient express the feelings of frustration and anger at the loss of the ability to perform and the loss of power over the situation.

3. **Depression.** As the patient begins to realize the reality of the situation, depression is the next stage. The patient's self-worth declines during this time. The patient feels he or she has no physical or emotional control. Not participating with the team can cause feelings of isolation, further adding to self-doubt and low self-esteem. Hope is questionable at best because the patient sees no good results forthcoming.

It is during this phase that rehabilitation becomes the most difficult for both you and the patient. It becomes difficult for the patient to comply with the rehabilitation program. The patient may not attend scheduled treatment sessions or may not fully participate in them.

4. **Acceptance.** In this final phase the patient begins the battle of fighting the physical limitations and psychological downswing experienced during the previous stages.

Progression Through the Stages

Throughout the grieving process there are no abrupt changes; rather, the patient goes through gradual transitions, and fluctuation between stages can occur. For example, a patient who has entered the depression phase may swing back into the anger phase in the beginning but later return to the depression phase. As the patient progresses through depression, he or she displays less and less anger. As the patient enters the acceptance phase, he or she may regress to depression before finally accepting the situation.

You must be aware that these swings occur and are natural. Seeing these stages on a continuum from the extreme ends of denial and acceptance, each phase overlapping with the adjacent one, may help you in dealing with the patient as he or she goes through these stages.

When a patient is unable to advance through the grieving process smoothly, or if you are concerned about the patient's emotional condition, it is your responsibility to support the patient and encourage him or her to seek additional psychological support from a counselor, psychologist, psychiatrist, or other psychological professional. You should never hesitate to refer a patient to an appropriate specialist.

The Rehabilitation Clinician's Role in Psychological Recovery

Supporting the patient in psychological recovery is vital to achieving goals of therapeutic exercise and rehabilitation programs. The rehabilitation clinician is crucial to this process because of the role he or she plays in the patient's response to injury and commitment to the rehabilitation program. A survey of certified athletic trainers (Fisher, Mullins, & Frye, 1993) revealed the most important variables influenced by certified athletic trainers in patients' compliance with rehabilitation programs. At the top of the list is education and communication. Whether you work with athletes or other populations prone to musculoskeletal injuries, if you educate the patient about the type and extent of the injury, inform him or her about the rehabilitation process, and communicate with him or her in a respectful, open, and honest manner, the patient will exhibit better compliance.

Communication

Using good communication skills throughout the rehabilitation process is important. Being a good and an active listener is a communication skill that every clinician should possess. Repeating the patient's uncertainties, worries, and goals is an active listening skill that demonstrates to the patient your interest and concern. Making good eye contact is a simple yet important part of communication. Being aware of the environment and realizing whether it is conducive to good listening and communication are also necessary. Simply being at the same eye level, instead of standing and looking down at the patient, encourages communication.

As discussed earlier in the section "Communicating With the Patient" (page 8), appropriate communication incorporates good judgment and interpersonal skills. Being timely with explanations and knowing how much to explain is often vital to patient acceptance. The information you provide the patient educates him or her, enhances compliance with your treatment program, and gives him or her hope for a foreseeable end to the injury and return to competition or normal activity.

Part of communication includes providing the patient with an appropriate level of information that enhances compliance with home programs. Studies have demonstrated that a patient's ability to recall instructions provided is dependent upon a number of factors such as the length of time between the instruction and the time of recall; the familiarity of the information presented; the age of the patient; the patient's gender (women generally recall better than men); the levels of anxiety, stress, and depression the patient may be feeling; and the complexity of the information provided (Wingfield & Byrnes, 1981). Therefore, when providing home instructions to patients, the clinician needs to be sensitive to these issues. Tests performed on subjects show that the number of words recalled range from five to nine

(Wingfield & Byrnes, 1981). A patient feeling stress because of the injury, concerned about his or her future in sports, or in pain will have a reduced ability to recall your instructions. Having the patient perform the home program activity before he or she leaves your clinic facility and providing written descriptions of exercises along with illustrations or photos ensures better patient recall and compliance with a home program (Quealy & Langan-Fox, 1998).

Offering encouragement for the patient's physical efforts throughout the therapeutic exercise program positively influences the patient's psychological response. Encouragement also improves compliance. When someone of authority and expertise whom the patient respects offers support and encouragement, the patient's performance and compliance are enhanced.

Goal Setting With the Patient

Goal setting is important in facilitating patient compliance and enhancing a positive attitude. The patient's assistance in setting goals offers two benefits: the patient feels he or she has some control over the situation, and working together to establish goals ensures mutual understanding of and agreement on those goals. It is natural for a patient to feel a loss of power or control when injured. Thus, regaining control is important.

You and the patient should have the same goals. If one has a goal that conflicts with the other's goals, failure is certain. You and the patient should understand each other's goals, agree with them, and work together to achieve them. For example, if an injured alpine skier has no desire to return to skiing but instead wants to become a recreational cyclist while your goal is to have the patient return to the slopes, you will be frustrated when the patient does not work as hard as you would like. The patient will also be frustrated that you are making her work harder than necessary to achieve her goal.

Monitoring the patient's progress, using goals, recording objective changes, and setting new and more challenging goals are all methods of providing the patient with additional incentives to adhere to the therapeutic exercise program. The patient may be able to feel some benefits from the program, but providing him or her with more objective, concrete measurements enhances his or her willingness and motivation to continue the rehabilitation program.

Supporting the Patient

Depending on the environment, the members of the patient's support system may vary. The rehabilitation clinician is central to this support system, however, and acts as the coordinator of the patient's support system to assist him or her in a successful outcome. Support team members can assist the patient with home exercises, provide encouragement, and share with the clinician observations or concerns noted outside the treatment environment.

Establishing Rapport With the Patient

Treating a patient on a frequent, if not daily, basis, the rehabilitation clinician develops a rapport with the patient. This rapport results from their interaction, mutual respect, and desire to achieve the same goals. Establishing rapport can be a challenge when patients are hard to manage or have difficult personalities. In these cases it is the clinician's responsibility to put aside his or her own prejudices and feelings and act in a professional manner. Fortunately, however, this type of uncomfortable situation is rare. Normally, the challenge of the situation and the common bond between the patient and clinician facilitate an easily established rapport. The patient is more compliant and willing to perform any activity requested when this rapport exists.

Making the Program Interesting

Personalizing the program, making its goals challenging yet achievable, and using your imagination to make it interesting are important to overall success and the patient's compliance. The therapeutic exercise program can be a treatment of drudgery or stimulation for both the patient and you. It is up to you to see to it that it is the latter so your common goals are achieved.

A patient may go through four stages of grieving: denial, anger, depression, and acceptance. To ensure compliance with the therapeutic exercise program, the rehabilitation clinician must recognize the importance of the patient's psychological state, communicate effectively, educate, provide support, set goals cooperatively, establish rapport, and make the program interesting.

SUMMARY

Athletic trainers play a crucial role in the rehabilitation of musculoskeletal injuries. As the clinician who has the most encounters with the patient and others affected by the injury, the athletic trainer is essentially the team leader for the rehabilitation team. The athletic trainer must know how to communicate effectively with others and provide appropriate communication with all persons involved to bring about a successful outcome of the rehabilitation process. The athletic trainer guides the patient throughout the rehabilitation program, providing planning and an overall understanding of the rehabilitation process to assure patient compliance, efficient recovery, and optimal function at the completion of the program.

KEY CONCEPTS AND REVIEW

1. Identify rehabilitation team members and their roles.

A rehabilitation team consists of individuals who are closely related to the rehabilitation program or who have peripheral roles. Some of these individuals are the patient, athletic trainer as rehabilitation clinician, physician, family members, health care students, coach or supervisor, team members or peers, and specialists.

2. Discuss the qualities of professionalism in athletic training.

The rehabilitation clinician is a health care provider who is responsible for looking, acting, and being professional. Being a professional means acting as a responsible clinician and contributing within the professional organization. Being a professional carries with it the responsibility of continuing to learn new techniques and applications that are pertinent to the profession. It also means always treating others in a respectful and courteous manner.

3. Discuss the principles, goals, and objectives of rehabilitation.

The mnemonic ATC IS IT can help you remember the principles of rehabilitation. The objectives of any therapeutic exercise program are to prevent deconditioning of the unaffected areas, including the cardiovascular system, and to rehabilitate the injured area safely, efficiently, and successfully.

The goals established for each patient are based on achieving these objectives and are divided into short-term and long-term goals. The long-term goal is to restore the patient to at least former levels of function to permit the patient to return to sport participation or normal activity. Short-term goals are used when the patient has a more severe injury and cannot participate in sports or normal activities for a while.

To achieve these goals and objectives, you must be sensitive to the patient and what the patient is going through psychologically.

4. Describe the relationship between goals, progression, and examination.

Short-term goals are based on measures as objective as possible, recorded to see the patient's progress, and changed when the patient achieves them until the final long-term goals are achieved. You must continually assess the patient's and the injured area's response to treatment. Using objective measures in this assessment and recording the results help the patient and you to realize the changes that are the product of the rehabilitation program and to know how the program should progress.

5. Outline the importance of outcomes-based rehabilitation.

Outcome assessment investigates whether a program that you design for a patient produces the expected response and whether the program meets expectations and goals.

6. Outline the basic components of a therapeutic exercise program and their interrelationships.

A rehabilitation program must progress in a sequential manner, since each parameter builds upon the components of the prior parameter so that a patient can ultimately return to full participation or normal activity. The sequential parameters include flexibility and range of motion; strength and muscle endurance; proprioception, coordination, and agility, leading to full functional activity.

7. Identify the stages of grief and the rehabilitation clinician's role in assisting the patient through the stages.

Although it has not been clearly demonstrated that an injured individual follows the four stages of grief, they follow this sequence: denial, anger, depression, and acceptance. To ensure the patient's compliance with the therapeutic exercise program, the rehabilitation clinician must recognize the importance of the patient's psychological state, communicate effectively, educate, provide support, set goals cooperatively, establish rapport, and make the program interesting.

CRITICAL THINKING QUESTIONS

1. How would you handle a situation in which an athletic trainer with whom you work did not properly complete the requirements established by the Board of Certification (BOC) to sit for the certification examination but was able to get his or her supervising certified athletic trainer to sign off on the required documents anyway? Would you report him or her to the BOC, discuss it with him or her or your supervisor, or ignore it?

2. If you were treating a patient whose injury was severe enough to doubt whether he or she would return to full sport participation at the preinjury level, how would you deal with the questions the patient would have regarding long-term goals? Would you tell the patient in the beginning that returning to his or her prior level of participation was questionable? Would you let the patient discover the reality him- or herself? Would you ease the patient into that reality?

LAB ACTIVITIES

1. Go to the NATA Web site at www.nata.org and perform the following functions:
   a. Identify the different membership categories.
   b. Calculate what your dues would be for national and state membership.
   c. Identify each of the districts and the states within each district.
   d. If your district has a Web site, identify its address.
   e. If your state has a Web site, identify its address.
   f. Locate information at each Web site that is of personal interest to you and indicate what that piece of information is.

2. Role-play a situation where you and your lab partner are the clinician and a patient. The patient is going through the grieving phases following a severe and debilitating injury. Act out how the patient may express himself or herself at each of the different grieving stages and how the clinician should respond to each of those stages.

3. Role-play a situation where one person is the athletic trainer and the other person is the injured athlete's coach. The coach wants to have the athlete ready to play by the weekend, but the athletic trainer knows that will not be possible. Act out how an athletic trainer should approach the coach so the coach is able to understand and accept that the athlete's injury will not allow the athlete to participate by the weekend.

Concepts of Healing

OBJECTIVES

After completing this chapter, you should be able to do the following:

1. Explain the differences between primary and secondary healing.
2. Identify the healing phases.
3. Describe the primary processes of each healing phase.
4. Discuss the causes for the signs of inflammation.
5. Explain the role of growth factors in healing.
6. Discuss the differences between acute and chronic inflammation.
7. Discuss healing characteristics of specific tissues.
8. Identify the relevance of tensile strength.
9. Discuss factors that can modify the healing process.
10. Explain the role NSAIDs play in inflammation.
11. Discuss the timing of treatment with the various stages of healing.

▶ Daniel Edwards has been assigned to work with gymnast Becki Gumble, who underwent an Achilles tendon repair seven days ago and is now in the athletic training clinic for her first day of rehabilitation. Daniel's knowledge of healing allows him to judge where in the healing process such an injury should be and what rehabilitation techniques can be safely applied to the Achilles tendon at this time. He understands the tendon's tensile strength and the precautions that apply for repairs such as Becki's. He also understands the status of the healing connective tissue and the processes that are now under way.

However, Daniel suspects that Becki has poor eating habits. Before applying rehabilitation techniques, Daniel decides to discuss the importance of proper nutrition and the role proteins, vitamins, and minerals play in tissue healing.

Although the world is full of suffering, it is also full of overcoming.

HELEN KELLER, 1880-1968, writer and lecturer, blind and deaf from birth

Understanding the entire healing process, like Helen Keller's life, is a triumph. Unfortunately, unlike Helen Keller, we have not yet accomplished our goal. However, having an appreciation of what is currently known of the healing process allows us to create safe and effective therapeutic exercise programs. As a professional who rehabilitates sport injuries, you have a duty to understand healing and realize the impact of the therex techniques you apply. There are many aspects to healing that are still unknown, even to experts. What is presented here is the most current information we have on the body's response to injury and the process it undergoes in an effort to return to normal.

It is common knowledge that an injury produces a scar when healing. Although there are occasions when the body actually replaces damaged tissue with normal tissue, more frequently in sport and orthopedic injuries, scar tissue is the end result of the healing process. This chapter provides an elementary focus on the essential elements of the healing process involved in scar tissue formation following injury.

In spite of all that has been written and investigated on healing, there is still a lot of information that eludes us. The information presented in this chapter has resulted from the research of a great many people. I have attempted to simplify this complex topic and to present what rehabilitation clinicians should know to safely apply therapeutic exercise and rehabilitation techniques.

This chapter introduces many terms that may be new and unfamiliar to you. To assist you in becoming familiar with these terms, table 2.1 defines the terms that appear in boldface in this chapter and indicates their most common function or their significance in the healing process. You can also find these terms in the glossary at the back of this text.

PRIMARY AND SECONDARY HEALING

There are many ways to classify injuries. Some refer to the type of injury as either primary (direct) or secondary (inflammatory) while others discuss injuries as either acute (from direct trauma) or chronic (from overuse), and still others may choose to use superficial (involving the epidermis and/or dermis) or deep (involving deeper structures).

Regardless of the term used to define an injury, when an injury occurs, the healing process that follows depends on the extent of the injury and the approximation of the wound site's stump ends. If the separation of tissue is small, a bridge of cells binds the ends together. This is called healing by **primary intention.** This type of healing commonly occurs in minor wounds. It also occurs in surgical incisions where the stump ends are sutured together.

TABLE 2.1   Terminology of Wound Healing

Term	Definition	Significance/function
acetylcholine	A neurotransmitter at the neuromuscular junction of striated muscles.	Causes vasodilation.
adrenaline	See *epinephrine*.	
angiogenesis	Formation of blood vessels.	Provides for subsequent scar tissue formation and normal healing events that follow.
arachidonic acid	An unsaturated essential fatty acid.	A precursor in the production of leukotrienes, prostaglandins, and thrombaxanes.
basophil	A white blood cell in the subgroup of polymorphonuclear leukocytes.	See *granular leukocyte*.
bradykinin	A local tissue hormone that is activated by the interaction of proteases with the Hageman factor.	A very potent local vasodilator. It increases vascular permeability and stimulates local pain receptors.
callus	Fibrous matrix formed at a bone fracture site.	Immobilizes the bone fragments and serves as the foundation for eventual bone replacement.
chemotactic factor	A chemical gradient. Also referred to as a chemotactin or chemo-attractant.	See *chemotactin*.
chemotactin	An agent that facilitates chemotaxis.	Must be present and function properly to promote the healing process.
chemotaxis	Movement or orientation of cells in response to a chemical stimulus after an injury, which occurs through complex and not totally understood processes.	Cells either become oriented along a chemical concentration gradient or move in the direction of that gradient. For example, chemicals attract platelets, red blood cells, and PMNs into an injured area.
collagen	Major type of protein in the body. There are five types: I is most abundant, high in tensile strength, and found in dermis, fascia, and bone. II is found in cartilage. III is found in embryonic connective tissue. IV and V are found in basement membranes.	Forms inelastic bundles to provide structure, integrity, and tensile strength to tissues.
collagenase	An enzyme produced by newly formed epithelial cells and fibroblasts.	Involved in degradation of collagen during tissue repair. Important in controlling collagen content in a wound.
complement system	Various proteins found in serum.	Act as chemotactic factors for neutrophils and phagocytes.
drug interaction	When one drug enhances or reduces the effectiveness of other drugs also being taken.	It is important to know what drugs an individual takes so that they are not rendered harmful or ineffective by each other.
duration of drug action	Amount of time the blood level of the drug is above the level needed to obtain a minimum therapeutic effect.	Determined by the drug's half-life.
elastin	An essential protein of connective-tissue elastic structures. Arranged in a wavy orientation.	Its wavy arrangement allows tissue to change shape with stress and resume normal conditions after stress removal. It plays an as yet unknown role in the remodeling phase.
endothelial cells	Large, flat cells that line blood and lymphatic vessels.	Are restored during angiogenesis.
endothelial leukocytes	Large white blood cells that circulate in the bloodstream and tissues.	Act as phagocytes to remove debris from an injured area.
eosinophil	A white blood cell in the subgroup of polymorphonuclear leukocytes.	See *granular leukocyte*.

(continued) ▶

■ **31**

Term	Definition	Significance/function
epinephrine	A hormone. Also called adrenaline.	A potent stimulator of the sympathetic nervous system and a powerful vasopressor. Increases blood pressure, stimulates the heart muscle, accelerates heart rate, increases cardiac output, and increases metabolic activities such as glycogenolysis and glucose release.
erythrocyte	An element of blood. Also known as red blood cell or corpuscle.	Used for oxygen transport.
extracellular matrix	The basic material from which tissue develops. Produced by fibroblasts in wounds. Composed of fibers and ground substance.	Serves as a foundation on which new tissue is cast.
exudate	Material that escapes from blood vessels following an injury. Contains high concentrations of protein, cells, and other materials from injured cells.	As PMNs die and decompose, exudate may resemble pus although no infection is present.
factor XII	See *Hageman factor.*	
fibrin	Insoluble fibrous protein formed by fibrinogen.	Important in clotting.
fibrinogen	A globulin present in plasma.	Converts to fibrin to form a plug at the injury site.
fibrinolysin	An enzyme in plasma released in later healing.	Converts fibrin into a soluble substance to unplug lymphatics system at injury site.
fibroblast	A connective tissue cell that differentiates into chondroblasts, osteoblasts, and collagenoblasts.	Forms the fibrous tissues that support and bind a variety of tissues.
fibrocyte	An inactive fibroblast. See *fibroblast.*	
fibronectin	An adhesive glycoprotein found in most body tissues and serum. Fibronectin is plentiful in early granulation tissue formation but gradually disappears during the remodeling phase.	Cross-links to collagen in connective tissue, thereby playing a role in the adhesion of fibroblasts to fibrin. Also involved in the collection of platelets in an injured area and the enhancement of myofibroblast activity.
glycoprotein	Protein–carbohydrate compounds. Elements of ground substance. Includes fibronectin.	Probably cross-links with collagen so tissue is able to withstand pressure.
Glycosaminoglycan (GAG)	Compounds occurring mostly in proteoglycans. Nonfibrous elements of ground substance in the extracellular matrix. Examples: hyaluronic acid, proteoglycans.	Different GAGs have different functions: stimulating fibroblast proliferation, promoting collagen synthesis and maturation, contributing to tissue resilience, and regulating cell function.
granuloma	Hard mass of fibrous tissue.	Occurs in chronic inflammatory conditions when the body produces collagen around a foreign substance to protect itself from that substance.
granular leukocytes	White blood cells, which are divided into three groups of polymorphonuclear leukocytes: neutrophils, eosinophils, and basophils.	Among their functions, they are chemotactic and phagocytic and release histamine and serotonin to produce vasoactive reactions following injury.
granulation tissue	Newly formed vascular tissue that is produced during wound healing. Consists of fibroblasts, macrophages, and neovascular cells within a connective tissue matrix of collagen, hyaluronic acid, and fibronectin. Has the appearance of small, red, velvety nodular masses seen in new tissue.	Eventually forms the scar of the wound.
ground substance	Gel-like material in which connective tissue cells and fibers are imbedded. Part of the connective tissue or extracellular matrix.	Reduces friction between the connective tissue fibers when forces are applied to the structure. Adds to the area's density.

Term	Definition	Significance/function
growth factor	Components released by platelets and macrophages. Also referred to as growth hormone factor.	Performs numerous complex roles, the stimulation of reepithelialization, and is chemotactic for macrophages, monocytes, and neutrophils. Its role is not thoroughly understood, but it is believed to play an important role throughout tissue repair.
Hageman factor	An enzyme present in the blood.	Initiates the blood coagulation process following trauma by converting prothrombin to thrombin.
half-life	Amount of time it takes for the level of a drug in the blood-stream to diminish by one half.	Determines the frequency with which a medication is taken.
histamine	A local tissue hormone released by mast cells and granulocytes.	Increases vascular permeability to proteins and fibronectin.
hyaluronic acid	A major component of early granulation tissue. Greatest amounts are seen in a wound during the first 4-5 days. See also *glycosaminoglycan (GAG)*.	Promotes cell movement and migration during repair. Stimulates fibroblast proliferation. Produces edema by absorbing large amounts of water to increase fibroblast migration.
kallikrein	A proteolytic enzyme found in blood plasma, lymph, and other exocrine secretions. Activated by the Hageman factor.	Forms kinins and activates plasminogen, a precursor of plasmin. Increases vascular permeability and vasodilation.
kinin	A generic term for polypeptides that are related to bradykinin. A potent local tissue hormone found in injured tissue, released from plasma proteins. Examples: bradykinin, kallidin.	Mediates the classic signs of inflammation. Acts like histamine and serotonin on the microvascular system in the early inflammation phase to cause increased microvascular permeability.
leukocytes	White blood cells or corpuscles. Different types include polymorphonuclear leukocytes and mononuclear cells.	Have phagocytic properties to remove debris from an injury site.
leukotriene	Compound formed from arachidonic acid.	Regulates inflammatory reactions. Some stimulate the movements of leukocytes into the area.
lipid	A heterogeneous group of fats and fatlike substances, including fatty acids and steroids.	Serves as a source of fuel and is important to the structure and makeup of cells.
lymphocytes	Non-phagocytic mononuclear leukocytes found in blood and lymph.	Serve as important structures in the body's immune system by producing antibodies.
macrophages	Mononuclear phagocytes that arise from stem cells in bone marrow.	Considered one of the regulators of the repair process. Serve to phagocytize injury areas of debris, kill microorganisms, and secrete substances into an injury site, including items such as enzymes, fibronectin, and coagulation factors. Play role in keeping the inflammatory process localized; enhance collagen deposition and fibroblast proliferation.
mast cells	Connective tissue cells. Also referred to as mastocytes and labrocytes.	Store and produce various mediators of inflammation. Through their release of histamine, enzymes, and other mediators, mast cells increase local blood flow, attract immune cells, stimulate cell production of fibroblasts and endothelial cells, and promote and control remodeling of extracellular matrix.
matrix	Substance of a tissue. Can refer to intracellular or extracellular structure.	Forms the basis from which a structure develops.
monocytes	Mononuclear phagocytic leukocytes. Formed in the bone marrow and transported to tissues to become macrophages.	Remove debris from an injury site.

(continued) ▶

Term	Definition	Significance/function
mononuclear phagocytes	Any cell capable of ingesting particulate matter. The term usually refers to macrophages (polymorphonuclear leukocytes) and monocytes (mononuclear phagocytes).	Migrate to areas of injured or infected tissue and develop into macrophages to ingest microorganisms and debride an injury site. They defend the body against many organisms and are one of the last cells to leave an area of inflammation.
myoblast	A cell formed from myogenic cells in muscle.	Forms myotubes, which eventually evolve into muscle fiber.
myofibroblasts	Fibroblasts that have a combination of the ultrastructural features of a fibroblast and the qualities of a smooth muscle cell.	Responsible for wound contraction.
myogenic cells	Cells arising from muscle that later become myoblasts.	See *myoblast*.
neurotransmitters	Hormones such as norepinephrine, epinephrine, and acetylcholine, which are found in capillary, arteriole, and artery walls.	Released at the injury site to enhance platelet and leukocyte adherence to the vessel surface.
neutrophil	White blood cell in the polymorphonuclear leukocyte group of WBCs.	Contain toxic chemicals that bind to microorganisms to kill them. See *polymorphonuclear leukocyte*.
norepinephrine	A hormone.	Acts as a powerful vasoconstrictor at the immediate onset of injury. It may last from a few seconds to a few minutes.
osteoblasts	Osteogenic cells from periosteum.	Lay down the callus of fractured bone. Convert later to chondrocytes.
osteoclasts	Large multinuclear cells.	Resorb dead, necrotic bone tissue.
osteocytes	Cells characteristic of adult bone.	Maintain new bone mineralization.
platelet-derived growth factor (PDGF)	Substance found in platelets.	Essential for the growth of connective tissue cells. Stimulates the migration of polymorphonuclear leukocytes.
PGE1	See *prostaglandin*.	Increases vascular permeability by causing vasodilation.
PGE2	See *prostaglandin*.	Is chemotactic to attract leukocytes to the area.
phagocyte	See *mononuclear phagocyte* and *polymorphonuclear leukocyte (PMN)*.	
phospholipids	Lipids that contain phosphoric acid. Found in all cells and in layers of plasma membranes.	Stimulate the clotting mechanism.
plasmin	An enzyme that occurs in plasma as plasminogen. It is activated by kallikrein and other activators.	Converts fibrin to soluble substances.
Plasminogen activator	See *fibrinolysin*.	
platelets	Irregular cell fragments found in blood.	The first cells seen at an injury site and considered one of the regulatory cells of healing. Release growth factors. Form a plug at the injury to stop bleeding.
primary intension	Healing that occurs with minor wounds or surgical wounds.	Re-epithelialization closes the wound within 48 hr. Scarring is minimal when healing by primary intention occurs.
polymorphonuclear leukocyte (PMN)	A type of white blood cell with more than one nucleus. One of the granular leukocytes. Also referred to as neutrophil.	Chemotactic and phagocytic in the healing process.

Term	Definition	Significance/function
prostaglandin (PG)	Hormone formed primarily from arachidonic acid as a result of cell membrane damage. Its release requires the Complement System and follows kinin formation. Specific PG compounds are designated by adding a letter, A through I, and a subscript number, 1 through 3, to designate the number of hydrocarbon bonds. Examples: PGE1 and PGE2.	Mediates cell migration during inflammation and modulates serotonin and histamine. Some PGs increase pain sensitivity, induce fever, and suppress lymphocyte transformation, thereby inhibiting the inflammatory reaction. Mediates myofibroblasts, initiates early phases of injury repair, and plays a role in later stages of inflammation.
protease	An enzyme.	Acts as a catalyst to split interior peptide bonds in protein. Activates kallikrein to release bradykinin, ultimately causing increased vascular permeability and an increase in concentration of proteins and cells in the wound spaces.
proteoglycan	Substance found in tissues, including synovial fluid and connective tissue matrix. Proteoglycan solutions are very viscous lubricants and are sulfated GAGs. See also *glycosaminoglycan*.	Provides a resilient matrix to inhibit cell migration. Regulates cell function and proliferation, and regulates collagen fibrillogenesis.
reticulin	Collagen-like fiber. Some consider it Type III collagen fiber.	Forms the early framework for collagen deposition in a wound.
satellite cells	Cells present in muscle.	Regenerate new muscle tissue.
secondary intention	Healing that occurs in large wounds associated with soft-tissue loss. The wound heals with granulation tissue from the bottom and sides of the wound. Epithelial tissue does not form until granulation tissue has filled the wound.	Larger scar formation occurs with healing by secondary intention. Wound contraction is evident with this healing.
serotonin	A hormone released by mast cells and platelets.	Produces vasoconstriction in small vessels after norepinephrine activity is complete; occurs only when blood-vessel endothelial walls are damaged. In later phases, initiates reactions leading to collagen cross-linking. Also involved in granuloma formation.
steady state of a drug	Occurs when the average level of drug remains constant in the blood, and the amount of drug leaving the body is equal to the amount being absorbed.	On average, occurs after about 5 doses; equals the drug's half-life.
tenocyte	Tendon cell.	Converts to fibroblasts during healing of tendons.
tensile strength	Maximal amount of stress or force that a structure is able to withstand before tissue failure occurs.	Varies as tissue healing occurs; must be taken into account when determining appropriate stress application during rehabilitation.
thrombin	An enzyme.	Converts fibrinogen to fibrin to form a fibrin plug early in the inflammation phase. In later inflammation, it stimulates fibronectin production and fibroblast proliferation.
thromboxane	A compound that is produced by platelets and is unstable. Its half-life is 30 s. Related to prostaglandins.	Acts as a vasoconstrictor and is a potent inducer of platelet aggregation.
white blood cells (WBCs)	Cells in the blood that fight infection and play an active role in wound healing.	There are subgroups of WBCs such as polymorphonuclear (PMN) leukocytes (multiple nuclei) and mononuclear leukocytes (one nucleus). Within the PMN subgroup are further divisions of WBCs: neutrophils, basophils, and eosinophils. Within the mononuclear subgroup there are two groups: monocytes and lymphocytes.

Healing by primary intention occurs through a bridge of tissue when the wound separation is small. Healing by secondary intention occurs by filling in the wound with new tissue from the sides and bottom when the separation is large.

In more severe wounds where the stump ends are farther apart and cannot be bridged by single cells, the wound heals by producing tissue from the bottom and sides of the wound to fill in the space created by the wound. This is called healing by **secondary intention.** This type of healing occurs, for example, in second-degree sprains where ligament tissue is separated by distance and not surgically repaired. Healing by secondary intention usually takes longer and results in a larger scar.

HEALING PHASES

Whether the body heals by secondary or primary intention, the process through which it proceeds is consistent and predictable in most situations. We do not entirely understand the process, but we can determine the outcomes of each phase.

Healing is a constantly changing continuum of events. To understand and clarify this process, researchers and clinicians divide the events into three different phases. Keep in mind, however, that as far as the body is concerned, the process is ongoing, without clear-cut delineations. The body merely continues the process until the end is achieved. The three phases designated by researchers and clinicians are

1. inflammation phase,
2. proliferation, or fibroplastic phase, and
3. remodeling, or maturation phase.

Inflammation Phase

When an injury occurs, the body immediately recognizes a problem and begins a series of defensive maneuvers to stabilize the injured site and protect it by rushing chemicals and cells into the area (Hildebrand, Gallant-Behm, Kydd, & Hart, 2005). These extremely complex processes take two to three days and sometimes up to a week to 10 days to complete. A simplified version of these processes is summarized in figure 2.1. The injured area is extremely busy during this phase in its attempt to protect the site and begin the return to status quo as well as possible.

Inflammation often has negative connotations. In reality, it is an important and necessary step in the healing process. Without inflammation, the body would be unable to complete the healing process. If inflammation did not occur, proliferation, maturation, and final resolution would not take place. The wound would remain unhealed. However, inflammation becomes deleterious when it is prolonged, extending beyond the normal healing time.

The goal of rehabilitation clinicians is to allow inflammation to happen but to minimize it. This goal is accomplished at the time of injury by applying initial first aid: ice, compression, elevation, and rest.

As the injury's status changes in the first few days, the clinician minimizes inflammation and encourages healing to continue along its normal path by using various treatment modalities that are discussed in the Athletic Training Education Series text *Therapeutic Modalities for Musculoskeletal Injuries* (Denegar, Saliba, & Saliba, 2010).

▶ **Figure 2.1** Immediate injury response.

To make appropriate decisions about when to employ modalities and therapeutic exercise techniques, the rehabilitation clinician must first understand the events that occur in the healing process. Let us examine the series of events involved in the first phase of healing, the inflammation phase.

Vasoconstriction and Vasodilation

When an injury occurs, blood and lymph vessel walls suffer damage. There is an immediate local vasoconstriction that occurs in the small vessels. This immediate vasoconstriction causes hypoxia in the local area to trigger the inflammation process. Vasoconstriction is quickly followed by vasodilation. You may have observed this when you suffered a laceration. At first there is no bleeding, but within a few seconds the wound starts to bleed.

Cellular Reactions

It is at this moment of injury that the inflammation phase begins. The vasodilation causes the release of blood and blood products into the injured site, including blood **platelets** and serum proteins as noted in figure 2.2a. As these products accumulate in the injury, chemicals are released, and other cells are attracted into the area. Platelets release **phospholipids,** which stimulate the clotting mechanism to stop the bleeding. Platelets also bind to the **collagen** fiber stumps that were exposed by the injury. Platelets release other important substances, such as **fibronectin, growth factors,** and **fibrinogen** (Hildebrand et al., 2005). Each of these substances is important in the healing process.

The three phases of healing are inflammation, proliferation, and remodeling. During inflammation, the injury is contained and stabilized and debris is removed. During proliferation, fibroblasts, myofibroblasts, and collagen peak to begin granulation tissue formation and angiogenesis. During remodeling, wound contraction is well under way, and Type III collagen is converted to Type I collagen to stabilize and restore the injury site.

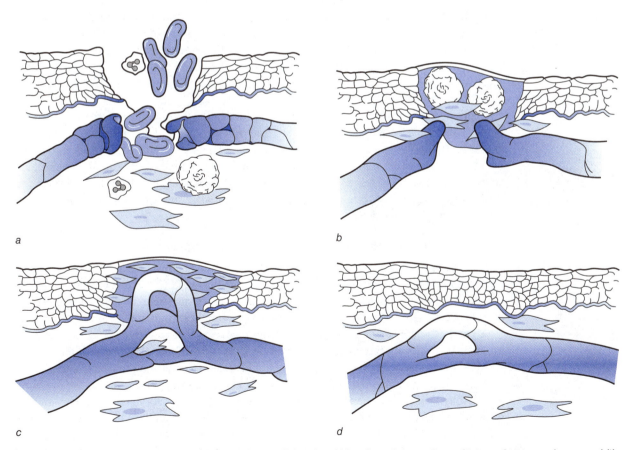

a

b

c

d

▶ **Figure 2.2** Epidermal wound healing. *(a)* Release of blood and blood products at time of injury. *(b)* Macrophages and fibroblasts in the area with capillary buds apparent. *(c)* Angiogenesis has caused anastamosis with new capillary growth. Fibroblasts are present in large numbers. *(d)* Reepithelialization has occurred. Regression of earlier established capillaries is noted.

Fibronectin binds together **fibrin** and collagen. Fibronectin and fibrin bind together in a cross-link arrangement with the exposed collagen ends to form a lattice-like complex, which acts as a plug to stop the bleeding. This plug is temporary and fairly fragile, but in these early hours it provides the wound's only **tensile strength** (Martinez-Hernandez & Amenta, 1990). As healing progresses, this plug is replaced by Type III collagen.

In addition to blood vessels, the more fragile lymph vessels are also damaged at the time of injury. Leakage from these vessels is also halted by the formation of the fibrin plug. Once fluid accumulates in the extracellular spaces, as it does during an injury, the only way it is removed is through the lymph system. Unfortunately, because the lymph vessels are plugged by the fibrin plug to stop leakage, their ability to remove the extra fluid from the area is compromised. Once the area becomes stable, **fibrinolysin** is released. Fibrinolysin is an enzyme that converts fibrin from an insoluble to a soluble protein to promote absorption of the fibrin plug and allow the lymph vessels to perform their normal function, draining the area of edema (excess fluid).

Within the first few hours of injury, the body attempts to remove debris from the site. This process is started by **neutrophils,** or **polymorphonuclear leukocytes (PMNs),** within 5 to 6 h of injury. PMNs contain toxic chemicals that allow them to bind to microorganisms and destroy them. The inflammation phase is named after these cells. Neutrophils are the most plentiful white blood cells in the body and migrate into the wound in great numbers, but their presence is short-lived. Other white blood cells in the granular leukocyte family include eosinophils and basophils.

The cells that replace the neutrophils are the **mononuclear phagocytes: monocytes** and **macrophages.** These become the predominant cells at the injury site within 24 to 48 h. Both PMNs and macrophages act as **phagocytes** to remove debris and dead tissue from the area.

As the inflammatory process proceeds, an inflammatory **exudate** is formed from the fluid escaping from the local vessels, dead tissue from the injury, and dying PMNs. Inflammatory exudate is commonly whitish and differs from the exudate seen in an infection, which contains bacteria. Although normally produced exudate is often referred to as pus, Peacock (Peacock, 1984) feels that this is a misnomer and prefers to refer to this uninfected substance as *cell aggregation centers,* not pus.

Debridement (removal of debris) is necessary for healing to continue. Before the subsequent phases can occur, the injury site must be cleared of excess fluid and other waste materials that have accumulated. For this reason alone, macrophages are vital to the healing process, but they perform other important functions as well. Once in the injury site, they recruit and activate other macrophages to assist in debridement. Macrophages also release growth factors and may trigger the termination of tissue growth when the healing process is complete (Diegelmann & Evans, 2004).

Chemical Reactions

There is an intimate interaction between cells and chemicals throughout healing. A cascade of events occurs because of these stimuli (Hildebrand et al., 2005). Some cells stimulate the production of chemicals, and certain chemicals at the injury site stimulate the arrival or production of specific cells in the area. This process of attraction or stimulation is called **chemotaxis.**

A good example of chemotaxis is the series of events that causes vascular permeability. Vascular permeability is a crucial event that initiates the inflammation phase. It allows cells and chemicals that normally remain in the bloodstream to enter the injury site and perform their functions to ultimately heal the injured tissue and return the area to as close to normal as possible. Vascular permeability is initially caused by **histamine** in the area. Histamine is released by cells that enter the area, such as platelets, PMNs and **mast cells.** Histamine is a **chemotactic factor** for **leukocytes,** or white blood cells, causing them to enter the area. Histamine is a short-lived, local hormone whose function of vascular permeability is continued by **serotonin** and **kinins** that also enter the area. Serotonin is released by mast cells and platelets, and kinins are released by plasma.

The presence of kinins in the injury site is short term, but they are followed by prostaglandin (PG) formation. Once kinins are released and a complement system is formed from serum proteins, PGs are discharged by cells that have been damaged. This stimulation of proteins that are normally inactive as they circulate through the system but enter the area of injury is also referred to as a complement cascade because of the surge of events that follow the activation of this system. These proteins are important to the healing process (Hildebrand et al., 2005).

There are two PGs that are most evident and perform important functions: PGE_1 and PGE_2. The function of PGE_1 is continuing the vascular permeability in the local area. PGE_2 is responsible for attracting leukocytes to the site. As healing progresses, they both appear to stimulate repair of the damaged area and permit advancement to the proliferative phase. They also seem to have a role in continuing inflammation at the same time (Wang, Iosifidis, & Fu, 2006). It is these compounds that are influenced by anti-inflammatory drugs, discussed later in this chapter.

During all of this activity, additional chemical reactions are also occurring. Hageman factor, sometimes referred to as factor XII, is produced in the area. It acts to stimulate production of the enzyme kallikrein, which increases vascular permeability and vasodilation (Peacock, 1984).

Signs of Inflammation

Many complex events go on during the inflammation phase. The injured area undergoes intense activity during this time. We see evidence of the degree of activity as common signs of inflammation, including localized redness, edema, pain, increased temperature, and loss of normal function. Edema is caused by the leakage of fluid, cells, and chemicals into the area because of the local vasodilation and increased vascular permeability. The increase in local cellular and chemical activity increases local temperature. Histamine and other released hormones and vasodilation cause redness. Edema is also the result of increased substances in the area and blockage of lymph vessels whose normal responsibility of drainage is restricted by the newly formed fibrin plug. The chemical substances that are released at the site, such as histamine, prostaglandins, and bradykinin (Butterfield, Best, & Merrick, 2006), make the local nerve endings hypersensitive and irritable, causing pain. Pressure from edema on nerve endings also causes pain. Pain causes a withdrawal reflex, which reduces the function of surrounding structures, limiting the patient's normal functional ability. Direct damage to tissues also prevents them from functioning normally.

Proliferation Phase

There is an overlap of phases as the injury site heals. Figure 2.3 demonstrates that there is no clear-cut delineation between one phase and another. Rather, as the body steadily accomplishes the tasks in one phase, the next phase evolves.

Although many cells and chemicals are involved during the inflammation phase, the macrophages (monocytes) are most responsible for removing debris and dead tissue from the area. Once this task is accomplished, the next step in the healing process is the development and growth of new blood vessels and granulation tissue. This transition from debridement to angiogenesis and formation of granulation tissue marks the beginning of the proliferation phase. Angiogenesis occurs at a rapid rate during this phase. This is important, for scar tissue formation requires vascular production and supply if subsequent events of healing are to follow.

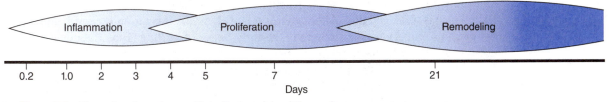

▶ **Figure 2.3** Tissue healing phases. Note the overlap of these phases.

The cells largely responsible for production of this new growth are **fibroblasts.** Fibroblasts are seen in greatly increased numbers three to five days following injury. Their increased numbers along with a decrease to minimal or nonexistent levels of PMNs are the hallmarks of the wound site's transition from inflammation to proliferation. Other activities that indicate that the injury has started the transition into the proliferation phase include a significant increase in extracellular collagen production, increased **proteoglycans,** and epithelial cell mitosis (cell division). The duration of the proliferation phase depends on factors such as the size and site of the injury and the tissue type involved. Generally, the phase is thought to last two to four weeks (Peacock, 1984).

As is true during the inflammation phase, during the proliferation phase there is an interactive response among cells and chemicals in the area. Growth factors, for example, enter into the area through chemotaxis produced by platelets and macrophages. In turn, these growth factors are responsible for the local migration and proliferation of **endothelial cells,** fibroblasts, and conversion of some fibroblasts to **myofibroblasts.**

The migration of fibroblasts is important during proliferation because these cells are primarily responsible for the development of new capillaries and the **extracellular matrix.** Although the initially formed matrix is not very strong, it holds the wound together and helps protect it from infection and stress. This wound matrix is soon replaced by a collagen matrix which is stronger and protects the new blood vessels that are forming during this time. Fibroblasts produce substances that will eventually make up this matrix. These substances, which include collagen, proteoglycans, and elastin, are required for ultimate scar tissue formation and maturation (Hildebrand et al., 2005).

Granulation tissue is the combination of the matrix and newly formed capillary buds. Granulation tissue is typically a bright, beefy red color. This is because the new capillary buds make up a significant part of the granulation tissue. Endothelial cells, the most important cell in the formation of these capillaries, contain a **plasminogen activator.** The plasminogen activator breaks down and removes the fibrin network that was formed during the inflammation phase so that lymphatic flow for removing local excess fluid can be restored.

The extracellular matrix has two components: fibrous and non-fibrous elements. The non-fibrous element is **ground substance.** This is a gel-like substance composed of **glycosaminoglycan (GAG),** proteoglycans, and **glycoproteins.** The ground substance fills in the spaces between the fibrous elements of the matrix and reduces friction between the fibers when stress is applied to the tissue.

Fibrous elements of the matrix include collagen, **reticulin,** and **elastin.** Collagen and reticulin are inelastic while elastin has elastic qualities. The combination of these types of fibers provides both tensile strength and some resilience to stresses applied to the tissue.

During the early proliferation phase, in the first five to seven days following injury, the fibroblasts produce these elements of the extracellular matrix. They form ground substance and rapidly lay down collagen. The activity during this phase is the result of new capillary growth by the fibroblasts. Capillary growth is followed by epithelial advancement across the granulating wound. As the epithelium progresses across the wound, epithelial cells and fibroblasts stimulated by the epithelial cells both release **collagenase.** Collagenase is an enzyme that prevents overproduction of collagen in the wound. This is an important process in normal tissue healing. An example of uncontrolled collagen production is keloid formations (excessive scar-tissue formations), a condition sometimes seen in dermal injuries.

Collagen produced in these early days of healing is Type III collagen. It is seen as early as 48 to 72 h after the injury occurs (Diegelmann & Evans, 2004). The fiber structure of Type III collagen is weak and thin. Although it is relatively weak, it is the substance that provides the wound's primary tensile strength in the early stages of healing. Type III collagen is laid down in a haphazard manner, without organized arrangement, further reducing its strength. It is later replaced by Type I collagen, a stronger and more durable collagen.

Tensile strength is directly related to the amount, type, and arrangement of collagen. By day 7 there is a significant amount of collagen in the area. By day 12 the immature Type III collagen begins to be replaced by the stronger Type I collagen. Both these occurrences add significant strength to the injury site.

While these processes are going on, a GAG known as **hyaluronic acid,** a part of the extracellular matrix, draws water into the area. This provides additional room for the proliferating fibroblasts in the wound site.

Although the proliferation phase generally occurs from 5 days following the injury to around day 21, this timeline can vary. The type of tissue damaged and the extent of the injury are factors that make this timeline variable. In slower healing tissue with extensive injury, proliferation is known to take much longer than three weeks.

External signs of this phase demonstrate this ongoing activity. The combination of increased capillaries and additional water volume accounts for the redness and swelling in the area. Pressure-sensitive nerve endings cause the site to be sensitive to pressure just as the tension-sensitive nerve endings make the area painful when it is stretched.

Remodeling Phase

During the remodeling phase, the wound tissue converts to scar tissue. Some of the activities that begin during the proliferation phase continue into the remodeling phase. One example of this is wound contraction. Myofibroblasts are responsible for this activity. They have been observed in wounds by the fifth day and have been seen longer than two months after the injury (Betz et al., 1992; Khan, Cook, Bonar, Harcourt, & Astrom, 1999). Some of the fibroblasts convert to myofibroblasts that migrate to the wound's periphery and pull the wound edges toward the center to contract the wound's size. The entire mechanism and function of myofibroblasts is very complex and yet to be fully understood. Contraction also occurs with continued remodeling because of collagen production, collagen cross-linking, and adhesions between collagen and adjacent tissues.

Wound contraction makes the scar smaller. This is advantageous, but it can be detrimental in situations in which joints are affected. If an injury occurs at or near a joint, scar tissue contraction and adhesions can cause a loss of motion at that joint. Indirect effects of wound contraction may occur if the wound is large and affects adjacent areas. The importance of preventing the adverse effects of scar tissue contraction is discussed later in this chapter in the section "The Role of Therapeutic Exercise in Healing."

Another activity that begins during the proliferation phase and continues into the remodeling phase is collagen transition. As Type I collagen is synthesized, Type III collagen is destroyed. When the construction rate equals the destruction rate, the healing process evolves to the final and longest phase, remodeling. This phase is generally about 12 months long, but may range from 6 months to 18 months (Connolly, 1988).

A number of activities diminish as the area becomes more stable and more permanent in its cellular and structural arrangement. The large number of capillaries produced during the proliferation phase to promote tissue growth is no longer needed and begins to recede. The extra capillaries will eventually disappear entirely (Peacock, 1984). Glycoproteins, GAGs, and the cells responsible for them — fibroblasts — in the extracellular matrix decrease significantly. Myofibroblasts also diminish.

With these cellular changes, visible changes can also be observed. These include the loss of the scar's red color with progressive change to white and eventually more normal skin tones. With the loss of extracellular matrix substances, swelling diminishes. Wound sensitivity also lessens.

As collagen is converted to predominantly Type I, it becomes more insoluble and more resistant to destruction. As fluid reduces in the area, the collagen fibers can produce more cross-links with each other, further strengthening the scar's structure. This collagen cross-linking becomes the primary source of the scar's tensile strength.

The maturation of the wound's collagen structure and arrangement is the primary activity during the remodeling phase, hence its name. Collagen strength is enhanced by the arrangement

TABLE 2.2 Chronology of Wound Healing

Phase	Time	Activity	Purpose or result
Inflammation	1 d	Neutrophil migration	Fight contamination. Release growth factors and biologically reactive substances.
Inflammation	1 d	Fibrin bridge creation	Area is red, warm, swollen, tender to touch.
Inflammation	1-2 d	→ Monocyte migration	Phagocytose bacteria
Inflammation	2 d	Angiogenesis	Ingrowing fibroblasts
Inflammation	2-3 d	Fibroblasts produce Type III collagen	
Proliferation	3-4 d	→ Rapid increase in fibroblasts Increased epithelial cell mitosis Increased synthesis of extracellular collagen Increased proteoglycans	
Proliferation	5 d	→ Myofibroblast production	Wound contraction
Proliferation	5-7 d	Collagen synthesis very active	
Remodeling	5-9 d	Reduction in fibroblasts Reduction in macrophages Reduction in wound vascularity → Reduction in fibronectin in proportion to the amount of Type I collagen formed	Less redness
Remodeling	10 d	Wound contraction	
Remodeling	12 d	→ Type III collagen converting to Type I	
Remodeling	6-18 wk	→ Reduction in capillaries	Reduced fluid content, increased scar density
Remodeling	6-18 mo	Completion of all healing	

→ = key activities of each phase

of collagen fibers. When collagen fibers align in an organized, parallel fashion, collagen can form the greatest number of cross-links and thereby possess optimal strength. The greatest degree of function and mobility occurs when collagen has this organized arrangement (Peacock, 1984). Properly applied external forces enhance this arrangement.

Table 2.2 summarizes in chronological order the phases of healing and identifies the primary activities and their timeline.

GROWTH FACTORS

Growth factors assist healing by causing cell proliferation and attracting fibroblasts, macrophages, and other cells needed for healing.

Growth factors are proteins that serve many functions. They interact with each other and other substances to promote the healing process. Their role is complex and not yet fully understood. One reason their function is difficult to understand is that their action in vitro is different than in vivo, so what is observed in the laboratory is not necessarily what occurs in the body. Another clouding factor is that what they are seen doing in laboratory animals is not necessarily what occurs in humans.

Specific growth factors perform specific tasks that affect specific cells to speed and enhance the healing process. Growth factors are named for the target cell they affect, their source, or their behavior. For example, the growth factor affecting the epidermis is called epidermal growth factor (EGF), the growth factor derived from platelets is called **platelet-derived growth factor (PDGF),** and transforming growth factors (TGFs) transform substances. Many of these growth factors work together to cause desired results in healing. Some of them are chemotactic, and others stimulate cell production.

Growth factors play a vital role in several key activities of healing (Angel, Sgaglione, & Grande, 2006; Best & Hunter, 2000; Breuing et al., 1997; Cromack, Porras-Reyes, & Mustoe, 1990). They control the migration and proliferation of cells vital to wound healing, including fibroblasts, macrophages, epithelial cells, and endothelial cells. Some growth factors are important in the early hours of inflammation, acting as stimulators of vasoconstriction and vasodilation. Growth factors also affect the formation of the fibrin plug. Others play roles in controlling macrophages and prevent phagocytization of healthy cells. In the proliferation phase, some growth factors assist and coordinate the capillary endothelial production. A number of growth factors are responsible for angiogenesis, granulation tissue, and collagen production. Growth factors in the remodeling phase stimulate the degradation of Type III collagen and the synthesis of Type I collagen.

A few growth factors stand out as primary players in healing and are worth identifying. One group is the EGFs. They stimulate production of a number of cells, including epithelial cells, endothelial cells, and fibroblasts. EGFs also draw epithelial cells into the damaged area and stimulate fibroblasts to produce GAG (Breuing et al., 1997).

Another important group of growth factors is the fibroblast growth factors (FGF). They are believed to be primarily responsible for formation of the new vascular and granulation tissue following injury. They promote angiogenesis by stimulating fibroblasts and capillary endothelial cell proliferation. They also stimulate production of chondrocytes (cartilage cells), keratinocytes (keratin-producing epidermal cells), and myoblasts (Breuing et al., 1997).

Platelets in a wound excrete a number of growth factors that aide in the healing process (Breuing et al., 1997; Cromack et al., 1990). These growth factors include platelet-derived growth factor (PDGF) and transforming growth factors, factor-alpha (TGF-a) and factor-beta (TGF-b). There is evidence that PDGF may stimulate events during the proliferation phase and may encourage healing of chronic ulcers (Breuing et al., 1997).

The primary TGF in wound healing is TGF-b. This growth factor has a number of responsibilities. Research has demonstrated that TGF-b stimulates healing during the inflammation and angiogenesis phases by increasing macrophage activity and stimulating epithelialization (Pandit, Ashar, & Feldman, 1999). It is involved in stimulating extracellular matrix production and coordinating the process of neovascularization (angiogenesis). TGF-b also coordinates other growth factors to regulate the healing process. Either directly or indirectly, TGF-b is responsible for causing the events that lead to granulation tissue formation.

The PDGF group is a family of growth factors that facilitate production of collagenase by stimulating fibroblast activity. The PDGFs are particularly active during the remodeling phase, when they prepare the extracellular matrix. They are produced by a variety of cells besides platelets, including macrophages, fibroblasts, epithelial cells, and vascular endothelial cells.

Keep in mind that many other growth factors play roles in wound healing. As mentioned, their function is not entirely understood, but their presence is vital if healing is to occur. Table 2.3 summarizes the most common growth factors in the healing process.

HEALING OF SPECIFIC TISSUES

Specific types and compositions of tissue show some variations in the healing sequence, although each tissue proceeds from inflammation to proliferation to remodeling generally following the timeline discussed. Given structural, cellular, and chemical differences, however, it is not reasonable to expect muscle tissue, for example, to proceed along the exact recovery timeline that bone or ligament follows. Let's take a look at some of the differences in tissues that we commonly see traumatized in athletic injuries.

TABLE 2.3 Common Growth Factors in Healing

Growth factor	Source	Target	Cell proliferation and chemotactic activity
EGF	Epithelial cells Macrophages Platelets	Fibroblasts Epithelial cells	Re-epithelialization Angiogenesis Collagenase activity
FGF	Macrophages Endothelial cells	Fibroblasts Endothelial cells	Angiogenesis Granulation tissue
PDGF	Platelets Macrophages Endothelial cells Epithelial cells	Fibroblasts	Fibroblast production Deposition of extracellular matrix
TGF	Macrophages Platelets Epithelium	Endothelial cells Fibroblasts Epithelial cells	Deposition of extracellular matrix Inhibition of epidermal proliferation

■ Chronic Inflammation

Normal healing of tissue occurs in the sequence just described. Occasionally, the injury does not progress along this normal timeline. It gets stuck in the inflammation phase and is unable to proceed in healing. This condition is referred to as *chronic inflammation.* Recall that in acute inflammation, the large number of granular leukocytes that initially invades the area is replaced with mononuclear phagocytes. The cells are transformed into larger macrophages and giant cells to debride the area. As the area is cleared of waste and foreign matter, these cells diminish in number, but in chronic inflammations they persist at the site.

Although we have much to learn about chronic inflammation, the presence of some substances have been identified as primary perpetrators of inflammation. It is known that large numbers of neutrophils are present in chronic inflammations (Butterfield et al., 2006; Diegelmann & Evans, 2004). It is thought that since they release enzymes like collagenase, they destroy collagen and prevent the matrix from developing (Butterfield et al., 2006; Diegelmann & Evans, 2004). It is also known that fibroblasts are stimulated during tendon activity, and these fibroblasts increase prostaglandin production, thereby creating an inflammatory condition (Wang et al., 2006).

In open wounds, the persistence of foreign substances, such as bacteria, causes continued inflammation. If an insoluble, nonphagotizable foreign substance, such as a sand grain or unabsorbed extracellular blood, is the cause of chronic inflammation, the area's response is the formation of a **granuloma.** The macrophages become chemotactic for fibroblasts to invade the area. The foreign substance becomes surrounded by the collagen that these fibroblasts produce to isolate the substance and form a granuloma.

It has been shown that chronic wounds have deficient growth factor levels (Hom, 1995). The introduction of growth factors such as PDGF, TGF-b, IGF-1, and others has improved healing (Hom, 1995; Scott et al., 2007). According to Hom (Hom, 1995), studies have also revealed that **protease** occurs at higher levels in chronic wounds. Protease degrades growth factors to prevent their presence in the wound. The studies that have investigated chronic wounds and growth factors have looked at several different effects, causes, and preventions and have all come up with one conclusion: Growth factors are necessary for proper healing; when they are not present, healing is impaired or prevented.

Although not technically a chronic wound condition, overuse injuries are frequently so classified. Overuse and overloading activities lead to cumulative trauma that exceeds the area's stress resistance. This is actually a continual re-injury, not a chronic wound. Overuse and overloading conditions are discussed in chapter 15.

Ligaments

When a ligament is torn, frayed stump ends are present where the ligament has been separated. The ligament undergoes the expected inflammation process, including local edema formation. The injured ligament stumps become surrounded with fluid, causing the ends to become friable, or fragile and easily damaged. Vascular permeability increases and permits the normal inflammatory products, including PMNs and **lymphocytes,** to invade the area. **Erythrocytes** and other cells accumulate to fill the gap between the stump ends. Within the first 24 to 48 hours, macrophages and monocytes enter the area to begin debridement. Macrophages also begin to secrete growth factors that begin epithelial growth and granulation tissue formation. Table 2.4 summarizes the timeline of ligamentous tissue healing.

Within 48 to 72 h after the injury, the proliferation phase begins with extra-cellular matrix development and proceeds through production of collagen and ground substance by the fibroblasts. Platelets in the area release a number of growth factors such as PDGF, TGF-b, and EGF. Macrophages are also producing PDGF, TGF-b, and FGF. These growth factors are chemotactic for cells (including fibroblasts) that produce collagen. This phase continues for up to six weeks (Andriacchi et al., 1988). Other routine processes occur during this phase, including capillary-bud formation that eventually joins with existing vessels. Phagocytosis also continues during this time. The quantity of collagen being synthesized is greater than the amount being degraded, so that there is an increase in net collagen during this time.

Several weeks later, the remodeling phase is heralded by the conversion of Type III collagen to Type I collagen and an increase in the number of collagen cross-links. There is also a reduction of edema, fibroblasts, and macrophages, and the area takes on a more normal appearance. This final stage may take eighteen months to complete (Tohyama & Yasuda, 2005).

Although all tissues follow the same general steps in healing, the course of healing in different tissues, such as ligaments, tendons, muscles, cartilage, and bone—varies and involves events specific to the tissue.

Tendons

As with ligaments, the tendon inflammatory phase is approximately three days (R. Gelberman, An, Banes, & Goldberg, 1988) to one week (Beredjiklian, 2003) long, depending on the specific tendon affected. Tendons have support from local structures that aid in the initial

TABLE 2.4 Ligament Healing Timeline

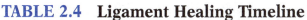

Phase	Time	Activity
Inflammation	First few hours	The injury site fills with erythrocytes, leukocytes, and lymphocytes. The ligament stumps become progressively more friable with the accumulation of serous fluid in the area.
	24 h	Monocytes and macrophages infiltrate the area. Fibroblasts begin to appear and eventually become significant in number.
	48-72 h	Fibroblasts produce the extracellular matrix.
Proliferation	1-2 wk	Fibrocytes and macrophages are numerous. Random collagen fibers and abundant ground substance are seen. Fragile vascular granulation tissue is seen at the injury site. The extracellular matrix continues to be synthesized by fibroblasts. Macrophages, mast cells, and fibroblasts continue to predominate. Vascular buds appear in the wound to communicate with existing capillaries. Elastin is seen in the area.
	2 d-6 wk	Proliferation phase occurs, during which cellular and matrix structures replace the blood clot formed during inflammation.
Remodeling	6 wk-12 mo	Macrophages and fibroblasts diminish.
	Up to 12 mo	Collagen concentration stabilizes with Type I collagen replacing Type III and collagen cross-links increasing in number. Ligament becomes more normal.
	40-50 wk	Near-normal tensile strength is restored.

TABLE 2.5 Tendon Healing Timeline

Phase	Time	Activity
Inflammation	First 3 days	Cells that originate from extrinsic peritendinous tissue and from intrinsic tissue from the epitenon and endotenon are active.
	5 d	Wound gap is filled by phagocytes.
	1 wk	Collagen synthesis is initiated, with new collagen fibers placed in a random and disorganized way.
Proliferation	10 d	Collagen synthesis is maximal.
	3 wk	The endotenon provides significant fibroblast proliferation in the injury site. Significant revascularization occurs. The synovial sheath is rebuilt, and a smooth gliding surface develops. Fibroblasts also start to become oriented in line with the tendon's axis.
	4 wk	Fibroblasts predominate in the healing area. Collagen content increases. Collagen is fully oriented with the tendon's long axis.
	35 d	Collagen synthesis is completed.
	42 d	Fibroblasts that have proliferated from the endotenon are the primary cells, simultaneously synthesizing collagen while contributing to collagen resorption.
Remodeling	2 mo	Collagen is mature and realigned along the tendon's axis.
	112 d	Fibroblasts have reverted to tenocytes, Type III collagen has been replaced by Type I, and maturation is complete.
	40-50 wk	Strength is 85%-95% normal.

healing process. These structures include the periosteum of underlying bone, the synovial sheath, the epitenon, and the endotenon. They provide the vascular supply and fibroblasts that are needed for healing. The epitenon and endotenon provide macrophage-like cells and fibroblasts to begin debridement. Table 2.5 summarizes the tendon healing timeline.

Within the first week, collagen synthesis begins and continues at a rapid rate for the first four weeks (Beredjiklian, 2003; R. Gelberman et al., 1988). During the second week, the collagen starts becoming more organized, so that by the end of the second week the cells are beginning to align themselves in the direction of stress. Collagen synthesis continues until day 35 (Peacock, 1984). Granulation tissue produced by fibroblasts migrating from surrounding connective tissue and from the tendon sheath is also present in rapidly forming quantities. By day 28, collagen and active fibroblasts producing the collagen are clearly aligned along the tendon's long axis. This assists the remaining collagen to form in a proper orientation.

During the first three weeks, the area undergoes a significant revascularization. With revascularization, it is possible to begin mobilization of a surgically repaired tendon by day 21. Immobilization prior to this time is important to allow reconstruction and restoration of local circulation because circulation is so vital to the tendon's successful recovery and function. Thus, immobilization is necessary not for the tendon to reconnect, but for the blood supply to be restored (Beredjiklian, 2003; R. Gelberman et al., 1988).

Also by three weeks, the synovial sheath is reconstituted. This is important so the tendon has a smooth gliding surface within which to move. When Type III collagen is replaced with Type I collagen and the fibroblasts revert to their original status as **tenocytes,** the remodeling phase is finished. This occurs by day 112 (R. Gelberman et al., 1988).

When a tendon is surgically repaired, the tendon and the surrounding soft tissue, including blood vessels, fascia, and skin, all become one wound. The area fills with a sticky gel. This gel is viscous and has the potential to become a thick, dense scar. If formed, the scar will limit the gliding of the tendon and thereby impede function of the muscle, ultimately limiting the success of rehabilitation (Beredjiklian, 2003). For normal function restoration, the scar tissue must not bind together normally separate structures but rather, permit tendon gliding within its sheath, the skin to move free from subcutaneous structures, and the blood vessels and nerves to have normal mobility. One major factor determining the success of this separation of elements is duration of immobilization. The effects of immobilization are discussed in further detail in chapter 5.

Muscles

Although muscle tissue may heal like the other tissues previously discussed and follow the same three phases to ultimately produce scar tissue, muscle also has unique structures within it that permit it to regenerate. These structures are **satellite cells.** These cells fuse with adjacent myofibers to repair and regenerate muscle tissue. It is believed that some destruction of muscle tissue occurs daily in routine activities. This destruction also occurs during regular exercises. The satellite cells restore and replace muscle cells routinely damaged during activity (Best & Hunter, 2000; Caplan, Carlson, Faulkner, Fischman, & Garrett, 1988). If an injury is sufficiently small, revascularized, and reinnervated and involves a muscle type that can regenerate, satellite cells replace injured muscle tissue with new muscle tissue. Table 2.6 summarizes the muscle's healing timeline.

In the early hours of healing, injured muscle tissue appears to follow the same route of other tissue: Phagocytes, primarily macrophages, invade the site within 6 h following an injury. Macrophages are the predominant cell in the area for the next 10 days; they debride the area. In the proliferation phase, muscle tissue regeneration begins as **myogenic cells** are activated. These evolve into **myoblasts,** which fuse together to form myotubes. Myotubes are in the injury site by day 13. Through a complex progression of events, these myotubes become muscle fibers and are apparent in the area by day 18. The final muscle regeneration is completed with the development of the neural aspect of the neuromuscular structure. When the process is complete, satellite cell levels return to normal and resume their daily function of less-intensive, ongoing muscle tissue replacement.

Larger muscle injuries are unable to repair by regeneration and must resort to scar tissue as the means of healing. When the mass of damaged muscle is larger than 3 g (0.1 oz), the muscle heals via the scarring process and goes through the sequence of healing we have discussed. Unfortunately, health professionals most often encounter these larger muscle strains in patients.

TABLE 2.6 Muscle Healing Timeline

Phase	Time	Activity
Inflammation	6 h	Fragmentation of injured muscle fibers begins. Macrophages appear.
	1-4 d	Fibroblasts appear.
	1 wk	Ability to produce muscle tension is progressively reduced. Scar tissue is seen in large muscle injuries. Muscle is able to produce near-normal tension.
Proliferation	7-11 d	Tensile strength reaches near normal.
	10 d	Large number of phagocytes, primarily macrophages, are seen at the injury site.
	13 d	Regenerating myotubes are seen.
	18 d	Cross-striated muscle fibers appear.
Remodeling	6 wk-6 mo	Contraction ability is 90% normal.

Articular Cartilage

There are many different types of collagen with cartilage. Hyaline collagen dissipates loads in joints. Commonly referred to as articular cartilage, it lines the surfaces of the diarthroidal joints. Fibrocartilage transfers loads between the tendons and ligaments and the bone. Examples of fibrocartilage are found in the intervertebral disks and the temporomandibular joint. Elastic collagen provides a flexible support to external structures and is similar to hyaline cartilage.

Although articular cartilage contains eight different types of collagen, it is composed primarily of Type II collagen (Lewis, McCarty, Kang, & Cole, 2006). When tissue healing occurs, Type I collagen is the primary resulting collagen. Cartilage does have some regenerative capability. The problem is that articular cartilage regenerates at a slower rate than scar tissue is deposited. Fibrocartilage seems to have a better capacity to regenerate than articular cartilage (Silver & Glasgold, 1995).

The differences between Type I and Type II cartilage are key in how an injured site manages stress post-healing. Articular cartilage is composed of 60-80% water, and 80% of its dry weight is Type II cartilage (Mosher & Dardzinksi, 2004). Its extracellular matrix holds a lot of water because of the proteoglycogans it contains. There is more water and fewer collagen fibers at the articular cartilage surface, and the reverse is true closer to the subchondral bone where the articular cartilage attaches. When an individual bears weight on a joint, the articular cartilage provides a dual system to protect the joint. When a joint first accepts a compression force such as body weight, the articular cartilage releases the water within the extracellular matrix to accept those forces. This is the fluid phase acceptance (Figure 2.4). If weight bearing continues, as in prolonged standing, the lower layers of articular cartilage where denser collagen is present provide for continued protection of the joint. This is the solid phase acceptance. Fibrocartilage does not have this structural arrangement, so it cannot offer the same protection to joints as does hyaline cartilage.

Whether or not an articular cartilage injury heals depends on three variables: the depth of the defect, the maturity of the cartilage, and the location of the defect (Gill, Asnis, & Berkson, 2006; Silver & Glasgold, 1995). Small, full-thickness defects repair with fibrocartilage via the blood supply in the bone adjacent to the lesion, but partial-thickness defects do not repair. Partial thickness lesions degenerate and do not heal because there is no vascular supply available.

In full-thickness lesions, the healing course of articular cartilage once again follows a sequence of events initiated with macrophages and fibrin-plug formation. Bone adjacent to

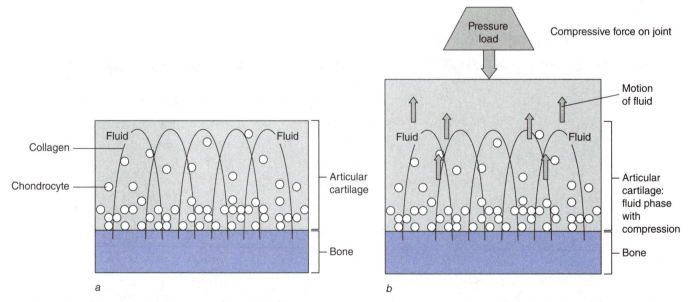

▶ **Figure 2.4** Schematic demonstrating the fluid phase of articular cartilage. *(a)* At rest without a load applied to cartilage. *(b)* Fluid phase of articular cartilage once a load is applied. Modeled after a schematic from Rheumaportal.com.

the full-thickness articular cartilage lesion bleeds into the area. Fibroblasts appear in the area to perform their rebuilding tasks. As the site advances into the remodeling phase, collagen becomes the prevalent structure. See Table 2.7 for a general outline of the sequence of events in cartilage healing.

Partial-thickness articular cartilage lesions are a source of concern for surgeons since many individuals experience these types of injuries. Partial-thickness articular cartilage injuries often become necrotic and lead to osteoarthritis because they lack a blood supply.

There are currently various surgical repairs used to delay this degenerative process. Most of these procedures have been to the knee since it experiences the greatest number of articular injuries. The surgical techniques are classified into three types: Cleaning the joint, repairing the joint, and restoring the joint. They all provide the patient with additional time before perhaps joint replacement is necessary. The first, cleaning, is ridding the joint of structures that produce pain in the joint; they are not reparative or restorative for the joint. These procedures include lavage and/or debridement. The goals of these procedures are to clean the joint and improve function by reducing pain for the patient. They are the easiest to perform by the surgeon and involve the relatively least cautious post-operative rehabilitation progression.

Reparative procedures include abrasion arthroplasty, drilling, and microfractures. All of these procedures are performed through an arthroscope. Abrasion arthroplasty, as the name implies, superficially abrades the articular surface without going down to subchondral bone to promote a healing response from the cells within the joint (Browne & Branch, 2000). Drilling and microfracture techniques repair the area of damaged articular cartilage by causing stem cells from the bone marrow of subchondral bone to migrate into the site via the bleeding that occurs with these techniques. A primary difference between these two techniques is the size and depth of the drill holes made in the subchondral bone to facilitate a bone marrow reaction. Smaller chondral destruction in the procedure with better results has brought microfracture repair to the forefront in recent years so it is fast becoming the favored reparative procedure (Detterline, Goldberg, Bach, & Cole, 2005; Steadman, Rodkey, & Briggs, 2003).

Results of the reparative procedures, especially the microfracture process, initially show evidence of normal articular cartilage in the lesion sites. Unfortunately, however, with time, the Type II cartilage is replaced with fibrocartilage. Fibrocartilage does not have the same ability to withstand stresses as articular cartilage since it has a higher friction coefficient. Hence, until more refined surgical procedures are developed, reparative procedures, as with cleaning procedures, will relieve pain and prolong the patient's need for additional surgery. The reparative procedures, however, may provide an individual with a longer period of pain-free and improved function post-operatively. There is some evidence to suggest that children may recover from articular cartilage injuries better than adults since children continue to produce articular cartilage during their growth years, especially if they are active (Jones et al., 2003). Caution and appropriate care are particularly important for young individuals who have many

TABLE 2.7 Articular Cartilage Healing Timeline

Phase	Time	Activity
Inflammation	48 h	Fibrin clot is formed to fill the defect.
	5 d	Fibroblasts are in the area and combine with collagen fibers to replace the clot.
Proliferation	2 wk	Fibroblasts differentiate, and islands of chondrocytes appear.
	1 mo	Fibroblasts have been completely differentiated.
Remodeling	2 mo	Satisfactory repair has occurred, with the defect resembling cartilage in appearance. The majority of collagen present, however, is type I.
	6 mo	A combination of type I and type II calcified cartilage has a normal appearance.

years before they may be eligible for joint replacement. Joint replacement rehabilitation is discussed in Chapter 16.

Two relatively new techniques that serve as restorative procedures include osteochondral plugs implantation and autologous chondrocyte transplantation (Miura, Ishibashi, Tsuda, Sato, & Toh, 2007). The osteochondral implantations use either the patient's healthy, non-weight bearing bone and cartilage or a cadaver donation. An **allogenic graft** is taken from another individual and is also referred to as a cadaver graft, homogeneous graft, or homograft. An **autologous graft** of articular cartilage and bone plug is taken from the individual's same joint as the damaged cartilage, but it is removed from a part of the joint that does not bear weight. Since this is a relatively new procedure, long-term results are not yet available, but early indications reveal good outcomes (Bartha, Vajda, Duska, Rahmeh, & Hangody, 2006). A procedure to replace articular cartilage with homogeneous cartilage, known as autologous chondrocyte transplantation was reported by Brittberg et al. (Brittberg et al., 1994) from the University of Gloteborg, Sweden. Autologous chondrocyte implantation is an expensive, complex process that involves at least two surgical procedures. The first surgery extracts healthy chondrocytes from the patient. The cells are then cultured in a lab for up to 21 days until a sufficient number of cells have replicated to fill the defect. The patient undergoes another surgery where the cultured cells are injected into the articular defect, and the defect is covered with a periosteal patch that is taken from the distal tibia (Brittberg et al., 1994).

For regeneration of articular cartilage to occur, the following conditions must be present (Buckwalter et al., 1988):

- Cells that will proliferate and differentiate into chondrocytes must be located in or migrate to the wound site.
- A mechanical stimulus that enhances articular cartilage formation must be present.
- Protection from excessive loads must be sufficient to allow cartilage repair without causing damage.
- A normal joint conformation must be maintained or restored.

These elements must be considered during the rehabilitation of chondral surgeries. Rehabilitation procedures for chondral surgeries are discussed in Chapter 23.

Autologous chondrocyte transplantation procedure is not yet widely used and is still being investigated. Other recent attempts have been made at the Stone Foundation for Sports Medicine and Arthritis Research in San Francisco (www.stoneresearch.org) using homogeneous grafts to transplant articular cartilage into arthritic joints without culturing the hyaline cartilage in a laboratory. This procedure is still at the experimental stage, but results have been promising.

Bone

As with other tissues, bone tissue has an inflammation phase that lasts three to five days (LaStayo, Winters, & Hardy, 2003), during which time fibroblasts and macrophages invade the area. The necrotic ends of the fractured bone and metabolic wastes are debrided by osteoclasts to clear the way and set the stage for the next phase.

During this next phase, the bone demonstrates its ability to regenerate. **Osteoblasts,** bone-generating cells, invade the area via the periosteum. As these cells go to work, a **callus** is formed at the site of each bone fragment end. This soft callus, whose formation takes three to four weeks, is a fibrous **matrix** of collagen that eventually becomes bone. The callus has an internal component and an external component. The external callus immobilizes the fragment ends, eventually bridges the two fragments, and allows stress to be applied to the bone without harming the fracture site before it completely heals. By the third week, the bony ends are united. It takes seven to 40 days from the time of injury for the fracture site to become mechanically stable with a soft callus (LaStayo et al., 2003). Table 2.8 demonstrates the healing timeline of bone.

TABLE 2.8   Bone Healing Timeline

Phase	Time	Activity
Inflammation	Immediately	PMNs, plasma, and lymphocytes occur.
	First few hours	Fibroblasts invade the area.
	3-4 d	Hematoma forms. Fractured edges become necrotic. Mast cells occur at the site. Macrophages remove debris. Osteoclasts mobilize in the area.
Proliferation	Up to 4 wk	Osteoclasts proliferate to form soft callus. Cartilage cells are seen.
	3-4 wk	Hard callus develops. Osteoclasts continue to remove dead bone. Endosteal blood supply continues to develop.
	4-6 wk	External blood supply dominates.
Remodeling	6-10 wk	Medullary circulation is re-established.
	3-4 mo	Fracture is healed, but remodeling continues.
	12 wk	Near-normal strength is attained.

As the osteoblasts move along the stump ends and farther away from the blood supply, they convert to chondrocytes, which produce a layer of cartilage. Osteogenic cells cover the chondrocytes. A fibrous layer covers these cells. This process occurs simultaneously on the external and internal layers in the bone's marrow cavity. The soft callus matures into a hard callus as the fibrous matrix converts into spongy bone. In a not fully understood process, the spongy bone converts to normal compact bone over time. In the long bones of adults, this routinely takes three to four months (Heppenstall, 1980).

During the remodeling phase, the callus size is reduced, the medullary canal is reestablished, the conversion to bone tissue is finalized, and normal oxygen and cellular alignment are restored (provided appropriate stresses are applied, via application of Wolff's Law) so the end product is as strong or stronger than the original bone (LaStayo et al., 2003).

TENSILE STRENGTH DURING HEALING

Tensile strength is the maximal amount of stress or force that a structure is able to withstand before tissue failure occurs. In other words, it is the amount of outside force applied to a muscle, tendon, ligament, or bone before it tears or breaks. Healthy tissue withstands high amounts of tensile force. Once injured, however, tissue's tensile strength seldom returns to 100% of its prior level.

This is about the only fact on which researchers of tensile strength agree. Disagreements arise because research techniques, the animals and specific structures investigated, the degrees of the injury, and the results of in vitro versus in vivo studies all vary. It is difficult to extrapolate findings of research with animals to humans, and it is even more difficult to obtain humans who are willing to suffer injuries to study the in vivo effects of injury on tensile strength. Studies often investigate only one structure or tissue. Results of these tensile strength studies are narrow because surrounding tissues that contribute to strength through their own framework, function, configuration, or attachment also contribute to tensile strength of an area.

The contributing strength of surrounding tissues may explain why athletes often return to full competition without becoming re-injured six months after reconstructive surgery, even though the tissue does not regain its full tensile strength for one year or more after injury. There are many unanswered questions about the tensile strength of healing and healed tissue; nevertheless, clinicians must be aware of current knowledge, incomplete though it may be.

Tensile strength takes a year or more to reach near-normal levels after an injury and seldom returns to its preinjury level, but the strength of surrounding tissues may permit a return to sport participation or normal activity sooner than that.

During the inflammation phase, normal tensile strength declines rapidly to 50% (R. Gelberman et al., 1988; R. H. Gelberman, Woo, Lothringer, Akeson, & Amiel, 1982). Depending on the tissue type involved, this decline occurs in 24 h to 48 h. In the very early stage of healing, the injured site's strength derives from the fibrin clot, which is insufficient to withstand much stress. Tensile strength is at its lowest during this time. Around day 5, tensile strength begins to increase. Without significant collagen, the injured tissue relies on other structures in the area, including the granulation tissue and ground substance, for this increase in strength.

As collagen becomes more plentiful and cross-links develop, the area's tensile strength becomes greater. Collagen conversion from Type III to Type I and the increased number of cross-links are the core reasons for tensile strength development.

Studies have demonstrated that time for tensile strength development in muscle varies, depending on the animal investigated. Rat studies show that by six weeks after injury, 90% of normal tensile strength is achieved, and in the cat, it takes six months (Caplan et al., 1988). Bone strength is the exception to the rule of not returning to normal strength; its strength returns to 83% of normal 12 weeks after injury (Grundnes & Reikeras, 1992) and to at least normal eventually, albeit months to years post-injury (LaStayo et al., 2003). Ligaments and tendons vary in the time it takes to achieve near-normal strength, depending on the specific structure. These tissues approach near-normal levels anywhere from 17 to 50 weeks after injury (Nordin & Frankel, 1980).

Researchers agree that once an injury occurs, the structure involved never regains full tensile strength. Tensile strength initially increases rapidly after an injury, then slows and even regresses as Type III collagen degrades and is replaced with Type I collagen. Depending on the structure, it may take a year or more for an injured part to regain maximal tensile strength.

FACTORS THAT AFFECT HEALING

A number of outside influences can profoundly or subtly affect the healing process. Clinicians can apply some of these factors to assist or stimulate the healing process. The patient, parents, or physician can control others. Still others, such as age and systemic diseases, cannot be controlled.

Figure 2.5 outlines the injury and healing process and the difference an effective rehabilitation program can have on tissue healing and its outcome. It is important for a clinician to know appropriate techniques that positively influence the healing process.

Treatment Modalities

Some of the treatment modalities most frequently used to enhance healing include electrical stimulation, and thermal modalities such as ice, superficial heat, and deep heat.

Ice is used during rehabilitation to reduce the signs and symptoms inflammation, especially in the early days of rehabilitation (Denegar et al., 2010). Occasionally in early rehabilitation after therapeutic exercises such as vigorous stretching or strengthening, signs of new inflammation, such as increased edema, may occur. Although ice will not affect existing edema, it can reduce new edema from overstretching or excessive-strengthening exercises. Remember that tissue irritation should be avoided; however, there may be occasions when it is unavoidable. At such times, ice used preemptively before signs occur may quell new pain and edema.

Electrical stimulation during the first week after injury enhances protein synthesis to help promote healing (Denegar et al., 2010). Because tendon and ligament structures are similar, electrical stimulation may also have the same effects when applied to ligaments.

Electrical stimulation applied to muscles may relax muscle spasm (Denegar et al., 2010). When facilitating muscle contraction, electrical stimulation may also assist in relieving local edema by pumping fluid into the lymph system, which reduces pain. With less pain, the patient may exercise more willingly.

Electrical stimulation is used to retard muscle atrophy following injury or prolonged inactivity. Electrical stimulation is used to facilitate muscle contraction and encourage reactivation

Factors that affect healing include the treatment modality, drugs, surgical repair, patient's age, systemic diseases suffered by the patient, injury size, infection, nutrition, spasm, and swelling.

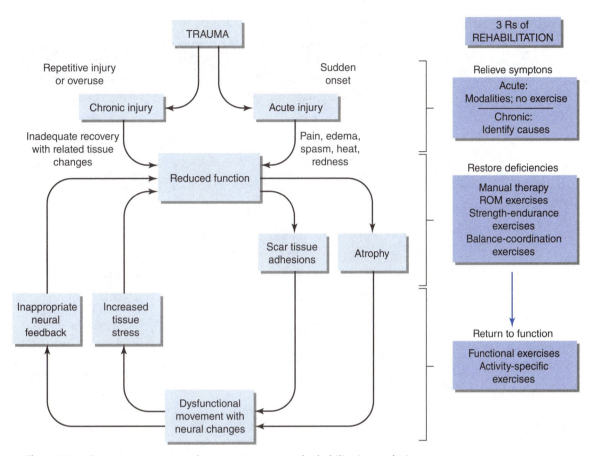

▶ **Figure 2.5** The injury process and appropriate types of rehabilitation techniques.

and recruitment of dormant fibers (Denegar et al., 2010). During short-term denervation, it may facilitate muscle contraction until nerve function is restored.

After the inflammatory phase, heat can be advantageous when applied prior to exercise. It may increase circulation to encourage healing and better exchange nutrients and waste products, relax muscles to allow better exercise execution with less pain, and reduce tissue viscosity to make an area more pliable for stretching (Denegar et al., 2010). It is believed that ultrasound and diathermy may speed healing and enhance effects of exercise by improving motion with less pain (Denegar et al., 2010).

Ultrasound has the benefit of producing thermal as well as mechanical effects. A contraindication to continuous ultrasound is in the acute inflammatory phase, when heat is deleterious. At that time, pulsed ultrasound is indicated. As a source of deep heat, ultrasound may be a useful pre-stretch application for tendon and capsular adhesions that lie deeper than superficial heat can reach effectively.

It is important for the rehabilitation clinician to know the desired results and choose a modality that best facilitates those results. As the patient progresses in the rehabilitation program, fewer modalities are required because the injury is more closely approaching normal function and metabolism. For example, as the patient enters the final stages of therapeutic exercise, ice is not needed following the therapeutic exercise program. If the patient continues to have swelling or pain that requires ice application following a therapeutic exercise routine, an examination for the cause for these symptoms is required since these symptoms should not occur late in rehabilitation. Table 2.9 provides a suggestion for possible modalities and manual therapy techniques to use throughout the rehabilitation process. This table should be used only as an example of suggestions for these applications; specific selections are individually determined and based on the patient's problems and needs.

TABLE 2.9 Modalities in Rehabilitation

Healing phase	Timeline	Possible modalities selection	Goal for modality application
Acute phase	Day 0-3	Cold: Ice pack, ice cup, cryobath, cold pack	Relieve pain, relieve swelling, promote blood clot formation
		Electrical stimulation	Relieve spasm, relieve pain
		Compression	Reduce swelling
		Elevation	Reduce swelling
		Low-power laser	Relieve pain
Early proliferation	Day 2-10	Cold: Ice pack, ice cup, cryobath, cold pack	Relieve pain, relieve swelling, promote blood clot formation
		Electrical stimulation	Relieve spasm, relieve pain, encourage healing
		Low-power laser	Relieve pain, encourage healing
		ROM activities	Gain motion, relieve pain, relieve spasm
		Joint mobilization, grades I and II	Relieve pain
		Cryotherapy	Reduce possible inflammatory effects from possible excessively aggressive treatment
Late proliferation	Day 7-21	Heat modalities	Encourage circulation, prepare tissue for other treatments
		High voltage electrical stimulation	Reduce edema, re-establish lymphatic flow
		Russian or interferential electrical stimulation	Muscle reeducation, muscle contraction
		ROM activities	Restore motion
		Joint mobilization, grades I and II	Relieve pain
		Selected massage techniques	Relieve swelling, re-establish lymph flow
		Cryotherapy	Reduce possible inflammatory effects from possible excessively aggressive treatment
Early remodeling	Day 14-48	Superficial or deep heat modalities	Prepare tissue for other treatments by improving deep or superficial circulation
		Russian or interferential electrical stimulation	Muscle reeducation, muscle contraction
		ROM activities	Restore motion
		Joint mobilization, grades I, II, III, IV	Relieve pain, restore mobility
		Selected massage techniques	Relieve swelling, re-establish lymph flow
		Strength, balance, coordination activities	Restore lost physical parameters
		Cryotherapy	Reduce possible inflammatory effects from possible excessively aggressive treatment
Late remodeling	Day 42 to 18 months	ROM activities	Maintain normal range of motion and mobility
		Agility, functional, performance-specific activities	Prepare patient for return to normal activities

Drugs

The injured athlete often consults with a rehabilitation clinician for information about the drugs that have been prescribed after an injury. Therefore, the rehabilitation clinician should have a basic understanding of medications, be aware of his or her own limited knowledge, and readily refer the patient to either the physician or the pharmacist for information beyond the scope of his or her knowledge.

Rehabilitation clinicians should remember certain general rules of thumb about medication. All drugs, even vitamins, have the potential to produce undesirable side effects. Any drug should be used with caution and taken according to recommendations of the physician, pharmacist, or manufacturer of over-the-counter (OTC) medications. If undesirable side effects occur, the physician should be contacted for instructions to either discontinue the medication or alter its administration. All drugs have a **duration of action,** the length of time that the amount of drug in the blood is above the level needed to obtain a minimal therapeutic effect. This length of time is determined by the half-life of the drug. The **half-life** is the amount of time it takes for the level of the drug in the bloodstream to diminish by half. The frequency with which the drug is administered is based on the half-life. The shorter the half-life, the more frequently the drug must be administered to obtain a minimal therapeutic effect. The example given in Houglum (J.E. Houglum, 1998) demonstrates this concept: Naproxen, with a half-life of about 14 h, is administered twice a day, whereas ibuprofen, with a half-life of around 2 h, is administered three to four times a day.

A goal of drug administration is to achieve a steady state. A **steady state** occurs when the average level of drug remains constant in the blood, that is, when the amount absorbed into the blood equals the amount removed through metabolism or excretion. After the first few administrations of the drug, the amount of drug in the bloodstream increases until this steady state is achieved. As a rule of thumb, a steady state is achieved after the dosing of the drug has continued for a time equal to 4-5 half-lives. For example, using 5 half-lives to calculate the time needed to reach steady-state, if a drug has a half-life of 12 h and is given twice a day, a steady state is achieved by the middle of the third day (5×12 h). If a drug has a half-life of 2 h and is administered every 6 h, a steady state occurs following the third dose (5×2 h), because the first dose is at time 0, the second is at 6 h, the third at 12 h, and so on. The difference between 4 and 5 half-lives is nominal: After 4 half-lives, a steady-state of 94% is reached, and is increased to 97% after 5 half-lives (J.E. Houglum, Harrelson, & Leaver-Dunn, 2004). A patient's compliance in taking medication is important for achieving a steady state and the desired results. If a patient fails to take prescribed medication, the intended results may not be achieved. By the same token, taking more than the prescribed dosage may not produce better results faster. In fact, it can be deleterious. "More is better" does not apply to drug dosages. Taking higher or more frequent doses of a drug causes higher concentrations and may cause toxic side effects. Taking two different anti-inflammatory drugs, whether they are prescription or OTC medications, should also be avoided because it is equivalent to increasing dosage and can be dangerous. These important precautions should be pointed out to the patient when medications are given.

Most drugs taken by mouth are absorbed in the small intestine. If medication is taken with liquid, a full glass of liquid is advisable, not just a swallow. The liquid helps dissolve the medication and also increases the speed with which the drug moves from the stomach to the small intestine. If a drug is to be taken with food, it is absorbed at a slower rate, but the food may reduce otherwise irritating effects on the stomach.

Other factors that alter drug absorption include exercise immediately following ingestion, since blood normally allotted to the gastrointestinal tract is shunted to working muscles. With delayed movement of medication from the stomach to the small intestine, irritation of the stomach lining may increase (J.E. Houglum, 1998). For this reason, it may not be a good idea to take an anti-inflammatory medication immediately before exercise, especially when the stomach is empty.

NSAIDs

Among the most commonly prescribed drugs in medicine today are anti-inflammatory drugs (Leadbetter, 1994). The most frequently used of these are the non-steroidal anti-inflammatory drugs (NSAIDs). Although research does not demonstrate a significant advantage of NSAIDs for athletic injuries, there is enough evidence to warrant their use, especially in the early days following injury (Mehallo, Drezner, & Bytomski, 2006). The NSAIDs are used to reduce pain and promote healing by minimizing inflammation in both acute and chronic athletic injuries. The NSAIDs reduce inflammation by inhibiting the enzymes cyclooxygenase-1 (COX-1) and cyclooxygenase-2 (COX-2). The primary reason for NSAID use in sport injury therapy is to reduce pain by inhibiting prostaglandin (PG) production. PGs stimulate local nociceptors (pain-receptive nerve endings) and enhance edema formation by increasing vascular permeability. By limiting PG production, NSAIDs can encourage healing progression from the inflammation phase to the proliferation phase. By reducing edema and pain, range of motion and other therapeutic exercises can begin sooner to promote recovery.

Several prescription and OTC NSAIDs are now available on the market. Refer to table 2.10 for a list of commonly used NSAIDs. Individuals respond differently to each of these

TABLE 2.10 NSAIDs

Generic name	Brand name	Doses/d	Maximum daily adult dose (mg)[1]
NONSELECTIVE COX INHIBITORS			
Aspirin[2]	many	4	6000
Fenoprofen	Nalfon	3-4	3200
Flurbiprofen	Ansaid	2-3	300
Ibuprofen[2]	Advil	3-4	3200
Indomethacin	Indocin	2-3	200
Ketoprofen[2]	Actron	3-4	300
Naproxen Na[2]	Aleve	2	1375
Piroxicam	Feldene	1	20
Sulindac	Clinoril	2	400
Tolmetin Na	Tolectin	3-4	2000
Diclofenac	Voltaren	2-4	150
Oxaprozin	Daypro	1	1800
SELECTIVE COX-2 INHIBITORS			
Celecoxib	Celebrex	1-2	400
Valdecoxib	Bextra	1-2	40
SLIGHTLY SELECTIVE COX-2 INHIBITORS			
Etokolac	Lodine	2-3	1200
Meloxicam	Mobic	1	7.5
Nabumetone	Relafen	1-2	2000

[1]Typical daily dose may be considerably less.
[2]Available without prescription.

Adapted, by permission, from J.E. Houglum, 1998, "Pharmacologic considerations in the treatment of injured athletes with nonsteroidal anti-inflammatory drugs," *Journal of Athletic Training* 33: 259-263.

drugs. As a rule, the amount of NSAID in the OTC dosage is half the equivalent prescription medication. One person may find better results from aspirin, whereas another may find aspirin ineffective but have great relief from ibuprofen. Another person may find that naproxen upsets the stomach but have no problem with tolmetin. Physicians commonly try a different NSAID if a patient does not respond appropriately to the first. Because each person responds differently, trial and error is often used to discover the medication that is most effective in achieving desired therapy goals.

Steroid medication is also used to control inflammation, but its use is currently limited because of its severe side effects. It is usually prescribed in large doses for a short amount of time. Administration is closely monitored by the prescribing physician because of the possible side effects.

Because NSAIDs inhibit the production of PGs through alteration of **arachidonic acid** metabolism, other physiological functions are also affected. Besides affecting the inflammation phase of local injuries, PGs play an important role in protecting the stomach lining. Therefore, one of the most common side effects of NSAIDs is stomach upset. For this reason, people with a history of ulcers or allergy to aspirin should not use NSAIDs. Stomach upset, nausea, and vomiting are possible side effects and may be reason for the patient to discontinue NSAID use. Generally, the tendency for stomach upset and ulcers increases the longer a person uses NSAIDs.

NSAIDs may also be harmful to kidney and cardiac functions. Arachidonic acid plays an important role in renal physiology, so people with renal disease may not be able to use NSAIDs. Because of the heart's relationship to renal function, people with congestive heart failure should avoid NSAIDs.

Like most drugs, NSAIDs should be avoided by women who are pregnant or nursing infants since NSAIDs may be harmful to the fetus or infant.

A family of NSAIDs was approved by the FDA in the late 1990s. These drugs primarily inhibit COX-2, by their influence on arachidonic acid metabolism. The more traditional NSAIDs are nonselective and affect both COX-1 and COX-2 to varying degrees. COX-1 enzyme is involved in many homeostatic processes in the body such as renal function, bronchial tone, platelet aggregation, temperature regulation, and gastric mucosa protection (Urban, 2000). On the other hand, function of the COX-2 occurs primarily in the inflammation process. While the nonspecific NSAIDs inhibit both COX-1 and COX-2, the Selective COX-2 inhibitors isolate their activity to the inflammation-producing activity of COX-2, so these newer NSAIDs reduce inflammation with less impact on gastric and kidney cells and other normal essential functions dependent upon COX-1. The unfortunate aspect of the selective COX-2 inhibitors is that a few individuals taking them have died from coronary problems.

As a rule, disregarding side effects, a drug should be continued as long as desired results are obtained. Researchers disagree about the length of time an NSAID should be administered. Generally, NSAIDs should be administered during the first two phases of healing. There is some indication that continued use of these drugs into the third phase may slow healing (Almekinders & Gilbert, 1986; Mehallo et al., 2006). It seems intuitive that the most effective time for using anti-inflammatory medication is during the inflammation phase, when production of PGs is the greatest. The use of NSAIDs during the first week following injury, therefore, may be most crucial. If an individual continues to respond to the medication beyond that time, however, it may be useful to continue it into the proliferation phase. The physician, of course, makes this decision.

Drug Interactions

Any drug can interact with other drugs also being taken to either enhance or reduce their effectiveness. This is known as **drug interaction.** For example, NSAIDs increase blood-clotting time by affecting the role of arachidonic acid in platelet aggregation and therefore magnify the results of drugs used in anticoagulant therapy. NSAIDs may also decrease the effectiveness of other drugs such as diuretics (medication to increase urine excretion, usually to relieve systemic swelling), beta blockers (medication to slow heart rate), angiotensin-converting enzyme inhibitors (medication to lower blood pressure), and oral hypoglycemic agents (medication taken orally to control non-insulin-dependent diabetes). Antacids delay the rate at which an NSAID is absorbed.

Other Drugs

Some medications may delay the healing process. Antibiotics, antineoplastic drugs, heparin, nicotine, and corticosteroids can all delay healing.

Other Modifying Factors

A number of other factors affect healing. Some of the factors over which the sport rehabilitation clinician has no control include surgical repair, patient's age, systemic diseases from which the patient suffers, and wound size. Other factors such as infection, spasm, and swelling, can be reduced by appropriate and timely treatment. Nutrition can be influenced through instruction and advice to the injured athlete.

Surgical Repair

The physician's surgical and sterile techniques have a direct effect on the healing of injuries that are repaired surgically. Infection complicates and delays the healing process. The quality of the surgeon's repair technique and follow-up care directly influences when rehabilitation can be started. If a surgeon's technique results in increased rather than decreased postoperative edema, tissue repair is delayed. If a surgeon immobilizes an injury for three months rather than three weeks, rehabilitation results will be slower.

Age

Age can be a factor that alters healing. A good blood supply is crucial for any injury to heal properly. A poor blood supply delays or prevents an injury from healing properly. Blood supply is often impaired with age. Diseases associated with age also can affect healing.

Disease

Certain systemic diseases can impede healing. If a patient has diabetes, HIV, arthritis, endocrine disease, connective tissue disease, carcinoma, or other systemic diseases, extra care should be taken with healing wounds. Additionally, conditions not often seen in athletes that can delay healing include renal, hepatic, cardiovascular, and autoimmune diseases. If a patient has any of these conditions, the athletic trainer is wise to be especially cautious.

Wound Size

Generally, the greater the injury, the more time necessary for healing to occur. If a patient suffers a first-degree ankle sprain, he or she may be able to participate in practice the next day. However, if a patient has a second-degree ankle sprain, he or she may be unable to return to practice for one week.

The larger the destruction of tissue and separation of tissue ends, the longer it will take for the body to debride the area and connect the stump ends. Similarly, the greater the injury, the greater the scar tissue. Scar tissue can impede rehabilitation, depending on where the scar tissue is and how long the injured site is immobilized before exercises begin.

Infection

Infection is a possibility any time an open wound occurs, whether it is an abrasion, a surgical wound, or a needle stick from an injection or aspiration. Precautions should always be taken to prevent infection, regardless of the source or size of the wound. Infection always delays healing. When an infection occurs, the wound site will have more scar tissue than it would otherwise have had.

Nutrition

Nutrition plays an important part in healing. The clinician should encourage the patient to have good nutrition through well-balanced meals to enhance healing. Diets lacking in protein, vitamins (especially A and C), or minerals (especially the trace minerals zinc and copper) make healing more difficult.

Muscle Spasm

Spasm is a reflex that occurs with injury as the body attempts to minimize the injury by immobilizing the area. Pain and muscle inhibition combine to diminish function. Spasms result in ischemia by restricting blood flow. Applying immediate first aid to the area is important in reducing spasm and ultimately improving the rate of tissue healing and the function of the injured part.

Swelling

The amount of swelling for similar injuries varies from one person to another. As a rule, however, the more severe the injury, the greater the swelling for all individuals. Swelling is caused by fluid in the interstitial spaces and can include blood, watery fluid from damaged cells, and plasma fluids. The body interprets extracellular blood as a foreign substance and works to rid the area of it. Edema also puts pressure on sensitive nerve endings, causes reflex muscular inhibition, and negatively affects nutrient exchange at the site of injury. These factors ultimately increase pain, reduce function, and slow healing. The greater the amount of accumulated extravascular blood and fluid, the greater the symptoms of inflammation and the longer it will take the body to progress from inflammation to proliferation. It therefore is crucial for the clinician to apply immediate treatment to minimize the edema and promote healing. Minimizing edema also reduces inflammation, pain, and loss of function.

THE ROLE OF THERAPEUTIC EXERCISE IN HEALING

Now that you understand the healing process, it is time to see how this knowledge can help in designing therapeutic exercise programs for patients. Your knowledge of the events and timing of the healing cycle should help you know what to do and when to do it to promote the patient's safe and timely return to competition.

The clinician can influence healing positively or negatively, depending on the treatment and when it is applied. Knowledge plays a vital part in the delivery of treatment. Knowing how to apply a treatment is the easy part. Knowing when to apply it, the intensity of its application, and the consequences or benefits of applying it is more difficult.

Although immediate treatment after an injury is considered first aid, it is really the first step in rehabilitation. Rehabilitation involves two aspects of treatment following on-field evaluation and immediate care. Therapeutic modalities are often first applied to promote healing, reduce spasm and pain, and allow the next phase of rehabilitation—therapeutic exercise—to begin. Therapeutic exercise allows the patient to resume full sport participation. Various aspects of therapeutic exercise are discussed in detail throughout this text. This section covers only general principles. It is important to realize that rehabilitation involves the use of both modalities and therapeutic exercise. Each component serves a very different purpose and together are used to achieve a common goal, the full recovery of the injured athlete. Table 2.11 provides a summary of the types of rehabilitation techniques that may be considered throughout the healing process. This table serves as only a suggestion.

Timing of Treatment

Once the injury is stabilized, efforts to control the edema and pain are important in the early rehabilitation phase. Even at this time, efforts can be made through therapeutic exercise to

Application of therapeutic exercise components must be carefully coordinated with the phases of healing. Respecting tissue healing must always be a dominant consideration when planning a successful rehabilitation program.

TABLE 2.11 **Healing and Rehabilitation Timeline**

Healing phase	Healing characteristics	Rehabilitation techniques
Inflammation	Fragile fibrin plug provides stability. Pain, edema, muscle spasm, loss of function.	Modalities to relieve pain, reduce muscle spasm and edema. No exercises to disrupt fibrin plug. May exercise non-involved body segments and cardiovascular conditioning.
Proliferation	Type III collagen forming. Angiogenesis. Less muscle spasm, but may have continued edema, pain, loss of function.	Continue with modalities and exercises for non-involved segments. Begin ROM to influence collagen arrangement: Mild PROM, AAROM, or some AROM. Mild isometrics may be possible.
Remodeling	Type III collagen being replaced with Type I collagen. Scar tissue becoming more permanent. Tensile strength increases with time. Improving function with less pain, edema in early phase with none of these seen with progression.	Modalities, only if indicated. Move from full motion exercises to resistive exercises. Progress to balance and agility exercises. Functional and activity-specific drills are incorporated at the end of rehabilitation. Aggressiveness of exercises is increased as tissue strength improves.

encourage the healing process. Care must be taken, however, not to disturb the newly formed, tenuous fibrin plug, which provides the injured site's primary stability and strength. Recall that in the first three days after injury, there is a lot of physiological activity at the injury site. Among other activities, macrophages are attempting to clear the site of debris so that the fibroblasts can start their task of rebuilding. Undue stress to the injury at this time re-injures the site, disrupts the fibrin clot, and causes additional edema. In severe injuries, the rehabilitation clinician must be cautious about the amount of stress applied to the area, especially in the early healing phases. During these phases even patients with surgical repairs can begin therapeutic exercise early. Even though the injury is unable to tolerate high stresses, the patient can work toward one of the goals of rehabilitation (discussed in chapter 1): maintaining the conditioning status of uninjured parts and the cardiovascular system. For example, if a patient has had surgery on the right knee, he or she can maintain cardiovascular conditioning by performing activities such as one-legged cycling or upper-body cardiovascular activities. Upper-body weight lifting and left lower extremity resistance exercises can also be a part of the program at this time. Some evidence indicates that exercising the contralateral limb provides some gains in strength in the involved extremity (Folland & Williams, 2007; Steadman, Forster, & Silferskiold, 1989).

By the end of the first week, the injured site is already entering the remodeling phase. Type I collagen is being produced, and the area becomes stronger and able to withstand more stress than in the first few days. The site of injury is still very weak compared to normal tissue, but it is able to tolerate some controlled stress. At this time, depending on the injury and the tissue involved, flexibility exercises and some early strengthening activities are used, although there are some exceptions to this general rule.

Tendon repair is one exception. Some physicians permit range of motion exercises but no strengthening exercises until the third week. Others prefer to wait six weeks or longer to begin strengthening. Some physicians allow strengthening exercises after one week because collagen fibers are being synthesized rapidly and reach their maximum levels by day 10. They feel that the collagen is strong enough at this time to start mild resistive exercises, often in the form of isometrics. Other physicians prefer to wait three weeks because it is then that the synovial sheath has been rebuilt to provide a smooth gliding surface for the tendon. Physicians who wait six weeks presumably do so because by then the new collagen is fairly mature and risk of rupture is significantly less. The risk of waiting too long to initiate activity following surgery is that the tendons becomes bound down by scar tissue formation following surgical disruption of skin, fascia, surrounding soft tissue, and the tendon itself. It is important to know the physician's preferred protocol regarding initiation of therapeutic exercise.

As mentioned in chapter 1, flexibility must be achieved before the other physical parameters. After reading this chapter, you should appreciate the reasons for this sequence. By the end of the first week of healing, collagen is transforming from weak Type III to stronger, permanent Type I. The cross-links are increasing, and the bonds between the collagen are becoming stronger. As a general rule, the most effective gains in range of motion are made during the first three weeks after injury. Changes in motion can be made relatively easily during the first two months following surgery or severe injury. After that time the collagen becomes more mature and resistant to change. This is the reason why an ankle that has been immobilized for three months is much more difficult to restore to its former range of motion than one that has been immobilized for three weeks.

Different techniques for achieving flexibility are used at different times in the rehabilitation process. Specific flexibility techniques depend on how mature the scar tissue is. These techniques are described and differentiated in chapter 5.

Once a therapeutic exercise program has begun and flexibility activities have been initiated, strength activities should begin when it is safe to do so. Depending on the severity of the injury and the status of the patient, early strength exercises may include only isometrics. Progression of strengthening exercises is discussed in more detail in chapter 7. The sport rehabilitation clinician must be cognizant of the stresses applied by strengthening activities. Care must always be taken to stress the tissues enough to provide the desired results without overstressing them and causing damage. The most dangerous time for strength activities is during the inflammation phase, when there is little tensile strength in the injured area except the fibrin clot securing the injury site. Care must also be taken during the remodeling phase, when collagen is converted from Type III to Type I, especially following surgical repair, when tendons and ligaments are particularly vulnerable.

The therapeutic exercise program should progress as described in chapter 1. Once flexibility is achieved, emphasis is placed on progressive strength and muscular endurance activities. These exercises become more intense as the injured area increases in tensile strength through healing and the muscles, tendons, ligaments, and bones themselves gain strength from the exercises.

As the injured area's supporting structures, especially the muscles that provide dynamic control, increase strength, exercises progress to improve the next parameter, proprioception. These activities emphasize balance, agility, speed, and coordination. The exercises are progressive and more advanced until the patient can transit into functional activities that replicate the motions and stresses of his or her normal performance demands.

The timing of the injured part's healing is always considered in determining when the patient should progress in the program. Stresses applied to the injured part must be assessed and correlated with tissue's healing timeline.

Overuse Injuries

Rehabilitation programs for overuse injuries involve somewhat different strategies from those for acute injuries because of the differences in causes. These differences are discussed in more detail in chapter 15. A rehabilitation program must always be designed with the healing of injured tissue in mind.

Often, an overuse injury is caused by continual or cumulative irritation to an area. The aggravating factor must first be changed before a successful treatment program can be instituted. Once the cause has been determined, healing can begin, although it is often slower than the healing of acute injuries.

For any injury, two considerations determine the appropriate course of therapeutic exercise. The first is the usual healing sequence and timing. Knowing when the tissue is most vulnerable and how long it takes for various tissues to go through their normal healing process determines what stresses can be applied safely.

The second consideration is the individual's unique response to injury and treatment. To evaluate each person's response, examine the area for negative and positive responses to treatment. Increased edema, increased pain, and diminished function are signs that the exercise was too severe for the injury to tolerate. Asking the patient for his or her response to exercise is helpful. "Did your knee have more swelling last night?" "Was there more pain in your shoulder after you left the athletic training facility yesterday?" "Was it easier or more difficult to walk on one crutch after the last treatment?" If you determine that an exercise produced undesirable effects, the appropriate action is to exclude that exercise until the injured area further improves. If no deleterious effects occur, the current course of treatment is appropriate.

SUMMARY

There are three phases of healing. Although healing proceeds moment by moment without clear delineations between the healing phases, these phases give health care providers a system to better understand and appreciate the healing process and the progression that must occur to complete it. Outside factors such as growth factors, diet, age, and injury severity will influence healing. Healing is also the factor with the greatest influence on rehabilitation progression. What the athletic trainer clinician is able to do with a patient and the success of that clinician's treatment are primarily dependent upon the clinician being able to accurately identify where the patient is in the healing process. Little activity outside of the application of modalities for pain, edema, and spasm relief is used during the inflammation phase, but once the injury enters the proliferation phase, activity begins with range of motion. From this point, the patient progresses to strength, balance, agility, and coordination, and then into functional and sport-specific activities before being tested to assess the patient's ability to return to normal function.

KEY CONCEPTS AND REVIEW

1. Explain the differences between primary and secondary healing.

Primary healing produces a minimal scar and occurs when the damaged edges of a wound are close to each other, whereas secondary healing produces a greater scar because the wound must heal by filling in tissue from the bottom and sides of the wound.

2. Identify the healing phases.

The body follows a very complex and not entirely understood process of healing, going through the three phases of healing: inflammation, proliferation, and remodeling.

3. Describe the primary processes of each healing phase.

During inflammation, neutrophil migration begins the process, fibrin-plug production prevents fluid and blood from escaping, monocyte migration rids the area of debris, angiogenesis restores blood flow, and Type III collagen is produced. Proliferation occurs when fibroblasts, myofibroblasts, and collagen synthesis are at their peak. During remodeling, healing slows, wound contraction is well under way, and Type III collagen is converted to Type I collagen.

4. Discuss the causes for the signs of inflammation.

Redness, localized warmth, swelling, pain, and dysfunction are all signs of inflammation. Redness occurs because of increased circulation and released chemicals, localized warmth and swelling are caused by interstitial fluid leakage and increased metabolic activity in the area, pain is caused by pressure on nerve endings from edema and damage to nerves in the area. Dysfunction occurs because of the physical restrictions of swelling, damage to structures, and the muscular inhibition from the pain.

5. Explain the role of growth factors in healing.

Growth factors are not well understood, but present knowledge indicates that they play an important role throughout tissue healing. They assist in causing cell proliferation and chemotactic activity that are vital to healing.

6. Discuss the differences between acute and chronic inflammation.

Acute inflammation occurs through a systematic progression of chemical and cellular activity. Chronic inflammation occurs when the site is unable to proceed from the inflammatory phase to the proliferation phase because leukocytes persist in the area and granulocytes are unable to fully debride the area so that mononuclear cells persist.

7. Discuss specific tissue healing characteristics.

Ligaments, tendons, muscle, bone, and cartilage all follow the general healing process, but their healing also has aspects unique to their own cellular makeup. For example, muscle has myogenic cells that are able to regenerate muscle tissue, bone has osteoblasts, and tendons have tenocytes.

8. Identify the relevance of tensile strength.

Tensile strength enables a structure to withstand stresses. Once an area is damaged, the tensile strength is not restored to 100% normal except in bone. In spite of this, a patient is able to safely return to normal participation if the injury has properly healed and a proper rehabilitation program has been followed.

9. Discuss factors that can modify the healing process.

Healing of any tissue is influenced by a number of factors. Factors that can be influenced include the use of medications (especially anti-inflammatory drugs), the use of various treatment modalities, the application of first aid, edema and pain, infection, and nutrition. Other factors over which the certified athletic trainer has no control include the physician's surgical technique and the patient's age and general health.

10. Explain the role NSAIDs play in inflammation.

NSAIDs reduce the effects of inflammation by altering chemical production or the impact of specific chemicals on the healing process. If administered correctly, they can positively reduce the inflammation phase to promote healing.

11. Discuss the timing of treatment with the various stages of healing.

Therapeutic exercise must be administered appropriately without causing harm to the healing tissues if the rehabilitation program is to be successful. It is important to use exercises carefully and watch for adverse effects from the exercises.

CRITICAL THINKING QUESTIONS

1. If you were Daniel in the opening scenario, how would you approach Becki to discuss whether or not she has anorexia? How could anorexia affect Becki's healing process? What could you do to counteract her anorexia? What precautions should you take to "do no harm"?

2. If a patient presented to you with Achilles tendinopathy that began two weeks ago, at what stage would you estimate the tendinopathy to be? What would be your criteria for determining whether it is acute or chronic?

3. A patient who undergoes an outpatient surgical repair of the elbow comes to you three days after the surgery to begin rehabilitation. Where in the healing process do you estimate this patient to be, and what healing activities are occurring? What would you do for treatment in the first three days of your treatment program? What would you do for treatment in the first three weeks of your treatment program? What factors would you consider to determine when to change the treatment program?

4. A patient with a second-degree ankle sprain that occurred four days ago comes to you for rehabilitation. If the patient was 50 years old; had diabetes, severe swelling, and cramps in the calf muscles; was on Coumadin and an oral hypoglycemic medication; and had been taking oral anti-inflammatories for the past three days, what would your treatment program include? How would your treatment be different if the patient was 22 years old, had severe swelling and cramps in the calf muscles, and had been taking oral anti-inflammatories for the past three days?

LAB ACTIVITIES

1. Identify three reliable Web sites to which you can refer for additional information on tissue healing, the stages of healing, or specific tissue healing.

2. List the types of rehabilitation techniques you would be able to use within each phase of healing.

3. Identify three medications kept either in the athletic training clinic or your own home, and list what influence, if any, they may have on healing.

4. Investigate the influences growth hormones have on healing. Where are they produced in the body, how are they attracted to an injury site, and during what stage of healing would you expect them to be most evident? Why?

CHAPTER 3

Concepts of Physics

OBJECTIVES

After completing this chapter, you should be able to do the following:

1. Define force and give an example of an internal and an external force.
2. Explain the relevance to therapeutic exercise of Newton's first, second, and third laws of motion.
3. Explain how center of gravity changes with movement.
4. Discuss how a change in base of support can change a person's stability.
5. Explain the relationship between line of gravity and base of support.
6. Explain two ways of increasing stability.
7. Identify the difference between stabilization and fixation.
8. Explain how torque can be altered in the body.
9. Identify how varying position changes a muscle's mechanical advantage.
10. Discuss the difference between mechanical and physiological advantage of a muscle.
11. Explain the importance of positioning in exercising two-joint muscles.
12. Distinguish between velocity and acceleration.
13. Discuss the relevance of elasticity, stress-strain, creep, and friction to therapeutic exercise.

▶ Joel Edgars is working to rehabilitate Reeda Skaalie, a swimmer with a shoulder injury. The facility where Joel works has an adjustable pulley system, and he wants to use it for the series of scapular strengthening exercises he has planned for today's program with Reeda. He wants to exercise the lower trapezius, middle trapezius, rhomboids, and serratus anterior on the pulleys. Joel realizes that the muscle's physiological length, lever-arm length, and angle of pull all influence the amount of work that is done by the muscles and understands that stabilization must be a consideration, but he is at a loss as to where the pulleys should be placed to obtain the best results. Reeda is scheduled to begin the program in 30 min, so Joel must quickly figure out the pulley placement for the exercises he has in mind for today's program.

You had better live your best and act your best
and think your best today; for today is the sure preparation
for tomorrow and all the other tomorrows that follow.

HARRIET MARTINEAU, 1802-1876, author

As Ms Martineau's words suggest, this chapter will prepare you by providing a foundation for future knowledge and understanding of therapeutic exercise technique applications. Knowing why we do what we do in therapeutic exercise is vital. Only with an understanding of theory and precepts can we adjust exercises to each injured individual's needs and develop soundly structured, knowledge-based therapeutic exercise programs. The concepts presented in this chapter provide what should be a review of basic physics principles that are frequently used in rehabilitation, specifically therapeutic exercise. Many of them may be review for you, but the clinical applications used in this chapter may help you understand why the concepts presented are important to remember.

The physics concepts in this chapter are not new; they have successfully endured the test of centuries. Many of the ideas that Sir Isaac Newton and other engineers and philosophers introduced during the 1600s have profound impact on the delivery of therapeutic exercise in musculoskeletal rehabilitation today. These concepts are another vital part of the foundation of knowledge that you will need to guide a patient through a therapeutic exercise program. Without this knowledge it is difficult to apply forces correctly for stretching and strengthening, use your own body efficiently and effectively, or develop a successful therapeutic exercise program.

As you read through this chapter, you should develop an appreciation of basic physics principles that will affect the application of your clinical skills daily. These principles are not complicated, but they are vital for rehabilitation clinicians. First, concepts are presented; then examples of direct applications to daily tasks in therapeutic exercise are provided.

FORCE

A **force** is a form of energy that causes movement and has direction and magnitude. A mass is moved in a specific direction when a specific amount of force is applied. In the human body, the force can be either internal or external and usually produces either a push or a pull. Internal forces, of course, are generated by the muscles. External forces can be applied by a wide variety of sources, the most basic being gravity.

Gravity is probably the most basic external force; we all deal with gravity continuously. Whether you realize it or not, it affects your every move. For example, if there were no gravity, activity as we know it would be drastically different. Although Sir Isaac Newton didn't formulate his law of gravity until the late 1600s, gravity has been around since before the beginning of earth.

Sir Isaac Newton's law of gravity states that every object attracts every other object with a force proportional to the product of their masses and inversely proportional to the square of the distance between them. Because the earth is so massive compared with the objects on its surface, gravity is commonly thought of as the force of attraction that the earth exerts on an object. Gravity is counterbalanced by the supporting surface on which a person is standing, sitting, or lying. In other words, without surfaces such as a floor, bed, or chair on which to balance our weight, we would simply fall. This concept leads us to Newton's third law of motion, which is discussed later.

A force causes movement and has direction and magnitude. Gravity is a pervasive external force that affects every movement.

NEWTON'S LAWS OF MOTION

The mathematician Sir Isaac Newton (1642–1727) formulated laws of motion and gravity that are used to explain movement. The three laws of motion discussed here are inertia, acceleration and momentum, and action-reaction.

Inertia

Newton's first law of motion deals with **inertia:** A body remains at a state of rest or remains in uniform motion until an outside force acts on it. This is one reason why it is difficult for a weak muscle to initiate the lifting of a limb, but once movement begins, it becomes easier for the muscle to continue the movement. The muscle must have enough strength not only to lift the weight of the limb but also to overcome inertia. For example, if you give assistance in the beginning of a weightlifting exercise, such as a straight-leg raise, the patient may be able to continue the exercise on his or her own once the motion has begun, provided there is enough strength to lift the limb. It is also why it is difficult to push something heavy, like a dresser or file cabinet, but once you are able to budge it, it is easier to move across the floor.

Acceleration and Momentum

Newton's second law of motion deals with **acceleration** and **momentum.** It states that the acceleration of an object is directly proportional to the force causing motion and inversely proportional to the mass of the object being moved. Momentum is the amount of motion a moving object has. The formulas used to calculate acceleration and momentum make it easy to understand:

Momentum = mass × velocity

Mass = weight ÷ acceleration due to gravity

Linear velocity = distance ÷ time

Newton's second law of motion is important in therapeutic exercise because it explains why a slow, controlled motion of an extremity requires more strength than a quickly executed movement. You can easily realize this fact if you lift a 10 lb dumbbell slowly then lift it quickly; it is much easier to lift it fast than slowly. If strength gain is the goal, it is better to have the patient move the extremity through the motion in a slow, controlled manner.

Action-Reaction

The force of gravity is commonly referred to as **weight.** If this force is counterbalanced, a body does not fall to the earth. This demonstrates **Newton's third law of motion:** An object reacts to a force with a force of equal magnitude in the opposite direction. Stated another way, for every action there is an equal and opposite reaction. Here are a couple of everyday

> ### ■ Newton's Three Laws of Motion
>
> Here is a summary of Newton's first three laws:
>
> 1. **Newton's first law of motion: inertia.** A body remains at a state of rest or remains in uniform motion until a force acts on it.
> 2. **Newton's second law of motion: acceleration and momentum.** The acceleration of an object is directly proportional to the force causing motion and inversely proportional to the mass of the object being moved.
> 3. **Newton's third law of motion: action-reaction.** For every action there is an equal and opposite reaction.

Newton's first and second laws of motion describe inertia, momentum, and acceleration. These laws explain that the faster an object already moves, the less force is needed to move it in the same direction. His third law, action-reaction, states that for every action there is an equal and opposite reaction.

applications of this law: If you hold a book in your hand, your muscle force counteracts the force of gravity and prevents the book from going to the ground. Another example is a patient lying on a treatment table: The force of gravity on the patient is counterbalanced by the upward force of the treatment table.

Let's consider the next step, what happens when a force that is stronger than gravity causes a body to move in the direction of that force. For example, a basketball being shot is propelled by a force strong enough to move the basketball up and toward the basket. The force must not only be applied with enough intensity to get the ball to the basket, but the force must be applied in the correct direction or angle to reach the target accurately. As another example, a volleyball player jumping to block at the net must produce enough force to overcome the force of gravity; the more force applied, the higher the volleyball player jumps. To perform a straight-leg raise, a patient must exert enough muscle force at the hip to counteract gravity's pull on the lower extremity.

CENTER OF GRAVITY

Every object has a **center of gravity.** It is the point in the body or an object around which its weight is balanced. If we look at a symmetrical, rigid pole, the center of gravity is easy to find; it is the point toward the middle at which the pole balances when suspended. Every body part and even the entire human body has its own center of gravity, as noted in table 3.1. Knowing the center of gravity's location is important for knowing where to apply force and how much force to apply to move or maintain a position.

The center of gravity is harder to find in the human body because of the body's irregular shape. In the anatomic position, the body's center of gravity is generally considered to be at about the level of the S2 vertebra. It is slightly higher in men than in women and varies with individual variations in shape. It also is different in children, because their weight distribution is different from that of adults.

As the body or part of the body moves, the center of gravity changes, as seen in figure 3.1. When a sprinter is in the starter blocks, the center of gravity is much lower than when running. When a rhythmic gymnast reaches out to catch a baton, her center of gravity changes as the arm extends forward and the baton's weight is added to her body weight.

The center of gravity also changes when weight is added to the body. For example, if a track and field athlete picks up a 15.9 kg (35 lb) hammer in his left hand, his center of gravity shifts to that side. If a 91 kg (200 lb) weightlifter jerks a 68 kg (150 lb) barbell overhead, his center of gravity becomes significantly higher than vertebra S2; this is why some weightlifters have a difficult time stabilizing themselves in this maneuver.

The lower the center of gravity, the more stable the object. We see this concept commonly in athletics. For example, a football lineman protects himself from being pushed by an opponent by lowering his center of gravity.

Center of gravity refers to the point in the body or object around which its weight is balanced. Knowing the center of gravity of a body of an object can lead to understanding how to increase its stability.

TABLE 3.1 Parts of the Human Body and Their Centers of Gravity*

Body part(s)	kg	lb	%	Location of center of gravity
Entire body	68.2	150	100	Anterior to second sacral vertebra
HEAD AND TRUNK				
Head	4.7	10.3	6.9	In sphenoid sinus, 4 mm beyond anterior inferior margin of sella (on lateral surface, over temporal fossa, on or near nasioiniac)
Head and neck	5.4	11.8	7.9	On inferior surface of basioccipital bone or within bone 23 ± 5 mm from crest of dorsum sellae (on lateral surface, 10 mm anterior to supratragic notch above head of mandible)
Head, neck, and trunk	40.1	88.5	59.0	Anterior to 11th thoracic vertebra
UPPER LIMB				
Arm	1.9	4.1	2.7	In medial head of triceps, adjacent to radial groove; 5 mm proximal to distal end of deltoid insertion
Forearm	1.1	2.4	1.6	11 mm proximal to most distal part of pronator teres insertion; 9 mm anterior to interosseus membrane
Hand	0.4	0.9	0.6	Axis of 3rd metacarpal; 2 mm proximal to proximal transverse palmar crease and between this palmar crease and radial longitudinal crease
Entire upper limb	3.4	7.4	4.9	Just above elbow joint
LOWER LIMB				
Thigh	6.6	14.5	9.7	In adductor brevis muscle; 13 mm medial to linea aspera, deep to adductor canal, 29 mm below apex of femoral triangle and 18 mm proximal to most distal fibers of adductor brevis
Leg	3.1	6.8	4.5	35 mm below popliteus, at posterior part of posterior tibialis; 16 mm above proximal end of Achilles tendon, 8 mm posterior to interosseus membrane
Foot	1	2.1	1.4	In plantar ligaments, or just superficial in adjacent deep foot muscles; below proximal halves of second and third cuneiform bones; on a line between ankle joint center and ball of foot in plane of metatarsal II
Entire lower limb	10.6	23.4	15.6	Just above knee joint

*Segmental weights and percentage of total body weight for a 68 kg (150 lb) man

STABILITY AND FIXATION

A number of factors determine a person's or object's stability. These factors all relate, however, to the relationship between the line of gravity and the base of support.

The **line of gravity** is an imaginary line that runs vertically through the center of gravity toward the center of the earth, so the line is perpendicular to the earth's surface. This line is used as a point of reference when discussing posture and is investigated in chapter 11. The line of gravity is also used to determine stability of an object. An object is most stable when the line of gravity falls within the object's base of support, as demonstrated in figure 3.2.

The **base of support,** simply referred to as the base, is the two-dimensional area between and including an object's points of contact with the supporting surface. As the example in figure 3.3 demonstrates, when you stand with your feet 15 cm (6 in.) apart, your base of support is the area of the surface that your feet contact and the area between your feet. If you spread your feet 46 cm (18 in.) apart, your base becomes larger.

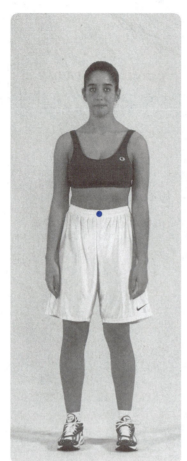
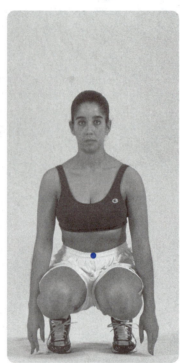
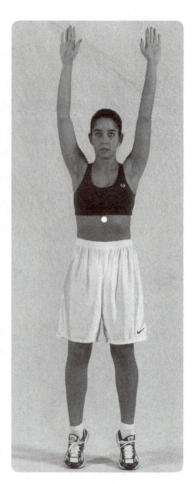

▶ **Figure 3.1** Center of gravity, as indicated by the dot, changes with changes in body position.

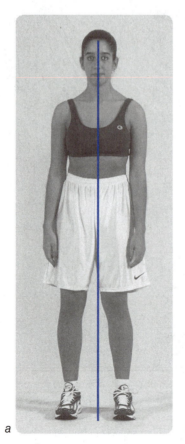
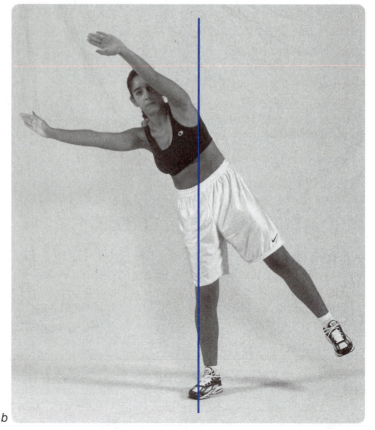

a   b

▶ **Figure 3.2** Line of gravity must fall within the base of support for the object to be stable. The larger the base of support is, the more stable the object is. According to the description above, is this patient more stable in *(a)* or *(b)*?

Stability

An object is **stable** when the line of gravity falls within the base of support. A person is stable when standing upright with the line of gravity within the base of support, but if the line of gravity falls outside of that base, it is difficult to maintain balance. For the hammer thrower in the earlier example to maintain his balance while holding the hammer with his left hand, his center of gravity must remain inside his base of support. So what must he do to keep himself upright? He leans to the right to shift the center of gravity over his feet. The size and shape of the base of support also determines stability. The larger the base of support, the more stable the object. If you stand with your feet together, it is relatively easy for someone to push you over. If you spread your feet to give yourself a larger base of support, it is easier for you to maintain your stability and harder for someone to push you over.

The shape of the base can give additional support against external forces. A football lineman has more success in resisting an opponent's force if his feet are spread apart and in line with the direction of the oncoming player so he will place one foot forward of the other. In this position he is more likely to keep his center of gravity within his base of support and maintain stability. Most of us make these unconscious adjustments when we ride the bus or train while standing; we position our feet depending on our relation to the forward motion of the vehicle, either standing with feet side by side if we are standing sideways or positioning them in a tandem stance (one farther forward than the other) if we are facing forward, as shown in figure 3.4. Likewise in therapeutic exercise, the shape and position of your base of support determines the ease with which you can provide manual resistance to a patient. For example, it is easier for you to provide manual resistance to a biceps curl while facing a seated patient if you position your feet in a forward-backward stance rather than a side-by-side stance.

Fixation

Fixation is a state of stabilization in which motion is restricted or prevented. Fixation provides a degree of stability optimal for efficient muscle function and is also desirable in certain therapeutic exercise situations. Fixation can be produced by either active muscle contraction or application of an external force. In performing an arm curl, fixation of the upper arm allows movement of the forearm to produce the desired goal of elbow flexion. When referring to the act of fixating a body segment to produce a desired motion, *stabilization* is the term often used, since the desired effect—stability—is the result of fixation of a body part.

Fixation is often needed in therapeutic exercise to produce a desired result. If fixation of a body segment and stabilization of the body are not applied during exercise, substitution of unwanted muscles or muscle groups can result in exercising a muscle other than the one intended, and desired results are diminished. For example, when you give manual resistance to hip abductors of a side-lying patient, it is important that the hip is stabilized to prevent the patient from using hip flexors or rotators during the exercise. On an isokinetic machine the thigh strap is the external fixator used to stabilize the thigh and prevent the patient from using hip flexors to lift the leg as the knee moves into extension.

Motion at both its proximal and distal attachments occurs when a muscle contracts, moving both ends towards its center. One end of the muscle must be fixated to achieve the desired

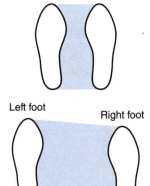

Left foot

Right foot

▶ **Figure 3.3** Base of support.

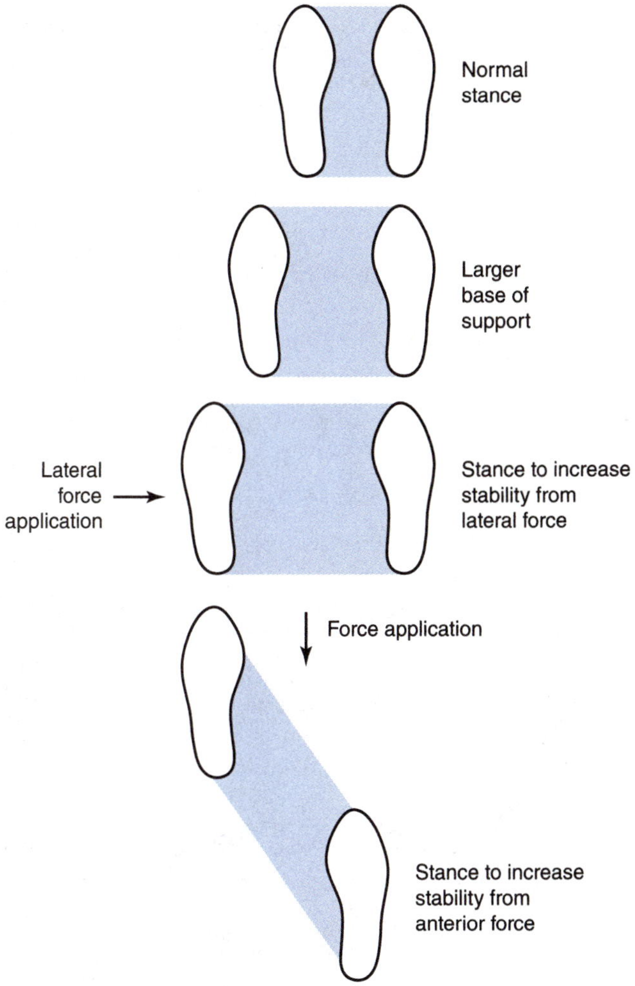

Lateral force application

Normal stance

Larger base of support

Stance to increase stability from lateral force

Force application

Stance to increase stability from anterior force

▶ **Figure 3.4** Changing base of support for stability.

Stability is a state in which a person or object is not easily thrown off balance. Fixation is a state of stabilization in which motion is restricted or prevented.

motion. For example, the upper trapezius can move its proximal end to produce cervical extension and rotation as well as its distal end to cause scapular and clavicular elevation. To provide the greatest cervical motion, the scapula must be stabilized, but if scapular elevation is the desired motion, the neck must be stabilized. This stabilization is usually performed by other muscles.

Using a muscle as a stabilizer to fixate a body segment can be one way of strengthening it, especially in the early stages of a therapeutic exercise program. For example, if injured abdominal muscles are too weak or painful to perform an abdominal curl, they may be able to work during a straight-leg raise; the abdominals exert force to fixate the trunk during this activity but do not work as hard as they would to perform a trunk curl.

BODY LEVERS

A lever is a simple machine that contains a rigid bar and a fulcrum, or point of movement. The body and its segments move because of their levers. It is important to know about the types of levers within the body and its segments since levers are used continually in therapeutic exercise to produce resistance or to enhance movement.

There are three classes of levers. Each lever, regardless of its classification, has three primary components (shown in figure 3.5): the force arm (and force point), the resistance arm (and resistance point), and the fulcrum. The fulcrum is the point at which the bar rotates. In the body, the fulcrum is the joint and the bar is the bone attached to the joint. The resistance point in the body's lever system is the center of gravity of the body segment being moved. If an external object such as a weight is attached to the segment, the center of gravity for that segment, and thus the resistance point, changes. For example, the center of gravity for an average forearm and hand is approximately 3/7 the distance from the elbow to the fingertips. If the patient grasps a weight in the hand, the center of gravity resistance point moves more distally; the heavier the weight, the more distally the resistance point's center of gravity moves. The resistance arm is the distance from the fulcrum to the resistance point. The force point is the point at which the force moving the lever is applied, and the force arm is the shortest distance from the force point to the fulcrum. The generic term for resistance arm and force arm is lever arm. Since joint movement is rotational, the lever arm is technically referred to as the moment arm; clinicians often interchange these two terms. Two lever arms and a fulcrum comprise a lever system. The relationship among the positions of these components determines the class of lever that is being used.

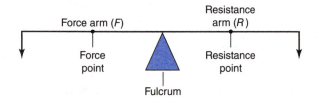

▶ **Figure 3.5** Basic lever system.

First-Class Lever

A first-class lever is one in which the fulcrum is located between the resistance and the force. A simple example is the seesaw. In the body an example of a first-class lever is the triceps, shown in figure 3.6: Its point of force is at its insertion on the olecranon process, proximal to the joint, and the resistance force is at the center of gravity of the forearm, down the forearm 3/7 of the distance between the elbow and the fingertips. If two equal forces act against each other, the advantage will lie with the force having the longer lever arm. For example, if two people, both weighing 100 lb, sit on opposite ends of a seesaw, they will balance the board in the middle; however, if one of them moves closer to the fulcrum, that individual's lever arm becomes shorter so he will be raised upward by the weight of the person who remains at the end of the seesaw (Figure 3.9).

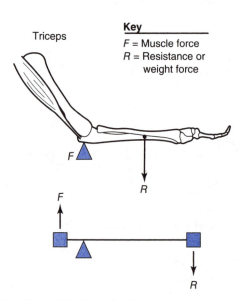

▶ **Figure 3.6** First-class lever.

Second-Class Lever

In a **second-class lever** the resistance point is between the fulcrum and the force. This class of lever always has a longer force arm than resistance arm. It is efficient in production of force, because the amount of force needed to move a resistance is always less than the resisting force. A typical example is the wheelbarrow. In the human body the brachioradialis, seen in figure 3.7, is an example of a second-class lever because it inserts on the forearm distal to the forearm's center of gravity.

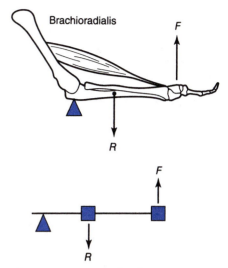

▶ **Figure 3.7**   Second-class lever.

Third-Class Lever

A **third-class lever** has the force between the fulcrum and the resistance. This is an inefficient lever since the force arm is always shorter than the resistance arm, so more force is always required to move the resistance. Many of the levers of the body fall into this class. The elbow can once again be used as an example of this class of lever: As seen in figure 3.8, the biceps tendon inserts on the forearm between the elbow joint and the center of gravity of the forearm.

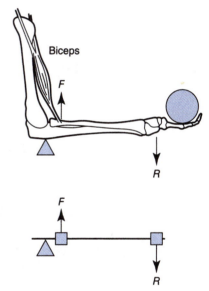

▶ **Figure 3.8**   Third-class lever.

Effects of Levers

These classes of levers determine the body's mechanical response. They can increase or decrease the forces produced, the speed of movement of a body part, and the range of motion of the joint. If one or more of these factors increases, the remaining factors decrease. Conversely, if one or more decreases, the others increase. Figure 3.9 shows two people of equal weight at opposite ends of a seesaw. If person A is 4 ft from the fulcrum and person B is 8 ft from the fulcrum, person B can exert more torque (discussed later in this chapter) than person A, and person A moves more slowly and over a shorter distance than person B.

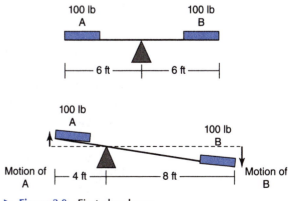

▶ **Figure 3.9**   First-class lever.

A lever is a simple machine consisting of a rigid bar that rotates about a fulcrum. Levers are classified as first class, second class, or third class, depending on the relative positions of the fulcrum and the points where resistance and force are applied. Levers in the body can affect the force, speed, or distance of a movement.

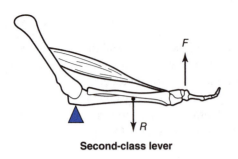

Second-class lever

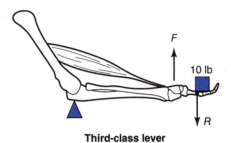

Third-class lever

▶ **Figure 3.10** Changing from a second-class to a third-class lever.

Adapted from R. Groves and D.N. Camaione, 1983, *Concepts in kinesiology* (Philadelphia: W.B. Saunders). 106. © McGraw-Hill Companies.

Levers are classified according to the relative position of the fulcrum, force point, and resistance point. Sometimes when an outside resistance—such as a weight in a hand—is added, the class of lever changes. Recall that the brachioradialis is normally a second-class lever. If a heavy enough weight is placed in the hand, however, as seen in figure 3.10, the center of gravity (resistance point) moves more distally and can change the brachioradialis from a second-class to a third-class lever.

LEVERS AND FORCE

Linear motion is movement in a straight line, whereas **angular motion** is rotational movement through an arc. All joints in the body produce angular motion, but movement of the entire body through space is often linear. In other words, the rotational movement of the hips, knees, and ankles causes the body to move forward linearly, a motion known as walking. Similarly, an individual in a wheelchair moves linearly forward because of the rotational movements of the chair's wheels.

Torque

The ability of a force to cause a rotational movement is referred to as **torque.** Torque is the product of the force and length of the force arm. Torque is commonly expressed in units such as Newton-meters (N-m), foot-pounds (ft-lb), or inch-pounds (in-lb). When torque is produced, the force arm is referred to as a moment arm, but as mentioned, clinicians commonly interchange the two terms.

An increase in the length of the moment arm increases the torque produced by a force ($T = F \times L$). For example, if you apply manual resistance at the thigh to a straight-leg raise, your torque is less (or you have to produce more force for the same torque) than if you positioned your hand at the ankle. With your hand at the ankle, your effort is less for the same torque production because your lever arm is longer (from the patient's hip to ankle vs. hip to thigh). Conversely, if a patient has a difficult time performing a straight-leg raise against gravity, bending the knee to shorten the leg's resistance-arm length may permit the patient to lift the leg without assistance.

Torque can also be altered by changing the force. Placing a 4.5 kg (10 lb) weight on an ankle produces twice as much torque as a 2.25 kg (5 lb) weight on a knee-extension exercise.

A muscle's torque changes as a joint moves through its range of motion. This is related in part to the change in the muscle's line of pull and the angle of pull causing the moment-arm length to change.

Line of Pull

The **line of pull** of the muscle is the long axis of the muscle. The **angle of pull** is the angle between the long axis of the bone (lever arm) and the line of pull of the muscle. The angle of pull and moment arm of the muscle change as the joint goes through its range of motion. As demonstrated in figure 3.11, the maximal amount of torque is produced when the angle of pull of the muscle is 90° and the moment arm is at its greatest length. In this position all the muscle's force is directed to produce only rotation. As the muscle's angle of pull increases or decreases from 90°, the part of the force that contributes to rotational motion (rotational force) decreases, and the part that does not contribute to rotation (non-rotary rotational force) increases, so the ability to produce rotational motion—or torque—diminishes. How much rotational force (vector) and how much non-rotational force (vector) each exists depend on the angle of pull and the moment arm. The non-rotational force will tend to either stabilize the joint by providing compression or destabilize the joint by providing a distracting force, depending on the angle of pull. The farther the angle of pull is from 90°, the more force is used to stabilize or destabilize the joint and the less force is used to rotate the joint. For example, the biceps, seen in figure 3.12, has a non-rotational force component that is pulling the ulna into the elbow and provides stability to the joint. It also has a rotational component causing the forearm to move through its arc of motion. In therapeutic exercise, the mechanics of each joint and the angle of pull of the muscles surrounding the joint should be appreciated. A recently dislocated shoulder, for example, should not be placed in positions that encourage surrounding muscle to destabilize it. For this reason, early rehabilitation of this condition warrants avoiding overhead or full-external-rotation positions where the non-rotational forces that distract the joint are significant.

▶ **Figure 3.12** Rotatory and non-rotatory components of a force application: (a) mechanical representation, (b) muscle representation. With one end of a stick anchored, a force applied will rotate the stick around the fixed end. In (a), the closer to vertical the force application to the stick is, the greater will be the amount of force applied only to rotation. The remaining force is applied as a compressive force toward the anchored end.

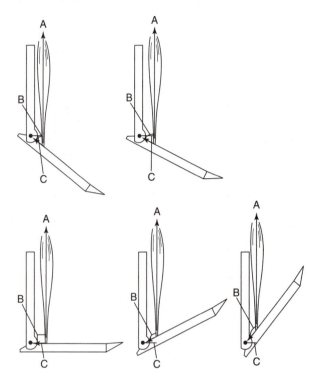

▶ **Figure 3.11** The angle of pull changes as range of motion changes. The most rotary force occurs when the muscle's angle of pull is 90°.

Adapted from R. Groves and D.N. Camaione, 1983, *Concepts in kinesiology* (Philadelphia: W.B. Saunders). 106. © McGraw-Hill Companies.

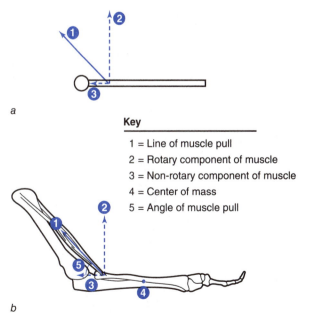

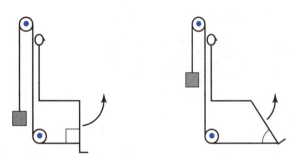

The ability of a force to cause a rotational movement, or torque, is affected by the angle at which the force acts on a body part.

Angle of Pull

Angle of pull of a muscle is an important concept in therapeutic exercise. If you want to produce the maximal torque from a muscle, the joint must be positioned so that the muscle being worked has a 90° angle of pull on the extremity.

This concept also works for external forces applied to the body. With pulleys, the maximal resistance occurs when the angle of pull of the pulley's rope is 90° to the extremity being resisted, as shown in figure 3.13. With free weights, the maximal resistance occurs when the pull of the weight is perpendicular to the ground regardless of the extremity's position. For example, when a supine patient performs elbow flexion with a weight, the greatest resistance is at the start of the motion when the patient's elbow moves from full extension to flexion, as seen in figure 3.14. If the patient is standing or sitting, however, the maximal resistance from the weight is when the elbow is at 90°.

▶ **Figure 3.13** With this pulley arrangement, the greatest resistance is produced at 90° of knee flexion.

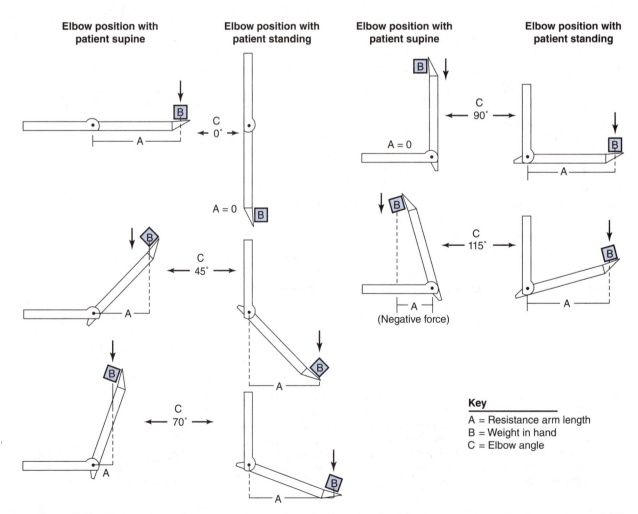

▶ **Figure 3.14** Changes in position cause changes in resistance arm. Resistance is greatest at 0° when supine and 90° when standing.

PHYSIOLOGICAL MUSCLE ADVANTAGES

What we have been discussing thus far is the mechanical advantage of muscles, which relates to the angle of pull and moment arm of the muscles and the amount of resistance a muscle must overcome to produce motion. **Physiological advantage** is a muscle's ability to shorten. This is an important functional concept in therapeutic exercise. A muscle has the most physiological advantage when it is at its resting length. The resting length of a muscle is the length to which a muscle can be lengthened in a relaxed condition without producing tension or any additional stretch. For example, the greatest physiological advantage of the brachialis is with the elbow in full extension, and the greatest physiological advantage for the soleus is with the ankle in dorsiflexion.

As a muscle shortens, its physiological advantage becomes progressively less until it is unable to produce a force, as illustrated in figure 3.15. A muscle is able to shorten to about 66% of its resting length (Smith, Weiss, & Lehmkuh, 1996). At that point, all the muscle's energy is used to shorten it, so no external force can be exerted.

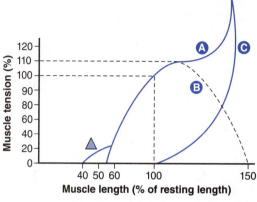

Key

A = Combination of stretch of connective tissue and muscle elasticity
B = Active tension of muscle fiber as it is stretched
C = Passive stretch of connective tissue

▶ **Figure 3.15** Physiological advantage of muscles.

Multi-joint Muscles

If a multi-joint muscle is shortened as far as possible, it will ultimately impact the position of all the joints it crosses. For example, if the hamstrings were maximally shortened, it would produce extension of the hip and flexion of the knee. However, since the muscle has used up its shortening ability, it cannot shorten any further. This condition is called *active insufficiency*. Likewise, if a multi-joint muscle is elongated over the joints it crosses to its maximum length, its antagonist muscle is unable to shorten any more. This condition is called *passive insufficiency*.

Because of active and passive insufficiency, when a two-joint or multi-joint muscle contracts, it should be elongated at the stabilized, unaffected joint so it can work optimally at the injured joint. For example, if you want to maximize efforts of the hamstrings during a knee flexion exercise, the best position for the patient is sitting so the hamstrings are lengthened at the hip to allow for a better contraction at the knee. If the patient is prone, the hamstrings are already shortened at the hip and will be unable to fully contract at the knee. When you want to produce as much force from a two-joint or multi-joint muscle as possible, the muscle should be placed on stretch at the stabilized joint(s) as it moves the joint at which the muscle's motion is needed. This permits all its available physiological length to be used at the desired site.

Summation of Forces

Summation of forces is especially important during the functional phase of a therapeutic exercise program. The **summation of forces** is a sequence of movements timed so that each movement contributes to the next movement to produce a desired outcome. For the summation of forces to be successful, the forces from each part must be correctly timed, and each successive joint from which the activity occurs must be stabilized. This is more easily understood with an example: A baseball pitcher goes through a series of sequential movements starting with the hips, progressing to the trunk, then the shoulder, the elbow, and finally the wrist and hand. Acceleration of the ball occurs by a series of rotations and extensions in each of the joints. If a ball is pitched with movement only from the wrist, it does not go as far as when it is thrown correctly using a summation of forces from all body segments. Even using only the upper extremity and not the hips and trunk produces a far less effective throw than a full summation of forces. The forces applied by the muscles in each of the joints must be precisely timed to build on the previous forces. If correct timing does not occur, the pitcher ends up using forces primarily from the arm, not the hip and trunk, and risks injury to the shoulder or elbow.

A muscle's ability to shorten is its physiological advantage. A two-joint muscle will have a better physiological advantage when it is placed on stretch at one joint while it is moving the other.

Additionally, for summation of forces to occur, each joint must be stabilized in correct sequence. If this does not occur, the transfer of forces generated fails because the forces are dissipated. Once a joint's desired motion is produced and the muscle's forces have been transmitted, the joint must be stabilized by a static contraction of the muscles for summation to occur. If the pitcher does not have good hip strength for stabilizing the hip and back during pitching, the pitch will be weak and demand higher forces from the upper extremity to compensate for the hip's weakness. This example not only demonstrates summation of forces but also points out the importance of two concepts in therapeutic exercise: (1) maintaining normal parameters in uninjured parts and (2) achieving normal parameters of factors, including strength, before functional activities can be resumed.

OTHER CONCEPTS IN PHYSICS

Many physics terms have been used in this chapter. To improve your understanding and because these terms are used in later chapters, words that are commonly used in therapeutic exercise and rehabilitation programs are defined here.

Strength

Strength is a muscle's relative ability to resist or produce a force. The greater the strength, the greater the ability to produce a force. The muscle's angle of pull, the angle of the resisting force, the muscle's length, and the speed of contraction and movement are factors that determine a muscle's strength.

The measure of a muscle's strength varies, depending on these factors as well as on the method of measurement used. Using free weights to determine strength assesses the strength of the muscle at its weakest point in the range of motion. For example, if a patient performs a forearm curl with a maximum weight of 14 kg (30 lb), this is the weight the forearm flexors can lift at their weakest point. Although the weight of the dumbbell does not change as the forearm goes through its range of motion, the muscles' strength changes with the changing angles of pull and lever-arm lengths of the muscles' force arm and dumbbell's resistance arm, and the changing physiological length of the muscles.

An isometric contraction can be used to evaluate the muscle's strength only at the specific joint position tested. The quantity of strength produced in an isometric contraction changes as the joint position changes in its range of motion because of the adjustments in the muscle's lever-arm length, angle of pull, and physiological length. A more complete discussion of strength is in chapter 7.

Work

Work is the product of the amount of force *(F)* and the distance *(d)* through which the force is applied:

$$W = F \times d$$

Work is measured in foot-pounds (ft-lb) in the English system and joules (1 J = 1 N·m) in the metric system. If you lift a 20 lb (89 N) weight from the floor to a shelf 6 ft (1.8 m) above the floor, you would do 120 ft-lb (about 160 J) of work (6 ft × 20 lb, or 89 N × 1.8 m). When a weightlifter lifts a 250 lb (1112.5 N) barbell overhead to a height of 6.5 ft (2 m), he produces 1625 ft-lb (2225 J) of work.

Power

Power is the work per unit of time, or how fast the work is produced:

$$P = Fd / t$$

Work is done regardless of how much time it takes to perform the work. Power is a measure of the work done in a specific amount of time. In the English system it is measured in foot-pounds per second or in horsepower (1 horsepower = 550 ft-lb/s). In the metric system it is measured in joules per second or Newton-meters per second. Power is sometimes incorrectly interchanged with force.

In sports, the most frequently used tests for power include the standing vertical jump and the softball throw. These activities require a sudden contraction of muscles to move the body or object in a short amount of time, thus generating a large force and great power.

Power requires strength to produce the force necessary to perform an activity with neuromuscular control to contract the muscles rapidly. Proprioception and functional aspects of therapeutic exercise programs should include power activities for patients involved in rapid activities. Keep in mind when working with athletes that power training is sport specific and requires you to understand the requirements of the patient's activity demands.

Energy

Energy is the capacity to do work. There are different types of energy. The law of conservation of energy states that energy can neither be created nor destroyed. Energy can, however, be converted from one form to another. For example, when a volleyball player serves the ball, some of the mechanical energy is converted to sound energy, but no energy is lost.

In therapeutic exercise and rehabilitation, we are interested primarily in two energy classifications: potential energy and kinetic energy. Potential energy and kinetic energy are often converted from one to the other. Potential energy is the capacity to do work that is stored in a body. Kinetic energy is the energy a body has because of its motion. When a moving body stops, kinetic energy is all converted to potential energy. It is important to absorb this energy in a way that prevents injury. For example, when a gymnast dismounts from the high bar, he bends his knees to absorb energy. When a patient performs plyometrics in the final stages of the therapeutic exercise program, the patient moves to safely absorb the energy produced by the movements in the exercise.

Velocity

Velocity is the rate of change of position. It is expressed in miles per hour (mph), feet per second (ft/s), or meters per second (m/s). *Velocity* is often interchanged with *speed,* which is not entirely accurate, but in most instances the difference is inconsequential. We use velocity to assess how well a sprinter runs the 100 m or how quickly a basketball player can get to the other end of the court on a fast break. Part of the functional examination before allowing a patient to return to activity may include an evaluation of the patient's velocity in functional activities.

Acceleration

Acceleration is the rate at which velocity changes. It is expressed in feet per second per second (ft/s^2) or meters per second per second (m/s^2). A sprinter coming out of the blocks at the start of a race accelerates, increasing velocity as she continues. In the final stages of a therapeutic exercise program, it is important for you to work on acceleration activities with patients for which acceleration is a factor. The therapeutic exercise program for an injured sprinter needs to include explosive strength development in the starting positions of hip flexion and knee flexion if the sprinter is to have the acceleration necessary to get out of the starting blocks.

Negative acceleration is called deceleration, the process of an object's slowing down rather than speeding up. After a baseball is pitched, the pitcher's arm goes from sudden acceleration to deceleration until the arm stops moving. It is the follow-through on an activity that provides as smooth a transition as possible from acceleration to deceleration. Poor follow-through increases the risk of injury because of the more rapid change from acceleration to deceleration. This is an important concept to recall in the final stages of the therapeutic exercise program, when activity-specific exercises are part of the program.

Gravity provides a constant acceleration of 9.8 m/s² or 9.8 m/s/s (32 ft/s² or 32 ft/s/s). In other words, every second that an object falls, it moves 9.8 m/s (32 ft/s) faster than it did during the previous second. If you drop a golf ball from a 10-story building, after the first second it falls at a velocity of 9.8 m/s (32 ft/s). After the next second it falls at a velocity of 19.6 m/s (64 ft/s), and after the third second it has a velocity of 29.4 m/s (96 ft/s). As Galileo discovered during the late 1500s when he dropped objects from the Tower of Pisa, this rate of acceleration occurs regardless of the object's weight if the effect of air resistance is disregarded. If you drop a ping-pong ball from the same height as the golf ball at the same time, its acceleration will be the same as the golf ball and they will hit the floor at the same time.

On the other hand, a diver who jumps off a 3 m board will not hit the water at as great a speed as one who jumps off a 10 m board. Their acceleration is the same, but the diver from the 3 m board has a shorter distance to go before hitting the water; therefore, the time during which he accelerates is shorter, so his velocity by the time he hits the water is less than that of the 10 m diver.

Elasticity

Elasticity is the ability of an object to resume its former shape after a deforming or distorting force is applied then released. A muscle has elasticity because it can be stretched but returns to its normal length when the deforming force is discontinued. All substances have some degree of elasticity. Rubber tubing or bands used in therapeutic exercise have a lot of elasticity. Steel has elasticity but less than asphalt. Ligaments have more elasticity than bone but less than muscles.

Stiffness

Stiffness is the ability of an object to resist deformation when a stress is applied to it. When a force is applied quickly to connective tissue, the connective tissue has more stiffness to resist the force than if the force is applied slowly over time. Tissue's tensile strength is related to its stiffness. Elasticity and stiffness are at opposite ends of the spectrum, so tissue that is more elastic doesn't have as much stiffness as tissue that is less elastic. Most human structures have a combination of elasticity and stiffness to provide them with both an ability to return to their former shape but also resist outside forces.

Stress and Strain

Stress is a force that changes the form or shape of a body. **Strain** is the amount of change in the size or shape of the object caused by the stress. **Hooke's Law,** developed during the 1600s by the physicist and mathematician Robert Hooke, deals with the relationship of stress and strain to elasticity: The strain is proportional to the stress producing it (so long as the strain is not too great—once the elastic limit is exceeded, permanent deformation occurs).

This concept is demonstrated in figure 3.16. The *OA* curve segment represents the elastic range. If a load is released in this range of the stress-strain curve, the object returns to its normal length. A is called the elastic limit, beyond which Hooke's law is no longer valid. Beyond the elastic range is the plastic range *AM*. When a load stresses an object into this range, a permanent change in the object's size or shape occurs. Any load that continues beyond the plastic range ultimately causes a failure of the object, *F*.

The size of these ranges varies from material to material and from structure to structure. In rehabilitation, it is important to

Key

A = Elastic limit
Y = Yield point
0A = Elastic range
M = Maximum strength
AM = Plastic range
F = Failure point

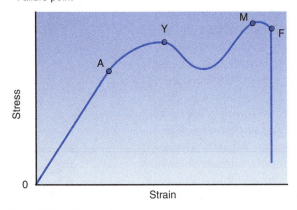

▶ **Figure 3.16**   Stress-strain curve.

realize the differences in the stress-strain curves of structures such as bone, muscle, tendons, cartilage, and ligaments. This knowledge is important in prevention and treatment of injuries. Some ligaments contain more elastic fibers than others, so they can withstand more stress, whereas others have fewer elastic fibers and provide more stability to a joint. Recently formed scar tissue has more elasticity than more mature scar tissue. Knowing the age and maturity of scar tissue determines the amount of stress and the amount of time the stress should be applied to affect a change in the scar tissue's length.

Creep

Creep occurs when a low-level stress, usually starting in the elastic range of the tissue, is applied over a long enough period to cause deformation of the tissue in its plastic range. Creep causes a realignment of tissue's collagen, proteoglycans, and water so a permanent change occurs (Nimni, 1983). Increasing the temperature of the tissue increases the rate of creep. For this reason, applying heat to an area before stretching may make the stretch more effective. This concept also explains why longer stretches produce better results. It also demonstrates why poor posture over time causes changes in muscles, joints, and connective tissue; sitting with your head forward for a prolonged time as you read this book will cause the ligaments and muscles of your posterior neck and upper back to lengthen, making it ultimately more difficult to resume a proper posture. Permanent changes in tissue length result over time with repetition of any position.

Structural Fatigue

All tissues and objects are subject to structural fatigue. Structural fatigue is the point at which a tissue or object can no longer withstand a stress, and breaks. This can occur in a sudden movement, as when a ligament is suddenly torn, or it can occur over time with an accumulation of stress. The point at which tissue failure results from long term stress is sometimes referred to as the endurance limit or fatigue failure. Breakdown of bone from cumulative trauma is called a stress fracture. Injuries caused by repeated stress, such as carpal tunnel syndrome, are called repetitive stress syndromes or overuse syndromes. Treatment of cumulative trauma injuries is different from that of acute trauma injuries and is discussed more thoroughly in chapter 15.

Friction

Friction is the relative resistance between two surfaces. It can be advantageous or deleterious, depending on the circumstances. A patient who is very weak may have difficulty abducting the thigh in supine because friction of the leg against the treatment table adds resistance. If the surface is made smoother by applying a friction-reducing agent such as talcum powder, the activity is easier.

Standing with a wide base of support, with the feet spaced wider than the hips, stabilizes the body but requires friction. If a person takes that same stance on ice, he or she will fall because ice provides less friction than many other surfaces.

Sometimes we want to increase friction to obtain more traction and apply more force. Cleats on football shoes or tread on basketball shoes are good examples of this. When decreasing friction is desirable, such as on the uneven parallel bars in gymnastics, a substance such as chalk is used to reduce friction and minimize the risk of blisters.

In therapeutic exercise, friction may not be desirable in pulley exercises because it wears out the equipment more quickly and makes exercises more difficult. On the other hand, it may be advantageous to have more friction to increase resistance in other exercises. For example, a patient sitting on a rolling stool and propelling it with one foot is exercising the hamstrings, as in figure 3.17a. A weight attached and dragged behind the stool increases friction and provides more resistance to movement (figure 3.17b).

Other concepts that relate to movement and the way the body responds to force include strength, work, power, energy, velocity, acceleration, elasticity, stress, strain, creep, structural fatigue, and friction.

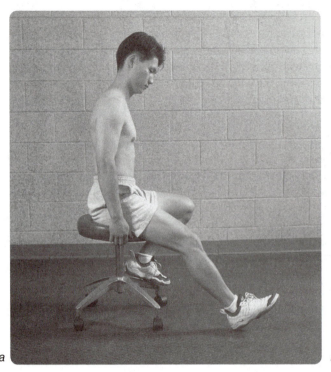
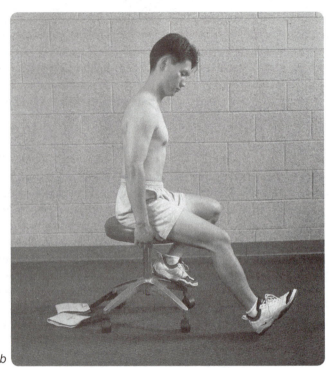

a   b

▶ **Figure 3.17**   Use of friction in therapeutic exercise.

SUMMARY

Before we can approach exercises in rehabilitation, we must first gain an understanding and appreciation of physics concepts that affect how exercises are used in rehabilitation. Some of these concepts include the laws of motion, body levers and how they change with changes in body position or resistance, changes in the center of gravity, stability, and how forces affect the body and how the body may affect force application or delivery. Once these concepts are put to functional applications, the clinician is able to adjust exercises as required for the individual.

KEY CONCEPTS AND REVIEW

1. Define force and give an example of an internal and an external force.

Force is energy that causes movement and has direction and magnitude. Internal forces are generated by muscles. An example of an external force is gravity.

2. Explain the relevance to therapeutic exercise of Newton's first, second, and third laws of motion.

Newton's first law of motion deals with inertia, the second law of motion deals with acceleration and momentum, and the third law of motion concerns action and reaction. All these laws govern how the body moves and reacts to forces applied to it.

3. Explain how center of gravity changes with movement.

The center of gravity is the theoretical center of mass of an object. When the object changes shape, the center of mass also changes. For example, the body's center of gravity becomes higher if the arms are raised overhead and lower if the body crouches. If a weight is carried at the side, the center of gravity shifts to the side with the weight; to maintain balance and keep the center of gravity over the feet, the body must lean away from the weight.

4. Discuss how a change in base of support can change a person's stability.

The narrower the base of support, the less stable is the object; the wider the base of support, the more stable it is.

5. Explain the relationship between line of gravity and base of support.

An object is stable when the line of gravity falls within its base of support.

6. Explain two ways of increasing stability.

A person can increase stability by aligning the feet in the direction of the applied force or lowering the center of gravity while keeping it within the base of support.

7. Identify the difference between stability and fixation.

Stability is a state in which a person or object is not easily thrown off balance. Fixation is a state of stability where motion is being restricted or prevented. When referring to the act of fixating a body segment to produce a desired motion, stabilization is the term often used, since the desired effect, stabilization, is the result of fixation.

8. Explain how torque can be altered in the body.

Torque produced by the body is altered most easily by changing the force-arm length, the amount of force applied, or the angle of pull.

9. Identify how varying positions change a muscle's mechanical advantage.

As a joint moves through its range of motion, the angle of pull of a muscle changes, altering the length of the muscle's lever arm, which changes its mechanical advantage.

10. Discuss the difference between mechanical and physiological advantage of a muscle.

A muscle's mechanical advantage has to do with its line and angle of pull and the forces it must produce to overcome a resistance, while the physiological advantage is the muscle's ability to shorten.

11. Explain the importance of positioning in exercising two-joint muscles.

The ability of a two-joint muscle to produce force is affected by its relative length at both joints. A muscle is able to shorten to no less than about 66% of its resting length, so its position at one joint affects its ability to produce force at the other joint. If it is shortened over the stable joint, the muscle is unable to produce as much force at the moving joint as when the muscle is lengthened over the stable joint.

12. Distinguish between velocity and acceleration.

Velocity is the rate of change of position, whereas acceleration is the rate at which velocity changes.

13. Discuss the relevance of elasticity, stress and strain, creep, and friction to therapeutic exercise.

Elasticity, stress and strain, and creep are all qualities that affect a tissue's ability to change its length or shape. These factors influence the type of stretch that is applied to a structure and the effectiveness of that stretch. Friction can be advantageous or detrimental, depending on the exercise and its goal.

CRITICAL THINKING QUESTIONS

1. Explain how Newton's first three laws of motion and gravity affect therapeutic exercise programs. In other words, how do inertia, acceleration, action-reaction, and gravity determine how you have a patient perform an exercise?

2. Using the concepts about base of support discussed in this chapter, describe how you can improve your base of support while giving manual resistance to hip flexion and extension on a patient who is supine. Use a partner and try the changes in your base of support to demonstrate how those changes give you an advantage or disadvantage in the manual-resistance exercise.

3. Explain how the different classes of levers apply to therapeutic exercise. Give an example of each class of lever with a different therapeutic exercise, and explain how the class of lever can change with a change in the exercise position or resistance application.

4. Describe how an elbow-flexion exercise changes when the technique or equipment used is manual resistance, rubber tubing, pulley, dumbbell, weight machine, and hydraulic machine. Does the type of resistance change? What about the kind of muscle activity? What advantage of each exercise makes it different from the others?

5. In what position would you put a patient to provide maximal muscle shortening during an exercise for the hamstring? In what position should the patient be to maximize hamstring activity at the knee? at the hip?

6. Throw a ball as far as you can while standing on one foot and then with both feet on the ground. In which position are you able to throw the ball farther? What mechanical concepts come into play here?

LAB ACTIVITIES

1. State the primary planes in which the following motions occur (assume the anatomical position unless otherwise noted):

   Stair climbing

   Wrist ulnar deviation

   Turning a door knob (using the forearm with the elbow flexed to 90°)

   Using a screwdriver with the elbow extended and the arm at the side

   Cervical rotation

   Jumping jacks

   Lumbar spine sidebending

2. The following exercises are to be performed in the sitting position with the elbow straight:

   Perform shoulder flexion to 90° with a 5 lb weight held in the hand

   Perform shoulder flexion to 90° with a 5 lb cuff weight placed above the elbow

   Which motion is easier to perform? Why?

3. With one person lying supine on a table as the patient and the other person standing beside the table as the rehabilitation clinician, have the patient lift the leg in a straight-leg raise and return to the start position. Now have the rehabilitation clinician apply resistance to the leg with a hand on the mid thigh as the patient lifts the leg as hard as possible and returns to the start position. Next, the rehabilitation clinician applies resistance force at the knee, and in the final repetition, the rehabilitation clinician applies force at the ankle. On each repetition, the patient should push against the rehabilitation clinician as hard as possible.

Answer the following questions:

    a. Which repetition was the most difficult for the patient? For the rehabilitation clinician?
    b. Why?
    c. Of what value is this information to you in performing a resistance exercise with a patient? In performing a manual muscle test?

4. Hold a 5 lb weight in your hand with your elbow bent and next to your side. Now hold it out so your shoulder is in front of you at 90° and your elbow is flexed to 90°. Now straighten your elbow so the elbow is fully extended in front of you.

Answer the following questions:

    a. Calculate the torque of the 5 lb weight for each position.
    b. How much torque do your muscles produce to hold the weight in each position?
    c. Of what value is this information to you in setting up a patient on resistance exercises?
    d. Have your partner perform a push-up in an easy, moderate, and then difficult position. What are the three positions? What is the principle upon which the difficulty increased with the exercise progression?

5. Position your partner to achieve passive insufficiency of the finger flexors. What joints do the long finger flexor tendons cross; into what position did you position each joint?

6. Position your lab partner to place the quadriceps in a passively insufficient position. Now resist the quadriceps in knee extension. What was the outcome? Why?

7. Have your partner create active insufficiency of the quadriceps. Now resist the quadriceps in knee extension. What was the outcome? Why?

8. What do the results of questions 7 and 8 demonstrate to you in terms of importance in exercises?

ADDITIONAL SOURCES

Cornwall, M.W. 1984. Biomechanics of noncontractile tissue. *Physical Therapy* 64:1869–1873.

Dumbelton, J.H., and J. Black. 1975. *An introduction to orthopedic materials.* Springfield, IL: Charles C Thomas.

Wilmore, J.H., and D.L. Costill. 2004. *Physiology of sport and exercise,* 3rd ed. Champaign, IL: Human Kinetics.

CHAPTER 4

Examination and Assessment

OBJECTIVES

After completing this chapter, you should be able to do the following:

1. Identify the primary factors of subjective examination.

2. Outline an objective examination procedure that includes all primary factors.

3. Explain the different types of end-feel and distinguish between normal and pathological end-feels.

4. Explain how a treatment plan is designed and upon what factors it is based.

5. Define the SOAP note and explain its significance to rehabilitation.

6. Identify two other records used in rehabilitation and demonstrate their importance.

▶ Catherine An instructs incoming athletic training students on rehabilitation examination procedures. She has found in the past that the students' primary point of confusion is identifying the difference between examination of an acute injury for first aid and examination of an injury for rehabilitation. Instruction with her new class begins today. Her first goal is to identify the differences between an acute-injury examination and a rehabilitation examination. Catherine will then introduce the procedures for a rehabilitation examination, explain how to identify the patient's problems, how to base goals on those problems, and how to develop a plan of treatment based on the problems and goals.

Although many of the students have been exposed to record keeping for initial injuries in the athletic training clinic, few of them know the record-keeping procedures for rehabilitation. Some of them have seen SOAP notes during their observations in their freshman year, but not many of them understand what these notes mean and their relevance. In addition to SOAP notes, Catherine will introduce students to the other records used in rehabilitation. Many new students are overwhelmed with their first sight of what seems like a mountain of paperwork, but Catherine knows from experience that the paperwork is an important part of patient care and is not the insurmountable task students initially think it to be.

Oh . . . I listen a lot and talk less.
You can't learn anything when you're talking.

BING CROSBY, entertainer, 1903-1977

Examination and assessment of an injury serve as the foundation for a treatment program. The patient must first be examined and results assessed before the rehabilitation clinician can design an appropriate therapeutic exercise program. Without an examination to know where deficiencies lie, the extent of the injury, and other factors that may affect a therapeutic exercise program, the rehabilitation clinician has no basis on which to decide what should or should not be incorporated into the rehabilitation program. The terms *evaluation* and *examination* are often interchanged. This text uses **examination** to indicate the means by which a rehabilitation clinician seeks information on the severity, irritability, nature, and stage of a patient's injury. The examination is composed of subjective and objective elements. The subjective examination is the history of the injury and the patient's experience of pain and other symptoms. It is obtained from the patient and serves to guide the objective portion of the examination. Like Bing Crosby, the clinician can learn a lot by listening to the patient. The **objective examination** reveals the observable signs and effects of the injury and involves observing, testing, and palpating the injury. The results of the subjective and objective examinations allow the rehabilitation clinician to assess the patient's injury and determine the most appropriate treatment for achieving whatever goals are established for the patient. An **assessment** is a conclusion based on the gathering of information. At the time of an initial examination, assessment is used to design a therapeutic exercise program. Once the program has been instituted, the results of the treatment are evaluated to assess the treatment's effectiveness. Finally, before the patient returns to full sport participation or normal activity, the patient is examined and assessed for readiness and ability to perform and withstand the stresses of the sport or activity. In short, an examination must precede an assessment, and both are required not only at the commencement and conclusion of a rehabilitation program, but frequently throughout the program as well.

This chapter is divided into three parts. The first part deals with subjective and objective aspects of an examination, the second part discusses assessments that are based on the examination, and the third part introduces records of these examination assessments that should be kept throughout the rehabilitation process. This chapter concludes the presentation of the basic concepts needed to understand the whys of therapeutic exercise.

EXAMINATION: MAKING A PROFILE

The first part of performing an initial examination to determine the extent and involvement of the injury, the patient's deficiencies, and a course of treatment is to create a profile of the injury. This is accomplished by performing a subjective and an objective examination.

It is important to take an accurate and complete history before the objective examination. As Bing Crosby indicated in the opening quotation of this chapter, listening is fundamental to learning, and obtaining a history includes listening to the patient's reports of the injury. A history is only as good as the questions asked. If you expect a thorough history from the patient, you must ask questions that will reveal all that is necessary to obtain a complete picture.

Once the subjective examination is completed, an objective examination follows. This includes observations of abnormalities, palpation, and measurements of deficiencies in range of motion, strength, proprioception, and other parameters, which provide you with a clear picture of problems. A treatment program cannot be planned and delivered until you identify and assess the problems and deficiencies that the injury has caused. Problems are identified by thorough and accurate subjective and objective examinations.

Subjective Examination

The subjective examination is essentially the history of the injury and the patient's report of pain and other symptoms. The subjective examination can assist in determining the extent of the injury, how aggressively the objective examination can be performed, and what to include in the objective examination. The specific questions to ask during the history vary, depending on a variety of factors such as the area injured and the severity and nature of the injury.

To obtain a thorough and accurate history, it is best to ask questions that do not lead the patient to an anticipated answer. For example, rather than ask, "Is it painful to walk?" a better question is, "What activities cause you more pain?"

The questions should be simple and straightforward. They should be presented in a logical and systematic sequence. It is best for each rehabilitation clinician to develop his or her own method or system of sequential questions that is consistent and easy to remember. This is not to say that the questions should be rigid and unchanging. Because each patient's history is different, the line of questioning will be different in each situation. The idea is to make history-taking procedures a habit that results in a consistent overall profile. When you first start out, you may need to write down questions to establish a routine for yourself, but listening to patients' responses and taking a logical and thorough history will become more automatic with experience.

History of the Injury

Allow the patient to explain in his or her own words how the injury occurred. The goal is to get an idea of the mechanism of injury, tissues involved, and extent of involvement. The patient should tell when the injury occurred, whether it occurred suddenly or gradually, immediate and later signs (e.g., immediate swelling or swelling only 24 h later), and what treatment has been provided. The patient should also say whether he or she was able to continue sport participation or normal activity, if the injured part remained functional (e.g., was the patient able to walk?), and what, if anything, has changed between the time of the injury and the time of your examination. Information of this type can help you determine the severity of the injury and the tissue type involved. Knowing whether ice or heat has been applied may change your impression of the injury. The involved area may be very swollen because no treatment was given, heat was applied, or the patient swells easily. If the patient has taken medication, it may mask pain or change the results of the tests you perform.

Medical History

Getting a medical history of previous injury is important. If a prior injury has occurred, what treatments were provided? Did the patient seek medical care? Did the patient receive treatment, and if so, what treatment was given, how long was it provided, and what was the outcome? How many subsequent injury episodes has the patient experienced? Is the pain the same this time as it was in the past?

Recurring episodes may affect your assessment of the current problem and the treatment program you establish. For example, recurring ankle sprains can produce additional scar tissue in or around the joint, restrict soft-tissue mobility, reduce strength and proprioceptive abilities, or increase laxity and instability of the joint. Repeated muscle strains may cause tendinopathy. Recurring knee meniscus lesions may lead to chronic synovitis. Repetitive injuries to a joint may eventually cause arthritis.

In the case of prior injuries, a report of the previous treatments provided is helpful to get a picture of prior injury management. Good management may have minimized previous injuries and left the patient with a good impression of rehabilitation, but poor management may prejudice the patient into having little confidence in rehabilitation outcomes and may also complicate the current picture. For example, if a patient presents with a knee injury and a history of prior similar injuries that were not treated, the current injury may have resulted from muscle weakness and other knee structure deficiencies that may prolong the current treatment. In these cases, you will need to deal with effects of both the current and prior injury.

Special Questions

Special questions, such as whether the patient is taking any medications and about the general health of the patient, can reveal factors that influence your understanding of the injury and your treatment plan. Does the patient have any systemic diseases that may affect treatment, such as diabetes, asthma, HIV? Has there been any unexpected weight loss lately? This may be a sign of unsuspected cancer and should be referred to the physician. Is the patient taking steroids? This can interfere with the healing process. Questions regarding difficulty with bowel or bladder control are important to ask with back injuries since a positive answer may indicate an injury to the cauda equina, a condition that requires immediate medical attention. Knowing what tests have been performed, such as X-rays or MRI, can help you further confirm or identify problems.

Additional Information

Additional information is also useful in completing an accurate profile of the injury and the patient's expectations of the treatment program. The patient's normal level of activity and the activities to which the patient wishes to return after rehabilitation give you an idea of the patient's expectations and the physical requirements for meeting those expectations. For example, if a runner presents with a knee injury that has been getting worse over time, what does he want to be able to resume doing once the treatment is over? How far, fast, and frequently was he running before the injury? Over what kinds of terrain was he running? What kind of shoes does he use? Has he had any changes in his workouts, terrain, or other activities? Questions like these help you create an accurate profile of the patient and determine the cause of injury.

Other general questions include the patient's sport and position in that sport, if the patient is an athlete. The answers give you an idea of the amounts and kinds of stresses that may have caused the injury and the stress level that the patient's body must withstand in order to return to the sport.

When working in a high school or college athletic program, the clinician often knows the age of the patient. In a clinic, however, the ages of patients can vary greatly. The patient's age is important in identifying certain injuries and in deciding what treatment to apply. For example, osteoarthritis is a common problem among individuals over the age of 40. Ultrasound is not a treatment choice for a 13-year-old knee injury patient because of the knee's immature epiphyseal plates at that age.

Does the patient hear **crepitus** (clicking or snapping) from the injured part? These are what I call the "rice krispy" sounds: the snap, crackle, and pop of injury. Crepitus in a joint can sound either light or coarse, depending on whether the roughening of cartilage surfaces is slight or significant. A fine crepitus sometimes can be palpated in a joint with synovial thickening, as in synovitis. Crepitus can also be felt or heard in tendinitis because of the increased thickening and friction between the tendon and its sheath. A creaking sound is heard in joints that are in the later stages of joint-surface degeneration. A clicking or popping sound can be heard with meniscal displacement in either the temporomandibular joint or the knee joint; if the clicking is painful, the meniscus may be torn. Non-painful clicks heard in joints, especially hypermobile joints, may be a normal vacuum click and of no consequence. Non-painful but sometimes loud snapping sounds are frequently the inconsequential result of a ligament or a tendon slipping over a bony prominence when a joint moves. A clunking sound is produced by a joint that is unstable and subluxes as it moves through a particular part of its motion. Repeated subluxation making this sound can eventually cause degeneration of the joint.

Pain Profile

A profile of the patient's pain assists in determining the nature and severity of the injury as well as what to include in your objective examination and initial treatment plan. Several questions are asked to obtain this profile:

■ **Where is the pain?** Can it be located with one finger, or is it over a larger area? Does it stay localized, or does it go to other areas? Is the pain deep or superficial? Is it in a joint or in the surrounding area? A small, pinpoint area of pain is probably a localized, minor injury or a chronic injury. A larger, more diffuse or deep area of pain probably indicates a larger or more serious injury or an acute injury.

Pain that radiates into other areas may be referred pain caused by pressure on a nerve or myofascial referral from stimulation of trigger points. This pain and its cause need to be identified and further examined during your objective evaluation.

■ **Did the pain come on suddenly or gradually?** This question helps determine the cause of injury. A sudden pain is most often seen in sport injuries and occurs with a sudden overstress of tissue, as occurs with a muscle strain or a ligamentous sprain. Gradual onset of pain occurs more often with tendinopathy and other repetitive injury conditions. With gradual pain, patients commonly do not seek medical assistance until the pain interferes with sport or work performance or less stressful daily activities.

If the pain occurred gradually, how long has the patient had the pain? This determines whether the problem is acute or chronic. Acute pain is treated differently from chronic pain.

■ **Is the pain constant or intermittent?** Most pain is intermittent or varies in intensity with either activity or time of day. The cause of pain that is constant and unchanging must be suspected as something other than musculoskeletal injury. Pain that is initially constant becomes intermittent with appropriate treatment.

■ **How intense is the pain?** Have the patient rate the pain on a scale of 0 to 10, where 0 is no pain and 10 is "take me to the hospital, I'm dying" pain. Pain is very subjective and varies greatly from one person to another. Trying to quantify pain by assigning a number to it does not make it an objective measure but does allow relative individual comparisons. The patient's pain rating gives you an idea of the patient's pain tolerance and can be used later to determine changes in the patient's pain. If a patient rates pain initially as 8 and three days later as 4, your treatment program is achieving its desired goal. This numerical system gives both you and the patient a method of gauging changes. It would be improper and useless to compare one patient's pain to another's, but there is some value in reassessing the patient's pain ratings as the treatment program progresses.

■ **How does the patient describe the pain? What kind of pain is it?** A variety of descriptors can be used to identify pain, such as sharp, dull, aching, burning, and tingling. Musculoskeletal pain is usually deep, dull, or an ache. The pain of more acute or severe muscle injuries is often sharp, stabbing, or throbbing.

■ **What are aggravating and easing factors? What does the patient do that causes or intensifies the pain? What relieves or reduces it?** In general, musculoskeletal pain occurs with movement and is relieved with rest. Pain from inflammation may not be relieved with rest. Prolonged positioning, such as poor sitting posture, can irritate soft tissues by applying prolonged or abnormal low-level stress to them.

■ **Does the pain vary with time of day? How does the area feel in the morning? As the day progresses? By evening?** Stiffness in the morning can be related to inflammation. If the pain increases as the day progresses, it may be that the injured area lacks sufficient strength and endurance to carry on activities and becomes fatigued. Spasm and pain may intensify as the day progresses, especially in acute injuries.

■ **Does the pain awaken the patient at night?** Musculoskeletal pain can worsen at night enough to disturb the patient's sleep. Inflammation and bone pain can also cause sleep disturbances. Inflammation pain that causes sleep disturbances indicates a bigger problem than pain that does not disturb sleep. If pain disturbs sleep, ask the patient how many times this occurs in a night and how long it takes to return to sleep. The answers to these questions give you an idea of the irritability of the injury. The more frequent the disturbances and the longer it takes the patient to return to sleep, the more irritated the injury.

The intensity of the pain, the kinds of activities that aggravate it, how long a patient can perform an activity before the pain increases, and how long it takes to reduce the pain once it has increased also indicate the **irritability** of the injury. The more irritable an injury is, the greater the pain, the more easily pain is increased with even low-level activity, and the longer it takes to ease. Corrigan and Maitland (1989) define an injury as being irritable when only a moderate amount of activity increases the pain and pain lasts for an hour. When an injury is not irritable, the patient feels only a momentary pain after stress.

Objective Examination

Once you have completed your subjective examination by taking the history of the injury, determining the patient's activity level and performance expectations, and profiling the pain and injury, it is time to perform your objective examination. Your goal is to determine exactly the structure or structures involved and the extent of the injury's effects so that you can determine your course of treatment.

Before you begin your physical examination, you already have a lot of information about the injury. This information guides your objective examination. From your subjective examination you have an idea of the nature of the problem, the severity and irritability of the injury, how aggressive or cautious you should be in performing your objective examination, which special tests to use, and which contraindications to consider. Although you may expect certain findings from your objective examination, it is important to keep an open mind and look at all possibilities for the injury and the tissues involved. Do not assume that you know what the diagnosis is until you have a total picture based on the accumulated information from both the subjective and objective segments. Narrowing your scope of vision may lead you to an inaccurate conclusion so you create an inappropriate rehabilitation program.

If an injury is irritable, your objective examination should be brief, relatively gentle, and less stressful to the injury. On the other hand, if an injury is not irritable, your examination can be more aggressive. A second degree sprain that occurred two days ago, that now exhibits a lot of swelling, causes persistent pain that increases with any active or passive range of movement, and causes pain with weight bearing is considered irritable and requires a gentle, brief examination to determine initial treatment. At a later stage when the injury is less irritable, a more aggressive and complete examination can be performed. Right now, however, your evaluation goal is to determine what treatment will best reduce current symptoms so that the patient's injury becomes less irritable so you can begin an effective rehabilitation process.

If a patient is able to walk without pain and has minimal edema, your objective evaluation can be more aggressive to determine the extent of the injury, the tissues involved, and the treatment approach that will most effectively and efficiently return this patient to normal activity.

A **comparable sign** is an active or passive movement that reproduces the patient's pain symptom (Maitland, 1991). Although it is not always easy to achieve a comparable sign in an objective examination, the rehabilitation clinician usually attempts to produce one.

Observation and Visual Inspection

Your visual inspection starts the moment you see the patient enter your facility. How is the patient walking? What is the posture and gait? General observations give you information about the severity of the injury and the items to inspect in your examination. For example, if the patient complains of medial knee pain and has excessively pronated feet, part of the problem may result from the feet and not the knee. If a patient has hip pain and genu valgus, weakness or structural anomalies at the knee may be contributing to hip pain.

Other general observations include noting whether the patient requires any assistive devices, such as a brace or crutches. Is the patient reluctant to move the injured part? Noting any abnormal movements, posture, or behavior helps you complete your picture of the injury. For example, if a patient enters your facility walking with crutches, you already know that gait training will eventually be a part of your treatment program. If you see a patient limping into the room, you should examine the entire lower extremity for weakness, because limping can cause weakness of improperly used muscles very quickly.

Your visual inspection of the injured area includes noting any abnormalities in the extremity that need more discriminate examination. Is there edema present, and if so, how much? Is there any discoloration, rash, wound, deformity, or atrophy present? If there is discoloration, does it appear distal to the injury, indicating that the patient probably did not elevate and correctly treat the injury when it occurred, or is the discoloration around the injury or proximal to it? Is there a scar, and if so, is it healed, does it look infected or excessive, and how recent does it appear to be?

Range of Motion

Range of motion of any joint can be normal, excessive (hypermobile), or less than normal (hypomobile). Normal ranges of motion for specific joints and how to measure them are discussed in chapter 5. Examination of the quality and quantity of available joint mobility investigates the capsule and ligamentous stability of the joint.

Active Range of Motion **Active range of motion (AROM)** is the amount of movement produced by an individual without assistance (figure 4.1). Active range of motion depends on the amount of pain caused by active movement of the part, the willingness of the patient to move it, the strength of the muscles moving the joint, and the available range of motion of the joint. Pain may not be the only reason a patient is reluctant to move a part through its range of motion. For example, the patient may be apprehensive of re-injury. When evaluating active range of motion, the rehabilitation clinician must consider the patient's position and be aware of gravity's effect on movement. For example, in a test of shoulder-flexion range of motion, a sitting patient has to overcome the greatest resistance to gravity at midrange, but in a supine position gravity's effect is

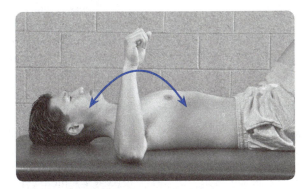

▶ **Figure 4.1** Active range of motion.

greatest in the initial stages of movement. If a patient is unable to raise her arm overhead when sitting, the rehabilitation clinician should have the patient lie supine to see whether additional active motion is possible when gravity has less impact on shoulder-flexor strength in that position.

Restricted joint motion may have a number of causes. Edema, tightened joint capsule or ligaments, loss of muscle flexibility, and mechanical blockage, such as a loose body or osteophyte, can, by themselves or in combination, prevent a patient from achieving full range of motion. As your examination proceeds, the cause should be revealed.

It is also important to observe the quality of movement. Is the movement full and fluid, or is it irregular, hesitant, or jerking? Does it occur through substitution of other muscles? If active motion causes pain, where in the motion does it occur? Is the pain in midrange of an arc of motion? This often indicates an irritated structure, such as the shoulder's supraspinatus tendon or a disc protrusion in the spine.

Information regarding the patient's ability to move helps you determine what to include in your rehabilitation program, such as pain-relief measures, joint motion and strength exercises, and coordination and functional activities.

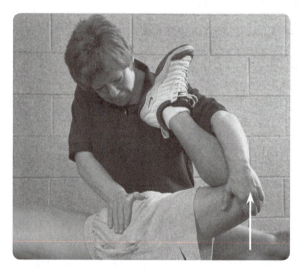

▶ **Figure 4.2** Passive range of motion.

Passive Range of Motion **Passive range of motion** is the amount of movement produced without any active participation by the patient (figure 4.2). Passive joint motion is divided into two categories: physiological and accessory. **Physiological joint motion** is movement that can also be performed actively by the individual. Physiological motion is also called cardinal motion. **Accessory joint motion** is motion that cannot be performed actively but is necessary for full active motion to occur.

Passive physiological range of motion is the motion a joint attains when someone other than the patient moves it while the patient remains relaxed. It is usually greater than the active range of motion in both injured and uninjured joints. As you move the joint through its motion, have the patient tell you when and where pain occurs in the motion. You should observe the patient's facial expressions, which also may indicate pain. The joint should be moved through the range of motion as far into the pain as the patient can tolerate it so you can get as good an impression of the amount of motion possible. If pain prevents you from moving the joint through its full motion, this should be recorded in your notes.

Once again, observe and record both the quantity and quality of the motion, whether passive motion causes pain, and if so, where in the motion the pain occurs. Pain that occurs with passive movement may be the result of stretching either inert structures, such as ligaments and capsules, or active structures, such as muscles. As you move the part through its motion, it is also important to note the end-feel of the movement.

If a joint's movement is normal and painless, **overpressure** is applied to truly assess full, painless motion. The pressure should be moderate and achieve slightly more motion as the joint is brought to its end range, but the motion should remain painless. To truly consider a joint as normal, firm overpressure must produce a painless and full range of motion (Maitland, 1991).

End-Feel of Movement The **end-feel** of a joint's movement is the nature of resistance palpated at the end of a range of movement. The end-feel can be normal or pathological, depending on the particular joint and the extent of its range of motion compared to what's expected. A number of authors have identified different end-feels (Cyriax, 1982; Kaltenborn, 2002; Paris & Patla, 1988). The most complicated system that uses tissue identification as end-feel labels is the Paris system (Paris & Patla, 1988). Cyriax (Cyriax, 1982) and Kaltenborn (Kaltenborn, 2002) both use a simpler system of identifying end-feels. Table 4.1 lists the Cyriax and Kaltenborn end-feel classifications.

TABLE 4.1   End-Feel Classifications

System	Normal end-feels	Abnormal end-feels
Cyriax	Capsular	Capsular in abnormal point in motion
	Bone-to-bone	Bone-to-bone in abnormal point in motion
	Tissue approximation	Springy block
		Spasm
		Empty
Kaltenborn	Soft	Any end-feel that either is of an abnormal
	Firm	quality for a joint or occurs at an abnormal
	Hard	point in the joint's range of motion

A capsular end-feel is a firm, leathery sensation when bringing a joint to the end of its motion. It is firm but not hard. If you move a normal, uninjured shoulder into full lateral rotation you will feel a firm, leathery end-feel. A capsular end-feel can also be felt in a pathological joint, such as a knee that has no edema or inflammation but does have joint restriction.

A common example of a normal bony end-feel is that of the elbow in full extension with the olecranon process moving against the olecranon fossa. It is a sudden-stop or a hard end-feel. In pathological states, the sensation is the same, but it occurs because of an abnormal condition, such as a bony growth or malunion fracture, and the total motion is less than normal.

Tissue approximation end-feels occur when two muscle bellies meet to prevent further movement and is considered a soft end-feel. A normal example is the anterior upper arm and forearm meeting in elbow flexion. The sensation is soft at the end of the movement.

A muscular end-feel is softer, less abrupt, and more rubbery than a capsular end-feel. It has a spring to it, much like what is felt when performing a straight-leg raise that is restricted by the hamstring muscles. The soft muscular end-feel is different from a muscle spasm end-feel in that the muscle spasm end-feel is more abrupt, usually causes pain, and does not allow full normal motion. A rebound of the muscle as it reflexes into a contraction in response to the stretch is felt in pathological conditions or if a normal muscle is stretched too quickly.

A type of abnormal soft end-feel is the boggy, mushy end-feel that is usually observed with joint effusion, when fluid within the joint prevents full motion. While the sensation of movement is boggy, the fluid's pressure blocks normal motion. It is common for this sensation to follow capsular joint movements, but this sensation occurs before the capsular end-feel is achieved.

An abnormal springy end-feel occurs from the mechanical block of a loose body and indicates an internal derangement. It is most commonly seen in the knee, where loose bodies of cartilage or meniscal flaps can stop normal joint movement. This end-feel can be considered soft or firm, depending on how intrusive into the joint is the loose body.

An empty end-feel is not common. There is no resistance to joint movement because the ligamentous and capsular restrictions are gone, and there is too much pain with muscular restriction for the patient to voluntarily stop the movement. In the absence of any ligamentous injury, acute bursitis or a neoplasm should be suspected with an empty end-feel.

Regardless of its description, an abnormal end-feel is usually also painful. The combination of pain with an abnormal end-feel aids in the identification of pathology within a joint.

Accessory Joint Mobility

The other portion of passive motion, accessory joint motion, must also be evaluated to determine overall joint mobility. Accessory joint motion is motion that cannot be produced actively by the patient but is necessary for full, normal motion of a joint. Accessory joint motion is

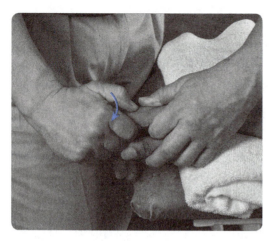

▶ **Figure 4.3** Accessory joint mobility.

evaluated by joint mobilization techniques. A good example of accessory joint motion is longitudinal rotation of the finger on the metacarpophalangeal joint (figure 4.3). It is not a motion that the patient can produce by any muscle activity, but you can rotate the phalanx easily by grasping the finger and rotating the proximal phalanx on its metacarpal. This accessory rotation must be present for full, active finger flexion-extension to occur. Specific joint mobilization techniques for treatment are the same as those used in examination and are discussed in chapter 6.

A joint can be normal in its mobility, hypermobile (excessive mobility), or hypomobile (restricted mobility). Joints that are hypomobile may be so because of muscle spasm protecting the area or because of restriction of ligamentous and capsular structures. Adhesions within the capsule can occur following injury, surgery, or immobilization. If you determine that a joint lacks full capsular mobility, part of your treatment plan should include joint mobilization techniques.

In examination of physiological and accessory joint mobility, you are looking for signs of stiffness in the joint, amplitude of available mobility, quality of motion, end-feel, and motion that is pain free. The best examination of the quality and quantity of stiffness and amplitude of motion is made by comparing the joint with its contralateral counterpart. Joint hypermobility is generally normal for the individual if it is bilateral. Normal accessory joint motions are pain free throughout the entire range of movement.

Resistive Range of Motion: Muscle Strength

Examining muscles surrounding the injured area involves investigation of their strength and endurance in addition to their motion. There are a number of procedures available that can examine muscular strength and endurance. The most common technique is isometric strength testing (figure 4.4). Other techniques can be used and are discussed in chapter 7.

Isometric testing for a quick determination of muscular strength is usually performed in a midrange or end-range joint position to measure gross muscle-group strength. This method of strength examination is called a **manual muscle test** and is discussed in detail in chapter 7 along with other methods of strength examination. Table 4.2 lists the muscle strength grades used in a manual muscle test. A more extensive table is seen in chapter 7.

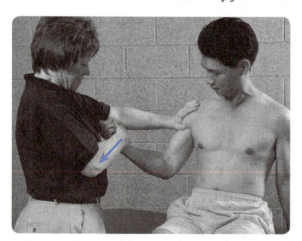

▶ **Figure 4.4** Muscular strength testing.

TABLE 4.2 **Muscle Strength Grades**

Numerical grade	Qualitative grade	Definition
5	Normal (N)	Able to resist maximum force throughout a full range of motion in a gravity-dependent position
4	Good (G)	Able to resist some force throughout a full range of motion in a gravity-dependent position
3	Fair (F)	Able to move the segment through a full range of motion against gravity but with no resistance
2	Poor (P)	Able to move the segment through a full range of motion but with gravity eliminated
1	Trace (T)	Palpation reveals a contraction of the muscle but no limb motion occurs
0	Zero (0)	No perceptible contraction is present

Special Tests

Special tests are used in the examination to determine the aggressiveness of the treatment program and where in the rehabilitation progression the patient should begin. For example, if a patient has an ankle sprain with a positive anterior drawer test, you should avoid aggressive dynamic proprioception examination in weight bearing until the patient's ankle has increased strength sufficiently to keep the ankle stabilized during those activities. If, on the other hand, a patient has a mild sprain and a negative anterior drawer sign, you can include those examination activities in the initial examination.

Neurological Tests

If your examination demonstrates neurological changes, neurological testing is warranted. These special tests include examination of sensory, motor, and reflex parameters (figure 4.5). Many professionals, including Corrigan and Maitland (Corrigan & Maitland,

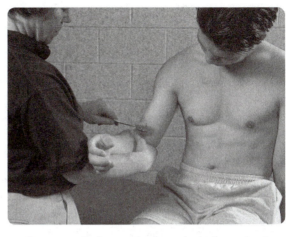

▶ **Figure 4.5** Reflex test for neurological examination.

1989), advocate using neurological testing when any signs or symptoms occur distal to the acromion in the upper extremity and distal to the gluteal fold in the lower extremity. This rule of thumb is especially warranted if you did not witness the injury incident and the patient is unsure of the nature of the injury. If neurological deficiencies are noted, impingement on the nerve root is possible and should be addressed in the treatment program.

Palpation

Palpation of the site is performed after the other tests are completed because palpation can irritate the tissues and can also lead to inaccurate conclusions. This sequence with palpation at the end of the rehabilitation examination is different from an examination made at the time of injury. One of the primary reasons for this is that it is not always clear during a rehabilitation examination what structures are involved until the examination is nearly complete, but when you see the injury occur, there is usually less question of what structures are involved. If palpation is performed early in a rehabilitation examination, before a good profile of the injury is obtained, the rehabilitation clinician may end up palpating a structure that is not actually injured, reducing the patient's confidence and wasting time.

Several structures are examined through palpation. Skin and subcutaneous tissue are examined by light touch for temperature, tone, and edema. Light movement of the skin and subcutaneous tissue against underlying structures is performed to reveal any excessive rigidity or adhesions of tissue, as commonly seen following prolonged immobilization or excessive edema with immobilization. If movement between the subcutaneous tissue and underlying structures is impaired, reduced mobility results. Deficiencies of these type warrant soft-tissue mobilization techniques as part of the treatment plan.

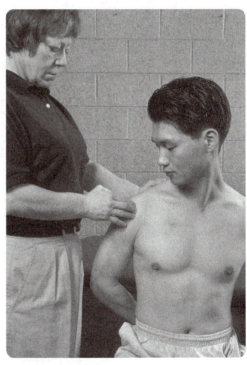

▶ **Figure 4.6** Palpation.

Palpation of fascia, muscles, ligaments, and tendons for tenderness, trigger points, and texture is important in examining causes of pain, motion restriction, and irritability (figure 4.6). Examination of these structures starts with light palpation of superficial structures; if the area's irritability permits, palpation pressure then increases to palpate deeper structures. Palpation of deeper structures requires a sensitive touch, not heavy pressure. For example, in palpating the midback area, light palpation is first performed to examine skin and subcutaneous mobility. Then slightly deeper palpation allows examination of the rhomboids and trapezius. Even deeper palpation is required to examine the paraspinal muscles. The deepest palpation in this region allows examination of the costovertebral joints. Palpate only as deeply as necessary to obtain the information you seek.

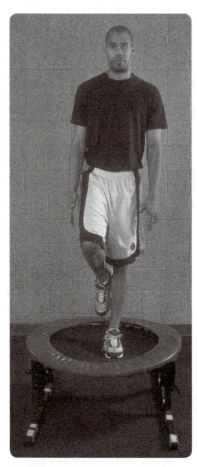

▶ **Figure 4.7** Functional testing.

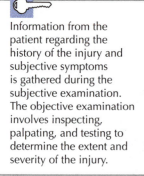

Information from the patient regarding the history of the injury and subjective symptoms is gathered during the subjective examination. The objective examination involves inspecting, palpating, and testing to determine the extent and severity of the injury.

Areas of tenderness are detected by palpation. Areas of spasm, crepitus, nodules, and scar tissue can also be palpated. Palpation reveals specific sites of tenderness and the tissue type involved. Palpation is also used to examine consistency, mobility, and abnormalities of underlying tissue. Gaps, rigidity, loss of normal mobility, woodiness, nodules, and other textures and tissue quality are recorded and used later to form the assessment.

Functional Testing

Functional tests are not always performed at the time of the initial rehabilitation examination. When they are used will vary. Sometimes they are used after palpation and after other factors have been examined, and sometimes they are incorporated before palpation to assist you in further identifying specific deficiencies. The irritability and severity of the injury dictate when these tests are appropriate. These tests determine whether specific activities produce pain, the injured part's ability to perform an activity, and the quality of movement during the activity. Agility, balance, coordination, and proprioception play key roles in a patient's ability to perform functional tasks. Simple functional tests include having the patient perform a squat while you look for smoothness of movement, full motion, and an ability to keep the feet flat on the floor.

Standing on one foot (figure 4.7), standing on toes, walking on toes, walking on heels, jumping, running, and cutting are other functional tests used to determine functional ability and quality. More advanced functional testing includes sport-specific or activity-specific skills.

Examination Results

Once you have accumulated all the information from the subjective and objective portions of your examination, you are ready to make a well-informed assessment and determine the diagnosis and problems that should be addressed in the treatment plan. The treatment program is designed to resolve these issues and achieve the goals that you and the patient set.

ASSESSMENT: PLANNING FOR ACTION

Once the subjective and objective examinations are complete, you interpret the information you have accumulated from these subjective and objective parts. This is where you express your opinions as a health care professional regarding the patient's problems, potential, and progress (Borcherding, 2000). Your judgment as to the patient's response to treatment, expected outcomes, functional limitations, and ability to perform is also included in this section.

Problems to Overcome

The rehabilitation clinician identifies the diagnosis and problems that the injured individual must overcome in order to return to full competition. Several simultaneous problems may need to be addressed, including subjective findings of pain and swelling or objective findings of reduced joint mobility or strength. Inability to perform can be an additional problem.

Progress and Potential

The assessment section is where the clinician expresses his or her opinion of the patient's progress, response to treatment, and potential for success in rehabilitation. Is the progress as expected, are the complaints of the patient reasonable or exaggerated from objective findings, is the patient working hard in his or her rehab program? Does the patient show enthusiasm or is the patient difficult to motivate? Is the patient's poor trunk stability contributing to poor agility? Any observations of the patient's performance, deficiencies, issues needing to be addressed, concerns, changes for the better or worse, or other points the clinician feels should be noted are recorded here. The assessment section is really the only portion of the SOAP note where you are able to record your professional opinions and judgments.

After the subjective, objective, and assessment portions of the examination or treatment are completed, the plan is next. Within the plan are included goals for treatment and what the clinician intends to do with the patient during the next session.

Goals for Treatment

This process includes creating a list of problems and a list of goals. The goals address the problems, and the problems are based on the findings of the examination.

Once the problems are identified, the treatment program and its goals can be outlined. The general goals most often are to remove or reduce the problems and return the patient to full competition. Specific goals may include relief of pain and swelling and restoring normal levels of joint mobility and strength. For every problem listed, there should be a goal to address and resolve it. A goal should not be listed if a problem associated with it has not been identified. For example, a goal to relieve spasm should not be listed if spasm is not a problem. There is a direct relationship between the problems identified by an evaluation and the goals of the treatment program.

Both short-term and long-term goals are set with specific objective aims regarding the activity to be accomplished (e.g., walk 2 flights of stairs), any conditions under which it may be achieved (e.g., without assistive devices), and the time frame within which it should be accomplished (e.g., in one week), as discussed in chapter 1. The goals should be objective and measurable. The time it will take to achieve short-term and long-term goals should be estimated. A common duration for a short-term goal is two weeks. You should estimate how far you expect the patient to progress in the next two weeks of your therapeutic exercise program and base your short-term goals on those estimates. The long-term goals are the final goals that the patient will achieve.

Some long-term goals are achieved sooner than others are during the course of the treatment program. For example, full flexibility is achieved before full agility and coordination. A short-term goal for week 6 of a rehabilitation program following ACL reconstruction surgery might be 100% range of motion of the knee, 50% normal quadriceps strength, and 30% normal agility. Once a goal is achieved, maintaining that goal becomes the next goal until all long-term goals are achieved. So, in the example just stated, the next short-term goal for week 8 may include: maintain full knee motion, 70% normal quadriceps strength, and 60% normal agility.

Plan for Treatment

After the goals have been outlined, a plan of action to achieve those goals can be designed. The **plan of treatment program** includes the frequency and duration of the treatment and the components included. The plan in a treatment note may change depending on the patient's response to the previous treatment. For example, the clinician may have recorded in the plan of the last treatment: "P: Begin jogging activities next treatment," but if the patient reports that the injury has been more painful since the last treatment, the clinician may choose to defer jogging activities and attend to the issue causing the increased pain first.

Various factors are involved in the treatment program, depending on the problems and goals that have been identified. For example, if goals include relieving swelling and pain and increasing range of motion and strength, modalities to reduce swelling and pain are included. Active range of motion may also be used to relieve these problems. Joint mobilization, range-of-motion exercises, massage, and home exercises may all be used to increase range of motion. Resistive exercises to increase strength may start with isometrics or more aggressive exercises, depending on the patient's ability and restrictions. Just as goals are designed to fit the problems, the plan is designed to achieve those goals.

A good therapeutic exercise program changes as the patient's problems decline and his or her status improves. As short-term goals are achieved, new short-term goals are set. To meet those goals, new treatment techniques must be planned. For example, if the patient achieves

For every problem listed, there should be a goal to address and resolve it. A goal should not be listed if a problem associated with it has not been identified.

a short-term goal of balancing in a stork stand for 30 s, a new goal should be established to further challenge the patient to achieve normal balance and progress to agility tasks.

The final short-term goals are actually the long-term goals. The patient progresses in the treatment plan until only the long-term goals are left. Once these are achieved through the treatment plan, the final treatment goal is returning the rehabilitated individual to full participation.

Continual Examination and Assessment

Examination and assessment take place before treatment, after treatment, and periodically throughout treatment to determine whether a specific technique is achieving its goals. For example, an examination before applying modalities determines the extent of muscle spasm present. An examination at the conclusion of the modality treatment assesses the success and efficacy of the modality. Similarly, an examination before applying a joint mobilization technique determines the quantity and area of joint restriction. An examination during the treatment determines whether joint mobility is improving as the mobilization technique is applied. An examination following the joint mobilization technique determines its effectiveness: Did your treatment achieve the improvements in pain reduction, range of motion, and joint mobility that you expected? How much more motion is there?

The only way to assess whether the treatment is producing the desired effects is to continually examine and reexamine. Examination and assessment are also performed after exercise. Sometimes the exercise effects are determined immediately: Was the patient able to perform the exercise correctly? Could the patient have tolerated a higher resistance or more repetitions? Did the patient favor the injured extremity during the exercise? At other times, the effectiveness and appropriateness of exercise are determined at the next treatment session: Did the patient suffer any unwanted side effects, such as more pain or edema after the exercise? Was there any muscle soreness without pain and edema? Your pretreatment findings determine your treatment for the day. These findings also denote whether you are providing the patient with an appropriate exercise program and what exercise and treatment changes are necessary to achieve your goals.

Rehabilitation program alterations are frequently necessary. Without ongoing examination and assessment, the rehabilitation clinician is unable to determine when to advance a patient, what techniques to use, how much force to apply in treatment techniques, and whether a treatment is beneficial or harmful to the patient. An examination and assessment occurs before, during, and after each treatment and from one treatment session to the next so optimal results occur with each treatment session.

Functional Examination

As the therapeutic exercise program advances, more and more functional activities are incorporated. Functional activities are covered in detail in chapter 10. As the patient nears the end of the therapeutic exercise program and is preparing to return to normal activity, it is important that the rehabilitation clinician examine the patient's abilities and readiness to return to normal, full participation. This is accomplished through functional testing. Specific functional activities vary from job to activity requirements, from sport to sport, and from one position to another within a sport. For example, a soccer offensive wing and a soccer goalie perform different activities. A gymnast has different functional requirements and is examined differently from a basketball player. A warehouse worker has different physical demands than an editor. It is your responsibility to appreciate these differences; know functional examination tools that appropriately test the necessary skills of different sports, positions, and occupations; and accurately assess the patient's readiness to return to full participation.

KEEPING REHABILITATION RECORDS

Record keeping sometimes can seem overwhelming to medical and allied health care professionals, but it is a crucial part of the treatment process. Records report the patient's initial levels

Assessment involves identifying problems based on information from the evaluation, setting goals to address those problems, and planning the treatment program for achieving those goals.

of ability and performance, the effects of treatments, and the final outcomes of a rehabilitation program. It is important to keep accurate records because they can be referred to later to determine progress, they can be used by other rehabilitation clinicians to provide consistent treatment, and they are legal documents. Because medical records are legal documents, all records that are not typed must be recorded clearly and legibly in pen, not pencil. Recorded items should not be erased, blacked out, or covered with correction fluid; an error should be corrected with one line drawn through it and your initials next to it, indicating that you have altered the record. You should always sign or initial and date the record after completing notes.

> Records are a legal document and are either typed or written in pen. Corrections are made with one line drawn through the error and initialed by the individual correcting the error.

Recording the Examination

Many different formats are used to record the examination. Most directors of athletic training clinics and other health care facilities develop their own forms for use in the facility. Preprinted forms are easy to use and provide consistency and thoroughness in examinations. Forms can offer a detailed list or a general outline, but they should include all the necessary information discussed in this chapter. A human figure on the form is also convenient so that the specific area of injury can be easily marked. Figures 4.8a (p. 103) and 4.9 (p. 107) are examples of detailed and general examination forms respectively. Figure 4.8b (p. 105) is a sample of a completed examination form.

The record should include information from the patient's subjective examination, including the injury site and onset; history and previous treatment of prior injuries; pain profile; additional medical problems; special questions; patient's activities, such as occupation or school demands; and if the patient is an athlete, the patient's sport and position. Any tests that have been ordered and their results should be included as well.

The objective portion of the form should include observations and inspections; examination findings on range of motion, strength, joint mobility, soft-tissue mobility, and neurological signs; palpation findings; and special test results.

A list of problems and a list of goals are a routine part of the examination form. The final portion of the examination form is the presentation of the treatment plan. A copy of the examination is frequently forwarded to the physician as a professional courtesy. It also completes the physician's records and helps the rehabilitation clinician and the physician communicate and coordinate their treatment plans and goals.

Recording the Treatment

Recording your treatment sessions is as important as recording your examination (figure 4.10, p. 108). A common method of record keeping is the SOAP (subjective, objective, assessment, and plan) note, which is thoroughly described in Borcherding (Borcherding, 2000). SOAP notes are the most commonly used system of problem-oriented record keeping in the medical profession. SOAP notes are clear, concise, and easily understood, and they provide a plan of action for medical care and treatment.

S: Subjective

Subjective notes are what the patient says. Direct quotations can be used. A common mistake is to put the clinician's impressions or assessments in this category. For example, a statement such as "The patient seems depressed" is incorrect. A more correct statement would be, "The patient states that he feels depressed," or "The patient states that he is having trouble sleeping, has lost his appetite, and doesn't feel like working on his rehabilitation program."

O: Objective

Objective notes record what is done in the treatment session today. They also include any objective measurements or examination and test results, for example, "ROM L knee = 115°. Leg press, L with 90 lb, 3 × 15. Heel raises on L only, 3 × 20 w/o wt. Ice L knee × 15 min. Home exercise program: Quad sets, 1 × 10, 4 times a day." You notice that if a home exercise program is given to a patient, it is included in the objective portion of the SOAP note since it something that was done at today's treatment session. Additionally, any objective measures that are made during this treatment session are placed in the objective portion of the SOAP note.

Many organizations use an exercise record sheet as part of their objective reporting. Figure 4.11a (p. 109) is a sample of an exercise record sheet, and 4.11b (p. 110) is an example of how an exercise record sheet could be filled out for a few treatment sessions. This is particularly useful in rehabilitation, where many exercises are included from one treatment session to the next. It saves time by reducing paperwork and needless repetition, yet still provides an accurate record of treatment.

A: Assessment

The assessment is your interpretation of the problems being addressed and how the patient and the injury responded to the treatment. Here is an example: "Patient continues to walk with an antalgic gait secondary to pain in the medial knee joint. His range of motion and strength are improving but remain deficient. He seems to be depressed about the injury but is willing to perform all activities in the treatment session."

P: Plan

This is the treatment plan. What will you do with the patient at the next treatment session? Continuing with the patient in the previous examples, the plan may be written like this: "Add early agility activities with stork standing and balance board next treatment. If pain persists, use electrical stimulation to reduce pain. Continue strengthening program progression as tolerated, add weight to heel raise, and increase repetitions on leg press. Patient to see ortho next Monday."

Additional Records

Additional records help to form a complete synopsis of treatment and progression for a patient. They provide a well-rounded perspective of progress, a summary of overall results, and a reference in the event of future injury.

Progress Note

When the patient is seen for follow-up visits by the physician, a brief progress report in a SOAP format is often sent with the patient, and a copy is kept in your records as well. An example of a progress note is seen in figure 4.12a (p. 111) and a completed progress note is seen in figure 4.12b (p. 112). The progress note provides the physician with a written record of the rehabilitation program and the patient's progress. It also allows communication between the rehabilitation clinician and the physician and helps to ensure that both are on common ground in the patient's care.

Additionally, the progress note provides you with a regular summary of the changes in the patient's condition. Objective and subjective changes that occur over time are sometimes difficult to assess when working with a patient regularly but are easily seen with a glance at your progress notes. You can judge more easily whether the patient is progressing appropriately.

Discharge Summary

When the patient achieves the long-term goals that were established at the outset of the rehabilitation program and is discharged from care, a brief discharge summary is completed, one copy is sent to the physician, and another is kept in your files (figure 4.13, p. 113). A discharge summary is important because it indicates the completion of the patient's rehabilitation program. It states the patient's condition at the time of discharge and summarizes the rehabilitation program and its duration. If the patient suffers another injury to the same area, the discharge summary also provides a quick reference to the patient's response to treatments, willingness to work in a therapeutic exercise program, and status at the time he completed the rehabilitation program.

REHABILITATION EXAMINATION

Name: _____ Date: _____

Medical Diagnosis: _____ DOI: _____

Age: _____ Occupation/Sport: _____ M.D.: _____

Activity level: _____

Current history:

Previous history:

Pain

Area:

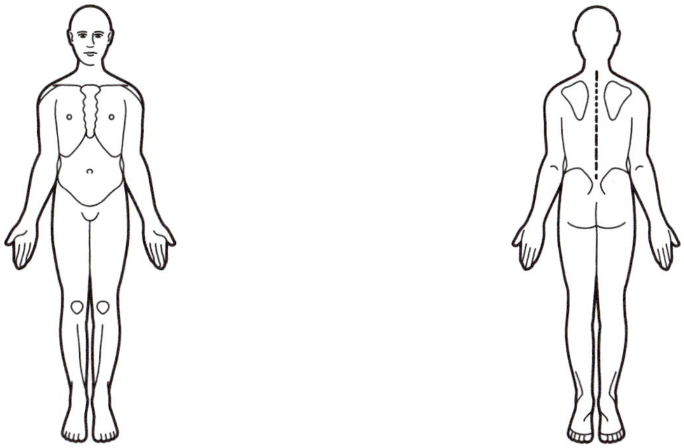

Description:

Intensity: (0 = no pain; 10 = "take me to the hospital, I'm dying")

Aggravating factors:

Easing factors:

24-hour profile

   AM:

   As day progresses:

   Evening:

   Night:

Special questions

GH: WL: X-rays: CE:

Steroids: Meds:

Patient's goals:

▶ **Figure 4.8a** Detailed examination form.

From P. Houglum, 2010, *Therapeutic Exercise for Musculoskeletal Injuries, Third Edition* (Champaign, IL: Human Kinetics).

OBJECTIVE EXAMINATION

Observation/Inspection:

Range of motion/Flexibility:

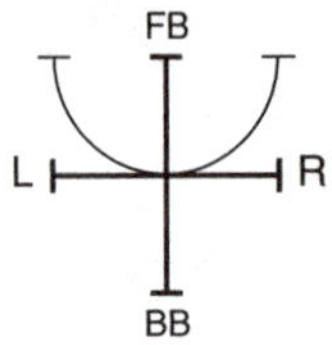

```
              FB
          L ──┼── R
              BB
```

Strength/Endurance: **Special tests:**

Tension signs: **Neurological signs:**

Accessory movements:

Palpation:

_____

Problems:

Goals:

Recommendations/Plan:

Initial treatment:

_____

Rehabilitation clinician

▶ **Figure 4.8a** *(continued)*

From P. Houglum, 2010, *Therapeutic Exercise for Musculoskeletal Injuries, Third Edition* (Champaign, IL: Human Kinetics).

REHABILITATION EXAMINATION

Name: _____ *Samuel Jole* _____ Date: _____ *5-16-09* _____

Medical Diagnosis: _____ *ACL reconstruction, left knee* _____ DOI: _____ *4-01-09* _____

Age: __ *20* __ Occupation/Sport: _____ *student/basketball team* _____ M.D.: _____ *E. Jesness* _____

Activity level: _____ *varsity BB until injured in game; currently going to class* _____

Current history: *Injured L ACL landing from a lay-up during game at home. Seen immediately by team MD; referred to Dr. Jesness for ortho consult. OP Sx: 4-16-09 for reconstruction with ipsilateral quad tendon. Immed post-op, WB to tol with 2 crutches, but now WB with 1 crutch. Brace set at 0°-90°; to ↑ today to 110°.*

Previous history: *No prior knee injury. Ankle sprain ×6 yrs with good post-injury rehab; no problems since.*

Pain

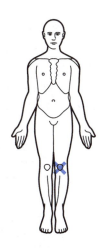 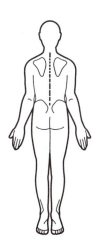

Area: *L Ant knee around patellar tendon surgical site.*

Description: *Normal post-op pain.*

Intensity (0= no pain; 10 = "take me to the hospital, I'm dying"): *2-4/10*

Aggravating factors: *Prolonged standing and walking.*

Easing factors: *Getting off the leg.*

24-hour profile

　AM: *Stiff.*

　As day progresses: *Loosens up and feels good by mid-day.*

　Evening: *Tired with some soreness, especially if swelling from doing too much is there.*

　Night: *No sleep disturbance any more. Had trouble sleeping first few days post-op. Still sleeping with brace but no problems; he's gotten used to it.*

Special questions

GH: *Neg*　　　　WL: *None*　　　X-rays: *MRI: +RACL*　　CE: *NA*

Steroids: *None*　　　Meds: *Pain meds given but none taken; denies other meds.*

Patient's goals: *Return to BB ASAP*

▶ **Figure 4.8b**　Completed detailed examination form.

OBJECTIVE EXAMINATION

Observation/Inspection: *Amb well c̄ 1 crutch, brace. Removes brace easily. Mod edema around knee, slightly warm. Well-healed surgical scars over P. tendon and arthroscopic window sites. Ecchymosis in distal knee and proximal leg. Edema 4 cm above joint line: L is 2 cm larger than R. Midbelly of calf is 1 cm smaller on L, and mid-thigh is 5 cm smaller on L. Unable to stand on L LE s̄ assist.*

Range of motion/Flexibility:

Knee Flex = 60°
Knee Ext = 10°

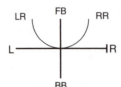

Strength/Endurance: *L hip: grossly 4/5; L ankle: grossly 4/5*   **Special tests:** *Deferred*

L knee flex = 4−/5; ext = 2+/5

R LE = WNL throughout

Unable to perform a complete quad set.

Tension Signs: *Deferred*   **Neurological signs:** *N/T*

Accessory movements: *L Patella: 50% restricted in all planes; L tibiofemoral joint: deferred for now*

Palpation: *Warmth around knee, as expected. Some tenderness over surgical sites. Swelling is boggy but no thickness palpated. Light spasm in gastroc-soleus, hamstrings.*

Problems: *Weakness and reduced endurance in L LE; Reduced motion in L knee; reduced mobility of L patella; reduced balance; mod edema around L knee; mild pain; abnormal gait; reduced level of activity.*

Goals: *Pt. to have: No pain, spasm in 1 week; No significant edema in 10 days; full AROM in 3 weeks; normal strength in 10-15 weeks; normal proprioception and balance in 4 weeks; normal ambulation s̄ assistive devices in 2 weeks. Good agility in 4-5 months. Return to full optimal function c̄ BB team in 6 months.*

Recommendations/Plan: *Per ACL protocol: relieve pain, spasm, edema within next 2 weeks. Patellar mobs for mobility; grade II tibiofemoral mobs for pain relief. Instructions in gait training with progression to ambulation without crutch. Progress as tol.*

Initial treatment:

O: *Pt seen for eval and initial rx.*

Rx: *Pulsed interferential current to R knee × 15 m for edema, spasm relief.*

Patellar mob for inf, sup, med, & lat: each II 1 × 30 s, III 2 × 45 s.

AROM with wall slides to tol × 5 m.

Assisted SLR, 2 × 5, then indep SLR 3 × 5.

Standing wt transfer L-R with verbal cueing for proper hip motion.

M.R. to L hip ab, ad, flex, ext; knee flex—all to fatigue ×1 set.

HEP: *instructed in quad sets; to perform 10 q 2 hr.*

Ice after ex. L knee AROM after rx: 15-95° and edema ↓ by 1 cm.

A: *Pt tired easily with strength ex; low endurance. Required some assistance with quad set, but was able to perform it well by end of rx. Pt appeared less apprehensive to move the R LE after rx. Spasm seems nearly resolved after rx.*

P: *Cont with modalities to ↓ pain, edema, spasm; add SAQ, IV patellar mobs next rx; if knee flex is 110°, start on stationary bike.*

Ella B. Grace
_____
Rehabilitation clinician

▶ **Figure 4.8b**   *(continued)*

EXAMINATION

Name:

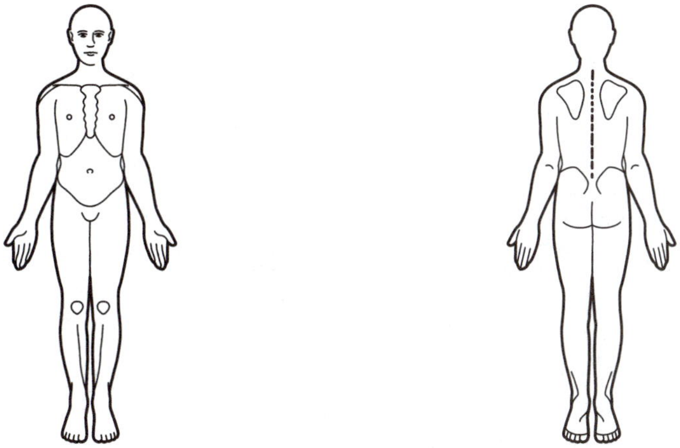

Subjective/History:

Objective/Findings:

Assessment/Problems:

Plan/Goals:

_____
Date

_____
Rehabilitation clinician

▶ **Figure 4.9** General examination form.

From P. Houglum, 2010, *Therapeutic Exercise for Musculoskeletal Injuries, Third Edition* (Champaign, IL: Human Kinetics).

TREATMENT NOTES

Patient: _____ Diagnosis: _____

Date: _____

S: _____

O: _____

_____

A: _____

_____

P: _____

_____

_____
Rehabilitation clinician

· ·

Patient: _____ Diagnosis: _____

Date: _____

S: _____

O: _____

_____

A: _____

_____

P: _____

_____

_____
Rehabilitation clinician

· ·

Patient: _____ Diagnosis: _____

Date: _____

S: _____

O: _____

_____

A: _____

_____

P: _____

_____

_____
Rehabilitation clinician

▶ **Figure 4.10** Rehabilitation treatment form.

From P. Houglum, 2010, *Therapeutic Exercise for Musculoskeletal Injuries, Third Edition* (Champaign, IL: Human Kinetics).

EXERCISES

Name: _____ DX: _____

M.D.: _____ Precautions: _____

Date												
Exercise												

▶ **Figure 4.11a** Exercise record sheet.

From P. Houglum, 2010, *Therapeutic Exercise for Musculoskeletal Injuries, Third Edition* (Champaign, IL: Human Kinetics).

EXERCISES

Name: _____ *Samuel Jole* _____ DX: _____ *L Bicipetal Rupture* _____

M.D.: _____ *E. Jesness* _____ Precautions: _____ *DOI 4-03-09* _____

Date	5/20		5/22		5/24		5/27		5/29		6/1		6/3										
Exercise	Reps	Wt	Reps	Wt	Reps	Wt	Reps	Wt	Reps	Wt	Reps	Wt	Reps	Wt	Reps	Wt	Reps	Wt	Reps	Wt	Reps	Wt	Reps	Wt
Biceps curl	2×15	15#	2×20	20#	2×12	20#	15,12	20#	2×15	20#	20,15	20#	2×20	20#										
French curl	2×10	8#	2×12	8#	15,12	8#	2×15	8#	20,15	8#	20,17	8#												
Wall pushup					2×20	0	3×15	0	3×15	0	2×20 15	0	3×20	0										
Military press-up					15,12	15#	2×15	15#	2×15	15#	20,18	15#												
Supination									2×12	4#	17,15	4#												
Pronation									2×12	8#	18,16	8#												

▶ **Figure 4.11***b* Partially completed exercise record sheet.

REHABILITATION PROGRESS REPORT

Name: _____ Date: _____

Diagnosis: _____

Number of treatments: _____

Subjective:

Objective:

Assessment:

Recommendations/Plan:

_____

Rehabilitation clinician

▶ **Figure 4.12a** Rehabilitation progress report.

From P. Houglum, 2010, *Therapeutic Exercise for Musculoskeletal Injuries, Third Edition* (Champaign, IL: Human Kinetics).

REHABILITATION PROGRESS REPORT

Name: _____ *Samuel Jole* _____ Date: _____ *4-15-09* _____

Diagnosis: _____ *L ACL reconstruction (3-31-09)* _____

Number of treatments: _____ *8 daily treatments* _____

Subjective: *Patient reports that he feels the treatments are helping him. He states he is now able to sleep the entire night without waking with pain.*

Objective: *Patient was started on treatments at 3 days post-op on 4-04-09. Initial treatments were provided to decrease post-op pain, edema, and muscle spasm in the quadriceps. At 10 days post-op active, active assistive ROM was started and is provided on a daily basis.*

AROM of L knee: 20° to 110°

Strength of LLE: Knee flexion = 4/5; knee extension = 3+/5; hip abduction, extension, and adduction = 4/5; hip flexion = 4−/5; ankle dorsiflexion and plantar flexion = 4+/5.

Gait: Pt is ambulating with the knee brace set at 15° to 120° as per MD orders. He is able to ambulate without the crutches for community distances.

Swelling: Girth at 4 cm proximal knee = 1 cm more on L, down from 3 cm at time of first treatment.

Pain: Decreased from 6/10 to 3/10 since initial treatment.

Assessment: *Pt is making gains with improvement in pain and edema levels. ROM is lacking more than is expected at this time, but patient appears reluctant to move the knee outside the brace without supervision.*

Recommendations/Plan: *Continue with ROM activities to gain full passive extension and flexion to 130° within 2 weeks. Encourage pt to perform home exercise program for ROM gains. Isometric exercises for knee muscles, manual resistance to the hip, and body weight resistance exercises to the plantar flexors will be initiated tomorrow as per ACL protocol.*

_____ *Ella B. Grace* _____

Rehabilitation clinician

▶ **Figure 4.12***b*   Completed rehabilitation progress report.

REHABILITATION DISCHARGE SUMMARY

Name: _____ Date: _____

Diagnosis: _____

Number of treatments: _____

Initial treatment date: _____ Final treatment date: _____

Discharge status

Pain/swelling: _____

ROM: _____

_____

Strength: _____

_____

Function: _____

_____

Recommended home program: _____

_____

Goals achieved: _____ Yes _____ No

Reasons for discharge: _____

_____

_____

Rehabilitation clinician

▶ **Figure 4.13** Rehabilitation discharge summary.

From P. Houglum, 2010, *Therapeutic Exercise for Musculoskeletal Injuries, Third Edition* (Champaign, IL: Human Kinetics).

> Record keeping is essential for judging the treatment's effectiveness, for communicating with other caregivers, as a reference in the event of reinjury, and as a legal document.

Outcomes

Assessment of outcomes is important in health care records. It can assist the clinician in providing useful information on patient perceptions of treatment quality and effectiveness. Outcomes can be especially valuable when clinicians bill for their services; third party providers often require evidence of outcomes for reimbursement. More detailed outcomes information is presented in chapter 1.

Diploma

An optional bit of paperwork that usually is a pleasure instead of drudgery is a rehabilitation diploma (figure 4.14). With today's software programs, diplomas are easily designed. A diploma printed on special paper for a patient who successfully completes a rehabilitation program is often well earned and coveted. It provides a bit of motivation for patients. Patients with whom I have worked have cherished and even framed their rehabilitation diplomas. Successful completion of a rehabilitation program involves dedication, hard work, and diligence, so a diploma is a well-deserved reward.

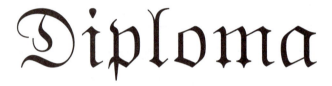

This is to certify that

_____

Has satisfactorily completed and endured the rigors of rehabilitation and the trauma of treatment prescribed for graduation from this facility, and is awarded this diploma for rehabilitation of _____

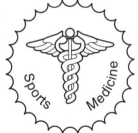

_____
REHABILITATION CLINICIAN

_____
DATE

State University of Science and Technology

▶ **Figure 4.14** Rehabilitation diploma.

SUMMARY

The examination serves as the starting point from which a rehabilitation program is designed. The clinician is similar to an investigator who works to identify the source of the patient's problem. This investigation includes a systematic process by which the patient's history and complaints are gathered, an objective examination is performed, and an assessment of the total picture is obtained from these elements. Once the assessment is completed, the clinician is able to identify the patient's problems and what will be done to resolve those problems. Both long- and short-term goals are then determined so that a planned approach for an optimal recovery is outlined. Record keeping includes records of examinations, progress, treatments, and discharge summaries.

KEY CONCEPTS AND REVIEW

1. Identify the primary factors of subjective examination.

The subjective portion of the examination should include a history of the injury, pain profile, medical history, special questions, and additional questions about factors that may affect the injury.

2. Outline an objective examination procedure that includes all primary factors.

The objective portion of the examination includes observation and visual inspection, examining active and passive physiological and accessory range of motion, strength tests, special tests, palpation, and functional tests if appropriate.

3. Explain the different types of end-feel and distinguish between normal and pathological end-feels.

Typical normal end-feels include capsular, bony, soft tissue, and muscular, although these can also be abnormal, depending on the tissue involved. Other abnormal end-feels are springy, boggy, and empty.

4. Explain how a treatment plan is designed and upon what factors it is based.

A treatment plan is developed after an assessment is made of the results of the examination. A list of problems based on the findings dictates a list of treatments to relieve those problems.

5. Define the SOAP note and explain its significance to rehabilitation.

A SOAP note is a common method of record keeping. It includes subjective reports from the patient, objective treatment provided, assessment of the results of and tolerance to the treatment, and plan of treatment for the next session. It provides a record of progress and allows consistency of treatment.

6. Identify two other records used in rehabilitation and demonstrate their importance.

A progress note to the physician, written when the patient returns to the physician for follow-up visits, and a discharge summary when the patient returns to sport participation are common rehabilitation records.

CRITICAL THINKING QUESTIONS

1. Describe the difference between an examination that occurs at the time of an injury and one that occurs before a rehabilitation program is started. Why are these differences important? What information may be different from one evaluation to the other?

2. Since pain is often the dominant complaint, an accurate pain profile provides you with a better idea of its source and how to proceed in your treatment program. Can you identify the most common types of pain and what they classically indicate? How does duration or intensity of pain influence the treatment you provide?

3. Your objective examination is based on the results of the subjective examination. How would your objective examination of a patient who reports severe pain most of the time compare with an examination of a patient who has minimal pain most of the time with occasional severe pain? If the patient's pain prevents you from performing all the tests you would like, what does your objective examination include, and what do you do for treatment?

4. Is it possible to have a goal without a problem? Is it possible to have a problem without a goal? How are these two factors related? If the goals change, does that mean the problem has changed?

5. You have been newly hired at a university that has not kept medical records beyond the initial injury incident report and daily athletic training clinic visitation record. How would you change the system to make it more compliant with record-keeping standards for medical facilities? What forms would you develop to make the process as simple as possible? What minimum record-keeping requirements would you put into place? What are the justifications for these changes?

LAB ACTIVITIES

1. Indicate which of the following statements are S statements, which are O statements, which are A statements, and which are P statements:

   a. Pt c/o L wrist pain.
   b. Pt will demonstrate a normal gait pattern 95% of the time within 3 wk.
   c. Flexion in lying reproduces pt's worst R LE pain.
   d. Pulsed US @ 1.5-2.0 W/cm2 to R upper trap for 5 min.
   e. States onset of pain was in July 2002.
   f. AROM: WNL bilat LEs.
   g. ↑ AROM R shoulder to WNL within 2 mo.
   h. Will inquire if pt can be referred to orthopedist.
   i. Pt was too groggy following pain medication and could not follow instructions well.

2. Write the two-week goals for each of the following scenarios:

Scenario A:

Dx: Fx R tibial plateau. Long leg cast applied 8/30/03

O: Amb: Not attempted; MD wants pt to begin with crutches, NWB R LE

A: Pt. has difficulty with standing; this may be a slow process based on pt's initial reaction to treatment.

P: Long-term goal: Indep amb c̄ crutches for unlimited distances on level surfaces & stairs within 1 mo.

Short-term goal: _____

You estimate that the pt will be able to ambulate 100 ft × 2 on level surfaces and require minimal assistance on stairs in 1 wk.

Scenario B:

Dx: Neck strain

S: c/o neck pain of an intensity of 9/10 with any movement of the neck.

O: AROM: 0-5° cervical rotation L & R

A: May have neck pain for a few weeks.

P: Long-term goal: ↑ neck AROM to WNL & pain free within 1 mo.

Short-term goal: _____

You judge that the patient will be able to move her head to ~10° of rotation to either side in 2 days.

3. Read the following report and convert it into a SOAP note:

When I saw the patient this morning he reported that he didn't sleep well after his last treatment session. He reported that the pain in his right shoulder was more intense than it usually was after the treatment, going from a 3 to a 6 on the 10-point scale, and thinks that it might be because of the new strength exercise that was added last time. Since he was more sore today I decided not to continue with the overhead lat pulldown exercise with 60 pounds we started last time and keep his shoulder exercises no higher elevation than 90°. I started out with ultrasound to the supraspinatus tendon at 1.5 w/cm2 for 5 minutes. The ultrasound was followed by some joint mobilization, grade II for distraction, then grade III for anterior-posterior glides and inferior glides for about 5 minutes, and then I finished with more grade II distractions. After the mobilization he did his stretching exercises. The stretching exercises included stretches for 30 seconds each to his shoulder lateral rotators, flexors, abductors, and horizontal abductors. The strengthening exercises I had him do today included wall push-ups for 2 sets of 20, shoulder medial rotation in sidelying on his right side with 7 pounds for 3 sets of 15, shoulder lateral rotation in sidelying on his left side with 5 pounds for 3 sets of 15, shoulder abduction with him in standing using 5 pounds and going to only 45° for 3 sets of 20. I finished his treatment today with ice to the shoulder for 15 minutes. I instructed him to do only his usual range of motion exercises for flexion, abduction, lateral rotation, and horizontal adduction for his home program until the pain subsides to where it was before the last treatment. I also told him to put ice on the shoulder at home if the pain increases again. He said he felt better after today's treatment and thought he would sleep better tonight. Next time I'll see how he feels before we start his program. If he is better, I will try the lat pulldown exercise again but with less weight. If he still has more pain, I think I should probably refer him to the doctor.

4. For two weeks you have been treating a soccer player with an old hamstring strain that has not resolved. He has been on your program for two weeks, and you want to examine how his progress has been with the treatments you have performed.

    a. What tests will you perform?

    b. How will you know if your treatment program has been effective?

    c. What soccer activities will you have him perform as part of his functional activities?

5. Three days ago a gymnast suffered a grade II ankle sprain. You are going to start her on rehabilitation today.

    a. What will you examine before you begin her program?

    b. What will be the determining factors in what to include in your program today?

    c. How will you know if you have provided an appropriate program for her?

6. An athlete comes to you, reporting that she has pain in her knee but she doesn't remember injuring it recently. What questions would you ask her? What is your reason for asking each question?

7. With your lab partner lying on the treatment table, go to the end range of the following motions and describe what you feel for each end-range position:

    a. Elbow extension

    b. Elbow flexion

    c. Knee extension

    d. Knee flexion

    e. Subtalar inversion

    f. Shoulder flexion

    g. #2 MCP extension

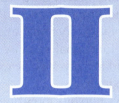

PART

II

Therapeutic Exercise Parameters and Techniques

*Continuous effort—not strength or intelligence—
is the key to unlocking our potential.*

WINSTON CHURCHILL, British Prime Minister, 1874-1965

The next six chapters delve into specific techniques for restoring range of motion and flexibility, muscular strength and endurance, coordination and agility, soft-tissue and joint mobility, and functional and activity-specific exercises.

Recall from part I that the parameters of normal function are emphasized in a logical sequence, each one building on the previous ones, throughout the therapeutic exercise program. This part follows that sequence in the presentation of topics. In chapter 5, range of motion and flexibility are discussed. What normal joint motion is and how to achieve it are presented. Chapter 6 extends the material of chapter 5 in that it deals with soft-tissue and joint pathology that may interfere with normal motion. The various techniques commonly used to resolve problems in these areas are discussed.

Progressing in the rehabilitation sequence, strength and muscular endurance are discussed in chapter 7. The various types of strengthening techniques, equipment used, program progressions, and precautions are also introduced.

Proprioception—including balance, agility, and coordination—is discussed in chapter 8. Progression from a static to a dynamic program is also included.

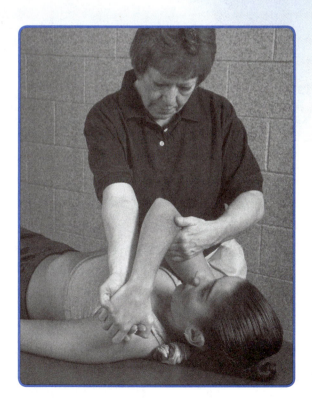

Chapter 9 presents information on plyometrics—activities that require flexibility, strength, endurance, and proprioception. Plyometrics are often incorporated into a rehabilitation program before functional exercises.

Chapter 10 presents functional exercise and activity-specific exercises and their concepts. Functional and activity-specific exercises are the final progression of a total therapeutic exercise program.

The words of Winston Churchill apply directly to your education in rehabilitation. As you read through the chapters of this part, the relevance of the information presented in part I will become clear. By the time you complete part II, you will have the knowledge of the 'what' needed for parts III and IV, where general and specific programs for injuries are presented. Parts I and II are your gateway to understanding and appreciating the 'how' of practical program applications and concepts in parts III and IV. By the time you have completed this book, you will be able to apply what you have learned to develop your own rehabilitation programs.

CHAPTER 5

Range of Motion and Flexibility

OBJECTIVES

After completing this chapter, you should be able to do the following:

1. Define the differences between range of motion and flexibility.

2. Explain the differences in structure of loose connective tissue and dense connective tissue.

3. List the deleterious effects of prolonged immobilization.

4. Discuss the mechanical properties of plasticity, elasticity, and viscosity of connective tissue.

5. Explain the physiological properties of creep and stress-strain and how they affect stretching techniques.

6. Discuss the neuromuscular influences of the muscle spindle and GTO on stretching muscle.

7. Explain the procedure for measuring range of motion with a goniometer.

8. Discuss the active and passive methods for stretching.

9. Identify two mechanical assistive devices used to increase range of motion.

10. List contraindications, indications, and precautions of stretching.

11. Discuss the progression of a stretching exercise program.

▶ As a senior athletic training student, Anthony Johns is on his first sports medicine clinical rotation. His first patient today is a new shoulder patient. Anthony knows from his experiences at his last clinical site that he will measure the shoulder, elbow, and wrist ranges of motion in all their planes of movement. He also knows that the patient had a rotator cuff repair, but he does not know when the surgery was performed, what specific repair was used, or the physician's post-operative restrictions on shoulder motion. He anticipates, though, that there will be some limitations and precautions. Although there should be no limitations on elbow and wrist motions, if the shoulder is immobilized in a sling, there may be some loss of motion in the elbow that must be evaluated and addressed.

Nobody can make you feel inferior without your permission.

**ELEANOR ROOSEVELT, U.S. Delegate to the United Nations
and wife of the 32nd president, 1884-1962**

By now you realize that a rapid restoration of range of motion and flexibility is important in a therapeutic exercise program. The aim of this chapter is to present ideas and techniques to regain and maintain flexibility by making the most of physiological principles that affect tissue length changes. Additionally, this chapter introduces the deleterious effects of prolonged immobilization, defines the differences between range of motion and flexibility, discusses the various methods and progressions for achieving full motion, identifies normal levels of motion throughout the body, and investigates the equipment used to evaluate motion.

At the conclusion of this chapter, the consequences of establishing or not establishing normal motion and of delaying the process should become clear. You will also know the techniques and skills needed for successfully restoring range of motion, and you will acquire an awareness of precautions and progression of flexibility in rehabilitation.

DEFINING FLEXIBILITY AND RANGE OF MOTION

Range of motion and flexibility are closely related. Although the terms are often used interchangeably, their definitions are different.

Flexibility refers to the musculotendinous unit's ability to elongate with application of a stretching force. The amount of flexibility of an area is related to its stiffness, suppleness, or pliability. Prolonged loss of flexibility can reduce range of motion.

Range of motion is the amount of mobility of a joint and is determined by the soft-tissue and bony structures in the area. The status of soft tissues—including muscles, tendons, ligaments, capsule, skin, subcutaneous tissues, nerves, and blood vessels—all affect the range of motion of a joint. If a patient has impaired flexibility, range of motion is also limited.

Clinically, range-of-motion measurements quantify both range of motion and flexibility. Although there is a technical distinction between the two, clinical interpretations make differences less clear. For this reason, range of motion and flexibility are used interchangeably in this text.

CONNECTIVE-TISSUE COMPOSITION

Mobility of the musculoskeletal system is determined by the composition of connective tissue and the orientation of the various soft-tissue structures. Connective tissue is composed of primarily two structures: cells and extracellular matrix. The cells of most interest in connective tissue are fibroblasts, the cells that create in connective tissue components of collagen, elastin, reticulin, and ground substance. These components comprise the extracellular matrix. The quantities of these substances vary according to the specific structure and determine the

🔑 Flexibility is a musculotendinous unit's ability to elongate, whereas range of motion is a joint's mobility, which is affected by the tissues in and around the joint.

characteristics of the structure. For example, there is more collagen in ligament and more elastin in skin.

Collagen provides tissue with strength and stiffness. Recall from chapter 2 that the collagen fibers bind themselves together; the more binding between the fibers, the greater the tensile strength and stability of the structure. Collagen fibers are five times as strong as elastin fibers.

Elastin fibers provide a structure with extensibility. Elastin fibers are able to withstand elongation stress and return to normal length. Tissues that have more elastin have more flexibility.

Reticulin fibers are essentially Type III collagen fibers. They are weaker than Type I. They are particularly important during repair following injury.

Ground substance is a structureless organic gel that serves to reduce friction between the collagen and elastin fibers, maintains spacing between the fibers to prevent excessive cross-linking, and transports nutrients to the fibers.

Three different kinds of connective tissue are present in the body and are classified according to their density and arrangement. The fiber arrangement of **areolar (loose irregular) connective tissue** is irregular and loose with relatively long distances between the cross-links. Loose connective tissue's open network is composed primarily of thin collagen and elastic fibers interlaced in several different directions. This arrangement provides the structure with tensile strength as well as pliability. Fascia of skin and that surrounding muscles and nerves are examples of areolar connective tissue. Loose irregular connective tissue lies between structures in areas where motion occurs, such as joint capsular fascia, intermuscular layers, and subcutaneous tissue. Areolar connective tissue permits movement in all directions.

Tendons are an example of a structure containing more highly organized connective tissue with regular parallel collagen fibers and more cross-links. This arrangement allows **dense regular connective tissues** to resist high-tensile loads and still provide some flexibility. Ligaments are similar to tendons in their structure except that their fiber arrangement is not quite as regular, but they are still within this category of dense regular connective tissue. Ligament collagen fiber arrangements are primarily parallel, but there are also spiral and oblique arrangements.

On a continuum between the structural extremes in the arrangement, orientation, and quantity of fibers and cross-links in skin and tendons are structures such as ligaments, capsules, and fascia. Even within these categories, fiber arrangements vary. For example, ligaments that must resist higher forces have more organized fiber arrangements with greater quantities of cross-links.

The third type of connective tissue, **dense irregular connective tissue,** is similar to dense regular connective tissue, but its arrangement is not parallel. Dense irregular connective tissue is multidimensional in its fiber pattern. Such an arrangement allows the tissue to provide resistance to forces in multiple directions. Such tissue provides for tensile strength but has little extensibility to deform. Examples of this connective tissue are found in joint capsules, aponeuroses expansions of tendons, and bone periosteum.

EFFECTS OF IMMOBILIZATION ON CONNECTIVE TISSUE

Connective tissue is continually replaced and reorganized as a part of normal body function. As a part of the reorganization process, connective tissue normally tends to shorten (F.J. Kottke, Pauley, & Ptak, 1966). To combat this tendency, normal motion is maintained through daily activity. If motion is restricted, either voluntarily or passively, rapid changes in the structure and function of connective tissue occur. Immobilization following injury is sometimes necessary to protect the area and permit the healing process to occur unimpeded. Immobilization, however, can also be detrimental. Depending on how long an area is immobilized, the changes in connective tissue can be either permanent or reversible. Although it does not take long for changes to occur, the longer the period of immobilization, the more difficult the restoration to normal becomes.

Connective tissue supports the body and provides it with its framework. It is composed of many different kinds of cells and fibrous and ground substances that form in various combinations, depending on the specific connective-tissue type. These connective tissues vary in the types, orientation, and linking of their fibers, which affect their ability to withstand stress.

To understand the problems involved in restoring normal range of motion and other lost parameters of an affected area, you must first be aware of the changes that occur with immobilization. Immobilization affects all tissue, from bone to skin.

General Changes in Soft Tissue

Soft-tissue changes are seen following even one week of immobilization and are increased by edema, trauma, and impaired circulation (F.J. Kottke & Lehmann, 1990). Immobilization causes a loss of ground substance, which, in turn, results in less separation and more cross-link formations between collagen fibers. The fiber meshwork contracts so the tissue becomes dense, hard, and less supple. Even if a normal joint is immobilized for four weeks, the dense connective tissue that forms prevents normal motion.

Following an injury, the newly formed fibrin and collagen fibers arrange in a haphazard way if the injury is immobilized. New formations of increased cross-links impair motion. Although cross-links are necessary for collagen strength, excessive cross-links can restrict normal movement of collagen tissue (figure 5.1). After two weeks of immobilization, an injured joint has reduced motion because of these connective tissue changes. Remember also that as scar tissue forms, the natural process of wound contraction augments the injured area's motion loss.

When edema combines with immobilization, fibrosis increases, probably because of more tissue fluid protein and metabolites in the area along with deficient local metabolism. The result is less tissue mobility. Fibrosis further increases when circulation is impaired, either because of age or local conditions. Edema acts like a glue to bind down tissue structures, especially if its presence is prolonged.

Although an area is immobilized, connective tissue still continues its normal process of remodeling and reorganizing. Without movement, as collagen is formed, it creates a dense, hard meshwork of sheets or bands with a loss of normal suppleness. Collagen fibers then form between the connective tissue's reticular fibers and from one structure to another, "gluing down" the area. The result is restricted motion where normal areolar connective tissue would have permitted one tissue type to freely move over another. Muscle tissue becomes restricted by fascia, tendons lose their ability to move against subcutaneous tissue, and ligaments adhere to capsules.

Immobilization produces structural weakness as well as a loss of tissue mobility. Weakness occurs because of a decrease in collagen mass. This is thought to occur because of the reduction in applied load or stress when a part is immobilized. Klein et al. (Klein, Heiple, Torzilli, Goldberg, & Burstein, 1989) demonstrated that if motion is allowed in a non-weight-bearing extremity, the integrity of the ligaments is not lost. Immobilized, non-weight-bearing limbs also lose bone density. When possible, therefore, activity in rehabilitation should be instituted for non-weight-bearing extremities until weight bearing and a full therapeutic exercise program are allowed.

Effects on Muscle Tissue

Changes in muscle tissue following immobilization include reductions in muscle fiber size, number of myofibrils in the muscle, and oxidative capacity. As these changes occur, there is an increase in the fibrous and fatty tissue in the muscle and a reduction in the intramuscular capillary density. These changes, which cause the muscle to become smaller

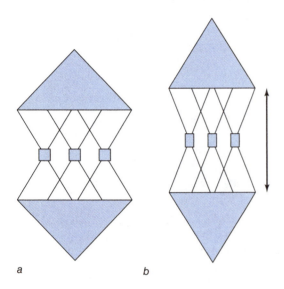

a   *b*

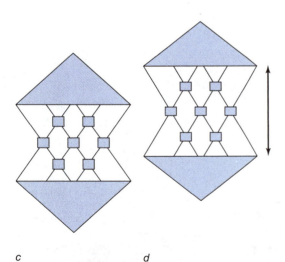

c   *d*

▶ **Figure 5.1** Collagen cross-links reduce mobility. Parts *a* and *b* are normal cross-links; *c* and *d* are excessive cross-links. Parts *a* and *c* are at resting length; *b* and *d* are stretched. Increased cross-links prevent full extensibility of tissue.

and weaker, occur after two weeks of immobilization (Montgomery & Steadman, 1985). The longer a muscle is immobilized, the greater the number of muscle fibers that degenerate and the greater the quantity of fibrous and fatty tissue. As the muscle becomes weaker, loses its motion, and is immobilized, the normal neural feedback system of movement is lost. The combination of these factors along with changes in the ligaments impairs proprioception (Hewett, Paterno, & Myer, 2002; Montgomery & Steadman, 1985).

Histological changes observed in immobilized muscle include decreased levels of adenosine triphosphate (ATP), adenosine diphosphate (ADP), creatine phosphate (CP), creatine, and glycogen. When the immobilized muscle works, more than the normal level of lactic acid is produced. These changes, along with a reduction in mitochondrial production and size, cause a reduction in the oxidative capacity of the muscle, which causes the muscle to fatigue more quickly and easily.

Several clinical observations can be made of immobilized muscle. The most obvious change is that the muscle is smaller in size. It is also unable to produce as strong a contraction and cannot sustain activity for as long a time as before immobilization. Additionally, the muscle is slower to respond to a stimulus when it contracts.

Many of these changes occur within the first few days of immobilization. A decrease in muscle size (atrophy) and mitochondrial production occur within the first five to seven days of immobilization. The rate of atrophy, however, varies from one muscle to another. For example, when the thigh is immobilized, the quadriceps becomes weaker and smaller at a faster rate than the hamstrings.

Effects on Articular Cartilage

Articular cartilage also suffers changes from immobilization. These changes depend on the position of immobilization, the duration of immobilization, and whether the joint bears weight or not during immobilization. With immobilization, the mechanical properties decay: The cartilage becomes thinner, the proteoglycan concentration decreases, and the matrix organization declines (Buckwalter, 1996). Articular cartilage of joint surfaces that are not in contact with each other also changes. In addition, necrosis of articular cartilage occurs when constant pressure between the joint surfaces is maintained during immobilization. Immobilization also increases the amount of fibrofatty tissue that ultimately becomes scar tissue within the joint.

Buckwalter (Buckwalter, 1996) indicated that with continued immobilization, joints suffer irreparable damage. These changes include contracture of the joint because dense, fibrous tissue forms around the joint and in muscles that cross the joint; reduction of the articular cartilage lining of the joint surfaces; and replacement of the normal joint cavity with fibrofatty tissue. The time required before the process becomes irreversible has not yet been definitively established in humans. In rats, it occurs after 60 days of immobilization (Evans, Eggers, Butler, & Blumel, 1960). In rabbits, irreversible changes were seen after immobilization for six weeks (Finsterbush & Friedman, 1975). Studies performed on animals also demonstrate that the longer an extremity is immobilized, the longer it takes to establish pre-immobilization parameters. Presumably, at least in this regard, human tissue is no different.

Effects on Periarticular Connective Tissue

Periarticular connective tissue is soft tissue surrounding the joint, such as ligaments, joint capsule, fascia, tendons, and synovial membranes. As with muscle and articular cartilage, all these structures are adversely affected by immobilization. The connective tissue becomes thick and fibrotic. As has been discussed, the ground substance, a viscous gel that contains GAGs and water, serves to separate the collagen fibers, lubricate the area, and keep the fibers gliding freely. During immobilization the GAG and water content in the ground substance is reduced, causing a diminution of extracellular matrix. The combination of changes in ground substance, increased collagen cross-links, and continued normal collagen processing diminishes tissue mobility. The clinical impact of these changes is a loss of motion of the affected joint.

Immobilization causes changes that result in loss of motion in all tissues. Increased collagen cross-links, loss of ground substance, and fibrosis all impair the flexibility of connective tissue.

With all these dramatic changes from immobilization, it makes sense to minimize the duration of immobilization. Immobilization is important and necessary after some injuries and surgeries. It is in the best interest of the patient, however, to base the time of immobilization on the time course of injury and healing that was discussed in chapter 2.

Recall that collagen formation is well under way after seven days following an injury. The injury has gone from inflammation to proliferation and is entering the start of the remodeling phase. By day 21, the remodeling phase is in full swing, and the permanent structure is emerging. Although there are exceptions, gentle range-of-motion activities may start by day 7 and certainly should be instituted by the third week following injury or surgery.

From a biological standpoint, the initiation of range-of-motion activities depends on the severity of the injury, the tissue and body part involved, and the surgical repair technique used. From a practical standpoint, it is also determined by the patient's ability and status, the philosophy of the physician, the physician's confidence in his or her own surgical repair, and the abilities of the rehabilitation clinician.

EFFECTS OF REMOBILIZATION ON CONNECTIVE TISSUE

Orthopedic injuries were commonly immobilized for several weeks following surgical repair in the late 20th century; our knowledge of the deleterious, long-term effects of this practice has eliminated prolonged immobilization in post-injury and post-operative care. Just as there are many disadvantages to prolonged immobilization, there are many advantages to early remobilization.

Collagen in all tissue is affected with remobilization. Immobilization causes collagen to be misaligned during its development; this causes a reduction in tensile strength (Provenzano et al., 2003). Remobilization effectively realigns collagen to improve its strength (Gomez et al., 1991). In addition to this important understanding of remobilization, specific tissues have additional specific responses to being moved after immobilization. The following few paragraphs summarize the advantageous effects of mobilization.

Effects on Muscle Fibers

Muscle fibers recover from immobilization if it has not been excessive. Initially, the recovery is rapid, but as it continues, the rate of change slows until full recovery occurs. Injured muscle responds best to a short period of immobilization followed by active motion. Movement causes a more rapid absorption of hematoma, an increase in tensile strength, and improved myofiber regeneration and arrangement for an effective overall recovery. Adhesions of muscle to fascia with immobilization will reduce the muscle's flexibility and affect joint range of motion. Techniques for treating these restrictions are discussed in chapter 6.

Effects on Articular Cartilage

Less articular cartilage degeneration occurs if both joint motion and weight bearing are allowed on a limited basis. Controlled weight bearing or loading of articular cartilage may even encourage repair of damaged cartilage (Heckmann, Barber-Westin, & Noyes, 2006). Overall, research findings consistently indicate that a joint, after injury, responds best to a rehabilitation program that provides controlled loading and movement, which stimulate proteoglycan and chondrocyte production.

Effects on Periarticular Connective Tissue

Remobilization of periarticular connective tissue prevents abnormal cross-link formation and helps to maintain the fluid content of the extracellular matrix so that proper fiber distance can be maintained (Donatelli & Owens-Burkhart, 1981). Fatty tissue buildup around the joint limits mobility and must be broken by techniques such as stretching and joint mobilization. Stretching techniques are discussed later in this chapter, and joint mobilization is introduced in chapter 6.

MECHANICAL PROPERTIES AND TISSUE BEHAVIOR IN RANGE OF MOTION

Remobilization enhances recovery. It prevents abnormal collagen cross-link formation and increases fluid content in the extracellular matrix of connective tissue.

Even when an extremity is not immobilized, injury or surgery causes scar-tissue formation, and this scar tissue can lead to adhesions of connective tissue and increased fibrosis. When loss of motion occurs, it is because connective tissue extensibility diminishes. Connective tissue is in joint capsules, ligaments, tendons, and fascia. Although muscles are not composed primarily of connective tissue as these other structures are, muscles are surrounded by an extensive fascial network that affects their flexibility and response to stretch. Therefore, flexibility of all tissues that rehabilitation clinicians deal with is influenced by connective tissue.

To determine the most effective ways to increase the range of motion of injured parts, it is important to review the physiology of connective tissue. Stretching exercises can affect the non-contractile element of all connective tissue. Because collagen gives a structure its tensile strength, resilience, and form, it is also the primary component restricting range of motion and, therefore, should be the primary target of stretching exercises.

Remember that body parts are three-dimensional and respond to forces in three dimensions. When stress is applied, a structure's response depends on the direction, duration, and magnitude of the force and the specific fibers involved.

Mechanical Properties of Connective Tissue

To effectively apply stretching forces to collagen, you must first understand its mechanical properties. Collagen is elastic, viscoelastic, and plastic. Connective tissue possesses all these qualities simultaneously. When connective tissue is stretched, all three qualities may be affected. If we separate the properties and look at them individually, it might be easier to understand how collagen functions and what we can do to influence it. Plasticity allows the connective tissue's length to change, while elasticity allows some restoration of normal length. The effectiveness of the stretch depends on the amount of collagen and elastin in the gross structure. The effectiveness of the stretch also depends on the amount of force applied, the duration of the stretch, and the temperature of the tissue. The physical properties of collagen also influence the effectiveness of a stretch.

Elasticity

Elasticity is the ability to return to normal length after an elongation force or load has been applied. This restoration of length occurs because of its stored potential energy. Elastic material is commonly symbolized by a spring in engineering models (figure 5.2a). A rubber band easily demonstrates elasticity. If you give a rubber band a brief pull, then release the force, the rubber band returns to its normal length.

Viscoelasticity

Viscoelasticity is in substances that have both elastic and viscous properties. **Viscosity** is the resistance to an outside force that causes a fluid-like, permanent deformation. Resistance occurs from a cohesion of molecules that provides a shearing force to resist change in shape. No potential energy is stored in a viscous object, so there is no energy to permit its return to normal length; the energy is released as heat before it can be stored. An example of a viscous substance is tar. A hydraulic cylinder represents viscosity, as in figure 5.2b. **Viscoelasticity,** then, is the ability of a structure to resist change of shape when an outside force is applied but an inability to completely return to its former state after changing shape. A combination of a spring and a hydraulic cylinder represents viscoelasticity (figure 5.2c). We see this mechanical feature occur when we stretch the hamstrings. After a stretch, there is an increase in hamstring length, but if we examine the hamstring a little later, some of the length that was originally gained is maintained because of the viscous component, but some is lost because of the elastic component.

Plasticity

Plasticity is the ability of a substance to undergo a permanent change in size or shape after a deforming force is applied. Viscosity and plasticity create similar effects in human tissue. An example of plasticity is pulling a ball of putty; the putty changes in length and does not return to its former condition when you release your force. Plasticity is represented by a block as seen in figure 5.2d. If the force applied to the block is greater than the structure is able to withstand, the structure will lengthen; if the applied force is less than the structure's resistance to change, no lengthening will take place. So it is with plasticity of collagen: Change in length occurs when the applied force is greater than the force holding collagen fibers attached to one another. Figure 5.2e diagrams the combinations of plastic and viscoelastic elements working against a resistance force, but it fails to identify how tissues with these characteristics resist deformation forces applied to them. Figure 5.3, on the other hand, is a more practical representation of biological tissue, which has both of these plastic and viscoelastic components. When a load is applied to the structure in this model (figure 5.3b), the tissue responds with its viscous and elastic elements first, followed by plastic deformation when the viscoelastic components are used up. When the load is released (figure 5.3c), there is some change in the

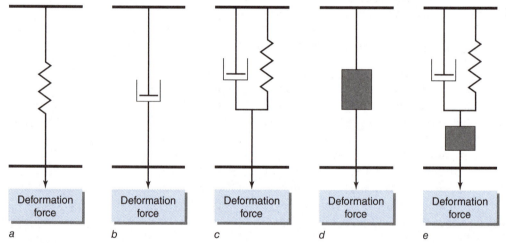

▶ **Figure 5.2** Models of tissue resistance against forces of deformation: *(a)* elasticity, *(b)* viscosity, *(c)* viscoelasticity, *(d)* plasticity, *(e)* viscoelasticity with plastic components.

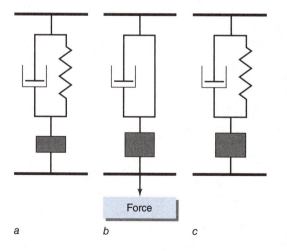

▶ **Figure 5.3** An illustration of the integration of plastic and viscoelastic qualities of tissue resistance working against a force to increase the tissue's length. *(a)* tissue without a force resisting its length; *(b)* tissue unable to withstand a force with plastic tissue changes occurring after viscoelastic tissue has been stretched; *(c)* plastic changes remain after the stretch is released and viscoelastic qualities are returned.

structure's length because of the plastic deformation, but there is some return toward normal length as well because of the elastic component of the tissue.

Physical Properties of Connective Tissue

The physical behaviors of connective tissue include force relaxation and creep. They are both time-dependent responses that rely on the duration of the outside force and the rate at which it is applied. **Force deformation** is the amount of force that is applied to maintain a change of length or other deformation of tissue. It results in a relaxation of the tissue. If the force is applied too quickly and viscoelastic and plastic changes occur that are faster or greater than the tissue can tolerate, an injury can result.

Creep

Creep is the elongation of tissue when a load, usually of low-level, is applied over an extended time to cause plastic deformation. The result is a permanent change in the tissue's length. Creep is time dependent, so a load that is applied for a longer time is more effective in causing a change in tissue length than a load that is applied and released quickly. Increasing the tissue's temperature increases the rate of creep. In functional terms, applying heat to a muscle before and while stretching it permits a better stretch.

If a load is applied in the elastic range, the structure gradually returns to normal length once the load is released. This does not cause a permanent change in tissue length.

A structure's length can also be affected by structural fatigue. Fatigue of a structure occurs when it is loaded repetitively below the failure point until the cumulative stress results in failure; the greater the load, the fewer the repetitions necessary for failure to occur. The point at which structural fatigue causes tissue failure is referred to as **fatigue failure** or **endurance limit.** When structural fatigue occurs in bones it is called a stress fracture; when it occurs in tendons, as an overuse injury, it is called tendinopathy.

Stress-Strain

As was discussed in chapter 3, the load required to change the length of connective tissue is directly related to the tissue's strength, and the tissue's strength is directly related to its ability to resist a load. This relationship is defined by **Hooke's law,** which states that the strain (deformation) of an object is directly related to the object's ability to resist the stress (load), and is illustrated by the stress-strain curve. **Stress** is a force that changes the form or shape of a body. Connective tissue is subject to three types of stress: tension stress (stretching force), compression stress (from muscle contractions and weight bearing on joints), and shear force (force applied parallel to the cross section of the tissue).

Strain is the amount of deformation that occurs when a stress is applied. All structures have a stress-strain curve that represents their own specific ability to resist deforming forces. Although various body tissues' stress-strain curves may differ in timing and magnitude, they share the same general characteristics. The specific reactions of a tissue to a load are illustrated in figure 5.4.

The initial portion of the stress-strain curve is the toe region. In connective tissue, the collagen fibers have a wavy crimp arrangement at rest. The toe region accounts for 1.5% to 4% of the total collagen fiber lengthening that is possible (Butler, Grood, Noyes, & Zernicke, 1978). As a force is applied, the fibers stretch into the elastic range. As the slack in the collagen is taken up, it loses its wavy appearance. At a macroscopic level, no resistance is felt until the tissue is brought to the end of the elastic limit. In the elastic range, a collagen fiber elongates 2% to 5% of its total possible elongation (Butler et al., 1978). The tissue's full normal range

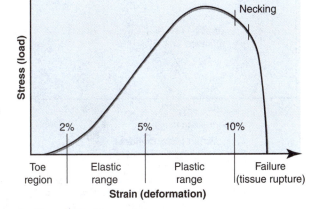

▶ **Figure 5.4** Stress-strain curve.

of motion is in the elastic range. If the force is released in this range, the tissue will return to its pre-stretch length.

At the yield strength point, the stress loads the tissue beyond its elastic range and into its plastic range. Tissue loaded into this range undergoes permanent elongation. This is the result of the failure of a few of the collagen fibers to withstand the stress, creating a disruption of some cross-links. Collagen fibers fail through a number of mechanisms, including a failure of the force-relaxation response when a load is applied too quickly for the collagen's viscoelastic and plastic adaptations to occur. Fibers also tear if the creep response causes too much deformation too quickly. This deformation can occur either in one episode or from accumulated stress from a number of lesser loads. This failure of isolated collagen fibers occurs unpredictably and results in an increase in range of motion.

Two factors beyond the plastic range should be mentioned. **Ultimate strength** is the greatest load that a tissue can tolerate. After this point, the fiber length changes without application of any additional load. The point of ultimate strength is not usually a goal in stretching. There may be a necking region prior to failure of the tissue, where the tissue's strength noticeably decreases so that less stress is needed to cause a change in the tissue's length. When this occurs, tissue failure or rupture is often imminent if the stress application continues.

Fatigue failure is the point at which the tissue is unable to tolerate continued stress and then ruptures. In collagen, this occurs when the fiber is stretched to 6% to 10% beyond its resting length (Butler et al., 1978; Smith, Weiss, & Lehmkuh, 1996).

The general shape of the stress-strain curve appears in figure 5.4, but the specific shape of the curve varies from one structure to another. Some additional factors influence the failure point of the whole structure rather than just the connective tissue. Tissue width is one of these factors. A structure's larger cross-sectional size indicates more fibers, so more stress is required to produce failure of the structure. The tissue's slack length is another factor. Longer tissues can withstand greater forces because they have more slack. For example, if two pieces of rope have the same number of fibers but one is twice as long as the other, the longer rope can tolerate greater deformation before breaking. The microstructure of the tissue and the orientation of the structure to the forces applied also influence the ability of the ligament or tendon to withstand deforming loads.

Given these physical and mechanical properties of connective tissue, some methods of stretching can be more effective than others for increasing range of motion. Using the principle of creep, a low load applied over time can effectively remodel collagen bonds to increase motion. Stretches that take advantage of creep are more effective in remodeling collagen and maintaining range of motion gains than other stretch methods. This type of stretch is a prolonged stretch and is discussed later in this chapter.

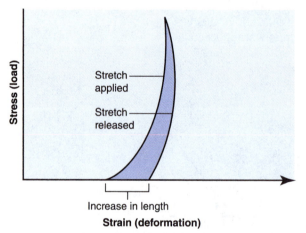

▶ **Figure 5.5** Hysteresis.

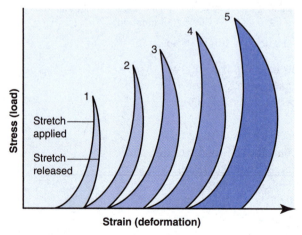

▶ **Figure 5.6** Deformation with hysteresis in repetitive stretching.

Hysteresis

Repetitive stretching with submaximal loads can also be effective in increasing range of motion. Energy in the form of heat releases when stress is applied to tissue. As local tissue is heated with repetitive stretches, the tissue is more easily stretched. When tissue is unable to keep pace with the forces, with each successive load application, it elongates more. This response is **hysteresis.** When a stress is released, the tissue returns to its normal length at a different rate from that of stretching it, as seen in figure 5.5.

As the tissue changes length and is heated with repeated stretches, higher-level loads are tolerated in subsequent repetitions, as seen in figure 5.6. In other words, the tissue's failure load increases, so a greater force can be applied to produce additional tissue deformation (lengthening). This principle is used when a **proprioceptive neuromuscular facilitation (PNF)** stretch is applied, released, and then reapplied to a patient's hamstrings; in the second stretch, the patient's hamstring is stretched farther and the patient can tolerate a slightly greater stretch force.

Rehabilitation and Utilizing These Physical Properties of Connective Tissue

So, now that we understand all of these physical properties of connective tissue, why is it important to us in rehabilitation? There are two good reasons why this information is important. Before we discuss these reasons, recall that tissue healing occurs over three phases. During the first phase, there is no collagen formation, but it starts to appear during the proliferation phase. In the first phase, injured tissue is at its weakest, relying only on the fibrin plug for tensile strength. As collagen forms, tensile strength increases, until in the third phase of healing, the remodeling phase, we see a conversion of Type III collagen to the stronger Type I collagen.

Here are the important rehabilitation points relative to the physical properties of connective tissue we have just identified. First, tissue does not have the strength to withstand stresses applied to it during the initial phase of healing. If we apply stresses during this time, we may further damage tissue. Second, once healing has approached the proliferation phase, we should begin mild mobilization of tissue since it is during this time that collagen is being laid down in a disorganized fashion but is pliable enough to be influenced by motion. As collagen becomes more mature in the later healing, it becomes less influenced by our attempts to increase motion. This resistance to change occurs as the collagen becomes more resilient to applied stresses and the adhesions that have formed between the newer fibers and the surrounding tissues become more permanent. The best time to influence collagen arrangement is during proliferation and in early remodeling. Figure 5.7 demonstrates the relationship between healing, the degree of risk to tissue when a force is applied to it, and the ability to influence and change collagen arrangement throughout the healing process.

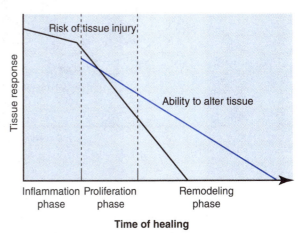

▶ **Figure 5.7** Relationship between danger of tissue mobilization and time to influence collagen change after injury occurs.

A tissue's mechanical properties, such as plasticity, elasticity, and viscoelasticity, affect its response to force and thus to stretching.

NEUROMUSCULAR INFLUENCES ON RANGE OF MOTION

In addition to the physical and mechanical properties of connective tissue, neurological factors influence the effectiveness of stretching techniques in increasing range of motion. Neurological components that affect a muscle's ability to respond to a stretch force include the muscle spindle and the Golgi tendon organ (GTO). The muscle spindle is much more complex than the GTO.

Muscle Spindle

There is a variation in the ratio of muscle spindles to muscle fibers in each muscle. The more precise the movement required of a muscle, the lower the ratio of muscle fibers to muscle spindles. A typical muscle fiber is an **extrafusal fiber.** Muscle spindles vary in length and diameter, but all lie between and are parallel to the extrafusal muscle fibers. The muscle fibers containing the muscle spindles are the **intrafusal muscle fibers.**

Entering the intrafusal muscle fiber are three efferent nerve fibers: alpha, beta, and gamma nerves, as noted in figure 5.8. Exiting the intrafusal fibers are the Ia, Ib, and II afferent, or sensory, fibers. The muscle spindle is composed of these nerve fibers, the intrafusal muscle

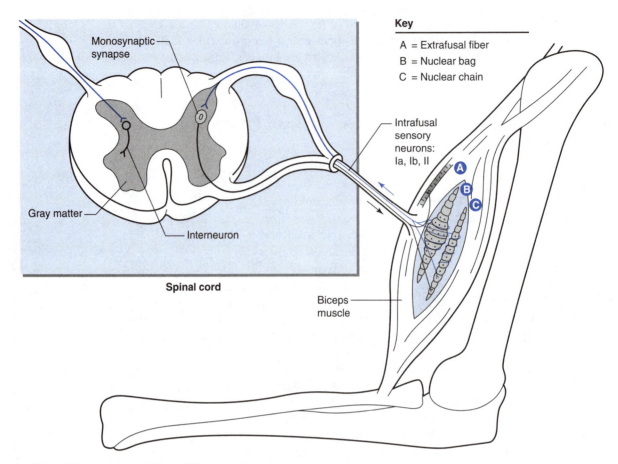

▶ **Figure 5.8** Muscle spindle and Golgi tendon organ.

fibers, and the sac that surrounds these structures. There are two types of intrafusal fibers, and each has a different function within a muscle spindle. One type, the **nuclear bag fiber,** has an enlarged center region with two or three nuclei stacked beside each other. The shorter, thinner fibers are **nuclear chain fibers,** and their nuclei are in single file in the center region. Although both are sensitive to stretch, the nuclear bag fiber has more elasticity and is, therefore, sensitive to the velocity of the stretch.

An afferent Ia nerve fiber wraps around the center region of the intrafusal fibers. This nerve ending is sometimes called a *primary ending* or an *annulospiral ending.* The secondary or II afferent nerve endings are at the ends of the intrafusal muscle fibers, primarily on nuclear chain, and are sometimes called *flower-spray endings* because of their appearance. Because of the structure of Ia nerve fibers, they respond much more quickly to stimulation than the II nerves. The Ia nerve fibers are sensitive to a quick stretch, while both Ia and II nerve fibers respond to a static stretch (Eldred, 1967; Lundberg, Malmgren, & Schomburg, 1977, 1987). Because the intrafusal fiber attaches to the connective tissue surrounding extrafusal muscle fibers, the intrafusal muscle fiber is sensitive to changes in the muscle's length. Both afferent nerve fibers in the muscle spindle transmit signals to the spinal cord regarding changes in the muscle's length and the velocity and duration of a stretch. An efferent response sent to both the intrafusal and extrafusal muscle fibers causes the muscle to react to the stimulation. Gamma efferent fibers transmit to the intrafusal muscle fibers, and alpha efferent fibers transmit to the extrafusal muscle fibers to produce a muscle contraction. Once the muscle contracts and shortens, stress and stimulation of the muscle spindles cease.

In addition to stimulating the muscle in which they lie, a muscle's group I nerve fibers send branches to synergistic muscles and antagonistic muscles. The result is simultaneous stimulation of synergistic muscles and inhibition of antagonistic muscles. Group II nerve fibers also transmit to the synergistic and antagonistic muscles, but they use another neuron link to complete the transmission. The impact of stimulating synergistic muscles will become more apparent in chapter 7 during the discussion of proprioceptive neuromuscular facilitation (PNF).

Muscle spindles and Golgi tendon organs are sensitive to tension in the muscle and its tendons, respectively, and protect these structures from abrupt changes in tension.

Golgi Tendon Organs

Like the muscle spindle, the Golgi tendon organ (GTO) also functions as a protective mechanism. Golgi tendon organs are not as sensitive to stretch as muscle spindles, but they are very sensitive to contraction and tension in a muscle.

Golgi tendon organs, located at the distal and proximal muscle-tendon junctions, are long, delicate, tubular capsules that contain a cluster of Ib nerve fibers. These nerve fibers originate on the tendon's fascicles. The protection performed by the GTO is known as autogenic inhibition. When the GTO is stimulated, its activity causes simultaneous inhibition of the alpha motor neuron of its own muscle and internuncial activation (between afferent and efferent neurons) of the antagonistic muscle.

The result of the combined reactions of the muscle spindle and the GTO is evident in functional activities. If a muscle stretches quickly, the muscle spindle produces a monosynaptic response, which is a rapid reflex motor response resulting from a direct neural connection between a sensory (afferent) and motor (efferent) nerve in the spinal cord without an intermediary neuron. A monosynaptic response is the most rapid response because only two nerves are involved. If a stretch force is applied too quickly, the muscle being stretched reflexively responds secondarily to stimulation of the muscle spindle. This potential problem occurs with ballistic stretching and is discussed later in this chapter. On the other hand, if a stretch occurs slowly, the GTO inhibits muscular contraction. This application may actually provide better relaxation of the muscle to improve the effectiveness of the stretch.

DETERMINING NORMAL RANGE OF MOTION

Before you can determine whether a joint has deficient range of motion, you must first know what is normal motion. Table 5.1 demonstrates that there is some dispute among authors as to what is considered normal, though all are within close range of one another. Differences are probably due to the populations each investigator measured to achieve the data. Measurement results are affected by age and sex of subjects and the positions in which measurements are taken. Regardless of whose data are used, they provide rehabilitation clinicians with a guideline for expectations of normal range of motion.

Each patient's normal range of motion is actually determined by comparison with the contralateral part. It is also based on the demands of the individual's activities. For example, normal range of motion for shoulder external rotation is different for a baseball pitcher and a football lineman.

It is important for you to become familiar with normal ranges of motion. Without this knowledge, it is impossible to determine when a problem exists. If problem areas are not identified, proper therapeutic exercise programs cannot be designed, and the rehabilitation program cannot be successful.

MEASURING RANGE OF MOTION

Now that you have been introduced to the physiological constructs that determine range of motion and to the normal values of range of motion, you are ready to learn how to measure range of motion.

Normal range of motion requirements are different for each joint, each patient, and each sport and position.

TABLE 5.1   Examples of Normal Ranges of Motion in Upper and Lower Extremities According to Various Authors

Joint Motion	Hoppenfeld (Hoppenfeld, 1976)	Daniels & Worthingham (Daniels & Worthingham, 1986)	A.A.O.S. (AAOS, 1965)	Kendall & McCreary (Kendall, McCreary, & Provance, 1993)	Kapandji (Kapandji, 1982, 1987)	Esch &Lepley (Esch & Lepley, 1974)	Gerhardt & Russe (Gerhardt & Russe, 1975)
Shoulder							
Flexion	180	—	180	180	180	170	170
Extension	45	50	60	45	50	60	50
Abduction	180	—	180	180	180	170	170
Lateral rotation	45	90	90	90	80	90	90
Medial rotation	55	90	70	70	95	80	80
Horizontal abduction	—	—	—	—	—	—	30
Horizontal adduction	—	—	135	—	—	—	135
Elbow							
Flexion	135+	145-160	150	145	145-160	150	150
Forearm							
Supination	90	90	80	90	80	90	90
Pronation	90	90	80	90	85	90	80
Wrist							
Extension	70	70	70	70	85	70	50
Flexion	80	90	80	80	85	90	60
Radial Deviation	20	—	20	20	15	20	20
Ulnar Deviation	30	—	30	35	45	30	30
Thumb, carpometacarpal							
Abduction	70	50	70	80	50	—	—
Flexion	—	—	15	45	—	—	—
Extension	—	—	20	0	—	—	—
Opposition			Tip of thumb to tip of 5th finger (all authors agree)				

Thumb, metacarpophalangeal							
Flexion	50	70	50	60	80	—	—
Thumb, interphalangeal							
Flexion	90	90	80	80	80	—	—
Digits 2-5, metacarpophalangeal							
Flexion	90	90	90	90	—	—	—
Extension	45	30	45	—	—	—	—
Digits 2-5, proximal interphalangeal							
Flexion	100	120	—	—	—	—	—
Digits 2-5, distal interphalangeal							
Flexion	90	80	—	—	—	—	—
Subtalar joint							
Inversion	—	—	35	35	52	30	40
Eversion	—	—	20	20	30	15	20
Ankle, talocrural							
Dorsiflexion	20	—	20	20	20-30	10	20
Plantar flexion	50	45	50	45	50	65	45
Knee							
Flexion	135	140-160	135	140	135	135	130
Hip							
Flexion	120	115-125	120	125	120	130	125
Extension	30	15	30	10	30	45	15
Abduction	45-50	45	45	45	45	45	45
Adduction	20-30	—	30	10	30	15	15
Medial rotation	35	45	45	45	45	33	45
Lateral rotation	45	45	45	45	60	36	45

Equipment

Range of motion is measured with an instrument known as a **goniometer.** It is essentially a protractor with a stationary arm and a movable arm, as shown in figure 5.9. It can measure up to either 180° or 360°. Many goniometric variations have been designed to measure different joints. Other devices have been designed either to measure specific body segments or to make measurement easier. For example, the Leighton flexometer has a weighted, 360° dial with an enclosed needle; it attaches with a strap to the body part that is being measured. An inclinometer is a device similar to a flexometer and is used to measure degrees of rotation on a 360° dial; it is used to measure spine motion. An elgon, or electrogoniometer, was developed by Karpovich et al. (Karpovich, Herden, Asa, & Karpovich, 1959) and uses a potentiometer rather than a protractor. It is used to measure primarily dynamic motion, as it is less accurate with static motion. The number of joints that it can be used to measure is also limited. Another electrogoniometer, the Penny and Giles, is shown in figure 5.10.

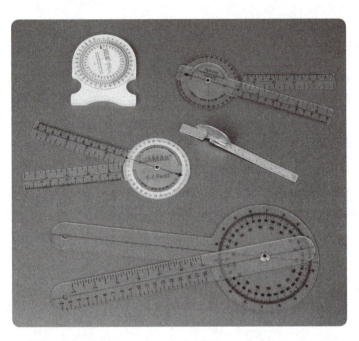

▶ **Figure 5.9** Goniometers come in different sizes to measure various body segments. They are most often 360° or 180°.

Spine motion is difficult to measure with a standard goniometer. Using the Moll and Wright (Moll & Wright, 1971) method (figure 5.11), marks are made at the top and bottom of the lumbar spine. A metal tape measure is used to measure the difference in distance between the two marks in flexion, extension, and normal standing. This measure is relative to the individual being tested and cannot be used to determine an individual's deviation from normal, because standards have not been established and would probably be difficult to determine.

A common method for measuring spine flexion is the fingertip-to-floor method, demonstrated in figure 5.12. The person stands with trunk flexed, and the distance between the finger-

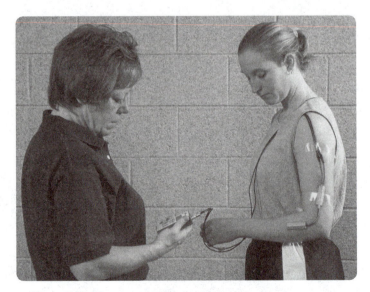

▶ **Figure 5.10** Penny and Giles electrogoniometer.

tips and the floor is measured. Side bending (figure 5.13) also produces a relative measurement, recorded as the distance from the fingertips to either the fibular head or the floor. Although this method may not be as accurate as others and does not isolate the structure being assessed (i.e., the spine), it can be reproduced in the same individual so that changes can be evaluated.

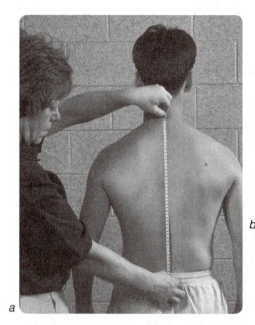

a

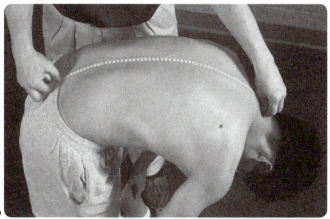

b

▶ **Figure 5.11** Moll and Wright spinal ROM method while spine is *(a)* stretched and *(b)* in flexion.

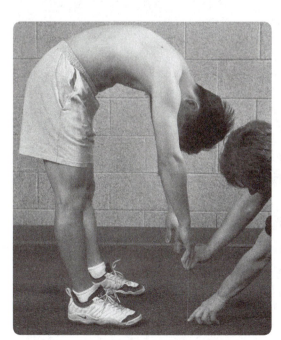

▶ **Figure 5.12** Measuring trunk flexion.

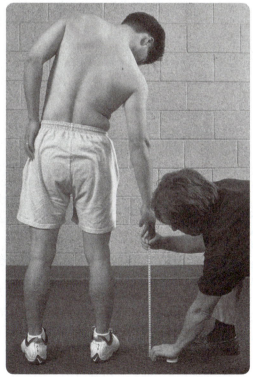

▶ **Figure 5.13** Measuring lateral trunk flexion.

Application

To measure accurately with a goniometer, the most common tool for evaluating range of motion, correct placement of the protractor and arms is very important. The arms of the goniometer are positioned along the length of the two limbs forming the joint. If placed correctly, the pivot point of the protractor is lined up over the axis of motion of the joint. For correct alignment, the limbs being measured should be exposed. With some exceptions, the goniometer is placed along the central lateral aspect of the limb. Figure 5.14 demonstrates measuring techniques for some joints.

Range of motion is measured in either a 180° or 360° system using either a 180° or 360° goniometer. In the 360° system, 0° is overhead and 180° is down, toward the feet. In the 180° system, 0° is at the start of the range in the anatomical position and 180° is at the end. Either

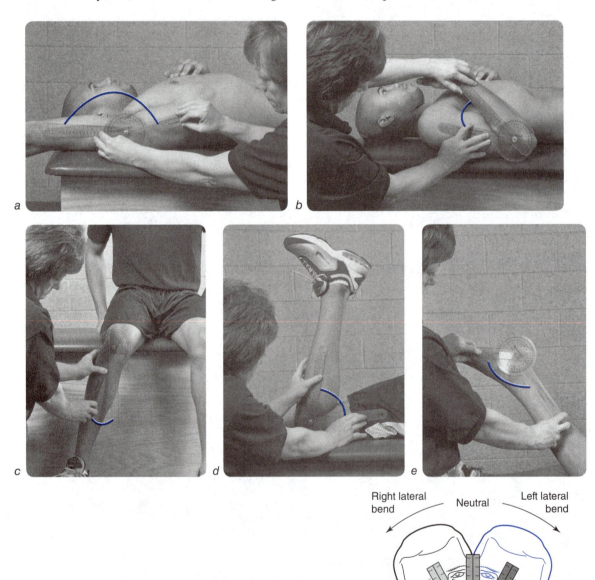

▶ **Figure 5.14** Goniometer placement for measuring *(a)* shoulder flexion, *(b)* elbow flexion, *(c)* hip medial rotation, *(d)* knee flexion, *(e)* ankle plantar flexion, and *(f)* cervical lateral flexion. The center of the goniometer is placed over the joint's center (axis of motion). Alignment of the goniometer's stationary and movable arms and fulcrum must be accurate for reliable measurements.

system is valid and may be used to measure range of motion. The most commonly used system for musculoskeletal injuries is the 180° system. There is some variation in both systems for measurements of inversion and eversion, forearm supination and pronation, and trunk lateral flexion. For these motions, 0° is the mid-position for each plane of motion.

Accuracy

A rehabilitation clinician's ability to accurately measure range of motion depends on his or her training, experience, and attention to detail. Even an experienced clinician with good equipment can expect accuracy only within 3° to 5° of true values (Cook, Baker, Cham, Hale, and Redfern, 2007). It is, therefore, vital to be as consistent as possible. Careful attention to the placement of the goniometer arms and making sure that the axis of the goniometer coincides with the joint's axis of rotation are very important to assure accurate measurements. Check the goniometer placement, adjust the patient's position if necessary to achieve correct body segment alignment, and then check again before recording your final measurement to help ensure accuracy. Consistent measurements depend on your attention to these details. If your technique is good, your measurements should be reliable. If your technique is inconsistent, your results will be unreliable and of no use to you, the patient, or anyone else. If your technique is accurate, other clinicians (assuming their technique is also good) should obtain measurements that are the same or within 5° of yours.

Interpretation of range-of-motion measurements can be clouded by a variety of conditions. The position in which the patient is placed, whether active or passive motion is measured, pain occurring with motion, spasm, voluntary resistance to movement, wounds, and the patient's willingness to move the part can all affect measurements. You should note such conditions in your record.

Recording Range of Motion

Range of motion is documented by the joint and motion measured, and then by the type of motion measured: active range of motion (AROM) or passive range of motion (PROM). Degrees are most often recorded based on a 180° scale, so if a 360° is used, it should be indicated as such. 0° is usually the position of neutral as in pronation-supination and plantar flexion-dorsiflexion or in full extension such as knee and elbow extension. If a patient is unable to achieve full extension (0°), the point at which the patient is able to move is recorded along with the end motion in the opposite direction. For example, if a patient was lacking 15° from full extension and was able to flex the knee to 100°, the record would show: knee extension-flexion = 15° to 100°. Sometimes a clinician will record the amount of degrees lacking from extension as a minus (–) number, such as –15°. This can be misleading, however, in that it may also be interpreted as 15° of hyperextension.

TERMINOLOGY IN GONIOMETRY

To ensure accurate interpretation of your results by those to whom your report is sent or by those who refer to your notes, you and your readers should use common terminology. The following section gives common terms used in goniometry.

Body motion is divided into three planes: sagittal, frontal or coronal, and horizontal or transverse. Their frame of reference is the anatomical position, which is the body standing erect with the hips and knees in extension, the feet facing forward, the elbows and wrists in extension, the hands at the sides, and the palms facing forward.

Motions of flexion and extension occur in the sagittal plane. Motions in the frontal plane include abduction and adduction at the shoulders and hips. Transverse plane movement includes hip and shoulder rotation, pronation, and supination in the anatomical position. Although discussions of range of motion refer to these planes, functional activities usually involve oblique planes of motion that include all three conventional planes.

Range of motion is typically measured with a goniometer. Good technique is essential for measuring accurately and consistently.

Standard terminology and frames of reference to describe bodily movements and range of motion make your records usable by others.

■ Goniometric Terms

- Sagittal plane: The anterior-posterior vertical plane through which the longitudinal axis passes and that divides the body into right and left halves.

- Frontal (coronal) plane: Any vertical plane that divides the body into front and back parts.

- Transverse (horizontal) plane: A plane that divides a section of the body into upper and lower parts. It is parallel to the horizon.

- Flexion: Moving a joint so that the two body segments approach each other and decrease the joint angle.

- Extension: Moving a joint so that the two body segments move apart and increase the joint angle.

- Abduction: Lateral movement of a limb or segment away from the midline of the body or part.

- Adduction: Lateral movement of a limb or segment toward the midline of the body or part.

- Medial rotation: Rotation of a joint around its axis in a transverse plane toward the middle of the body. Also called *internal rotation*.

- Lateral rotation: Rotation of a joint around its axis in a transverse plane away from the midline of the body. Also called *external rotation*.

- Supination: Movement of the palm forward or upward into the anatomical position. Also, the multiplanar rotation of the subtalar and transverse talar joints that includes plantar flexion, adduction, and inversion.

- Pronation: Movement of the palm backward or downward so that the palm faces in a posterior direction, opposite the anatomical position. Also, a multiplanar rotation of the subtalar and transverse talar joints that is the combination of dorsiflexion, abduction, and eversion.

- Inversion: Inward turning motion of the foot that causes the bottom of the foot to face medially.

- Eversion: Outward turning motion of the foot that causes the bottom of the foot to face laterally.

- Dorsiflexion: A flexion of the ankle that causes the dorsum (top) of the foot to move toward the lower leg so that the angle of the ankle decreases.

- Plantar flexion: An extension of the ankle that causes the dorsum (top) of the foot to move away from the lower leg so that the angle of the ankle increases.

- Radial deviation: A movement of the wrist toward the thumb side of the forearm. Also called radial flexion.

- Ulnar deviation: A movement of the wrist toward the little-finger side of the forearm. Also called ulnar flexion.

- Opposition: A diagonal and rotational movement of the thumb across the palm of the hand to permit it to make contact with one of the other four fingers.

- Depression: A downward movement of the scapula.

- Elevation: An upward movement of the scapula.

- Protraction: A forward movement of the scapula on the thorax. Also called *scapular abduction*.

- Retraction: A backward movement of the scapula on the thorax. Also called *scapular adduction*.

- Upward rotation: A movement of the scapula that causes the glenoid to face forward and upward. The inferior angle of the scapula moves laterally away from the spine, and the scapula slides forward on the thorax.

- Downward rotation: A movement of the scapula that causes the glenoid to face downward and backward. The inferior angle of the scapula moves medially, and the scapula slides backward on the thorax.

- Horizontal flexion: A motion of the upper extremity in a transverse plane toward the midline of the body. Also called *horizontal adduction*.

- Horizontal extension: A motion of the upper extremity in a transverse plane away from the midline of the body. Also called *horizontal abduction*.

STRETCHING TECHNIQUES

When an individual has an injury that results in deficient range of motion, several techniques may be applied to restore range of motion, depending on your preference and skill, the type of tissue restriction involved, the extent of the injury, and the duration of the loss of motion. Continuous passive motion machines and other mechanical devices are discussed later in this chapter. Joint mobilization and various techniques of soft-tissue mobilization are presented in chapter 6.

Probably one of the most common methods of increasing range of motion is stretching exercises. Many researchers have investigated various methods and techniques in search of the best and most effective way to gain range of motion. Studies performed on normal populations have disputed the advantages of pre- and post-exercise stretching as to whether there is any benefit (W. E. J. Garrett, 1996; Sexton & Chambers, 2006; Shellock & Prentice, 1985) or not (Kovacs, 2006; Thacker, Gilchrist, Stroup, & Kimsey, 2005). Unfortunately, research has not yet provided an answer to the benefits of flexibility exercises in rehabilitation. One of the problems is that most of the research studies investigating stretching have been performed with normal, uninjured subjects or with animals. Some of the investigations are not sound, objective, or reproducible. Studies, thus far, have failed to provide answers regarding the best method of stretching damaged and healing tissue. Therefore, we must rely on our knowledge of injury, healing, and the physiology of connective tissue more than on research evidence to determine the best way to stretch an injured area. The other factor we rely upon to present us with positive benefits of flexibility exercises in rehabilitation is anecdotal information of experienced clinicians; these professionals have consistently indicated positive effects of flexibility exercises following injury. Therefore, although research data is lacking, we can confidently conclude that stretching does improve the status of injured body segments.

Regardless of the type of stretch used, the application of heat before (Swenson, Swärd, & Karlsson, 1996) or during (Shrier & Gossal, 2000) the stretch produces a better result. Heat can be applied either passively or actively. An example of a passive heat application is the application of a hot pack before stretching. A better method is active heat application, in which the patient performs a warm-up activity, such as exercising on a stationary bike, stair climber, or upper-body ergometer, before stretching. A hot pack provides superficial heat, but an active exercise increases the deeper tissues' temperature more effectively and more safely than a passive modality (Saal, 1987).

Active Stretching

Stretching exercises can be divided into active stretching, passive stretching, and a combination of the two. Active stretching includes flexibility exercises performed by the patient without outside assistance from either another person or equipment (figure 5.15). Depending on the duration and repetitions of the active stretch, it affects the elastic range of connective tissue and may have some effect on the plastic range. Conclusive studies on the parameters of stretching on injured patients have yet to be identified (Shrier & Gossal, 2000). Although a stretch duration was not recommended, evidence has demonstrated that second degree hamstring strain injuries achieve quicker and better restoration in range of motion with increased frequency of flexibility exercises than with one stretch (Malliaropoulos, Papalexandris, Papalada, & Papacostas, 2004). Based on the results of this study and four other studies on normal subjects (Bandy, Irion, & Briggler, 1997; W. E. Garrett, Jr. , 1990; McNair, Stanley, & Strauss, 1996), (Taylor, Dalton, Seaber, & Garrett, 1990) along with my clinical observations and experience over the years, I feel the best application of an active stretch is

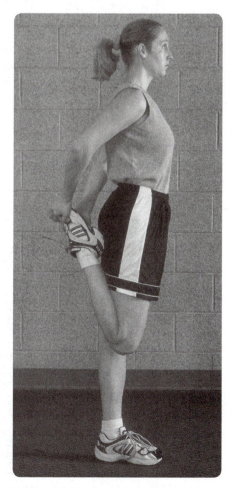

► **Figure 5.15** Active stretch.

one that is performed for a 15 to 30 s hold for four to five repetitions and repeated at least three times a day. For patients who have significant loss of motion, repeated stretch sessions throughout the day may be beneficial; although there have not been any studies other than the one by Malliaropoulos et al. (Malliaropoulos et al., 2004) demonstrating that repeated sessions are beneficial, intuitive reason indicates the possibility that they may be, especially during scar-tissue formation and wound contraction. If the individual is participating in sport activities, the stretches should also be performed after the activity.

Because of the phenomenon of antagonist inhibition, if the individual contracts the opposing muscle, relaxation of the stretched muscle increases. This contraction of the antagonist results in a more effective stretch of the agonist. For example, a better stretch occurs when the patient actively contracts the quadriceps as the hamstrings are stretched.

It is believed that a strong relationship between muscles and their antagonists affects muscle flexibility. When a muscle becomes tighter, its antagonist becomes weaker It is believed that an agonist muscle is shortened when its antagonist is weak, presenting an imbalance between the two and resulting in a loss of motion (Sahrmann, 2002). If the antagonist is facilitated, the agonist becomes inhibited, which allows a restoration of normal flexibility. You can perform this quick experiment on yourself to see the impact of agonist inhibition on increasing muscle flexibility. Do not perform this activity if you have a lumbar disc injury. In a standing position, first evaluate your hamstring flexibility by bending over to touch your toes while you keep your knees straight. Return to an upright position. Now, bend over at the waist to touch your toes but with your knees bent to prevent a stretch of the hamstrings. While in this flexed position and with your hands on your toes, straighten your knees by tightening the quadriceps. Repeat this activity three or four times. Now return to a full standing position, and reevaluate your hamstring flexibility by attempting to touch your toes, keeping your knees straight. You should be able to reach farther than on your initial attempt. This improvement occurs because the contraction of the quadriceps causes a reciprocal inhibition of the hamstrings, so the hamstrings are able to relax and allow elongation to occur.

The effects of this reciprocal inhibition demonstrate the need to accompany any stretching technique with strengthening exercises to maintain newly acquired muscle length. Strengthening exercises also assist in restoring balance between agonist and antagonist muscle groups. This topic is discussed in later chapters.

Passive Stretching

Passive stretching includes a variety of methods, including short-term and long-term stretches. Passive stretching involves the use of equipment or another person, and the patient does not assist in the stretch activity (figure 5.16). A typical example of a short-term passive stretch is when the clinician moves the patient's injured part through its range of motion and applies a stretch at the end of the motion.

When applying a stretch, the part is be moved to the end of its motion (Flowers & LaStayo, 1994). The proximal segment of the joint being stretched is stabilized to prevent its movement while a firm pressure is applied to the joint's distal segment. A steady pressure is applied until the soft tissue's slack is taken up and the muscle is taut. The joint is then moved slightly beyond this point. The patient should feel a stretch or tension, but not pain. If a two-joint muscle is stretched, first one joint is

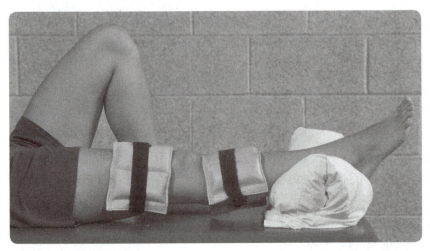

▶ **Figure 5.16** The patient does not assist in passive stretch. The stretch here is provided by gravity and further assisted with weights on the leg.

positioned in the muscle's lengthened position, then the second joint, until maximum muscle length is achieved. The stretch is repeated four to six times.

The most effective stretches involve the steady application of force over a length of time. This prolonged passive stretch produces a better plastic deformation of connective tissue, primarily because of the length of time it is applied. Although research has yet to define how long a prolonged stretch should be applied, Kottke, Pauley, and Ptak (F.J. Kottke et al., 1966) suggested 20 min in clinical applications and Ono et al. (Ono et al., 2007) suggested 30 minutes. Although prolonged stretching is the most effective of all stretching techniques, it seems to be the least investigated (Light, Nuzik, Personius, & Barstrom, 1984).

A prolonged stretch is applied with a reduced load. Two articles by Warren, Lehmann, and Koblanski (Warren, Lehmann, & Koblanski, 1971, 1976) reported that the amount of time required for a prolonged stretch to change connective tissue length is inversely proportional to the amount of force used. As with short-term stretches, research is lacking on prolonged-stretching effectiveness on scar tissue. One study investigated normal subjects with a prolonged stretch of 3 min but used full body weight as the force; they found significant linear increases in motion because of the great amount of force applied over a 3 min period (Pratt & Bohannon, 2003). Most of the time, however, prolonged stretches applied to healing tissue are not that intense, so to influence changes in the scar tissue's plastic range, stretch time is increased. A prolonged stretch is effective in increasing motion because of its impact on tissue's stress-strain curves and the creep phenomenon, discussed earlier in this chapter.

When using prolonged stretches, the segment must be stabilized to permit the load to stretch the correct tissue. This stabilization can be provided either by the weight of the body or segment or by a mechanical device such as a weight or strap. The stretch is applied slowly and steadily to the point of tightness. The segment is then secured in this position and held for the desired amount of time. If a two-joint muscle is stretched, the secondary joint should be placed in a position that elongates the muscle. For example, if the hamstring is stretched with the knee in extension, the patient should sit to elongate the hamstrings at the proximal end where it crosses the hip joint. The patient commonly does not feel much, if anything, when the stretch is first applied. Within 5 to 10 min, however, the patient will feel the stretch's effect. The minimal prolonged stretch duration is usually 15 to 20 min; if the patient cannot tolerate the stress, the force should be reduced to allow the patient to stretch for the desired time.

The part placed in a prolonged stretch can feel very stiff when the stretch load is removed. The patient should be cautioned about this prior to releasing the stretch. The stretch should be released slowly. As the stretch is released, the patient is advised to simultaneously contract the stretched muscle to reduce the discomfort. Gentle, active range-of-motion activities following the stretch release helps relieve the stiffness.

Proprioceptive Neuromuscular Facilitation

The unique combination of active and passive stretching is sometimes referred to as neuromuscular facilitation or proprioceptive neuromuscular facilitation (PNF). Although PNF is also used as a strengthening technique, it is useful for gaining range of motion. A more extensive discussion of PNF principles is presented in chapter 7. Of the various PNF techniques used to increase motion, the most frequently used are the hold-relax, contract-relax, and slow reversal-hold-relax techniques (figure 5.17).

There are two technique patterns used in PNF: agonistic and antagonistic. The *agonistic muscle pattern* occurs when the muscle is contracting toward its shortened state. The *antagonistic muscle pattern* is diagonally opposite to the agonistic pattern and occurs when the muscle is approaching its lengthened state.

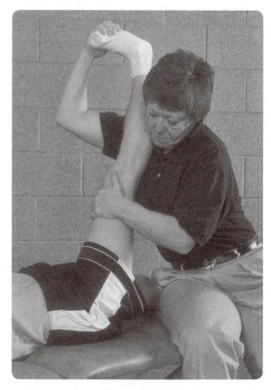

▶ **Figure 5.17** PNF stretch.

In each of the descriptions that follow, it may be easiest to visualize an example. Think of a hamstring muscle that is tight and you want to improve its flexibility. In this example, the hamstrings group is the antagonist and the quadriceps group is the agonist.

The *hold-relax* technique is a maximal isometric contraction of the antagonist (hamstrings) in all three planes of movement at the end range of the agonist (quadriceps) that is followed by a relaxation of the hamstrings. After the hamstrings relax, the agonist (quadriceps) contracts to actively increase motion of the antagonist (hamstrings). Rotation must be a component motion of the movement pattern.

This technique is used to relax muscle spasm. For example, if a biceps is in spasm and limits elbow extension, the hold-relax technique can be used to facilitate biceps relaxation. To begin the technique, the elbow is extended to its end range by the triceps, and then the biceps performs an isometric contraction with a simultaneous maximum effort by the biceps against a pronation and flexion resistance for 5 to 10 s. The patient then relaxes the biceps and actively extends the elbow using the triceps without any resistance. This process is repeated four to five times or until the desired results are achieved. The isometric contraction of a muscle facilitates a better relaxation of that muscle.

The *contract-relax* technique is used with patients who have limited range of motion. We will use a tight hamstring as an example. With the patient's knee and hip placed at the end-range (knee extension and hip flexion) in the agonistic (quadriceps and iliopsoas) pattern, the clinician provides isotonic resistance against the antagonist muscles (hamstrings) to allow diagonal and rotational motion to the end range (knee flexion and hip extension with hip rotation). When the patient relaxes the muscle, the clinician moves the part passively into the agonistic muscle pattern to stretch the antagonist (hamstrings). The process is repeated several times.

The *slow reversal-hold-relax* technique uses concentric contraction of the agonist (quadriceps and iliopsoas) into the range-limited motion of the antagonist (hamstrings) followed by an isometric contraction of the antagonist (hamstrings). Relaxation of the antagonist (hamstrings) then concentric movement by the agonist (quadriceps) follow the isometric hold. The clinician also provides maximal isometric resistance against the rotational component.

All the PNF stretch techniques are useful when the primary resisting factor is a shortening of the antagonist caused by muscle spasm or loss of motion. Table 5.2 summarizes the three PNF techniques for improving flexibility.

Various investigations have compared the different types of short-term passive, active, and combination stretching procedures. Many investigators conclude that PNF stretches are more effective than other active or short-term passive stretches (Prentice, 1983; Sady, Wortman, & Blanke, 1982; Sharman, Cresswell, & Riek, 2006). Others conclude that PNF techniques are either no different or less advantageous than other stretching techniques (Bradley, Olsen, & Portas, 2007; Church, Wiggins, Moode, & Crist, 2001; Davis, Ashby, McCale, McQuain, & Wine, 2005; Sullivan, Dejulia, & Worrell, 1992). The body parts stretched, duration of stretches, frequency, and duration of studies vary widely among the investigations. With so

TABLE 5.2 PNF Techniques to Gain Flexibility

Technique	Muscle activity
Hold-relax	Muscle is brought to end-motion, isometric of tight muscle, relax, stretch via contraction of opposing muscle.
Contract-relax	Muscle is brought to end-motion, isotonic contraction of tight muscle, relax, passive movement to end-range.
Slow reversal-hold-relax	Opposing muscle contracts to bring tight muscle to end-range, isometric contraction of tight muscle, relax, stretch via unopposed contraction of opposing muscle.

many variables, it is not surprising that little or no consensus has been reached on specific methods, duration, and frequency of these stretching techniques.

Ballistic Stretching

Ballistic stretching is the use of quick, bouncing movement through alternating contraction and relaxation of a muscle to stretch its antagonist. This type of stretch is not used in rehabilitation because of the damage it can cause to already injured tissue. The physiological characteristics of connective tissue and muscle discussed previously in this chapter provide an understanding of the dangers of ballistic stretching in therapeutic exercise:

- Ballistic stretching stimulates both the muscle spindles and GTOs. These structures normally oppose stretch reactions to protect the muscle from injury, but with uncoordinated firing, their protective mechanisms are ineffective.
- Control of the stretch is limited by the velocity of the force applied in the stretch. Plastic deformation is related to the magnitude and duration of the force. A greater force over a shorter period of time is likely to cause failure of the structure, risking injury to the connective tissue. Injury will result in more scar tissue formation that ultimately decreases flexibility.

Ballistic stretching is used most often by normal, healthy people in sport activities and serves well to increase dynamic flexibility. In unhealthy tissue, however, the risk of causing further injury is too great for ballistic stretching to be a safe technique in rehabilitation.

Assistive Devices

In addition to equipment such as weights, pulleys, and straps for providing prolonged stretch to areas of limited motion, other devices are also used to facilitate range of motion gains.

Continuous Passive Motion Machines

A continuous passive motion (CPM) machine is sometimes used following surgery to restore range of motion. A CPM can help counteract the deleterious effects of immobilization and reduce pain and edema after surgery. Because range of motion is more quickly restored with the use of a CPM (Brander & Stulberg, 2006; O'Driscoll & Nicholas, 2000), the patient is able to begin active exercises sooner to ultimately shorten the recovery and rehabilitation time following surgery (Brander & Stulberg, 2006). There is also some evidence to demonstrate that CPMs improve joint proprioception following ACL reconstruction surgery (Friemert, Bach, Schwarz, Gerngross, & Schmidt, 2006). CPMs are designed for a variety of joints, including the knee, ankle, elbow, wrist, and shoulder. An example of a knee CPM is seen in figure 5.18.

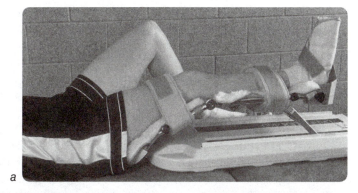

a

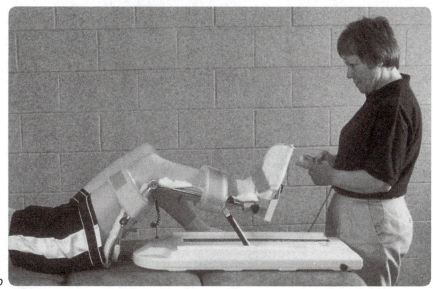

b

▶ **Figure 5.18** CPM machine: range-of-motion limits for extension *(a)* and flexion *(b)* can be set at desired levels as necessary.

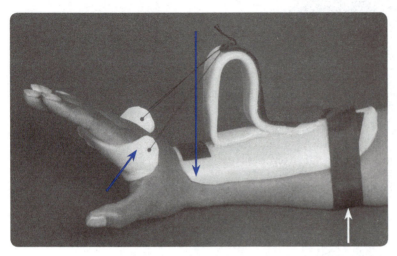

▶ **Figure 5.19** Splint to increase range of motion. Notice the 3-point system used to provide the stretch force.

Splints

Specifically designed splints also assist in prolonged stretching of restricted joints. After injury, the collagen and connective tissue that result in scarring become progressively more difficult to stretch as the cross-links become more numerous and the collagen more mature with time (figure 5.7). Prolonged stretching for more than 20 min is often needed with very mature or restricted scar tissue. In such instances, various splints that apply a very low-level, continual stretch force for several hours are often very beneficial. They commonly use a three-point lever-and-spring system to provide a low-level, continual load (figure 5.19). These devices are designed to stretch connective tissue surrounding joints but do not change muscle length. The magnitude of the load and the angle at which the stretch is applied is adjusted to meet the individual patient's needs. A splint is worn for several hours at a time, most often overnight, to cause effective plastic deformation of connective tissue.

Indications, Contraindications, and Precautions

Before applying a stretch to increase range of motion, you must first know when stretching is indicated, when you should not use stretching, and precautions for its use.

Indications

As part of the patient evaluation performed prior to rehabilitation treatment, the clinician determines deficiencies in range of motion, identifies the structures causing the loss of motion, and assesses the status of the tissue. Is the loss a result of recent scar tissue formation, adherent and mature scar tissue, spasm, edema, postural deformities, or weakness of opposing muscles? If ligaments, capsules, muscles, fascia, skin, or other soft tissues are shortened because of scar tissue adhesions, stretching exercises are indicated. Stretching is also indicated in the presence of contractures and structural deformities from injury or posture changes over time. If weak muscles are overpowered by opposing tight structures, flexibility of the restricted structures must accompany strengthening of the weak muscles for the treatment program to be optimally effective. If muscle spasm or edema contributes to reduced motion, the rehabilitation program must include modalities and activities to address these problems first.

Contraindications

Although stretching is usually safe, it is contraindicated when certain conditions are present. These conditions include recent fractures when immobilization is necessary for healing and movement is detrimental to it, a bony block that restricts motion, infection in a joint, acute inflammation in a joint, extreme or sharp pain with motion, and when tightness of soft tissue actually contributes to an area's stability.

Precautions

Precautions are taken to ensure the most effective application of the stretch and to prevent harm from a stretch. Before applying any treatment, you should always explain to the patient what you will do and the sensations and outcome to expect. A patient who is apprehensive and unable to relax will not receive an effective stretch treatment.

The force applied in a stretch should cause sensations of tension, perhaps unpleasant, in the segment stretched but there should be no residual pain following release of the stretch. This is true for both active and passive stretching. It is important that the patient understands that during active stretches the sensation of a stretch is necessary, but it should be without pain. Residual pain beyond a brief transitory tenderness, especially accompanied with new edema within a 24-hour post-treatment period, is an indication that the stretch has been too aggressive. In this instance, the stretch force is reduced in the subsequent treatment to still induce the proper plastic changes but without these undesirable post-stretch symptoms.

The release of a stretch force is as important as its application. Both should be done slowly. A quick application or release of a stretch, especially release of a prolonged stretch, can be very uncomfortable. Begin applying the stretch slowly, and do not apply more force until you know the patient can tolerate it. Some pain and stiffness are normal after release of a stretch, especially a prolonged stretch. As mentioned earlier, these symptoms can be relieved by contracting the agonist as the stretch is released and following the stretch with gentle, active range of motion exercises.

If a stretch is painful, gentle traction applied to the joint during the stretch may relieve the pain. If this is not successful in relieving the pain, reduce the stretch load. A stretch should not be painful.

A stretch force affects all soft tissue in the area where the force is applied. Knowing exactly which tissues are affected has thus far eluded researchers. Just like tissues affected by scar tissue, the structures affected by a stretch may include joint capsule, ligaments, surrounding tendons, muscles, fascia, nerves, skin, and subcutaneous tissue.

Vigorous stretching of areas that have been immobilized for a while should be used with extreme caution and even avoided in the early stretching stages. Recall that immobilization reduces the tensile strength of many connective tissue structures, including tendons and ligaments, so caution must be used.

Stabilization of the area is necessary to properly apply the stretch force in the correct direction and to the correct structures. During both active and passive stretches, the part is positioned so the stretch force affects only the targeted structures. For example, if a patient is stretching the left hamstrings in a standing position with the left foot on a chair or bench, the foot should be facing the ceiling, not rotated; in the rotated position, the hip adductors, not the hamstrings, are stretched.

When stretching a muscle that traverses two or more joints, the other joints must be positioned so that the muscle is elongated throughout its entire length. In other words, every joint a muscle crosses is placed such that the muscle is stretched at that joint for an appropriate elongation of the muscle to occur. For example, to stretch the quadriceps, place the hip in extension with the knee in flexion so the rectus femoris portion of the quadriceps is fully lengthened.

In active and passive stretches, the muscle stretched should be relaxed for optimal results. If a muscle tenses, it will resist the stretch and make it ineffective. For this reason, careful positioning and understanding of positional biomechanics is important. For example, standing bent over from the waist to touch the floor with the fingertips is an ineffective position to stretch the hamstrings, since the hamstrings must tense to hold the position and cannot relax. Likewise, if a passive stretch is too forceful and causes a reflex or voluntary muscle contraction, the stretch will be both ineffective and painful to the patient.

Once full range of motion is achieved following an injury, maintenance flexibility exercises are used. With the ongoing healing process and contraction of connective tissue as scar tissue matures, loss of motion will also continue. This is why a patient can achieve full range of motion in one rehabilitation session and return for treatment the next day with less than full range of motion. Until the healing process is complete, maintaining full range of motion, once it is achieved, is important.

Stretching can be active, passive, or a combination of the two. Knowing the indications, contraindications, and proper precautions for stretching is necessary to safely and effectively use any stretching technique.

The choice of stretching technique depends on the tissues involved, the stage of healing, the patient's motivation, the time and facilities available, and other factors of the injury.

EXERCISE PROGRESSION

Common questions regarding therapeutic flexibility exercises include concerns such as, when is the best time to use stretching exercises, and which stretching exercises should I use? The information presented in this chapter and in chapter 2 provides the answers.

If motion is permitted immediately following an injury, active range of motion may be all that is necessary to regain motion. Active motion is the first choice because it does not require outside assistance, so the patient can perform it frequently and independently throughout the day when it is convenient. Frequent flexibility exercise sessions throughout the day can be an effective way to increase flexibility.

Following major surgery, the physician may prescribe the use of a CPM machine for an involved area that requires close monitoring. A CPM machine does not harm the surgical site yet provides immediate postoperative motion, reduces pain, and lessens edema that can otherwise limit post-operative motion. The use of CPM machines is not as prevalent today as it was when they were first introduced; surgeons have discovered that active motion within safe bounds can also produce similar beneficial results.

Other techniques may be needed after immobilization. To some extent, the method of stretching depends on the length of immobilization, the tissues affected by the immobilization, the patient's motivation, and the rehabilitation clinician's facilities and availability. Recall that collagen appears in a wound as early as three to five days following an injury. By the seventh day, collagen may abound, and the forming scar tissue begins to contract. As has been mentioned, this contraction continues into the final phase of healing and requires stretching exercises to maintain range of motion even after full motion has been achieved.

If scar tissue is relatively new and still pliable, active and short-term passive stretches are effective to increase motion. PNF stretching techniques can also be utilized with success, assuming the patient has the muscle control for these types of exercises. When scar tissue is more mature and well into the remodeling phase, however, prolonged-stretching techniques should be the main part of the stretching program. Short-term and active stretches accompanying the prolonged stretches help to reinforce the effects.

In particularly difficult situations where scar tissue is more than three to four months old and range of motion is still deficient, prolonged-stretch machines are more beneficial to achieve maximal range of motion. The degree of plastic deformation of connective tissue required at this point to effect change in range of motion requires a very prolonged stretch.

SPECIAL CONSIDERATIONS

As with application of any therapeutic exercise technique, application of stretching techniques requires common sense and consideration of the specific structure to be stretched.

Trunk

The most important consideration in stretching the trunk is to avoid any stretch that causes pain or a change in sensation down either leg.

Upper Extremity

When stretching the glenohumeral joint, the scapula must be stabilized. If it is not, the stretching force is distributed into the scapular muscles, and gains in motion may not be actual gains in the intended area.

When stretching the elbow, remember that several muscles acting at the elbow also cross the shoulder, so the shoulder should be positioned and stabilized before stretching the elbow. Because the elbow flexors and extensors work in both supination and pronation, stretches for those muscles should be performed in both positions. One possible side effect of vigorous elbow stretching is myositis ossificans, especially in youth. For this reason, elbow stretches should be performed with caution. Active stretches and reciprocal inhibition techniques may help prevent this problem.

When stretching the wrist, the distal force is applied over the metacarpals, not the fingers. The patient's fingers should remain relaxed during the stretch since the extrinsic finger flexors and extensors cross the wrist and can affect the stretch if they are not relaxed.

Lower Extremity

The ankle and foot contain many joints and soft-tissue structures. When stretching these areas, the location where the joint's tendons cross and the appropriate force application must be considered.

The position of the hip affects stretching the knee. Since both the knee flexors and extensors cross the hip joint, the effectiveness of the stretch is determined by the position of the hip during the stretch.

When stretching the hip, the pelvis must be stabilized. If the pelvis is not stabilized, as with the scapula during shoulder stretching, movement occurs in this segment, and an increase in hip range of motion is sacrificed to the pelvis.

Caution must be used when stretching hip rotators with the knee in flexion and the force applied at the tibia. This position offers the clinician a tremendous lever arm advantage and reduces the force required to cause hip joint subluxation, especially in patients who have undergone prolonged immobilization, recent fracture, or recent dislocation.

> The anatomy of the specific structure to be stretched determines the most appropriate stretch application.

SUMMARY

Many factors influence an individual's range of motion and flexibility both normally and following injury. One of the major issues after injury is scar tissue formation and adhesions of that scar tissue to adjacent and surrounding tissues. If this is not managed properly, long-term loss of motion may result in long-term effects on an individual's ability to perform. Other factors influencing an individual's mobility include tissue viscosity, elasticity, plasticity, and neural input. The clinician must be aware of how to influence these factors to obtain optimal rehabilitation results. Accurate measurement of joint motion is necessary for reliable outcomes. There are many types of stretching techniques to increase flexibility and mobility. Each has its advantages and indications, so the clinician must be aware of which techniques are most appropriate for each patient if optimal results are going to occur.

KEY CONCEPTS AND REVIEW

1. Define the differences between range of motion and flexibility.

Range of motion is the amount of mobility of a joint, and flexibility is the musculotendinous unit's ability to elongate with application of a stretching force. Both are closely related and are often used interchangeably.

2. Explain the differences in structure of loose connective tissue and dense connective tissue.

The primary tissue that determines range of motion is connective tissue. The fiber arrangement of loose connective tissue, such as skin, is unorganized and loose with relatively long distances between the cross-links. Dense connective tissue, such as tendons and ligaments, is highly organized with parallel collagen fibers and more cross-links.

3. List the deleterious effects of prolonged immobilization.

Immobilization affects different tissue types differently, but some generic changes are seen in all tissues. These include a loss of ground substance, which in turn results in less separation and more cross-links between collagen fibers. The fiber meshwork contracts, so the tissue becomes dense, hard, and less supple. The more severe effects occur with more prolonged immobilization. If a normal joint is immobilized for four weeks, the dense connective tissue that forms prevents normal motion.

4. Discuss the mechanical properties of plasticity, elasticity, and viscosity of connective tissue.

Connective tissue's plastic quality allows its length to change, while its elasticity allows some return toward normal length. Viscoelasticity is a combination of elastic and viscous properties that allows either a change in length or a return to former length after stretching, depending on the speed, duration, and magnitude of the stretch force applied.

5. Explain the physiological properties of creep and stress-strain and how they affect stretching techniques.

Creep permits a gradual change in tissue length with the prolonged application of a low-level stretch force. The stress-strain curve describes a tissue's ability to withstand stresses and the subsequent strains they produce on the tissue. If a stretch force is applied beyond a tissue's elastic limits, deformation occurs.

6. Discuss the neuromuscular influences of the muscle spindle and GTO on stretching muscle.

The muscle spindle and GTO are neuromuscular protective mechanisms that attempt to reduce the stress-strain forces on the musculotendinous unit. The muscle spindle is more sensitive to stretch, and the GTO is more sensitive to muscle shortening.

7. Explain the procedure for measuring range of motion with a goniometer.

To measure a joint's range of motion, the goniometer's stationary arm is placed along one segment, and the movable arm is aligned along the segment on the other side of the joint. The protractor portion of the goniometer is placed over the joint's axis of rotation.

8. Discuss the active and passive methods for stretching.

Active stretching uses the antagonistic muscles to provide the stretch force to the agonist. In passive stretching, outside assistive devices or another person provide the force to gain additional range of motion.

9. Identify two mechanical assistive devices used to increase range of motion.

CPMs and splints are commonly used as external devices to gain additional motion. CPMs are sometimes used after surgery to counteract the deleterious effects of immobilization. Splints can be used to apply prolonged stretch to joints restricted by mature or very restricted scar tissue.

10. List contraindications, indications, and precautions of stretching.

Indications for stretching include a shortening of ligaments, capsules, muscles, fascia, skin, and other soft tissue by scar tissue or adhesions. Some precautions include explaining to the patient the technique and expected sensations before application, applying and releasing the force slowly and steadily, and avoiding pain. Contraindications include recent fractures, inflammations, infections, and extreme pain.

11. Discuss the progression of a stretching exercise program.

The type of flexibility exercise applied depends on a number of considerations, including the age of the scar tissue, the stage of healing, available equipment, the patient's motivation and pain tolerance, and the tissue involved. If the scar is in the early remodeling phase of repair, active exercises may be sufficient. If the scar tissue is more mature, a more prolonged stretch that affects the plastic range of the tissue is indicated.

CRITICAL THINKING QUESTIONS

1. How would you stretch the quadriceps muscle if you did not want to fully lengthen the rectus femoris? In what bodily position is the rectus femoris included in the quadriceps stretch? Try these two positions with a partner. Does the knee motion change in the different positions? If so, what does that tell you?

2. Over the course of a week, stretch a partner's hamstrings using a different technique each day: a passive technique with a 15 to 30 s hold, a contract-relax-stretch PNF maneuver, a ballistic stretch, and a prolonged stretch for 15 to 20 min. Measure the hamstring length each day before you begin the stretch exercise and again immediately after the stretch is released. Record each day's findings and which stretch technique is used each day. Which technique gives you the greatest change in hamstring length? Why does this occur? Do any of the physical properties of creep, stress-strain, or hysteresis influence the changes?

3. If you are measuring a patient's shoulder range of motion, in what position should he or she be for the most accurate measurements? Why? What position would provide the least accurate measurements when measuring a weak shoulder? Why?

4. Explain why active range of motion is not usually as great as passive range of motion. Can you think of exceptions to this generalization and explain why they occur?

5. If a patient had a condition in which the GTOs did not respond to stimuli, what would be the result? Could this be harmful during normal activity?

6. If you did not have a goniometer small enough to measure finger joint range of motion, what could you use to record flexibility in each finger joint? How can you measure trunk motion without a goniometer?

7. What is the most effective stretch for a patient who has a tight Achilles tendon? Why would you select that stretch?

LAB ACTIVITIES

1. Measure active and passive range of motion with a goniometer on the following motions. Watch for substitutions as you measure to be sure the patient is going through the range of motion correctly.
   a. Ankle dorsiflexion
   b. Knee extension
   c. Hip abduction
   d. Shoulder flexion
   e. Elbow flexion
   f. Wrist lateral flexion
   g. #1 MCP abduction

2. Measure active and passive range of motion of knee flexion with the patient in seated and prone positions. Why do the measurements change with position changes?

3. What is normal motion for the following movements?
   a. Shoulder abduction
   b. Elbow flexion
   c. Wrist extension
   d. Supination
   e. PIP flexion
   f. Hip lateral rotation

g. Knee flexion

h. Ankle inversion

4. Measure hip abduction with the patient lying supine and the foot facing the ceiling so there is no lateral rotation. Now have the patient laterally rotate the leg, and then abduct it. Which position provides the greatest motion? Which measure should you record as the patient's motion? Why?

6

Manual Therapy Techniques

OBJECTIVES

After completing this chapter, you should be able to do the following:

1. Discuss the three techniques of massage and their indications, precautions, and contraindications.
2. Explain the progression of myofascial restriction after an injury.
3. Discuss the techniques for myofascial release.
4. Explain the theory of the mechanism of myofascial trigger points.
5. Discuss the spray-and-stretch trigger point release theory.
6. Explain the concave-convex and convex-concave rules.
7. Define joint mobilization grades of movement.
8. Discuss the direction of glide and traction in relation to the treatment plane.
9. Explain the double-crush syndrome.
10. Discuss the dangers of neural mobilization.
11. Describe one neural self-mobilization technique for the upper extremity and one for the lower extremity.

▶ Michael Turner, athletic trainer for a Division III college, had never seen scar tissue adhesions like the ones he encountered in his most recent rehabilitation case. Over 6 months ago, one of the softball players, Emilie, had suffered a severe cleat laceration along her entire forearm when an opposing player sliding into second base ran the bottom of her shoe into Emilie's forearm. The forearm required over 30 stitches. Although Emilie hadn't suffered any immediate loss of motion from the scar, she was now losing some elbow and wrist motion because the scar tissue was pulling on both joints. When Michael palpated the forearm, he could feel a lot of hard, unyielding scar tissue adhesions below the skin. He knew he had to soften the scar tissue and mobilize the tissue below the skin if Emilie was to have normal elbow and wrist motion. He also knew he would have to show Emilie some soft-tissue techniques that she could perform on her own throughout the day to reinforce his efforts in the athletic training clinic.

Beyond all doubt, the use of the human hand, as a method of reducing human suffering, is the oldest remedy known to man.

JAMES MENNELL, *Manual Therapy*

Manual therapy is the use of hands-on techniques to evaluate, treat, and improve the status of neuromusculoskeletal conditions. A variety of structures, including joints and soft tissue, are affected by procedures that come under the category of manual therapy. The various procedures in this category are defined according to the tissues and structures they influence. This chapter discusses some of the more commonly used manual therapy procedures and techniques. Manual therapy techniques are subjective and vary from one clinician to another; because clinicians are different and patient conditions are also different, quantitative research on the efficacy of such treatment techniques is difficult to obtain. It is challenging to create an objective research design of these treatments because the specific application, direction, duration, and amplitude of a force can vary from one health care provider to another. With these variations comes a variety of outcomes, so a truly objective assessment of treatment effectiveness is difficult, if not impossible. Most of the benefits recorded are anecdotal because of their subjective, rather than objective, basis. Manual therapy techniques, however, deserve attention and application because of the overwhelming clinical reports of successful outcomes. Certain common principles apply to all manual therapy techniques if they are to be used successfully.

The manual therapy techniques we may have heard about include those most commonly used. These techniques are joint mobilization and soft tissue mobilization. Other manual therapies include techniques such as massage, trigger point release, myofascial release, muscle energy, strain-counterstrain, and neural mobilization. Even exercises such as proprioceptive neuromuscular facilitation, manual resistance, stretching, and stabilization may be considered manual therapy techniques. It should be mentioned that many manual therapy techniques are sometimes collectively classified under the umbrella term of *alternative medicine* or *alternative therapy*. Alternative therapy is a clinical practice in the western world that is not universally accepted as conventional treatment. Oftentimes, the types of care that fall into this category lack evidence-based documentation of their effectiveness. As has been mentioned, because of the subjectivity involved in manual therapy, evidence outside of case studies is lacking in this form of patient care.

Manual therapy techniques essentially address soft tissue, and more specifically, collagen of soft tissue. Even joint mobilization impacts joint motion by affecting changes in the soft tissue (capsule and ligaments) that surrounds the joint and not the bone ends that form the joint. Although various manual therapy techniques are applied with goals of altering specific soft tissues, it should be understood that other local tissues may also be affected. For example, neural tissue mobilization techniques likely affect other soft tissues in the local area in addition to the connective tissue surrounding nerves. Likewise, myofascial release techniques may also impact skin and subcutaneous tissue.

Manual therapy can be divided into two large categories: direct techniques and indirect techniques. **Direct techniques** are manual therapy maneuvers that load or bind tissue and structures (Giammatteo & Kain, 2005). These techniques move toward the point of limitation of tissue mobility. Techniques such as stretching, joint mobilization, trigger point release, and muscle energy fall into this category. The goal of these techniques is to move the point of restriction closer to the normal range of motion. For example, if a patient had a tight hamstring, the clinician would move the hip into flexion with the knee in extension, toward the point of restriction to gain additional motion in hamstring flexibility.

Indirect techniques are the opposite of direct techniques. They move the tissue away from the direction of limitation. Positional release therapy, or strain-counterstrain, is an example of this technique. The theory in this technique is to allow tissue to "let go" or release its restriction and allow more motion (Giammatteo & Kain, 2005). The basis for this theory is that there is relatively greater motion in the non-restricted direction of movement, so a re-establishment of balance between the restricted and non-restricted directions of motion is necessary. For example, if a patient has a tight hamstring, the knee is placed in flexion with the hip in extension to reduce the hypertonicity in the hamstrings. Once the hamstrings relax, more motion is gained.

As we go through this chapter, some techniques will be explained in detail while others will be merely introduced. The more commonly used and the ones I prefer in my own practice will be presented in more detail. It is impossible to devote enough time to all the different manual therapy techniques in this text, but if one is of particular interest to you, I suggest that you obtain additional textbooks and attend workshops on the topics.

Although there are many types of manual therapy, there are several principles they all have in common. It is important for you to keep in mind these common principles when you apply any manual therapy technique:

- Position the patient in a comfortable position.
- Place yourself in a comfortable position.
- Always use good body mechanics.
- Obtain feedback from the patient throughout the treatment so you can better provide proper application of the technique with appropriate pressure.
- Your fingernails should be clean and trimmed. As a general rule, the nail should not extend beyond the end of the fingertip.
- Before you apply the technique, explain what will be done and what sensations to expect. Warn the patient in advance when any discomfort may be felt and ask her to tell you when less pressure or discomfort is desired during the treatment.
- Assess the patient's condition before, during, and at the conclusion of the treatment.
- The appropriate manual therapy technique must be correctly applied for a successful result.
- Always respect precautions and contraindications.
- If you are unsure, do not perform the technique.

Likewise, for all manual therapy techniques, having the skill to apply and deliver the technique is only half the requirement in effective use of the skills. The other half is possessing the ability to critically analyze in order to know not only what to do but also why it should be done and to understand the outcome before it is achieved.

Evaluation and assessment are important for selecting appropriate manual therapy techniques.

CRITICAL ANALYSIS

The foundation of any manual therapy technique is your ability to think critically and to analyze the patient's condition to determine the best and most appropriate course of action. This practice involves understanding the injury and healing process, identifying the structures and problems involved, analyzing the situation and all its parameters to decide on a plan of action, and critically appraising the results of the treatment plan to determine its effectiveness or the need to change it. Critical analysis and examination with continual reassessment are keys to effective manual therapy application and outcomes.

There is no cookbook method for applying manual therapy. You must be able to use your skills of observation, palpation, analysis, and technique application. As with other aspects of rehabilitation, analysis and deductive reasoning are skills vital to a successful treatment outcome. The rehabilitation clinician is a detective in search of answers to problems. Detective skills in the assessment of clinical findings and deduction of logical expectations are continuously used throughout the manual therapy process.

Depending on the specific injury and resulting impairments, you may choose to use more than one manual therapy technique. Evaluation and deductive reasoning allow you to select treatment techniques that can best reduce the impairment and improve the functional ability of the injured athlete.

Whatever techniques you choose, your selection is based on individual findings, not on rote or cookbook decisions. Always approach an injury with an open mind and maintain flexibility in your treatment options. Each patient is individually and objectively assessed to determine the best course of treatment. Two patients may have shoulder pain and loss of motion, but the causes and courses of treatment may be very different for each of them. A successful treatment program depends on your evaluation skills as much as on your treatment skills.

MASSAGE

Many types of massage are used in a number of applications to achieve a variety of goals. A sports massage is frequently used either before or after competition in what is known in non-medical circles as a rubdown. Even though massage is used in non-medical situations, it still produces a physiological effect. The use of massage for non-pathological conditions, however, is not discussed in this text. The range of techniques most commonly used in the injury treatment is briefly described in this section.

Definition of Massage

Massage is the systematic and scientific manipulation of soft tissue for remedial or restorative purposes. Massage affects various systems of the body through its influence on reflex and mechanical processes to produce desired results.

Effects of Massage

Massage produces reflex physiological and mechanical effects in the area treated. Repetitive pressure stimulation without irritation to the skin causes transmission from peripheral receptors to the spinal cord and brain, which results in relaxation of muscles and dilation of blood vessels. Mechanical effects improve blood and lymph flow, promote mobilization of fluid, and stretch and break down adhesions to ultimately assist in reducing edema and improving tissue mobility (DeDomenico, 2007). The overall end result is relaxation of muscles, dilation of local capillaries, increase in lymph flow to reduce edema, reduction of pain, and improvement in soft-tissue movement. The specific effects vary, depending on the type of massage given.

Types of Massage

Although there are many different massage techniques, three primary techniques are used in treating injuries to achieve the effects mentioned earlier. The French terms for many of these techniques were first introduced by Peter Ling of Sweden, who traveled widely in Europe (DeDomenico, 2007).

Effleurage

Effleurage, or stroking, is a massage that is performed by running the hand lightly over the skin's surface. The direction of the stroke moves distally to proximally (figure 6.1). Effleurage is used to assist in venous and lymphatic flow to decrease edema and aid in muscle relaxation. If the technique is used primarily to treat edema, it should be performed with the body segment in an elevated position so gravity can assist the flow. The pressure should be applied firmly and deeply but not heavily. The direction of stroking should be toward the heart.

Pétrissage

Compression and kneading fall under the category of pétrissage. In this technique the soft tissue is grasped between the thumb and fingers and manipulated intermittently so that there is movement between the skin's underlying structure and the muscle (figure 6.2). Pétrissage can also be performed with the whole hand, both hands, or one hand. Although the stroking movement is constant, the pressure is intermittent. The tissue can be lifted, pressed, rolled, or squeezed in pétrissage, depending on the specific method used. The tissue is grasped and released with varying degrees of pressure so that the action's mechanical effects reduce edema.

This technique is often preceded and followed by a stroking technique for relaxation. Pétrissage is used to promote circulation, relax muscle, mechanically assist fluid exchange, and improve mobility of muscle tissue.

Friction

Friction is a deep-pressure movement of superficial soft tissue against underlying structures (figure 6.3). Sometimes the underlying structure is bone or other hard surface, and sometimes it is soft tissue, such as muscle or fascia. The intent is to loosen small areas of scar tissue and adhesions of deeper parts, such as tendons, ligaments, and joint capsules, to improve movement and gliding of these structures. Friction also helps to stimulate circulation of the local area. It usually is applied through firm pressure by either the thumb or finger pads in a crisscross or circular motion. Elbows or knuckles can also be used. Little or no massage medium is used in friction massage, and the technique is usually applied transversely in short strokes across the targeted underlying structure.

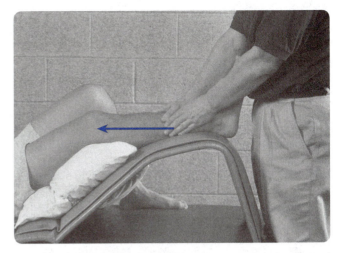

▶ **Figure 6.1** Effleurage: Stroking motion begins distally and moves proximally toward the heart. Elevating the segment during treatment further assists in edema reductions.

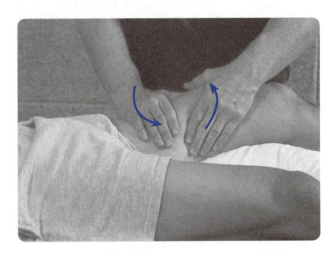

▶ **Figure 6.2** Pétrissage: Skin and underlying tissue are kneaded and lifted to improve tissue mobility, relax muscle, and promote circulation.

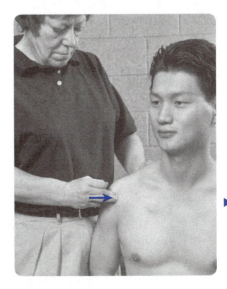

▶ **Figure 6.3** Friction massage across the biceps tendon will loosen adhesions and stimulate circulation.

Effleurage, pétrissage, and friction massage are techniques that can relax muscles, improve blood and lymph flow to reduce edema, reduce pain, and improve soft-tissue movement.

Indications and Contraindications

The indications for massage are related to its effects. Relief of pain, muscle relaxation, reduction of swelling, and mobilization of adherent scar tissue are all appropriate indications for the use of massage. The specific technique selection is based on the evaluation findings. Recent edema secondary to trauma is an indication for effleurage and pétrissage massage techniques. Friction massage is indicated when scar tissue restriction of superficial tissue can be palpated and in inflammatory conditions where adhesions play a role in continued symptoms, such as tendinitis and bursitis.

Massage is contraindicated when the technique may aggravate the condition or cause additional harm to the patient. Contraindications include the presence of infection, malignancies, skin diseases, blood clots, and any irritations or lesions that may spread with direct contact.

Precautions

When you apply massage to the patient, both the patient's skin and your hands should be clean. Your hands should be warm and your nails trimmed so as not to cause a laceration or abrasion. Rings, watches, and wrist jewelry should be removed for the same reason. A lubricant is used to reduce friction when using effleurage. Less lubricant is used with pétrissage, and even less is used with friction massage. Too much lubricant with friction massage does not allow the presence of enough friction to be effective, and too much lubricant with pétrissage makes it difficult to lift or grasp the tissue.

Application

Massage is a direct soft tissue technique. Before beginning the massage, position the patient comfortably with the body segment to be massaged properly exposed. If the massage is to reduce edema, elevate the part to enhance lymphatic flow. Explain the procedure to the patient and instruct the patient to inform you if he or she feels pain with the massage.

When using effleurage or pétrissage, the pressure of the massage strokes should be toward the heart, and the hands should not lose contact with the skin. On the return stroke, continue lightly touching the part. Keep your hand in good contact with the part and your fingers together, not spread apart. The rhythm of the stroke should be even and slow to promote relaxation. Maintain a comfortable position during the treatment and use proper body mechanics.

When using friction massage, it is important to warn the patient that some discomfort may be felt but that it will not be lasting. The thumb or finger pads are used on a small, localized surface in a cross pattern. A firm, consistent pressure and rhythm are also important. A small area at a time is massaged until the discomfort of the massage subsides and you can palpate an increase in tissue mobility. The massage is applied in a "cross" pattern perpendicular to the tissue's fiber arrangement.

MYOFASCIAL RELEASE

Myofascial release is a close relative to massage. Depending on the specific myofascial release method used, it can be either a direct or an indirect method. Myofascial release involves manual contact with the patient and uses the sense of touch to evaluate the problem and the effectiveness of the treatment, just as massage does. Massage and myofascial release also both include the use of pressure and tissue stretch to produce soft tissue results.

There are many different techniques of myofascial release, but they all are essentially variations of the same principle: The use of manual contact for evaluation and treatment of soft-tissue restriction and pain with the eventual goal of the relief of those symptoms to improve motion and function. There are different names for these techniques: myofascial release, myofascial stretching, strain-counterstrain, Rolfing, soft-tissue mobilization. Because of the individual variations in application, forces, duration, and precise technique, reliable research results on the efficacy of myofascial release remain elusive. Clinical observations and anecdotal reports of those who have recorded treatment results is currently the best barometer by which to judge the results of this type of treatment. Ultimately, treatment effectiveness must be assessed by the results of your own applications on the patients you treat. In this section, some of the more commonly used myofascial techniques are introduced briefly.

Before describing the various myofascial release techniques, their theoretical basis is discussed. The different myofascial release systems cannot be appreciated without understanding their basis.

Fascia

Fascia is a continuous structure that surrounds and integrates tissues and structures throughout the body. Fascia varies in density and thickness and is interconnected with the structures it surrounds. It can affect the relationship among the structures it encompasses (their physical orientation to each other, their chemical relationship, or their physiological relationship, e.g., what tissues are served by which blood vessels or nerves). Fascia is vital for tissue form, lubrication, nutrition, stability, integrity, function, and support.

Throughout the body, fascia is divided into three layers. The superficial layer is attached to the undersurface of the skin. Within this superficial layer lie capillaries, lymph vessels, nerves, and fat. Because this layer is a loosely knit structure made of fibroelastic and loose connective tissue, it permits the skin to move in many directions over the underlying structures. It is also an area where edema accumulates following injury.

Deep fascia is dense connective tissue that surrounds and separates deeper structures, such as muscle, tendon, joints, ligaments, and bone. Because of its stiffer, firmer structure, deep fascia is less able to accommodate edema, which can cause problems, such as compartment syndromes in the lower leg.

The final layer is subserous fascia, which surrounds internal organs. Its loose areolar connective tissue contains channels where fluid assists in providing the organs with lubrication. Myofascial release techniques do not treat fascia surrounding visceral organs.

Fascia contains collagen, elastin, cellular components, and ground substance. The elastin within fascia allows the structure to return to its original shape when applied stresses are released. Fascia also responds with plastic deformation when prolonged forces are applied. Creep and hysteresis, discussed in chapters 3 and 5, are properties of fascia and are impacted with myofascial release techniques.

Although fascia has high tensile strength and is able to tolerate multidirectional compression, stretch, and sheer forces, an injury can profoundly affect fascia. The fascia's normal biomechanics can be altered to cause either a temporary or a permanent deformation, depending on the load, duration, and type of stress applied to the fascia. Injury to fascia causes a change in the biochemical structure of the ground substance, and the scar tissue that forms after injury can interfere with normal fascia functions. When fascia either restricts normal motion or does not provide skin, subcutaneous, muscle, and other tissue with support, lubrication, and other functions, fascial dysfunctions can result in extended disability and prolonged symptoms following injury and the subsequent recovery process if not managed properly.

Myofascia maintains an intimate relationship with the muscle it covers and surrounds. The muscle and its surrounding fascia provide the combined contractile and non-contractile properties of muscle. Myofascia assists in increasing muscle strength during eccentric contractions. It helps provide structure and form to the muscle, lubrication between muscle fibers and muscles, and nutrition for the muscles. It also bears the blood and lymph vessels and nerves for the muscles. In short, myofascia provides vital support to permit normal muscle function.

Nonacute Biomechanical Forces

When injury or unbalanced biomechanical forces are applied to myofascia, its ability to support normal muscle function is impaired. This impaired myofascia eventually leads to pain,

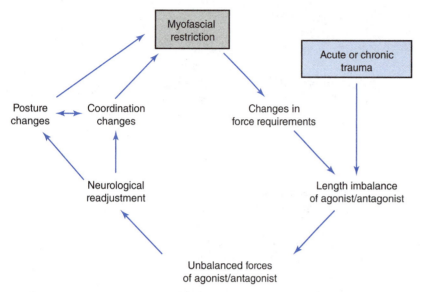

▶ **Figure 6.4** Pathology of myofascial restriction: Myofascial restriction can occur within a short time from acute injury and scar-tissue formation or gradually from minor but progressive alterations from repeated low-level trauma.

loss of motion, and reduced functional performance. Muscle dysfunction causes additional changes in the myofascia.

In pathology that occurs over time—for example, the swimmer who has developed poor posture—muscle imbalances occur. As noted in figure 6.4, the process may start with a minor trauma or injury. It causes a change in the muscle, perhaps as a part of its withdrawal reflex to the injury. This muscle change eventually causes an imbalance of muscle strength between an agonist group and its antagonist group. Muscle imbalances lead to changes in neuromuscular response and coordination, which lead to further imbalances, until the structure reaches a point where the imbalance and resulting increased tissue stress cause symptoms that impair performance and require treatment.

The patient can inadvertently start this cycle through the activities he or she performs. If the swimmer with poor posture concentrates on pectoralis strengthening without also working on antagonist strength, or uses only strokes that emphasize anterior and not posterior muscles, eventually a muscle imbalance will occur. Awareness of muscle imbalance is important in treating patients with loss of motion. Muscle imbalances are discussed more thoroughly in chapter 7.

There are a number of other factors that result in fascial changes and ultimately affect performance or produce pain. Some of these factors include a leg length difference; inadequate rehabilitation from previous injuries; worn, poorly constructed, or ill-fitting shoes and protective equipment; prolonged activities that overstress supportive structures; and poor ergonomics (Hunter, 1998). If any of these factors are present but not addressed, they eventually will produce imbalances of strength, flexibility, and fascial mobility so the body or segment is abnormally stressed and creates an environment that makes the individual susceptible to injury.

It is also important to realize that exercise is a vital collaborative adjunct of myofascial release treatments in a successful rehabilitation program. Myofascial techniques release restricted areas, but exercises for flexibility and strength reset neurological programming. Together they cause permanent positive changes in the affected tissues.

Acute Biomechanical Forces

Previous chapters have already addressed the biomechanical causes of fascial restriction following acute injury. Scar tissue is less extensible and creates a localized connective tissue meshwork that extends tentacles outward, much like a shattered plate glass window, to adjacent locations and can limit normal tissue mobility. Recall from the discussion of immobilization in chapter 5 that the scar tissue matrix can restrict neurovascular and lymph vessels and reduce local metabolism. With reduced metabolism a fluid imbalance further adds to the area's reduced mobility and continued inflammation. Less motion causes a loss of GAGs and promotes increased cross-link formations. Mobility between fibers becomes restricted through this process.

In addition to the scarring that occurs with acute injury, spasm can also influence the fascial system by producing prolonged tightness in one area that causes another area to compensate with prolonged looseness, initiating a cycle of imbalance and fascial pathology. It is important to evaluate for fascial restrictions in both acute and nonacute injuries.

Terminology

The term *myofascial release* is common and is frequently used in the techniques described here, but it is actually a misnomer. Myofascial release implies the treatment to myofascia. Although myofascia can certainly be the target of treatment, it is not always the targeted tissue nor the only tissue treated. For example, to relieve fascia contractures and restriction of skin and subcutaneous tissue mobility following edema and immobilization, myofascial release techniques actually commonly treat the fascia associated with skin, subcutaneous tissue, and other superficial structures that have limited mobility, not the muscle's fascia.

Even when the target tissue is myofascia, other structures may also be affected by treatment because of secondary restriction in the area. With subcutaneous restriction following edema and immobilization, for example, myofascial structures may be restricted and require myofascial release treatment, but the area's restricted subcutaneous and skin structures are also treated when the myofascia is treated.

Palpation

Palpation is fundamental in myofascial release. Not only is it required for an examination of the area, but continual palpation is performed during the treatment. The soft tissue's extensibility, movement, end-feel, and response to treatment are continually palpated during and after the treatment. Adjustments are made as the area is palpated and examined during the treatment.

Normal tissue has no tenderness when palpated. Normal tissue also has a springy end-feel that can be palpated when pressure to the tissue is released. This springy end-feel is present in normal tissue regardless of the tissue's excursion. Tissue mobility varies according to the body part and tissue type, but the springiness of the end-feel is consistent. In myofascial techniques, palpation also includes feeling the release in the tissues during the treatment. This release is the treatment goal and is necessary for restoring tissue mobility and balance. The release that is palpated has been described as the tissue giving way, letting go, relaxing, or melting as ice with a hot knife going through it.

Superficial to Deep Structures

When examining and treating with myofascial release techniques, you should move from superficial structures to deeper structures to avoid a mistake in identifying the structure or tissues that are restricted. Techniques should be applied with the least amount of force that is appropriate for achieving the established goals. More force is often indicated when scar tissue adhesions and reduced mobility are present, but the additional force is applied only after examining and assessing the area and determining the patient's tolerance.

Autonomic Effects

Neuroreflex changes can sometimes result from the use of myofascial techniques. Fascial restriction can cause autonomic changes, so it is not surprising that when restriction is released, the autonomic system can be affected. If pain and fascial restriction cause changes in skin color, moisture, temperature, and sensation, then their release will also cause changes in those signs and symptoms.

Afferent sensations are transmitted to the dorsal horn of the spinal cord. The dorsal horn is a processing center that receives and redirects information. It can send an impulse directly out the spinal cord as a reflex efferent response, or it can send the information to the subcortical or cortical level of the brain, where it is interpreted and a response is formulated and returned down the spinal cord to the appropriate locale.

The patient may experience an autonomic response when the myofascial treatment is particularly effective. The patient's sympathetic system is stimulated, and the patient demonstrates symptoms such as increased pulse rate, sweating, and blood pressure changes. Less intense responses include sensations of burning, tingling, stinging, or heat in the area being treated

(Sutton & Bartel, 1994). Although these sympathetic responses are unusual, you should be aware that they may occur and be prepared to respond appropriately.

Treatment Techniques

Because there are many different ways to apply myofascial techniques, only general application techniques regarding time, frequency, pressure, and palpation are introduced here. This is by no means an exhaustive list of myofascial techniques. It is, however, a list of the more commonly used techniques.

General Guidelines

In the beginning, it may be necessary to restrict the treatment time to 3 to 5 min and increase it as the patient's tolerance and the response of the area indicate. Daily treatment can be beneficial. If bruising occurs, the technique is too aggressive. Because bruising causes additional scarring and adhesions, it should be avoided. Bruising is not a desirable reaction, but a short-term redness of the skin in the area should be expected.

There are many different ways to apply myofascial release techniques (Manheim, 1994). Palpation and relaxation by the rehabilitation clinician are basic to applying myofascial techniques. If you are relaxed you will have more sensitivity in your hands and fingertips to palpate the area being treated. An exercise to illustrate this idea is to take a dime in your fingertips, close your eyes, tense your arm from the shoulder to the fingers, and try to feel the nose on the portrait. Then relax your entire arm and try to feel the nose. It should be easier to locate the nose when your arm and hand are relaxed. To ensure both the patient's and your relaxation, you should both be in comfortable positions.

In one of the most frequently used techniques, both hands move longitudinally in opposite directions while stretching the tissue (figure 6.5). In another variation, only one hand applies the treatment while the other hand stabilizes or supports the tissue. The treatment hand applies pressure through the finger pads, thumb, knuckles, or heel of the hand (figure 6.6). The pressure can also be applied by the forearm or elbow, depending on the size and location of the area being treated. The stabilizing hand anchors the tissue so that the pressure can be applied in the direction of the restriction. The tissue's slack is taken up, and a steady pressure into the restriction is continued until the area releases or for about 90 s.

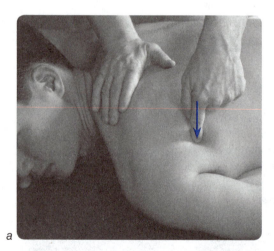

▶ **Figure 6.5** In longitudinal myofascial release, fascial tissue between the hands is stretched.

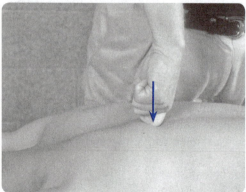

a

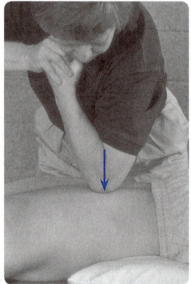

b

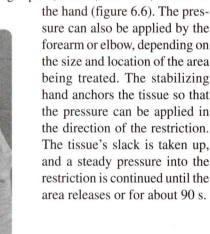

c

▶ **Figure 6.6** Alternative myofascial release applications using *(a)* finger pad, *(b)* knuckle, or *(c)* elbow.

The amount of pressure applied is determined by the tissue involved and the sensitivity of the area, but it is generally a low-load, sustained pressure.

J-Stroke

A J-stroke is a common direct technique that is used on limited areas of tightness and on longitudinal scars. The technique is used in these situations because of its multidirectional stretch. As shown in figure 6.7, the treatment hand draws short Js across the restricted area.

Oscillation

When muscle spasm is present, a direct technique, an oscillating pressure technique, can be used. This technique involves a rhythmic, back-and-forth application of a low-load pressure while maintaining constant contact.

It is designed to relax the muscle by reducing the spasm and relieving the patient's guarding of the area. It can be applied with finger pads for small areas, as shown in figure 6.8, or with the palms for larger areas.

Wringing

In areas of generalized or multidirectional restriction, a direct technique referred to as *wringing* can be effective. In this technique both hands are used for treatment. The hands are placed on the area in similar positions. They are then rotated on the extremity in opposite directions to twist or wring the tissue, as in figure 6.9. This same technique can be used on smaller areas using the two thumbs in the same manner.

Stripping

The stripping technique is used as a deep-tissue release. It is similar to the general technique described earlier, but it is applied directly to restricted deeper tissue. Knuckles and elbow are frequently used in this technique (figure 6.10) but, the finger pads can also be effective over small areas. The pressure is slow, consistent, and deep. It is uncomfortable for the patient, but if it can be tolerated, it is effective in breaking up deep adhesions.

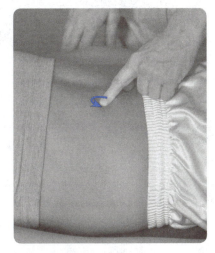

▶ **Figure 6.7** J-stroke.

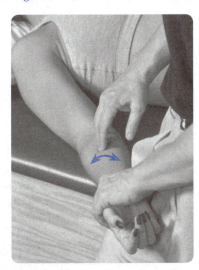

▶ **Figure 6.8** Oscillation.

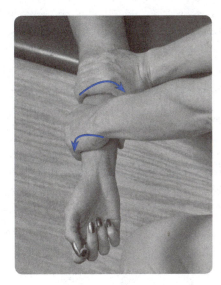

▶ **Figure 6.9** Wringing: a generalized, multidirectional release technique.

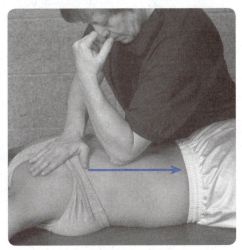

▶ **Figure 6.10** Stripping: a deep tissue release using one hand to stabilize and the elbow to treat.

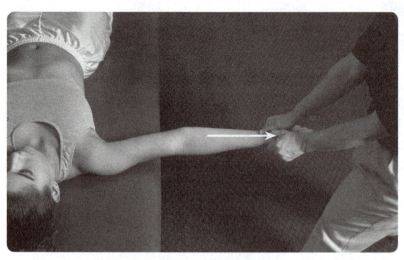

▶ **Figure 6.11** Arm pull: a generalized technique in which traction is applied to the arm while moving it into abduction and rotation to the point of resistance. Movement through an arc of motion continues following the resistance after the extremity releases.

Arm Pull and Leg Pull

The arm pull and leg pull are gross techniques applied to generalized tightness in the upper and lower extremities, respectively. These techniques involve the application of longitudinal traction to the arm or leg from the hand or foot with the patient lying supine (figure 6.11). As the traction is applied, the extremity is slowly moved into abduction and rotation. When tissue resistance is felt, the motion is stopped, and the position is maintained until you feel the extremity release. Once the area releases, the extremity is passively moved through its arc of motion into the new area of restriction, and the sequence is repeated until an end position is reached.

> Myofascial release involves manual contact to evaluate and treat soft-tissue restriction and pain, relieve symptoms, and improve motion and function. It is commonly used to treat the restricted fascia associated with the skin, subcutaneous tissues, and other superficial structures.

Precautions

As with any treatment, you should take precautions with this application. Myofascial release is used cautiously on new scars. The new tissue is fragile because of its reduced tensile strength. It also may have increased sensitivity and limited tolerance to pressure.

Care should also be used on patients with complex regional pain syndrome (CRPS), or reflex sympathetic dystrophy (RSD). RSD is exacerbated with pain, so treatments should avoid pain.

Bruising is also avoided. This is especially true when the purpose of the treatment is to improve scar tissue mobility, because bruising produces more scar tissue.

The patient is warned in advance of the treatment that sensations of pain, tingling, burning, and warmth may occur and are normal with this technique. The patient should also be instructed to inform you if any additional sensations are felt.

Contraindications

Myofascial technique contraindications include malignancy, hypermobile joints, recent fractures, hemorrhages, sutures, osteoporosis, local infections, and acute inflammations (Sutton & Bartel, 1994). As always, contraindications should be respected, and treatment in the presence of these conditions should be avoided.

MYOFASCIAL TRIGGER POINTS

Two of the most recognized names in the study of myofascial trigger points are Janet Travell and David Simons. They devoted their professional lives to understanding and treating trigger points. Most of the information presented here is the result of their findings. For additional information on trigger points, see Travell (J. Travell, 1976), Simons (Simons, 1981), and Travell and Simons (J. G. Travell & Simons, 1983, 1992).

Myriad terms are often used interchangeably with myofascial trigger point. Some of the more commonly used terms include myalgia, fibrositis, muscular rheumatism, fibroplastic syndrome, myositis, and myofasciitis.

Definition of Trigger Point

Travell and Simons (J. G. Travell & Simons, 1983) define a **trigger point** as a "focus of hyperirritability in a tissue that, when compressed, is locally tender and, if sufficiently hypersensitive, gives rise to referred pain and tenderness, and sometimes to referred autonomic phenomena and distortion of proprioception." Trigger points can be located in cutaneous, fascial, myofascial, ligamentous, and periosteal tissue. The discussion here is limited to myofascial trigger points.

A myofascial trigger point involves a taut band of muscle tissue and its surrounding fascia, hence the name. A central focal point of local tenderness can be palpated as a nodule within the taut band. Compression of this point often refers pain to other areas or causes an autonomic response.

Travell and Simons (J. G. Travell & Simons, 1983, 1992) identify two types of trigger points: active and latent. An **active trigger point** is one that is always tender and can produce referred pain whether the muscle is active or inactive. The muscle can also display weakness and reduced motion. When an active trigger point is palpated with a rolling pressure crosswise against the muscle fibers, the muscle fibers are stimulated to produce a localized twitch response. This palpation technique is called a snapping palpation and is performed using firm, constant pressure and moving the fingertips across the muscle fibers as if plucking a guitar string. The local twitch response is an involuntary contraction of the muscle fibers in response to the snapping palpation (J. G. Travell & Simons, 1983). Sometimes this response is incorrectly called a *jump sign*. A **jump sign** is also a reflex response but is a reaction of wincing or withdrawal.

A **latent trigger point** is painful only when it is palpated. Normal muscles do not have areas of tenderness, sites that elicit a local twitch response, or palpably taut bands.

Trigger Point Characteristics

Trigger point tenderness is often described as a dull ache and can be merely uncomfortable or very intense. Pressure on the trigger point can elicit a referred pain pattern that is unique for each muscle. The more irritable the trigger point, the more severe and extensive is the referral pattern. For detailed trigger point referral patterns, refer to the two texts that Simons and Travell (J. G. Travell & Simons, 1983, 1992) have written on this topic. The earlier publication deals with referral patterns of the upper extremities, and the more recent text addresses lower-extremity referral patterns.

The referral patterns do not follow neurological referral patterns; this is an important distinction. The sensation of trigger-point referral pain is also different from neurologically referred pain. Trigger-point pain is often a deep ache. Occasionally, a trigger-point pain is a sharp or stabbing pain, and rarely is it described as burning. Referred sensation from peripheral nerve entrapment or nerve root irritation, however, is evidenced by prickling, tingling, or numbness.

Myofascial trigger-point pain becomes amplified by muscle activity (especially strenuous activity), passive stretch of the muscle, direct pressure of the trigger point, prolonged stationary periods followed by moving (such as getting up in the morning or standing after prolonged sitting), repeated or sustained muscle activity, and cold. On the other hand, myofascial trigger points are relieved with short periods of rest; heat accompanied by slow and sustained stretches; short-term, low-level activity; and specific treatment techniques that are discussed later in this chapter.

Trigger Point Causes

Travell and Simons (J. G. Travell & Simons, 1983) have put together the most comprehensive compendium of trigger points to date, mapping common trigger points and their referral patterns throughout the body. Their theories on causes and creation of trigger points have been disputed but not disproved (Huguenin, 2004). Trigger points can be activated by various factors, including injury, overload, fatigue, and cold. Acute conditions that can activate trigger points include fractures, sprains, dislocations, muscle impact injuries, and the stress of excessive or unusual exercise that the body is unable to tolerate. Overload of the muscles from a prolonged stationary posture, prolonged muscle immobilization in a shortened position, and nerve compressions are the most common causes of gradual trigger point onset.

The exact mechanism of trigger point production, however, is only theoretical at this time. Travell and Simons (J. G. Travell & Simons, 1983) have proposed a theory that involves the contractile activity of a muscle: During contraction of a normal muscle fiber, calcium that is stored in the fiber's sarcoplasmic reticulum is rapidly released when the contraction begins and then reabsorbed in the presence of ATP when the contraction terminates. This process is triggered by a brief nerve impulse called an action potential. A contraction is the result of the shortening of the sarcomere when its cross-bridges pull the actin and myosin filaments over each other (figure 6.12). If an injured muscle fiber's sarcoplasmic reticulum is damaged, its calcium is released to simulate the sarcomere, producing a sustained contraction. Ischemia occurs with this sustained contraction, so the muscle cells, deficient in oxygen, are unable to produce enough ATP to relax the contraction. Without any ATP, the sarcomere's filaments cannot release from each other and remain fixed in their contracted position. In partial support of Travell and Simons' theory, there has been some evidence to suggest that there is present in trigger points a metabolic pathology of local tissue (Bengtsson, Henrikkson, & Larsson, 1986). These findings did not support ischemia as the basis for pain, but it did agree with the presence of some metabolic issue affecting trigger points.

Investigators who dispute Travell and Simons' theory of ischemia favor a theory based on neurological pathology causing trigger points and associated sensory, motor, and autonomic changes (Gunn, 1997; Quintner & Cohen, 1994). Supporters of this theory feel that this theory explains the referral of pain to distant sites and treatment should focus on nerve roots rather than on muscle. This theory is yet to be proven.

In spite of other theories, Travell and Simons' theory of trigger point pathology remains pertinent and most popular (Huguenin, 2004). It gains further support when combined with the convergence projection theory (Gerwin, 1994; Huguenin, 2004). This theory indicates that a noxious stimulation in one area is interpreted by the central nervous system as coming from a different source of pain. So what may start as a local reaction can escalate and refer pain to other regions.

When trigger points occur because of either injury or increased demands placed on the muscle, irritating or noxious chemicals are released (J. G. Travell & Simons, 1983, 1992). The release of nerve-sensitizing substances such as histamine, serotonin, kinins, and prostaglandins (mentioned in chapter 2) may be the cause of continued, localized, runaway metabolic activity. Travell and Simons (J. G. Travell & Simons, 1983, 1992) propose that these substances, which are released following an injury, increase the metabolic demands and sensitize afferent nerve endings to make them hyperirritable to mediate referred pain, autonomic and motor neutron responses, and cause trigger points.

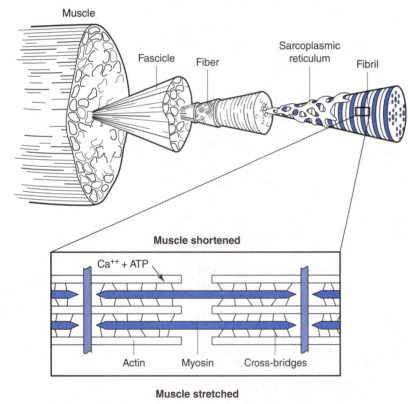

▶ **Figure 6.12** Normal skeletal muscle structure and a sarcomere in shortened and lengthened conditions.

Trigger Point Examination

As part of the total treatment plan, the causes of the patient's pain must be accurately assessed to rule out trigger points as a possible factor. Observation and examination of the patient's posture, range of motion, weakness patterns, pain areas, and history are all required to determine the patient's injury and rehabilitation needs. It is sometimes easier to identify patterns if the patient indicates the areas of pain on a figure drawing like the one in figure 6.13.

A compression test over the muscle can detect taut bands, nodules, and local and referred pain. A local twitch response confirms the presence of a trigger point. A taut band is palpated by stretching the muscle until the taut fibers are pulled to the point of discomfort without pain while the overall muscle remains slack. The taut band feels like a cord within the muscle. Begin at the band's distal attachment and palpate with either the pad of the thumb or two or three fingers along the taut band toward the fibers' proximal attachment to locate the trigger point within the band. It is an area of increased tenderness and feels like a hard ball within the taut band.

A local twitch response is elicited along the taut band with a snapping palpation of the band. A snapping palpation is produced by first placing the muscle in a relaxed, neutral position and then strumming the fibers with pressure perpendicular to the fiber alignment, much like strumming a guitar. In a positive response, the taut band twitches. The more closely the pressure is applied to the trigger point of the taut band, the more vigorous is the response. This technique works most effectively on superficial muscles.

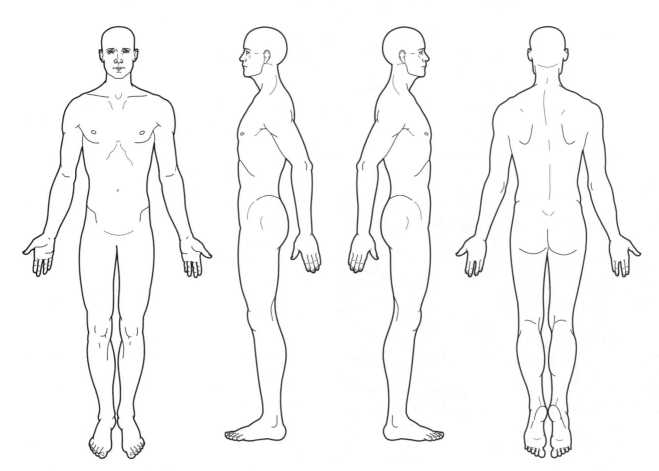

▶ **Figure 6.13** Pain-referral figure.

Trigger Point Treatment

Travell and Simons (J. G. Travell & Simons, 1983, 1992) and Cyriax (Cyriax, 1977) advocate the use of trigger point injection as an effective method of treatment, but this treatment is neither appropriate nor legal for rehabilitation clinicians. When an active trigger point does not respond to the treatment techniques presented here, it may be useful to refer the patient to a physician who can inject the site.

Trigger point treatments using Travell and Simons' techniques are direct methods. Three primary methods of myofascial trigger point treatments are discussed briefly here. For additional information, refer to the Travell and Simons texts (J. G. Travell & Simons, 1983, 1992), the source of the techniques described next.

Spray/Ice-and-Stretch

Fluorimethane as a vapocoolant spray was formerly used as a common treatment for myofascial trigger points. Now that we are more aware of the harm that chlorofluorocarbons cause to the atmosphere, fluorimethane is no longer used. A cold spray without fluorimethane is commercially produced and available. Some clinicians who are environmentally concerned have replaced cold spray with ice stroking using an icicle. An "icicle" is made by placing a tongue depressor in a cup of water and freezing the water. Before applying the icicle to the skin, the paper or styrofoam cup is torn back and covered with thin plastic wrap to avoid getting any cold water drips on the patient's skin; keeping the skin dry throughout the treatment maintains the contrast between the warm skin and the cold ice. Travell and Simons (J. G. Travell & Simons, 1983) indicated that this technique of applying ice or vapocoolant followed by a stretch was the most effective technique to treat trigger point pain.

Before application, the patient should be instructed to relax. Applying just enough pressure on the trigger point area to produce the referred pain may help the patient understand why your treatment is not being applied directly to the area of pain. The patient is placed in a comfortable position with the skin exposed and the body part supported to permit full relaxation. Before treatment, the part is moved through its range of motion so you and the patient can judge changes made by the treatment. With the muscle anchored at one end, the ice or vapocoolant spray is applied in a sweeping motion in parallel strokes in only one direction over the length of the muscle and then over the referred pain pattern. As the ice or vapocoolant is applied in a rhythmic, unhurried fashion, a slow, continual, passive stretch is applied progressively to the muscle. Any one area of the skin should receive only two to three strokes of cold before rewarming to achieve optimal results of the ice-and-stretch technique (figure 6.14). The rate at which the ice or vapocoolant is moved over the skin is approximately 4 in/s (10 cm/s). The stretch force should be light enough that it does not elicit a stretch reflex from the muscle but strong enough to be effective. As a muscle releases, you must be able to detect the relaxation and place the muscle in a new stretch position that takes up the slack and provides the same level of tension on the muscle. The application and release of the stretch force should be done smoothly and gradually, not quickly. A hot pack can be immediately applied to further relax the muscle. The patient can also assist the stretch by contracting the antagonist, but you must monitor the contraction so as to prevent a co-contraction of the agonist and antagonist. The cold-and-stretch technique can be repeated for several cycles after the skin has been rewarmed, depending on the results of treatment, the patient's response, and desired goals.

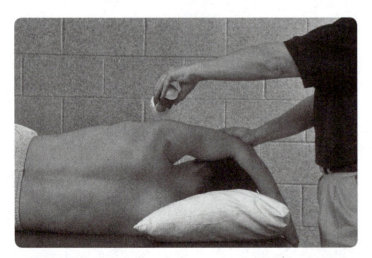

▶ **Figure 6.14** In the ice-and-stretch technique, ice or vapocoolant strokes are applied in sweeps that include the muscle, its trigger points, and its referred pain areas. The ice is applied in a rhythmic fashion while a gentle stretch is applied to the muscle.

Theory of Effectiveness

It is believed that this technique is effective because of two mechanisms, although they have not been confirmed through research. The gate theory of pain presented by Melzak (Melzack, 1973) and the modified gate control theory advanced by Castel (Castel, 1979) postulate that sudden cold and touch sensations inhibit the pain cycle by blocking transmission of pain signals. Active trigger points activate the pain-spasm response. Ice stroking inhibits the pain-spasm cycle and allows the muscle to respond to the stretch (figure 6.15).

The second factor is mechanical: If a muscle is stretched, its sarcomere elongates and releases the actin and myosin elements enough to end the sustained muscle fiber contraction.

Ischemic Compression

Another myofascial trigger point release is ischemic compression. In this technique, pressure is applied slowly and progressively over the trigger point as the tension in the trigger point and its taut band subsides (J.G. Travell & Simons, 1983). Pressure is maintained until the tenderness is gone or the tension is released. This is followed by stretching the muscle. Before application, the patient should be informed that some discomfort may occur. Hanten et al. (Hanten, Olsen, Butts, & Nowicki, 2000) found that this technique of ischemic compression followed by stretching provided the best and most effective decrease in trigger-point pain levels.

Stripping

A third technique is stripping massage, a deep-stroking massage applied with minimal lubrication on the fingertips. A firm pressure is used along the length of the taut band (J.G. Travell & Simons, 1983). The pressure increases progressively with each successive pass along the muscle. A milking movement from the distal to proximal end of the muscle goes over the trigger point at the rate of about 1 in. (2.5 cm) every 3 s. As the effects of the technique become apparent, the taut band relaxes, the trigger point nodule softens, and the area ceases to be tender and no longer refers pain.

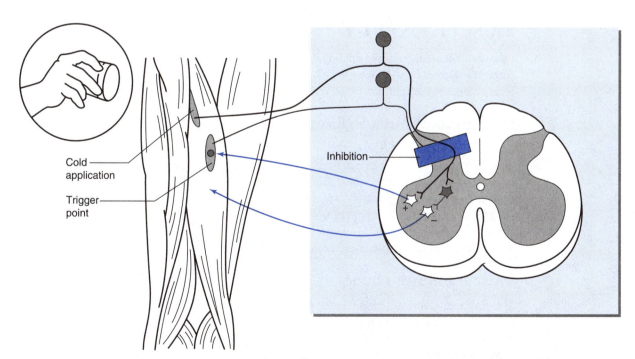

Cold application

Trigger point

Inhibition

▶ **Figure 6.15** Effect of trigger point release on neural pathways: The sudden cold and touch afferent stimulation facilitates a presynaptic inhibition to "close the gate" to pain transmission. The cooling sensation moves along the faster beta fiber to reduce pain and reduce spasm via the autonomic reflex system.

A myofascial trigger point is an area of tenderness in a muscle or its fascia that can cause referred pain and is palpated as a taut band with a nodule. Ice stroking, ischemic compression, stripping, and PNF are techniques often used to treat trigger points.

The ischemia produced by the pressure of the ischemic compression or stripping massage techniques is believed to cause a reflexive hyperemia that returns the site to a normal condition (J.G. Travell & Simons, 1983).

Proprioceptive Neuromuscular Facilitation

The PNF techniques of contract-relax and reciprocal inhibition, which were introduced in chapter 5 and are discussed further in chapter 7, are also effective when combined with soft tissue mobilization in relaxing myofascial trigger points (Godges, Mattson-Bell, Thorpe, & Shah, 2003). In addition, various other techniques are used in the treatment of myofascial trigger points. Modalities such as hot packs, ultrasound, and electrical stimulation are also frequently used as adjuncts to enhance the effectiveness of treatments.

Precautions

Before application, an accurate history should be taken and the patient's condition assessed to determine whether trigger point therapy will be effective. Trigger point therapy is not as effective on scar tissue adhesions as on myofascial restrictions.

The patient should relax for optimal treatment results. The stretch applied should be passive without any contraction of the agonist. If the patient is able to isolate the antagonist, and if you can monitor the patient's response, contraction of the antagonist may improve treatment results, as long as the stretched muscle remains relaxed. Cold is not as effective if it is applied too quickly or repetitively over the same area. The stretch should be applied slowly and should not cause painful spasm or prevent the patient from relaxing, but it should be sufficient to produce the desired results.

The cause of the myofascial trigger point must be corrected for the treatment to be successful, particularly if the cause is poor posture or chronic stress of the muscle. In these cases, the cause is corrected with flexibility and strengthening exercises and patient education and instruction.

Prolonged direct pressure over nerves and blood vessels should be avoided. Ischemic compression pressure should not be used if the patient complains of tingling or numbness.

MUSCLE ENERGY

Like many manual therapy techniques, muscle energy techniques have their origin in osteopathic medicine. Fred Mitchell, DO, originally developed muscle energy techniques that others have since modified.

Definition of Muscle Energy

According to Greenman (Greenman, 1996), "muscle energy is a manual technique that involves the voluntary contraction of a muscle in a precisely controlled direction, at varying levels of intensity, against a distinct counterforce" applied by the clinician. Essentially, muscle energy is the use of muscle contraction to correct a joint's malalignment. Muscle energy is a direct or an indirect technique, depending on which muscle is activated to produce a treatment result. When it is a direct technique, it is not usually as aggressive as the trigger point techniques of Travell and Simons, so it is more comfortable for the patient.

Muscle Energy Theory

Muscle energy theory is based on the premise that joint malalignments occur when the body becomes unbalanced. Malalignment may be the result of a muscle spasm, a weakened muscle overpowered by a stronger muscle, or restricted mobility. The muscle contraction used to correct a malalignment may be **isometric, concentric,** or **eccentric.** The patient controls the magnitude of contraction, and the clinician positions the patient and provides the resistance to change the treated joint's alignment.

In malalignments, movement is restricted by what Mitchell (Mitchell, 1958) identifies as a barrier. A **barrier** is not the end of the existing range of motion, but a resistance that is felt when a part is moved through its passive range of motion. For example, you can passively move the leg of a patient with a tight hamstring in a straight leg raise. Although the hip may be able to go through its full motion, you will feel a resistance because of tightness in the hamstring at some point before the end of its motion. Where in the motion this resistance is felt depends on how tight the hamstring is.

Isometric muscle contraction is most commonly used when treating the spine with muscle energy techniques, whereas isotonic or isometric contractions are used in the extremities. Briefly reviewing muscle physiology principles can help you understand how muscle energy techniques work. When the patient contracts a muscle against an external resistance, the contracting muscle causes the neurological response of reciprocal inhibition. In other words, the contracting muscle causes relaxation of the antagonist and contraction of synergists through responses of Golgi tendon organs and muscle spindles via spinal cord and cortical reflexes. After the isometric contraction, the antagonist relaxes enough to permit a stretch. Its relaxation also impedes its inhibition of the contracting muscle to permit a more normal force-counterforce balance between the agonist and antagonist. Repeated contractions combined with passive stretches then provide additional motion gains and improved muscle balance.

It is believed that these muscle contractions and changes in muscle length affect the surrounding fascia and connective tissue (Greenman, 1996). Since the technique is an active one, requiring the active participation of the patient, muscle physiology is affected and can result in post-exercise soreness secondary to metabolic waste build-up and a change in the fascial length. You should warn the patient that muscle soreness may occur and avoid overpowering the patient or overdoing the activity. Because the forces used are relatively low and the techniques involve an active motion and a passive stretch, the only contraindications to muscle energy techniques are recent or nonunion fractures.

Components of Muscle Energy Technique

The components necessary for muscle energy techniques are an accurate determination of the cause and best treatment of the malalignment, a specific joint position, a precise active muscle contraction performed by the patient, an appropriate counterforce produced by the rehabilitation clinician, and an applied stretch force that results in increased motion without pain.

Before you can determine the appropriate muscle energy technique to apply, you must determine through an examination the presence of a malalignment and the cause of the malalignment.

Once you determine that muscle energy would assist in correcting the deficiency, you must determine the most effective position for the muscle energy technique. The patient's injured segment is then positioned at the end of the barrier, and the patient is instructed on the type of muscle contraction desired. While the patient actively contracts the muscle, you apply the appropriate resistive force with the correct direction, duration, and magnitude.

Isometric contractions are used for muscle energy techniques. The force of the isometric output is only about 2 ounces of force. The isometric contraction is not strong but should be sustained. It should be sustained for 5 to 10 s, and the muscle's length does not change.

When an isotonic contraction is used, enough counterforce occurs to allow motion at an even, controlled speed. The muscle contraction should be forceful and through the muscle's full range of motion.

For either an isometric or an isotonic contraction, it is important for you to allow full relaxation of the muscle following the contraction before stretching the segment to a new barrier position. This allows the muscle to enter its refractory period (time of relaxation) following its contraction and achieve optimal stretch results. The technique is repeated three to five times for the best results. The greatest changes occur after three repetitions; clinical observations indicate that more than five repetitions produce little additional benefit.

Muscle energy techniques are used to treat joint malalignments. These techniques involve the precise and controlled voluntary contraction of a muscle against a counterforce provided by the rehabilitation clinician, followed by relaxation and then a passive stretch.

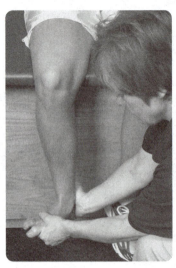

▶ **Figure 6.16** Muscle energy release to gain knee extension: With the lower leg in lateral rotation and the foot in dorsiflexion, the patient rotates the tibia medially while you provide a smooth resistance throughout the full movement. Once the patient relaxes the muscles, the tibia is laterally rotated to its new barrier.

Application

A couple of examples can demonstrate the application of muscle energy techniques. In the first example, an isotonic contraction is illustrated. Let us look at a basketball player who has undergone rehabilitation after an ACL reconstruction. After many varied attempts to attain full motion, she still lacks full extension. You investigate possible alternative methods for relieving the problem:

1. **Assessment of the problem.** You determine that the lack of extension is the result of restricted lateral rotation of the tibia on the femur.

2. **Specific joint position.** The patient sits with the tibias hanging over the table. You position the ankle in dorsiflexion and the leg in lateral rotation to its barrier (figure 6.16).

3. **Precise active contraction by the patient.** The patient contracts the medial hamstring to move the tibia into medial rotation through the full range of motion.

4. **Appropriate counterforce.** While the patient contracts the medial hamstrings to rotate the joint, you offer resistance that permits a smooth, controlled movement into medial rotation for 5 s. Guide the tibia through the correct plane of motion while offering resistance.

5. **Stretch force.** Instruct the patient to relax while holding the distal tibia at its end position, wait to feel the hamstrings fully relax, then apply a stretch into lateral rotation to a new joint position until a new barrier is felt. This technique is repeated three to five times. Re-examine for range-of-motion changes after the final repetition.

In the next example, isometric contractions are used in a muscle energy technique applied to a soccer player who collided with another player and suffered a direct blow to the right anterior ilium. The contusion is resolved, but he continues to complain of groin pain that goes down his right leg. The physician has ruled out a disc injury and reports to you that the problem may be coming from his pelvis. You prepare to evaluate and treat the patient's injury:

1. **Assessment of the problem.** Your examination reveals that there is an inflare of the right ilium. Other tests for lumbar dysfunction have ruled out injury to the low back. You determine that muscle energy techniques would be an appropriate treatment.

2. **Specific joint position.** With the patient lying supine, the right leg is placed in a figure-4 position with the right knee flexed, the hip abducted and flexed, and rotated so the outside of the ankle is placed on the distal left thigh to the barrier point. Stabilize the patient's pelvis by placing your left hand on the left anterior superior iliac spine and the right hand on the patient's medial right knee. Then apply enough pressure on the knee to move the right hip to its end position of lateral rotation.

3. **Precise active contraction by the patient.** Ask the patient to contract isometrically in an attempt to move the leg into medial rotation, pulling the knee toward the left shoulder as you provide resistance to prevent the motion from occurring. The isometric contraction is held for 5 to 10 s.

4. **Appropriate counterforce.** The amount of resistance applied by the patient is not great: two ounces of resistance. Since the contraction is isometric, you must instruct the patient to match your force and not to overpower the resistance you provide (figure 6.17).

5. **Stretch force.** As in the previous example, instruct the patient to relax while you support the extremity at its end position, wait to feel the muscles fully relax, then apply a stretch into lateral rotation and abduction by pushing the right knee toward the table to the new barrier. The process is repeated three to five times. After the final repetition, passively return the leg into hip and knee extension. Re-examine for alignment and pain.

The majority of muscle energy techniques must be accompanied by exercise to effectively treat the problem. You must understand the mechanics of the change that occurs with muscle energy treatment to correctly use accompanying active stretches. As an example, you could instruct the soccer player with the iliac inflare to perform a stretch on his own that is similar to the position used in the treatment. It is also necessary for the patient to progress to strengthening exercises that support the stretching exercises, such as hip lateral rotation and hip abductor strengthening exercises.

Muscle energy will be addressed again in the spine and sacroiliac chapter. In that chapter, specific examination, assessment, and application of muscle energy will be introduced as part of the sacroiliac treatment regimen

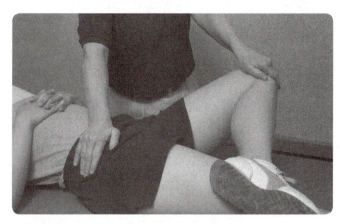

▶ **Figure 6.17** Muscle energy release to correct ilium inflare.

OTHER MANUAL THERAPIES

As has been mentioned, there are many other manual therapy techniques. A few of them will be briefly discussed here.

Strain-Counterstrain

Lawrence Jones, an osteopath, initiated strain-counterstrain (S-CS) during the 1960s after several years of clinical application and technique modifications (McPartland & Goodridge, 1997). Strain-counterstrain was first called "spontaneous release by positioning" and later, "positional release." It is an indirect soft tissue treatment technique because the dysfunctional segment is placed in a position of ease rather than into the restricted movement pattern (Lewis & Flynn, 2001).

Theory

The goal of Dr. Jones' strain-counterstrain treatments was to relieve what he called "tender points." These points are small areas of tenderness that are located in subcutaneous, muscle, tendon, ligament, or fascial tissue (Mesequer, Fernández-de-las-Peñas, Navarro-Poza, Rodríguez-Blanco, & Gandia, 2006). Like trigger points in Travell and Simons' (J.G. Travell & Simons, 1983) descriptions, they are areas of local tenderness, but unlike trigger points, they do not evoke any referred pain, do not have a taut band, and do not produce autonomic reactions (Mesequer et al., 2006). Some clinicians feel that tender points, trigger points, and acupuncture points are all similar and occur because of trauma or dysfunction (D'Ambrogio & Roth, 1997). The goal of each of the therapies that address these differently labeled points all aim to reduce tissue tenderness and thereby improve the patient's condition (D'Ambrogio & Roth, 1997).

Dr. Jones theorized that myofascial tender points, created by body dysfunctions, caused incorrect neural output from muscle spindles and resulted in pain at the tender point sites. By placing the segment in a position of ease, the affected muscle spindles relax. A slow return to a normal position from the position of comfort prevents the muscle spindle reflex from recurring so pain is relieved (Stone, 2000). Related to these tender points are other tender points. Some of them may be in the local area and others may be remote to it. Most tender areas are located in tissues that undergo mechanical stress, most notably, those undergoing increased postural demands (D'Ambrogio & Roth, 1997). The clinician must find these tender areas and treat them for all pain to be relieved. Dr. Jones spent several years creating a mapping of tender points throughout the body and identifying the positions required to ease them (Jones, Kusunose, & Goering, 1995).

The "mobile point" is the position into which the patient is passively positioned and is the point of maximum ease; this is a position where any change in position from it produces an increased tissue tension that can be palpated by the clinician (Lewis & Flynn, 2001).

Treatment Principles

An assessment of the patient is required prior to a S-CS treatment application. The patient's history reveals problems that may have caused the somatic (body) dysfunction. Factors such as prolonged sitting in poor posture, an acute injury, or a leg length difference may be the source of dysfunction. The clinician identifies this source of somatic dysfunction and locates the tender points associated with the problem. Once these factors are identified, the clinician finds the mobile point and passively places the patient in that position. While maintaining the patient in this mobile point, the clinician applies a mild pressure on the tender point. The mobile point and mild pressure over the tender point are held for up to 90 s. When the treatment is completed, the patient slowly returns to an upright posture.

Fine-tuning the position of either the mobile point or the tender point pressure is sometimes required for an effective treatment. Other treatment regimens to keep in mind can also improve efficacy. These factors include identifying and treating the most sensitive tender points first; treating more proximal tender points before more distal ones; and when tender points are in rows, treat the middle ones before the peripheral ones (Stone, 2000).

There are research investigations of S-CS techniques and applications that have been published. Unfortunately, most of them are case studies that deal with pain reduction or range of motion gains in isolated subjects. Additionally, these studies do not produce experimental results but are more reflective of anecdotal reports (Wong & Schauer, 2004).

Strain-counterstrain is not a manual therapy in which proficiency comes quickly. Dr. Jones did not feel an individual became proficient with strain-counterstrain techniques until he or she had practiced 8 hours a day for two years (Stone, 2000).

Rolfing

Ida P. Rolf, an American with a PhD in biochemistry, lived during the first half of the 20th century when women with doctorates in the sciences were rare. She developed an interest in homeopathic medicine while on a leave of absence from her work and studying mathematics and atomic physics in Switzerland. Her interest and work evolved into what she referred to as "structural integration." By the middle of the 1900s, her treatment techniques became known worldwide. She eventually opened a school in Boulder, Colorado, The Rolf Institute; there are now five institutes around the world teaching what is now known as Rolfing. The technique that became known as Rolfing intertwined Dr. Rolf's observations, knowledge, and exposure to a range of topics beyond biochemistry including osteopathic manipulation and yoga control of body motion.

Theory

Dr. Rolf based her techniques on the realization that fascia surrounded all tissue and body structures, so it also influenced those tissues and structures when it was modified. She observed that the body centered around a vertical line of pull created by gravity. It was her theory that the body was most efficient and healthy when it was able to function in an aligned and balanced arrangement. With gravity's continuing pull, stresses and injuries occur to pull the body out of its normal alignment; imbalance occurs and causes the body to become painful, malaligned, and inefficient. Dr. Rolf's intent in her philosophy and techniques was to improve the body's posture so all functions including breathing, flexibility, strength, and coordination were optimally efficient.

Gravity and the body have a constant relationship. The body is in constant battle with gravity, and unless the body is optimally conditioned, gravity is the victor. Factors such as fatigue, injury, age, and body configuration are factors that encourage the body to develop an imbalance and lose its war with gravity. Dr. Rolf was a strong believer in the intimacy between form and function. If the body is to perform its normal functions, then it must have an appropriate form within which to perform its functions (Smith, 2005). The goals of Rolfing are to align the body's large anatomical segments, the head, neck, shoulders, trunk, pelvis, and legs, in line with gravity and to integrate each of those segments with each other in both structure and function (Bernau-Eigen, 1998). Dr. Rolf believed that integrating these segments would also better influence function of the mental, emotional, and spiritual aspects of an individual (Bernau-Eigen, 1998).

Finally, Dr. Rolf based her treatments on the notion that her treatment interventions were required in a specific series of events, and once a change in the body's structure occurred, changes in other arenas such as metabolism, emotion, psychology, and function would follow (Smith, 2005).

Treatment Principles

The treatment techniques of Structural Integration include ten sessions, each one focusing on a central theme, goals, and a sequence of structural interventions (Smith, 2005). The ten sessions are divided into three categories, sleeve sessions, core sessions, and integrating sessions.

The goals of the treatments are to balance and realign the body in all planes. If these goals are accomplished, pain is resolved, imbalance is no longer an issue, and the body performs most efficiently. The first three of the ten sessions are the sleeve and include, in order of sequence, sessions on respiration, balance through the legs and feet, and sagittal balance. The second group of sessions, the core sessions, include base of the core (midline of the legs), abdomen (psoas for pelvic balance), sacrum (weight transfer from head to feet), and the relationship of the head to the rest of the body (primarily the occiput–atlas relationship, then to the rest of the body). The final sessions are the integrating sessions and include two sessions on balance between the upper and lower girdles and a final session on balance throughout the whole system.

Goals for each session are different and progressive (Bernau-Eigen, 1998):

Session 1: Release the fascial layer below the skin's surface

Session 2: Free up and reorganize fascial planes in the feet and legs

Session 3: Reorganize the lateral alignment, using this session as a transition between superficial and deep fascial layer treatments

Session 4, 5, 6: Release the deep fascia closest to the spine and balance the pelvis and back structures

Session 7: Balance head and neck

Session 8, 9, 10: These are the integrative sessions where superficial, middle, and deep fascial layers are worked with and integrated.

Dr. Rolf thought that since gravity tends to shorten fascia, Rolfing techniques should lengthen fascia. Once an evaluation is completed to identify the shortened segments, part of the Rolfing technique involves application of firm strokes with gentle pressure to affect fascial restrictions. This procedure is sometimes identified as "mildly uncomfortable" (Molinary, 2006). Other Rolfing strategies include active stretches and instruction in proper realignment of body segments by enhancing awareness of bad movement patterns, imbalances, and providing instructions on ways to make changes and improve. Changes vary within individuals but common changes include a sense of increased height; improved general well-being; greater strength, flexibility, and coordination; increased energy levels; and enhanced confidence.

JOINT MOBILIZATION

Joint **mobilization** is one of the most commonly used manual therapy techniques in the treatment of restricted joint motion. **Manipulation** and mobilization are not new concepts. Hippocrates (460–355 B.C.) used these techniques in his medical practice and recorded various methods of manipulating bones and joints. In the modern age, chiropractors are most noted for commonly using manipulation techniques in their practices.

Through the years, a variety of approaches to manipulation and mobilization have been developed. More recent schools of thought have been influenced by the teachings of manual clinicians such as Geoffrey Maitland (Maitland, 1991), Freddy Kaltenborn (Kaltenborn, 2002), James Cyriax (Cyriax, 1982), James Mennell (Mennell, 1964), and Stanley Paris (Paris & Patla, 1988). Table 6.1 identifies the main distinctions of each of these manual clinicians' approaches.

Definition of Joint Mobilization

Joint mobilization is on a continuum with manipulation. They both involve passive movement of a joint, but mobilization is under the patient's control in that voluntary contraction of a muscle will stop the movement. Manipulation is at such a speed that the patient is unable to stop the passive motion produced by the clinician. Mobilization is frequently performed by rehabilitation clinicians, but manipulation is not. Manipulation is most commonly performed in chiropractic applications, and is beyond the scope of this book.

Joint Motion

There are two types of joint motion: physiological and accessory. **Physiological joint motion** is movement that the patient can do voluntarily, such as flexion and abduction. **Accessory motion** is necessary for normal joint motion but cannot be voluntarily performed or controlled.

There are two types of accessory motion: joint play and component motion. Both component motion and joint play are necessary for full motion. Component motions are not capsular,

TABLE 6.1 Manual Therapy Schools of Thought

Sources	Key distinction
James Cyriax (Cyriax, 1982)	Uses selective tension techniques to identify faulty structures in the examination. Emphasizes the need for soft-tissue massage and frequently uses injection of muscle trigger points. Believes the disc is the primary source of low-back pain and uses nonspecific spinal techniques designed to move the disc to relieve nerve root pressure.
Freddy Kaltenborn (Kaltenborn, 2002)	Arthrokinematics. The techniques incorporate the influence of muscle function and soft-tissue changes in the manifestation of the patient's loss of function. The techniques are eclectic and very specific.
Geoffrey Maitland (Maitland, 1991)	Uses primarily passive accessory movements to restore function after an extensive assessment based on information from the patient's subjective examination (history) and the evaluator's objective assessment. The movements are oscillations, the techniques are specific, and the goal is to relieve what he terms "reproducible signs."
James Mennell (Mennell, 1964)	Feels that "joint play" is key to normal joint function. Emphasizes the importance of the small accessory movements as necessary for full joint motion to occur. Techniques are more specific for the extremities than for the spine.
Stanley Paris (Paris & Patla, 1988)	Incorporates both chiropractic and osteopathic orientations in his eclectic approach to normalization of arthrokinematics, especially joint play and component motions. As a general rule, the patient's pain is not used to guide treatment.

but they accompany physiological motion. The rotation of the clavicle during shoulder flexion is an example of a component motion. Joint play occurs within the joint and is determined by the joint capsule's laxity. If you grasp and twist a finger, you can feel the joint play of the metacarpophalangeal joint.

Arthrokinematics

Arthrokinematics refers to the motions between the bones that form a joint. There are five types of arthrokinematic motion that occur within a joint: roll, slide, spin, compression, and distraction. These motions permit greater motion of a joint and can occur only with appropriate joint play. This concept is vital to understanding how joint mobilization works and how it can be applied.

Most joint surfaces are concave, convex, or both. Joints that have one concave and one convex surface are called *ovoid* (figure 6.18a). Joints that have a surface that is concave in one direction and convex in another with the opposing surface convex and concave in complementary directions are called *sellar* or *saddle joints* because of their similarity to a saddle (figure 6.18b). The shape of the joint determines its arthrokinematic motions.

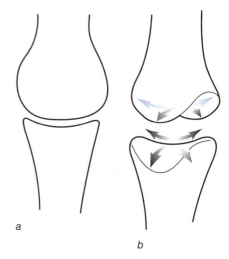

▶ **Figure 6.18** Joint surfaces of *(a)* ovoid and *(b)* sellar joints.

Roll

Roll occurs between joint surfaces when a new point of one surface meets a new point of the opposing surface (figure 6.19). Rolling occurs with sliding or spinning in a normal joint. Roll occurs in the direction of bone movement.

Slide

Slide occurs between joint surfaces when one point of one surface contacts new points on the opposing surface (figure 6.20). Like rolling, sliding does not usually occur by itself in normal joints. When a passive mobilization technique is applied to produce a slide in a joint, the technique is referred to as a glide. The more congruent a joint is, the better it responds to gliding mobilization techniques to gain mobility. Slide and roll occur together, sometimes moving in the same direction, and sometimes moving in opposite directions, depending on the joint's configuration and which joint surface is moving.

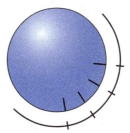

▶ **Figure 6.19** Roll: different points on one surface come in contact with different points on the second surface.

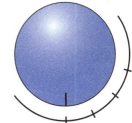

▶ **Figure 6.20** Slide: one point on a surface comes in contact with different points on a second surface.

Spin

Spin occurs in a joint when one bone rotates around a stationary axis (figure 6.21). Like roll and slide, spin does not occur by itself during normal joint motion.

Compression

Compression is a decrease in the space between two joint surfaces (figure 6.22). Compression adds stability to a joint and is a normal reaction of a joint to muscle contraction. During roll, some compression occurs on the side in the direction of the motion.

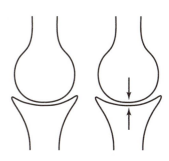

▶ **Figure 6.22** Compression.

Distraction

Distraction of a joint occurs when the two surfaces are pulled apart (figure 6.23). A gentle distraction can relieve pain in a tender joint. Distraction is often used in combination with joint accessory mobilization techniques to further stretch the capsule.

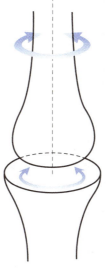

▶ **Figure 6.21** Spin: a segment rotates about a stationary mechanical axis.

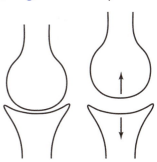

▶ **Figure 6.23** Distraction.

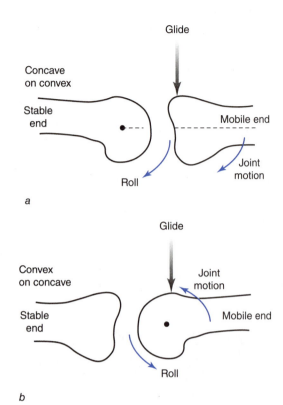

▶ **Figure 6.24** Rules for concave and convex joint surfaces. *(a)* Concave-convex rule: Joint mobilization glide force is applied in same direction of bone motion. *(b)* Convex-concave rule: Joint mobilization glide force is applied in the opposite direction of bone motion.

Concave and Convex Rules

Knowing which type of joint is being treated and keeping in mind the concave and convex rules (figure 6.24) is basic to the application of correct mobilization techniques. In these rules, one joint surface is mobile, and the other is stable. The concave-convex rule states that concave joint surfaces slide in the same direction as the bone movement (figure 6.24). The convex-concave rule states that convex joint surfaces slide in the opposite direction of the bone movement. For example, if the thigh is stabilized to prevent the femur from moving at the knee, the tibia's concave joint surface slides posteriorly when the tibia moves posteriorly from extension to flexion. In contrast, if the glenoid is stabilized at the shoulder, the convex humeral head surface slides inferiorly as the humerus is moved superiorly into abduction. In other words, if you want to increase knee flexion, your mobilization force on the tibia is in an anterior-to-posterior (AP) direction. If you want to increase knee extension, you apply a posterior-to-anterior (PA) mobilization force. On the other hand, when mobilizing a convex surface such as the humeral head of the shoulder, if you want to increase shoulder flexion, you apply an AP force, and to increase extension you apply a PA force.

Capsular Patterns of Motion

As discussed in chapter 5, all joints have expected, or normal, ranges of motion, and various problems can prevent normal motion. When loss of motion results from tightness within the joint capsule, specific characteristic changes occur in the joint's pattern of motion loss and are referred to as a **capsular pattern.** Table 6.2 indicates the capsular pattern for most joints. When you examine a joint's range of motion, knowing both the joint's normal degree of motion and the typical pattern of capsular restriction is crucial. When a capsular pattern is present, full joint motion will not be attained until the capsular tightness is treated. A capsular pattern indicates that at least some of the loss of motion is due for a joint mobilization treatment program. A non-capsular pattern indicates that structures other than the capsule are preventing normal motion, so joint mobilization may not be necessary.

Effects of Joint Mobilization

Of the manual therapies, joint mobilization has had the greatest amount of scientific evidence of its efficacy in recent years. Studies performed on patients with spine (Flynn, Wainner, & Fritz, 2006), lower extremity (Konradsen, Holmer, & Sondergaard, 1991; van der Wees et al., 2006), and upper extremity (Johnson, Godges, Zimmerman, & Ounanian, 2007) demonstrate the beneficial effects of joint mobilization. Additionally, many clinicians anecdotally report consistent, positive results from their treatments. Although the reason for these benefits is yet to be verified, it is presumed that beneficial biochemical, biophysiological, or biomechanical alterations are produced by joint mobilization techniques.

Neurophysiological Effects

Although there is no evidence to demonstrate how joint mobilization relieves pain, anecdotal evidence indicates that it does. One theory is that joint mobilization facilitates the gait-control mechanism (Vicenzino, Collins, Benson, & Wright, 1998). Small-amplitude joint mobilization oscillations stimulate the mechanoreceptors that inhibit the transmission of nociceptive stimulation from the spinal cord and brain stem. Small-amplitude and mild joint mobilization oscillations also affect muscle spasm and muscle guarding (Brander & Stulberg, 2006). Inhibition of nociceptive stimulation results in relaxation.

TABLE 6.2 Capsular Patterns

Joints	Capsular pattern
Glenohumeral	Lateral rotation is more limited than abduction. Abduction is more limited than medial rotation.
Elbow	Flexion is more limited than extension.
Forearm	Supination and pronation are equally limited at the proximal radioulnar joint. Pronation and supination are equally limited at the distal radioulnar joint.
Wrist	Flexion and extension are equally limited.
Finger	Abduction is more limited than adduction of the thumb CMC. Flexion is more limited than extension of the MCPs and IPs.
Hip	Medial rotation is more limited than flexion. Flexion is more limited than abduction. Extension and abduction are equally limited. Generally, no limitation of lateral rotation.
Knee	Flexion is more limited than extension.
Ankle	
Talocrural	Plantar flexion is more limited than dorsiflexion.
Subtalar	Inversion is more limited than eversion.
Foot and toes	
1st MTP	Extension is more limited than flexion.
2nd-5th MTP	Variable.
IP joint	Extension is more limited than flexion.
Lumbar spine	If a left facet is limited: Forward bending (FB) produces a deviation to the left. Side bending right (SBR) is limited. Side bending left (SBL) is unrestricted. Rotation left (RL) is limited. Rotation right (RR) is unrestricted.
Cervical spine	If a left facet is limited: FB produces some deviation to the left. SBR is unrestricted. SBL is comparatively unrestricted. RL is comparatively unrestricted. RR is most limited.

CMC = carpometacarpal; MCP = metacarpophalangeal; IP = interphalangeal; MTP = metatarsophalangeal.

Nutritional Effects

Distraction or small gliding movements can cause synovial fluid to move within the joint (Yoder, 1990). The avascular articular cartilage within a joint depends on synovial fluid movement for its nutritional needs and nutrient-waste exchange. In edematous and painful joints, these movements can improve nutrient exchange to prevent deleterious effects of joint swelling and immobilization.

Mechanical Effects

More aggressive mobilization techniques can improve the mobility of hypomobile joints (Michlovitz, Harris, & Watkins, 2004). Immobilized joints that have lost their normal range of motion develop collagenous adhesions and thickened connective tissue. Mobilization techniques that stretch collagen structures into their plastic range of deformation increase the tissue's mobility and improve the joint's motion (Maitland, 1991). Mobilization not only stretches capsular tissues but also effectively loosens or breaks down adhesions to improve mobility (Kaltenborn, 2002).

Cavitations

Occasionally, a mobilization or joint movement produces a cracking sound. The sound is called "cavitation" (Unsworth, Dowson, & Wright, 1971). When tension is produced in a synovial joint, increased pressure within the joint causes a vaporization of gas within the synovial fluid. When the gas is liberated as the gas bubble forms then collapses, the joint space expands. The collapse of the gas bubble causes the noise (Corrigan & Maitland, 1989). It takes about a half-hour for the gas to be reabsorbed into the synovium; until then, the joint cannot be cracked again (Unsworth et al., 1971). Initial reports indicated that the gas formed was nitrogen, but it is now believed to be carbon dioxide.

Following this cracking, joint mobility often increases. This is believed to occur because of the expansion of the joint capsule from the increased pressure and the reflex relaxation of surrounding muscles through stimulation of inhibitory mechanoreceptors (Paris & Patla, 1988). This increased joint mobility can be advantageous or disadvantageous. It is advantageous for hypomobile joints. For hypermobile joints, a reduction of muscle tone along with an increase in joint laxity can lead to increased joint stress and pain; the muscles reflexively tighten and cause additional discomfort. Although "cracking" one's back or neck may offer temporary relief, Paris and Patla (Paris & Patla, 1988) believe that such joint cracking may increase the risk of spinal disc injury. When cracking occurs repeatedly in the spine, the joints become unstable. Conversely, when it occurs repeatedly in the extremities, as when cracking the knuckles, the joint capsule eventually becomes thickened and increases the joint's stiffness.

Application of Joint Mobilization

Before you apply joint mobilization, you must identify the forces and excursions that can and should occur as well as what is considered "normal" for a joint and the individual. These issues are discussed in the following sections.

Grades of Movement

According to Maitland (Maitland, 1991), movements used in joint mobilization are divided into four grades, indicated I, II, III, and IV. Manipulation uses grade V. The grading is based on the amplitude of the movement and where within the available range of motion the force is applied. Grades I and IV are small-amplitude movements performed at the beginning and end of the range, respectively. Grades II and III are large-amplitude movements. Grade II movement does not reach the limits of the range, whereas grade III movement is performed up to the limit of the available range. These grades overlap somewhat, as seen in figure 6.25. Grade V is the manipulation grade and is a small amplitude thrust beyond the end range of a joint's restriction.

The amount of motion within each grade is relative to the specific joint and to the available motion within that joint. For example, a normal glenohumeral joint has larger grade I, II, III, and IV movements than a severely restricted glenohumeral joint and certainly larger movement than a normal metacarpophalangeal joint.

Grades I and II are used to relieve joint pain. Oscillations in these grades stimulate joint mechanoreceptors to inhibit nociceptive feedback into the joints (Maitland, 1991). These grades often are also used before and after treatment with grades III and IV, beforehand to

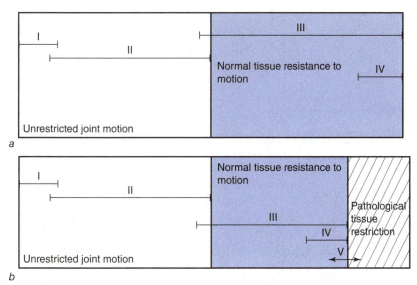

a

b

▶ **Figure 6.25** Grades of movement in a normal and a restricted joint: Grades I and II do not reach the limits of movement. Grades III and IV do reach the limits of movement. Grades I and IV are small amplitude, while grades II and III are large amplitude.

Adapted from G. Maitland, 1991, *Peripheral manipulation,* 3rd ed. (Woburn, MA: Butterworth-Heinemann).

relax the joint and afterward to relieve discomfort that the more aggressive grades may have caused.

Grades III and IV are used to gain joint motion. These grades stretch the capsule and connective-tissue structures that limit joint mobility (Maitland, 1991). They can be uncomfortable but are not necessarily so.

Oscillatory motions are frequently used with the various grades of movement. However, sustained joint-play motions can also be used. The sustained techniques involve only three grades: I, II, and III. Their grade definitions are slightly different from those of oscillatory motions: Grade II goes to the end point of resistance, and grade III is essentially a stretch of the joint, going toward a normal joint's limit (figure 6.26). The techniques discussed here use the oscillatory motions, since they are the most common.

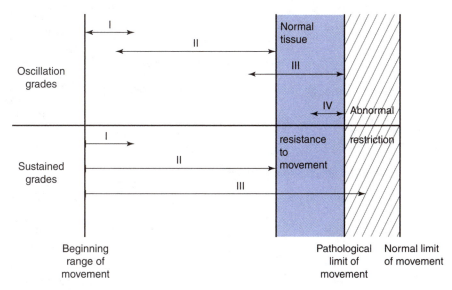

▶ **Figure 6.26** Sustained versus oscillation mobilization.

Movement Diagram

A movement diagram is a visual aid that can sometimes be helpful in determining which mobilization grade to use in a treatment. Either physiological or accessory movements can be diagrammed. A movement diagram is shown in figure 6.27. **AN** is the normal range of motion of a joint; **A** is the beginning of motion, and **N** is the normal limit of a motion. **L** is the abnormal limit of motion. **H** indicates a joint's hypermobile range. **B** is the intensity of a treatment technique.

Key

A = Beginning of movement
N = Normal limit of ROM
L = Abnormal limit of ROM
H = Hypermobile range
B = Intensity

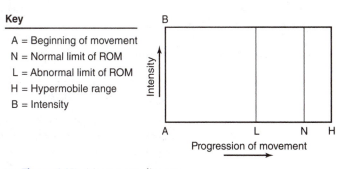

▶ **Figure 6.27** Movement diagram.

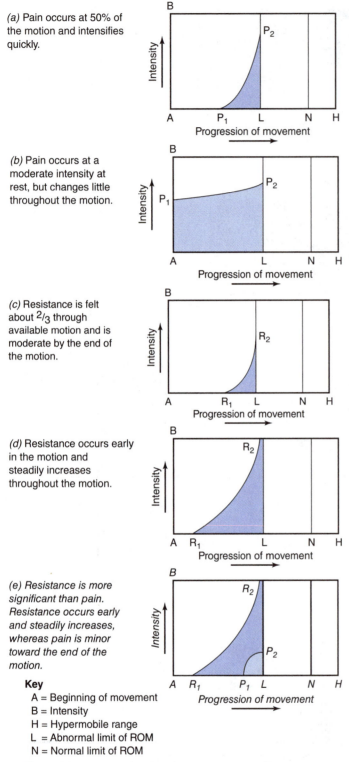

(a) Pain occurs at 50% of the motion and intensifies quickly.

(b) Pain occurs at a moderate intensity at rest, but changes little throughout the motion.

(c) Resistance is felt about 2/3 through available motion and is moderate by the end of the motion.

(d) Resistance occurs early in the motion and steadily increases throughout the motion.

(e) Resistance is more significant than pain. Resistance occurs early and steadily increases, whereas pain is minor toward the end of the motion.

Key
A = Beginning of movement
B = Intensity
H = Hypermobile range
L = Abnormal limit of ROM
N = Normal limit of ROM

▶ **Figure 6.28** Pain and resistance on movement diagrams.

You mark on the movement diagram where the patient reports pain. P in figure 6.28 represents where within the range of motion the patient reports pain and the intensity of the pain; P_1 indicates where the pain starts, and the P line is drawn according to the patient's description of changes in the pain throughout the motion. P_2 is the intensity of pain at the end of motion. R_1 indicates where you first feel resistance during a passive movement of the joint, and R_2 is the intensity of the resistance at the end of the motion. The path of R is drawn to reflect the resistance changes as you move the joint through its motion. If the patient has pain at rest before your assessment begins, the P curve begins at A and is placed at a height on the vertical scale (AB) that corresponds to the intensity of pain reported by the patient. If the pain is mild, the mark is placed low on the AB line; if pain is moderate, the mark is placed higher (figure 6.28b). If the patient reports the start of pain at 50% of possible motion, P_1 is placed at the midpoint of the AL line (figure 6.28a). If the pain occurs gradually but progressively over the length of the motion, a gradually sloping upward line is drawn, but if pain begins suddenly and quickly intensifies, a steep line is used.

To determine where R is drawn, you passively move the joint through its available accessory range and indicate on the graph where the start of the restriction can be palpated. If the restriction begins abruptly and provides a rapidly progressive restriction of motion, a steep, rapidly climbing line is drawn. If restriction is more gradual, a line with a gentler slope is drawn.

Once you complete a movement diagram, you can easily assess the treatment needs and determine whether to attend to the patient's pain or to joint restriction first. If the pain is not significant, you may choose to treat the restriction first, but if pain appears more intense and increases more quickly than resistance on the movement diagram, pain should be addressed before restriction is treated.

Until you understand joint mobilization techniques, mobilization grades, and develop the skill to palpate and evaluate pain and resistance, it is a good idea to draw a movement diagram on paper or in your head. It will help you determine what you need to treat first and what grades of mobilization are most appropriate.

Normal Joint Mobility

Determining normal and abnormal joint mobility requires practice and familiarity with the patient. Because joint mobilization is a manual therapy, you must develop your sense of touch so that you can detect what is normal for any particular joint. This is done only through practice on normal subjects. Once normal mobility is identified, abnormal mobility is easier to recognize. Additionally, mobility that is normal for a glenohumeral joint is not normal for a wrist joint.

Normal mobility also varies for different populations and depends on factors such as age, disease, occupation, sport, and position in a sport. For example, a 40-year-old man will not have the same normal lumbar spine mobility as his 15-year-old son has. Even though they may both have normal vertebral mobility, what is considered normal for the father is not normal for the son. Age plays a role in determining normal joint mobility.

Athletes from different sports also demonstrate various degrees of normal joint mobility. For this reason, it is important to compare the joint being treated with the contralateral side to assist in determining normal mobility for that individual. For example, a baseball pitcher may have a hypermobile anterior glenohumeral joint when compared with a football lineman. A ballet dancer may have a hypermobile hip compared with a shot-putter. You must consider the specific needs and demands of a sport or activity and even of a position within the sport when determining an individual's normal joint mobility.

Close-Packed and Loose-Packed Positions

The relative position of the joint surfaces must be considered prior to applying joint mobilization techniques. In a **close-packed position,** the joint surfaces are most congruent with each other (table 6.3, p. 185). The convex surface of one bone is at its maximum congruence with the opposing concave surface of the other bone. The ligaments and capsule are taut, and the joint surfaces cannot be easily separated with traction. Joints are not usually mobilized in a close-packed position, but this position can be used to stabilize an adjacent joint before applying mobilization forces to another joint. For example, if you want to mobilize a proximal interphalangeal joint, the metacarpophalangeal joint can be positioned in full flexion, its close-packed position, to stabilize the proximal segment.

A **loose-packed position** is any position that is not close packed. The articular surfaces are not completely congruent, and some portions of the capsule are lax. Examinations and early mobilization techniques are both performed with a joint in its maximum loose-packed position. This position is a joint's **resting position.** See table 6.3 for a list of resting and close-packed positions for the joints. As a rule, extremes of joint motion are close-packed positions, and midrange positions are loose-packed positions.

Indications

There are two main indications for the use of joint mobilization techniques. The first is joint pain. Grade I and II oscillations relieve pain (Maitland, 1991). The other indication is a hypomobile joint, which is determined by a capsular pattern of joint motion and less mobility than the contralateral joint. Grades III and IV improve joint mobility(Maitland, 1991).

Precautions and Contraindications

Absolute contraindications to joint mobilization grades III and IV include hypermobile joints, malignancy, tuberculosis, osteomyelitis, osteoporosis, recent fracture, ligamentous rupture, and herniated discs with nerve compression. Joint effusion is a contraindication, since the capsule is already swollen from the extra fluid in the joint. Grade I and II mobilizations may be used to relieve pain, but grade III and IV techniques are avoided for these conditions. The rehabilitation clinician's skill ability and the individual patient's specific situation determine relative contraindications. Relative contraindications are also precautions and include osteoarthritis, pregnancy, flu, total joint replacement, severe scoliosis, poor general health, and a patient's inability to relax. Precautions should also be taken when treating hypermobile joints using the pain-relieving grades. If you doubt whether to use joint mobilization, err on the side of caution and refrain from its use.

Joint mobilization involves passive movement of a joint to relieve pain or restore mobility. Proper application requires knowledge of joint mechanics, normal range of motion, and proper technique.

Rules for Application of Joint Mobilization Treatments

As with other manual therapy techniques, you should understand the following rules before applying the techniques and use them as guidelines for all joint mobilization treatments:

1. The patient should be relaxed.

2. Before application, explain to the patient the purpose of the treatment and what sensations to expect.

3. Joint physiological and accessory mobility are assessed before and after the treatment. It may be necessary to check accessory mobility at various points within the physiological range.

4. Compare the joint to be treated with the contralateral joint to determine what is normal for the patient.

5. Determine treatment goals before treatment.

6. Grades I and II are used to relieve pain. Grades III and IV are used to increase mobility.

7. Stop the treatment if it is too painful for the patient.

8. Initial mobilization is performed in a resting position.

9. One segment, usually the proximal joint segment, is stabilized, while the other is mobilized.

10. Your hands should be as close to the joint as possible.

11. The larger the surface area of contact, the more comfortable the force application for the patient. When you use the entire hand, the fingers should be together, and as much of the finger and palm surface as possible should contact the patient's extremity.

12. Always use good body mechanics, and use gravity to assist the mobilization technique whenever possible.

13. The direction of the mobilization force is either parallel or perpendicular to the treatment plane. The treatment plane lies on the concave articulating surface, perpendicular to a line from the center of the convex articulating surface (figure 6.29). Traction is applied perpendicular to the treatment plane, and gliding is applied parallel to it. The treatment plane can change with a change in a joint's position. Carefully determine the joint's treatment plane before application.

14. Always apply the concave-convex and convex-concave rules when determining in which direction to apply the mobilization force.

15. Emphasize one plane of motion at a time, although more than one plane may be treated in a session.

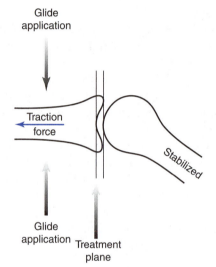

▶ **Figure 6.29** Direction of force application. The application is either perpendicular or parallel to the treatment plane.

16. The patient's response determines the selection of oscillating or sustained techniques. Oscillation is used more often than sustained techniques for pain relief. Gains in range of motion can be achieved by either oscillation or sustained techniques.

17. The patient's comfort and tolerance determine the duration of treatment. Oscillation techniques should be applied smoothly and regularly at the rate of two to three oscillations per second and should be repeated for 1 to 2 min for pain and 20 to 60 s for tightness. Sustained techniques are applied for only about 10 s in painful joints and repeated several times between bouts of rest. For tightness, sustained techniques are held for 10 to 30 s, depending on the patient's tolerance, and repeated three to five times.

18. Begin and end mobilization treatments for increasing range of motion with grade I or II distraction oscillations to facilitate relaxation at the start of treatment and relieve pain following treatment.

19. Progression is individually determined by the patient's response to the treatment. You must assess the patient's response to treatment in terms of pain, changes in joint mobility and range of motion, and the patient's psychological reaction to determine whether changes in the mobilization techniques are warranted. Progression can involve increasing the length of the treatment, increasing the grade if treating a hypomobile joint, or changing the joint to a less loosely packed position.

20. Mobilization techniques to improve motion should be accompanied by therapeutic exercise to reinforce the gains made with the manual treatment. Flexibility exercises after joint mobilization help to reinforce the gains made with mobilization.

TABLE 6.3 Resting and Close-Packed Joint Positions

Joints	Resting	Close packed
Fingers and thumb		
Metacarpophalangeal	1: Mid-flexion/ext & mid-abduction/add	1: Full opposition
	2-5: 20° flexion	2-5: Full flexion
Interphalangeal	20° flexion	Full extension
Wrist	0°	Full flexion or full extension
Forearm		
Proximal Radioulnar	70° elbow flexion with 35° supination	Full pronation or full supination
Distal Radioulnar	10° supination	Full pronation or full supination
Elbow		
Humeroulnar	70° elbow flexion with 10° supination	Full extension, forearm supination
Humeroradial	Full elbow extension with full supination	90° flexion, 5° supination
Shoulder girdle		
Glenohumeral	55° flexion with 20°-30° horizontal abduction	Full abduction with full lateral rotation
Sternoclavicular	Relaxed arm at side	Full shoulder elevation
Acromioclavicular	Relaxed arm at side	90° shoulder abduction
Hip	30° flexion, 30° abduction with slight lateral rotation	Full extension, medial rotation, and abduction
Knee		
Tibiofemoral	20°-30° flexion	Full knee extension with tibial lateral rotation
Patellofemoral	Full knee extension	Knee flexion
Tibiofibular	10° plantar flexion	Full dorsiflexion
Ankle and midfoot		
Talocrural	10° plantar flexion	Full dorsiflexion
Subtalar and midtarsal	Midrange of inversion and eversion	Full inversion
Forefoot and toes		
Metatarsophalangeal 1	20° dorsiflexion	Full dorsiflexion
Metatarsophalangeal 2-5	20° plantar flexion	Full dorsiflexion
Interphalangeal	20° plantar flexion	Full dorsiflexion

NEURAL MOBILIZATION

Of all the manual therapy techniques, neural mobilization is the most dangerous and must be used with care and precision. The rehabilitation clinician must not take its use lightly. Neural mobilization is discussed here so that you can be aware of its proper use and possible consequences.

Fascial Connection

Like the myofascial system, the neural system is continuous throughout the body. It too is surrounded with fascia and can be affected by direct and indirect injuries to fascia and adjacent tissues. The effects of neural injury, like those of fascial injury, can refer to distant areas. The referred pain of neural injuries is different from myofascial pain referral patterns, however.

Afferent System

Referred pain from nerve-tissue injury follows the neural pathways and is described as tingling or burning. It can also jump from one area to another or progress along a neural pathway. The type of pain the patient reports is related to the nerve fiber carrying the impulse. Peripheral afferent nerve fibers that carry painful signals are called nociceptive fibers. The stimuli that activate pain fibers include mechanical forces, chemical irritants, and hot or cold temperatures. The A-delta and C fibers respond to pain stimuli that result in a pain-reflex withdrawal. They are myelinated afferent fibers that are excited by a mild mechanical stimulus. The A-alpha afferents are high-threshold mechanoreceptors that can also respond to temperature stimuli. The A-delta fibers are stimulated in sudden injuries, such as an ankle or knee sprain. About 75% of peripheral pain receptors are C fibers and respond to both mechanical and chemical stimuli. They can also spark the release of histamine through their excitation of mast cells and action as vasodilators. An insect bite, for example, can cause this activity. C fibers are also stimulated by swelling and stiffness and cause the aching sensation that occurs with these conditions. C fibers and A-delta fibers both respond to inflammation.

Once these fibers enter the dorsal horn of the spinal cord, many connections to both inhibitory and excitatory neurons are possible. The impulse can travel up the spinal cord to the thalamus and cortex. Stimulation of the cortex registers conscious pain sensation. Stimulation of the midbrain produces an inhibitory response through the release of endogenous analgesics (pain relievers that the body produces). Normal neural tissue does not refer pain at rest or during normal movement or activity. Pathological conditions, however, can produce referral patterns both proximally and distally from the site of pathology. This pain-referral pattern is referred to by Butler (Butler, 1994) as pathoneurodynamics. The source of **pathoneurodynamics** can be either intraneural or extraneural, coming from injury either to the nerve itself or to the surrounding tissue that interacts with the nerve. In either situation, the physiology and mechanics of the nerve can be disrupted.

Susceptible Sites

Given that the nervous system, like the fascia system, is in intimate contact with other tissues throughout the body, it makes sense that when an area suffers an injury, neural tissue may also be affected. Certain nerves are susceptible to injury because of their location or pathway. Butler (Butler, 1991) has identified these five susceptible sites:

1. In soft tissue or bony tunnels. A good example of this is the median nerve as it passes through the carpal tunnel at the wrist.

2. Abrupt neural branches, particularly in areas where the nerve's ability to move within the surrounding structures is limited. For example, the common plantar digital nerve in the web space between the third and fourth toes has limited movement, is formed from an abrupt junction of the lateral and medial plantar nerves, and is a common site for Morton's neuroma.

3. In areas where the nerves are relatively fixed. The common peroneal nerve as it traverses around the fibular head is an example of a relatively fixed nerve with little mobility.

4. High-friction areas where nerves are close to unyielding interfaces. Two examples are the nerves passing through the plantar fascia in the foot and the brachial plexus passing over the first rib.

5. Tension points, such as the tibial nerve in the popliteal fossa, where abnormal stress can be placed on the nerve.

Previous Trauma

Previous trauma can predispose an area to neural symptoms later. Like all other tissue, nervous tissue is surrounded by layers of fascia that serve to support and supply nutrients to the nerves. If a nerve is injured, it undergoes the healing process discussed in chapter 2. Scar tissue forms as a result of healing by the nerve, its surrounding fascia, and any other structures involved in the injury. Scarring binds down the nerve to affect its neurobiomechanics and neurophysiology.

Even an injury not directly involving neural tissue can affect the nervous system. Locally damaged blood vessels and ensuing edema can cause neural changes. The nervous system is very dependent on a continuous blood flow for survival and for functioning. Although the nervous system constitutes only 2% of the body's mass, it uses 20% of the circulating blood's oxygen supply (Dommisse, 1975). Because nerve tissue has no means of storing reserves, if a nerve's blood supply is interrupted, damage to the nerve tissue can result from a lack of adequate oxygen and nutrients.

Either edema or vascular insufficiency causes nerve tissue damage, and nerve damage results in connective tissue fibrosis. A tethering effect on the nerve by the restriction of the scar tissue can reduce the flexibility and mobility of the neural tissue. Ultimately, symptoms of abnormal neural tension can occur in locations along the nervous system other than the site of injury. According to Butler (Butler, 1991), this transpires because the mechanical alterations in one nerve location can alter tissue tension throughout the nervous system, impaired neural stimulation at one site can affect the entire neuron, mechanical changes from an injury are accompanied by vascular changes, and an abnormal nerve impulse can cause abnormal neural firing elsewhere in the nervous system.

Double-Crush Syndrome

The condition in which an injury at one site produces signs and symptoms at another site is sometimes referred to as the **double-crush syndrome** or phenomenon (Upton & McComas, 1973). An example of this is carpal tunnel syndrome. In some cases of carpal tunnel syndrome, the cause is actually a neural lesion in the cervical spine. This neural source should be ruled out, especially in cases of bilateral carpal tunnel syndrome. In patients who have a history of cervical injury and present with complaints of elbow or wrist pain bilaterally or unilaterally, a double-crush syndrome should be ruled out. Likewise, if a patient complains of bilateral shin splints or foot pain, you should investigate prior low-back injury and suspect a possible central lesion. Multiple-crush syndromes can be seen in patients who report more than one area of pain. For example, a patient who has a history of neck injury and reports mid-thoracic, elbow, and wrist pain should be evaluated for a multiple-crush phenomenon.

The term *crush* is a misnomer, since the injury is not necessarily a crush injury. The syndrome is actually caused by scarring and fibrosis, restricted blood flow, alterations in neural stimulation, or some combination of these. This pathology progressively increases pressure and friction on the nerve until symptoms distal to the site of origin occur.

Symptom Profile

Although a patient may use many unique adjectives to describe neural pain, it is usually described as a deep, burning, aching, or heavy sensation. It can occur along the nerve's pathway, jump from one area to another, or clump around joints or tension areas. It can be constant or intermittent, although a constant pain is more indicative of inflammation or compressive pathology. Sometimes the pain is worse at night, and sometimes it is worse at the end of the day.

Pain that occurs because of local neural ischemia is sharp or knifelike. Ischemia-related pain lessens with easy motion and worsens with overuse. Sometimes an inflammation can cause a sharp pain, but it generally presents as an ache at the end of the day with stiffness in the morning or after prolonged inactivity. An inflammation-based pain feels better with gentle activity and worse with rest.

A good history of injuries and evaluation of the location and patterns of pain can help detect the source of the patient's pain. The following types of pain should be examined for neural origins: pain that occurs in susceptible neural-tissue areas, such as the carpal tunnel and fibular head; symptoms that do not match the common pain patterns; and pain that follows a dermatome, or sensory-nerve distribution.

Treatment

Treatment can be either direct or indirect. Direct treatment techniques are the same as those used in the examination of neural tissue. Indirect treatment techniques can be as simple as changing posture and often involve altering a soft-tissue structure, which affects the nerve. A hamstring stretch can affect the sciatic nerve, and a cervical stretch can affect the brachial plexus.

There are several different direct neural mobilization techniques. Only a few of the more common ones are discussed here. Before these techniques are presented, however, you should understand that neural mobilization is not a common treatment and should be used only as a last resort. Any neural technique can easily injure the patient, so extreme caution must always be used in deciding whether and when to apply the technique and in applying the treatment. It is impossible to overstate this point. Even the most experienced rehabilitation clinicians use neural mobilization only after all other modes of treatment have failed and only when benefit to the patient from its application is strongly indicated. Precautions and contraindications are discussed later in this chapter.

Techniques

There are seven basic neural tension tests: one for the spine, three for the lower extremity, and three for the upper extremity. The spine test is passive neck flexion (PNF). The lower-extremity tests include straight-leg raise (SLR), slump test, and prone knee bend (PKB). The upper-limb tension tests are ULTT1, 2a, 2b, and 3. The lower-extremity tests assess the sciatic and femoral nerves, while the upper-extremity tests assess the median, radial, and ulnar nerves, respectively. These test procedures are also used as treatment techniques. You must accurately apply the mobilization technique and assess for symptoms, responses, range of motion, and resistance before and after the treatment. All these techniques can be applied either proximally to distally or vice versa. The direction of application may produce varying results, depending on the location and cause of the irritation or restriction. The positions described here are based on and described in detail by Butler (Butler, 1991). His text and courses are recommended for readers who have an interest in pursuing neural mobilization techniques.

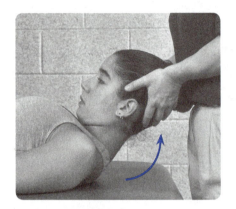

▶ **Figure 6.30** In passive neck flexion the patient's head is supported as the neck is passively flexed.

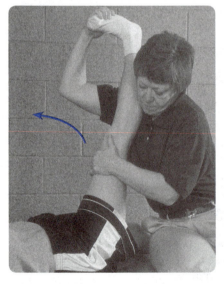

▶ **Figure 6.31** Straight-leg raise: Tension is applied to the sciatic nerve. With the knee extended, additional neural stress can be applied with ankle dorsiflexion, hip adduction and internal rotation, and neck flexion.

Passive Neck Flexion

PNF can be used by itself or along with the lower-limb or upper-limb tests. PNF is performed with the patient either sitting or lying supine. In the supine position, the patient does not use a pillow. The patient initiates the motion by lifting the head off the table (figure 6.30). The rehabilitation clinician places his or her hands under the head to support it and moves the neck into flexion while the patient remains relaxed.

Straight-Leg Raise

Straight-leg raise (SLR) is sometimes referred to as Leseague's test or Lazarevic's test. The patient lies supine without a pillow, and the rehabilitation clinician places one hand on the foot and the other on the quadriceps just proximal to the patella. The extremity is lifted by the hand on the foot, while the hand on the quadriceps keeps the knee from flexing. If enough flexibility is present, the patient's leg may be placed on the rehabilitation clinician's shoulder (figure 6.31). Neural tension may be increased in the SLR with the addition of passive ankle dorsiflexion, ankle plantar flexion with inversion, hip adduction, hip medial rotation, or passive neck flexion, individually or in combination.

Prone Knee Bend

Prone knee bend (PKB) is similar to a quadriceps stretch. With the patient prone and the head turned to the side being treated, the rehabilitation clinician grasps the leg above the ankle and flexes the knee, moving the heel toward the buttock while maintaining slight hip extension (figure 6.32). PKB is used to examine or treat anterior thigh and groin pain.

Slump Test

The slump test should not be used on patients who have an irritable disorder. With the patient sitting on a table in a slumped or sagging position and the hands behind the low back, the rehabilitation clinician applies pressure to the shoulders to bow the spine without changing the hip position. The patient then brings the chin down to the chest, and the rehabilitation clinician applies slight overpressure to the head (figure 6.33a). The patient then

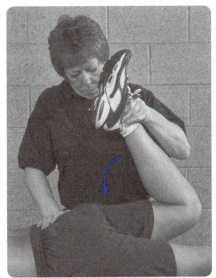

▶ **Figure 6.32** Prone knee bend: Tension is applied to the femoral nerve with passive hip extension and knee flexion.

extends one knee and follows this motion with ankle dorsiflexion while keeping the knee extended (figure 6.33b). Neck flexion pressure is released slowly. This technique must be applied with extreme caution; because of its forceful application, it is used as a test, not a treatment. It assesses the response of the nervous system to treatment. If the patient reports symptoms before the entire technique is applied, it is not necessary to go through the full procedure. This procedure is not recommended for patients with a suspected disc injury.

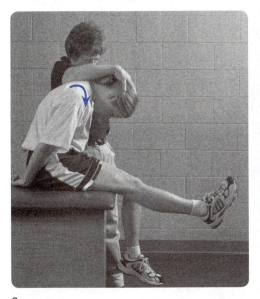
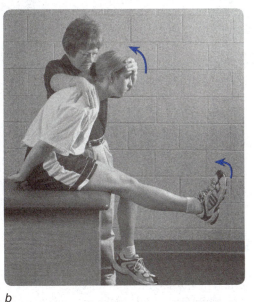

a   b

▶ **Figure 6.33** Slump test: (a) The shoulders are passively pushed downward to bow the spine and the chin is brought to the chest. While in this position, one knee is extended with the ankle dorsiflexed. (b) Maintaining is lower limb position, the neck pressure is slowly released.

Upper-Limb Tension Test 1

ULTT1, also known as the brachial plexus tension test or Elvey's test, is used to test the median nerve and to treat symptoms in the thoracic spine, neck, and arm. The patient should have full range of motion of the entire upper extremity and neck and should not have an irritable disorder. The patient lies supine; if treating the left upper extremity, you hold the patient's left hand with your right and place the patient's left upper arm along your left thigh. Place your left hand on top of the patient's shoulder and apply a stabilization force on the shoulder girdle to prevent elevation throughout the treatment (figure 6.34a). Then, abduct the patient's arm to about 110° while keeping it in contact with your thigh (figure 6.34b). Laterally rotate the patient's shoulder, then supinate the forearm, and extend the wrist, thumb and fingers, and elbow, in that order (figure 6.34c). The patient then actively flexes the neck laterally away from the left side.

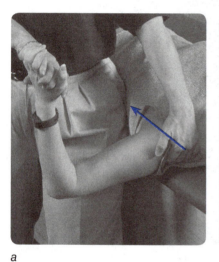
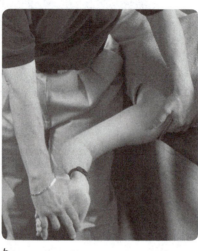
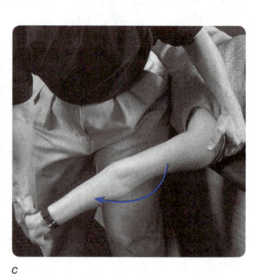

a b c

▶ **Figure 6.34** Upper-limb tension test 1 for the median nerve.

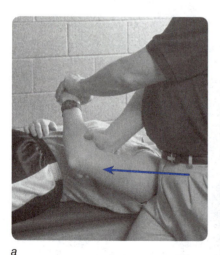
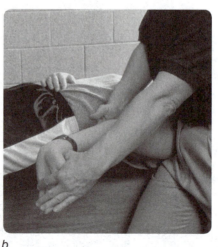

a b

▶ **Figure 6.35** Upper-limb tension test 2a for the median nerve.

Upper-Limb Tension Test 2a

Because shoulder girdle depression has such a significant impact on the brachial plexus, this position was developed by Butler (Butler, 1991). He feels that ULTT2a is a more effective position than ULTT1. If the left arm is being treated, the patient lies on a slight diagonal on the table, with the head toward the left side and the left scapula off the table. You stand at the top of the patient's shoulder with your right thigh against the patient's shoulder. Your right hand holds the patient's elbow and the left hand crosses over to hold the wrist. Your thigh depresses the patient's shoulder girdle (figure 6.35a). Bring the patient's arm to about 10° of shoulder abduction, extend the elbow, and laterally rotate the arm. Slide your right hand down to the patient's hand and extend the patient's wrist, fingers, and thumb (figure 6.35b).

Upper-Limb Tension Test 2b

ULTT2b tests the radial nerve and treats cervical, thoracic, and upper-extremity disorders, especially those involving the radial nerve. The patient and rehabilitation clinician are positioned as for ULTT2a. The hand placement, shoulder girdle position, and elbow extension are the same (figure 6.36a). You then medially rotate the patient's shoulder, pronate the forearm, and after moving your left hand to the patient's hand, flex and ulnarly deviate the patient's wrist and flex the patient's fingers and thumb (figure 6.36b).

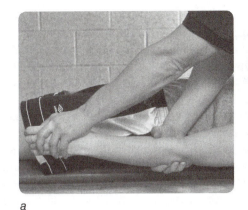 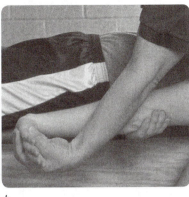

a   b

▶ **Figure 6.36** Upper-limb tension test 2b for the radial nerve.

Upper-Limb Tension Test 3

ULTT3 tests the ulnar nerve and treats ulnar-nerve restrictions. To treat the right shoulder, the patient is supine and you as the rehabilitation clinician stand on the patient's right side facing the patient's right shoulder with the patient's right shoulder girdle depressed and the patient's right arm resting on your right thigh (figure 6.37a). Laterally rotate the patient's shoulder, then abduct the shoulder, flex the elbow, extend the wrist, and extend the fourth and fifth fingers (figure 6.37b). The patient can additionally actively flex the neck laterally away from the arm being treated.

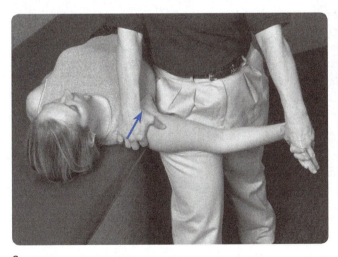 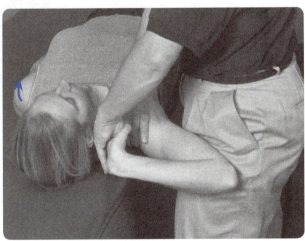

a   b

▶ **Figure 6.37** Upper-limb tension test 3 for the ulnar nerve.

Application

Tension tests should be performed before all neural mobilization treatments to determine the appropriate force to apply during treatment. Pre-treatment and post-treatment tension tests should be used to assess the patient's symptom response and the resistance of the tissue. Symptom responses include pain, numbness, and tingling; the rehabilitation clinician must know when and where in the motion these symptoms may occur to avoid them during the treatment. Identifying where tissue resistance occurs determines the extent of application for the mobilization technique and helps the clinician evaluate the treatment results.

Neural mobilization is used to treat non-irritable conditions. These conditions are likely to have pathomechanical causes with secondary fibrosis, connective-tissue adhesions, and restriction of normal tissue mobility. Neural mobilization techniques to treat these conditions enter into the resistance range of grade III and IV motions, but you should still try to avoid pain. As a rule, grade III motions produce less pain than grade IV. Throughout the treatment, the patient's symptoms must be monitored. Initial treatment should not cause or increase symptoms. A constant dull ache and sensations of pins and needles should be avoided. The patient should be relaxed throughout the treatment.

The duration, amplitude, and number of repetitions can be changed as the treatment progresses and the patient responds positively to treatment. A sequence of slow oscillations can last 20 to 30 s, followed by a reassessment of the patient's condition. A sustained movement should be released if symptoms occur and should last no longer than 10 seconds, even without symptoms. Sustained movement and oscillations can be repeated a number of times as the treatment progresses so that the treatment lasts for several minutes. As treatments progress, the amplitude can also be increased until some symptoms are produced, although the minimal force that achieves a positive response is all that is necessary. Complementary techniques, including muscle energy, myofascial mobilization, cross-friction massage, and neural self-mobilization, can also be added to the program.

Self-Mobilization

If neural mobilization techniques provide positive results, it may be beneficial for the patient to perform self-treatment techniques as part of a home exercise program. Along with these techniques, the patient's rehabilitation program should include therapeutic exercises and corrective techniques that resolve the problem's precipitating factors.

Self-mobilization techniques for the lower extremities are easier to apply than those for the upper extremities. One of the more difficult tasks in self-mobilization of the upper limb is maintaining scapular depression during the activity. Specific instructions on correct application and proper sequencing given to the patient ensure the best results. It is important that the patient demonstrate proper execution of the technique to the rehabilitation clinician before he or she attempts the technique without supervision. Figure 6.38 demonstrates lower- and upper-extremity self-mobilization tension techniques.

Precautions

Again, neural mobilization techniques should be applied only as a last resort after other treatment techniques have been unsuccessful. Continual feedback from the patient about the area's response to the treatment is required. Avoid reproduction of painful symptoms, especially numbness and tingling sensations. The slump test and the upper-limb tension tests are complex maneuvers that involve many structures and, therefore, require consistent care and discretion. It is much easier to irritate upper-limb nerves than lower-limb nerves, because the upper-limb nerves are smaller and traverse more complicated paths around bones and through muscles than those of the lower limbs.

A worsening disorder, indicated by increased symptoms, is an indication to stop the technique. Always apply treatment carefully and err on the side of caution if there are any doubts about the treatment.

Diabetes, AIDS, and other systemic diseases can weaken the nervous system. Take extra care when applying neural mobilization techniques to patients with these conditions.

Whereas the circulatory system closely follows the nervous system throughout the body, take care with individuals who have circulatory system disturbances. Remember that if a nerve is mobilized, the circulatory structure next to it is also mobilized.

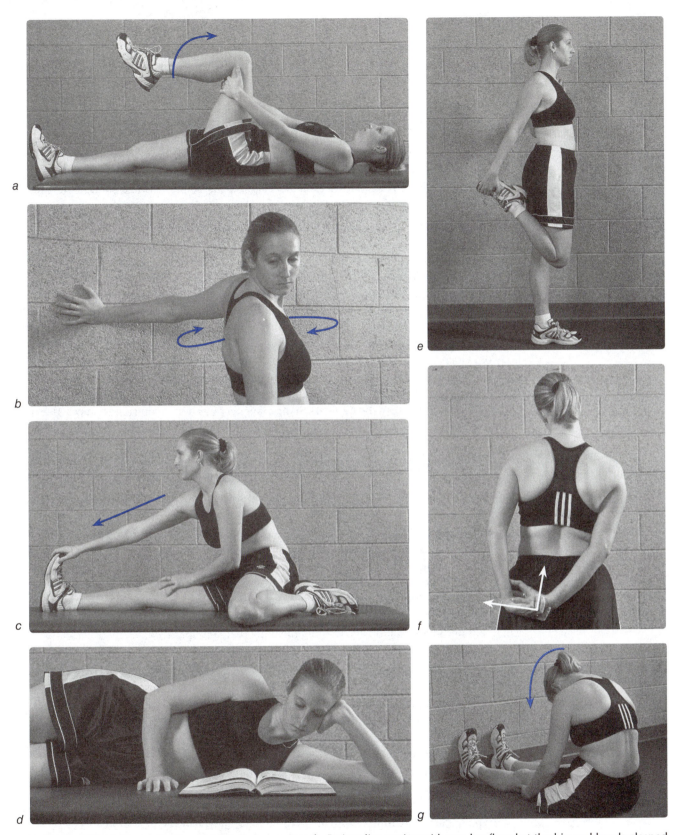

▶ **Figure 6.38** Self-mobilization. *(a)* Sciatic nerve stretch: Patient lies supine with one leg flexed at the hip and hands clasped behind the thigh. In this position, the lower leg is raised into a straight-leg position. *(b)* Brachial plexus stretch (median nerve): Patient places the hand on the wall at shoulder level with the elbow straight. Maintaining the hand flat on the wall, the patient rolls away from the hand. *(c)* Combined straight-leg raise and prone knee bend stretch: Patient assumes a seated hurdler's stretch position with one leg flexed behind and the other extended in front. The patient reaches forward toward the foot. *(d)* Ulnar nerve stretch: Sidelying, the patient supports the head with the hand. The elbow is flexed and elevated above the shoulder. *(e)* Femoral nerve stretch: Standing, the patient flexes the knee and grasps the foot behind the buttock. *(f)* Radial nerve stretch: With both hands behind the back and the elbows straight, the uninvolved hand grasps the involved hand and passively moves the wrist into extension and pulls the arm across the body. *(g)* Slump: With feet positioned in neutral against a wall, the patient sits with knees extended and slumps the shoulders, moving the chin to the chest.

Neural mobilization should be used with extreme caution and only as a last resort when other treatment techniques have failed.

Contraindications

Contraindications to neural mobilization include malignancies of the nervous system or vertebral column, acute inflammatory infections, areas of instability, and spinal cord injuries. Suspected disc lesions, cauda equina lesions (suggested by changes in bowel or bladder function or changes in perineal sensations), dizziness related to vertebral artery insufficiencies, and any central nervous system disorder, such as spina bifida or multiple sclerosis, are also contraindications. Worsening neurological signs are another important contraindication.

SUMMARY

A clinician who uses his or her hands to affect tissue is performing manual therapy. There are many different kinds of manual therapy that affect different tissues and structures. Only a few manual therapy techniques were presented in this chapter: massage, general myofascial release techniques, trigger point treatments, joint mobilization, and neural mobilization. Other alternative therapy techniques were briefly introduced. Although the evidence that demonstrates the effectiveness of manual therapy techniques remains sparse, it is a growing body of evidence, especially in the arena of joint mobilization where objective measures are more easily made than for some of the other manual techniques. Each of these techniques has precautions, indications, and contraindications the clinician must respect. Each technique also has a specific method of application which the clinician must both understand and practice in order to become proficient at utilizing these techniques to affect a patient's outcome.

KEY CONCEPTS AND REVIEW

1. Discuss the three techniques of massage and their indications, precautions, and contraindications.

The primary massage techniques used in rehabilitation include effleurage, or stroking; pétrissage, or kneading; and friction. They relieve pain, relax muscles, reduce swelling, and mobilize adherent scar tissue. Massage should be avoided in the presence of infection, malignancies, skin diseases, blood clots, and any irritations or lesions that may spread with direct contact. Precautions include clean hands and body surface to be treated, explaining the procedure before application, removing jewelry that may interfere with the application, using warm hands and massage medium, and draping the body part appropriately.

2. Explain the progression of myofascial restriction after an injury.

Myofascial restriction occurs following an injury as scar tissue forms and adhesions occur between the newly formed tissue and adjacent structures. Immobilization following an injury can also lead to myofascial restriction and loss of tissue mobility.

3. Discuss the techniques for myofascial release.

The primary techniques for myofascial release include J-stroke, oscillation, wringing, stripping, and arm or leg pull.

4. Explain the theory of the mechanism of myofascial trigger points.

The theory of myofascial trigger points is that a damaged sarcoplasmic reticulum interferes with normal muscle fiber activity. The calcium of the damaged sarcoplasmic reticulum stimulates the sarcomere to produce a sustained contraction as long as ATP is present. The sustained contraction no longer needs an action potential to continue, as long as the calcium and ATP are present together. Ischemic-causing substances also make afferent nerve endings hyperirritable to mediate referred pain, autonomic response, and motor-neuron response.

5. Discuss the ice (spray)-and-stretch trigger point release theory.

According to the gate theory of pain, the sudden, brief application of cold inhibits the pain-spasm cycle and provides muscle relaxation and pain relief, especially when accompanied by a stretch.

6. Explain the concave-convex and convex-concave rules.

Joint mobilization techniques are based on these rules. The concave-convex rule states that concave joint surfaces slide in the same direction as the bone movement, and the convex-concave rule states that convex joint surfaces slide in the opposite direction of the bone movement.

7. Define joint mobilization grades of movement.

Movements in joint mobilization are divided into four grades. Grade I is small-amplitude movement in the beginning range of motion, grade II is large-amplitude movement in the middle of the non-restricted range of motion, grade III is large-amplitude movement to the restricted range of motion, and grade IV is small-amplitude movement to the restricted range of motion.

8. Discuss the direction of glide and traction in relation to the treatment plane.

Glide movements during mobilization should be parallel to the treatment plane, and traction is perpendicular to the treatment plane.

9. Explain the double-crush syndrome.

A double-crush syndrome occurs when an injury at one site produces signs and symptoms at another site, so although a patient reports pain at one area, the actual injury is in another area. For example, patients with neck injuries commonly report pain in the arm.

10. Discuss the dangers of neural mobilization.

Neural mobilization is used very carefully and only as a last resort. Incorrect use can result in nerve injury.

11. Describe one neural self-mobilization technique for the upper extremity and one for the lower extremity.

Examples of neural self-mobilization techniques include the prone knee bend for the femoral nerve, the straight-leg raise for the sciatic nerve, and sidelying on the elbow with the hand on the face for the ulnar nerve.

CRITICAL THINKING QUESTIONS

1. What problem would you suspect if, during a myofascial release treatment, a patient began to sweat and became pale? What steps would you take to relieve the symptoms? Why might this occur?

2. A patient you are treating for a shoulder injury has range-of-motion measurements of 120° flexion, 90° abduction, and 40° lateral rotation. What techniques would you use to improve range of motion? Why? If the patient's motion was 120° flexion, 125° abduction, and 70° lateral rotation, what techniques would you use to improve motion? Why?

3. A patient who had surgery on his ankle three months ago has severe joint and soft-tissue restriction of all motions. There is more loss of plantar flexion than of dorsiflexion, and the soft tissue around the ankle feels very stiff. What techniques would you use to improve motion and why? Which techniques would you emphasize the most and why?

4. You instruct a patient in a straight-leg-raise exercise to stretch the hamstrings and she complains of calf pain when performing it. What are the possible causes of the patient's complaints, and what precautions should you take? What instructions would you provide to relieve the pain?

5. A patient complains of shoulder-blade pain with some arm movements and has head-aches. What are the possible causes of the patient's complaints? What treatments would you initiate, and why would you select those techniques? Would you give the patient any home program, and if so, what would it include?

6. If you were Michael, the athletic trainer in the scenario described at the beginning of this chapter, what techniques would you use to relieve the soft-tissue adhesions of Emilie's forearm? What home activities would you give her to increase soft-tissue mobility on her own?

LAB ACTIVITIES

1. Apply grades I, II, III, and IV to the tibiofemoral joint in anterior-posterior glides on your lab partner. Feel what the relative amounts of force and motion are for each grade. Now apply the same grades to your lab partner's #2 MCP joint. What are the relative amounts of force and motion for this joint? How do they compare with those of the knee joint? Where in the mobility of the joint do you feel the resistance begin?

2. Apply grades I, II, III, and IV to your lab partner's glenohumeral joint. Feel for where the resistance begins. Does it get greater as you move the humerus through the glenoid fossa or does it stay at a relatively same level of resistance throughout the mobilization? How does the amount of mobility for each of the grades compare with those you found in the knee and MCP joints?

3. Apply a posterior–anterior joint mobilization glide on the talocrural joint of each member in your class. Can you feel a difference among the different individuals? How are they different?

4. Actively and passively abduct and adduct the MCP joints in various positions of flexion and extension. Describe the difference in motion available at the joint. Which position would you classify as closed packed and which position would you classify as the resting position?

5. An athlete suffered a fracture of the mid-radius when he was tackled in football three weeks ago. The forearm, wrist, and elbow were in a cast for the past three weeks, but the physician wants you to begin joint mobilizations on him today. What is the purpose of the joint mobilizations? What are you feeling for as you examine the mobility in his elbow and wrist joints? How do you determine whether joint mobilization is appropriate for this patient?

6. Apply myofascial release to your lab partner's back using a J-stroke. What type of injury or fascial restriction would benefit from this technique? Give an example of a condition that would not benefit from this technique but would from another myofascial technique. Why?

7. Apply an oscillation myofascial technique to your lab partner's forearm. What type of injury or fascial restriction would benefit from this technique?

8. Apply a wringing myofascial technique to your lab partner's forearm. What type of injury or fascial restriction would benefit from this technique?

9. Apply a stripping myofascial technique to your lab partner's hamstring. What type of injury or fascial restriction would benefit from this technique?

10. About mid-thigh on the medial aspect you are likely to find trigger points in your lab partner's hamstrings. Locate a trigger point in this area and apply a trigger point pres-

sure technique. How much pressure should you apply? What will be your guidelines in determining the amount of pressure used? Are you able to feel the trigger point relax as you continue to hold the pressure on it? How does this type of manual therapy compare to the myofascial techniques investigated in questions 6-9 above? What kinds of problems would lend themselves to each technique?

11. A patient with rotator cuff repair has had the left arm in a sling for the past 3 weeks. He comes to you today, 3 weeks after the surgery because his physician wants him to begin rehabilitation today. How can you determine if the patient will need manual therapy? How can you determine what type of manual therapy he will need? What kinds of problems would you expect him to have at this stage? What would today's treatment include? What would you avoid doing with him today? How will you know if your techniques are beneficial? Justify each of your answers.

ADDITIONAL SOURCES

Åstrand, P.O., and K. Rodahl. 1977. *Textbook of work physiology.* New York: McGraw-Hill.

Breig, A. 1978. *Adverse mechanical tension in the nervous system.* Stockholm: Almqvist & Wiksell.

Grieve, G.P. 1984. *Mobilisation of the spine.* New York: Churchill Livingstone.

Kenneally, M., Rubenach, H., and R. Elvey. 1988. The upper limb tension test: The SLR of the arm. In *Physical therapy of the cervical and thoracic spine,* ed. R. Grant. New York: Churchill Livingstone.

Lee, D. 1986. Principles and practice of muscle energy and functional techniques. In *Modern manual therapy of the vertebral column,* ed. G. Grieves. New York: Churchill Livingstone.

Mackinnon, S.E. 1992. Double and multiple crush syndromes. *Hand Clinics* 8:369.

Rubin, D. 1981. Myofascial trigger point syndromes: An approach to management. *Archives of Physical Medicine and Rehabilitation* 62:107–110.

Muscle Strength and Endurance

OBJECTIVES

After completing this chapter, you should be able to do the following:

1. Describe the sarcolemma and its function in muscle activity.
2. Identify the elements of a motor unit.
3. Explain how an action potential is transmitted.
4. Explain the characteristic differences between fast-twitch and slow-twitch muscle fibers.
5. Discuss the relationship between muscle strength, endurance, and power.
6. Identify the various types of dynamic activity.
7. Discuss the differences between open and closed kinetic chain activity.
8. Identify the various grades of manual muscle testing.
9. Discuss the grades of muscle activity.
10. List the PNF techniques commonly used in rehabilitation and their purposes.
11. Identify four principles of strengthening exercises.

▶ Now that Matthew Carlson, athletic trainer for the local high school, has achieved good range of motion in Kamryn's knee, he is ready to begin a more aggressive strengthening program. Early in the season, Kamryn injured her right knee during gymnastics practice. She underwent rehabilitation but continued to have difficulties with the knee throughout the season. Three weeks ago she underwent an arthroscopy for a partial meniscectomy.

Matthew wants Kamryn to progress in a good rehabilitation program with effective, efficient, and appropriate strengthening exercises, but he's having difficulty deciding what equipment to use. Fortunately, the high school's booster club has been very generous to his athletic training program and has furnished his athletic training facility with a nice variety of rehabilitation equipment. He wants to do a combination of open and closed kinetic chain activities. Until now, he has used manual resistance and body-weight resistance to provide strengthening activities, but at this point in Kamryn's program, more resistance would be beneficial.

It's what you learn after you know it all that counts.

JOHN WOODEN, basketball coach, 1910–

Coach John Wooden's words are worth considering as you begin reading about a topic that you may think you already know well. Even if you possess a good deal of knowledge, you cannot assume you will know best how to apply that knowledge. As you read this chapter, you will discover that much about muscle strength is yet to be learned. This text does not come close to presenting the body of knowledge available; however, the discussion covers the importance of having muscle strength, the methods of achieving it, and the ways in which rehabilitation clinicians can maximize muscle strength and endurance development in a therapeutic exercise program for injured individuals.

As you read this chapter, keep in mind that many of the concepts presented are not black and white but shades of gray. There is not necessarily a single answer for even simple questions such as *What is the best number of repetitions for increasing muscle endurance?* The "best" answer will emerge through your ability to combine the knowledge you obtain from this text, your coursework information, and your own observation skills and common sense. This combination will enable you to determine your own best answers about what strengthening program will be most effective for each individual patient you rehabilitate.

One can never have too much knowledge. Knowledge leads to understanding, understanding leads to appreciation, appreciation leads to respect, and respect leads to appropriate application. The greater your understanding of the "whys" and "hows," the more effective will be your application of the knowledge you possess.

Accordingly, then, the chapter begins with physiological and biomechanical information to help you achieve a true understanding of the rationale for muscle strengthening techniques. The progressions provided throughout this chapter will provide you with additional skills so that you can design and build your own therapeutic exercise program for any patient, regardless of any obstacles or complications associated with the patient's injury.

MUSCLE STRUCTURE AND FUNCTION

Before you can learn how to affect strength and muscle endurance, you must understand muscle structure and function. Such awareness serves as a foundation for understanding how strength changes occur, why certain techniques are applied, and what procedures will provide the best results.

Structure

Previous chapters have addressed the intimate relationship between connective tissue and other tissue throughout the body. Muscle also contains layers of connective tissue. The outer connective tissue layer covering the entire muscle is the **epimysium;** the layer covering muscle fascicles or groups of fibers is called the **perimysium;** and the connective tissue layer covering each muscle fiber is the **endomysium.** The endomysium is continuous with the muscle fiber's membrane, the **sarcolemma.** This macrostructure of muscle appears in figure 7.1.

As mentioned in previous chapters, a **motor unit** is composed of the nerve, or motor neuron, and the muscle fibers that it innervates (figure 7.2). The number of motor units in any healthy muscle depends on the size and the function of that muscle. For example, in a small muscle that performs primarily finely tuned activities, such as the intrinsic muscles of the hand, the ratio of muscle fibers to neurons is small. Larger muscles used primarily for gross motor activities, such as the gastrocnemius, have a much higher ratio of muscle fibers to neurons. The sidebar on p. 203 provides some examples of average numbers of muscle fibers in motor units of various muscles.

The **sarcomere** is the smallest contractile element of a muscle fiber. The **extrafusal fibers,** or myofibrils, contained within the sarcomere are **actin** and **myosin.** Myosin fibers are the thicker filaments—with diameters about 1/10,000 that of a hair strand (16 nm)—and are surrounded in a hexagonal pattern by smaller actin filaments. A three-dimensional model shows that the myosin filaments form a triangular pattern in relationship to each other—so in a sarcomere there are six actin filaments around each myosin filament and three myosin filaments around one actin filament (figure 7.3).

Within a sarcomere, the actin and myosin are arranged longitudinally from Z-disc to Z-disc, where the actin filaments are anchored on either end of the sarcomere. The myosin filaments are in the equatorial center of the sarcomere and anchored with each other at the M-bridge in the center of the H-band (figure 7.4). The A-band contains myosin and actin filaments, whereas the I-band contains only actin filaments. Because of the myosin filaments, the A-band is darker; the combination of the A-band and the I-band gives skeletal muscle its striped appearance—hence the name, striated muscle.

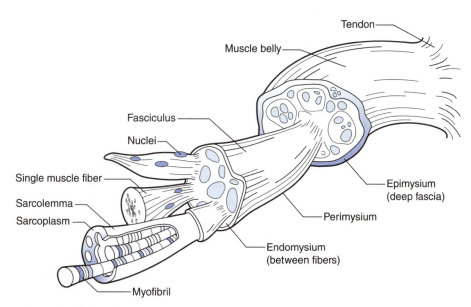

▶ **Figure 7.1** Muscle structure.

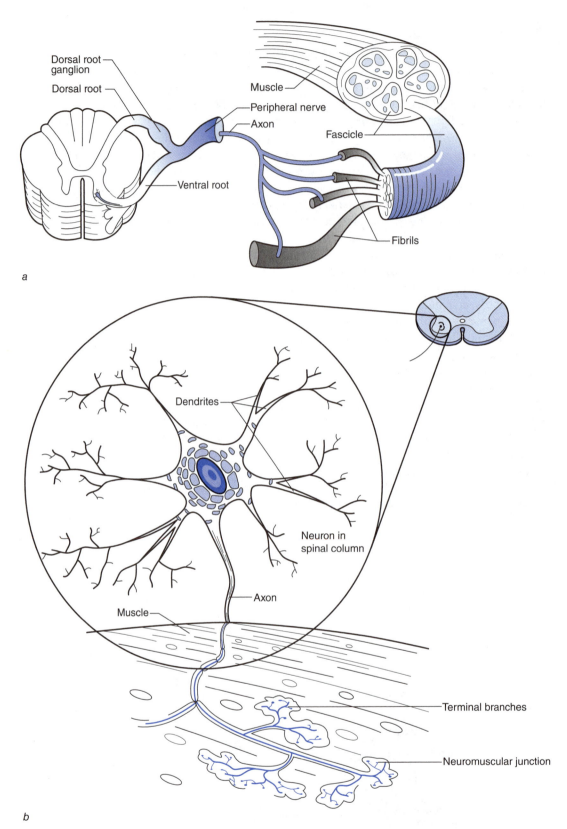

Dorsal root
ganglion

Dorsal root

Ventral root

Muscle

Peripheral nerve

Axon

Fascicle

Fibrils

a

Dendrites

Neuron in
spinal column

Axon

Muscle

Terminal branches

Neuromuscular junction

b

▶ **Figure 7.2** Motor unit: *(a)* schematic drawing of the components of a motor unit—the anterior horn cell, its axon and terminating branches, and the muscle fibers it innervates; *(b)* one neuron from the spinal cord with its axon extending into the muscle. The number of muscle fibers a single motor unit innervates can range from a few to several thousand (R. M. Enoka et al., 2003; Johnson & Wiechers, 1982).

Muscle Fibers in a Motor Unit in Different Skeletal Muscles

The number of muscle fibers in a motor unit varies greatly depending on the size and function of that muscle. Examples of muscles that have a relatively high number of muscle fibers per motor unit include

Medial gastrocnemius, approximately 1600-1900 fibers/unit

Biceps brachii, 750 fibers/unit

Opponens pollicis, 595 fibers/unit

Tibialis anterior, approximately 560-660 fibers/unit

Brachioradialis, more than 410 fibers/unit (Enoka, 1995).

By contrast, the platysma muscle of the neck has only about 25 muscle fibers per motor unit and the tensor tympani muscle of the middle ear has only about eight muscle fibers per motor unit (Enoka, 1995).

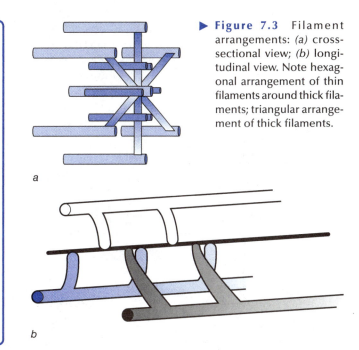

► **Figure 7.3** Filament arrangements: *(a)* cross-sectional view; *(b)* longitudinal view. Note hexagonal arrangement of thin filaments around thick filaments; triangular arrangement of thick filaments.

a

b

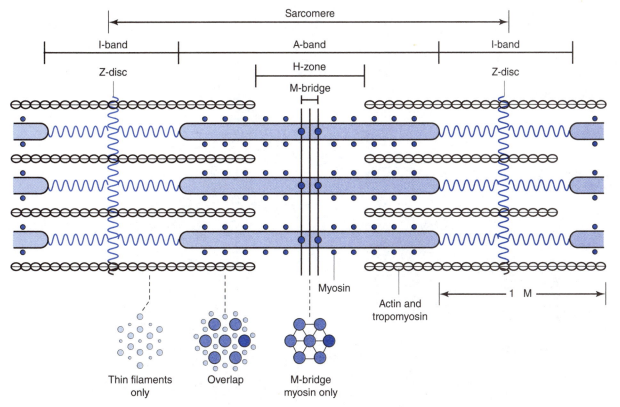

► **Figure 7.4** Longitudinal *(top)* and cross-sectional *(bottom)* diagrams showing the principal elements of the sarcomeric cytoskeleton *(black)* and the thick and thin filaments *(blue)* forming the contractile apparatus.

Function

When a motor unit is stimulated by an excitatory impulse called an **action potential,** the myosin cross-bridges flex and pull the actin filaments toward the center of the sarcomere. During this process, the H-band becomes smaller and the Z-discs move toward the sarcomere's equatorial center to produce a shortening of the sarcomere. The theory that describes this process is the *sliding filament theory*. The sarcomere's length changes because the actin and myosin filaments slide over each other, not because they change length.

When the sarcomere is lengthened, the H-band gets larger; when it shortens, the H-band gets smaller. During lengthening and shortening of the sarcomere, the length of the filaments does not change. Only the relative sizes of the areas of the sarcomere that do not contain myosin (I-band) or actin (H-band) change (figure 7.5).

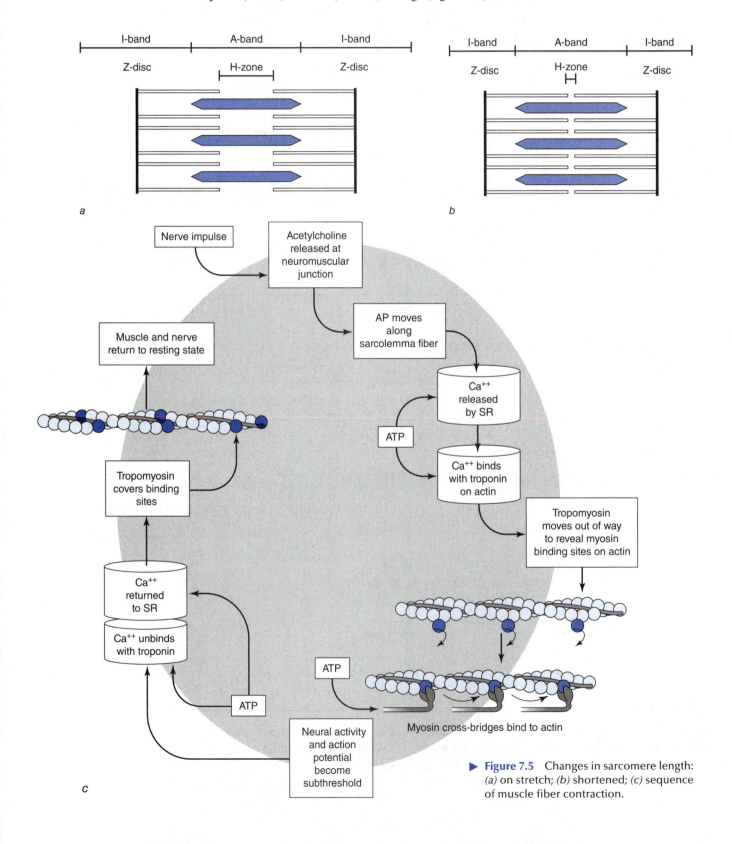

▶ **Figure 7.5** Changes in sarcomere length: (a) on stretch; (b) shortened; (c) sequence of muscle fiber contraction.

The biochemical process that causes this shortening is rather complex and occurs instantaneously. There are two tubular systems vital to the activity of the sarcomere. The **sarcoplasmic reticulum** is an internal tubule system that is arranged parallel to and surrounds the sarcomere in a fishnet mesh arrangement that terminates near the Z-discs. The transverse tubule (T-tubule) system extends into the inner aspects of the fiber to encircle the myofibrils and runs perpendicular to the sarcoplasmic reticulum. The T-tubules terminate near the Z-discs between two sarcoplasmic reticulum tubules in a triad arrangement (figure 7.6).

In addition to the sarcoplasmic reticulum and T-tubules, other elements also are vital in producing a muscle contraction. The cross-bridges of the myosin filaments attach to and detach from the actin filaments via hinge-like mechanisms. This process is regulated by two proteins in actin, **tropomyosin** and **troponin.** Troponin is a protein that is attached to tropomyosin, and troponin attaches directly to actin. When a muscle is relaxed, tropomyosin prevents the cross-bridges from connecting the actin and myosin filaments. Troponin is the protein that attaches the actin and myosin together, so in order for it to do its job, the tropomyosin must first shift out of the way.

When an action potential is released from the nerve, the point of contact between the muscle and its nerve, the motor end plate, is the point where chemicals (e.g., acetylcholine) are released. The T-tubules transmit a signal to the sarcoplasmic reticulum. The sarcoplasmic reticulum's calcium ion stores are then released. The calcium is then released and binds to the troponin. This binding, in turn, causes the tropomyosin to shift out of the way, allowing the troponin to bind to the cross-bridges. The cross-bridges then undergo a power stroke to move the filaments over each other (figure 7.7).

The parts of the sarcomere can be summarized as follows: The A-band is dark and contains both actin and myosin filaments; the H-band is the section of the A-band that contains only myosin filaments. The I-band is lighter and contains only actin filaments, and it is transversely bisected by a Z-disc. The M-bridge is the equatorial center of the sarcomere that anchors myosin filaments; this is also the center of the H-band. The Z-disc serves as the border of the sarcomere and the site where actin filaments on either side of the H-band are anchored.

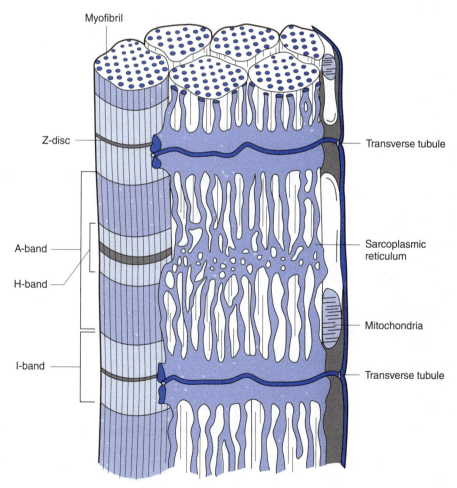

▶ **Figure 7.6** Tubule system.

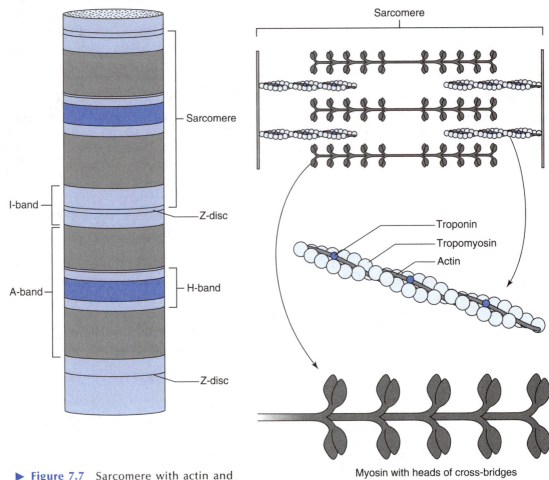

I-band

A-band

Sarcomere

Z-disc

H-band

Z-disc

a

Sarcomere

Troponin

Tropomyosin

Actin

Myosin with heads of cross-bridges

b

▶ **Figure 7.7** Sarcomere with actin and myosin filaments.

The motor units in muscle consist of the nerve (motor neuron) and muscle fibers. Within the fibers are small contractile elements called sarcomeres, and within the sarcomere are filaments called actin and myosin. Muscle function involves various processes that occur when a motor unit is stimulated by an excitatory impulse.

The cross-bridges contain an enzyme, myosin **ATPase,** which is a catalyst that breaks down the **adenosine triphosphate (ATP)** into **adenosine diphosphate (ADP)** and phosphate for energy production. This is the energy source for the sarcomere activity. As long as calcium ions are present and ATP hydrolysis occurs to permit the cross-bridges to re-cock, the activity continues and muscle activity is sustained. This series of attaching and releasing occurs at an asynchronous rate along fibers, with some attaching while others are releasing during muscle activity.

Because the positively charged calcium is stored in the sarcoplasmic reticulum and not the actin, when muscle is inactive, the actin and myosin are not bound by cross-bridges. At rest, they are separated from each other because the negatively-charged ATP is bound to the myosin filament's cross-bridges and the actin filaments are also negative. When an excitatory impulse releases the calcium ions, the calcium ions bind with the ATP on the myosin filaments' cross-bridges and neutralize the ATP's negative charge. Since the myosin remains negatively charged, the actin now binds with the myosin. When the cross-bridges fold in toward the trunk of the myosin, the ATP comes into contact with the myosin's ATPase. When this enzyme breaks down the ATP, the actin and myosin break contact as the ATP becomes negatively charged once again. Through a variety of energy systems, the ADP that is released from ATP breakdown is reformed again into ATP. If an excitatory stimulus continues, this cycle is repeated.

The sarcoplasmic reticulum also contains **mitochondria.** Mitochondria are the most metabolically active part of the sarcomere because they contain the substances needed for metabolism. They store the glycogen used for energy production. They also contain the enzyme that is used to metabolize lactic acid for energy to form ATP. The more mitochondria present in the sarcoplasmic reticulum, the more active the muscle.

We know that one motor unit can innervate several muscle fibers in a muscle. These fibers are spaced throughout the muscle and are not necessarily in proximity to one another. Because the lengths of the nerve's end plates vary according to the distance between the motor point and the muscle fiber that the nerve stimulates, the impulse does not reach all of the muscle fibers at the same time. This causes an asynchronous firing of the muscle fibers. Although it may sound counterintuitive, this asynchronous firing of a single motor unit produces a smooth muscle contraction.

NEUROMUSCULAR PHYSIOLOGY

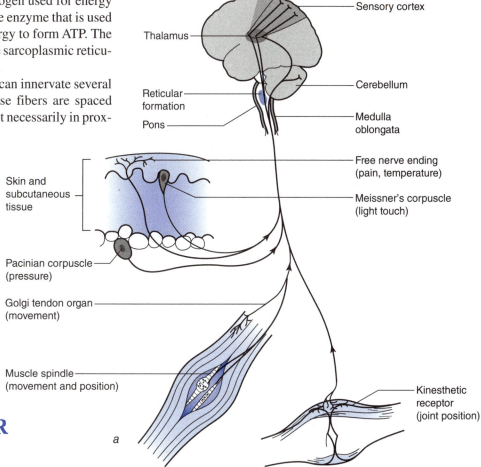

As mentioned in the preceding chapter, many sensory receptors provide input to the central nervous system and can influence the neuromuscular system. Figure 7.8 indicates that various sensory receptors on the skin—including the free nerve endings that perceive pain and temperature, the Meissner's corpuscles that receive light touch sensation, and the Pacinian corpuscles that perceive pressure sensation—all transmit afferent impulses to the central nervous system. These impulses are interpreted at various levels within the central nervous system, including the spinal cord, brain stem, cerebellum, and cerebral cortex. Once received and interpreted, a response is transmitted down the spinal cord through appropriate spinal pathways to the anterior horn, along efferent nerves to the motor structures that respond to the impulses they receive.

When an impulse is strong enough to produce an action potential, the motor neuron fires and all of the muscle fibers that it supplies respond; this response is in accordance with the **all-or-none principle.** Within the entire muscle, a few or many motor units are facilitated to fire at one time. As a rule, the more motor units recruited, the stronger the muscle's response. The stimulation of an electrical impulse, an action potential, moves along the motor neuron to the neuromuscular junction. At this junction, the action potential causes the release of acetylcholine, which stimulates the sarcolemma to release its calcium ions, beginning the muscle activity just described. When this occurs just once, the result is a muscle twitch.

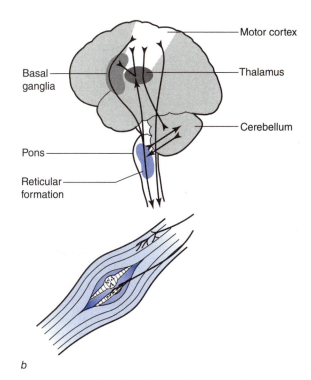

▶ **Figure 7.8** Neural pathways: *(a)* sensory; *(b)* motor.

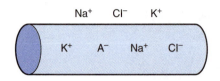

▶ **Figure 7.9** Resting membrane potential.

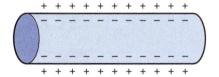

▶ **Figure 7.10** Arrangement of charges on the membrane of an axon.

Resting Potential

The wall of a nerve or muscle cell membrane has a **resting potential.** There are positive and negative ions in the intracellular and extracellular fluids of the nerve and muscle cell membranes. The extracellular fluid contains many sodium (positive) and chloride (negative) ions. Inside the cell are many potassium (positive) ions, protein molecules (A^-), and some chloride (negative) ions (figure 7.9). This distribution of ions produces a cell's resting potential. If microelectrodes are placed on the inside and the outside of a cell, they will show that an axon's intracellular fluid is 70 to 90 mV. Figure 7.10 is a diagrammatic image that demonstrates the interior negative charge and exterior positive charge of the cell membrane. There is a natural tendency to attempt to attain ion equilibrium. The task of keeping the ion concentration balance in check—because the potassium tends to "want" to leak out of the cell and sodium to leak into it—is the responsibility of the sodium-potassium pump. This constant activity level produces a net resting membrane potential average of approximately –85 mV.

When an excitation impulse occurs, a change in the electrical charge along the cell membrane occurs and produces an action potential. The membrane potential goes from negative to positive and quickly returns to negative once the impulse has passed. This process takes probably no longer than 0.5 ms (Clark, 1975) and is much like throwing a rock into water and producing one wave. The rock serves as the initial stimulus, and the wave is the depolarizing impulse that moves along a nerve axon or muscle fiber, creating a brief change and then returning the water to its original calm. The process continues until the wave hits the shore, its final destination.

Physiological Properties

Skeletal muscle physiological characteristics are unique to skeletal muscle and are vital for normal functions of muscle. It is important to know how a muscle works at its cellular level to appreciate how it responds to demands we place on it during therapeutic exercise. It is also important to know the normal responses of muscle so that when an injury occurs, we are able to recognize what alterations in therapeutic exercises will provide appropriate demands but not aggravate the injury. The following sections provide a brief look at some of muscle's physiological properties.

Irritability

Irritability of the motor unit determines the amount of stimulation required to initiate the response of a muscle fiber. Irritability is a physiological property of skeletal muscle. To cause a response, a minimum amount of stimulation—called **threshold stimulation**—is necessary. A sub-threshold stimulation level causes no muscle activity. If the stimulus is above the threshold level, the reaction is greater because either more motor units respond or the duration of discharge of impulses along one motor unit is increased.

If a muscle fiber is stimulated for about 1 ms (Brown, 1980), the membrane depolarizes and is unable to be immediately restimulated. This is the **absolute refractory period.** In other words, a muscle fiber cannot respond to two stimuli that are less than .001 s apart. There is a **relative refractory period** when the membrane becomes partially re-polarized and can respond if the stimulus is greater than the normal threshold level.

The **refractory period** includes a latent period during which there is a momentary cessation of activity as the area prepares to fire. The latent period not only occurs in the electrical phase of contraction, but also occurs in the energy production and mechanical results of the response, as shown in figure 7.11. Once the depolarization of the membrane occurs, the energy changes are facilitated and the mechanical response of the muscle is produced.

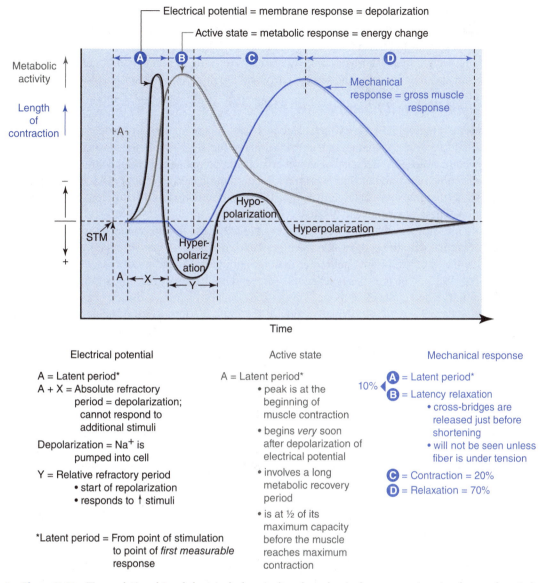

Electrical potential = membrane response = depolarization

Active state = metabolic response = energy change

Electrical potential

A = Latent period*
A + X = Absolute refractory
period = depolarization;
cannot respond to
additional stimuli

Depolarization = Na⁺ is
pumped into cell

Y = Relative refractory period
• start of repolarization
• responds to ↑ stimuli

*Latent period = From point of stimulation
to point of *first measurable*
response

Active state

A = Latent period*
• peak is at the
beginning of
muscle contraction
• begins *very* soon
after depolarization of
electrical potential
• involves a long
metabolic recovery
period
• is at ½ of its
maximum capacity
before the muscle
reaches maximum
contraction

Mechanical response

10% ◄ Ⓐ = Latent period*
Ⓑ = Latency relaxation
• cross-bridges are
released just before
shortening
• will not be seen unless
fiber is under tension
Ⓒ = Contraction = 20%
Ⓓ = Relaxation = 70%

▶ **Figure 7.11** Time relationship of electrical, chemical, and mechanical responses in a simple muscle twitch.

Contractility

After depolarization, the mechanical response is the contraction. This is the second physiological property of skeletal muscle—simply the ability to contract. In a muscle fiber, it is a simple twitch response. One contraction, or twitch response, occurs for each stimulus. If a muscle is to sustain a contraction, multiple succeeding stimuli must occur. The **contraction phase** of a mechanical response follows a 10% latency period and occurs through the next 20% of the cycle. As seen in figure 7.11, the mechanical response is delayed longer than the electrical and metabolic responses because of the series elastic component of the muscle fiber.

Viscosity

Viscosity is the internal resistance that limits the rate of muscle contraction. The general rule of viscosity applied to muscle activity is that the faster the rate of muscle contraction, the greater the internal resistance and the less the external force that can be exerted by the muscle. At faster speeds, more force is required to lift the same weight. Water provides a good example of viscosity. If you put your arm under water, you will find that moving your hand slowly through the water is relatively easy. However, if you move your hand as fast as you can, you'll notice that you need much more strength.

This is an important property to recall when you are instructing a patient in a therapeutic exercise program. Let us take an example of a wrestler with an injured ankle. He is able to lift 22.5 kg (50 lb) in a slow heel-raise exercise. You should not expect him to be able to lift the same weight in a faster heel-raise exercise, performing the same number of repetitions at the faster speed while using the same control and moving through the same range of motion.

Extensibility and Elasticity

A muscle's individual fibers follow Hooke's law: Stress applied to stretch a body is proportional to the strain (change in length) that is produced as long as the elasticity limit of the body is not exceeded. Because of the fiber's elastic components, when a stretch is applied, there is some return to the fiber's original length; but because the fiber also contains plastic elements, there is some change in length if the force applied is of sufficient magnitude or duration. These principles are discussed in chapter 5.

As a muscle is stretched, it becomes more **extensible** because its connective tissue is heated and stretched with the activity. On the other hand, if a part is inactive, it gets stiff. The connective tissue around joints gel rather than remaining fluid, and motion becomes restricted (Kottke, 1982). If an area has reached this state and is stiff, overstretching it can cause tearing of capillaries and connective tissue. This stiffness can be overcome by active exercise. Active exercise before stretching helps to increase the muscle's temperature, reduce its viscosity, and relieve the stiffness. Overall, a stretch is more effective if done after a warm-up of active exercise.

Stiffness

All tissues and structures have **stiffness.** Stiffness is the resistance of tissue or a structure to deformation or change in shape or length. If tissue is stretched quickly, the tissue's stiffness, or resistance to change, is greater than if it is stretched slowly (Threlkeld, 1992). The greater stiffness tissue has, the more force it will take to change the tissue's length. Tissue stiffness depends on how well connected the tissue's structures are to each other and to the tissue's matrix. We are concerned about stiffness in tissue in rehabilitation because of the resistance to stretch increased tissue stiffness can cause. For example, we already know that immobilization causes an increase in cross-links between collagen and reduces intracellular matrix fluid so protein fibers become more adherent to one another; this process increases tissue stiffness. On the one hand, we want injured tissue to become more resistant to outside forces, but on the other hand, excessive resistance to outside forces can make restoration of normal motion difficult when we stretch stiff tissue. This is especially true when efforts to regain motion are delayed and tissue becomes stiffer as it heals.

As tissue becomes stiffer and more resistant to outside forces, the clinician must be aware of these tissue changes and apply alternative flexibility-restoration techniques to regain lost motion. These techniques will be presented later in the chapter.

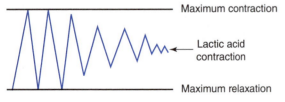

Maximum contraction

Lactic acid contraction

Maximum relaxation

▶ **Figure 7.12** Contracture.

Contracture

Contracture is a failure of relaxation of a muscle. Relaxation is a normal metabolic process of a muscle following contraction. Many believe that the onset of fatigue causes both a decrease in the ability to produce an initial maximal contraction output and a decrease in the ability to reach a maximum relaxation level. One theoretical explanation is a lactic acid buildup in the muscle as demonstrated in figure 7.12. As the muscle fatigues, the resting length shortens.

Contracture is one reason for the importance of stretching after exercise. As the muscle fatigues with activity, the fibers shorten and do not resume their normal resting length. One theory is that over a period of time, the gross muscle loses flexibility if stretches are not performed to regain the normal resting length of the fibers.

Contracture is also the reason you should have the patient perform more-strenuous and more-demanding therapeutic exercises early in the day's rehabilitation session. As the patient fatigues and the muscle fibers' resting length decreases, the muscle's ability to perform the activity correctly becomes limited, so the risk of injury increases. The more difficult and challenging activities should be performed early in the day's session to ensure good results.

It is important not to confuse muscle contracture with an orthopedic contracture, which is a connective-tissue shortening that causes a reduced range of motion. Nor should you confuse contracture with a **muscle spasm,** which is a prolonged reflex muscle contraction.

The physiological properties of skeletal muscle include irritability, contractility, viscosity, extensibility and elasticity, fatigue, and summation.

Fatigue

The property of **fatigue** is closely related to contracture. Fatigue can result either from exhaustion of a muscle with prolonged activity or from failure of the circulatory system to provide the necessary nutrients to continue muscle activity. One agent responsible for local muscle fatigue is **lactic acid.** A by-product of muscle activity, lactic acid buildup in muscle increases after intense or prolonged muscle contraction because there is not enough oxygen available to oxidize the lactic acid at the rate to which it is produced. In a resting muscle, the quantity of lactic acid is 0.5 to 2.2 mmol/kg of muscle, but in a muscle that is exercised to exhaustion, the lactic acid level is 25 mmol/kg of muscle (Kraemer, 2000). Lactic acid is measured as small amounts leak from the muscles into the blood. As activity increases, the lactic acid amount in the blood increases and serves as an index for calculating how vigorously the patient is working. Lactic acid buildup is associated with muscle tiredness and pain. The ability to tolerate increased levels of lactic acid varies from one person to another and is to some extent a determining factor in endurance. When working at the same level, people who are better conditioned have lower levels of lactic acid in their bloodstreams than individuals who are not as well conditioned (Conley, 2000).

Lactate levels are influenced by activity intensity, the exercise duration, the state of training, initial glycogen levels, and muscle fiber type. The type II, fast-twitch fibers produce lactic acid at a higher rate than the type I, slow-twitch fibers. High-intensity activities such as sprints and weight lifting produce higher levels of lactic acid in a shorter time than low-intensity prolonged activities such as distance running and aerobic exercises. Individuals who are conditioned tolerate higher levels of lactate better than untrained individuals (Conley, 2000).

If you are working with a patient who has become severely deconditioned because of prolonged inactivity, you need to keep these factors in mind, especially in the early sessions of the therapeutic exercise program when the patient's deconditioning level is more severe. Since the patient's ability to tolerate exercise intensity changes in severe deconditioning, earlier exercise sessions require more rest periods than later sessions.

The muscle's circulation is impeded more with sustained isometric activity than with either isotonic or brief isometric activity. The sustained activity of the muscle restricts blood so that fatigue occurs more quickly than with other types of muscle activity. You need to consider this when designing a therapeutic exercise program. The section "Relationship Between Muscle Strength and Muscle Endurance" deals more extensively with recovery from fatigue.

Summation

If a second twitch is produced before a muscle fiber completely relaxes, a greater force is produced. This phenomenon, known as **summation of forces,** is similar to what occurs when a moving car is hit from behind—the car will move forward with a greater total force than it did before it was hit. If a series of stimuli is delivered to the muscle fiber at a rapid frequency, the muscle fiber produces a **tetany,** a sustained maximal contraction (figure 7.13). While tetany is a sustained muscular contraction, **tetanus** is an intermittent contraction that is noted by a fibrillating tremor (figure 7.13, C).

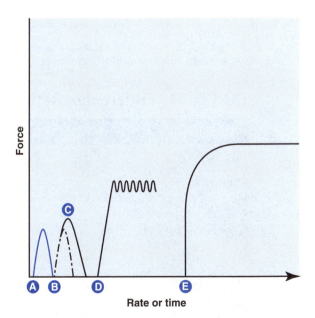
▶ **Figure 7.13** Twitch, twitch summation, tetanus, and tetany of a motor unit: A and B, single twitches; C, force resulting from summation of two twitches; D, tetanus; E, tetany, sometimes called a sustained maximal contraction.

FAST- AND SLOW-TWITCH FIBERS

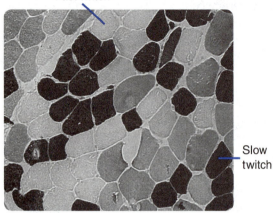

▶ **Figure 7.14** Fast- and slow-twitch fibers.

Reprinted, by permission, from J.H. Wilmore and D.L. Costill, 2008, *Physiology of sport and exercise,* 4th ed. (Champaign, IL: Human Kinetics), 36.

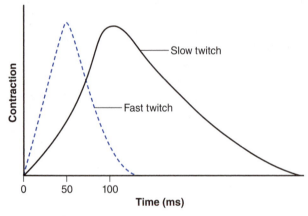

▶ **Figure 7.15** Contraction-relaxation curves for fast-twitch and slow-twitch skeletal muscle fibers.

Skeletal muscle contains **fast-twitch** and **slow-twitch fibers.** The ratio of these fiber types varies within the individual from muscle to muscle, and from individual to individual for the same muscle. In other words, one sprinter may have more fast-twitch fibers in the quadriceps than another sprinter does, and may have more fast-twitch fibers in the quadriceps than in the hamstrings. The ratio is determined by genetics and muscle demands. Whether or not a fiber can convert from one fiber type to another is an unresolved question; but a muscle that is considered an antigravity muscle, such as the soleus, tends to have more slow-twitch fibers than a muscle that is used more for locomotion and fast or powerful movements, such as the quadriceps, which has a combination of fast- and slow-twitch fibers.

The two fiber types have different appearances, metabolic capacities, and contraction characteristics. Their names are based on their relative speed of activity. The slow-twitch fibers, sometimes referred to as type I fibers or slow oxidative fibers, are darker and take about 110 ms to reach their peak tension when stimulated (figures 7.14 & 7.15). The fast-twitch fibers, sometimes called type II fibers or fast oxidative fibers, are lighter in color and reach their maximum tension approximately 50 ms after being stimulated (Wilmore & Costill, 2004) (figures 7.14 & 7.15). The slow-twitch fibers have a slower-acting myosin ATPase, and the fast-twitch fibers have a faster-acting myosin ATPase, so the ATP is converted more quickly to produce energy faster for the fast-twitch fibers than for the slow-twitch fibers. The fast-twitch fibers also have a more extensive sarcoplasmic reticulum, allowing a more efficient

TABLE 7.1 Differences Between Type I and Type II Muscle Fibers

Characteristics	Type I	Type II
Speed	Slowest	Fastest
Axon size	Smaller	Larger
Color	Red	White
Conduction velocity	Slow: 110 ms	Fast: 50 ms
Fatigue resistance	Greatest	Least
Recruitment threshold	Lower	Higher
Firing rates	Lower minimum and maximum	Higher minimum and maximum
Myosin ATPase	Slow acting	Fast acting
Mitochondria	Greater number	Smaller number
Activity	Endurance	Brief bursts

delivery of calcium ions to permit a quicker fiber response to stimulation. The slow-twitch fibers have a greater quantity of mitochondria, more myoglobin, and more glycogen stores, so they are better equipped for prolonged or sustained activity (table 7.1).

Fast-twitch fibers have three sub-classifications: type IIa, IIb, and IIc. Very little is known about type IIc. These fibers are in very small quantities in muscles, approximately 1% to 3% on average. Type IIa and type IIb fibers are approximately equal in quantity in an average muscle (Wilmore & Costill, 2004). Although the differences between these fast-twitch fibers are not yet understood, the type IIa fibers are more often recruited during muscle activity than the other type II fibers. Since type IIb fibers require a greater stimulus to fire, they are not recruited in low- or medium-intensity activities but are used in high-intensity activities such as the 100 m swim. Type IIb fibers are the fastest, and type IIa fibers are a transition between type I and IIb fibers since type IIa fibers have qualities of both.

The slow-twitch fibers have more mitochondria than the fast-twitch fibers. Since mitochondria are the primary energy-storage facilities for the cells, they give the fibers a greater potential to produce a greater oxidative capacity. The higher mitochondria count and related increased myoglobin and blood supply account for the cells' red color. With a greater energy source available, the slow-twitch fibers are able to sustain activity for a longer time than the fast-twitch fibers. For this reason, they are considered endurance fibers and are the fibers primarily responsible for an individual's ability to perform low-intensity endurance activities such as a marathon.

Fast-twitch fibers have fewer mitochondria and less ability to sustain activity. Their activity is anaerobic, so they fatigue quickly. However, they are capable of producing a more powerful output and are responsible for high-power, short-term activities such as a 400-m sprint (figure 7.16). A factor that allows fast-twitch fibers to produce stronger forces is the fast-twitch motor unit's higher content of muscle fibers in comparison to a slow-twitch motor unit. The greater number of responding muscle fibers causes a greater force production.

The fast-twitch and slow-twitch fibers of skeletal muscle differ in appearance, metabolic capabilities, and contraction characteristics.

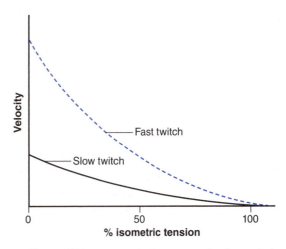

▶ **Figure 7.16** Force-velocity curves for fast-twitch and slow-twitch skeletal muscle fibers.

MUSCLE STRENGTH, POWER, AND ENDURANCE

Before discussing how to improve muscle function, it is necessary to identify the components involved.

Muscle Strength

Strength is the maximum force that a muscle or muscle group can exert. In healthy individuals. In healthy individuals, it is measured in 1RM, the one-repetition maximum. A 1RM is the weight that a muscle or muscle group can lift for only one repetition. If an individual can perform only one repetition of a forearm curl with 20.5 kg (45 lb), that is his 1RM, or strength, for the forearm curl. A person who can lift 22.5 kg (50 lb) for 1RM in a forearm curl has twice the strength of someone who has a 1RM of 11.3 kg (25 lb).

Rehabilitation assessment of strength, however, does not use a 1RM system. Since this system is too demanding for injured or weak muscles, there are other strength assessments that are more appropriate. One of the more common rehabilitation systems is a 10-RM maximum. This is the amount of weight an individual can lift for 10 repetitions but not 11 or more repetitions; this method of determining muscle strength is similar to the 1RM system, but the weight is not as heavy, so the stresses on the tested muscle are not as severe.

Power

Power is strength applied over a distance for a specific amount of time. Power is involved in most athletic events and is strength incorporated with speed. The volleyball player who can leg press 180 kg (400 lb) in half the time it takes a basketball player to lift the same weight has twice the power of the basketball player. Power is represented mathematically by this formula:

$P = F \times d / T,$

where P = power,

F = force,

d = distance, and

T = time.

You may recall from chapter 3 that work is force × distance. In essence, power is work performed over a specific amount of time. Power increases by either performing the same amount of work in less time or increasing the amount of work performed in the same amount of time.

Speed, however, depends on coordination, efficiency of movement, and timing (Kotzamanidis, Chatzopoulos, Michailidis, Papaiakovou, & Patikas, 2005; Stamford, 1985). In a rehabilitation program, these elements are developed after strength because, to some extent, they depend on the patient's strength. Since power involves the element of speed, ways of improving power are discussed in chapter 9.

Muscle Endurance

Muscle endurance is the ability of a muscle or a muscle group to perform repeated contractions against a less-than-maximal load. A muscle's endurance, or ability to prolong activity, depends on the status of the energy systems available and the quantity of forces resisted. With advanced conditioning levels, circulatory and local metabolic exchanges improve. The greater the forces resisted, the more quickly fatigue occurs. If a person's 1RM on a bench press is 136 kg (300 lb), the person will be able to lift 68 kg (150 lb) for more repetitions before fatiguing than if that individual lifts 113 kg (250 lb).

Relationship Between Muscle Strength and Muscle Endurance

Muscle strength and muscle endurance lie on a continuum of exercise. High-intensity, low-repetition exercises, at one end of the continuum, emphasize primarily strength gains. Low-intensity, high-repetition exercises, at the other end of the continuum, produce primarily muscle endurance gains.

Although he has been the only one to perform this study, Berger (Berger, 1962) determined that high-intensity exercises performed for 3 to 9 repetitions appear to best emphasize strength. A high-intensity exercise is one that is at least 90% of the 1RM (Baechle, Earle, & Wathen, 2000). Low-intensity exercises performed for 20 or more repetitions at an intensity of 70% of the 1RM emphasize primarily muscle endurance improvement. Exercises that are moderate intensity—at 70% up to 90% of the 1RM—and are performed for 6 to 12 repetitions provide gains in both strength and muscle endurance, although not as much as when either strength or muscle endurance is emphasized individually (ACSM, 1998). Most researchers have found that in order to produce strength gains, an exercise must provide resistance levels of at least 66% of the muscle's maximum.

Endurance gains can be made by increasing strength through high-resistance, low-repetition exercises, but not as effectively as by increasing the repetitions of an exercise. Conversely, some strength gains can be achieved with high-repetition exercises, but not as well as with high-resistive, low-repetition exercises. As a general recommendation, if your primary emphasis is strength, perform no more than 10 repetitions; but if your goal is primarily endurance increases, repetitions from 15 to 20 are advised. The closer the exercise resistance is to the maximum resistance, the fewer repetitions performed in the exercise; the further from the maximum resistance the exercise resistance is, the more repetitions performed. The relationship between muscle strength and muscle endurance, relative to the repetitions used to make gains in each of the parameters, is visually demonstrated in figure 7.17.

The amount of work performed by a muscle during an exercise program is referred to as training volume. Training volume is based on the number of sets of each exercise, the number of repetitions completed of each set, and the amount of resistance (Feigenbaurm & Pollock, 1999). In the early-1960s, one study was performed that demonstrated three sets of an exercise was beneficial in increasing strength (Berger, 1962). Although this study has not been replicated since, other investigators have questioned Berger's results. Most recently, the American College of Sports Medicine published a position statement on strength gains (ACSM, 1998). Based on their investigations of current literature, they recommend that one set of 8 to 12 repetitions, or to fatigue is adequate to increase strength (ACSM, 1998). We must remember, however, that most research investigating training volume has used normal subjects; the response differences between healthy and injured subjects and the optimal recommendations for training volume for injured patients undergoing rehabilitation are yet to be determined.

Working a muscle optimally and to fatigue requires a recovery period between sets. Several studies have addressed the relationship between fatigue and recovery of muscles, in both isometric and isotonic activities. The recovery following fatigue from isotonic exercise is slower than that from isometric exercise, but the recovery curves have similarities. As seen in figure 7.18, the recovery rate is rapid within the first 30 to 90 s. The rate of recovery then declines slightly over the next couple of minutes before making another rate change to a very gradual return to full recovery that takes place over a longer time period. The exact time of recovery depends on the study design and the type of exercise investigated, but all researchers have found a similar curve for the recovery pattern. When the activity is isokinetic, it takes approximately 4 min for a muscle to recover to 90% to 95% of its initial torque levels following an exercise bout to fatigue (Sinacore, Bander, & Delitto, 1994). Recovery from isometric and isotonic exercises to fatigue occurs most rapidly in the first minute—58% and 72%, respectively. After the first minute, the recovery from isometric activity occurs at about a 35% faster rate than from isotonic activity (Clarke, 1971). In all of these types of exercise recovery, there is an initial burst of recovery within 30 to 90 s. This recovery burst is followed by a slightly slower but still rapid recovery. In the final phase of recovery, it takes more than 40 min for the muscle to return to pre-fatigue strength levels. On the basis of his findings in a classic study, Lind (Lind, 1959) extrapolated the probability that it would take more than 90 min for a muscle to fully recover.

Because of these differing recovery rates, a presumption has been that there are different recovery systems that lead to the muscle's overall recovery following exercise to fatigue (Lind, 1959). The initial rapid recovery is thought to occur because of the removal of lactic acid and other buildup of metabolites that took place during the activity. The slower recovery may involve replacement of the muscle's metabolic reserves that were depleted during the activity.

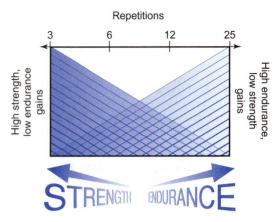

▶ **Figure 7.17** Relationship between muscle strength and endurance. Greater strength gains are achieved with lower repetitions and higher resistance, whereas greater endurance gains are achieved with higher repetitions and lower resistance.

Key

A = Initial rapid recovery
B = Less rapid but still quick recovery
C = Prolonged time to full recovery

A + B = Metabolic waste removal
C = Reserves replacement

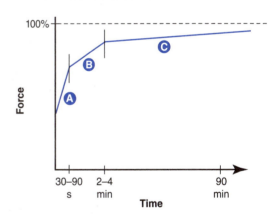

▶ **Figure 7.18** Recovery following fatigue.

Muscle strength is the maximum force a muscle can exert, and power is strength over a distance for a specific time. Endurance is the ability to prolong an activity. Exercises for muscle strength and endurance lie on a continuum from low to high repetitions with high to low resistance.

These fatigue recovery findings have an impact on your therapeutic exercise program design. For example, if you are treating a hockey player with a quadriceps strain and he or she performs a leg press to fatigue, you should allow a 1/2 - to 1-min recovery before the next exercise set. If you are using an isokinetic machine to rehabilitate the quadriceps, the recovery time should be 2 to 4 min. With the use of isometric exercises, the rest between sets should be about 1 min.

Sometimes it is not possible to employ high-intensity exercises even though strength gains are needed. This situation is common, especially in early stages of therapeutic exercise when the patient's pain limits the resistance tolerated. In such cases, it helps to remember that the patient can still achieve strength gains using low-resistance, high-repetition exercises. For example, if a gymnast develops a patellar tendinopathy and is unable to tolerate much weight on a leg press exercise, he or she can use less weight and lift it for more repetitions and still make gains in quadriceps strength. Later in the program as the quadriceps strength improves and pain is reduced, the patient can use higher-resistance and lower-repetition exercises.

The number of repetitions a patient performs depends on several factors, including the patient's pain tolerance, the phase of the healing process, and the demands on the patient after return to competition. For example, a football defensive lineman's therapeutic exercise program is primarily strength based; a soccer player's program involves endurance exercises; and a basketball player—whose sport demands both strength and endurance—will have a program that emphasizes both strength and endurance exercises. If a patient begins a therapeutic exercise program one week after surgery, the resistance exercises are mild so as not to cause undue stress on newly forming tissue.

High-resistance, low-repetition exercises produce **hypertrophy** of the fast-twitch, type II muscle fibers. Moderate-resistance, higher-repetition exercises produce a more general increase in hypertrophy by affecting the size of both type I and type II fibers (Conroy & Earle, 2000).

As a rehabilitation clinician, you must possess knowledge of injuries and activity performance requirements and must use good judgment to determine what level of resistance exercises to incorporate into the patient's therapeutic exercise program. Appreciating the demands to which the patient will eventually return provides a good basis for designing appropriate rehabilitation programs.

FORCE PRODUCTION

Some of the concepts in this section were introduced in chapter 3, but they are worth a brief review here. Putting together all the factors that determine strength output of a muscle not only helps clarify the concepts discussed in chapter 3, but also enables you to appreciate the therapeutic exercises that can improve a patient's strength.

Muscle strength is determined by the angle of the joint, the length of the muscle and the sarcomere, the size and fiber arrangement of the muscle, the speed of contraction, and the number and type of muscle fibers activated. Let's look at each of these factors briefly.

Joint Angle

As you recall from chapter 3, joint movement is the result of a muscle's pull on the joint. The amount of force directed to cause rotation of the joint (movement) and the amount of force directed at compression or distraction of the joint (stability or instability, respectively) are determined by the angle of the joint and the vector forces that are produced. Since movement around a joint is rotational, the force is **torque.** Remember that torque is determined by the amount of applied force and the length of the moment arm: $T = F \times D$ (torque = force × distance). As the joint moves through its motion, the moment arm length changes, causing a change in the muscle's torque. For example, when a patient performs a biceps curl, as the elbow moves from 90° flexion to 125° flexion, the lever arms of the resistance and the biceps shorten. Since the lever arm of the resistance (weight) undergoes a greater change than the lever arm of the biceps, the weight gets easier to lift by the time the patient reaches the end of elbow motion, as seen in figure 7.19. In terms of joint angle, the greatest force production occurs when the tendon's moment arm is at its greatest length.

Length-Tension

A muscle's strength production involves both active and passive elements. The active component is the motor unit; the passive component is the connective tissue surrounding the whole muscle, its fascicles, and its fibers. A muscle's ability to shorten actively lessens as the length of the muscle diminishes. In shortening, the muscle uses only its active component. At a muscle's shortest position, all of the cross-bridges between the fibers' actin and myosin filaments are used up. If, however, the muscle is lengthened before it shortens, its passive component, the surrounding connective tissue, becomes taut and produces an additional resistive force because of its elasticity. The optimal length of a muscle to produce increased strength—because of the combined release of elastic energy from the passive elements and the actin-myosin cross-bridges from the active elements—is slightly beyond its resting length (figure 7.20). However, if we stretch the muscle beyond that point, separation between the actin and myosin occurs and reduces available cross-bridges so that less force, rather than more, results.

Therefore, when it is desirable to achieve a maximum muscle force, it is advantageous to produce a quick stretch of the muscle to use its elastic energy component. This factor is frequently utilized in

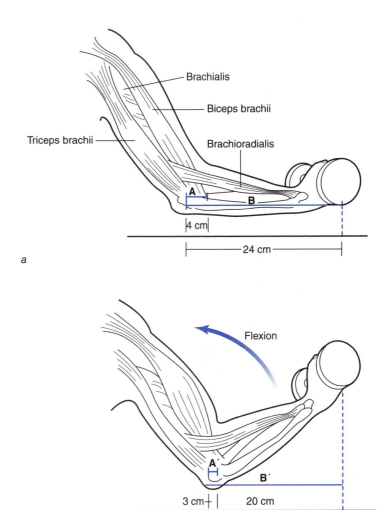

▶ **Figure 7.19** Change in biceps lever-arm length (A to A') and change in resistance lever-arm length (B to B') with different joint angles.

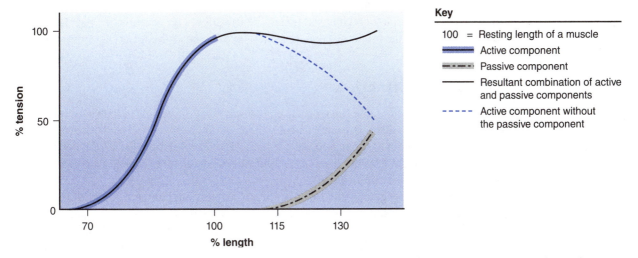

▶ **Figure 7.20** Length-tension factor: Because of the active and passive muscle-tissue elements, a muscle produces its greatest strength slightly beyond its resting length.

activities such as proprioceptive neuromuscular facilitation and plyometric exercises, both of which are discussed later.

The length-tension factor requires additional consideration for multi-joint muscles. The performance of a muscle that crosses more than one joint is profoundly affected by the position of both joints. For example, if you are working with a patient's injured knee and want to obtain a maximal contraction from the hamstrings, the beginning position to the hamstrings on stretch is with the hip in flexion and the knee in extension. If the exercise is performed with the patient prone, the hip is extended and the hamstring is already in a partially shortened position. In this position, it is impossible to apply a pre-exercise stretch to the hamstring muscle.

Although it is commonly known that as a muscle fiber shortens, its ability to create force diminishes, how short a fiber is able to become is unanswered. Studies have looked at muscle fiber length and determined that a fiber can shorten to about 70% of its longest length (Lieber, 1992). However, these studies used isometric contractions, not isotonic contractions, so the information obtained from these studies cannot be extrapolated to functional motion (Lieber, 1992).

Muscle Size and Fiber Arrangement

Muscle fibers are arranged in series or in parallel with each other. Those muscles with series arrangements are longer muscles that are able to produce a greater shortening velocity. The muscles with parallel fiber arrangement have a larger cross-sectional area and are able to produce a greater force. As a simplified example, if a muscle is composed of three muscle fibers that are placed end to end and are stimulated to contract simultaneously, the muscle will shorten three times as much as a muscle with one fiber (figure 7.21). The muscle with the three fibers in a side-by-side (parallel) arrangement, however, will produce a contraction three times as powerful as a muscle with one fiber.

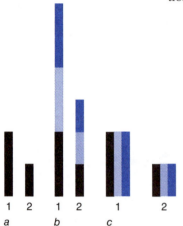

▶ **Figure 7.21** Fiber arrangement: *(a)* one fiber, *(b)* three fibers in series, *(c)* three fibers in parallel. Three fibers in series are able to shorten much farther than only one fiber, but three fibers in parallel are able to produce much more force than three fibers in series. 1 for each muscle is the resting length; 2 is the shortened length.

There is a direct correlation between a muscle's cross-sectional size and its strength. The cross section is the width of the muscle taken at an angle perpendicular to the length of the fiber. The cross section is greater when muscle fibers are arranged at angles to the axis of the muscle. Because of its featherlike appearance, this is called a pennate arrangement. The more pennates in a muscle, the greater the cross section. Those muscles with pennates tend to be force-producing muscles, not shortening-velocity muscles. Whereas the sartorius is an example of a shortening-velocity muscle, the gastrocnemius is an example of a multi-pennate muscle. The angle of pennation of any specific muscle varies from one person to another. Hunter (Hunter, 2000) believes that even if two people have the same size muscle, the angle of pennation may be a factor in the differences between their strength and speed.

Speed of Contraction

When a muscle shortens, the force produced is inversely proportional to the velocity of shortening. It is assumed that this occurs because there are fewer cross-bridges between actin and myosin filaments with a higher velocity shortening (Billeter & Hoppeler, 1992). For example, a patient who lifts 22.5 kg (50 lb) quickly finds that same weight relatively easy to lift when performing the activity more slowly.

When a muscle lengthens, the force is directly proportional to the velocity of movement. For example, when using a lengthening activity in therapeutic exercise, the patient is able to tolerate more resistance than with muscle-shortening activities. A variety of studies have addressed the relationship between force production and muscle length. One study (Hortobágyi & Katch, 1990) showed that force production using a muscle-lengthening activity is 120% to 160% more than with a muscle-shortening activity. Other investigators (Wilmore & Costill, 2004) believe that this figure is close to 130%.

Number and Type of Muscle Fibers

As mentioned earlier, larger muscles are able to produce more force than smaller muscles. Fast-twitch fibers are able to produce more force than slow-twitch fibers because there are more muscle fibers in each motor unit of the fast-twitch fibers. If you are rehabilitating two patients with knee injuries, the patient with more fast-twitch fibers is able to produce a stronger output of the quadriceps than the patient with fewer fast-twitch fibers in the muscle. This is one reason that it is fruitless to compare one patient to another and expect the two to be able to perform equally, even if they are the same size and have similar injuries.

Muscle force production is determined by the angle of the joint, the size of the muscle and its fiber arrangement, the speed of contraction, and the type and number of muscle fibers that are activated.

TYPES OF MUSCLE ACTIVITY

Although some authors refer to the types of muscle activity as muscle contraction, it is not entirely accurate. Contraction implies a shortening of the muscle, but as you will see, a muscle does not always shorten when it acts. Therefore "muscle contraction" is referred to here as *muscle activity* or *movement*. There are two types of muscle activity, static and dynamic. **Static activity** is **isometric. Dynamic activity** is divided into **isotonic** and **isokinetic.** Isotonic activity is further divided into **concentric** and **eccentric** movements.

Static Activity

Static, or isometric, activity is produced when muscle tension is created without a change in the muscle's length. Static activity is not only used in therapeutic exercise but is also part of daily activities and sport participation. Trunk muscles act statically to provide a stable base for arm and leg movements. The shoulder muscles act as a shoulder stabilizer when a patient moves the elbow and hand.

The advantage of isometric exercise is that this type of activity can strengthen a muscle without imposing undue stress on injured or surgically repaired structures. For example, in situations such as a recent fracture or a surgical repair in which movement is restricted or limited, isometrics are used early in the therapeutic exercise program until motion is permitted. Isometrics can also be used when the muscle is too weak to offer sufficient resistance against gravity or other outside forces. The disadvantage of isometrics is that strength gains are isolated to no more than 20° within the angle at which the isometric is performed. It is important to remember to caution the patient to avoid a **Valsalva maneuver** during isometric exercises. Valsalva occurs when the patient holds his or her breath, causing an increase in intrathoracic pressure. In turn, this can impede venous return to the right atrium, leading to an increase in peripheral venous pressure (increasing blood pressure) and reducing cardiac output because of lowered cardiac volume. If you see a patient holding his or her breath during exercise, remind the patient to breathe in order to avoid the valsalva maneuver risk.

If a maximal effort is exerted in an isometric exercise, tension within the muscle progressively decreases because of fatigue. At 5 s the tension is 75% of the tension exerted at the start of the isometric activity. By 10 s, the strength drops to 50% of the original tension (figure 7.22). Because of this fatigue factor, no one has the ability to produce a sustained maximal contraction. An example of this is when you assist in carrying a stretcher with an injured person on it. As the upper extremity muscles performing the isometric activity of grasping the stretcher begin to fatigue, the muscles start to burn, and the transport team has to stop because someone will request a rest if it takes more than a short time to carry the patient.

This concept is important to remember when a patient performs isometric exercises in a therapeutic exercise program. It is unnecessary for a maximal isometric activity to be performed for more than 5 to 10 s at a time; 6 s is the recommended duration for one maximal isometric exercise (Hettinger & Müller, 1953). The number of repetitions and

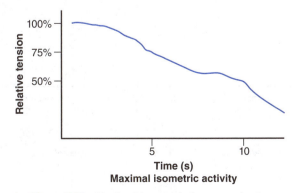

▶ **Figure 7.22** Maximal isometric force production.

frequency of exercise throughout the day depend on the condition of the muscle, the ability of the body part to move, and the phase of the healing process.

Strength gains are achievable if the muscle's effort is 66% to 100% of its maximum output. Efforts at 35% to 66% of maximal isometric output produce some gains in strength, but the increase is slow. Most daily activities, apart from sport activities, produce periodic tensions of 20% to 35% of maximum. This level of output maintains strength. If a muscle is immobilized and rendered inactive, there may be a range in loss of strength from 8% a week (MacDougall, Elder, Sale, Moroz, & Sutton, 1980) to 5% a day (Müller, 1970).

Keep in mind that it takes about one week to increase strength by 5% (MacDougall et al., 1980) to 12% (Müller, 1970). These numbers may vary from one study to another because of the different protocols researchers use, but all the data make a similar point: The rate of strength lost is much quicker than the rate of strength regained. In essence, it may take up to a week to recover the strength lost in one day of inactivity. This realization highlights how important it is to keep a muscle active if activity causes no deleterious effects. If an injured part must be immobilized, isometric exercises can become very important in retarding atrophy and weakness.

Dynamic Activity

The term *dynamic* in relation to activity implies a change in the position of a muscle. Dynamic activity is further defined by the specific types of activity that occur.

Isotonic Activity

Isotonic activity is dynamic in that it involves a change in the muscle's length. If the muscle shortens, the activity is called *concentric*. If the muscle lengthens, the activity is called *eccentric*. Although you can isolate muscle activity to produce either concentric or eccentric motion, most sport and daily activities involve the use of both concentric and eccentric actions. For example, lifting a weight during an elbow curl is a concentric action, and lowering the weight is an eccentric action. Likewise, jumping for a basketball rebound is a concentric action that is preceded and followed by an eccentric action.

An eccentric action can produce anywhere from 20% to 40% more force than a concentric action (Hortobágyi & Katch, 1990). Wilmore and Costill have averaged out that range and indicate that eccentric activity produces 30% more force than concentric activity (Wilmore & Costill, 2004). For example, if an 18 kg (40 lb) weight can be lifted in a curl exercise concentrically, the same muscle can lift 23.5 kg (52 lb) eccentrically when the arm is lowered. It is believed that the muscle's noncontractile elements provide the additional forces during eccentric activity that permit increased muscle loading.

There are several other differences between concentric and eccentric activity. Although it takes more energy to perform a concentric action, there does not seem to be any difference in strength gains between the two types of exercise. As the speed of a concentric activity increases, the muscle's ability to produce force decreases. The opposite is true for eccentric exercises: As speed increases with eccentric exercise, the force increases initially, then eventually levels off or decreases. The differences in speed and force production of concentric and eccentric activity are demonstrated in figure 7.23.

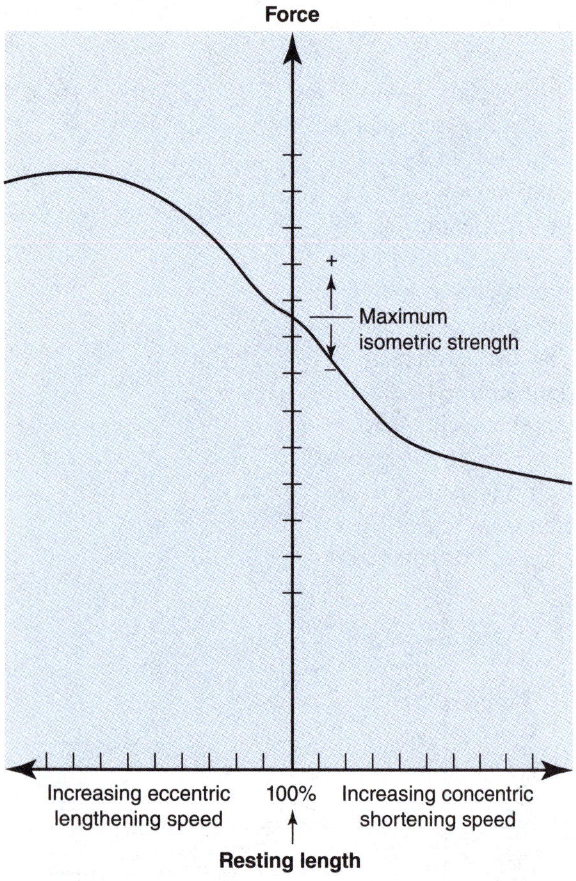

▶ **Figure 7.23** Concentric-eccentric force-length relationship.

There is also a greater likelihood of delayed-onset muscle soreness (DOMS) with eccentric exercise. Although the research is not conclusive, some believe that this is the result of a combination of damage occurring to muscle membranes and a secondary inflammatory reaction within the muscle (Wilmore & Costill, 2004).

You can reduce DOMS by taking a few precautionary steps when providing a therapeutic exercise program that incorporates eccentric activity. One way is to avoid eccentric exercises early in the program when the muscles are particularly weak. Another way is start at a lower level of intensity and gradually increase the intensity as the patient is able to tolerate higher-level exercises. Delayed-onset muscle soreness may occur but it is generally better tolerated as the patient becomes stronger and more accustomed to higher levels of activity intensity. The occurrence of DOMS does not necessarily mean you should limit therapeutic exercise in subsequent sessions, but you should realize that the patient may not be able to offer as great an effort if DOMS is present. You should make a decision regarding the use of eccentric activities in advance and determine whether risking a reduced-intensity session the next treatment day outweighs the benefits of providing eccentric exercises and risking muscle soreness. This is an individual determination that you make based on the patient's tolerance and motivation, the goals for therapeutic exercise, the level of healing, and the patient's current status.

The term *isotonic* means "having the same tension." It is, in fact, inaccurate, because the amount of tension produced by a muscle varies throughout the range of motion. The amount of tension produced depends on moment arms and the physiological principles previously discussed. The greatest amount of tension created during an isotonic activity is actually the force that the muscle or muscle group can produce at its weakest position in the motion. For example, if a patient lifts 18 kg (40 lb) in an elbow curl, that weight is the maximum the elbow flexors can exert at their weakest point. If the patient performs the exercise while standing, the weakest point occurs when gravity is at its greatest, with the elbow at 90° flexion. The elbow flexors can lift more than 18 kg at the beginning of the motion and at the end of the motion as gravity's lever arm length shortens. They can also lift more in the beginning of the motion, where the muscles are at their greatest physiological length, than they can at the end of the motion when they are at a physiological disadvantage. Because the elbow flexors can lift no more than 18 kg at 90°, the maximum weight the patient can lift through the full range of motion is 18 kg. Similarly, because the weight feels relatively lighter in the beginning and at the end of the motion, the patient is able to lift the weight at a faster speed during those parts of the motion. As the weight becomes more difficult to move around the 90° range of motion, the patient's movement slows down.

Isokinetic Activity

Isokinetic activity is a dynamic activity in that it involves motion. It differs from isotonic activity, however, in that the velocity is controlled and maintained at a specific speed of movement. Isokinetic means "having the same motion" and refers to the unchanging speed of movement that occurs during these activities. Whereas the speed of motion remains constant, the amount of resistance provided to the muscle varies as the muscle goes through its range. To return to the example of the elbow curl, if the exercise is isokinetic the patient's elbow moves through its motion at a uniform speed, but maintaining that uniform speed requires varying the amount of resistance. In that part of the motion where an isotonic exercise would be easy, the resistance in an isokinetic exercise is greater; and where the isotonic exercise would be normally more difficult, the resistance offered isokinetically is less in order to accommodate the varying strength of the muscle group as it goes through a constant motion. It is assumed in isokinetics that the patient provides a maximal output throughout the exercise. Isokinetics is sometimes called **accommodating resistance** exercise because of the change in resistance given throughout a range of motion. Today's equipment makes it possible to perform isokinetic activities both eccentrically and concentrically. Although isokinetics was very popular during the 1970s and 1980s, closed kinetic chain activities are the current trend.

Muscles perform several types of activity: Static activity occurs when there is tension but no change in the muscle's length. Dynamic activity occurs when there is a change in the muscle's length. Isotonic and isokinetic activity are particular types of dynamic activity.

OPEN AND CLOSED KINETIC CHAIN ACTIVITY

A kinetic chain is a series of rigid arms linked by movable joints. This is a mechanical description of the body. **Open kinetic chain (OKC)** and **closed kinetic chain (CKC)** activity within the body are identified in terms of the distal segment of the extremity, the hand or foot. The kinetic chain is open when the distal segment moves freely in space. Kicking and throwing a ball are open kinetic chain activities. A kinetic chain is closed when the distal segment is weight bearing and the body moves over the hand or foot. Running and a handstand are closed kinetic chain activities. Generally, open kinetic chain athletic activities produce high-velocity motions such as throwing a ball or swinging the distal leg during running. Closed kinetic chain activities are functional activities that place lesser shear forces on the joints, so they are generally safer to use earlier in a therapeutic exercise program.

Both OKC and CKC activities involve a relationship between one joint and the others within the chain. This is important to remember in therapeutic exercise, because if you ignore the other joints within the chain, rehabilitation success will be elusive. Function of one joint is not exclusive: The function of one joint determines the function of the other joints within the chain. Abnormal stresses applied to an injured joint are transmitted to and absorbed by other structures within the chain and have the potential to cause additional problems if those stresses are not tolerated by those other areas. For example, if a baseball pitcher has weak shoulder muscles and is unable to keep the arm elevated correctly during the pitch, he may develop elbow pain because of the additional stress transmitted by the abnormal forces directed from the shoulder.

Lower-extremity activities in sport are primarily CKC events. They involve isometric, concentric, and eccentric activities. Closed kinetic chain exercises are used to improve strength, power, stability, balance, coordination, and agility and are capable of generating large forces but relatively low velocities of movement. Lower extremity closed-kinetic chain activities are functional in that they occur in normal activities from walking and standing to running and jumping. In a CKC, no link within the chain can move independently of the others; movement of one segment affects all. For this reason, the inadequacies of a weak link in the chain can be compensated for by other links within the chain, but additional stresses are subsequently applied to those other links. When extremities are weight bearing, they function in a closed kinetic chain.

Open kinetic chain activities are also used in daily activities and in sport. Examples of OKC activities are kicking, throwing, and lifting lower body weights in a seated position, as in performing knee extensions. Even part of the running or walking cycle involves an OKC activity. In an OKC, any link in the chain is free to move independently of the other links. Generally, the forces generated by an OKC are small but the velocities are large. Body parts that operate in an OKC are non-weight bearing.

Open and closed kinetic chain activities are produced in both upper and lower extremities (figure 7.24). But different stresses are applied to the body by the two types of activities. The differences in stresses occur because the motion is different. In OKC activity, the proximal segment initiates the movement for the distal segment. For example, the shoulder motion initiates the movement at the hand. In CKC activity, there is compression of the joints, and stabilization occurs because of co-activation of opposing muscle groups. In a squat, the quadriceps work eccentrically while the hamstrings activate to counteract knee flexion movement. The result is stabilization of the knee through simultaneous activity of opposing muscle groups.

If we continue our focus on the knee, only the hamstrings work in OKC knee flexion. In OKC knee extension, the quadriceps perform the motion while the hamstrings remain quiet. This exercise increases the moment force of the leg as it goes from flexion to extension. Moment force is the product of the amount of force (weight of the leg) and the perpendicular distance from the joint to the distal end of the limb (lever arm). In other words, as the leg moves into extension, the work required to lift the segment increases because the moment arm of the resistive force (gravity) increases. This change not only requires more quadriceps strength as the knee reaches terminal extension, but in an OKC, the knee suffers a high shear

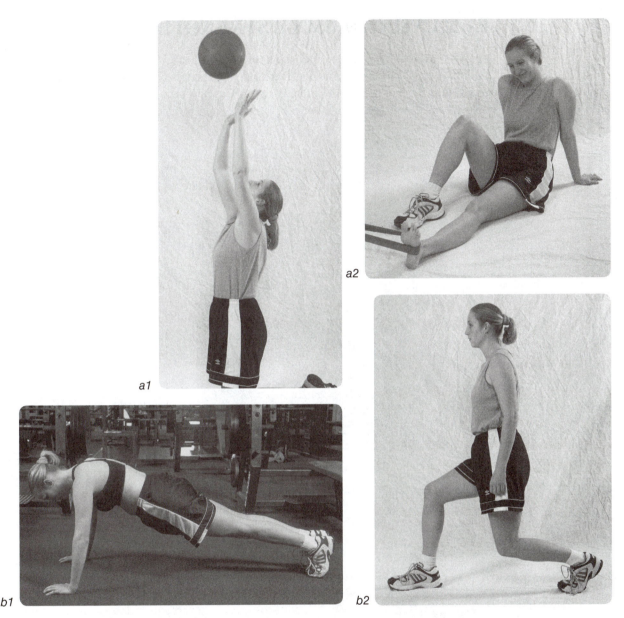

a1

a2

b1

b2

▶ **Figure 7.24** Open *(a)* and closed *(b)* kinetic chain activities for the upper *(a1, b1)* and lower *(a2, b2)* extremities.

force with an active contraction of the quadriceps as the muscle moves the knee from flexion to extension, especially during the last 30°. The quadriceps tendon creates this shear force by causing an anterior translation of the tibia as it pulls the knee into extension. In a CKC, the shear force is counteracted by a co-contraction of the hamstring. Co-contraction produces less stress on the knee during terminal extension and increased stability of the joint through the simultaneous contraction of the hamstrings and quadriceps in a closed kinetic chain exercise.

Although CKC exercises may provide more joint stability, in situations when the patient is unable to bear weight it may be necessary to use open kinetic chain exercises. The advantage of OKC activities in this situation is that strengthening activities are not delayed until weight bearing occurs. Another advantage of open kinetic chain exercises is that they also isolate muscles that are weak, so that emphasis on weaker muscles occurs. This point presents one precaution in the use of CKC exercises: Because more than one muscle group is active during CKC exercises, substitution of stronger muscles rather than correct use of weaker muscles is always a possible pattern and must be corrected when observed. A therapeutic exercise program should include a combination of open and closed kinetic chain exercises for optimal results.

The differences between open and closed kinetic chain activities relate to whether the distal segment moves freely in space (open) or not (closed).

EVALUATING MUSCLE STRENGTH

Chapter 3 addressed the idea that muscle activity produces joint motion. The amount of force a muscle exerts is determined by its lever arm length and its angle of pull. In functional situations, you may not need to calculate the exact force produced, but you should have an idea of the relative strength of the muscle.

Evaluation Equipment

Strength can be objectively determined in a variety of ways. Isokinetic devices, discussed later, can evaluate isokinetic strength; cable tensiometers can measure isometric strength; and free weights or weight machines can measure 1RM maximum isotonic strength (figure 7.25).

Instruments that measure strength of specific areas or muscle groups are also available. For example, the grip dynamometer and the pinch dynamometer (figure 7.26) measure grip and finger pinch strength, respectively.

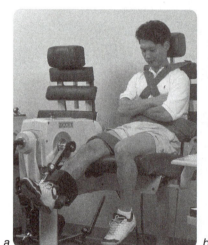
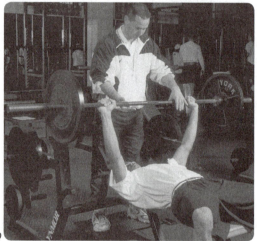

▶ **Figure 7.25** Strength evaluation: *(a)* isokinetic testing, *(b)* 1RM.

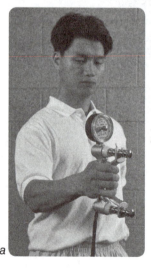
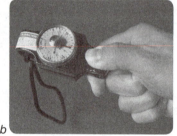

▶ **Figure 7.26** Special test equipment: *(a)* Grip dynamometer measures hand-grip strength, and *(b)* pinch dynamometer measures finger-pinch strength.

Manual Muscle Test

Not everyone has an isokinetic machine or cable tensiometers, and establishing a 1RM for an injured extremity is usually not appropriate. The 1RM is an isotonic measure used most often with healthy individuals; 1RM is not used to assess strength in therapeutic exercise because it imposes too much stress on an injured part and may aggravate the injury.

The more universal, efficient, and readily available method of evaluating strength is the manual muscle test (MMT). The basis of this test is assessment of the muscle's ability to move a joint through its normal range of motion in as isolated a manner as possible. Depending on the muscle's strength, gravity is an important factor, eliminated, used by itself, or used in conjunction with an outside manual force applied by the clinician. The muscle's strength is graded numerically from 0 to 5; sometimes qualitative grades, from "no function" to "normal," are used instead.

Manual muscle testing grew out of the need to identify and grade muscle strength in patients with polio. Robert Lovett, a New York physician, developed the MMT, a system based on strength relative to gravity and resistance, and first used it in 1912. Lovett later collaborated with a physiologist, Dr. E. G. Martin, and published the tests in 1916. These first tests used the verbal scoring system. During the 1920s and into the 1950s, others further refined and redefined Lovett's MMT. In 1932, Dr. Arthur Legg, in collaboration with physical therapist Janet Merrill, published a book on muscle testing using the numerical scale with plus and minus designations for all except the two lowest strength grades (Hislop & Montgomery, 2002). Over the years, the MMT scale has evolved and been redefined as clinical trials and studies provide clearer pictures of its clinical value and limitations. The currently used grades are summarized and defined in table 7.2.

TABLE 7.2 Muscle Strength Gains

% Normal strength	Number grade	Letter grade	Qualitative grade	Definition
100%	5	N	Normal	Full range of motion against gravity and is able to tolerate full manual resistance to movement.
	4+	G+	Good +	Full range of motion against gravity and is able to tolerate nearly full resistance to movement.
75%	4	G	Good	Full range of motion against gravity and is able to tolerate moderate, but not full, resistance.
	4–	G–	Good–	Full range of motion against gravity and is able to tolerate some resistance.
	3+	F+	Fair +	Full range of motion against gravity and is able to tolerate minimal resistance through a partial range of motion.
50%	3	F	Fair	Full range of motion against gravity. The muscle is unable to go through its full range of motion if resistance is provided in an antigravity position. It may be able to tolerate resistance when gravity is eliminated.
	3–	F–	Fair–	Full range of motion against gravity but with difficulty.
	2+	P+	Poor +	Full range of motion with gravity eliminated. The muscle is unable to go through its full range of motion in an antigravity position. It may be able to tolerate mild resistance through a partial range when gravity is eliminated.
25%	2	P	Poor	Full range of motion with gravity eliminated. The muscle is unable to tolerate resistance in a gravity-eliminated position.
	2–	P–	Poor–	Full range of motion with difficulty in a gravity-eliminated position.
	1+	T+	Trace +	Partial range of motion is possible with gravity eliminated.
10%	1	T	Trace	There is evidence of a muscle contraction but no joint motion occurs. A flicker of tension in the tendon may be seen or palpated, but the joint does not move.
0%	0	0	Zero	No evidence of contractility of the muscle. Facilitation produces no voluntary muscle response.

Since the development of these grades, it has become common practice to further define the scoring using plus (+) and minus (–) signs. Just as with school grades, the +/– system in muscle grading defines the gray areas into which scores sometimes fall. For example, a deltoid that offers minimal resistance to antigravity with resistance is less than a grade 4 and more than a grade 3, so the clinician grades it as 4–. The grade is recorded as 4–/5, indicating that the strength of the muscle is 4– on a 5-point scale. If a muscle has some motion against gravity but not full range of motion, the rehabilitation clinician may give it a 3–/5 grade. If it has full motion in a gravity-eliminated position and is able to tolerate some resistance in this position but still is unable to go through a full range of motion in an antigravity position, its grade is 2+/5. The plus (+) and minus (–) system is not usually used within the average population for any grades except grades 2 and 3 (Hislop & Montgomery 2002); however, in the athletic population where there may be a significant difference between grades 4 and 5, the plus and minus system is commonly used.

When the clinician provides manual resistance to a muscle, the muscle's position for grade 4 and 5 manual muscle tests is an antigravity (against gravity) position. Before resistance is given to a muscle, the muscle actively moves the joint through its full range of motion. If that is successful, the clinician then applies manual resistance to determine the strength grade. Resistance can be applied either through the full range of motion or at specific positions within

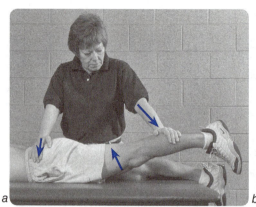

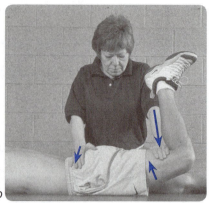

the motion to determine strength. If isometric resistance is offered and the muscle is a single-joint muscle, then the resistance is provided at the muscle's end motion position. If the muscle crosses more than one joint, then the isometric resistance is provided in the muscle's mid-range position. If testing positions are different from the standard positions, this is noted on the record.

When applying a resistance force, you should exert the pressure in a direction that is opposite to the muscle's line of pull, providing stabilization if needed to permit isolated testing of the specific muscle or muscle group you are evaluating. Give the resistance on or near the joint distal to the joint tested. Avoid placing your hand on the belly of the muscle tested. Give the resistance gradually, building it up as you feel that the patient is able to accept more resistance until you have determined the maximal resistance tolerated. Provide the maximum resistance possible to obtain an accurate result: If the muscle is able to tolerate more resistance than you have provided, your assessment is inaccurate. Compare to the opposite side to determine what is normal for the patient. What is normal for a golfer

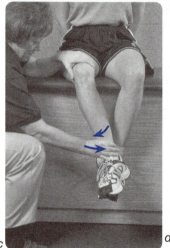

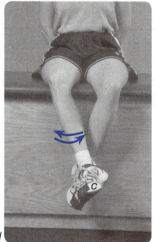

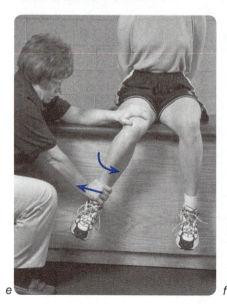

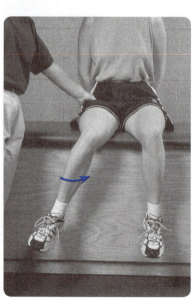

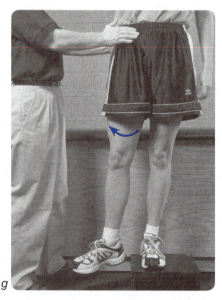

▶ **Figure 7.27** Manual muscle tests. *(a)* Grade 4 and 5 test for hip extension with gluteus maximus and hamstrings. Note stabilization of hip to prevent pelvic rolling or hip flexion. *(b)* Grade 4 and 5 test for hip extension with isolation of gluteus maximus. Stabilization of hip and pelvis is necessary to isolate hip extension motion. *(c)* Grades 4 and 5 test for hip medial rotators: While stabilizing the thigh, resistance is applied to the leg against medial rotation movement. *(d)* Grade 3 test for hip medial rotators: Patient should not lower the knee or roll the pelvis as the hip is moved through lateral rotation. *(e)* Grade 4 and 5 test for hip lateral rotation: the thigh is stabilized while resistance is applied to the lower leg against hip rotation movement. *(f)* Grade 3 test for hip lateral rotation: While stabilizing the pelvis, the hip is moved through a full range of external rotation. *(g)* Grade 2 test for hip lateral rotation: As the patient moves the hip through a full range of motion, the pelvis is stabilized to isolate movement.

may not be normal for a football lineman; what is normal for a recreational sprinter may not be normal for a competitive sprinter.

If a muscle is unable to perform a movement through its full range of motion in an antigravity position, place the segment in a gravity-eliminated test position to determine whether the muscle has at least grade 2/5 strength. If full motion in an antigravity position is possible, resistance is provided in this position to determine whether a 2+/5 strength is present. Figure 7.27 presents examples of strength testing of the hip, knee, ankle, shoulder, elbow, and wrist muscles.

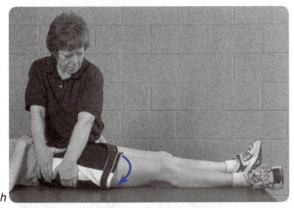

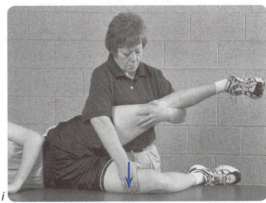

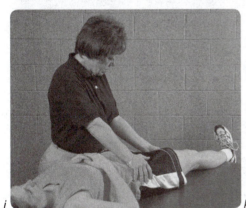

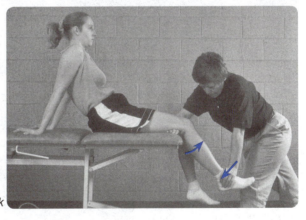

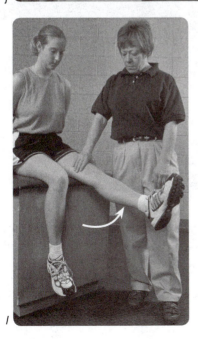

▶ **Figure 7.27** *(continued) (h)* Grade 1 test for hip lateral rotation: Hip lateral rotators are palpated as the patient performs the movement. The upper hand stabilizes the pelvis. *(i)* Grade 4 and 5 test for hip adduction: Resistance is applied to the thigh during movement into adduction while avoiding hip flexion or rotation substitution. *(j)* Grade 1 and 2 test for hip adduction: While stabilizing the pelvis and palpating the hip adductors, movement into adduction is attempted. Watch for hip rotation or flexion substitution. *(k)* Grade 4 and 5 test for knee extension: With one forearm under the thigh to elevate the thigh and protect it against the table surface, resistance is provided against knee extension motion. *(l)* Grade 3 test for knee extension: While the thigh is stabilized, the knee is extended through a full range of motion without resistance.

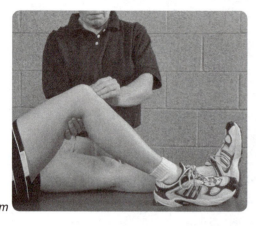

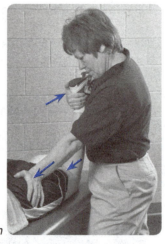

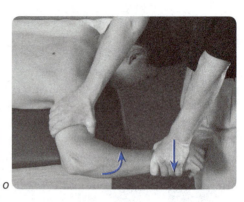

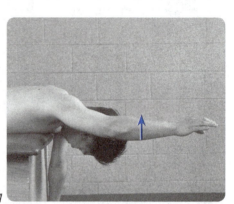

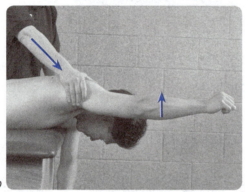

▶ **Figure 7.27** *(continued)* (m) Grade 1 test for knee extension: With the quadriceps on stretch in knee flexion, the quadriceps tendon is palpated as the knee is actively extended. *(n)* Grade 4 and 5 test for knee flexion: With the hip and pelvis stabilized, resistance at the ankle is provided to knee flexion. Resistance to leg rotation can be simultaneously provided to isolate medial and lateral hamstrings. *(o)* Grade 4 and 5 test for shoulder lateral rotators: While stabilizing the arm, downward resistance is applied at the forearm. *(p)* Grade 4 and 5 test for lower trapezius. *(q)* Grade 3 test for lower trapezius. *(r)* Grade 3 test for tibialis anterior: While the hip is stabilized, the foot is moved into dorsiflexion and inversion through a full range of motion. The test may be performed in sitting or standing. *(s)* Grade 4 and 5 test for plantar flexion: Full heel elevation should occur 20 times for normal strength. Watch for body rocking and knee flexion substitutions.

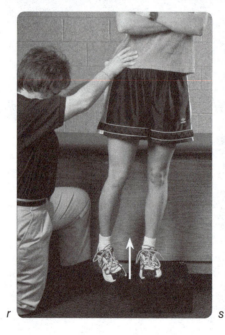

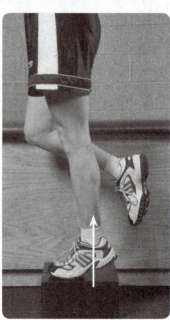

On rare occasions, you may encounter a patient who does not offer a smooth resistance during the muscle strength test. The resistance is a series of catch-and-release tensions of the muscle as it goes through its range of motion. Called **cogwheel resistance,** this response occurs in individuals who are not producing a maximal effort. Reasons for this response may include fear, pain, and malingering. When you see a patient who provides this form of resistance, you should be aware that it is not a normal response but rather a voluntary response that produces an inaccurate test result.

GRADATIONS OF MUSCLE ACTIVITY

Just as there are grades of muscle strength, there are grades of muscle activity. The kind of muscle activity possible is, in part, determined by the muscle's strength.

Passive Range of Motion

Passive range of motion (PROM) is an activity that requires no active work on the part of the muscle. The motion is produced by an outside force, either a machine or another person. The intent is to maintain range of motion in situations in which either the muscle is incapable of moving voluntarily or it is desirable that the muscle not perform actively. Continuous passive motion machines, discussed in chapter 4, are sometimes used after surgery when motion is beneficial, but active motion is not possible because of limitations such as pain, swelling, or spasm or because restricted muscle activity is desirable. The rehabilitation clinician can also perform PROM by moving the extremity through its motion without the patient's assistance.

Active Assistive Range of Motion

Active assistive range of motion (AAROM) is performed either when the muscle is incapable of producing the full motion without assistance, or when it is desirable for the individual to perform limited voluntary activity with assistance from an outside source to achieve the objective of the exercise. For example, if a patient has undergone reconstructive surgery on the shoulder, it may be desirable for him or her to perform actively through part of the motion, but not in the portions of the motion that may impose risk of shear stress or possible detachment of recently repaired tendons.

Active Range of Motion

Active range of motion (AROM) occurs when the patient is able to produce full range of motion of the segment, with no assistance. No resistance is applied. These types of exercises are also sometimes referred to as range of motion (ROM) exercises. Following surgery, the physician may permit a patient to perform full AROM exercises but may not want any outside resistance to be applied. These exercises are performed to maintain or increase range of motion and help reduce atrophy of the muscles involved in the motion.

Resisted Range of Motion

Resisted range of motion (RROM) falls into the broad category of dynamic exercises. Motion with resistance applied to the muscles is permitted. These types of exercise are commonly referred to as strengthening exercises or progressive resistive exercises. A later section of this chapter introduces the variety of progressive resistive exercise programs used in the rehabilitation of musculoskeletal injuries.

STRENGTH EQUIPMENT

Many types of equipment are available to provide strength gains in both rehabilitation and conditioning programs. Most equipment can be used for both purposes. Cost varies greatly also—from very little to several thousand dollars. What you decide to use in your therapeutic exercise programs depends on your familiarity with the equipment, availability, budget, and the specific needs of your patient population. Regardless of the amount or kind of equipment you have, you can design a very comprehensive, progressive, and appropriate therapeutic exercise program for every patient you treat. Your imagination and knowledge are ultimately the determining factors in the quality of the program you create.

The following sections deal with the most common items of equipment available on the market. Most are items you will become familiar with before you complete your curriculum.

A thorough presentation of strength-testing positions and techniques for all grades of movement is available in various muscle-testing textbooks. Two suggestions are *Muscles, Testing and Function, Fourth Edition* (Kendall, McCreary, & Provance, 1993) and Daniels and Worthingham's *Muscle Testing: Techniques of Manual Examination, Seventh Edition* (Hislop & Montgomery, 2007).

Rehabilitation clinicians evaluate the strength of muscles with various types of machines or through manual muscle testing.

Muscles perform various gradations of muscle activity; from the least active to the most active, these are passive range of motion, active assistive range of motion, active range of motion, and resisted range of motion.

Manual Resistance

Manual resistance equipment is the least expensive therapeutic exercise equipment. The only requirement is you. Manual resistance exercise is an exercise in which the rehabilitation clinician applies manual force to produce either static or dynamic resistance. Manual resistance can be applied isometrically if movement is not desirable, if pain occurs with motion, or if the patient's muscle has a specific area of weakness within a range of motion.

Manual resistance can also be applied concentrically or eccentrically, through part of the motion or the full motion. It can be applied in a straight plane of movement or in a more functional diagonal plane.

Technique

Once you have assessed strength and identified deficiencies, you can determine how much resistance to apply during the exercise. You can also determine whether you should provide additional special considerations such as an isometric hold at a specific position in the range of motion to focus on a site of weakness.

Before performing the exercise, the rehabilitation clinician explains to the patient the exercise, the sensations to be expected, the number of repetitions or qualifications for the duration of the exercise, and any necessary precautions. For example, I sometimes tell the patient that the goal is 15 repetitions or I'll state that we will continue the exercise until "one of us gets tired, or I start to sweat." If I want to deliver an isometric in the middle range, I tell the patient ahead of time to prepare him or her that at that point the motion will stop but the exercise will continue. It is also a good idea to take the extremity passively through the range of motion in the desired plane in advance of the exercise to let the patient know exactly what is expected during the exercise.

The resistance is applied in a manner that permits the patient to perform the desired motion smoothly. The motion should not be jerky or uncontrolled. During the activity (AAP & fitness, 2001; Akihiko & Shinichi, 1997), the patient should produce a maximal effort and continue to breathe throughout. Occasionally, as already mentioned, a verbal reminder to breathe is necessary to prevent a Valsalva maneuver.

The clinician should watch carefully to see that substitution and unwanted movement patterns do not occur. It is important to correct the patient's motion if there is any substitution so the exercise is properly performed and facilitation of the appropriate muscle occurs.

Like in manual muscle testing, the force application should be near the joint distal to the joint exercised. If you cannot control the resisted movement because the patient's muscle is stronger than you are, as can be the case when you apply manual resistance to the hip, you can apply the resistance even more distally, at the ankle rather than the knee; this is permissible only if pain is not produced at the knee when the force is applied at the proximal ankle. The more distal application gives you a longer lever arm so you can do less work yet offer the same amount of resistance to the hip. Exercises should be pain free and offer enough resistance to produce the desired results.

Advantages

As already suggested, the greatest advantage of manual resistance is that it requires no equipment. It is also a good way to establish rapport with the patient, because a hands-on technique usually results in the patient's developing trust and confidence in the clinician. This often leads to a greater desire to work harder. It also gives you immediate feedback about the patient's progress. You assess the changes and improvements each time you perform the exercises, and you can make immediate changes according to the patient's response to a specific exercise. As the patient gets stronger, you can immediately increase the resistance or repetitions. The ability to modify the speed of the exercise within a set, the ability to change from concentric to eccentric activity or to include both, and the ability to incorporate isometric resistance into the weaker points of the motion are all unique to manual exercises. A progression of exercises is easily incorporated into a therapeutic exercise program by increasing either the manual resistance or the number of repetitions or sets.

Disadvantages

There are some unique disadvantages to the use of manual resistance. Because it requires one-on-one work with the patient, this method may be more time consuming than others and may not easily fit a situation that necessitates working with several patients at one time.

Another disadvantage is that manual resistance does not provide an objective measure for changes in strength. As a subjective method, it relies on consistent performance and reliable recall by the same clinician to reflect the patient's strength changes. If the rehabilitation clinician is not sensitive to the amount of force he or she is applying, judgment about the amount of force and about subsequent changes in the patient's condition may not be dependable. If you are more fatigued than usual on a given day, you may provide less force than on other days; without good awareness of how you feel you may incorrectly perceive a significant increase in the patient's strength.

Body Weight

Exercise using body weight also requires no equipment. The patient's own body weight provides the resistance. A variety of exercises for the upper and lower extremities and the trunk can be used, along with progressions, to offer an adequate system of therapeutic exercises.

Technique

You can provide a progression by increasing the amount of body weight used in an exercise, by prolonging the time of the exercise, or by increasing the number of repetitions or sets. For example, if a patient has a weak serratus anterior, a progression to increase the amount of body weight for a push-up exercise starts with a wall push-up, as seen in figure 7.28a and progresses to an incline, perhaps in a position with the hands on the back of a chair or a countertop (figure 7.28b), then to the hands on a chair seat (figure 7.28c). An even more advanced position is a modified push-up. As strength improves, the patient changes to a regular push-up position (figure 7.28d). If additional resistance is desirable, the patient can move to a decline push-up in which the feet are higher than the hands (figure 7.28e). The most advanced push-up is a handstand push-up. This is one example of a progression from easy to most difficult, providing the patient with a body-weight resistance exercise.

Examples of additional progressions include increasing the number of repetitions and/or sets the patient must perform, having the patient perform an isometric at the middle or end of the motion, and increasing the time of the hold as strength increases. A change of speed also changes the effort of the exercise.

You must impress on patients that performing an exercise through a full range of motion is necessary for maximal benefit. Partial range of motion execution provides for strength gains only in the portion of the motion exercised. In the beginning, the patient should do the exercises slowly and in a controlled manner so that he or she executes them correctly without substitution of the wrong muscle. As strength and control improve, the speed of the exercise may increase to mimic functional activities.

It is also important to instruct the patient in the correct execution of the exercise, providing information about common substitution patterns to avoid. This helps to minimize incorrect technique and to produce better results.

Once the patient has demonstrated the correct technique, he or she can perform the exercises without your assistance. This builds a sense of independence and control over the therapeutic exercise program and requires the patient to demonstrate initiative.

It is beneficial to give patients handouts illustrating these exercises. Such information serves as a reminder of correct exercise execution and also helps the patient comply with the therapeutic exercise program.

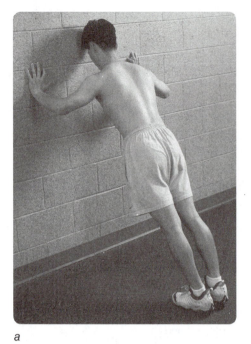

a

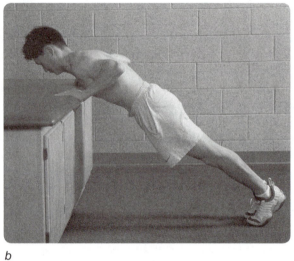

b

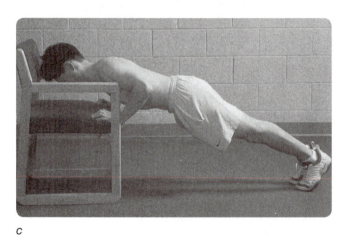

c

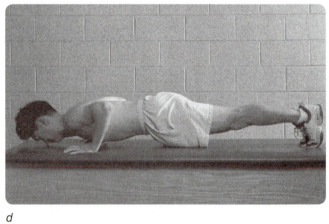

d

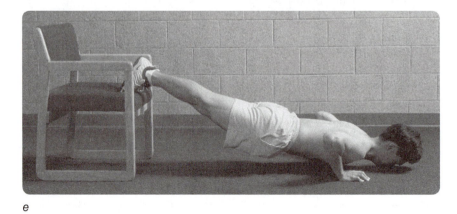

e

▶ **Figure 7.28** Body-weight resistance push-up progression: The easiest push-up is performed using a wall (a). Progression then moves to an incline (b and c), to the floor (d), to an inverted position (e). The positions shown in figures b-d increase difficulty by increasing the lever-arm length of the body. The position shown in figure e increases the difficulty by forcing the arms to bear more of the body's weight.

Pilates is a type of body weight resistance program that many people use for both conditioning and rehabilitation. Pilates is introduced in chapter 11 with the Feldenkrais Method and Alexander Technique, two other body awareness techniques.

Advantages

The most obvious advantage of body-weight resistance exercises is that they require no equipment. They can be performed anywhere, whether the patient is in the clinic, in the weight room, at home, or on the road. A related advantage is that there is no expense, although handouts provided to improve compliance may add minimal costs.

Another positive feature is that once the patient can perform the exercises correctly and continue them independently, treatment sessions can focus on other activities that require the expertise of the clinician, making optimal use of the treatment session.

Many weight-resistive exercises, such as the standing squat, are actually functional activities. They can be used as a progression of activities that naturally lead to those specific activities performed in the patient's sport or occupation.

Disadvantages

A disadvantage of body-weight exercises is that if the patient is performing them independently, there is no guarantee that he or she is doing them correctly or even doing them at all. On the other hand, it is not difficult to assess whether or not is complying with the home treatment program. If there are gains, chances are that the patient is complying, and, obviously, the converse is just as true.

Occasionally, a patient is unable to tolerate body-weight resistance exercises either because the muscle is too weak or because performing the exercises is too painful. In this situation, it is better to begin with activities that provide less body-weight resistance—such as a wall push-up, or even isometrics. Once strength has improved, body-weight resistance activities are incorporated.

Some areas of the body lend themselves better than others to body-weight resistance and progressive exercises using body weight. For example, the fingers and wrists are difficult to exercise with body resistance, especially in the beginning when the patient may not be able to perform an activity such as fingertip push-ups.

Rubber Tubing and Bands

Rubber tubing and bands provide dynamic resistance exercises. They are available in large and small rolls, so strips can be cut to varying lengths. They also come in a range of resistance levels, indicated by different colors. Although various companies market the bands with their own color indicators, the most familiar spectrum corresponding to resistance levels from lightest to heaviest is tan, yellow, red, green, blue, black, silver (gray), and gold (butterscotch). The color-coding scheme for tubing is similar.

Rubber tubing and bands provide resistance via the elastic elements of their makeup. The resistance provided is in direct relation to the amount the band or tubing is stretched (P. A. Page, Labbe, & Tropp, 2000). They can be stretched up to five times their original length; since most clinical use of rubber tubing and band does not stretch them more than 3 times their length, we can assume that as the band stretches, the resistance will change directly according to the amount of stretch (P. Page, 2003).

When selecting the length of a rubber band or tubing, it should be close to the length of the part being exercised. For example, if an elbow is to be exercised, the length of the forearm to the hand should be measured, and rubber tubing or band of that length should be selected.

Technique

Rubber tubing and bands can be used both in straight-plane exercises and in functional patterns. Depending on the specific activity, the patient may use his or her own body to secure the band or an object such as a door or table leg.

The bands and tubing can be used to mimic exercises performed with other equipment that is available in the clinic but not available for the patient at home. For this reason, tubing and bands are useful for home exercises.

Because of the variety of types of exercises that one can perform with tubing and bands, it is difficult to discuss specific application techniques. Provide the patient with general guidelines, however, before providing bands or tubing to use for home exercises. Instruct the patient to perform the exercise slowly and in a controlled manner so the targeted muscles are used correctly. Going through a full range of motion is necessary for developing strength throughout the muscle's range. In addition, instruct the patient how to stabilize the exercising segment to ensure correct performance. Inadequate stabilization causes substitution and strengthening of the wrong muscles.

To determine which color band or tubing to use, you will first perform a MMT on the muscle. Trial and error may be necessary to become proficient at judging the correct resistance band to provide the patient, but after the test, you should be able to narrow down the choice of colors. You have selected the appropriate color when the patient can perform the activity through an appropriate range of motion for the desired number of repetitions and feels that the muscle has been at least moderately exercised.

As with body weight resistance, to ensure better compliance, it is advisable to give patients handouts that include drawings or photos along with providing oral explanations of the exercise. As mentioned in chapter 1, studies show consistently that if an individual receives both written and oral instructions, the likelihood of correct performance of the exercise and of compliance increases significantly.

Advantages

The cost of rubber tubing and bands is relatively low. In some clinics, it may be possible to recuperate the costs by billing the patient or the patient's insurance company. These items are easy to transport; because they weigh little and are not bulky, patients can take them home or can easily pack them into suitcases and exercise almost anywhere.

Since exercises using bands or tubing are easily converted to home exercises, they need not be repeated during clinic treatments. Treatment time can then be better spent on other activities that require the expertise of the rehabilitation clinician. This allows the patient to gain a sense of responsibility, independence, and control over the injury recovery process.

The color-coded bands and tubing offers an easy-to-implement system of progression. As the patient's strength increases, you can provide progressive colors to achieve greater resistance with the same exercise. Additional instruction is not necessary, because the exercise itself is the same.

Exercises that mimic functional motions can be used with the tubing and bands. This provides for strength gains in functional patterns. This method is especially convenient for upper-extremity muscle groups that may not easily lend themselves to body-weight resistance and other exercise systems.

Disadvantages

Since the patient performs rubber tubing and band exercises independently, you do not have control over compliance. It is the patient's responsibility to perform the exercises. This can be an advantage or a disadvantage, depending on the patient's attitude, dependability, and motivation.

Another disadvantage is that as the band or tubing stretches during the exercise, the resistance increases, causing more resistance to the muscle as it reaches its weaker point in the motion. The resistance is then greater at the end than at the beginning of the motion when the muscle is at a stronger physiological length. So, although the band offers resistance to the muscle, the amount of resistance provided does not coincide with the muscle's ability to produce force.

If the clinic cannot recuperate the cost of bands and tubing, the expense can add up quickly. The heavier bands are more expensive than the lighter bands, so as a patient's strength increases, the cost of distributing the bands and tubing also increases. If a facility provides tubing and bands for patients but is unable to recover the costs, additional budget allowances are necessary.

Although it is possible to design exercises for the hip and knee using bands and tubing, the greater number of exercises using these items involve the upper extremities. Figure 7.29 provides examples of some rubber band exercises for the upper and lower extremity muscles.

Free Weights

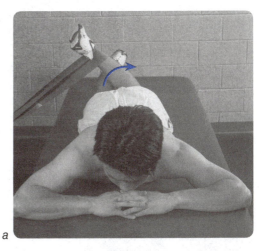

When most people think of strengthening, they think of free weights. Free weights include cuff weights, barbells, and dumbbells. They come in a variety of sizes and styles. The weight is either attached to the body segment or held by the patient during the exercises. Cuff weights typically cannot be changed in size. Some cuff weights can be modified by the addition of preset weighted tubes or packets that are placed in a pocket on the cuff. The cuffs are attached to ankles or wrists.

Some dumbbells and barbells are adjustable: Weight plates are placed on the bar and secured with collars. Other dumbbells and barbells are fixed and their weight cannot be changed. *Dumbbells* refers to weights that are used in one hand, are usually smaller, and are either fixed weights or adjustable. *Barbells* refers to a larger free-weight system that requires using both hands. Barbells are used for lower- and upper-body strengthening. The bars vary in length from 1.5 m to 2.1 m (5-7 ft). A bar that has become popular in the past several years for conditioning and later-stage rehabilitation is the standard Olympic bar, which weighs 20.5 kg (45 lb) and is about 2.2 m (87 in.) long. The collars used to secure the weight plates to an Olympic bar weigh 2.25 kg (5 lb) each. The sleeves on which the plates are mounted are larger than more conventional plates and rotate so that the plates do not stick to the bar when it is lifted. The plates are also larger in diameter than the traditional plates so that a patient who drops the bar is not crushed or otherwise injured by the bar.

Technique

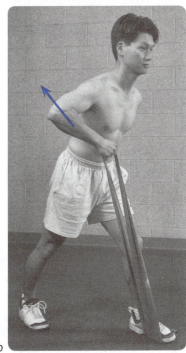

As with any exercise, proper instruction in execution is necessary in order to achieve appropriate strengthening without substitution of activity by incorrect muscles. It may be helpful, especially in the beginning, to have the patient use a relatively light weight so that he or she can perform the technique correctly and learn what muscle is to be used during the activity. Stabilization of the part exercised is necessary and is more difficult with free weights than with machine weights. Once you are confident that the patient is able to perform the exercise correctly and understands the proper procedure, you can increase the exercise resistance to an appropriate resistance level for strength gains.

The patient should have control of the weight throughout the entire range of motion. A full range of motion during the exercise is necessary to provide for strength gains throughout the motion. The patient should perform the activity in a slow, controlled manner. As the muscle's strength improves and more functional activities are appropriate, the speed of the motion may increase, depending on the goals you have determined for the exercise.

Free weight exercises are more difficult to perform than machine weight exercises, because while the weight is being lifted, it must also be controlled. The exercising extremity must stabilize itself with the added weight and control the weight simultaneously. This requires work not only of the specific muscle being exercised, but also of the surrounding muscles.

▶ **Figure 7.29** Rubber band exercises: *(a)* hip medial rotation exercise; *(b)* shoulder horizontal extension (or bent-over row) exercise.

One selects the exercise weight according to the strength of the muscle being exercised, while also considering the repetition and set goals. The weight should be heavy enough to challenge the patient yet light enough to allow him or her to accomplish the goals.

What determines the position in which the patient performs the exercise is the point in the motion where the greatest resistance is desired. For example, in an elbow curl, the greatest resistance in standing occurs when the elbow is at 90°. If the patient performs the exercise in supine, the greatest resistance is in the beginning of the exercise when the elbow begins moving into flexion from full extension. Here is a lower extremity example: If a cuff weight is attached to a patient's ankle for a hamstring curl exercise, the maximum resistance occurs in the beginning of knee flexion if the patient is lying prone, but it occurs at 90° knee flexion if the exercise is performed in standing. This change in position of maximum resistance occurs since the maximum resistance is determined by the relationship between the pull of gravity on the weight and the position of the segment being exercised. As mentioned in chapter 3, when the pull of gravity is perpendicular to the lever arm, the resistance is at its greatest. The rehabilitation clinician must determine where in the motion to place the primary emphasis for strength before selecting the proper position for the exercise.

When a muscle's position changes to acquire a maximum resistance at a different angle, the stresses to the muscle change. For example, if a patient performs an elbow curl with 4.5 kg (10 lb) in a supine position, then changes to a sitting position, the weight tolerance will change. The maximum stress is applied in the middle of the motion in the seated position rather than at the beginning as it was in supine, so the muscles may not have the strength to lift 4.5 kg by the time the elbow moves to 90° in the seated position. This is a consideration when determining the patient's exercise position.

A pulley system is a form of free-weight system. A pulley board or other unit includes a cable to which a weight is attached. The cable runs through at least one, or most often two, pulleys. The pulleys can be adjustable to provide more variety in exercise positions. The position of the pulley and rope determines where in the range of motion the greatest resistance is provided to the muscle. Maximum resistance occurs when the line of the rope from the pulley to the extremity forms a 90° angle with the extremity. Figure 7.30 demonstrates this concept.

Again, you can change the maximum resistance by changing the angle of the force. In this case, the angle of the force is determined not by gravity but by the pulley position. These lever arm concepts are presented in chapter 3.

The equipment is secured before the patient lifts the weight. This means checking that the dumbbell and barbell collars are secure so the weight plates will not fall off during lifting. If the patient is using cuff weights, the straps should be in good shape and secured so that the weight will not fall off when the patient moves the extremity.

The amount of weight lifted increases as the patient's strength improves. Once strength improves, the weight's proportional resistance declines, the exercise becomes easier, and additional changes in strength do not occur unless the weight is increased. You routinely reevaluate strength to determine when the patient is ready for a weight increase.

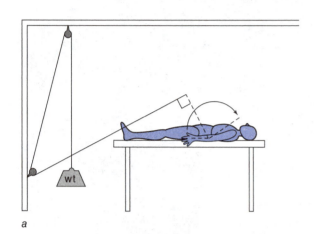

a

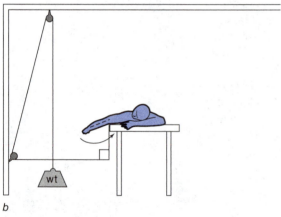

b

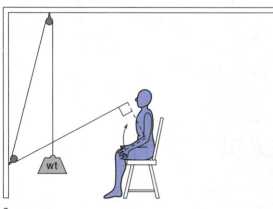

c

▶ **Figure 7.30** Different pulley angles for an elbow flexor strength exercise: *(a)* supine, *(b)* prone, and *(c)* seated. Maximum resistance occurs when angle of pulley cable to the arm is 90°.

Advantages

With free weights, the amount of resistance offered to the patient is not limited by the rehabilitation clinician's strength. This is the most obvious advantage of free weights over manual resistance.

There is a variety of free weight equipment on the market today, ranging from the plain, simple, and inexpensive to the complex, "gadgetized," and expensive. Selection depends on budget, space, needs, preference, and ability to use the equipment.

Free weights are used in a number of ways to increase muscle strength, and they can be used in different positions to provide maximum resistance at varying angles. This can add variety to the therapeutic exercise program.

Another benefit is that free weights make it is easy to determine quantitative measures of strength and of improvement in strength. This gives the clinician an evaluative tool and provides the patient with an automatic motivating factor. The clinician can document objective improvements when the patient's weights change. The patient is motivated to increase the amount of weight lifted and feels a sense of accomplishment when achieving weight goals.

The cuff weights can be used in a functional activity when attached to the wrist or ankle. For example, an injured soccer player can add resistance to kicking during the activity by attaching a weight cuff to the ankle.

Disadvantages

The greatest disadvantage of free weights is safety, which you must always consider when using this equipment. The risk of injury if the weight is too great or is not used properly is a consistent danger. The patient should be instructed to use the weights correctly and to return them to their proper place when finished with the exercise. A patient cannot control a weight that is too heavy.

Because lifting free weights is an isotonic activity, the amount of weight lifted is no greater than that which the muscle is able to lift at the weakest part of its motion. The amount of resistance changes as the lever arm length changes when the segment moves through its motion.

Finally, lifting weights can be boring. Bored patients are less likely to work as hard during an exercise. It is also more difficult to become motivated if the exercise is not interesting, and compliance may be more difficult.

Isotonic Machines

In addition to free weights, a variety of machines can be used for isotonic exercises. Some have a fixed lever system that offers different amounts of resistance. Changes in resistance occur differently, depending on the machine. The most commonly used machines provide altered resistance with weights, resistance bands, or hydraulic pressure. This category of equipment includes a long list of machines made by many companies. A list of generic examples includes hydraulic devices, multiple-station units, individual freestanding stations, and rubber cord resistive machines.

Isotonic machines provide a constant load during an exercise. As with free weights, the load lifted is whatever the muscle at its weakest point is able to manage.

The design of some machines is such that you can control the allowable range of motion by placing a weight key at different positions on the weight's arm. This can change the excursion of the exercise and the weight lifted. For example, you can change a range of motion excursion on a bench press machine by first elevating the bench press arm and then inserting the key at the desired weight load.

Isotonic machines can also be used for isometric exercises. To use the machine this way, you place the weight key at a weight that is too heavy for the patient to lift, or lock the lever so that movement is not possible.

Other simple isotonic "machines" fall into this category because they offer isotonic activity against a mechanical resistance. This group includes a large variety of equipment such as the N-K table (named after its two designers R. B. Noland and F. A. Kuckhoff), hand putty, and grip exercisers.

Technique

As always, instruction in proper use of the equipment and proper execution of the exercise is necessary. You should not assume that patients are able to perform an exercise correctly merely because they state that they have done the exercise before. Patients often either perform an exercise incorrectly prior to their injuries or, because of weakness, use the wrong muscles to perform an exercise that was easy before they were injured. You should first demonstrate the exercise for the patient and then have the patient do the exercise while you observe for correct execution.

It is important to watch the speed of the exercise to observe for and caution against muscle substitution. Educate the patient regarding the proper speed and performance. This is especially important if you intend to have the patient perform the exercises independently later in the program. Changes in speed can occur with strength advances. As indicated with other exercises, the patient should perform exercises through a full range of motion.

Advantages

The greatest advantage in the use of isotonic machines is safety. The weight is guided and controlled by the machine, so the chances of injury resulting from the weight's dropping or the patient's losing control of the machine are very slim.

The multiple-station units allow many patients to work simultaneously. You can easily establish a circuit program on the machine so that either one patient or several can exercise at one time.

Once exercises are established, the patient can exercise without assistance. The rehabilitation clinician can perform periodic reevaluation with increases in repetitions, sets, or weights. The treatment time can then be used for other, more directed activities.

It is easy to establish a machine exercise progression by changing the number of repetitions or sets, the speed of the exercise, or the resistance. Changing these parameters can also add some variety to a therapeutic exercise program.

Weight machines most often have either a specific weight indication or a progressive number indication on the plates. This permits an objective measure of improvement. Quantifying gains introduces a motivating factor and is an objective measure of progress for both the patient and the rehabilitation clinician.

Some pieces of equipment are not expensive; some can even be handmade and modified to fit specific clinic or individual patient needs. For example, a wrist exerciser can be made from a weight disk, dowel, and rope.

Disadvantages

Some of the disadvantages of isotonic machines are the same as for free weights. One is that the muscle's weakest point determines the maximum weight that can be lifted.

Using equipment can be boring. It may be difficult to motivate patients to perform daily exercises on the machines.

Additionally, some isotonic machines are very expensive and require considerable facility space. This is particularly true for the individual freestanding machines. The multi-unit machines may require less space, but they are also expensive, and many still require a relatively large space for installation and operation.

Isokinetic Machines

Isokinetic exercise machines have been available since the early 1970s. They were very popular during the 1970s and 1980s. Several manufacturers produced isokinetic equipment during the 1980s. Today, emphasis has moved away from isokinetic equipment, and the demand has dwindled drastically. Today, there are only two manufacturers—Biodex (Biodex Corporation, Shirley, NY) and Cybex (Henley Health Care, Cybex Medical Division, Sugarland, TX). A Biodex is shown in figure 7.31.

Isokinetic machines offer resistance at a constant speed, so the amount of resistance varies through the range of motion. This is sometimes referred to as *accommodating resistance*. To produce a constant speed, the machine offers a matching resistance when the patient attempts to push the arm of the machine as hard as possible. For an isokinetic exercise to produce the desired results, the patient must resist the machine with maximal effort.

Technique

Isokinetic machines today offer resistance concentrically, eccentrically, and isometrically. The type of exercise used depends on the settings established on the machine by the rehabilitation clinician. The settings are determined according to the specific goals and the type of exercise the rehabilitation clinician decides is the best method of achieving those goals.

The isokinetic machine's speed is preset before the exercise begins. Settings range from very slow (less than 30°/s) to very fast (over 300°/s). Even at the fastest settings, the speeds do not mimic the speeds of motion during functional activities. For example, forearm speeds greater than 9,000°/s occur with throwing a ball (Braatz & Gogia, 1987). Even normal walking produces a tibial swing-through phase speed of about 48 kph (30 mph). One of the early claims of isokinetic advocates was that the isokinetic machines could mimic functional speeds; now that we can measure true joint speeds we know that this is not the case.

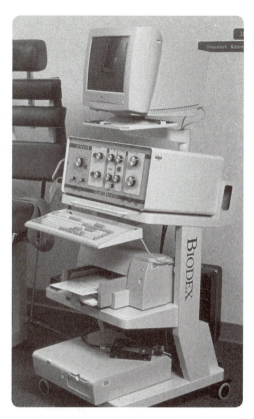

▶ **Figure 7.31** Isokinetic machine.

It is necessary to instruct the patient in proper exercise execution on the equipment. The exercise sensation is not necessarily one that the patient has experienced before, since other equipment provides a variation in resistance and speed whereas isokinetic equipment forces the patient's speed to remain constant throughout the motion.

Isokinetic equipment can be used at submaximal levels. This is particularly important if the patient's injury is recent or if the patient has too much pain to permit a maximal resistance output. It is important to explain to the patient the goal of the exercise if that goal is less-than-maximal output.

The equipment should be properly set before the exercise begins. Isokinetic machines can be placed in a variety of positions to be used on a variety of joints. Proper alignment of the machine's joint is necessary to avoid placing undue torque on the patient's joint. Correct machine lever arm length should also be determined before the beginning of exercise.

Instructions should include precautions about avoiding pain during the exercise and eliminating substitution by other muscle groups. Stabilization straps should be applied to ensure minimum substitution. If the patient experiences pain, changes in the exercise parameter settings are indicated.

Advantages

Isokinetic equipment provides a constant-speed, accommodating-resistance exercise to produce a maximum muscle resistance throughout the range of motion.

The machines can be used for maximal and submaximal muscle output. Less-than-maximal output can be controlled to permit exercise without increasing injury. Likewise, use of a maximal muscle output can provide increased stress to the muscle as healing progresses and the muscle's tolerance improve.

Diagonal patterns can be performed on the equipment to produce a more functional form of exercise. This can assist the muscles in relearning functional patterns of motion.

The machine produces measurable and reproducible results and can be used for testing as well as exercising. The machine's computer records the muscle's output throughout the range of motion and can correlate the strength with a specific degree within the motion.

The computer's visual readings provide immediate feedback to the patient and to the clinician. Goals can also be indicated on the screen. This information serves to motivate the patient as a goal is established and results of efforts toward it can be seen. The clinician also receives immediate information about the patient's effort, areas of weakness through the range of motion, and points at which there should be greater emphasis in other exercises.

Comparison of records between one session and another also provides feedback on progress. Maintaining a record reveals concrete and objective changes in the patient's progress.

The machine's speeds can be varied, so a patient can exercise at slower or faster speeds to work on fast-twitch and slow-twitch muscles in the same session. Exercises can be used to improve strength, muscle endurance, coordination, and speed of movement.

Disadvantages

Isokinetic machines have two primary disadvantages. One is cost: An isokinetic machine, with the equipment and computer, costs over $40,000. Many facilities find this price prohibitive. The other clear disadvantage is that the exercises are primarily OKC exercises. Since lower-extremity activities are primarily CKC, functional application is minimal.

Another disadvantage is that in performing evaluations, the rehabilitation clinician must remain consistent with respect to speed, settings, and positions from one session to another in order to obtain consistent results. Changing anything during the activity, even the motivating commands, can alter the results.

Some clinicians find the setup of the machine and the need to change its position and pieces of equipment too complicated and too time consuming to be practical. This is the case especially if the machine is used infrequently.

Isokinetic computers can offer a great deal of information on the patient's performance. This can be an advantage or a disadvantage. It can be advantageous if the rehabilitation clinician understands the information and its significance for the therapeutic exercise program. It is disadvantageous, however, if he or she does not understand the data and does not take time to learn their significance. In this case, the clinician may be frustrated and intimidated by the information so instead of using the machine, discards it as impractical.

If many patients are using the machine for therapeutic exercise, they may need to wait their turns. One patient may use the machine for several bouts of exercise or for various positions. This takes time and can prohibit its use by others for extended periods. In situations in which a clinician has limited time to spend with a patient, this may not be a piece of equipment that is available at the right time or convenient to use.

Other Equipment

Other accommodating-resistance machines provide variable resistance through the range of motion. One type of equipment, familiar in gyms, is known as Nautilus (Nautilus, Deland, FL)—so named because its cam resembles the cross section of the shell of the sea mollusk nautilus. Machines of this type offer a variable resistance through a cam system. The cam allows the lever arm length of the machine to change so that the amount of resistance changes. These changes are supposed to coincide with the change in the muscle's lever arm, so that as the muscle's strength changes, a concomitant change in the resistance is offered to it by the machine; however, because these machines are not designed for all body sizes, the machine's resistance may not match the individual's muscle-length changes through its range of motion. Smaller men and many women may find that the machines do not correlate with their extremity lengths. In these cases, using the machines may cause injury.

Other machines and exercise equipment are available for strengthening. Some of these devices are mentioned in other chapters in connection with such topics as proprioception. Nautilusä and other machines may not be indicated for therapeutic exercise use, especially

The primary methods of increasing strength include use of body weight, rubber tubing and bands, free weights, and isotonic and isokinetic machines. Each has its own advantages and disadvantages.

in the earlier stages of rehabilitation. The rehabilitation clinician must understand the functions, the weight minimums and increments, and the way in which each machine operates before determining whether or not a piece of equipment is appropriate for a patient's use. The patient's abilities, healing phase, size, injury limitations, and restrictions are all factors to consider before advocating the use of any machine.

PROPRIOCEPTIVE NEUROMUSCULAR FACILITATION

Sherrington, a neurophysiologist, provided the basic concepts that were used by Herman Kabat, MD, during the late 1940s and early 1950s to develop **proprioceptive neuromuscular facilitation (PNF)** exercise techniques. The underlying significance of this technique was in the use of combinations of primitive movement patterns performed with a maximum amount of resistance applied throughout the range of motion. The techniques were originally found to be useful in the treatment of neuromuscular disorders, but over time they have also proven beneficial for application to orthopedic disorders. Proprioceptive neuromuscular facilitation has been helpful in restoring flexibility, strength, and coordination of injured muscles and joints.

Facilitation

It is in this sense—restoration—that rehabilitation clinicians use PNF today. Proprioceptive neuromuscular facilitation incorporates the inhibitory and excitatory impulses from the afferent receptors of skin, muscle, tendon, visual, and auditory neurons that facilitate a response from the motor neurons, resulting in a desired action. For example, the rehabilitation clinician's hands on the patient's leg provide a stimulus from the skin receptors; a stretch force applied by the rehabilitation clinician on the muscle stimulates the muscle spindle and Golgi tendon organs; the patient's ability to see where the leg is going provides additional input to produce the desired motion pattern; and the verbal cueing and guidance of the clinician during the activity stimulate the patient's auditory receptors to send messages to increase or decrease muscle activity.

Each of these afferent stimuli influences the motor response. To see the significance of this point, you can easily perform a simple test. With a person lying supine, place one hand on the hamstring and one hand on the quadriceps. Ask the person to maximally resist you in a straight-leg raise, and judge the amount of resistance the person provides. Now place your hands only on the quadriceps and have the patient repeat the maximally resisted movement. You should experience greater resistance with both of your hands on the quadriceps surface and less resistance with one hand on the hamstrings and one on the quadriceps. With tactile input of both surfaces, the afferent stimulation is a mixed one, producing both facilitation in and inhibition to the anterior muscles. When both hands are on the same surface, facilitation to the muscles performing the action is provided without inhibition from sensory nerves of the hamstring surface.

A quick stretch provided in a PNF movement immediately before the exercise produces a stretch reflex from stimulation of the muscle spindles and Golgi tendon organs. This causes increased response from the muscle.

Taking the patient's leg passively through the activity before performing the actual exercise gives the patient the visual and proprioceptive feedback to realize the direction and pattern that the leg should traverse. If you do not do this before the exercise, you will find not only that the patient is confused about what to do, but also that the output of the muscle is significantly less. The more confidence the patient has about being able to perform the pattern correctly, the stronger the motion will be.

Verbal input is used commonly in athletic events. We do it when we cheer a team or player during competition. When we want a patient to perform an exercise at a maximal output, we use verbal cues to encourage him or her to do the most work possible. Verbal cues in PNF provide the same stimulus. They are also necessary for permitting the patient to correctly perform the pattern of activity desired. Cueing with brief, well-timed words and phrases facilitates an improved muscle response.

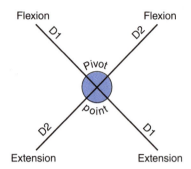

▶ **Figure 7.32** PNF patterns: Neural motion occurs in diagonal planes of component motions.

Patterns of Movement

The premise underlying PNF is that central nervous system stimulation produces mass movement patterns, not straight-plane movements. Natural motion does not occur in straight planes but in mass movement patterns that incorporate a diagonal motion in combination with a spiral movement. In other words, all major parts of the body move in patterns that have three components. These diagonal patterns include the components of flexion and extension. Because the patterns are diagonal, they also include motions either toward & across the midline (adduction) or away from & across the midline (abduction). Rotation is the third component of PNF patterns. Figure 7.32 demonstrates these components. Although PNF can be used for the trunk as well as the extremities, discussion of PNF here is limited to the upper and lower extremities, since these are the areas primarily treated with PNF in musculoskeletal rehabilitation.

The movement patterns are referred to as D1 and D2. D1 flexion and D1 extension patterns are moving into flexion and moving into extension, respectively. D2 patterns are divided in the same way.

This pattern designation is easier to remember if you recall that in the upper extremity, lateral rotation always goes with flexion, and in the lower extremity, lateral rotation always goes with adduction. For example, in the upper extremity as the shoulder goes from extension to flexion it always laterally rotates whether the movement is adducted or abducted (figure 7.33a). Therefore, when the arm goes into extension, the shoulder medially rotates, and the varying motion is either adduction in a D1 pattern or abduction in a D2 pattern.

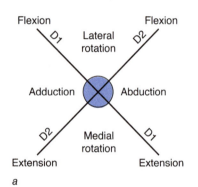

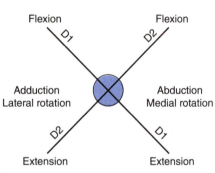

▶ **Figure 7.33** *(a)* Lateral rotation is associated with flexion while medial rotation is associated with extension in the upper extremities. *(b)* In the lower extremities, adduction and lateral rotation occur together as do abduction and medial rotation.

Because lateral rotation accompanies adduction in the lower extremity, the variables are flexion and extension. When the hip moves into flexion and adduction, the rotational movement is lateral rotation (D1), but when it moves into flexion with abduction, medial rotation (D2) also occurs (figure 7.33b). Likewise, when the hip moves into extension, either lateral rotation with adduction (D2) or medial rotation with abduction (D1) will also occur, depending on which pattern is used.

When you think about it, these are natural patterns that you see every day in sport and daily activities. For example, when throwing a ball overhand, the shoulder starts in abduction, flexion, and lateral rotation. As the ball is thrown, the follow-through ends with the shoulder in extension, adduction, and medial rotation. Kicking a soccer ball also demonstrates the PNF pattern: As the ball is kicked, the leg moves from extension, abduction, and medial rotation to a follow-through position of flexion, adduction, and lateral rotation. When you sit in a relaxed position with your feet up and hands behind your head, the shoulder is in flexion, abduction, with lateral rotation, and your legs are extended in front of you, crossed, in adduction and lateral rotation.

If you remember these natural positions, the patterns of movement for the part of the extremity beyond the shoulder and hip should make sense. Figures 7.34 and 7.35 diagram and illustrate the positions of the other joints in D1 and D2 patterns.

In each position, the joints go from one extreme to the other by the time the movement is complete. For example, if the patient begins with the shoulder extended, abducted, and medially rotated, the elbow extended, the forearm pronated, the wrist ulnarly extended, and the fingers and thumb extended, the end position will be the D1 flexion position—in shoulder flexion, adduction, and lateral rotation, elbow flexion, forearm supination, wrist radially flexed, and fingers and thumb flexed and adducted. Note that the elbow and the knee can be

Joint	D1 flexion	D2 flexion
Shoulder:	Flexion	Flexion
	Lateral rotation	Lateral rotation
	Adduction	Abduction
Forearm:	Supination	Supination
Wrist:	Radial flexion	Radial extension
Fingers:	Flexion	Extension

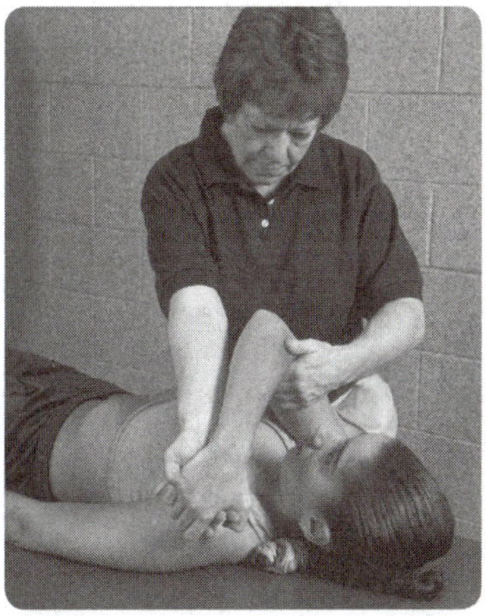

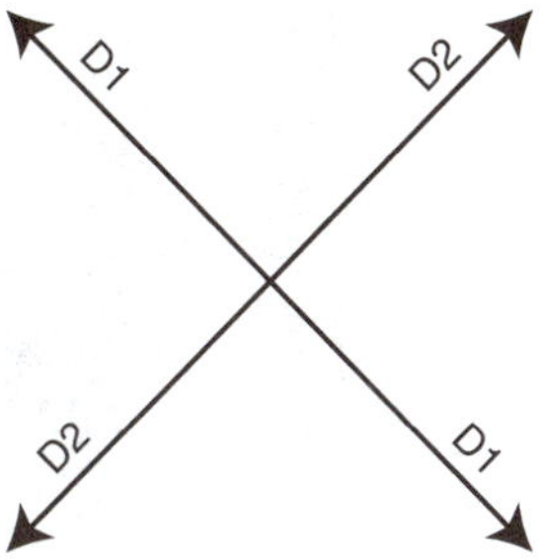

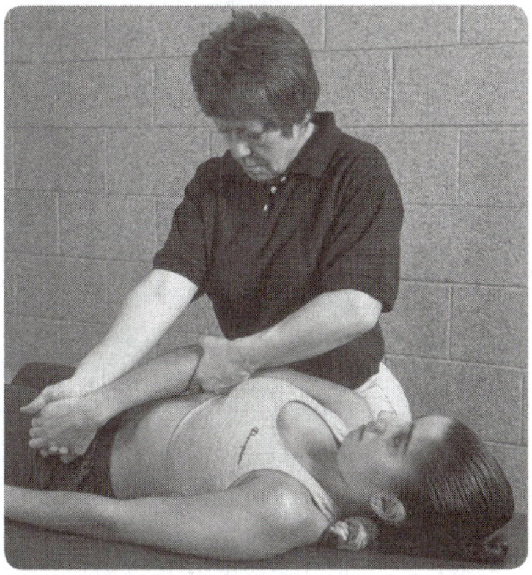

Joint	D2 extension	D1 extension
Shoulder:	Extension	Extension
	Medial rotation	Medial rotation
	Adduction	Abduction
Forearm:	Pronation	Pronation
Wrist:	Ulnar flexion	Ulnar extension
Fingers:	Flexion	Extension

▶ **Figure 7.34** Upper-extremity PNF patterns.

moved from flexion to extension or extension to flexion with any of the patterns. The position the elbow or knee is in at the end of the motion is the opposite of the joint's position at the beginning of the movement.

Essentially, all that has been written about PNF in recent years has been based on the works of Knott and Voss (Knott & Voss, 1968). The patterns of movement, techniques, and principles most commonly used today center on the information these authors have provided to the medical community. For the best results, they advocate the use of basic principles in the application of PNF.

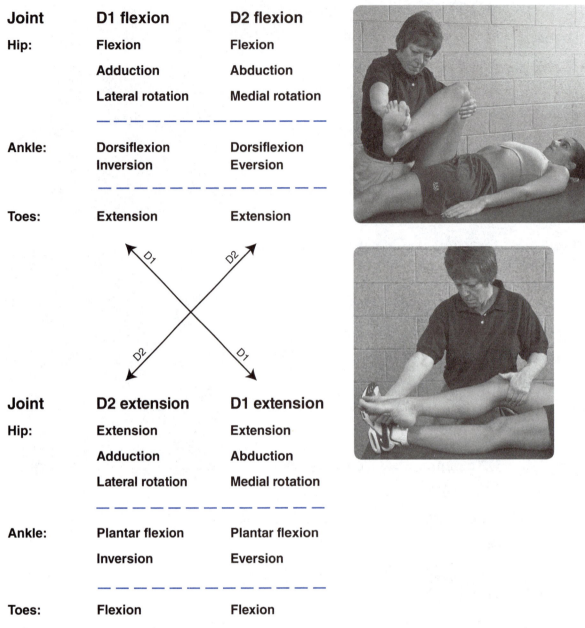

Joint	D1 flexion	D2 flexion
Hip:	Flexion	Flexion
	Adduction	Abduction
	Lateral rotation	Medial rotation
Ankle:	Dorsiflexion	Dorsiflexion
	Inversion	Eversion
Toes:	Extension	Extension

Joint	D2 extension	D1 extension
Hip:	Extension	Extension
	Adduction	Abduction
	Lateral rotation	Medial rotation
Ankle:	Plantar flexion	Plantar flexion
	Inversion	Eversion
Toes:	Flexion	Flexion

▶ **Figure 7.35** Lower-extremity PNF patterns.

Principles

The principles of application incorporate the physiological facilitation and inhibition responses of the body to stimuli. Effective use of these responses produces an optimum result. The primary principles of application are the following:

1. *The clinician's hand placement is important for providing appropriate facilitation of the deep-touch and pressure receptors.* The hands are placed on the surface side toward which the extremity is to move to stimulate those muscles. For example, if the patient's hip is moving into extension, the knee is flexing, and the foot is plantar flexing, the hamstrings and plantar foot should be the points of contact.

Manual contact using appropriately applied pressure also helps guide the patient's extremity in the correct direction. The contact is firm and reassuring, not painful or hesitant.

2. *Verbal cues are given in a moderate tone if the patient is providing a maximal output.* If additional force is desired, a stronger, sharp verbal command is given. The wording should be one- or two-word phrases, simple and meaningful. For example, "push" or "pull," "hold" or "relax," and "rotate" or "across" are all simple commands that give the patient easy-to-understand, clear instructions. The commands are timed correctly in relation to the activity.

3. *The technique should not be painful.* Pain will produce a reflex withdrawal and cause an inhibition of activity rather than facilitation.

4. *Proper instruction in the PNF pattern before the start of exercise is important if the muscles are to receive optimal facilitation.* The patient should receive simple instructions that include the sequencing of activities, the diagonal pattern, and appropriate speed of activity. If the patient knows before execution what is expected and understands the exercise, the patient is better able to perform the activity and elicit a stronger response from the muscle. The visual stimulation of seeing the movement before performance of the exercise provides additional feedback for the patient's increased facilitation of the muscles.

5. *Rotation is an important component of the diagonal motion.* It begins distally and progresses toward the proximal muscle groups as the patient continues through the motion. Rotation begins the pattern so by mid-ROM, rotation movement should be finished. Proper verbal cueing for correct distal-to-proximal movement assists the patient in proper execution of the exercise.

6. *Providing traction to separate the joint surfaces or approximation to compress the joint surfaces stimulates the joint's proprioceptive nerve endings.* As a rule, traction occurs with pulling motions and approximation occurs with the pushing motions. If a joint is very irritable, traction or approximation may aggravate it; the clinician must use caution and good judgment before applying this technique.

7. *A quick stretch applied immediately before the beginning of the movement pattern uses the stretch reflex to facilitate the muscle into a stronger initial response.* In some injuries, a stretch may be contraindicated. Once again, caution and good judgment are needed before a quick stretch is applied.

8. *The motions are performed precisely and through a smooth range of motion.* The movement is not jerky. Isometric contractions should build until maximal output from the patient's muscle is achieved. No motion is produced during an isometric activity, and the rehabilitation clinician does not break the isometric hold.

9. *The clinician must use good body mechanics.* Application of manual resistance in PNF techniques requires that the rehabilitation clinician use his or her own body efficiently and safely and conserve energy. Proper body mechanics makes this possible.

Techniques

Stretching techniques of PNF, including hold-relax, contract-relax, and slow reversal-hold-relax, are discussed in chapter 5. The techniques used for strengthening are rhythmic initiation, rhythmic stabilization, slow reversal, and slow reversal-hold. Whether a PNF technique is used to gain mobility or strength, the principles and movement patterns presented above hold true.

PNF techniques can be confusing if correct terminology is not understood. There are two patterns in PNF: agonistic and antagonistic. The *agonistic muscle pattern* occurs when the muscle is contracting toward its shortened state. The *antagonistic muscle pattern* occurs when the muscle is approaching its lengthened state. The location of the antagonistic pattern is diagonally opposite of the agonistic pattern of motion.

Rhythmic initiation is used to increase a muscle's ability to initiate movement and stabilize. It includes voluntary relaxation, passive movement, and repeated isotonic activity in the agonistic pattern. The extremity is moved by the clinician to the shortened range of the antagonistic pattern. The patient is then asked to move the extremity through the agonistic muscle pattern. The exercise may start as an active-assistive exercise in a very weak patient and progress to resistive motion. In more advanced procedures, an isometric activity in the weaker portion of the motion can be incorporated within the isotonic movement. Athletes are usually at a higher level than patients who most benefit from this technique, so it is not used often with patients seen by rehabilitation clinicians working with athletes.

Reversal of antagonists techniques are the ones most commonly modified and used in rehabilitation. They most mimic normal activity because they incorporate the use of first one muscle group and then its opposing muscle group, much as daily activities and sport performance activities do. These techniques begin in the end range of the agonistic pattern with resisted motion occurring first in the antagonistic pattern of motion. This is immediately followed by resistance through the agonistic pattern. These techniques include rhythmic stabilization, slow reversal, and slow reversal-hold.

Rhythmic stabilization uses isometric activity of agonists and antagonists. The rehabilitation clinician offers resistance that does not break the isometric activity of the antagonist and then offers resistance to isometric activity of the agonist. This produces a co-contraction to improve stabilization. The technique is repeated several times without movement of the extremity with no pause between the contractions. It can be repeated at several points within the range of motion. Isometric contractions are first performed in an antagonistic pattern and then in an agonistic pattern.

Slow reversal is a technique that provides a maximum resistance in an antagonistic pattern from the rehabilitation clinician throughout a range of motion. This is followed by resistance in the agonistic pattern of motion. For example, if hamstrings were the weak muscle group, the clinician applies resistance to the lower extremity D1 pattern going into hip flexion-adduction-lateral rotation. At the completion of the antagonistic movement pattern, the rehabilitation clinician reverses hand positions on the patient's lower extremity to provide resistance to D1 going into hip extension-abduction-medial rotation moving into an agonistic pattern. In the *slow reversal-hold* technique, the procedure is the same except that an isometric hold is performed at the end of the motion.

These techniques can be applied individually or in combination. Their use is determined by the patient's deficiencies and needs.

> ■ **PNF Techniques**
>
> | Stretching | Strengthening |
> | --- | --- |
> | Hold-relax | Rhythmic initiation |
> | Contract-relax | Rhythmic stabilization |
> | Slow reversal-hold-relax | Slow reversal |
> | | Slow reversal-hold |

Exercise techniques based on proprioceptive neuromuscular facilitation use impulses from the afferent receptors in various parts of the body to stimulate the desired motion. One such technique, reversal of antagonists, is common in rehabilitation because it mimics daily and sport performance activities.

STRENGTHENING PRINCIPLES

When do strengthening exercises begin in a therapeutic exercise program? The answer depends on the severity of the injury, the tissue injured, healing timeline, the physician's preference, and the patient's tolerance. Once a therapeutic exercise program starts, strengthening exercises at some level should begin. At first, they may be no more than isometrics or exercises that concentrate on other areas or those adjacent to the injured site. Chapter 2 addresses the importance of rest and the importance of activity. The rehabilitation clinician makes a careful judgment and considers the variable factors to determine when the strengthening exercises should occur and how intense they should be.

The rehabilitation clinician should have a sound reason for using any strengthening exercise in a patient's therapeutic exercise program. Use of many exercises that have the same goal and that work the same muscle may be a waste of time unless the specific goal is to increase muscle endurance and provide variety to prevent boredom. The rehabilitation clinician should design a therapeutic exercise program specific to the needs of the patient as determined by analysis of the patient's deficiencies and knowledge of the demands of the patient's activities. A strengthening program may emphasize primarily strength or muscle endurance or a combination of these.

Progression of a patient in a therapeutic exercise program is individually determined. Each patient is different. Expectations based on other patients' progression or the clinician's hopes are unrealistic and unfair. You should periodically examine the injury during the treatment program so that you can accurately determine the response to treatment and maintain an optimal course of treatment.

A strengthening program is designed according to four principles. The acronym **SNAP** stands for the primary concerns in the establishment of any strengthening program:

Specific exercises

No pain

Attainable goals

Progressive overload

Let's look at each of these issues individually.

Specific Exercises

A therapeutic exercise program contains specific exercises to achieve the long-term goal, the patient's return to normal activity or sport performance. This concept is based on the **SAID** principle: Specific Adaptations to Imposed Demands (Wallis & Logan, 1964). This means that the muscle will adapt and perform according to the demands placed on it. For example, if a patient lifts low weights for high repetitions, the muscle will gain endurance. If a patient wants to gain strength, resistance should be closer to his or her maximum resistance and consist of about six repetitions. The SAID principle also means that exercises should mimic stresses placed on a muscle during functional activities to produce appropriate strength gains. If a patient's sport calls for a specific activity, such as holding a pike position on the parallel bars in gymnastics, then the strength exercises for that patient should include isometric hip flexor and abdominal exercises. If the patient's sport is soccer, which does not demand sustained movements, the therapeutic exercise program for that patient requires more isotonic endurance and power-related activities. If an individual's job is to lift and move boxes, then his therapeutic exercise program should be repetitive in nature.

Since a muscle's greatest recovery occurs in the first 30 to 90 s following exercise to exhaustion, the design of the therapeutic exercise program should take this into account (figure 7.36). As a muscle continues an activity, the maximal output declines as fatigue occurs with more repetitions. Exercise sets should include a rest period of 30 to 60 s between each set. A rule of thumb is a 1:1 ratio between the time it takes to perform the exercise and the rest time. Later in the program, the patient may need more or less rest, depending on the intensity of the exercise and the patient's goals.

In the early stages of a therapeutic exercise program, rapid gains in strength are commonly seen in a debilitated or deconditioned muscle. This occurs during the first three to five weeks of a therapeutic exercise program without a change in the muscle's atrophy (Moritani & DeVries, 1979). Many believe that these initial strength gains are primarily the result of neural adaptations within the muscle's neuromuscular system (Gabriel, Kamen, & Frost, 2006).

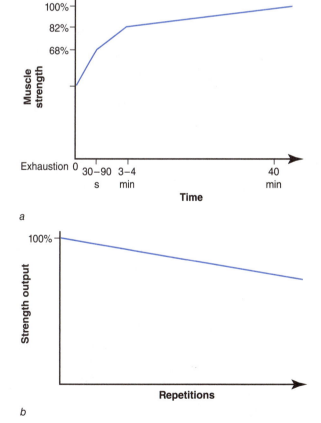

▶ **Figure 7.36** Effects of fatigue on strength and recovery: *(a)* recovery from fatigue, *(b)* maximal output declines with fatigue from repetitious activity.

Reflex inhibition of the muscle occurs with injury or inactivity. Immediate weakness is present after surgery as well. These sudden declines in strength are attributable to decreased neural activity. Because neural adaptations occur quickly with injury, it is postulated that they are also affected with attempts to restore the injured part (Hale, Hertel, & Olmsted-Kramer, 2007).

Strength is determined by both muscle fiber and neural control. The initial rapid gains in strength are attributed to improved neuromuscular recruitment, efficiency, coordination, and motor unit re-education (Gabriel et al., 2006; van der Hoeven, van Weerden, & Zwarts, 1993). Many researchers believe that improved neural activation results in an increased activation of synergists with a better coordination and co-contraction of the synergists, an inhibition of the antagonists, and improved activation ability and sensitivity to facilitation of the prime movers (de Ruiter, Van Leeuwen, Heijblom, Bobbert, & de Haan, 2006). A learning factor also affects the neural element of muscle activity.

Evidence to date appears to be anecdotal only; clinical observation has indicated that the rate of strength gains decreases as a therapeutic exercise program advances in time and duration (Houglum, 1977) (figure 7.37). Once the neural components are retrained, the gains are primarily made through muscle fiber hypertrophy. The greatest gains in strength occur in the early stages of a therapeutic exercise program—presenting the probability that neural changes are more significant than muscle size changes, especially in rehabilitation. Primary hypertrophic changes occur more commonly in patients who have lifted weights over a longer period of time or who use drugs to enhance hypertrophy (Folland & Williams, 2007).

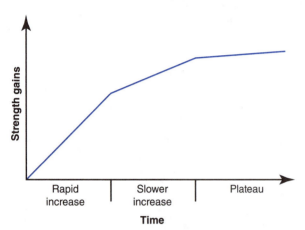

▶ **Figure 7.37** Rate of strength gains in a rehabilitation program.

In the early stages of a therapeutic exercise program, especially in cases in which muscle inactivity has been prolonged, the initial exercise efforts emphasize facilitation of the neural elements of the atrophied muscle. In addition to active exercise, electrical stimulation to assist in the facilitation of these neural pathways and in facilitation of proper muscle response may expedite recovery.

If a therapeutic exercise program following severe injury or surgery is prolonged, you will see a sequence in recovery that includes first, a rapid increase, and then a slower increase that is followed by a plateau. This sequence of change can occur over one cycle or more than one cycle. The pattern is individually determined and not predictable. If the patient reaches a plateau early in the program before achieving final goals, you should explain that this is common and that gains will come if the patient persists in the program. This situation during times of plateau can be difficult for the patient, since it may seem that no amount of effort produces gains. Patience and perseverance are essential to maintaining a good motivation level during this time. Sometimes the psychological lift of having a day off from the therex program can have a rejuvenating effect.

No Pain

There should be no pain during strengthening exercises. If a patient reports pain following a treatment session, questions regarding the site of pain are asked to clarify the site of pain. The patient's complaint of pain may actually be the result of working a weak muscle and not overstressing the injury site. Delayed pain or post-exercise pain at the injury site should be avoided. Post-exercise pain accompanied by post-exercise edema is an indication that the exercises have been too severe. It is advisable to reduce the severity of the exercise or even postpone the application of a strengthening exercise if you observe these symptoms. Pain produces a reflex withdrawal of muscle activity so that the muscle will not produce a maximal output. Progression of strengthening exercises should be progressive and within the patient's tolerance. If you increase resistance too much too quickly, the injury site may experience an inflammatory response, displayed by increased edema and pain.

Attainable Goals

Goals for the patient should be challenging but attainable. This means that it should be possible for the patient to move the amount of selected weight for the desired number of repetitions and sets. Most patients are goal oriented and are determined to achieve any goal set for them by themselves or by others. If goals are not achievable, the unrealistic expectations placed on the patient will serve only to frustrate both you and the patient. If you discover during the course of the exercise routine that you have set a goal too high, it is best to adjust the goal. However, setting unachievable goals is not to be confused with establishing challenges for the patient. For example, you may set a goal for a patient to lift a weight in a leg press for three sets of 20, and the first time he or she performs the exercise, the first set is performed to 20 repetitions, but in the second set, the patient can lift the weight 15 times and in the final set, only 10 times. You know that as his or her strength improves, the goal of three sets of 20 reps will be achieved. An unattainable goal is one that cannot be achieved by the patient, regardless of how strong he or she becomes. As an example, women are not usually capable of leg pressing 500 pounds, so that is not a goal you would set for any female patient you rehabilitated.

Estimating a patient's ability is something that is acquired with experience. Even seasoned clinicians sometimes miscalculate a patient goal but may not realize it until the patient's next treatment session. As with any clinician, if you find that you have made an error in setting a goal, you will occasionally need to adjust that goal based on the patient's response to the previous exercise session. This is more often the case early in the rehabilitation program when you may not yet know the patient's abilities, motivation level, and response to treatments.

Progressive Overload

Providing a progressive overload of exercises is fundamental to muscle strengthening. To continue to produce strength gains, the load must progressively increase. This concept is sometimes referred to as the **overload principle:** As a muscle's strength adapts to a resistance, the muscle must be additionally overloaded. For example, if a biceps is able to lift 8 kg for 10 repetitions, it must lift more than 8 kg for 10 repetitions to achieve additional strength. If the muscle lifts 8 kg repeatedly from one exercise session to the next, its strength will be maintained but will not increase.

When a muscle is not able to actively exercise or the patient is restricted from moving the injured area, **cross-training** can produce strength gains (Gabriel et al., 2006). Cross-training occurs when the contralateral part is exercised, resulting in strength gains on the opposite extremity. This form of training, sometimes also referred to as *cross-education,* has been around since the 1800s and has been used with varying degrees of success. The results depend primarily on the amount of resistance provided to the exercising extremity: The greater the effort of the extremity, the greater the results. This is a useful technique that you can apply in therapeutic exercise programs when the patient's injured area is restricted, perhaps because it is in a cast or splint, and exercise of the part is limited.

EXERCISE PROGRESSION

A progressive overload can be applied using various systems of progression. Several programs, advocated by a number of professionals over the years, have been used rather widely in rehabilitation.

DeLorme and Watkins (DeLorme & Watkins, 1948) provided a system that serves as a basis of progressive strengthening in many rehabilitation circles still today. They used 10 RM as a maximum strength determination. They advocated the use of three bouts, or sets, of

The rehabilitation clinician should be deliberate about when in a program to start strengthening exercises and should follow the principles of specificity, no pain, attainable goals, and progressive overload.

exercise, 10 repetitions each: The first set is performed at 50% of maximum, the second set at 75% of maximum, and the final set at 100% of the 10 RM (table 7.3).

Zinovieff, a physician who worked at England's United Oxford Hospitals, published a revision of the DeLorme program that he named the Oxford Technique (Zinovieff, 1951). Zinovieff found that with the DeLorme system his patients were too fatigued to complete the final set of 10 RM exercises. He suggested reversing the system, starting with the 10 RM on the first set of 10 repetitions and progressively reducing to 75% and then 50% on each successive set of 10 repetitions (table 7.4).

A number of authors have advanced a variety of other resistive exercise progressions. One of the more frequently used systems is the DAPRE (Daily Adjusted Progressive Resistive Exercise) technique (Knight, 1985). This is a complex system of daily exercise (six days a week) progression that meets the individual's ability to tolerate increased resistance. Table 7.5 illustrates the establishment of an RM and number of repetitions along with the determination of the next session's exercise weight.

TABLE 7.3 DeLorme and Watkins Strength Progression

Set	Repetitions	Weight
1	10	50% of 10 RM
2	10	75% of 10 RM
3	10	100% of 10 RM

TABLE 7.4 Oxford Technique of Strength Progression

Set	Repetitions	Weight
1	10	100% of 10 RM
2	10	75% of 10 RM
3	10	50% of 10 RM

TABLE 7.5 DAPRE System of Strength Progression

TECHNIQUE

Set	Repetitions	Weight
1	10	50% of working weight
2	6	75% of working weight
3	As many as possible	100% of working weight
4	As many as possible	Adjusted from 3rd set*

ADJUSTMENT GUIDELINES

Number of repetitions performed during prior set	4th-set weight adjustment based on 3rd set	Next-day weight adjustment based on 4th set
0-2	wt; redo set	wt; redo set
3-4	by 0-5 lb	Keep the same
5-7	Keep the same	by 5-10 lb
8-12	by 5-10 lb	by 5-15 lb
13 or more	by 10-15 lb	by 10-20 lb

*See Adjustment guidelines.
The number of repetitions performed on the third set determines the weight used on the fourth set. The next treatment day's starting weight is determined by the number of repetitions performed on the fourth set of the previous treatment.
Based on Knight 1985.

The essential element of DAPRE is that in the third and fourth sets of exercise, the patient performs as many repetitions as possible. The number of repetitions the individual can perform on the third set determines the amount of weight added for the fourth set of the day as well as for the start of the next treatment session.

The intent of the program is to have the patient perform as many repetitions during the set as possible. The goal is 5 to 7 repetitions. If the patient does 8 to 12 repetitions, the weight change is minimal; but if the patient performs 15 to 20 repetitions, the weight change is significantly larger. This program continues until the strength of the injured part is within 10% of the strength of the non-injured counterpart. At that time, the emphasis shifts to other deficiencies such as muscle endurance or coordination, and the DAPRE program is continued twice a week to maintain strength.

Most rehabilitation clinicians develop an exercise routine that seems to work best for them in achieving progression of a patient's strength. In the early stages of strengthening, the program I prefer has the patient lifting a weight that can be controlled for 6 to 15 repetitions for two sets. That weight is continued, with the patient attempting to perform as many repetitions as possible, until he or she is able to perform the exercise successfully for three sets of 20 to 25 repetitions each. At this point the weight increases and the patient reduces the number of repetitions. It is important, though, for the patient to perform as many repetitions as possible during each exercise session. The number of sets and repetitions depends on the demands of the patient's normal activity. Once the desired base-strength level is achieved, the number of sets, repetitions or exercise speed changes to meet the patient's sport demands.

As mentioned earlier in this chapter, Conroy and Earle (2000) advocate the use of high loads with low repetitions for strength gains. Figure 7.38 shows the relative gains in muscle strength and endurance with varying numbers of repetitions.

The program that the rehabilitation clinician chooses depends on individual preferences, his or her judgment about which program would benefit the patient most, and time availability. All the programs we have considered have been shown to be beneficial for making strength gains. As you gain experience with many patients who have varied therapeutic exercise needs, you will find a system that works best for you. Until then, I recommend that you keep an open mind, try different programs, and investigate the systems presented here as well as others to see what produces the best results for you. Whether you use an existing program or design one yourself, the key element for success is that it must be progressive; it must continue to stress the patient's muscles for continued improvement toward the specific rehabilitation goals. Experienced professionals often adjust programs according to what produces the best results.

> Several commonly used progressive overload systems are available.

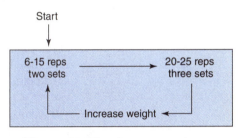

▶ **Figure 7.38** Houglum progression.

SUMMARY

The motor unit is the engine that produces motion. Intimate cooperation and coordination between the muscular and neural systems provide the body with a very complex physiochemical mechanism that creates movement. These mechanisms allow muscles to exert strength and build endurance. How we develop these two abilities is determined in part by how the injured muscles are rehabilitated. The clinician must be aware of sets and repetitions of muscle activity and of resistance levels used that will produce either one or the other. Additionally, the clinician must realize how changes in body positions may affect resistance and the body's ability to withstand that resistance. There are many ways to provide resistance for rehabilitation. Several factors such as cost, space, and versatility assist the clinician in determining what method may be best for rehabilitation. Selection of appropriate equipment is also determined by the advantages and disadvantages of each type and the patient's abilities. Muscles perform to different levels and in different manners, to provide movement, slow movement, or stabilize while motion occurs. The clinician must be aware of a muscle's function and rehabilitate it to function optimally at its required tasks.

KEY CONCEPTS AND REVIEW

1. Describe the sarcomere and its function in muscle activity.

The contractile element of a muscle fiber is the sarcomere. Actin and myosin filaments and their relationship to each other via cross-bridges determine the length of the sarcomere and its activity status. A complex system of biochemical processes and the stimulation of an action potential produce muscle activity through the release of calcium and ATP to cause a sliding of actin and myosin over each other, shortening the sarcomere's length.

2. Identify the elements of a motor unit.

A motor unit consists of a number of muscle fibers and the nerve that innervates the fibers. When stimulated, a motor unit behaves according to the all-or-none law in that all muscle fibers of the motor unit contract.

3. Explain how an action potential is transmitted.

The sarcoplasmic reticulum releases calcium to the muscle fibers through its T-tubules to the Z-discs where the calcium binds to the troponin on the actin filaments. This causes the tropomyosin on the actin filaments to shift and allow the head of the myosin cross-bridges to attach to the actin, shortening the sarcomere. The ATPase on the cross-bridges breaks down ATP for energy to allow the cross-bridges to re-cock and continue muscle activity. As long as calcium is present, the activity can continue.

4. Explain the differences between fast-twitch and slow-twitch muscle fibers.

Compared to fast-twitch or type II fibers, the slow-twitch, type I fibers are smaller, are red, have a slower conduction velocity, have a lower recruitment threshold, have lower minimum and maximum firing rates, have slower-acting myosin ATPase, have a greater number of mitochondria, and function in endurance activities rather than in rapid, brief bursts of activity.

5. Discuss the relationship between muscle strength, endurance, and power.

Muscle function includes strength, endurance, and power. Athletic activity involves all these factors to different degrees, depending on its specific demands. Muscle strength and endurance are closely related. Strength is the ability to produce force, and endurance is the ability to produce less forceful activities over a longer period; power is the strength output related to time.

6. Identify the various types of dynamic activity.

Dynamic activity includes muscle tension with movement. Dynamic activity is divided into isotonic and isokinetic activity. Isotonic activity is further divided into concentric and eccentric activity.

7. Discuss the differences between open and closed kinetic chain activity.

Open kinetic chain activity occurs when the distal aspect of the limb is not fixed and joints in the chain are able to move independently of each other; closed kinetic chain activity occurs when the distal aspect is fixed or anchored and movement of one joint impacts motion of the others in the chain.

8. Identify the various grades of manual muscle testing.

Muscle strength is rated from 5 (normal) to 0 (no function). A grade 4 muscle is one that offers some resistance beyond gravity but not normal resistance; a grade 3 muscle is able to lift the limb against gravity but unable to offer any additional strength; a grade 2 muscle is one that is able to move the limb through a full range of motion in a gravity-eliminated position; and a grade 1 muscle provides some voluntary activity but is unable to move the segment through a range of motion.

9. Discuss the types of muscle activity.

Passive motion is performed by an outside force without voluntary muscle activity; active assistive motion is motion that occurs through a combination of voluntary and assistive mechanisms; active motion occurs without the aid of any outside mechanism; and resistive motion occurs through a range of motion within which resistance to that motion is present.

10. List the PNF techniques commonly used in rehabilitation and their purposes.

Rhythmic initiation, slow reversal, slow reversal-hold, and rhythmic stabilization are the PNF techniques most commonly used for strengthening. The techniques used to gain motion include hold-relax, contract-relax, and slow reversal-hold-relax.

11. Identify four principles of strengthening exercises.

Development of a therapeutic exercise program must include consideration of SNAP guidelines: specific exercise, no pain, attainable goals, and progressive overload.

CRITICAL THINKING QUESTIONS

1. If you provide manual resistance to a patient's shoulder flexors, will the position in which the patient has been placed make any difference? Why or why not?

2. What steps could you take to improve performance if a patient were unable to perform a straight-leg raise without assistance because of weakness? How would your selection improve the patient's performance? How would it enable the patient to perform a straight-leg raise independently?

3. Explain four techniques that you could use to change the resistance without changing the amount of weight in a shoulder flexion exercise.

4. For a patient who has weakness in the quads, explain three progressive open kinetic chain and three progressive closed kinetic chain exercises you could use to strengthen the quads. What, if anything, would determine whether you started with the open or closed kinetic chain exercises?

5. If a patient were unable to bear weight on the lower extremity, not because of medical restriction but because of apprehension, what progression of activities would you select so that the patient could progress to weight bearing? What obstacles would you have to overcome for the patient to gain confidence that the leg would support him or her?

6. Is a patient able to lift a heavier dumbbell in elbow flexion in a seated or supine position? Where in the motion is the weight the most difficult for the patient to lift? Why? Is it a good idea to have the patient perform an elbow curl in both positions? Why? What other elbow-curl exercise would be an adequate substitute for a dumbbell exercise?

7. List six progressive exercises you would give Kamryn in the chapter's opening scenario. What is your justification for each exercise, and what are your criteria for progression?

LAB ACTIVITIES

1. Have your lab partner lift 5 lb in shoulder flexion in a standing position, supine position, and prone position. Where in the range of motion for each exercise did the patient encounter the most difficulty? Why? Of what relevance is this to you in setting up a patient on a strengthening program?

2. With your lab partner in supine and one leg abducted and in extension, place your hand on the top of her foot. Place your other hand on the calf and have your partner move the hip into flexion and adduction up and across the body. Instruct your partner to provide as much resistance moving into hip flexion as possible. Now repeat the resistive motion but remove your hand from the calf. What difference did you detect in the amount of

resistance offered by your partner? What do you think is the reason for this change in resistance?

3. Have your lab partner perform a lateral step up. Identify all the possible ways she could substitute and not use the muscles correctly for this exercise. For each error, indicate what suggestion you would provide the patient to perform the activity correctly.

4. Perform a step-up exercise and then return to the start position. What muscles are being used going up the step? What muscles are used going down? What type of muscle contraction is used to go up and to go down?

5. With your forearm on a table grasping a bar with a weight at its end, move your forearm all the way from full pronation to full supination and back to the start position. Explain which muscle and what type of muscle contraction is occurring throughout the range of motion in both directions. How would this information influence a rehabilitation program for the elbow or wrist?

6. Have your lab partner lie prone and isometrically contract the hamstrings at 0°, 45°, 90°, and 120° of knee flexion while you provide maximal resistance against your partner at each position. Compare the force production at each of these angles. Describe these differences. Consider the length-tension curve and the moment arm of the hamstrings. How does this information impact how you might set a patient on an early strength program?

7. Perform the following activities and identify the primary muscle(s) performing the activity and what part of the motion is concentric and what part is eccentric for that (those) muscle(s):

   a. Getting up from a chair
   b. Sitting down into a chair
   c. Doing a modified push-up
   d. Doing an abdominal curl
   e. Doing an elbow curl
   f. Doing a French curl
   g. Walking up stairs
   h. Walking down stairs
   i. Performing a vertical jump

   What realization has this given you regarding activity or performance? Of what relevance is this in establishing a strengthening program for a patient?

8. Identify how you could have a patient perform a quadriceps strengthening exercise using the following methods:

   a. Manual resistance
   b. Body weight resistance
   c. Rubber band or tubing
   d. Free weight
   e. Machine weight
   f. Isokinetics

9. A shot putter suffered a rotator cuff strain and has been undergoing a rehabilitation program. This will be his first day of strength exercises. How will you determine what exercises and number of repetitions he should start with today? Provide a justification for each exercise. What is the determining factor in the number of repetitions he will perform for all of his strength exercises? Indicate a progression of strength exercises for the rotator cuff for this patient. How will this patient's program differ from that of a baseball pitcher who has also suffered a rotator cuff strain and is at the same stage in his rehabilitation program? Why?

CHAPTER 8

The ABCs of Proprioception

OBJECTIVES

After completing this chapter, you should be able to do the following:

1. List the afferent receptors involved in proprioception.
2. Identify the CNS sites that relay proprioceptive information to the motor system.
3. Discuss the ABCs of proprioception.
4. Identify the systems that control balance.
5. Describe the components involved in coordination.
6. Explain a progression of proprioceptive exercises for the lower or upper extremity.

▶ Proprioception has always been a topic of interest for athletic trainer Amanda Lizbett. Even as a student in college, any topic related to the neurophysiology of proprioception fascinated her. She understood the interrelationship between balance, coordination, and agility, and was fascinated by how they must all work together to allow simple to complex motions, from standing and walking to highly skilled sport activities.

Amanda had started Tony, the school's star decathlete, on simple agility activities early in a hip rehabilitation program, but now he was ready to begin more intensive agility and sport-specific activities. Before he came into the athletic training clinic for his program this afternoon, Amanda would design an agility program that would progress Tony to a full and successful return to his sport.

Anybody can grab a tiger by the tail.
You only survive by knowing what to do next.

AUTHOR UNKNOWN

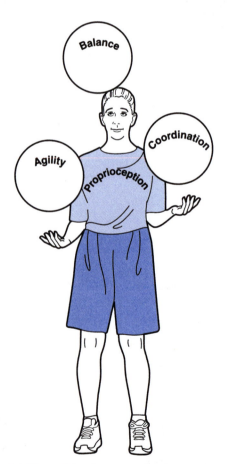

▶ **Figure 8.1** Components of proprioception.

Agility, balance, and coordination together allow an individual to move accurately, quickly, and efficiently. These three parameters are a complex unit that is dependent upon strength and flexibility for its foundation. If a muscle is too weak to move a body part, it cannot be expected to control the movement of that part. Likewise, an extremity must have the flexibility and muscle endurance necessary to allow it to function and meet the demands of athletic activity. If a muscle has limited flexibility so that it lacks the full motion required for an activity, or if a muscle is unable to work long enough to perform an activity accurately, the muscle will be unable to coordinate the segment properly for that activity.

Agility, **B**alance, and **C**oordination are also controlled by what are collectively referred to as proprioceptors (figure 8.1)—which is why this chapter refers to the **ABCs of proprioception.** Proprioception is fundamental to correct performance, and correct performance requires good agility, balance, and coordination. In other words, proprioceptors play a vital neurosensory role in the patient's motor skills and are a key factor in the ability to perform tasks with dexterity, mastery, and proficiency. It is certainly necessary for people to have good flexibility as well as muscle endurance and strength to perform well, but proprioception is crucial if the person is to execute any skill with accuracy, consistency, and precision. To know how to optimize proprioception in any activity, we must first understand what proprioceptors are and how they affect execution and skill.

Proprioception is the body's ability to transmit position sense, interpret the information, and respond consciously or unconsciously to stimulation through appropriate execution of posture and movement. Neuromuscular control of proprioception is produced by the input received from receptors within skin, joints, muscles, and tendons. These proprioceptors play an important role in the maintenance of posture, the conscious and unconscious awareness of joint position, and the production of motion. Proprioception is what allows us to know what position our fingers are in without looking at them. It is what maintains our balance when we stand. It is what enables us to write smoothly. It is what enables us to jump, run, and throw. It is what permits us to change our delivery when we miss the goal on a jump, to move from an asphalt to a gravel surface, and to correct the overshoot of our target with our throw. Although we must first have the flexibility, muscle strength, and endurance to be able to perform these activities, it is proprioception that gives us the agility to change the direction of movement quickly and efficiently, the balance to maintain our stability, and the coordination to produce the activity correctly and consistently.

Proprioceptors are afferent nerves that receive and send impulses from stimuli within skin, muscles, joints, and tendons to the **central nervous system (CNS).** Some of these impulses transmit information regarding the tension of a muscle and the relative position of a body part to control muscular activity. Some of these proprioceptive receptors, such as Golgi tendon organs and muscle spindles, have been discussed in previous chapters. Other afferent receptors also provide input to the CNS and determine a patient's performance ability.

An individual's agility, balance, and coordination are determined by the reception, interpretation, and response initiated by proprioceptors. Proprioceptors can be classified according to their location. A brief look at these receptors will enhance your ability to develop appropriate therapeutic exercise programs for patients.

NEUROPHYSIOLOGY OF PROPRIOCEPTION

Proprioceptors are located in the skin, muscles, tendons, and joints. There are several different receptors that have unique abilities to respond to different stimuli (figure 8.2).

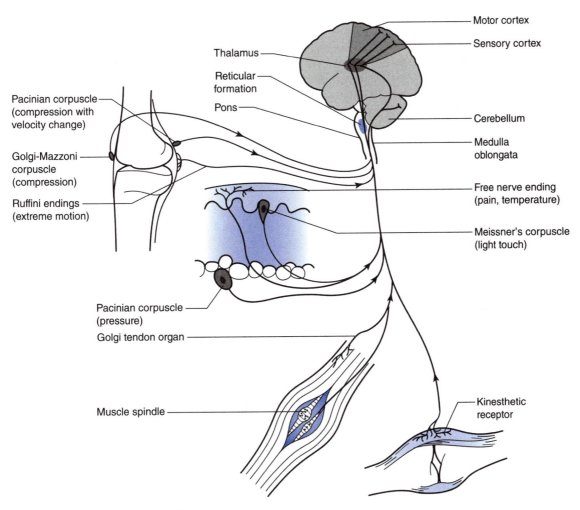

▶ **Figure 8.2** Proprioceptive afferent receptors.

Cutaneous Receptors

Isolation of skin and subcutaneous proprioceptive **afferent receptors** has been primarily confined to investigations of the hand. The receptors in the skin are fast-adapting afferents, slow-adapting I afferents, and slow-adapting II afferents. The fast-adapting afferents are responsible for vibration sense, and the slow adapting I and slow adapting II afferents are responsible for sensory perceptions such as skin stretching. Most researchers believe that these receptors do not play a major role in proprioception (Hewett, Paterno, & Myer, 2002). Evidence suggests that they provide cues regarding skin stretching and fingertip touching but do not have a major impact on joint proprioception in normal subjects (Grigg, 1994). However, evidence does indicate that injured subjects have an increased reliance on cutaneous receptors for proprioception (Callaghan, Selfe, Bagley, & Oldham, 2002). This newer information suggests that although non-injured individuals do not utilize cutaneous receptors for proprioception, body segments that are injured rely on local cutaneous receptors to "take up the slack" for those joint and ligament proprioceptors that are damaged. Much as blind individuals rely on other sensory feedback for information on their surroundings, injured people call their cutaneous proprioceptors into action when their normal proprioceptive receptors are damaged and unable to provide needed information on a joint's position.

Rapidly adapting receptors produce a rapid burst of impulses that quickly erodes. These receptors detect sudden changes in speed and movement such as acceleration and deceleration. On the other hand, slowly adapting receptors produce a constant maintenance level of stimulation. They are responsible for providing information regarding joint and limb position and slow changes in position.

Muscle and Tendon Receptors

The **muscle spindles** and **Golgi tendon organs (GTOs)** are the primary afferent receptors of muscles and tendons. These sensory structures are discussed in chapter 7. They are complicated structures that produce complex neuromuscular responses not only from the muscles and tendons where they are located, but also in the corresponding **antagonistic** and **synergistic** muscles. The GTO detects tension within a muscle and responds to both the contraction and the stretching of a muscle. Its stimulation results in muscle relaxation. The muscle spindle, on the other hand, responds to the stretch of a muscle. Its stimulation leads to a contraction of the muscle. Stimulation of these structures also causes facilitation to opposing muscles and to synergists to assist in accomplishing the desired movement. The GTO and muscle spindle are able to determine joint position because of their muscle length sensitivity. This capability also allows them to facilitate limb stabilization.

Joint Receptors

Afferent receptors primarily lie within the connective tissue of a joint's capsule and surrounding ligaments and influence proprioception. They are divided into fiber type Groups II, III, and IV. Group II afferents are large-diameter axons that have high-speed conduction and Group III and IV afferents are thinly myelinated or non-myelinated, small-diameter axons that have slower conduction of stimuli. The small-diameter nerves do not conduct as fast as the large-diameter nerves because they are not myelinated and/or their size offers more resistance to conduction than the larger-diameter fibers.

The large-diameter myelinated afferents are Group II afferents. There are two types of nerve endings in this group, Ruffini endings and Pacinian corpuscles. Both types are located in the joint capsule. Although the two types are sensitive to different stimuli, they both measure joint motion. The Ruffini endings, located in the joint capsule on the flexion side of the joint, are slowly adapting. They respond more to loads on the surrounding connective tissue than to displacement of that connective tissue. These receptors are stimulated by extreme joint motion when the capsule is stressed in extension with rotation. They are thought to be limit-detectors and protectors of unstable joints (Ellaway, 1995).

Pacinian corpuscles lie throughout the capsule, joint, and periarticular structures. Because they are rapidly adapting receptors, they are thought to be compression sensitive, especially during high-velocity changes when the joint accelerates or decelerates as it moves into its limits of motion (Ellaway, 1995).

Golgi-Mazzoni corpuscles, another afferent nerve ending, are located in joint capsules. They are stimulated by joint compression but not by joint motion. Any weight-bearing activity stimulates these slowly adapting receptors. They do not appear to play a role in proprioception except in identification of joint compression.

The small-diameter non-myelinated axons are divided into Group III and Group IV afferents. Group IV afferents are C fibers and Group III afferents are small diameter A fibers. These fibers are grouped together because they are both pain receptors and are called free nerve endings because of the appearance of their nerve terminals. Located throughout soft tissue and articular structures, they are **nociceptors** that are stimulated by pain and inflammation when a joint is placed in an end position. They do not play a role in proprioception, but can evoke a flexion response to cause a joint to unload and thereby protect it (Leroux, Bélanger, & Boucher, 1995).

The major categories of proprioceptors are cutaneous receptors, muscle and tendon receptors, and joint receptors. To varying degrees, they all influence proprioception.

Other Receptors

Ligaments also contain receptors. Although receptors have been identified in knee and shoulder ligaments, the most thoroughly investigated ligament receptors are those in the knee's anterior cruciate ligament. These receptors are generally not active in the middle ranges of movement but become stimulated when the ligament is stressed. When stimulated by ligament tension, they produce an inhibitory response of the **agonistic** muscles (Gabriel, Kamen, & Frost, 2006).

As important as it is to realize that many different afferent receptors in many structures are affected by joint movement, it is also important to understand that they do not work independently (Strasmann, van der Wal, Halata, & Drukker, 1990). There are afferent nerves that collaborate with each other throughout the body. Local afferent nerves work together to produce a complete picture of joint position and motion for the CNS. Such input allows the CNS to process and interpret the input to produce an accurate response. To make this easier to understand, think about what it would be like to try to correct a baseball pitcher's delivery if you watched only the pitcher's hand. You could not accurately identify necessary changes in the delivery unless you had the complete picture of the pitcher's performance—by watching the entire delivery and analyzing all of the joint movements and positions. Similarly, the CNS cannot determine the position of an extremity unless it receives input from all sensory, motor, and joint receptors.

CENTRAL NERVOUS SYSTEM PROPRIOCEPTOR SITES

Once the afferent nerves have sent their input to the CNS, the body's motor response is determined by the location within the CNS that interprets the stimuli and initiates the efferent reaction. There are three areas within the CNS that will react to the stimuli: **spinal cord, brain stem,** and **cerebral cortex.**

Spinal Cord

If an impulse goes from a dorsal root afferent nerve either to an internuncial connecting nerve or directly to an efferent nerve in the spinal cord and then immediately out the ventral root to the muscle, it is called a **spinal reflex.** This is a response in its simplest form. The reflexes that do not use an **internuncial neuron** produce a more rapid response than those that use an internuncial nerve. This is because of the additional time it takes to transmit from one nerve to another. The fewer the connections, the more rapid the reflex response. These proprioceptive reflexes are often used to protect an area through muscle splinting or rapid withdrawal motion. For example, a joint that is under excessive stress is protected by the sudden activation of the muscle's reflex flexion response to suddenly reduce the load on a joint. Reflexes provide joint stability, especially when there is a sudden change of direction or position. The joint proprioceptors, the muscle spindles, and GTOs all work together to produce a reflex response that provides the joint with stabilization to prevent injury.

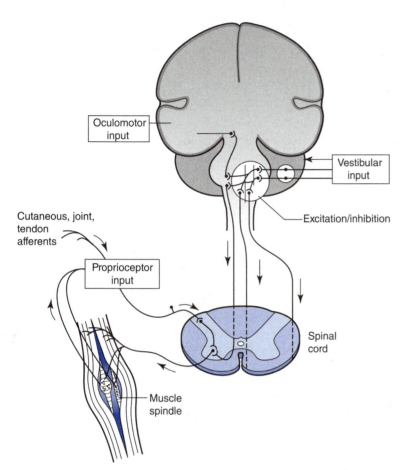

▶ **Figure 8.3** Balance pathways include oculomotor, vestibular, and proprioceptor pathways. These three neural pathways for balance result in inhibitory and/or excitatory stimulation to affect the body's motor response.

After the afferent nerves send their input to the CNS, the body's motor response depends on which of three CNS sites has received the impulse—the spinal cord, the brain stem, or the cerebral cortex.

Brain Stem

The brain stem is the primary proprioceptive correlation center. The proprioceptors relay information via interneurons in the spinal cord that maintain desired position or posture and either connect to or are part of the ascending pathways to the brain stem (figure 8.3). The brain stem also receives input from other areas such as the eye's visual afferent centers and the ear's vestibular afferent centers to assist in maintaining balance. The brain stem then sends excitatory or inhibitory efferent stimulation to produce an appropriate response. We will consider the importance of these sensory systems in the section "Balance."

Cerebral Cortex

Sensory pathways travel to the cortex of the **cerebrum** (figure 8.3). This is the highest level of the brain and the location of conscious movement—the center of volitional control of movement. It is here that correct movement is learned and consciously controlled before it becomes an automatic response. To understand this process, think about how you learned to type. When you were first learning, you were very conscious of what your fingers were doing and where they were on the keyboard. Now, after several years of typing, you do not have to think about what you are doing because the activity has become automatic. You make fewer mistakes and perform the activity faster than you did as a beginning typist. This is what occurs with any activity that is practiced repeatedly; conscious performance becomes automatic performance, and cognitive awareness of the activity is not required.

The ABCs of proprioception include a range of functions from simple to complex. Complexity is relative, though, since even the simplest function involves complex neuromuscular connections. Agility, balance, and coordination are all interrelated. This is the case simply because they have a similar root, the body's proprioceptors. These functions are discussed here in order of their complexity, beginning with the simplest and progressing to the more highly challenging functions.

BALANCE

Balance is fundamental to most activities. Balance is required to perform a simple activity such as standing. Correct performance requires the maintenance of balance. An individual who does not have good balance is in danger of injury. If balance is not restored following an injury, the risk of re-injury significantly increases (Verhagen et al., 2004).

Balance is the body's ability to maintain equilibrium by controlling the body's center of gravity over its base of support. Balance is important in both static and dynamic activities. Standing and sitting are static balance activities. Examples of dynamic balance activities include walking, running, and dancing.

Balance is influenced by strength and by input from the CNS. It is because strength influences balance that strength is emphasized before proprioception in a therapeutic exercise program. As already mentioned, the brain stem receives sensory input from the vestibular system, the visual system, and the proprioceptors (figure 8.4). The combination of input from the ears, eyes, and proprioceptors is crucial to maintaining good balance and posture. If you have ever had an inner ear infection, you may remember the difficulty you had in maintaining balance. A simple test to highlight the importance of visual input for balance is to stand on one leg with your eyes open and then close your eyes. You will discover that without visual input, it is more difficult to maintain balance. So, too, when proprioceptors are damaged following surgery or injury, balance is impaired since one of the three balance input systems is damaged.

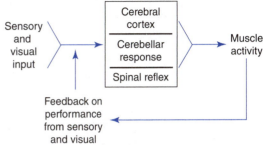

▶ **Figure 8.4** Feedback system for coordination.

Other factors can influence balance, but they depend on the visual, auditory, and proprioceptive systems. For example, a patient's ability to focus on the balance task is basic to the cognitive portion of the proprioceptive system, and a patient's ability to perform skills on different playing surfaces is directly related to the proprioceptive system. It stands to reason, then, that to further develop balance, providing the patient with distracting activities during balance or placing the patient on different surfaces will further engage proprioceptors.

Vestibular System

The **vestibular system** within the inner ear is responsible for sending messages to the CNS regarding static position and motion. The vestibular system includes three semicircular canals within the inner ear in the three different planes that detect changes in position and aid the body in maintaining an upright posture. The inner ear also has two sacs. One sac, the saccule, regulates equilibrium; the other, the utricle, senses forward-backward head motion. Both sacs respond to gravity and are sensitive to head and body motions. The inner ear provides a vestibular-ocular reflex. This allows the eyes to remain steady when the body is in motion.

Oculomotor System

Vision assists in providing feedback about the relative position of the body in space. This feedback system is the **oculomotor system.** As already noted, with your eyes closed it is more difficult to maintain good balance than with your eyes open. If you dive under water with your eyes closed or are in water in which vision is impaired, you can be disoriented and not know whether you are upright relative to the water's surface and bottom. If you sit in an environment that contains a lot of activity, the oculomotor and vestibular systems work together to determine whether you or the environment is moving. Sometimes the oculomotor system does not interpret the feedback correctly and you have a sense of moving when, in fact, you are staying still and it is the environment that is moving. This may occur when your car is stopped at a light but the car next to you is moving forward—you may have a sense that you are moving backward.

Patients who must perform activities requiring rapid change of position, such as ice skaters, gymnasts, or dancers, must learn to disregard the visual input so they do not get dizzy. The vestibular system provides rapid feedback about the change in position that occurs in these athletic events, but the athlete uses the technique of visual fixation, focusing on one object and disregarding other moving objects, to prevent dizziness and loss of balance.

Balance involves three systems—the vestibular system, the oculomotor system, and the proprioceptive system. The rehabilitation clinician can perform simple tests to evaluate balance.

Proprioceptive system

The proprioceptive system is sometimes referred to as the **somatosensory system.** We have already discussed the importance of a good proprioceptive system for balance. When proprioceptor nerves are damaged in injuries, the system's ability to function is impaired. Joint proprioceptors in the knee and ankle are commonly injured in sport, resulting in a reduction of balance and an increase in reaction time.

Balance must be restored and exercises must be included as part of the therapeutic exercise program if the individual is to have good performance stability and safety following rehabilitation. There are exercises that begin at a basic level and progress to more complex, functional activities as the patient's balance improves. These specific exercises and functional activities are discussed in later chapters.

Balance Evaluation

There are simple tests to determine a patient's balance deficiencies. The difficulty of these tests changes as the patient's ability improves, proceeding from static to dynamic and from simple to more complex. The simplest test is the **Romberg test,** in which the patient stands with feet together and eyes closed. No loss of balance is a normal response. Most individuals should be able to perform this test without difficulty. A slightly more difficult test is the stork stand, or single-leg stance, in which the patient stands only on the injured leg. The patient should be able to maintain this position for 30 s without touching the other foot to the floor or using arm support. If the patient is able to perform this test satisfactorily, you can use another test that is slightly more difficult, a single-leg stance with the eyes closed. The patient should also be able to perform this activity for 30 s. Difficulty with any of these static tests indicates a balance deficit and is addressed in the rehabilitation program.

COORDINATION

Coordination is another proprioceptive function fundamental to functional and sport-specific activities. **Coordination** is the complex process by which a smooth pattern of activity is produced through a combination of muscles acting together with appropriate intensity and timing. Several muscles are involved in a coordinated activity. These muscles are connected by a complex neurological network of sensory receptors, internuncial neurons, ascending and descending corticospinal pathways, and efferent receptors. Some muscles are stimulated to provide an activity while others are inhibited to permit the activity, and still others are stimulated to provide synergistic or stabilizing responses to permit the desired motion to occur. Each muscle must provide an accurate response both in timing and in intensity in order for the activity to be coordinated. If a muscle is too weak to provide the appropriate response, the activity will be uncoordinated and undesirable. For example, if a volleyball player does not have an appropriate amount of strength in the scapular rotators, the arm cannot be positioned correctly to hit and place the ball accurately. A soccer player who has weak hip abductors on the standing leg does not have the stability needed for holding the body firm and providing the base necessary to kick the ball well enough with the opposite leg. An archer does not have accuracy in shooting without the strength in the deltoids to control the weight of the bow or the pull on the string.

If muscles are weak, those muscles must work harder than they should to achieve a specific output. This causes an irradiation of stimulation, called **overflow,** to other muscle groups. We see this in a simple activity such as opening a jar. If the cover comes off with little effort, minimal activity of the hand and arm is required. However, if the cover is stuck and more effort is needed, the arm muscles tighten, the grip gets stronger, the jaw muscles contract, and the entire body tenses as we attempt to open the jar. Likewise, when the muscle is performing an activity but is not strong enough to provide the appropriate motion, it tries as hard as it can to perform the activity and in so doing stimulates otherwise inactive muscles to assist.

This overflow causes an undesired motion. For this reason, it is important to have the patient achieve strength gains before you include advanced coordination activities in a therapeutic exercise program.

Coordination Components

There are specific requirements for coordinated movement. Let's briefly look at them so that the logical progression of therapeutic exercises for improved coordination becomes clear.

Activity Perception

Probably the most basic of all elements within coordination is the awareness of **volitional** muscle activity. An awareness of joint position and movement is fundamental to the ability to perform activity. Proprioceptors are key to this awareness. Vision is also important, for it gives the patient feedback about the result of the activity: Has the activity been performed as desired? Vision slows down the response to activity, but especially in the beginning when a new activity is being learned and motor patterns are being established, vision is important to the development of motion accuracy.

Feedback

The learning process involved in the development of coordinated movement is similar to programming a computer. An activity is performed; the CNS evaluates the quality of the performance; the body sends information to the CNS to make adjustments for undesired activity; and the activity is repeated with the adjustments made. The proprioceptors are the most important elements in this feedback process. The sensory afferents send information to the cerebrum where input of the activity is received, to the **cerebellum** where automatic adjustment of muscle position and length is made, and to the spinal cord for reflex adjustments (figure 8.4). Cognitive-response information is relayed to the brain stem where it is integrated with other response feedback and sent down the spinal cord to provide an adjusted performance.

Repetition

As the activity becomes more accurate with repetition and adjustments, the performance becomes more consistent. To visualize this, we could use an analogy from cross-country skiing. The more the tracks on a trail are used, the deeper they get and the easier it becomes to stay within them. Deviation from the tracks becomes less likely the more the trail is used.

Repetition is a requirement for development of accuracy and coordination. As the activity is repeated, the effort decreases and there is less chance of overflow to the wrong muscles. Eventually, an activity engram that can be repeated precisely and accurately is developed. An **engram** is an effect or performance that is impressed upon the CNS through repetition. At this point the coordinated activity becomes automatic and is no longer a conscious process.

Inhibition

In the development of coordination it is important to inhibit undesired muscle activity. **Inhibition** cannot be trained directly (Kottke, 1982). It must be facilitated by precise, slow, and controlled activity until the engram is developed and the patient can increase speed of execution without producing unwanted muscle responses. In the early developmental stages of coordination, the activity should not be so difficult that the patient's performance causes an overflow and unwanted muscle responses. Given that early coordination requires cognitive awareness and conscious correction, it is best that the patient not be distracted with too many activities. Such distractions will lead to imprecise patterns of movement because the patient will not be able to concentrate adequately on any one activity. It is better to alternate attention if the situation calls for performance of more than one activity at a time.

Inhibition is part of the computer-like adjustment process that eventually results in coordinated activity. The patient should start with low-level, basic activity to eliminate the overflow

The components of coordination include perception of activity, feedback, performance adjustment, and repetition. Development of coordination involves progression of activities from simple to more complex, as well as repetition.

to other pathways until a coordinated pattern is established. As the desired motion becomes an engram, the activity can become more difficult, because the capacity to inhibit undesired activity becomes greater with improved coordination.

Coordination Development

Precision of motion, speed of motion, and strength are fundamental to coordination in many activities. As previously mentioned, once strength is achieved, coordination development through repetition of activity is the next rehabilitation step. The patient needs to perform activities that are simple in the beginning and become more complex as abilities progress. In the beginning, simple static exercises may be enough of a challenge. Coordination development progresses from static activities to dynamic activities. For example, once the patient is able to stork stand on an unstable surface such as a foam roller or trampoline, he or she can begin dynamic activities such as balance-board and jumping activities for the lower extremities or ball tossing at a target for the upper extremities.

Progression of coordination starts with simple activities and moves to ones that are more complex. Increasing the speed of the activity, increasing the force, or increasing the complexity are all ways to advance the difficulty of coordination exercises. All coordination activities require repetition. This means that any coordination exercise in a therapeutic exercise program should include many repetitions. This is especially important as the exercises progress to resemble the patient's normal activities.

Accuracy of performance is vital to coordination development. The rehabilitation clinician must be cognizant of this when the patient is performing therapeutic exercises. Once the patient begins to fatigue and coordination becomes less accurate, the activity should be discontinued. Continued execution of uncoordinated motions will engram undesired movement. This is also an important consideration with regard to the placement of coordination exercises within a therapeutic exercise session. The patient should perform coordination activities early in the treatment session when fatigue is not as much of a factor as it will be toward the session's end.

AGILITY

Agility is the ability to control the direction of a body or segment during rapid movement. Athletic agility requires a number of qualities: flexibility, strength, power, speed, balance, and coordination. It involves rapid change of direction and sudden stopping and starting.

Most sports require agility of the lower extremities. A football receiver must be able to cut suddenly to the left or right to evade a defensive player; a soccer forward must zigzag down the field to move the ball around an opponent; and a basketball player must sprint down the court and then suddenly stop to perform a jump shot. Upper-extremity agility is required of a piano player who moves the fingers rapidly across the keyboard, a water polo player who attempts to fake out an opponent and then score a goal, the hockey goalie who suddenly blocks a shot with his hands, and the racquetball player who moves quickly from a backhand to a forehand shot.

Agility is a highly advanced skill that requires a base of flexibility, strength, and power. Adequate flexibility provides a base for speed and power. Since power is needed for agility and power is force times distance divided by time ($F \times D/T$), one can increase power by increasing the distance through which the body part moves. Greater flexibility produces greater power. Power is important because the greater the power, the more quickly a patient is able to move.

Strength is also a component of agility. A patient who has good strength can control the inertia that forceful movement creates. If a 90 kg (200 lb) patient is unable to control his weight during movement, the movement will be ineffective. Strength is a controlling factor in a patient's maneuverability.

To be effective, speed must be accompanied by coordination. Coordination, as we have seen, is important for proper execution of an activity.

As with coordination activities, therapeutic exercise for agility should begin with simple exercises and progress to more complex activities as skill level improves. The ultimate goal of agility exercises is for the patient to perform all agility activities involved in that patient's sport or normal activities. Execution of simple activities using simple drills is used in the early stages of agility exercises. These activities are usually components of an athletic skill or specific job requirement and are performed at slower-than-normal speeds. As the patient improves, the activity becomes more complex and the speed more closely resembles normal.

Activities that can test a patient's agility should resemble the patient's sport or work activities. It is your responsibility as a rehabilitation clinician to understand the demands of the patient's sport position or occupation so you can provide appropriate agility exercises. For example, agility activities for a basketball player should include exercises such as lateral-line running, figure-8 cone running, sudden-stop activities, and running backward. Agility exercises for an assembly-line worker may include rapid eye-hand coordination activities to pull an object off the assembly belt, package it, and send it to be boxed before the next object appears. Performance of these activities is graded by speed of the activity, ability to suddenly change direction, ability to use the injured and non-injured leg equally in all directions, and smoothness of execution.

Agility is an advanced skill that is built on flexibility, strength, and power first, followed by coordination and balance.

THERAPEUTIC EXERCISE FOR PROPRIOCEPTION

Agility, balance, and coordination are parameters that naturally follow flexibility and strength within a therapeutic exercise program. Balance and agility are often intimately related and can be difficult to separate except in very basic exercises that are elementary static balance activities and the more complex pre-participation agility exercises. There is a general progression of proprioception exercises that is important, whether you are working with upper- or lower-extremity injuries. Proprioception exercises should be a routine part of a therapeutic exercise program.

General Concepts

Some concepts related to exercise for proprioception have already been introduced but are important enough to be repeated. Balance is achieved first, followed by coordination, and finally agility. The order is important because agility depends on coordination and coordination depends on balance. Balance exercises start with static activities and progress to dynamic activities as balance improves.

All exercises for proprioception progress from simple to complex. Simple exercises include activities in which the patient has only one or two items of concentration. Simple exercises also include activities that require only enough muscle activity to produce the desired result without overflow to unwanted muscles. Simple exercises involve activities performed slowly and deliberately in controlled situations and environments. Distractions should be avoided when a high level of concentration is required of the patient.

Progression from simple to complex occurs only after the patient has mastered the simple exercise. You can make the activity more complex by having the patient perform the simple activity at a faster pace or by requiring a more powerful output with control. Progression from simple to more complex can also include exercises requiring the patient to perform more than one task simultaneously. A task becomes more complex when one of the feedback mechanisms is restricted, as when the patient performs the simple activity with eyes closed. Progression to exercises that mimic sport or work participation occurs as soon as the patient's abilities allow.

The patient must perform the activity accurately. To encourage this, the difficult proprioceptive activities occur early in the therapeutic exercise session rather than later; when the patient is more fatigued and coordination is more difficult.

Repetition is always necessary to develop performance accuracy. Repetition is successful only if the patient is able to improve execution with repeated attempts. The rehabilitation clinician must carefully observe the patient for signs of fatigue to prevent an inaccurate engram from developing.

Lower-Extremity Progression

Although specific exercises are addressed in part IV as specific therapeutic exercise programs for the various areas of the body, a brief description of proprioceptive programs is presented here.

Static balance activities begin with the single-leg stance with eyes open. The patient stands on the foot of the involved leg with arms at sides. The goal is to stork stand for 30 s without touching the elevated foot to the floor. If a patient has difficulty with the stork stand, he or she can begin with stance in a tandem position with the toe of one foot touching the heel of the foot in front of it (figure 8.5a); this is more difficult with the injured leg in the back position. Without using arms to balance, the patient stands in this position 30 s with eyes open. After accomplishing either the single-leg stance or tandem position with eyes open for 30 s (figure 8.5b), the patient performs it with the eyes closed for 30 s. Balance activities progress from single-leg stance with eyes closed to single-leg stance on an unstable surface such as a mini-trampoline, foam rubber pad, or 1/2 foam roller, eyes open and eyes closed (figure 8.5c).

You can also create increased difficulty in single-leg stance by having the patient perform a distracting activity such as playing catch. This can become even more challenging if the ball is weighted.

The patient can also perform static balance activities in a sport-specific position. For example, a gymnast can perform the single-leg stance on a balance beam or with the hip in lateral rotation. A tennis player can perform static balance activities on the balls of the feet

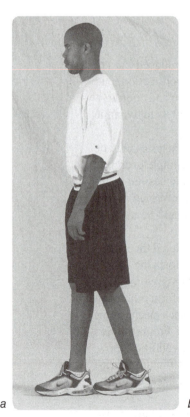
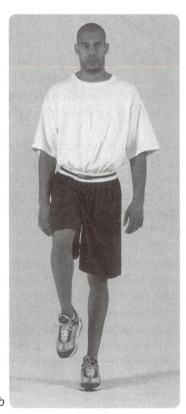
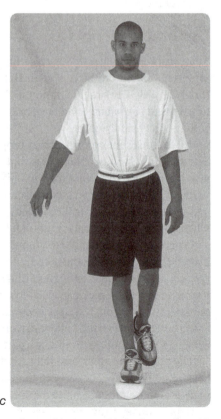

a   b   c

▶ **Figure 8.5** Static balance progression: *(a)* tandem stance balance, *(b)* stork stand balance, *(c)* stork stand on 1/2 foam roller.

with hip and knee flexion. A wrestler can perform static balance activities on the unstable surface of a mat.

After having mastered static balance, the patient progresses to dynamic balance. These activities include sport-specific demands such as running, lateral movements, and backward movements. More advanced dynamic activities include jumping, cutting, twisting, and pivoting. They begin as low-level activities, performed at a slow speed with balance and control, and progress to faster speeds. Some activities, such as jumping, can begin with the use of both legs but then progress to unilateral activities as the patient gains skill and confidence in execution. Plyometrics can be incorporated into the later stages of proprioceptive exercises within a therapeutic program. Plyometrics is a specialized system of exercises used only in the final stages of a program when the patient has good strength, flexibility, and control. Plyometrics are discussed in chapter 9.

In the final stages of these dynamic movements, the exercises are advanced to mimic specific sport situations. These exercises represent the true agility activities required of the patient in sport participation. You must know the component activities and understand the stresses applied in the sport to be able to design this part of the therapeutic exercise program. These activities fine-tune the patient's agility skills and restore the patient's confidence in his or her ability to return to the sport. Many of these activities are functional exercises and are discussed in chapter 10.

The use of braces, sleeves, and tape to enhance proprioception of ankle and knee injuries is still a matter of some dispute. There is evidence that proprioception input from skin and subcutaneous sensory receptors assists in perception of motion (Lephart, Kocher, Fu, Borsa, & Harner, 1992). There is also evidence that elements of proprioceptive function may be improved with bracing (Beynnon, Good, & Risberg, 2002; Willems, Witvrouw, Verstuyft, Vaes, & De Clercq, 2002). Other information indicates that the benefit of joint support is inversely proportional to the proprioceptive ability of the joint (Perlau, Frank, & Fick, 1995). The proprioceptive influence of these devices on functional activities is controversial (Risberg, Beynnon, Peura, & Uh, 1999), but this may be because many of the studies have been performed either a while after patients completed rehabilitation (Risberg et al., 1999) or on normal subjects (Blackburn, Guskiewicz, Petschauer, & Prentice, 2000). Recently, it has been demonstrated that individuals with proprioceptive deficient knees rely on their cutaneous proprioceptors more than non-injured individuals (Callaghan et al., 2002); it may be that tape or braces work by stimulating these cutaneous receptors to act as position sense monitors. Most studies on proprioception and kinesthesia have been able to demonstrate an improved awareness of the patient as to joint position or joint sense, but no evidence demonstrates that joint stability is enhanced during functional activities with use of such devices (Barrack, Lund, & Skinner, 1994).

Lacking strong evidence to support or discourage the use of braces and sleeves, you must decide about using them on an individual basis. If the patient feels more confident and better able to perform athletic activities, these devices may provide sufficient psychological benefit to warrant application.

Upper-Extremity Progression

Although most lower-extremity sport activities are closed chain activities, upper-extremity activities are both open and closed chain. The patient's performance requirements in relation to open or closed chain activities will determine the extent of the proprioceptive exercises to be used in the therapeutic exercise program. A well-rounded program should include both open and closed kinetic chain activities, but end-program emphasis is determined by the demands of the particular sport. For example, a pitcher's demands are open-kinetic chain, so the majority of proprioceptive exercises for a pitcher should be of this type. A gymnast performs open and closed kinetic chain activities and thus should do a combination of open and closed kinetic chain proprioceptive exercises, but a cyclist performs closed kinetic chain activities, so the program for this patient should include primarily closed kinetic chain exercises.

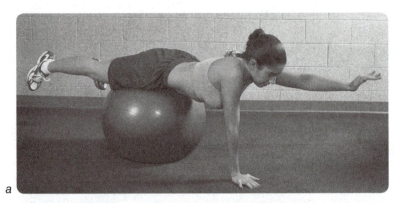

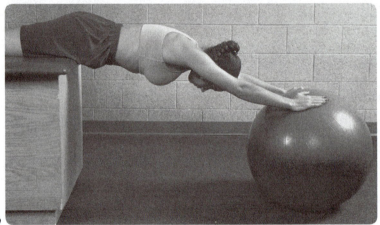

a

b

▶ **Figure 8.6** Proprioception exercises for the upper extremity on the Swiss ball: *(a)* Patient is supported by Swiss ball only, and *(b)* patient is supported by a table while moving a Swiss ball.

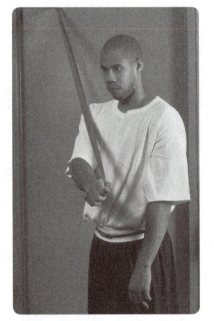

▶ **Figure 8.7** Resisted proprioceptive exercise.

Initial open kinetic chain proprioceptive exercises can include proprioceptive neuromuscular facilitation rhythmic stabilization. Rhythmic stabilization can progress to closed kinetic chain exercises. In a closed kinetic chain, the exercise can progress from co-contraction without movement, to movement on a stable surface, to movement on an unstable surface. For example, the patient can either be positioned on a Swiss ball and move his or her body with the hands on the floor, or be positioned with hands on the ball and the body supported on a table (figure 8.6). The activity can start with bilateral support and then advance to using only the involved arm.

1. Patient lies prone on a Swiss ball with feet off the floor. Patient begins with both hands on the floor and then raises the uninvolved arm to balance for 30 s (figure 8.6a).
2. Patient lies prone on a table with lower extremities on the table and hands on the Swiss ball. The Swiss ball is rolled outward and the position is held for 30 s (figure 8.6b).
3. Progressions for both exercises can include the patient's moving the ball using only the arms to propel the ball forward and backward and from side to side.
4. Further progression can include resistance to movement, for example on a Fitter or with manual resistance (figure 8.7).

Active and passive repositioning can be useful for early proprioceptive gains. Passive repositioning occurs when the rehabilitation clinician passively moves the patient's uninvolved upper extremity into a position and the patient then moves the injured upper extremity into the same position. This activity can progress from eyes open to eyes closed. When a mistake occurs, the patient visually compares to correct the position and repeats the exercise.

In active repositioning, the rehabilitation clinician moves the injured arm into a position and then returns it to the starting position. With eyes closed, the patient then reproduces the position the arm was placed in.

Both these activities can be performed in straight plane and in functional positions. The best response will be achieved in functional positions near the end of the joint's range of motion.

Functional exercises can be easily incorporated into an upper-extremity program. Proprioceptive neuromuscular facilitation exercises using manual resistance, machines, and tubing provide for strength and proprioceptive gains. Proprioceptive exercises start slowly and increase in speed as the patient is able to maintain control of the arm throughout the activity.

Plyometric exercises for agility can also be used for the upper extremity. Plyometric exercises for the upper extremities can include the use of body resistance and medicine balls as discussed in chapter 9.

As with lower-extremity functional exercises, upper-extremity agility exercises should be designed with knowledge of the requirements of the patient's specific sport. For example, functional exercises for a throwing sport patient should progress from throwing activities that initially include short distances and easy throwing, to longer distances with an increase in speed, and finally a full speed throw for functional distances.

SUMMARY

Proprioception is the body's perception of where it is in space relative to its environment. Receptors in muscles, tendons, ligaments, capsules, and skin send information into the central nervous system where it is processed before impulses triggering a response occur. Proprioceptors are important for balance; balance is important for coordination; and coordination is important for agility. Proprioception, then, is fundamental to these ABCs of activity. When an injury occurs to a joint or other body segment, the proprioceptors for that segment are also injured. If the ABCs are to be restored, the rehabilitation program must include progressive exercises that facilitate the proprioceptors and restore them to their optimal function.

Therapeutic exercises for developing balance, coordination, and agility follow exercises for flexibility and strength gains. Exercises for the lower and upper extremities progress from simple to complex and emphasize accuracy through repetition.

KEY CONCEPTS AND REVIEW

1. List the afferent receptors involved in proprioception.

Proprioception, an important part of therapeutic exercise programs, is determined by the input of several afferent receptors in skin, muscles, tendons, joints, and other areas.

2. Identify the CNS sites that relay proprioceptive information to the motor system.

The afferent receptors transmit information to one of three CNS sites: the spinal cord, the brain stem, or the cerebral cortex. The most rapid reflexes involve quick transmission and response from the spinal cord. The slower responses are sent from the cerebral cortex where conscious execution of the response is initiated.

3. Discuss the ABCs of proprioception.

The ABCs of proprioception are agility, balance, and coordination. Balance is fundamental to coordination and agility. A patient must have good balance, coordination, and agility to fully meet the demands of his or her sport. Specific exercises are used to restore these functions. These exercises can be initiated early in a program with simple activities and progressed to more complex activities as the patient advances in the therapeutic exercise program.

4. Identify the systems that control balance.

Balance is influenced by three systems: the vestibular, oculomotor, and proprioceptive systems. These all provide input to the CNS to maintain both static and dynamic balance.

5. Describe the components involved in coordination.

Coordination includes the process of perceiving an activity, getting feedback from the CNS about the result of the activity, and correcting the activity through a series of repetitions and alterations until the activity is performed correctly and without the need for cerebral cortex input.

6. Explain a progression of proprioceptive exercises for the lower or upper extremity.

Therapeutic exercise for proprioception progresses from easy to difficult, from static to dynamic, from slow to fast, and from simple to complex. As a rehabilitation clinician you must understand the complexity and requirements of the patient's sport in order to include appropriate proprioceptive exercises that will eventually permit the patient to return to full sport participation.

CRITICAL THINKING QUESTIONS

1. If a patient stands on one leg with eyes shut, which balance system is eliminated? How can the other two balance systems be eliminated in a stork-stand activity?

2. Would you expect a patient with an ankle sprain to have difficulty balancing on one leg? Why? List three progressive exercises that you could use to improve balance. What would be your criteria for advancement from one exercise to the next?

3. Coordination exercises are more effectively performed in a therapeutic exercise program before the patient becomes fatigued. Why is this? When, during the day's program, would new coordination exercises make any difference in performance? Why?

4. Identify three criteria that should be met before a patient advances from balance to coordination activities, and from coordination to agility activities. You should be able to explain to the patient why you are setting these criteria.

5. List three agility exercises you would provide Tony on his first day of agility training in the chapter's opening scenario. Provide two progressions for each exercise and your criteria for each progression.

LAB ACTIVITIES

1. Use a five-exercise progression, beginning with the easiest and progressing to the most difficult, to challenge your lab partner's lower-extremity proprioception. The first exercise should be a static balance activity; subsequent activities should progress to the final exercise in agility. Grade your lab partner's ability to perform each exercise level as you would in a patient's note. Indicate with each exercise selection what makes the exercise more challenging than the previous exercise. How will you determine when the patient is ready to proceed to the next level?

2. Use a five-exercise progression, beginning with the easiest and progressing to the most difficult, to challenge your lab partner's upper extremity proprioception. Grade your lab partner's ability to perform each exercise level as you would in a patient's note. Indicate with each exercise selection what makes the exercise more challenging than the previous exercise. How will you determine when the patient is ready to proceed to the next level?

3. With your lab partner seated on the table's end, instruct your partner to keep his or her eyes closed and move the leg into 45° of knee flexion. Measure the knee with a goniometer and record the position. Repeat this activity three times. Now instruct your partner to move the opposite leg to 45° and hold the position for 5 sec. While keeping the eyes closed have him or her extend the knee to 45° again. Measure the knee with a goniometer and record the position. Repeat this activity three times.

4. Have your lab partner stand on one leg, the arms at the sides, and the NWB thigh hanging comfortably but not adducted to the WB extremity. With eyes open, have your partner stand for 30 sec. An error occurs if the arms come away from the sides, the NWB extremity moves away from the body or the ankle wraps around the other leg, trunk moves out from alignment with the hips, or the NWB foot touches the ground. Count the errors. Repeat the exercise with the eyes closed. What is the difference between the two activities? Why? Identify two other ways the stork-stand exercise can be made more challenging for a patient. How would you determine when the patient is able to advance from one exercise to the next?

Plyometrics

OBJECTIVES

After completing this chapter, you should be able to do the following:

1. Identify the mechanical and neurological components of the neuromuscular principles involved in plyometrics.

2. Describe the factors involved in plyometric program design.

3. List three considerations for plyometric program execution.

4. List the precautions and contraindications for plyometrics.

5. Outline a progression of four plyometric exercises for either a lower- or an upper-extremity program.

▶ Athletic trainer Larry Carrell has been recently hired by the local athletic training clinic to head up its plyometric rehabilitation program. Once patients are sufficiently rehabilitated, Larry establishes the final phase of their sport rehabilitation program, the plyometric phase. Larry comes to the clinic with extensive experience and is well qualified to design and manage such a program to advance patients in this final portion of their rehabilitation.

Larry's most recent patient is his most challenging patient to date. Ed is a 70-year-old gold-medal track athlete who competes in the senior Olympics and has the endorsement of several companies. Ed strained his hamstrings several weeks ago and is now nearing the end of his rehabilitation program. Although Ed is energetic and enthusiastic, he also has a history of other lower-extremity injuries and underwent cardiac bypass surgery eight years ago. The cardiac surgery and his postoperative cardiac recovery program were what originally piqued his interest in track.

Larry sees Ed as an exciting challenge and is looking forward to designing a plyometric program to enable Ed to fully return to his competitive level of participation.

Arriving at one goal is the starting point to another.

JOHN DEWEY, American philosopher, psychologist, and educator, 1859-1952

Now that the patient has achieved goals in flexibility, strength, balance, coordination, and agility, the next step is to finely tune his or her abilities in preparation for specific sport and other skills. Most sports activities require explosiveness, rapid changes in direction and speed, and the ability to absorb and produce forces quickly—all performed automatically, economically, and efficiently. Goals that successfully demonstrate these parameters must be achieved before the patient moves on to sport-specific activities. A patient possesses the same inherent talent he or she has always had, but the effects of pre-injury training diminish following injury and inactivity. The ability to perform skills at pre-injury levels must be restored through therapeutic exercise and retraining before the patient is able to return safely to sport competition or the normal work environment.

Execution of activities of this magnitude requires the neuromuscular system to relearn skills. This is where plyometrics comes into play. Plyometrics is not only a precursor to functional activities but also a transition between strengthening and activity-specific exercises and can include specific functional or sport activities. **Plyometrics** is the use of a quick movement of eccentric activity followed by a burst of concentric activity to produce a desired powerful output of the muscle. In other words, a plyometric exercise is one that facilitates a muscle to produce a maximum strength output as quickly as possible. It is a brief, explosive exercise. Maximum power production is the ultimate goal in plyometrics. You will recall from previous discussions that power is calculated as force times distance divided by time ($F \times d / T$). The quicker the time, the greater the power. For example, if a patient weighing 80 kg (176 lb) jumps 0.6 m (2 ft) in the air and takes 1 s to perform the activity, he produces 352 ft-lb of power (176 lb $\times$ 2 ft $\div$ 1). If, however, he is able to jump the same distance in half the time, he will produce 704 ft-lb of power (176 lb $\times$ 2 ft $\div$ 0.5).

The term *plyometrics* was not used until 1975 when an American track and field coach, Fred Wilt, originated the term (Chu, 1998). Its Greek origins are *plio* and *metric,* which mean "more" and "measure," respectively. Before Wilt coined the term, plyometrics was referred to as "jump training." Although plyometric activities have been used since people first ran and jumped, plyometrics became popular in the late 1960s when people attributed the high performance abilities of Olympic athletes from the Eastern European countries to the jump-training exercises used by their coaches.

Because of the muscle activation involved in plyometrics, sometimes it is referred to as stretch-shortening activities. Although it has been primarily used in conditioning for healthy individuals, more and more rehabilitation programs are also incorporating plyometrics (Chmielewski, Kauffman, Myer, & Tillman, 2006). Unfortunately, most of the published research has investigated normal individuals, not patients, so the effects and purported benefits of plyometrics on the patient population has been anecdotal, not scientific. Therefore, the references used in this chapter refer to normal individuals, not patients. Considerations for patients in adaptations of plyometric exercises are discussed later in the chapter.

Many daily activities such as walking are essentially stretch-shortening activities. Plyometrics, however, is a more aggressive activity with the express purpose of improving a patient's output or performance through the utilization of several physiological and neuromuscular constructs.

NEUROMUSCULAR PRINCIPLES

The theory of how plyometrics works is based on information about the neuromuscular system and its response to stress. Many of these principles have been discussed in previous chapters. Putting these principles into practical application in plyometrics helps the rehabilitation clinician understand the "whys" and "hows" of incorporating plyometrics into a therapeutic exercise program.

Plyometrics involves the technique of first lengthening, then shortening the muscle to produce an increased power output. Thus, plyometrics is a **stretch-shortening exercise.** Stretch-shortening exercises are based on stretch-shortening principles, which in turn are based on knowledge of the mechanical and neurological components of the neuromuscular system.

Mechanical Components

The mechanical components can be divided into contractile elements and non-contractile elements. Both are important elements that play a role in plyometrics and will be briefly presented here.

Contractile Components

The **contractile components (CC)** are the myofibrils. As discussed in chapter 7, the myofibrils contain the sarcomeres, the contractile element of the muscle. Muscle is the only structure in the body that actively shortens or lengthens to cause motion. The contractile elements of the muscular system control the non-contractile elements.

Studies have demonstrated that when an active muscle is lengthened, two things happen: the speed with which the cross-bridges detach increases and the number of cross-bridges between actin and myosin increase (Rassier & Herzog, 2005; Rimmer, 2005). The end result is greater strength with a quicker release of connections between the two fibers occurs. These activities are important if the muscle is to be able to move quickly during a rapid lengthening but still maintain good strength.

Non-contractile Elements

The non-contractile elements, or components, include the muscle's tendons and the connective tissue surrounding the muscle and its fibers. The non-contractile elements are identified according to their arrangement and include a **series elastic component (SEC)** and a **parallel elastic component (PEC).** The tendons, sheath, and sarcolemma are the primary structures that make up the SEC, and the muscle's connective tissue composes the PEC (Dean, 1988).

Interaction of the Series Elastic Component, Parallel Elastic Component, and Contractile Component

When a muscle actively shortens, the component responsible for the muscle's ability to move the extremity or resist a force is the CC. As the muscle continues to shorten, a stretch is applied to the SEC.

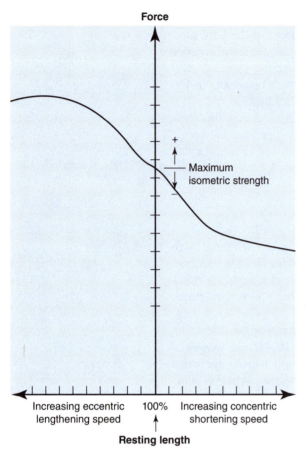

▶ **Figure 9.1** Concentric-eccentric force-production relationship.

When a muscle actively lengthens as in an eccentric activity, the components responsible for producing the force are the CC, SEC, and PEC. The SEC and PEC offer resistance to the movement as the muscle is elongated. The CC controls the speed and quality of the movement. When a muscle elongates, the contribution of the passive component force makes it unnecessary for the active component to produce the same total force as was produced during the shortening activity. To use a theoretical example, if a force of 4.5 kg (10 lb) is needed to lift a weight during a shortening activity, the active components must produce all 4.5 kg of force in order for the weight to be lifted. If the same weight is moved during a lengthening activity, only 3 kg (7 lb) of force needs to be produced by the active component, because 1.3 kg (3 lb) is produced by the passive components. The muscle works less to produce the same force during the lengthening activity. Although the exact differences in eccentric and concentric forces vary depending on the muscle groups investigated, this example demonstrates that less active force is required of the muscle during eccentric activity than during concentric activity. Since less work is required from active components during eccentric exercise, less energy is used during eccentric exercises—so if equal active muscle force is generated in concentric and eccentric activity, greater total force will be produced during eccentric activity.

As discussed in chapter 7, force production is different for concentric and eccentric activity (figure 9.1). At faster speeds of eccentric activity, a muscle is able to produce greater forces than at lower speeds, but the opposite is true for concentric activity. The importance of this principle will become apparent later in the discussion of specific plyometrics.

Neurological Components

The proprioceptors that play important roles in plyometrics are the muscle spindles and Golgi tendon organs (GTOs). The muscle spindle is stimulated by sudden changes in the muscle's length, as during an eccentric movement. It produces a stretch, or **myotatic reflex,** to facilitate a muscle shortening. The **stretch reflex** is the most basic sensorimotor response system because it does not involve an internuncial neuron, but instead goes directly from the afferent sensory nerve (muscle spindle) to the spinal cord where it makes contact with the efferent motor neuron to permit a rapid response by the muscle. Because no additional nerves are involved in the relay process, the stretch reflex is one of the fastest reflexes in the body. It is also referred to as a **monosynaptic response** because only one neural connection is involved.

Normally, the GTOs play an inhibitory role in muscle activity. As the muscle shortens, the GTOs are stimulated to send impulses to the spinal cord that relay, via an internuncial neuron, facilitation to limit muscle force production. Because of the internuncial neuron, this reflex is slightly slower than the muscle spindle reflex.

It has been believed that during plyometric training, the GTO excitatory level is elevated so that more stimulation is necessary to facilitate a response from the GTO, and this allows for an increased tolerance for additional stretch loads in the muscle (Wilk et al., 1993). As the stretch loads are better tolerated, there may be the ability to create a stronger stretch reflex, which results in additional power during the concentric phase of motion (Lundin, 1985).

The theory of the GTO playing an inhibitory role has been challenged more recently by evidence that demonstrates the GTO is stimulated during sub-maximal outputs and may actu-

Plyometrics works on the basis of specific mechanical and neurological components of the neuromuscular system. The mechanical components are contractile and non-contractile elements; the neurological components are the muscle spindles and the Golgi tendon organs.

ally store energy that is released during plyometric activity (Roberts, 2002). Therefore, the GTO may add to rather than detract from plyometric results.

PLYOMETRIC PRODUCTION

Plyometric results are facilitated through the mechanical and neurological systems that have been described. Combined, these produce the desired results of increased strength and power for athletic activity. The non-contractile, elastic elements are important in force production of stretch-shortening exercises. A simplified example of the way non-contractile elements work is a rubber band model: If the rubber band is stretched and then released, it shortens rapidly. The more it is stretched, the greater its force when the stretch is released. This is so because the greater the stretch, the greater the quantity of stored (potential) elastic energy within the rubber band. When the stretch is released, the stored elastic energy converts to kinetic energy to produce the rubber band's recoil.

Plyometric exercises provide an increased output of power during concentric activity. This has to do with transfer of the elastic energy that is produced during eccentric activity immediately prior to concentric activity. In a muscle that moves eccentrically, the load that is produced in the muscle during its lengthening is stored as elastic energy in the non-contractile elements. As the muscle moves from eccentric to concentric activity, the elastic energy is released and assists in producing the force during the concentric action. It is believed that a muscle's increased output during plyometric exercise training may be the result of improved synchronization of muscle activity rather than either strength or power (Toumi et al., 2001). This finding demonstrates that an individual's best performance is likely to occur when he or she is able to properly coordinate muscle firing activity to provide optimal results. Although muscle synchronization is important, strength and power also provide some influence—after all, they are required before synchronization can be optimized.

Range of motion cannot be forgotten as a contributing factor to optimal plyometric performance. If a muscle is able to go through a greater range of motion, the ability to produce greater function improves (Sexton & Chambers, 2006). For example, the patient who squats to only 30° of knee flexion does not jump as high as when he or she squats to 90° of knee flexion prior to takeoff. Greater forces can be produced when greater lengthening prior to concentric activity is permitted.

Another factor in improved performance with plyometric activity is the improved neuromuscular coordination. As speed increases and the activity is performed more accurately, the strength to perform the activity is improved. Energy and movement are not wasted on ineffective activity. Neuromuscular training involves development of the engram as discussed in chapter 7. Better coordination permits greater power production since the activity can be performed more efficiently and in less time.

When speed and coordination of activity are improved, greater power can be produced, as follows from the force-velocity relationship of increased strength with increased speed during eccentric activity (figure 9.1). The greater the eccentric activity, the greater the concentric response will be; and the less time it takes a patient to perform an activity, the more power the patient will produce.

PLYOMETRIC EXERCISE PHASES

Plyometric exercises can be divided into three phases: the eccentric phase, the amortization phase, and the concentric phase. All three phases are important to plyometric performance. The eccentric phase prepares the muscle, the amortization phase transitions the muscle, and the concentric phase is the outcome.

Working together, the components of the mechanical and neurological systems that operate in plyometric activities increase strength and power output.

Eccentric Phase

The eccentric phase is also called the stretch phase or cocking phase and occurs when the muscle is pre-stretched as it actively lengthens. The slack is taken out of the muscle, and its elastic components are put on stretch. This is the preparatory phase that "sets" the muscle as the individual gets ready to perform the activity. This phase utilizes muscle spindle facilitation so that the quality of the response is determined by the rate of the stretch. The muscle's activity directly correlates with the quantity of the stimulation: the greater the stimulation, the greater the muscle's response. The eccentric phase is the most important phase of plyometric activity because it increases the stimulation to provide for this increased muscle response.

The muscle spindle responds better to a rapid stretch and accommodates to a slow one. For this reason, the rate of the stretch is a more important factor than the amount of stretch. If a muscle lengthens quickly, it is able to produce more tension than if it is forced to elongate slowly (Koutedakis, 1989). The best results occur when the eccentric phase is performed quickly and through a partial range of motion.

Amortization Phase

The eccentric phase is followed immediately by the **amortization phase,** which is simply defined as the amount of time it takes to change from eccentric to concentric motion. Of all the phases, this is the most varying in plyometric descriptions. Some label this the transition phase or coupling phase (Chmielewski et al., 2006). The primary concern about the term *amortization* is that it is not an accurate description of what happens between the eccentric and concentric phases of plyometrics. This phase should be quick. In order to produce optimal results, the average duration for this phase during jumping is 23 ms (Bosco, Komi, & Ito, 1981). Contrary to this relatively "long" time, the ideal amortization phase is considered to be under 15 ms (Siff, 2004). If too much time is spent here in this transition phase, the elastic energy is dissipated as heat and is wasted. A prolonged amortization phase also inhibits the stretch reflex. The amortization phase is the transition phase. The quicker the transition from eccentric to concentric activity, the more forceful the movement will be.

Concentric Phase

The final phase, the concentric phase, is the result of the combined eccentric and amortization phases. The concentric phase is the outcome phase. It is also referred to as the shortening phase, unloading phase, or propulsion phase. If the eccentric activity has been quick and the amortization has occurred rapidly, the concentric phase will produce the desired powerful outcome.

If these phases are performed precisely, the end-result should be a higher jump, a greater distance, or an improved speed of execution. Over time, with practice and neurological facilitation, this speed-strength production becomes more efficient because the plyometric exercises lead to an improved synchronous activity of motor units and an earlier recruitment of the motor units. Plyometrics bridges the gap between strength and explosive power by integrating the mechanical and neurological factors that influence these sport performance elements (Wilt, 1975).

PRE-PLYOMETRIC CONSIDERATIONS

Development of power is important in most sports. For example, it is an important element of basketball, volleyball, gymnastics, track and field, baseball, softball, and skating. Since power is crucial for sport performance and plyometrics promotes neuromuscular efficiency, plyometric exercises should be considered for patients who are returning to sport. Before plyometrics can become part of a therapeutic exercise program, however, specific parameters must be present, because plyometrics places great demands on the body.

Plyometric activities occur in three distinct phases. In the eccentric or lengthening phase the muscle is pre-stretched; in the amortization or transition phase it makes a transition to the third, or concentric or shortening phase; and in the concentric phase it produces the powerful outcome.

Strength

Strength is basic to plyometric exercises. The patient should have enough strength to adequately control the activity. As the difficulty of the plyometric exercise increases, the patient needs to have even greater strength. One can minimize the potential for overuse injuries from plyometric activities with good pre-plyometric strength levels.

A greater strength provides for a better output during the plyometric exercise. Again, if $F \times d/T = P$, then the greater the force, the greater the power. Additionally, if a muscle has a greater cross section because of its hypertrophy following strengthening, it will have greater elastic elements to provide additional eccentric strength. Minimum strength requirement recommendations for plyometric exercises vary and depend on the severity of the plyometric exercise. For more severe lower-extremity plyometric exercises, the recommendation for healthy individuals is that the person be able to perform a squat with 60% of body weight for five repetitions within 5 s (Chu 1998). Unfortunately for patients, parameters have not been established. Logic, common sense, and knowledge of the injured site's healing status and impact of the stresses applied with any exercise are required of the rehabilitation clinician who is determining the use of plyometric exercises. Starting with less-impact and low-stress plyometrics, then progressing as the patient responds appropriately is a logical approach.

Flexibility

Flexibility is another pre-plyometric exercise requirement. As mentioned earlier, greater flexibility permits a greater lengthening of the muscle. A greater lengthening provides for a better eccentric phase that will lead to better concentric activity. A muscle that lacks good flexibility is unable to generate the forces for optimal plyometric results. The muscle is also at risk for injury because the reduced flexibility leads to a diminished level of force absorption, needed especially for impact and deceleration stresses. For example, the patient who is able to flex his knee to only 60° will be unable to absorb the forces imposed on him when he jumps from a 40 cm (16 in.) box. However, the patient who is able to fully flex her knees can absorb the impact stresses much more effectively to prevent the forces from being transmitted up the extremity.

Each patient must be individually determined for his or her flexibility readiness for plyometrics. The clinician must evaluate a patient for his or her actual flexibility and determine the minimal flexibility requirements needed to safely perform each plyometric exercise in the patient's program.

Proprioception

Another pre-plyometric consideration is the ABCs of proprioception as discussed in chapter 8. The patient must have agility, balance, and coordination to control the rapid and forceful movements in plyometric activities. The amount of control required depends on the complexity and severity of the plyometric activity. For example, a plyometric activity such as jumping rope is not as complex or as severe as the plyometric activity of bounding with vertical jumps. Although both activities require agility, balance, and coordination, the patient's abilities are more challenged with the bounding and vertical jump activities. For this reason, it makes sense not to include even simple plyometric exercises in a therapeutic exercise program until the patient is able to perform some of the basic dynamic ABC activities discussed in chapter 8.

Because flexibility, strength, and proprioceptive elements are prerequisites to plyometric exercises, the sequential progression of a therapeutic exercise program is important. As noted in chapter 1, each component builds on the previous one and serves as a foundation for the next one. Likewise, there are progressions within each parameter. Plyometrics is no different from any other type of exercise we have considered and must move in a progression from the simplest to the more difficult.

Patients must have certain levels of strength, flexibility, and proprioception in order to participate safely in plyometric exercises.

PLYOMETRIC PROGRAM DESIGN

A plyometric program is designed to improve the patient's overall coordination, efficiency, speed, and power output in preparation for sport participation. Most sports require high-power outputs and involve repetitive stretch-shortening muscle activity. Plyometric activities are the bridge between therapeutic exercise and functional performance. As has been mentioned, these exercises utilize the components of flexibility, strength, and proprioceptive elements that the patient developed in earlier exercise sessions and put these components to functional use through the further development of power, speed, coordination, and efficiency of movement. Some plyometric exercises mimic sport skills and others serve as building blocks for progression from simple functional activities to complex skills.

Just as a patient with a 4/5 grade muscle strength cannot be expected to lift the same weights as a patient with a 5/5 grade muscle strength, a patient should not be expected to perform high-level plyometric exercises when beginning plyometric activities within the therapeutic exercise program. A progression is crucial to avoid injury and provide a successful outcome. The progression is from general exercises to more sport-specific activities, from simple to complex, and from low-stress to high-stress activities.

One can use a number of variables to provide a plyometric exercise progression: intensity, volume, recovery, and frequency.

Intensity

Intensity is the degree, extent, or magnitude of effort applied during an exercise or activity. In strengthening, it is the amount of weight used; in flexibility, it is the force applied to the stretch; in proprioception, it is the complexity of the agility, balance, or coordination activity. In plyometrics, it is the stress of the activity. You can change stress in plyometrics by using weights during the activity, increasing the height of the vertical jump, increasing the distance of the horizontal jump or the throw, increasing the weight of the medicine ball, or increasing the speed of the activity. You can also increase stress by changing the complexity of the exercise. For example, hopping with one leg is more intense than hopping with two legs, and hopping side to side is more challenging than hopping in place.

Volume

Volume is the total quantity of work performed during one session. Volume in lower-extremity plyometric exercises is measured in total number of foot contacts for jumping activities and in distance for bounding activities during the session. Volume in the upper extremity and in medicine ball exercises is measured in the total number of repetitions and sets. Selection of the volume of plyometrics depends on the intensity and goals of the session.

Although no guidelines have been established for therapeutic exercise, for normal athletic conditioning the lower-extremity guidelines for beginners at low-intensity levels are 60 to 100 foot contacts (Chu 1998). The rehabilitation clinician must have knowledge of the patient's ability and of the stresses applied to the healing tissue by the activity, and must combine this knowledge with observation of the patient's performance quality, in order to determine the appropriate volume of plyometric exercises for the therapeutic exercise session.

Recovery

Recovery is the amount of rest time between sets or exercise groupings. The amount of rest time determines whether the plyometric exercises will be more effective in improving power or improving muscular endurance. The less rest time between exercise sets, the more the emphasis is on endurance; longer rest times will provide for more improvement in power. As a general guideline, rest periods of 45 to 60 s between sets or exercise groupings promote power increases (Chu 1998). This translates to a work-to-rest ratio of 1:5 to 1:10 (Chu 1998).

For example, if an exercise set takes 5 s to perform, the recovery could be 25 to 50 s. If the exercise set takes 10 s to perform, the recovery could be 50 to 100 s. Again, these recommendations are based on normal individuals and may have to be adjusted in rehabilitation.

If muscle endurance is a goal with plyometric exercise, the recovery time between exercise sets is less; the general guideline is 10 to 15 s. This amount of rest time does not allow an optimal recovery of the muscle, so muscle endurance improves.

Plyometric exercises can also be used to develop aerobic conditioning through use of a circuit program in which the patient performs various exercise groupings for 12 to 20 min with less than a 2 s rest between the exercises. A circuit program can develop aerobic, power, and muscle endurance levels.

A plyometrics progression for a sport rehabilitation program uses a number of variables: intensity, volume, recovery, and frequency.

Frequency

Another variable is the frequency with which plyometric activities are used in a therapeutic exercise program. Frequency depends on the exercise intensity and the patient's tolerance and ability to recover. As a rule of thumb, you should allow at least 48 h between plyometric exercise sessions. The research is very unclear about the time it takes healthy patients to recover from plyometric exercise and is essentially nonexistent on frequency of plyometrics in therapeutic exercise programs. Your judgment, common sense, and knowledge of stresses and the patient's abilities are essential to determining frequency for an individual patient's program.

PLYOMETRIC PROGRAM CONSIDERATIONS

Because plyometric activities are generally more intense than other types of exercises, you must consider several special issues regarding their application in therapeutic exercise programs. If the patient has satisfied the pre-plyometric considerations and has the flexibility, strength, and proprioceptive elements required for plyometric activities, he or she must also meet other criteria in order to participate safely. In addition, plyometric exercises must be performed on an appropriate surface, and progression and goals must be determined appropriately.

Age

Although most children use plyometric activities in their everyday activities such as running, jumping, hopping, and skipping, one must use plyometrics carefully with children and youth from ages 8 to 13. Plyometric activities for pre-pubescent and early-pubescent patients should remain at low volume and low intensity. As an example, jumping with both feet and without the use of boxes or weights is low-intensity jumping. Children are at higher risk than older individuals for injury during plyometrics because their central nervous systems are not mature and their GTO activation threshold is lower than in adults. The proprioceptive feedback mechanism is unable to provide necessary safeguards against the high stresses of plyometrics. Muscles and bones of pre-pubescent patients are also not strong enough to tolerate the moderate and high stresses of more advanced plyometric exercises (Gambetta 1986). Because of variability in physical maturity, it may be a safe rule of thumb to restrict patients under age 16 from participating in moderate- to high-intensity plyometrics.

Body Weight

The design of a plyometric program must take into account the patient's weight. Patients weighing 100 kg (220 lb) or more are not able to participate in the same plyometric exercises as lighter patients (Allerheiligen & Rogers, 1995). The stresses imposed on tendons and joints may be too great for safe participation by these patients in higher-intensity plyometric activities. For example, a 113 kg (250 lb) patient may perform single-leg hops for only half the distance that a 68 kg (150 lb) patient can. The intensity of plyometric exercises for heavier patients should be selected cautiously.

Competitive Level

Patients involved in competitive sports are more appropriate candidates for moderate- and high-level plyometric exercises than those in recreational activities are. The competitive patient has more advanced performance goals than the recreational patient and typically has more intense sport participation requirements. Although therapeutic exercise programs for all patients should include some level of plyometric exercises, only the competitive patients require higher-intensity plyometric activities.

Surface

The best surfaces for plyometric lower-extremity activities are those that have "give" to them. Although it can be indoors or outdoors, the surface should be one that yields to absorb some of the impact stress of the plyometric activity. Ideal surfaces include spring-loaded floors, Resiliteâ mats, and grass. Harder surfaces such as asphalt, concrete, and carpet or rubber over concrete should be avoided. Although the surface should be able to absorb some of the impact forces produced during the activity, it should not be so yielding that it reduces the elastic recoil, the crucial element of plyometric activity. If the surface prevents sufficient amortization and impedes the individual's concentric phase, the surface is probably too soft. For the higher-stress plyometric activities, this becomes a key consideration.

Footwear

Shoes that offer good support and provide some cushion for shock absorption are the best shoes to wear for plyometrics. A shoe can offer too much absorption and thus be too spongy, causing instability instead of providing stability in landing. If this is the case, the individual may report a sense of instability or find that he or she is unable to execute the exercise properly, or you may be able to observe instability at the foot landing or takeoff during the exercises. Shoes should be in good condition, not be excessively worn, be tied properly, and fit well.

Proper Technique

Technique is probably the most important among the special considerations. Foot position is an essential factor in jumping activities. The patient should land on the midfoot and then roll forward to push off from the balls of the feet (Gambetta, 1986). The patient should not land on the balls of the feet or the heel, since these landing techniques increase the impact forces and thereby increase stress applied at the foot, ankle, and knee. The midfoot landing also allows a shorter amortization time so that a more powerful concentric motion can occur.

The trunk should remain upright with a straight back so that summation of forces from the back, abdominals, and arms can be utilized. The arms can contribute 10% of the force of the plyometric jump, so both timing of activities and posture are important factors (Gambetta, 1986). Keeping the back straight will permit this transmission of forces and avoid back injuries.

The quality of the execution is important. As a rehabilitation clinician, you must carefully observe the patient's quality of performance. As the patient fatigues, performance quality declines. This can result in two problems: risk of injury and development of an improper engram. It is important to know the proper exercise technique and to observe the patient's performance closely so that you can discontinue the exercise when performance begins to deteriorate.

Progression

A gradual progression from simple to difficult, from few to more, and from general to specific is vital to avoid injury in plyometric activities. The patient's body must be allowed time to adapt to new stress levels in order to avoid overstress injuries. As we have seen, there are a variety of ways to implement progression into a program. The clinician must monitor the injury and note undesirable responses to activity and activity progressions. Continually aware that stresses applied to the injured site may cause an inflammatory response, the clinician should have alternative plans if unwanted responses occur.

Goals

The program's goals are individually dictated by the patient and the demands of the patient's sport. The specific exercises within the program are determined by the sport-specific requirements of each patient. For example, a long jumper will have a different plyometric jumping program than a basketball player, and a volleyball player will have a different jumping program than a wrestler. You must understand the stresses, skills, and demands of the patient's sport so that you can incorporate appropriate plyometric exercises into the therapeutic exercise program at the proper time.

You should assess the patient's plyometric performance at certain times during the therapeutic exercise program. Any time you initiate a plyometric activity, you should take initial measurements of the patient's performance. For example, in a standing jump, you should measure the jump height the first time the patient attempts the jump. As the patient progresses through the program, more intensive plyometric activities are introduced. Each time the patient performs a new activity, record initial performance values and establish new goals. Additional measurements can be taken either at specific intervals, such as every week, or when the patient is ready to advance to a more difficult activity. These recordings help the rehabilitation clinician maintain objective measures of improvement. They also provide additional motivation and goals for the patient.

PRECAUTIONS AND CONTRAINDICATIONS

As you realize, there are precautions for any therapeutic exercise program. Because plyometric activities can be vigorous, you must consider additional precautions before deciding to incorporate them into an individual's therapeutic exercise program:

- **Time.** Because plyometric activities place such high stresses on the body, they should not be performed for extended periods of time. They also should be performed in the early part of the therapeutic exercise session before the patient becomes fatigued and his or her strength, flexibility, and coordination are less than optimal. The time to perform the plyometric activities is after the warm-up but before fatigue increases and with it the risk of injury.

- **Post-exercise delayed onset muscle soreness.** It is important to caution the patient that because plyometric activities are more strenuous than other exercises, he or she may experience post-exercise soreness. Delayed onset soreness is common, especially at the time plyometric exercises are introduced into the program or when the intensity changes.

In addition, you must be aware of several clear contraindications to plyometric activity:

- **Acute inflammation.** Plyometric exercises should be avoided in acute inflammatory conditions. The intensity of these exercises can increase the inflammation.

- **Post-operative conditions.** Persons with immediate post-operative conditions should not engage in plyometric exercise. The tissues are unable to tolerate the stress of such exercises and are highly vulnerable to injury.

- **Instability.** Gross joint instability, until strength is sufficient to control the joint, is a contraindication. Strength is a prerequisite to any plyometric exercise. Strength permits the control necessary for safe and effective plyometric exercise execution.

A number of special considerations must enter into the decision of whether and how to use plyometrics within a patient's therapeutic exercise program. Plyometrics is appropriate for patients with certain characteristics and not others. Plyometric activities require particular types of surfaces and footwear. Other considerations involve progression and goals for this type of exercise.

Precautions concerning the use of plyometrics relate to the time the patient spends on these activities and to vulnerability to post-exercise soreness. There are also a few frank contraindications to the use of plyometrics in a therapeutic exercise program.

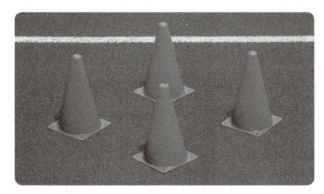

▶ **Figure 9.2** Plyometric cones.

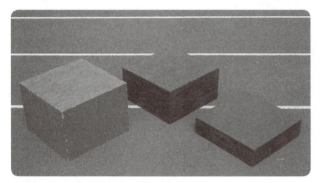

▶ **Figure 9.3** Plyometric boxes.

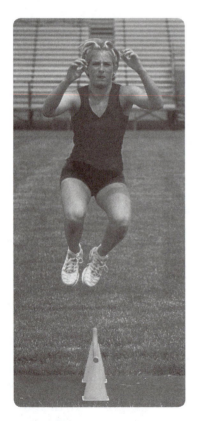

▶ **Figure 9.4** Plyometric hurdle constructed from cones and a dowel.

EQUIPMENT

Equipment for plyometric activities need not be elaborate or expensive. In fact, most plyometric exercises require little or no equipment. In the following sections we review some of the most commonly used items.

Cones

Plastic barriers or traffic cones are used as jump obstacles or for sprint activities. Their plasticity makes them safe for patients to land on. These cones come in various sizes from 20 to 60 cm (8 to 24 in.) (figure 9.2).

Boxes

Boxes come in a variety of heights, ranging from 15 to 106 cm (6 to 42 in.), and various designs. The top should have a non-slip surface. The lower boxes are used for less intense activities and the higher ones for more intense activities (figure 9.3).

Hurdles

Hurdles are used for more advanced plyometric exercises. Some are adjustable within ranges of 15 to 100 cm (6 to 40 in.). A low hurdle can be easily constructed from two cones and a dowel (figure 9.4).

Medicine Balls

Medicine balls are useful in plyometric activities for the upper extremities and trunk, and also provide additional resistance for lower extremity plyometrics. They come in a variety of sizes, weights, and surfaces. The leather-covered balls are limited to indoor use because moisture shortens the life of the cover. Balls should be of a manageable size and should have a surface that permits the patient to maintain an adequate grasp. If one-hand activities are required for the exercise, the ball should have a diameter that will accommodate the patient's hand size (figure 9.5).

Other Equipment

A variety of other equipment can be used for various plyometric activities. Jump ropes, stairs, and barriers are examples of items that are usually readily available. Their specific use depends on the goals of the exercise and the imagination of the rehabilitation clinician.

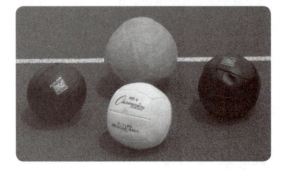

▶ **Figure 9.5** Medicine balls.

LOWER-EXTREMITY PLYOMETRICS

Once the patient has the prerequisite strength, flexibility, and coordination, and the tissues have healed sufficiently to tolerate the stress of such activity without incurring damage or additional inflammation, plyometric exercises can become a part of the therapeutic exercise program.

> Some plyometric exercises require no equipment, and others use a variety of items that are easy to obtain or to construct.

Progression

A lower extremity plyometric exercise progression involves six types of exercises: jumps-in-place, standing jumps, multiple jumps and hops, bounding, box drills, and depth jumps (Chu 1998).

Jumps-in-Place

Jumps-in-place are repeated jumps that begin and end in the same place. They can range in intensity from low to high. The low intensity jumps are good activities for developing a brief amortization phase. The specific goal, to develop a short amortization phase with a rapid rebound, often serves to develop the patient's jump technique. Jump-in-place exercises should relate to the patient's sport. For example, a two-foot ankle hop is suitable for a basketball player, and a hip-twist ankle hop is well suited to a skier. As the patient progresses, he or she can perform more difficult jumps-in-place or can advance to another type of jump exercise.

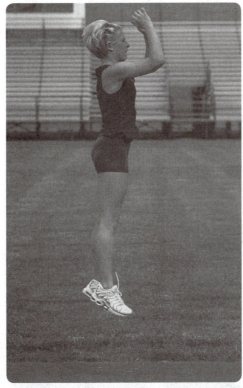
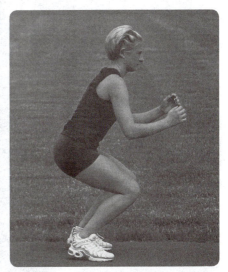

a

Two-Foot Ankle Hop   Have the

patient jump in place using only the ankles. The patient should jump as high as possible. The knees will bend, but only slightly (figure 9.6a). This exercise is particularly good for patients who play basketball.

Hip-Twist Ankle Hop   Have the

patient, with feet together, jump and twist 90° to the left, return to start position, and then repeat to the right. The patient should twist from the hips, not the knees (figure 9.6b). This exercise is particularly good for patients who ski.

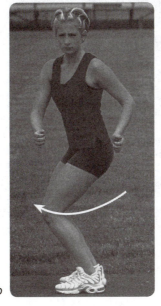
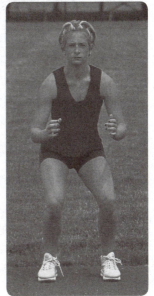
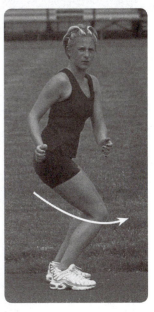

b

▶ **Figure 9.6**   Jump-in-place plyometric exercises: *(a)* two-foot ankle hop; *(b)* hip-twist ankle hop.

Standing Jumps

Standing jumps are single jumps that emphasize a maximal effort with motion occurring either vertically or horizontally. Recovery between each attempt is necessary for a maximal effort each time. A progression of this type of jump could consist, for example, of beginning with a standing long jump, progressing to a jump over a cone, and advancing to a standing long jump with a sprint. Standing jumps can go forward or laterally and can involve barriers.

Patients can combine standing jumps with multiple jumps, running, or sprinting in different directions.

Standing Long Jump The patient's feet are shoulder-width apart. Have him or her explode from semi-squat position to jump as far forward as possible. The patient should use arms to assist (figure 9.7a). This exercise is particularly good for patients who swim or participate in track.

Standing Jump over Barrier Have the patient, with feet shoulder-width apart, jump upward and over cone, landing on both feet simultaneously. The patient should keep hips over knees and feet (figure 9.7b). You can add cones from 0.9 to 1.8 m (3–6 ft) apart

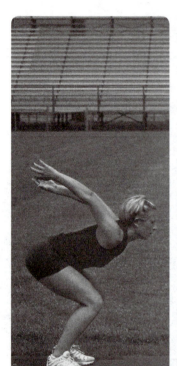
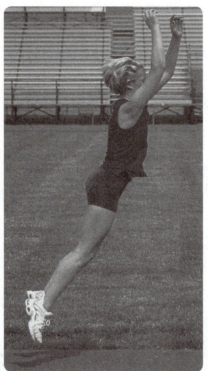

a

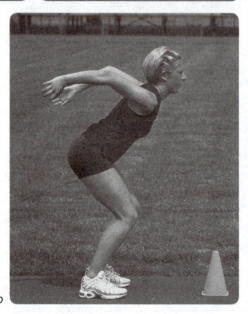

b

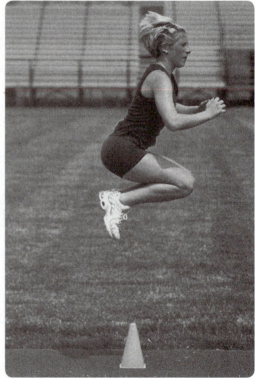

▶ **Figure 9.7** Example of a standing jump progression: *(a)* standing long jump, *(b)* standing jump over barrier.

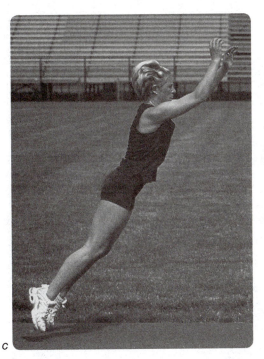
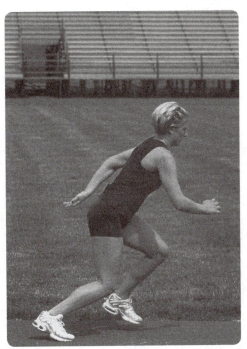

Refer to examples of plyometric jumping exercises for the lower extremities in Don Chu's *Jumping into Plyometrics, Second Edition* (1998). It is advisable for you to refer to this book for additional suggestions for plyometric exercises and progression programs.

▶ **Figure 9.7** *(continued) (c)* standing long jump with sprint.

for multiple jumps. This exercise is particularly good for patients who are figure skaters or basketball players.

Standing Long Jump with Sprint Using arms to assist, the patient should jump as far forward as possible. Immediately after landing, have him or her sprint forward as fast as possible for 10 m (figure 9.7c). Add sprints to left and right for additional activities. This exercise is particularly good for patients who play hockey, participate in track, or play football.

Multiple Jumps and Hops

Multiple hops and jumps combine the skills of jumps-in-place and standing jumps. The patient attempts to jump maximally and repeats the jumps without resting. The total distance in each set of exercises is usually kept under 30 m (Chu 1998). The jumps can be performed with one or two legs, in a straight line or in multiple directions, with or without barriers. A front cone hop is an example of a simple multiple-hop exercise. The single-leg hop and a series of stadium-step hops are examples of more difficult multiple hops.

Single-Leg Hops Have the patient jump from left leg, propelling as far upward and forward as possible, using arm movement to assist, and then land on the same leg. The patient should use forward movement of the right non-weight bearing leg to propel forward for the next jump, landing on right leg. Remind the patient to keep hips and knees directly over the landing foot (figure 9.8a).

Stadium Hops Have the patient jump one step at a time using both legs. The movement should be rapid, light, and continuous up the stairs, without stops or hesitation. The patient can progress to taking two steps at a time or using one leg and alternating (figure 9.8b). This exercise, as well as the single-leg hops on the previous page, is particularly good for patients who wrestle or play hockey.

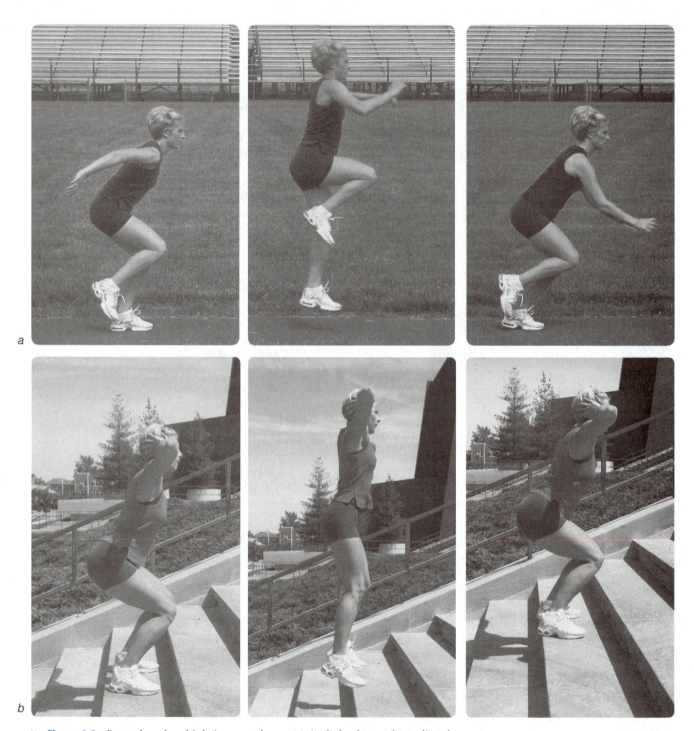

▶ **Figure 9.8** Examples of multiple jumps or hops: *(a)* single-leg hops, *(b)* stadium hops.

Bounding

Bounding exercises are an exaggeration of the running stride. They are used to improve stride length and speed. These exercises are most commonly used for patients in track and field events. Distances usually exceed 30 m (Chu 1998). A simple bounding exercise is skipping; an advanced bounding exercise is single-leg bounding. Skipping and bounding are explosive activities with the patient exploding quickly from landing and jumping upward and forward.

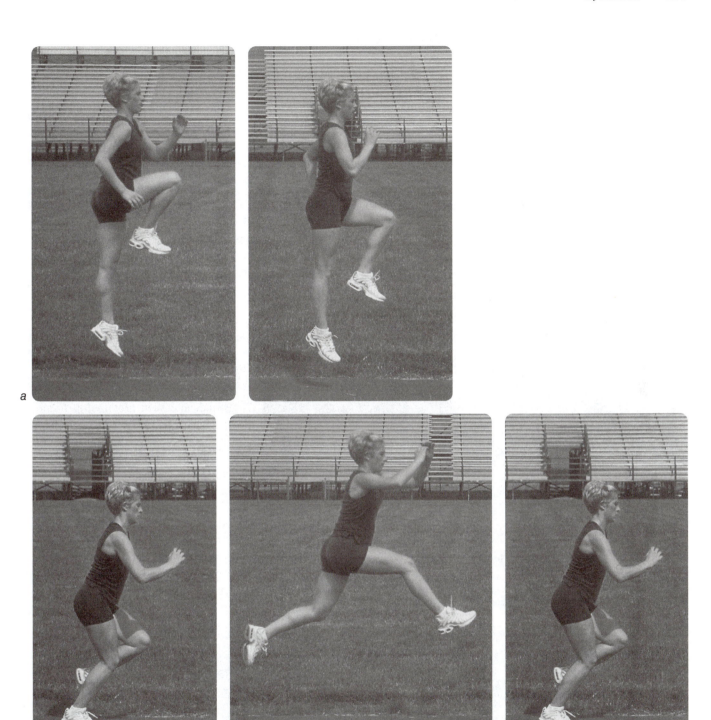

▶ **Figure 9.9** Examples of simple and more difficult bounding exercises: *(a)* skipping; *(b)* bounding.

Skipping   Have the patient lift the right leg with the knee bent 90° while also lifting the left arm with the elbow bent 90°. Then the patient should alternate with opposite extremities (figure 9.9a).

Single-Leg Bounding   While on the right leg, the patient should move forward and upward as far as possible by using the momentum of the left leg and both arms to propel forward, landing on the right leg. Have the patient continue the forward and upward movement, this time landing on the left leg (figure 9.9b).

Box Jumps

Box drills involve the more advanced skills required for multiple jumps and hops because the jumps and hops are performed onto and off boxes of varying heights. These exercises can be low or high intensity, depending on the box height. They use both vertical and horizontal jumps. Examples of box jumps are shown in figure 9.10.

Front Box Jump Begin with a box about 30 cm (12 in.) high. Jump onto the box with both feet. Step down and repeat. The difficulty can be increased by increasing the box height or using one leg, alternating left and right (figure 9.10a).

Pyramiding Box Hops Place up to five boxes of increasing height about 0.6 to 0.9 m (2-3 ft) apart in a line. Jump onto the first box, onto the floor on the other side, and then onto the next box, repeating to the end of the row. Use the arms to assist in the motion (figure 9.10b).

Depth Jumps

Depth jumps are the most aggressive plyometric exercises. They are box jumps of greater intensity in that the patient is challenged by his or her own weight and the acceleration of gravity. The motion in depth jumps includes stepping off a box, dropping to the ground, and then rebounding immediately upward. These are intensive exercises that the patient must perform with caution. Jumping off the box is avoided in these exercises because a jump will increase the distance to the floor and significantly increase the stresses applied to the patient.

An example of progression using depth jumps consists of starting from a simple depth jump in which the patient steps down from a box and jumps verti-

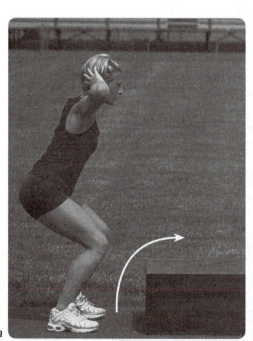

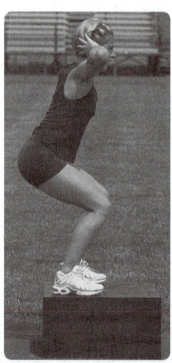

a

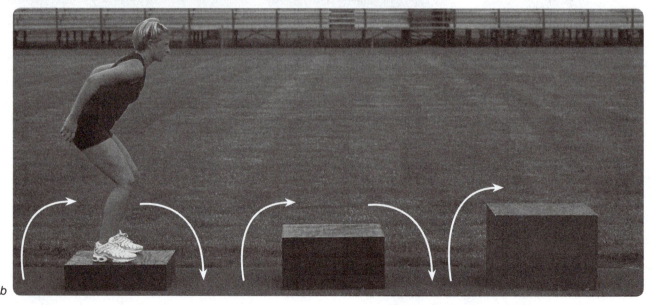

b

▶ **Figure 9.10** Examples of box jumps: *(a)* front box jump; *(b)* pyramiding box jumps.

cally, using both feet. The patient subsequently advances to a much more difficult depth jump—a single-leg depth jump in which the patient lands on one foot and jumps as high as possible from the one leg. A more challenging progression can include using a higher box or using more than one box and jumping onto the second box from the ground.

Depth Jump Have the patient step off a 30 cm (12 in.) box, landing on the floor with both feet. As rapidly as possible, the patient should jump upward as high as possible, using the arms to reach upward (figure 9.11a).

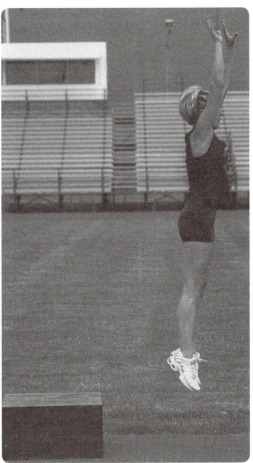

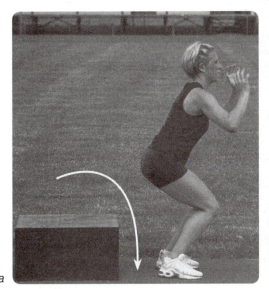

Single-Leg Depth Jump Have the patient step off a 30-cm box, landing on the left leg only. The patient should spring upward as high as possible from the left leg. Then have him or her repeat the exercise with the right leg (figure 9.11b).

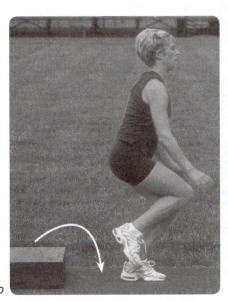

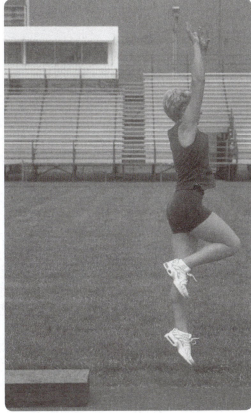

▶ **Figure 9.11** Examples of depth jumps: *(a)* depth jump; *(b)* single-leg depth jump.

Lower-extremity plyometric exercises use various types of jumps, as well as bounding and box drills, in various combinations to provide a progression of intensities.

Box Height   You must select a box height for depth jumps carefully. If the height is too great, the risk of injury increases. A height that is too great also requires the muscles to absorb the impact of the drop, and the time required to absorb the force makes the amortization time too long to be effective. Care must be taken in assigning a maximum box height for depth jumps. At a point when the patient takes too much time during the transition phase to move from eccentric to concentric, the height of the box is too high. Although boxes up to four feet high are available, rarely are these heights necessary for plyometric rehabilitation programs.

Chu (1998) recommends determining a box height for depth jumps using the following procedure. The individual performs a standard jump-and-reach test, and the target point the individual achieves is marked. The person then performs a depth jump from a 45-cm (18-in) box and attempts to reach for the same point as attained on the test. If the mark is attained, the box height increases by 15 cm (6 in) increments until the person is unable to achieve the target. The first box at which the person is unable to achieve the target point is the depth-box height. If the individual cannot reach the target point from the 45-cm box, either the box should be lowered or the person should not perform the activity until he or she achieves greater strength.

Selection

Although all the types of plyometric exercises provide a progression of difficulty from low to high intensity, you must analyze the exercise to determine its relative intensity. For example, a high-level standing jump may be more intense than a moderate-level box jump.

The selection of exercise for a patient's program depends on the demands of the patient's sport and the level of participation of that patient. For example, you may give one patient appropriate plyometric exercises with varying intensities of multiple jumps and hops; another patient may be more appropriately stressed with box jumps and depth jumps. Two patients in the same sport, one at a recreational level and the other at an intercollegiate competitive level, have different requirements because of the different competitive demands. This is a prime consideration in exercise selection.

UPPER-EXREMITY AND TRUNK PLYOMETRICS

We will consider upper-extremity and trunk exercises together, because many of the upper-extremity exercises with medicine balls strongly influence the trunk muscles and vice versa. Some exercises are specific to either the upper extremity or the trunk, as indicated. Because the trunk plays a vital role in stabilization during upper-extremity activities, the strength of the muscle groups in the trunk is important to the strength of the upper extremity. The trunk muscles also perform trunk movement during upper-extremity activities.

Plyometrics for the upper extremity and trunk have essentially the same considerations as those for the lower extremity. The exercises should be specific to the sport demands, should provide a progression of difficulty so that there is a challenge and the patient makes the desired gains, and should be performed with controlled speed of movement.

You can provide progression by changing the intensity. This can be done by changing the weights of the medicine balls, the speed of the activity, and the distance the medicine balls are passed. Passing medicine balls includes tossing and throwing. Tossing is defined as passing a ball a short distance with the arm below 90° of shoulder flexion; throwing is defined as passing the ball a long distance with the arm above 90° of flexion (Chu, 1989).

Passing exercises can be performed with either a partner or a Rebounder—a trampoline inclined so that it returns the ball to the patient (figure 9.12).

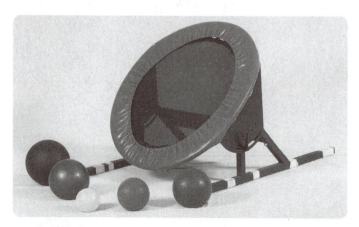

▶ **Figure 9.12**   Rebounder and medicine balls.

Figure 9.13 provides examples of medicine ball plyometric exercises for the upper extremities and trunk. The chest pass photo shows the patient executing a chest pass from a distance of about 3 m (10 ft), using the forward movement of the legs to coincide with the snap of the ball. Follow-through should continue until the arms are fully extended in front of the body and the backs of the hands face each other. In the overhead throw, once again the patient uses leg movement to coincide with arm motion so that as the ball is released from behind the head. The patient moves from the back to the front leg. Follow-through is with the arms straight, upward, and forward. During both activities, the trunk muscles are kept taut and the back is held straight to allow force from the legs to be transmitted through the trunk to the arms.

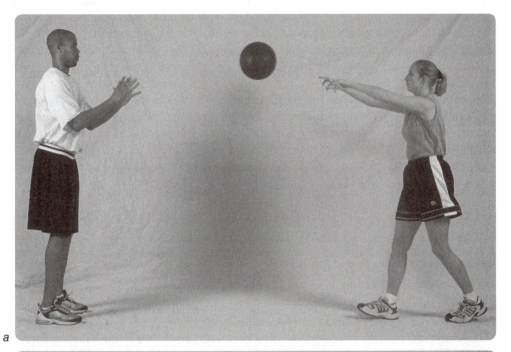

a

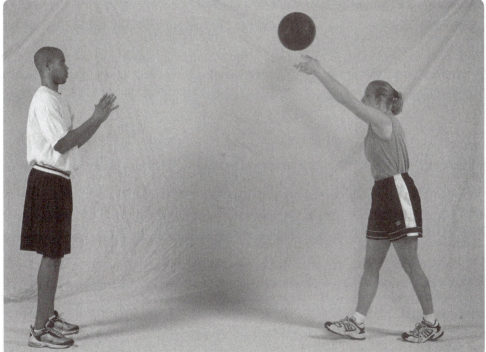

b

▶ **Figure 9.13** Upper-extremity and trunk plyometrics: *(a)* chest pass; *(b)* overhead throw.

Plyometrics for the upper extremity and the trunk use tossing and throwing activities with medicine balls.

As with lower-extremity plyometrics, upper-extremity and trunk plyometrics should be specific to the patient's needs. They should provide specific challenges that will permit the patient to make gains in the muscles most challenged by the patient's sport. The SAID principle is as important in plyometric exercises as it is in strength exercises. As was mentioned in chapter 7, the SAID principle is an acronym for Specific Adaptations to Imposed Demands and refers to the body's ability to adapt to stresses applied through exercise.

SUMMARY

Plyometrics utilizes both mechanical and neurological effects to optimize muscle performance. The mechanical principles involve making use of both the contractile and non-contractile elements of muscle composition to create more potential energy and convert it to mechanical energy. The neurological principles maximize the Golgi tendon organ and muscle spindle responses to obtain optimal results from the neurological system. These components are combined in a three-phase process to produce a plyometric movement. The three-phase process includes an eccentric phase, an amortization phase, and a concentric phase. Not all patients are candidates to use plyometrics in their rehabilitation programs. Factors such as age, weight, and competition level must be taken into consideration before plyometric exercise is included in the program. A variety of equipment may be used in plyometrics for the upper extremity, lower extremity, and trunk; the equipment chosen may be determined by cost, goals of the program, and space availability.

KEY CONCEPTS AND REVIEW

1. Identify the mechanical and neurological components of the neuromuscular principles involved in plyometrics.

Plyometrics involves the technique of first lengthening, then shortening the muscle to produce an increased power output. This type of exercise is based on the stretch-shortening principles. It is believed that a muscle's increased power during plyometric exercise training may result from a combination of an increased level of muscle elasticity and the adaptations that occur in the muscle spindle and GTO.

2. Describe the factors involved in plyometric program design.

Every plyometric exercise includes three aspects—the lengthening or eccentric phase, the amortization phase, and the contracting or concentric phase. The lengthening phase prepares the muscles for the rapid change, or amortization, and allows a greater contraction to produce greater results.

3. List three considerations for plyometric program execution.

When designing a plyometric program, one must consider the patient's physical condition and the sport's demands. Specifically, the patient should have adequate flexibility, strength, and proprioception before beginning a plyometric program. Special considerations also include factors such as the patient's age, weight, level of competition, footwear, the surface, proper technique, progression, and goals.

4. List the precautions and contraindications for plyometrics.

Precautions include factors such as the amount of time involved in plyometrics and the possibility of delayed-onset muscle soreness post-exercise. Contraindications include an acute inflammation, postoperative conditions, and instability.

5. Outline a progression of four plyometric exercises for either a lower- or an upper-extremity program.

A lower extremity plyometric exercise progression for a basketball player might begin with a two-foot ankle hop and progress to a single-foot ankle hop, side-to-side hops, standing jump-and-reach, long jump with lateral sprint, and box depth jumps.

CRITICAL THINKING QUESTIONS

1. If a plyometric jump is not executed quickly from the eccentric to the concentric phase, the patient is unable to jump as high during the concentric phase. What could the reasons be? What can be done if a patient does not understand the concept of a rapid change from eccentric to concentric and insists on pausing between the two phases? What cues or instructions can you provide to improve performance?

2. A patient with an ankle sprain is now ready for plyometric exercises. What are the criteria that he or she has to meet before these exercises can be added to the therapeutic exercise program?

3. A gymnast with a wrist sprain is ready for plyometric activities before returning to functional activities. Identify three plyometric activities that would prepare him or her for functional activities. What would your criteria be for progression from plyometric to functional activities?

4. The chief rehabilitation clinician of the university where you are working has asked you to write a sheet of instructions that the clinicians will hand out to patients before they begin the plyometric phase of their rehabilitation programs. What instructions will you include on the sheet? What precautions will you list? Are there any criteria that you will include for determining whether a patient is eligible for a plyometric program?

5. In the chapter's opening scenario, what precautions is Larry concerned about with Ed? What first-day plyometric activities would you recommend that Larry have Ed perform, and what should Larry look for when Ed performs them? How would you determine when Ed can progress in his plyometric program?

LAB ACTIVITIES

1. Have your lab partner perform each of the following jumps once, measure the height achieved with each jump, and record the results. Instruct your partner to begin each jump from the standing position. Allow a few practice jumps before doing the test jumps.

   a. Jump 1: Quickly bend the knees to approximately 60° and jump.
   b. Jump 2: Slowly bend the knees to approximately 60°, hold for 3 sec, and jump.
   c. Jump 3: Quickly bend the knees to approximately 120° and jump.
   d. Jump 4: Quickly bend the knees to approximately 120°, hold for 3 sec, and jump.
   e. Jump 5: Step off a step stool or box, then immediately jump up.
   f. Jump 6: Jump up onto a box, then immediately jump off and jump upward.

   Which jump produced the greatest height? What is the physiological reason for your results? What is the importance of how these results relate to a plyometric rehabilitation program?

2. Have your lab partner perform a series of long jumps to determine the most advantageous body position and arm movement during the jump, as well as proper foot placement on landing for optimal force production. Repeat each jump from the preceding exercise, adding the conditions listed below. Perform three jumps using each condition. Record the subject's average jump height for each of the conditions. The jumps for each set should be performed rapidly with little or no rest between jumps.

   a. Condition 1: No arm movement; lands on the balls of the feet.
   b. Condition 2: Uses arm movement; lands on the balls of the feet.
   c. Condition 3: Uses arms and lands on the midfoot.

Which jump produced the greatest distance? What is the physiological reason for your results? What is the importance of how these results relate to a plyometric rehabilitation program?

3. Have your lab partner select a sport he or she likes to play. Assume your lab partner is a patient who is now to the point where he is ready to perform plyometric exercises in the rehab program. Design a progression for the lower or upper extremity (using jumps in place, standing jumps, multiple jumps, box drills, and so on for LE; boxes, medicine balls, and so on for UE) to fit your individual patient's needs. Be sure to include how the patient would progress through the program and your outline of sets, reps, recovery, and intensity. Indicate your logic in why you selected these exercises, why you decided on this intensity level, and how you will determine when to advance the patient.

CHAPTER 10

Functional and Activity-Specific Exercise

OBJECTIVES

After completing this chapter, you should be able to do the following:

1. Explain the difference between functional exercise and activity-specific exercise.

2. Identify the contributions of functional and activity-specific exercise to a therapeutic exercise program.

3. Discuss the differences between basic and advanced functional activities.

4. List factors that can be varied in a progression of functional and activity-specific activities.

5. Identify precautions for functional and activity-specific exercises.

6. Outline a sample of functional exercise to activity-specific progression for either the lower or the upper extremity.

▶ Dawn Misty is a certified athletic trainer working with the university's tennis team. At the end of last season, Christian, the star singles player, underwent a shoulder capsular shift repair. He has progressed well through his rehabilitation program and is now ready to begin functional activities. Dawn knows that the functional activities will quickly progress to activity-specific activities before Christian returns to his regular tennis routine. It has been several weeks since Christian has swung a tennis racket, and he has a lot of apprehension about whether he will be able to return to competition. Dawn is confident that he will do well once he has completed the activity-specific phase of his rehabilitation program.

For the past few weeks Dawn has had Christian get used to holding a tennis racket by having him bounce a ball on the ground and in the air with his elbow near his side. Now it is time for Christian to begin ground strokes. Dawn has outlined the progression of the program she has designed for Christian, informing him that the program will move at his own pace and allow him and his shoulder to become accustomed to one level before advancing to the next level. Christian has confidence in Dawn's ability and judgment because she has done an excellent job of bringing him this far along in his rehabilitation program. He knows that if she feels he can do an activity, he probably can do it.

Be such a man, and live such a life, that if every man were such as you, and every life a life like yours, this earth would be God's Paradise.

PHILLIP BROOKS, American Episcopal bishop, 1835-1893

This chapter addresses an important but often forgotten aspect of therapeutic exercise: functional and activity-specific activities. Too frequently the patient's program focuses on restoring flexibility, strength, power, and endurance, while the functional and activity-specific demands are forgotten. During the later stages of the therapeutic exercise program it becomes important to prepare the patient to withstand the specific stresses of his or her normal activities and meet the skill demands; it is also essential for the patient to have confidence that he or she can return to full and regular participation.

Like the example in Reverend Brooks' quote above, most healthy individuals want to perform at exceptional levels. The presence of that pre-injury attitude is critical if a patient is to return successfully to full participation. To restore that attitude, the rehabilitation clinician must include functional and activity-specific exercises in the therapeutic exercise program.

The rehabilitation clinician must understand and appreciate not only the patient's sport or occupation but also his or her responsibilities or activities. Offensive and defensive football players encounter different stresses and demands, just as the defensive lineman and defensive halfback position requirements are different. A volleyball setter and a volleyball hitter have different needs; a warehouse manager and a warehouse worker experience different stresses. The clinician should know the patient's specific sport or job requirements and also know how to incorporate those requirements into the therapeutic exercise program.

Once the basic parameters of flexibility, strength, endurance, and proprioception have been restored, specific exercises mimicking necessary skills are added to the program. This will restore the patient's confidence in his or her performance ability and will also provide an avenue for renewing the skills lost following the injury.

DEFINITIONS, FOUNDATIONS, AND GOALS

Before we can discuss specific functional and activity-specific programs and exercises, we must understand what functional exercises and evaluations are, and what their basis and goals are. Once you realize how a therapeutic exercise program progresses to its functional exercise portion and then to the activity-specific phase, it will be easier to develop functional and activity-specific exercises during this final phase.

Definitions

Functional exercises or activities are exercises that precede activity-specific activities in a rehabilitation program. They commonly involve multi-planar activities and provide increased stresses and demands greater than strength exercises. They may include precursor activities to activity-specific exercises such as walking prior to running or underhand tossing prior to throwing. They prepare the patient for the more advanced skill demands they will experience in activity-specific activities. **Activity-specific exercises** are exercises that include drills or mimic tasks found within a specific sport or job. They differ from functional activities in that activity-specific exercises are specific to sport or work performance. For example, while an underhand toss is a functional activity for a baseball outfielder, throwing overhand by 50% force for a shortened distance is an activity-specific exercise since that is the specific activity required of an outfielder albeit with less force and distance than normal. Activity-specific exercises are included in the final phase of the rehabilitation program to mimic the stresses, demands, and skills of the sport or job and advance a patient toward a safe and prompt return to sport participation or normal activity demands.

In the rehabilitation of athletes, sport-specific exercises are used instead of activity-specific exercises. Athletes in the final phase of their rehabilitation program go through a sport-specific phase; this is the equivalent of an activity-specific phase. When we rehabilitate an injured worker, activity-specific exercises include a range of activities from sitting at a desk properly to lifting and transferring heavy boxes. Although "sport-specific" is not the correct term for terminal rehabilitation exercises for a person returning to work, keep in mind that the most important concept is that the final phase of any rehabilitation program includes the addition of *specific* activities that the individual performs in his or her normal environment, be it a sport or a job. Therefore, activity-specific exercises and sport-specific exercises are essentially the same thing, but the specific exercises involved are individually determined and based upon the specific needs of the individual patient.

Performance evaluation occurs throughout the therapeutic exercise program. **Performance evaluation** is an assessment of the patient's ability to perform and complete an exercise or skill drill safely and accurately before he or she is allowed to advance to the next level. The final performance evaluation takes place before the patient resumes full participation. In order to safely advance to each therapeutic exercise level, the patient must pass the functional tests. The functional tests vary according to the patient's level within the therapeutic exercise program. Examples of these tests are discussed later.

Goals

Functional exercise has three goals. The first goal is to attain full functional levels of flexibility, strength, endurance, and coordination. The second is to achieve full functional ability so that normal speed, power, control, and agility are restored. The third goal of functional exercise is to restore the patient's self-confidence in his or her own performance as well as confidence in the injured body segment. Activity-specific exercises achieve the final goal of the entire rehabilitation program: Return the patient to full participation safely and efficiently at a level at least equivalent to that of pre-injury performance.

The first and second goals are achieved through the therapeutic exercise program for basic and advanced functional activities. These are discussed in the next section. The third goal occurs through the advancement to functional exercises and the success the patient experiences at each level. Success builds self-confidence, and failure makes self-confidence elusive; so it is important that the clinician provide exercise goals that are challenging yet achievable. Both being injured and being unable to participate in normal activities often cause a patient to become unsure of his or her abilities. Not participating in normal activities also leads to loss of some of the skills that were so natural before the injury. To re-establish in the patient a pre-injury level of self-confidence in his or her athletic skills, it is necessary to incorporate into the therapeutic exercise program a progression of activity-specific exercises that mimic the skills the patient will need to resume normal-level functions.

The final goal is achieved when all the other goals have been met. This goal is the result and final goal of any therapeutic exercise program. To achieve it, the rehabilitation clinician must include both basic and advanced activity-specific exercises in the therapeutic exercise program. A final performance evaluation takes place before the patient returns to full participation, but it is the patient's ability to participate successfully in the normal activities that is the final test of a therapeutic exercise program.

CONTRIBUTIONS TO THERAPEUTIC EXERCISE

Functional exercises are a part of the total rehabilitation process. In that sense, they make a vital and unique contribution to the preparation and return to competition of the patient. They must place unique combinations of stresses on the patient to produce unique results. The following sections deal with eight of these demands and the corresponding results.

Normal Motion

Functional exercises are designed to reproduce the specific motions of the patient's normal activity. They are individually designed for the demands of each patient so that they mimic the normal activity that the patient will perform. Normal activity requires normal motion. If normal motion is lacking, the patient places undue stress on areas that must compensate for needed motion, and these areas are at risk for additional injury. For example, if a tennis player does not have the normal shoulder flexion and lateral rotation needed to serve, he or she may develop a low back injury by hyperextending the lumbar spine to hit the ball overhead.

Multifaceted Muscle Activity

Several different types of strengthening activities are used in functional exercises. They commonly include a mixture of isometric, concentric, and eccentric activities, because most functional activities include these types of movements. The muscle must have the strength, coordination, and control to quickly change from one type of movement to another and to effectively produce the summation of forces. Even in the simple activity of running, the lower-extremity muscles undergo a rapid change of concentric and eccentric activity in their roles as accelerators, decelerators, and stabilizers during different parts of the running cycle.

Multiplanar Motion and Multiple Muscle Group Performance

Functional activities are not performed in straight-plane movements. They involve the simultaneous use of all three planes of motion. They also include the use of many muscle groups that are recruited at one time to produce the desired activity. Functional exercises must mimic these functional activities by incorporating many muscle groups working in multiple planes.

Multiplanar motion is performed in a coordinated manner through the simultaneous facilitation and inhibition of many muscles. Even an activity like throwing a ball not only involves the shoulder, elbow, wrist, and hand muscles but also requires coordinated multiplanar motions from trunk and lower-extremity muscle groups.

Stabilization and Acceleration Changes

Functional motion requires that some muscles work to stabilize a part while other muscles work either to accelerate or decelerate or to change from stabilization to acceleration or deceleration quickly. If functional exercises are to mimic functional activities, muscles must be trained to perform these fluid functional changes that are part of even basic activities. To use the example of a throw, the trunk must be stabilized if the shoulder is to have a platform from which to propel the ball. Even during an activity such as walking, the hip and leg muscles stabilize and limit lateral movement as the body is propelled forward.

Proprioceptive Stimulation

Proprioception is the awareness of body movement and position. As discussed in chapter 8, proprioception is vital to performance. Proprioceptive skills, basic and advanced, must be finely tuned and must be prepared to meet the activity demands to which the patient will be returning. Performance of functional exercises requires the use of proprioception, and improvement of the patient's functional performance directly correlates to his or her proprioceptive development.

Agility and Power Development

Agility and power are essential requirements for most sports. Agility is necessary in order for the basketball player to dribble the ball downcourt, or the volleyball player to dive and pass the ball to the setter, and for the hurdler to time each jump correctly. Power allows the sprinter to reach the finish line before the other competitors, the football defensive lineman to sack the quarterback, and the crew team to sprint to the end of the race. Agility and power are required in a gymnast's floor exercise routine, an ice skater's triple-Lutz jump, and a water polo player's scoring a goal. Agility and power must improve as the patient increases his or her ability to perform functional activities. Progressive functional exercises provide a graduated increase in stress and, therefore, improve the patient's ability to perform at an agility and power level sufficient for appropriate skill execution within the sport and at the patient's level of competition.

Activity-Specific Skill Development

Functional exercises—from the basic exercises to the more advanced—have as their goal the patient's return to normal function. The advanced functional exercises evolve to the activity-specific exercises used in the later stages of rehabilitation. These late-stage activities are specifically designed with this goal in mind. The activity-specific exercises mimic the sport activities and place the same demands on the patient that he or she will encounter when returning to participation. The specific skills needed to perform the rehabilitation exercises are the same skills that are needed to perform within the sport, so many of these exercises are drills used in practice of the sport.

When a patient is unable to perform normal activities for a time, the ability to perform those activities declines (Kottke, 1980; Monfils, Plautz, & Kleim, 2005). To change the neural events that provide for accurate skill execution and create the right engram, there are steps the performer and clinician must take to assure those neurophysiological changes. These steps include the following: (1) instruct the patient in the desired performance; (2) make sure that the patient understands the task to be performed; (3) have the patient perform the activity slowly, precisely, and without resistance; (4) add more complex tasks once basic tasks are successfully performed; (5) as the patient's performance improves, increase the activity's intensity; and (6) remember that repetition of an activity is essential to its desired outcome (Kottke, 1980). Therefore, as we have progressed in other parameters, skill development also requires a progressive, planned, and coordinated system of therapeutic exercises. Starting with basic and simple skills and progressing to more complex activities as the simple ones are mastered until the patient performs specific-sport activities is the course of the sport-specific section of the therapeutic exercise program.

The basic functional exercises that begin an injured athlete's therapeutic exercise program are multi-planar activities that follow a progression to build the foundation for improvement in more specific skill activities.

Confidence Development

As the patient succeeds in performing those activity-specific exercises that mimic the demands of the sport or job, confidence returns. By the time the patient is ready to resume full participation, he or she has demonstrated an ability to perform the skills that participation requires. This gives the individual the self-confidence to perform without hesitation and meet the demands of the sport or job with confidence in the injured part.

BASIC FUNCTIONAL ACTIVITIES

In a good therapeutic exercise program, functional exercise and functional evaluation take place from the very beginning of rehabilitation and become more functional as the patient progresses in the program. The program starts with exercises for achieving basic parameter goals such as flexibility, strength, endurance, and proprioception. These parameters are prerequisite to complex functional activities because they are used to attain goals that are necessary for functional performance. For example, in order to jump hurdles, a runner has to gain a functional degree of flexibility in the hamstrings. In order to compete, a wrestler must have full functional flexibility in the shoulders. A pitcher needs functional muscle endurance to pitch a game. A gymnast must be able to stork stand on the ground before he or she can stand on a balance beam.

As has been mentioned, functional exercises are activities that require multi-planar abilities. Basic functional exercises such as a single-leg stance may occur early in a patient's therapeutic exercise program, provided the individual is bearing full weight, has sufficient strength to balance, and is able to recover from loss of balance, regardless of the plane in which the balance is lost.

As the therapeutic exercise program progresses with improvements in the required parameters, more complex functional activities are added to the program. These exercises may include lower extremity activities such as side shuffles, cariocas, hops, backward running, or exercising on a slide board. More complex upper extremity functional exercises include juggling, PNF movement with rubber tubing, throwing or dribbling a ball against a wall, or playing "rock, paper, scissors."

The primary difference between functional exercises and exercises for gains in range of motion or strength is that functional exercises are multi-planar while exercises intended to make specific gains in isolated muscles or muscle groups are not usually multi-planar. The primary difference between functional exercises and activity-specific activities is that while both are multi-planar, the activity-specific activities are drills that are used in a specific sport and involve skills required within that sport. Some sports have overlapping activity-specific and functional activities. These are primarily running sports such as track or cross-country.

ACTIVITY-SPECIFIC EXERCISES

Progression from complex functional to more specific skill activities requires the clinician to break down the specific skills required in a sport to provide the patient with fundamental skill review first. Once the fundamental skills are mastered, combining these basic skills into more complex performance activities is the next step. In addition to flexibility, strength, muscle endurance, and proprioception, these skill activities require the more advanced competence that includes combining agility, speed, power, and control. Depending on the requirements of the advanced skill, some basic skill exercises can be started earlier in the program while the patient is still working to achieve proficiency in other factors. For example, the patient can start basic coordination exercises such as bouncing a basketball before he or she has achieved full range of motion or full strength.

The patient should be able to perform plyometric exercises before specific skill activities are incorporated into the therapeutic exercise program. The skill of the rehabilitation clinician is a factor in determining exactly when the progressions should occur and what they should be. This skill is based on knowledge about tissue healing; knowledge of the influences of the stresses applied by various exercises and activities; observation of the patient's reaction to the stresses; knowledge of an exercise sequence; and knowledge of the specific demands, skills, and requirements of the injured patient's sport or work tasks. The rehabilitation clinician's ability requires good judgment and common sense about how much stress to apply and when during the therapeutic exercise program to apply that stress.

FUNCTIONAL TO ACTIVITY-SPECIFIC EXERCISE PROGRESSION

Functional exercises build on fundamental skill functions that the patient has already achieved and often include plyometrics. Activity-specific exercises focus on the specific functions and skills required for normal sports or job participation.

You may have noticed that some proprioceptive parameters are included in basic functional exercises and that agility is in the advanced functional exercises category. This is because proprioception is a transition parameter. Because of the wide range of complexity of proprioception, one of its simplest efferent results, balance, becomes a basic functional activity. Since agility requires a great deal of skill, it is a more advanced functional activity.

Some basic functional exercises actually mimic activity-specific activities in that they are performed during a specific task. Examples of basic functional activities in various sports are stork standing in ice skating, standing on the unstable surface of the edge of a diving board, and walking on a gymnastics balance beam. These examples of basic functional activities serve only as a reminder that it is sometimes difficult to draw the line between functional and sport-specific exercises.

When a patient is unable to use a specific skill, the ability to perform that skill rapidly declines (Monfils et al., 2005). Such is the case when an individual is unable to participate because of the injury suffered. Clinicians can accurately make the assumption that any patient who does not participate in his or her regular sport or work activity will lose his or her skills required of that normal activity. This loss of skill necessitates relearning the skill before the patient returns to full and normal participation. Progression of this skill acquisition is a methodical and systematic increase in physical and neurological demands, one building upon the previous, until skill is fully restored. Progression of the various parameters of these demands are presented here.

Force and Intensity

Force and intensity are the amount of resistance that an activity provides. Forces and intensities vary in type depending on the specific activity and the outcome desired. The intent is to provide an overload in accordance with the SAID principle that has been described in chapter 7. The force or intensity starts light and increases as the patient is able to tolerate increased loads. For example, in an upper-extremity functional exercise such as a volleyball pass, the patient may begin without any equipment and concentrate on the technique. As the skill is acquired, a light medicine ball such as a 0.9 kg (2 lb) ball may be used, then, increasing to 1.8 kg (4 lb) and so on until the desired medicine ball weight is achieved.

Speed

Speed is the rate of a functional exercise. In the beginning, the speed is slower so that the patient can master correct execution of the exercise. As skill improves, the speed requirement increases. For example, an injured track athlete may begin running at half normal speed for a specific distance but then increase the speed as his or her ability to handle increased stresses improves. In an upper-extremity exercise such as throwing, the patient may begin throwing at one quarter to one half normal speed and increase the speed of the throw as technique improves.

Specific speeds for initial functional exercises are individually established and are determined by a variety of factors. These factors include the length of time the patient has been out of full participation, the severity of the injury, the individual's competitive level, pre-injury distances, motivation level, and goals for return to participation. As a rule of thumb, initial functional exercise speed may be one quarter to one half the normal or pre-injury speed and progress to three-quarter speed and then to full speed. This is a very general rule, however, and you must always take into consideration the individual patient's condition and abilities, as well as the demands of the exercise.

Distance

Distances for functional activities range from short to long. The greater the distance, the greater the requirements of the activity. In the lower extremity, increasing distance may include increasing the patient's running distance or jumping distance. In the upper extremity, it may include throwing or hitting a ball farther or swimming farther.

As in determining functional exercise speeds, one sets specific distances in initial functional exercises individually and according to the factors already discussed. A general guideline, though, not a fixed rule, is to start with no more than one quarter to one-half the pre-injury distance. Initial distance, however, may be significantly less for a patient such as a marathoner who has been out of competition for four months and had a pre-injury running distance of 16 km (10 miles) per workout, or for an outfielder who must throw a ball 55 m (180 ft). The rehabilitation clinician uses his or her best judgment and knowledge of healing and performance demands to determine the most appropriate distances for initial functional exercises. It is better to underestimate than to overestimate the patient's ability to withstand stresses. You can avoid aggravation of an injury when you underestimate but provoke it when you overestimate.

Complexity

Complexity of an exercise refers to how involved the activity is and how challenging it can be. Functional and activity-specific exercises progress from simple to complex. Each level of progression places more demands on the patient's ability and skill. For example, in the lower extremity, a jumping progression may begin with a simple standing jump activity and progress to multiple jumps-in-place, to a forward or backward jump, and to multiple forward or backward jumps. Upper-extremity functional exercises may begin with a simple activity such as bouncing a tennis ball into the air from the racket. From these functional activities, the patient can progress to an activity-specific activity such as a forehand stroke, to a backhand stroke, to a combination of backhand and forehand strokes against a backboard, and to a combination of backhand and forehand strokes with another player across a net.

You can also increase complexity by having the patient perform a simple functional exercise and then progress to performing a number of simple activities at one time. For example, a stork stand with eyes open becomes more complex when you have the patient catch a ground ball while stork standing. The progression continues when you have the patient catch the ground ball while stork standing on an uneven surface.

The rehabilitation clinician determines on an individual basis how complex the initial functional exercise should be and how quickly the complexity should increase and when progression occurs to activity-specific exercises. You must consider the factors already outlined and make the best judgment. Remember, it is always better to err on the side of caution when advancing the patient so that progression continues consistently forward, without regression.

Support

Support refers to the number of extremities that are bearing weight during the activity. In simple standing, support is bilateral; in a stork stand, support is unilateral. Unilateral stance is more difficult than bilateral stance. Jumping on one leg is a progression from performing the same activity on two legs. Throwing a ball with one hand overhead is more difficult than throwing a ball with two hands overhead; performing a push-up with one hand is more difficult than performing it with two hands.

Type of Exercise

The type of exercise is what determines whether the level of activity is basic or advanced. Once the exercise mimics a specific skill or is a component of a skill, it is an activity-specific exercise. The progression of activity-specific exercises follows the same principles as for other types of exercises. For example, a common functional exercise progression for an injured cross-country athlete may include walking on toes on a treadmill, carioca on a treadmill, and then a combination of walk-jog for time or distance on a treadmill. When goals for these activities are achieved, activity-specific exercises include running a mile at half speed, increasing distance or intensity until the patient has attained near-normal levels, and then increasing to three-quarter speed with the patient maintaining the previously achieved intensity and distance. Once normal speed and distance on level ground are achieved, hill work may proceed.

Early activity-specific activities are light so that the patient concentrates on the quality of performance. Once performance is accurate and appropriate, the difficulty of the activity increases. Goals move from performance accuracy to other parameters such as speed, intensity, distance, or other competition requirements.

Throughout the progression, the exercises should be difficult enough to challenge the patient without causing failure. For this reason, the judgment and evaluative skills of the rehabilitation clinician are crucial in the decisions about the nature and pace of the progression of functional exercises. As the patient nears the end of the therapeutic exercise regimen and realizes that return to full participation is near, he or she must have self-confidence in his or her performance ability, as well as confidence in the injured part, in order to be able to return to competition without hesitation or doubts. A progression of functional exercise to the final stages of activity-specific exercises must be severe enough to impose demands on the patient but simultaneously build the necessary self-assurance.

Some exercises in a treatment session may be at different demand levels than others. For example, one exercise may be at half-speed while another is at three-quarter force. The session may include a simple exercise and one that is much more complex. Selection of each exercise level is based on the individual's ability to execute each specific skill.

PRECAUTIONS

Activity-specific exercises are more complex, more challenging, and more rigorous than functional exercises. This is generally so because multiple planes of motion, more muscle groups, more complex and simultaneous movements, and more accuracy are required for correct execution. Because of the increased demands such activities impose, there are also precautions that one must respect in assigning advanced therapeutic exercises to a patient.

Each day you work with the patient, the goals for the session are presented to the patient. The exercises for that session are designed to achieve those goals. Do not move to skills that are more complex until the basic skills are relearned by the patient. If the patient performs skill patterns incorrectly, the patient must be corrected to avoid making an incorrect engram of poor skill execution. Movements and activities you design for the rehabilitation session should mimic the movement requirements of the patient's sport and position within the sport. The patient warms up prior to performing the activity-specific program you have outlined for the day. At the end of the day's session, it is advisable to provide the patient with your feedback regarding his or her performance and inform the patient of general expectations for the next treatment. If you want the patient to work on any specific technique or maneuver before your next session, be specific in your instructions as to intensity, frequency, duration, and expected outcomes of the home program.

Explain the Exercise to the Patient

Before executing the exercise, the patient is made aware of how to perform the exercise, what its goals are, and what positions or movements to avoid. For example, the clinician demonstrates or explains a single-leg stance on a trampoline by telling the patient that the eyes should remain open, the arms are kept at the sides, and the position should be maintained for 30 s. During execution, cues are provided to correct the patient's performance. The cues should be constructive and should include specific suggestions about how to improve the execution. Having the patient perform the exercise on the uninvolved extremity first may provide the individual with internal feedback of the correct performance. This is particularly helpful if the clinician tells the patient to note how the muscles feel when standing on the uninvolved leg and then attain the same feeling when standing on the injured leg. Instructing the patient to tighten the gluteal and thigh muscles may help to enhance stability.

Avoid Pain and Swelling

Residual pain and swelling, especially on the following day or evening, should be avoided. Any increase in pain or swelling indicates that the exercise level is too severe for the injured area. If this occurs, the patient returns to the previous level of exercise until the injured part is able to tolerate additional stress.

When a patient advances in a program, the clinician should observe for pain and edema and instruct the patient to report any symptoms.

Understand Tissue Integrity

The rehabilitation clinician must be aware of the healing sequence and the time necessary for tissue to complete the healing process. He or she must consider the tissue's structural integrity and understand the amount of stress involved in each specific functional exercise before including any functional activity in the therapeutic exercise program.

Know the Patient's Confidence Level

Performance of functional exercises requires the patient's confidence in his or her ability to perform the activity and in the ability of the injured part to tolerate the stress of the activity. If the patient is not prepared mentally or emotionally to handle a particular functional or activity-specific exercise, you will start with a less stressful, less complex activity that the person feels able to perform before advancing to more complex, more stressful exercises.

Be Aware of Progression Tolerance

Activity-specific exercises are introduced at lower-than-normal speed, intensity, and difficulty. Increases in parameters occur one at a time until the exercise is equivalent to functional performance levels. The body must be allowed to adapt to increased levels of exercises before each change is are made. This will ensure that the patient's confidence increases and that tissue overload is not excessive, thereby preventing additional injury.

FINAL EVALUATION

Evaluation is an ongoing process. Throughout the therapeutic exercise program the rehabilitation clinician evaluates the patient's ability to perform both functional and activity-specific exercises. Advances in the program take place only after the patient is able to successfully perform to expected levels at each evaluation step. With the stork stand, for example, the patient does not progress until he or she is able to stork stand with eyes open for 30 s. Only after the patient passes that evaluation does the next phase of balance proceed. Then the patient may

Since activity-specific activities increasingly challenge the patient's skills, it is important to observe several important precautions within this part of the rehabilitation program. The patient must understand the exercise; the rehabilitation clinician must be aware of the patient's healing process and of his or her confidence and tolerance levels.

stork stand on an uneven surface or on the ground with eyes closed. The specific exercise used next depends on the demands of the patient's activity.

The final evaluation occurs before the patient returns to full participation. The patient's performance in the evaluation determines his or her readiness to return to normal and full participation. Final examination includes highly specific drills and tests the person's performance skill. These tests should be as objective as possible and mimic the individual's sport or work as much as possible. For a gymnast, the examination may include dismounts, tumbling skills, or apparatus skills. For a basketball player, the examination includes dribbling, shooting, cutting, or passing drills. For a warehouse worker, the examination includes lifting specific weighted objects and moving them within a specified distance using proper body mechanics and safety techniques. Because specific activities vary greatly from job to job or sport to sport and positions within a sport, you must be familiar with the specific requirements for the patient. You may need to obtain the supervisor or coach's help in defining functional exercises and tests for some specific activities. It is the goal of the final examination, however, to demonstrate to the patient, the medical team, and the supervisor or coach that the individual is able and ready to withstand the stresses of full participation.

The tests for determining readiness to return to full participation must fulfill certain criteria, some of which have been previously mentioned. One criterion is that the examination tool should be as objective as possible. The tests should be repeatable so that they can be used both in initial examination and in final examination to measure changes and assess whether or not the patient has achieved the appropriate goals. The tests should provide useful information to the patient and medical team about the progress and status of the patient's performance. They should also be able to show whether the exercise program is providing the advancement of parameters necessary for return to participation.

In the final examination, your observation and assessment of the patient's performance is critical. All activities are performed without hesitation, and the use of each extremity should be appropriate, without favoring of the injured limb. The patient moves quickly, stabilizes appropriately, and demonstrates self-confidence with all maneuvers. Based on the patient's performance, you should be unable to identify which extremity has been injured.

Step-by-step evaluation determines when the patient should advance to the next stage in the functional and activity-specific exercise program. The final evaluation, whose purpose is to determine whether the patient is ready to return to sport participation, is highly individualized.

A LOWER-EXTREMITY FUNCTIONAL AND ACTIVITY-SPECIFIC PROGRESSION

This section presents functional and activity-specific exercises for the lower extremity and then describes testing that could be included as part of the assessment before the patient is allowed to return to unrestricted activity.

Functional Exercises

Any functional exercise should be preceded by a simple warm-up activity. Simple functional exercises for the lower extremity can begin relatively early with a non-weight bearing exercise such as proprioceptive neuromuscular facilitation. Partial weight bearing use of the BAPS board can also begin early in the therapeutic exercise program. As the patient becomes weight bearing, he or she can start to do the single-leg stance, first with eyes open and then with eyes closed. This activity can progress from the floor to a BAPS board (figure 10.1), trampoline, 1/2 foam roller, or balance board (figure 10.2) and then to combining the balance activity with another activity such as ball catching. Single-leg stance activities will then progress to dynamic movement activities such as lunges, step-ups, and step-downs. Treadmill activities such as cariocas, backward walking, or sideways walking are also functional activities. Plyometric exercises such as jumping, hopping, and bounding exercises can be used in advance of activity-specific exercises.

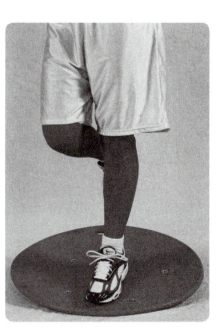

▶ **Figure 10.1** BAPS board.

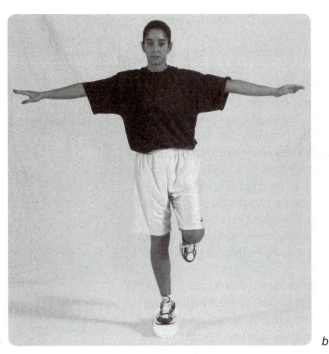
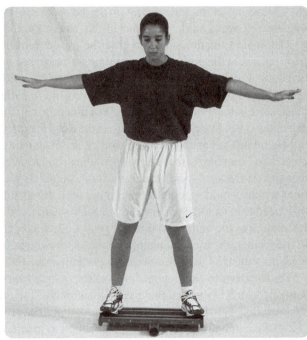

▶ **Figure 10.2** Balance activities: *(a)* stork stand on 1/2 foam roller, *(b)* balance board. It is best to leave the arms at the side, rather than extend them, while holding the positions.

Activity-Specific Exercises

Walking, walking combined with jogging, and jogging without walking intervals are included in activity-specific exercises. From jogging, the patient progresses to running. Running activities begin with a forward jog on a flat surface, progress to increased speed and distances, and then move on to lateral runs and cuts and sudden changes in direction. In figure 10.3a, the patient pushes forward from the left foot to the right foot and then moves laterally to the left foot before retracing the steps to the starting position, moving from one position to the next

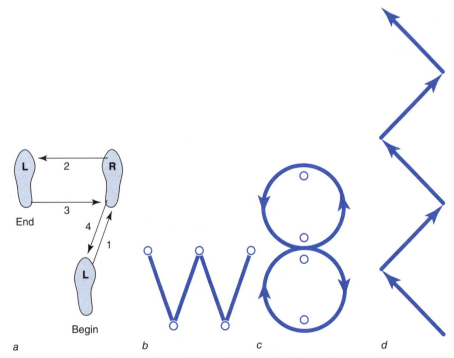

▶ **Figure 10.3** Agility drills: *(a)* 90° lunge, *(b)* W-sprint course, *(c)* figure-8 course, *(d)* Z-course (zigzag).

as quickly as possible. Figure 10.3b shows W-sprints requiring the patient to sprint forward to the first marked spot or cone, then backpedal to the second marker, and then sprint forward to the next, repeating the series as illustrated to completion of the exercise. These could be used for basketball players. Figure 10.3c shows a figure-8 run, which uses markers or cones around which the patient runs in a figure-8 pattern. These could be used for a soccer player. The exercise in figure 10.3d is similar to the W-sprint except that the patient runs straight ahead, pivots on the right outside leg to cut sharply to the left, runs straight ahead for a designated distance, and pivots on the left outside leg to cut sharply to the right until the end of the course. These could be used for lacrosse players. Each of these exercises can become more difficult if you require either a faster pace or smaller distances between the sudden motion changes.

Figure 10.4 shows examples of jumping exercises that can be used for basketball, soccer goalies, baseball players, volleyball frontline players, or football receivers. In the jumping exercise in figure 10.4a, the patient faces a platform, places one foot on top of the platform, and then jumps as high as possible, switching foot placement so that the opposite foot ends up on the platform. This is a continuous and rapid jump-and-switch maneuver for a specified time or number of repetitions. A lateral jump is displayed in figure 10.4b; here the patient jumps from side to side over a dowel, ball, or other object, attempting to stay within the cones. Difficulty can be increased by spreading the outside cones and having the patient jump over the ball and toward the cones, or by placing a number of balls and cones in a line and having the person perform a series of lateral jumps in both directions.

A progression of jumping activities includes starting with jumping forward on a flat surface, then progressing to jumping backward and jumping laterally, first with both legs and then with only the involved leg. Jumping then can progress to box jumps, starting with low boxes and advancing to higher ones. Progressions for these lower-extremity and running activities are presented in figures 10.5 and 10.6.

Specific exercises are determined by the patient's activity demands. As much as possible, running and jumping exercises should mimic the activities that the patient will be performing once he or she returns to full participation.

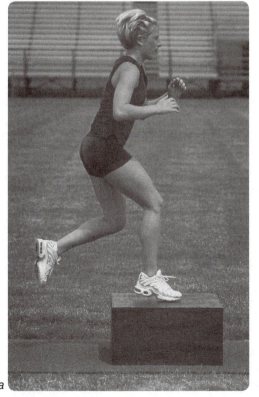
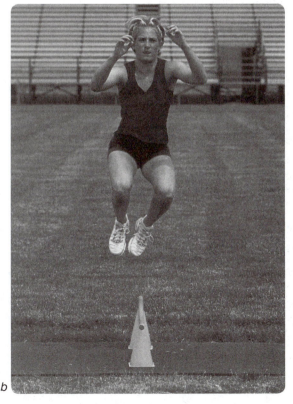

a   *b*

▶ **Figure 10.4** Agility drills: jumping.

BALANCE AND AGILITY PROGRESSION PROGRAM

1. **Beginning level**

   a. Double-weight support for balance: static

   1) Stand with eyes closed, feet together, 30 s
   2) Stand in tandem-stance position, 30 s each
      - eyes open
      - eyes closed

   b. Single-weight support for balance: static

   1) Stork stand with eyes open, 30 s
   2) Stork stand with eyes closed, 30 s
   3) Stork stand with eyes open on unstable surface, 30 s each
      - trampoline
      - 1/2 foam roller
   4) Stork stand with eyes closed on unstable surface, 30 s each
      - trampoline
      - 1/2 foam roller
   5) Stork stand with complex activity
      - Stork stand on ground while playing catch
        – sport ball
        – medicine ball
      - Stork stand on uneven surface while playing catch
        – sport ball
        – medicine ball

2. **Intermediate level: dynamic activities**

   a. Two-leg support: balance board, wobble board
   b. One-leg support: trampoline jumping
   c. One-leg support: hopping
   d. Treadmill retrowalking
   e. BAPS board
   f. Fitter
   g. Step-up exercises

3. **Advanced level**

   a. Running activities (start at reduced speeds and distances, and progressively advance to normal speeds and distances)

   b. Jumping activities (bilateral support)
   1) Lateral jumping
   2) Forward-backward jumping
   3) Command jumping

   c. Hopping activities (unilateral support)
   1) Lateral hopping
   2) Forward-backward hopping
   3) Command hopping

   d. Cariocas

   e. Plyometric box jumping

4. **Pre-injury level**

   a. Sport-specific running, jumping, cutting activities at full speed
   b. Normal sport-specific drills
   c. Resumption of sport participation
   d. Mimic work activities (start at low reps, advance to more reps or more time)

Note: Jumping and hopping activities may start as exercises performed in place, but then can progress to line, target, and zigzag jumping and hopping exercises.

▶ **Figure 10.5** Example of a balance and agility progression program.

LOWER-EXTREMITY FUNCTIONAL EXERCISE PROGRESSION

1. **Non-weight-bearing exercises**
   a. Proprioceptive neuromuscular facilitation
   b. Joint reposition sense activities

2. **Partial weight-bearing exercises**
   a. Aquatic exercises
   b. BAPS board
   c. Stationary bike

3. **Full weight-bearing exercises**
   a. Lunges
      - partial depth
      - full depth (90°)
   b. Running
      - running on level surface 50% maximum speed, 1/4 normal distance
      - running on level surface 75% maximum speed, 1/4 normal distance
      - running on level surface 100% maximum speed, 1/4 normal distance
      - running on level surface 100% maximum speed, 1/2 normal distance
      - running on level surface 100% maximum speed, full normal distance
      - running on incline surface 75% maximum speed, 1/2 normal distance
      - running on incline surface 75% maximum speed, 3/4 normal distance
      - running on incline surface 75% maximum speed, full normal distance
      - running on incline surface 100% maximum speed, full normal distance
   c. Sprinting
      - sprinting on level surface 50% maximum speed, 1/4 normal distance
      - sprinting on level surface 75% maximum speed, 1/4 normal distance
      - sprinting on level surface 100% maximum speed, 1/4 normal distance
      - sprinting on level surface 100% maximum speed, 1/2 normal distance
      - sprinting on level surface 100% maximum speed, 3/4 normal distance
      - sprinting on level surface 100% maximum speed, normal distance
   d. Jumping/Hopping
      - jumping rope, both feet
      - jumping rope, one foot
      - jumping lines, both feet forward, backward
      - jumping lines, one foot forward, backward
      - jumping lines, both feet zigzag forward, backward
      - jumping lines, one foot, zigzag forward, backward
      - box jumps, 6-in. boxes, two feet, forward
      - box jumps, 6-in. boxes, two feet, sideways
      - box jumps, 6-in. boxes, one foot, forward
      - box jumps, 6-in. boxes, one foot, sideways
      - box jumps of increasing heights with sequences above repeated
   e. Agility
      - cariocas, 50% speed, both to left and to right
      - cariocas, 75% speed, both to left and to right
      - cariocas, 100% speed, both to left and to right
      - circle-8s with same sequence as cariocas, starting with large circles and reducing the size to tight circles
      - zigzag sprints with same sequence as cariocas
      - command drills with sudden changes in direction of any agility exercise on command

Note: Any of these exercises can be made more difficult by increasing distance or number of sets, or using weights with the exercise.

▶ **Figure 10.6** Example of a lower-extremity exercise progression.

A progression for lower-extremity function may begin with non-weight-bearing exercise and proceed to stork-standing exercises, dynamic movement activities such as lunges, and activity-specific activities such as jogging and running activities. Lower-extremity testing reflects the patient's sport activity as much as possible and should be as objective as possible.

Final Testing

Several different tests for lower-extremity function can be used. The tests chosen should reflect the patient's sport activities as accurately as possible and should be as objective as possible. To measure gains in performance, you should use the same test to evaluate performance at the time the patient begins the functional exercise and before he or she returns to full activity.

Lower-extremity tests can be classified as running tests for time and distance, jumping tests for height and distance, and agility tests. The running tests can be sprints or can be timed long-distance runs, depending on participation demands.

Jumping tests can include a standing vertical jump, a step-and-jump, a repeated jump for distance, and a single jump for distance. A volleyball player's jump test is more functional if it is either a standing or a step-and-jump test, whereas a field athlete's test is more functional if it is a multiple or run-and-jump-for-distance test.

Agility tests use cariocas, zigzag runs, figure-8 runs, shuttle runs, and box runs, to name a few. Whatever activities are selected, the distances, angles, and sizes of the turns and circles should be the same on the pretest as on the posttest for accurate comparisons. Goals should also be predetermined. The specifics of these goals may be defined either with reference to established norms or by the athlete's pre-injury performance ability.

AN UPPER-EXTREMITY FUNCTIONAL AND ACTIVITY-SPECIFIC PROGRESSION

As in the discussion of the exercise program for the lower extremity, this section describes functional exercises and functional assessment for the upper extremity.

Functional Exercise

Like lower-extremity functional work, upper-extremity functional exercises may begin early in the program with proprioceptive neuromuscular facilitation (figure 10.7). Partial weight-bearing activities on a Swiss ball can sometimes be used early in the program as well. Closed

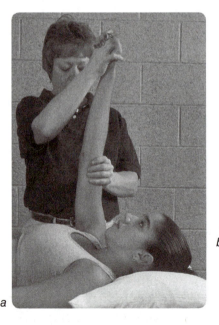

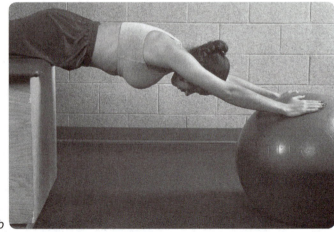

▶ **Figure 10.7** Functional exercise progression for the upper extremity: *(a)* open kinetic chain, *(b)* closed kinetic chain.

kinetic chain activities such as weight-bearing exercises, first on a stable surface and then on an unstable surface, can be used once full weight bearing is permissible. A patient in a push-up position with hands on a BAPS board or wobble board is an example of a closed kinetic chain activity on an unstable surface. Both hands are on the board while the patient moves the board. In a push-up position, the patient can start with two arms and advance to one, while the hands move side to side by bouncing. In another example with the patient in a push-up position, the patient moves the Fitter platform side to side. All push-up positions can progress from a modified push-up position on hands and knees to a full push-up position on hands and feet. The patient must attain scapular muscle strength, rotator cuff strength, and large shoulder muscle and other upper extremity strength gains, along with proper range of motion, before beginning more complex functional exercises.

Complex functional exercises for the upper extremity may include a variety of shoulder, elbow, or wrist and hand activities, depending on the sport demands to which the patient will return and his or her functional deficiencies. Examples of these types of activities include PNF-pattern movements using rubber tubing, throwing a rolled sock at a mirror to watch for follow-through motion, bouncing a ball between the legs and around the back, lying prone on a roller stool and using the arms to propel the stool, or juggling. As with lower extremity functional exercises, the upper extremity exercises involve multiple joints and planes of movement and require the individual to perform complex activities in preparation for advancement to activity-specific exercises.

Activity-Specific Exercise

Having achieved proper stabilization, strength, range of motion, and control, the patient progresses to specific exercises required for competitive shot putting, javelin throwing, golf, tennis, or swimming. A progression of throwing begins with shortened distances for reduced speed and with power throwing at reduced repetitions. Early activity-specific sessions emphasize correct technique and advance to increased sport demands once the skill is retrieved. These parameters include progressive increases in distances, numbers of throws, and severity of throws. See figure 10.8 for an example of a throwing progression program.

A golf progression may begin with the putter and short irons for putting and chipping activities and progress to longer irons, fuller swings, and then to the woods with a full swing. For each club the swing begins as a partial swing and increases to a full swing as the patient gains progressive control of the club. Repetitions also increase as the patient's endurance improves. See figure 10.9 for an example of a golf progression program.

We have already briefly looked at a progression of tennis exercises. A simple stabilization exercise such as bouncing the ball on the floor with the racket can begin once the scapular stabilizers and rotator cuff are able to maintain proper control. This activity advances to bouncing the ball in the air with the racket. More advanced exercises progress from a forehand to a backhand to overhead and serve strokes. See figure 10.10 for a general outline of a progression.

A swimmer's progression may begin with the use of a stroke for a short distance or with alternating strokes for short distances and performing the stroke for no more than half normal speed. Distances and speed increase as tolerated. See if you can develop an example of a swimmer's progression program using these guidelines.

I want to emphasize that the progressive functional and activity-specific exercise programs presented here are only examples. Specific programs vary depending on the patient's needs, abilities, level of competition, length of time away from the activity, and degree of injury. The programs described in this chapter offer only general guidelines and are a means of demonstrating how to progress and change parameters of functional and activity-specific exercise programs.

SPORT-SPECIFIC BASEBALL/SOFTBALL PITCHING/ THROWING PROGRESSION PROGRAM

1. **Beginning level**
   a. 40-45 ft distance
      50% normal speed
      30 throws, 2 sets
   b. 40-45 ft distance
      50% normal speed
      30 throws, 4 sets
   c. 40-45 ft distance
      75% normal speed
      30 throws, 3 sets
   d. 40-45 ft distance
      75% normal speed
      30 throws, 5 sets
   e. 60 ft distance
      75% normal speed
      30 throws, 3-4 sets
   f. 60 ft distance
      75% normal speed
      30 throws, 5 sets

2. **Intermediate level**
   a. 60 ft distance
      100% normal speed
      30 throws, 3-4 sets
   b. 100 ft distance
      75% normal speed
      30 throws, 3-4 sets
   c. 100 ft distance
      75% normal speed
      30 throws, 5 sets
   d. 100 ft distance
      100% normal speed
      30 throws, 3-4 sets
   e. 100 ft distance
      100% normal speed
      30 throws, 5 sets

   f. 150 ft distance
      75% normal speed
      30 throws, 3-4 sets
   g. 150 ft distance
      75% normal speed
      30 throws, 5 sets
   h. 150 ft distance
      100% normal speed
      30 throws, 5 sets

3. **Advanced level**
   a. 180 ft distance
      75% normal speed
      30 throws, 3 sets
   b. 180 ft distance
      75% normal speed
      30 throws, 5 sets
   c. 180 ft distance
      100% normal speed
      30 throws, 3 sets
   d. 180 ft distance
      100% normal speed
      30 throws, 5 sets

4. **Precompetition level**
   a. Throw off mound
      100% normal speed
      30 throws, 3-4 sets
   b. Throw off mound
      100% normal speed
      30 throws, 5 sets

Note: All throwing sessions begin with a warm-up and end with a cool-down. Warm-up and cool-down throws are performed as light, arcing tosses. A rest of 3 to 5 min between sets is allowed. If the patient experiences pain with an increase to the next level, he or she should return to the previous level for another session. If the patient is not a pitcher, throwing progression follows the same routine as listed, but the distances vary according to the sport (e.g., discus, javelin, football) and are determined by the distances and weights used within the sport.

▶ **Figure 10.8** Example of a baseball or softball pitching/throwing progression program.

SPORT-SPECIFIC GOLF PROGRESSION PROGRAM

1. **Beginning level**
   a. Putts and chips
      20 putts, varying distances
      10 chips
   b. Putts and chips
      20 putts, varying distances
      20 chips
   c. Putts and chips
      20 putts, 3 sets
      20 chips, 2 sets
   d. Putts and chips
      20 putts, 3 sets
      20 chips, 3 sets

2. **Intermediate level**
   a. Short irons, no more than three clubs
      partial swing, 1 × 20 each
   b. Short irons, no more than three clubs
      partial swing, 2 × 20 each
   c. Short irons, no more than three clubs
      partial swing, 3 × 20 each
   d. Short irons, no more than two clubs
      full swing, 1 × 20 each
   e. Short irons, no more than two clubs
      full swing, 2 × 20 each

   f. Short irons, no more than two clubs
      full swing, 3 × 20 each
   g. Long irons, no more than three clubs
      partial swing, 1 × 20 each
   h. Long irons, no more than three clubs
      partial swing, 2 × 20 each
   i. Long irons, no more than three clubs
      full swing, 2 × 20 each
   j. Long irons
      full swing, 3 × 25 each
   k. All irons
      full swing, 1 × 20 each

3. **Advanced level**
   a. Woods
      partial swing, 2 × 20 each
   b. Woods
      full swing, 2 × 20 each
   c. Woods and irons
      full swing, 1 × 20–25 each

4. **Preparticipation level**
   a. Par-three course
   b. Nine-hole course
   c. Return to regular play

Note: All sessions begin with a warm-up and end with a cool-down. A rest of 3 to 5 min between sets is allowed. If the patient experiences pain with an increase to the next level, he or she should return to the previous level for another session.

▶ **Figure 10.9** Example of a golf progression program.

Final Testing

It is more difficult to examine the upper extremity and obtain objective and measurable criteria than for the lower extremity. This is because of the variety of uses of the upper extremity in activities. If a speed gun is available, it is relatively simple to measure the speed of a patient's throw. However, if you do not have a speed gun or the patient's activity does not involve throwing, measuring skill objectively is more difficult.

Final goals are individually determined and based on the patient's pre-injury performance. For a golfer, it may be his or her score on 18 holes of golf. For the swimmer, it may be the ability to perform a specific swim event within the same time he or she had in pre-injury performances. For the tennis player, measurement using a speed gun for a serve is simple, but evaluating participation performance may be more difficult. Establishing goals such as hitting a specific target across the net on a given number of consecutive forehand and backhand shots, and using that number for pretest and posttest performance guidelines, may be a way of establishing an objective measure. When establishing any goal in this manner, it is important for you to consult with the supervisor or coach to arrive at realistic and achievable goals.

As with lower-extremity exercises, upper-extremity activities should resemble the activities of the patient's sport. Final testing for the upper extremity varies greatly because use of the upper body differs markedly from one sport to another.

SPORT-SPECIFIC TENNIS PROGRESSION PROGRAM

1. **Ball bounce**

   Bounce the tennis ball on the racket into the air. Start by grasping the racket on the neck and advance to the handle.

   a. 50 bounces with a palm-down grip
   b. 50 bounces with a palm-up grip
   c. 50 bounces alternating between palm down and palm up

2. **Forehand strokes**

   Forehand strokes only against a backboard or wall

   a. 50% power: 5 × 10
   b. 75% power: 3 × 20
   c. 100% power: 3 × 40

3. **Backhand strokes**

   Backhand strokes only against a backboard or wall

   a. 50% power: 5 × 10
   b. 75% power: 3 × 20
   c. 100% power: 3 × 40

4. **Alternate strokes**

   Alternate between backhand and forehand strokes against a wall or backboard

   a. 75% power: 5 × 15
   b. 100% power: 3 × 30
   c. 100% power: 4 × 40

5. **Overhead serve**

   Overhead serve against a wall or backboard

   a. 50% power: 5 × 10
   b. 75% power: 3 × 20
   c. 100% power: 3 × 40

6. **Game**

   a. Play one set of tennis
   b. Play two sets of tennis
   c. Play three sets of tennis
   d. Play full match of tennis

Note: All sessions begin with a warm-up and end with a cool-down. The patient should attempt to hit a specific target or targets on the backboard or wall. If the patient experiences pain with advancement to the next level, he or she should return to the previous level for the next 2 to 3 sessions before returning to the higher level.

▶ **Figure 10.10** Example of a tennis progression program.

RETURNING THE PATIENT TO FULL PARTICIPATION

Once the therapeutic exercise program, including activity-specific exercises, has been completed and the patient is ready to return to full participation, specific criteria must be fulfilled before the individual is actually allowed to return. The entire therapeutic exercise program has been designed and administered by the rehabilitation clinician for this very goal. The true test of the success of the program comes with the patient's return to his or her performance level.

In order for that to happen, the patient must meet four specific criteria:

1. The acute signs and symptoms of the injury have resolved, and no pain or edema is present.
2. The patient is able to demonstrate full range of motion; normal strength, muscle endurance, and cardiovascular endurance; and appropriate proprioception, agility, and coordination in relation to the required performance skills.
3. The patient is able to perform all activities at least as well as he or she could before the injury. As has been mentioned, you should be unable to identify the area that has been injured if the patient is performing the activities appropriately.
4. The patient has the confidence in both his or her own ability and the ability of the injured area to perform, without any hesitation or doubt, or any modification of performance or mechanics.

If these criteria are met and the patient is able to pass all tests, the rehabilitation clinician has accomplished the goals established at the start of the therapeutic exercise program.

Four criteria are used to determine that the patient has completed the rehabilitation program and is ready to return to sport participation. These relate to the status of the injury itself and to patient's functional levels, activity-specific skills, and degree of confidence.

SUMMARY

There is a difference between functional and activity-specific exercise. Functional exercises are those that precede activity-specific activities in a rehabilitation program. They commonly involve multi-planar activities and provide greater stresses and demands than strength exercises. They may include precursor activities to activity-specific exercises, such as walking prior to running or underhand tossing prior to throwing. They prepare patients for the more advanced skill demands they will experience in their specific activities. Activity-specific exercises include drills utilized for a specific sport or specific tasks performed within a job. Functional activities prepare the patient for specific activities to be performed in the activity-specific portion of the rehabilitation program. The clinician must understand the physical requirements of both functional and activity-specific tasks and be able to relate them to the specific demands the patient will face when he or she returns to normal activities. Whether the patient is a basketball player or a steel mill worker, a soccer player or a computer analyst, a tennis player or a plumber, the clinician must understand the elements and skills that are required to perform the specific tasks so they can be appropriately integrated into the rehabilitation program.

KEY CONCEPTS AND REVIEW

1. Explain the difference between functional exercises and activity-specific exercises.

Functional exercises are used in a therapeutic exercise program from its early stages to its final stages. Functional exercises are activities that precede activity-specific exercises in a rehabilitation program. They commonly involve multi-planar activities and provide increased stresses and demands greater than strength exercises to prepare the patient for more advanced skill activities. In later rehabilitation stages, activity-specific exercises advance the patient to the final activities, those that mimic normal activity. Final testing uses activities or drills that are specific to the patient's sport or work demands and activities to mimic the maneuvers and movements that will be required when the patient returns to full participation. This testing assesses whether the patient is ready to resume normal activities.

2. Identify the contributions of functional exercise and activity-specific exercise to a therapeutic exercise program.

Both exercises are used to ready the patient physically for the stress and demands of his or her activity and to prepare the patient mentally. The effects of successful execution of functional and activity-specific activities come through the patient's discovery that the injured segment is able to withstand normal stresses.

3. Discuss the differences between basic and advanced functional activities.

Basic exercises begin early in the therapeutic exercise program to assist in achieving flexibility, strength, endurance, and proprioception. Advanced exercises, however, include more complex functional performance exercises that prepare the patient for activity-specific exercises. More complex functional activities are usually tri-planar in nature.

4. List factors that can be varied in a progression of functional activities.

Functional exercises proceed from slow to fast, simple to complex, low force to high force, short distance to long distance, and bilateral support to unilateral support. A progression of functional exercises includes a steady change to allow for SAID principle advancement. Functional exercises include some characteristics unique to functional exercises and some characteristics common to most exercises.

5. Identify precautions for functional and activity-specific exercises.

Some precautions are those discussed in prior chapters and include explaining the exercise to the patient, avoiding pain and swelling, considering tissue integrity when designing exercises, knowing the patient's confidence level, and being aware of the patient's progression tolerance.

6. Outline a sample of functional to activity-specific progression for either the lower or upper extremity.

The specific progression and selection of exercises depend on the patient's specific task demands, especially as he or she nears the final stages of the program. A lower-extremity program may include a progression from non-weight-bearing use of the BAPS board that can start early in the therapeutic exercise program. As the patient becomes weight bearing, stork standing first with eyes open and then with eyes closed can begin. A progression of this activity can go from using the floor to using either a trampoline or a 1/2 foam roller or balance board to combining the activity with another activity such as ball catching. Stork-standing activities can then progress to dynamic movement activities such as lunges, step-ups and step-downs, walking, and jogging. Running activities begin with a forward jog on a flat surface, proceed to increased speed and distances, and then to lateral runs and cuts and sudden changes in direction.

CRITICAL THINKING QUESTIONS

1. On the basis of the scenario at the beginning of this chapter, what would you do to improve Christian's confidence in his tennis abilities? What activities would you have him do on the first day of his functional program? List three levels of progression and give your criteria for advancement. When would you have him start overhead activities and serves?

2. When would you decide that Christian is able to return to full participation? What would your criteria be for this, and why have you set these criteria?

3. A volleyball player who injured his knee and has completed the rehabilitation program up to the activity-specific exercises level is very anxious to return to full sport participation. You estimate that it will be another week before he has successfully completed the activity-specific exercises portion of the program. What will your first day's activities include, and how will you establish a progression of activities? What are your criteria for each level of progression? What specific activities must he be able to perform before he may resume full volleyball participation?

4. A cross-country competitor is now ready for activity-specific exercises. She has been running short distances of no more than 2 min without difficulty. What distance, speed, and terrain progression will you give her over the course of the next two weeks? Write up a two-week progression of functional activities that will move her to full sport participation.

LAB ACTIVITIES

1. Design a functional upper-extremity program of five exercises for your patient who is a computer programmer. Identify the goals for each activity, have her perform the activity, and score the performance. Explain your scoring criteria and report your lab partner's score. Identify how you would know when to progress from one exercise to the next exercise.

2. Design a sport-specific upper-extremity program for your lab partner who is a baseball outfielder. Identify the goals for each activity, have him perform the activity, and score the performance. Explain your scoring criteria and report his or her score. Identify how you would know when to progress from one exercise to the next exercise. How does this program differ from the one you set up for the computer programmer? Why?

3. Design a functional lower-extremity program for your partner who is a volleyball player. Identify the goals for each activity, have her perform the activity, and score the performance. Explain your scoring criteria and report your partner's score. Identify how you would know when to progress from one exercise to the next exercise.

4. Design a sport-specific lower-extremity program for your lab partner who is a 4 × 400 m relay runner. Identify the goals for each activity, have him perform the activity, and score the performance. Explain your scoring criteria and report his score. Identify how you would know when to progress from one exercise to the next exercise. How does this program differ from the one you set up for the volleyball athlete? Why?

5. You are in the final phase of a rehabilitation program for a basketball forward who is recovering from a lateral ankle sprain. Design a progressive functional and sport-specific exercise program in preparation for return to play. Have your partner perform each exercise you include in the program to see if you have provided a progression of the exercises, moving from the easiest to the most difficult. Assuming no delays or backward steps in ability to perform the exercises, outline how you would progress her in the program and what criteria you would use to determine when to progress.

ADDITIONAL SOURCES

Cordova, M.L., and C.W. Armstrong. 1996. Reliability of ground reaction forces during a vertical jump: Implications for functional strength assessment. *Journal of Athletic Training* 31:342–345.

Kegerreis, S. 1983. The construction and implementation of functional progressions as a component of athletic rehabilitation. *Journal of Orthopedic and Sports Physical Therapy* 5:14–19.

Kegerreis, S., Malone, T., and J. McCarroll. 1984. Functional progressions: An aid to athletic rehabilitation. *Physician and Sportsmedicine* 12:67–71.

Kegerreis, S., and T. Wetherald. 1987. The utilization of functional progressions in the rehabilitation of injured wrestlers. *Athletic Training* 22:32–35.

Keskula, D.R., Duncan, J.B., Davis, V.L., and P.W. Finley. 1996. Functional outcome measures for knee dysfunction assessment. *Journal of Athletic Training* 31:105–110.

Lephart, S.M., Perrin, D.H., Fu, F.H., and K. Minger. 1991. Functional performance tests for the anterior cruciate ligament insufficient athlete. *Athletic Training* 26:44–50.

Tippett, S.R., and M.L. Voight. 1995. *Functional progressions for sports rehabilitation.* Champaign, IL: Human Kinetics.

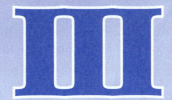
General Therapeutic Exercise Applications

If you nurture your mind, body, and spirit, your time will expand.
You will gain a new perspective that will allow you to accomplish much more.

BRIAN KOSLOW, author

As you progress through this text, you should continue to grow in your knowledge of therapeutic exercise and your appreciation of the complexity, expanse, and intricacy of the information that a rehabilitation clinician must possess. In reading part I, you obtained information vital to understanding the material in part II. Now that you have a basic knowledge of the physical and physiological concepts that underlie the principles of therapeutic exercise, we can investigate some general applications of this information.

Part III deals with general concepts that are important in themselves but also serve as the final foundational elements for part IV. Part III presents information on topics such as posture, body mechanics, and ambulation with and without aids. It also presents information on therapeutic

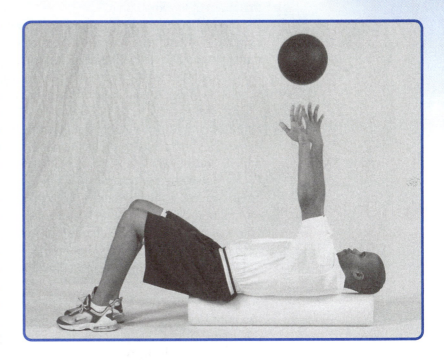

exercise techniques and applications that can be used with many different injuries and for most body segments. Part III also includes chapters that contain multi-segment conditions or problems that must be considered, regardless of the body segment affected.

Two new chapters in this category include chapter 16 on joint replacement and chapter 17 on age and how it impacts therapeutic exercise programs. This last group of chapters includes information on injuries or conditions that affect more than one joint. For this reason, they are included in part III rather than in part IV where specific body segments are addressed. Instead of needlessly repeating information from one chapter to the next in part IV, these conditions are addressed in part III and approached from a pathology and treatment perspective rather than a body segment perspective.

Chapter 11 presents information about posture and body mechanics. It is common to find that posture abnormalities, the ways that people use the body in physical activity, and muscle imbalances are key to an injury or are the reason an injury does not respond readily to treatment. Learning about posture, body mechanics, and body awareness will help you become more knowledgeable about often-undetected sources of injury.

Chapter 12 presents an overview of normal walking and running. This is followed by information on ambulation with assistive devices and correct methods of using the devices. You will also read about how to instruct the patient in the correct use of assistive devices, a critical topic for ambulation safety.

The next two chapters include information on commonly incorporated therapeutic programs using aquatics and aquatic equipment (**chapter 13**) and foam rollers and Swiss balls (**chapter 14**). Increasingly, therapeutic exercises include these items, so they are included as part of the total picture of therapeutic exercise.

Chapter 15 deals with therapeutic exercise for tendinopathy. Tendinopathy can affect several different regions of the body. Although it would have been possible to discuss tendinopathy in part IV, which covers therapeutic exercise of specific body parts, I have chosen to devote a separate chapter to tendinopathy. Tendinopathy is a complex problem that can nag a patient for an extended time and delay resumption of full activity. Specific techniques and procedures can alleviate the problem. Considering the uniqueness of tendinopathy in comparison to acute athletic injuries, I have given special attention to relevant principles, concepts, and precautions and to recent developments in the treatment of tendinopathy.

Since joint replacement surgeries are occurring more often in younger individuals, **chapter 16** identifies the recent evidence regarding rehabilitation following total joint replacement. Longer-lasting artificial joints and patients prematurely suffering degenerative joint disease are factors that are moving surgeons to opt with joint replacement surgery as the treatment of young athletes.

The final chapter in part III, **chapter 17**, identifies the concerns regarding rehabilitation of patients in different age groups. As individuals begin sports participation at earlier ages and adults continue their activity participation well beyond retirement years, athletic trainers are seeing a wide range of age groups in their athletic training clinics. Each group has its own unique characteristics that may affect rehabilitation. These issues are presented in the chapter. As with the tendinopathy information in chapter 15, the information from this chapter could have been inserted into the chapters in part IV, but I have provided a separate chapter for the age topic since much of it would be repetitious if placed in the part IV chapters.

Once you have completed part III, the remaining section, part IV, should simply be a matter of putting all the information gathered from parts I, II, and III together to create your own therapeutic exercise program. As you proceed through part III, continue to use your deductive reasoning skills, the knowledge that you have acquired from the previous chapters, and your common sense to see if you can anticipate the information presented in each chapter of part III. Although some of the material will be new, much of it is based on what you have already learned.

Posture and Body Mechanics

▶ Dan Maki is the certified athletic trainer who was hired by the local furniture-manufacturing company to rehabilitate the company's injured employees. Dan has provided the employees with in-service training on proper lifting mechanics, and injuries have decreased as a result. Nonetheless, some injuries still occur.

His most recent patient, Dee, is about to begin functional activities before returning to her workstation at full duty. Dee injured her back about three weeks ago when she lifted a box incorrectly. At the time of the initial examination, Dan noticed that Dee's posture in both sitting and standing was poor, so he corrected her posture very early in the program. The postural changes that Dee has made have improved her condition considerably. Dan wants to be sure that another injury does not occur, so he will instruct Dee on how to lift properly before allowing her to return to full duty.

> *Great and noble are those scientific judgments*
> *that preserve the health and lives of their creatures.*
>
> MOSHE BEN MAIMON (MAIMONIDES), Rabbi, physician, and author, 1135-1204

This chapter opens the door on the topic of posture and body mechanics. Now that you have become familiar with basic concepts and therapeutic exercise program parameters, it is time to see how they can be applied. Part III begins with this chapter on posture and body mechanics because these factors affect performance and risk of injury. If you are to improve an individual's posture or body mechanics, you must first identify what is normal. This chapter deals with normal standing and sitting posture, common causes and effects of pathological posture, and correct body mechanics. Body mechanics, as discussed here, relates to daily activities, sport activities, and activities that you as a rehabilitation clinician perform during your treatment sessions with patients. Two of the more commonly used body-awareness techniques are also introduced. Pilates exercises are introduced in this chapter since Pilates deals with balance of strength and flexibility to produce body control.

Once you have an appreciation for proper posture and correct body mechanics, it will become easier for you to examine injuries, especially chronic injuries, and develop the appropriate therapeutic exercise programs. Use of proper posture for you as the rehabilitation clinician is important if you are to conserve energy, prevent injuries for yourself, and provide efficient and effective manual therapy and manual-resistance applications.

POSTURE

Posture is the relative alignment of the various body segments with one another. When a person has good posture, the body's alignment is balanced so that stress applied to the body segments is minimal. When a person has poor posture, the body's alignment is out of balance, causing exaggerated stresses to various body segments. Over time, this continual stress, even at relatively low levels, causes anatomical adaptations. These changes alter the individual's ability to perform and affect the body's overall efficiency.

Although people seldom stand still, static standing posture is used as the reference for posture evaluation. Static posture can reveal abnormalities in relative balance and alignment of body parts that can affect structure and function during motion. Before we can discuss improper posture, we must identify normal posture.

Correct Standing Alignment

Standing posture is assessed in three planes: sagittal, frontal, and transverse. A plumb line is used as a point of reference. This term is derived from the Latin word, *plumbum*, meaning "lead." A **plumb line** is a string with a weight (formerly a lead weight, but any slightly heavy object will do) at the end. When suspended, the string forms a vertical line. The patient stands behind the plumb line as posture is assessed.

Anterior View

From the anterior, or front, view, the plumb line bisects the body into symmetrical left and right sides (figure 11.1). The patient should stand so that the feet are equidistant from the plumb line. The arms should be relaxed with the palms of the hands facing the sides of the thighs. In this position, the line should bisect the nose and mouth and run through the central portion of the sternum, umbilicus, and pubic bones. The earlobes should be level with one another, as should the shoulders, fingertip ends, nipples, iliac crests, patellae, and medial malleoli. The patellae should point straight ahead with the feet straight or turned slightly outward. The knees and ankles are in line with each other, with the knees angled neither inward nor outward.

Posterior View

The posterior, or back, view should demonstrate alignment similar to that observed from the anterior (figure 11.2). The plumb line should bisect the head and follow the spinous processes from the cervical through the lumbar spine. The earlobes, shoulders, scapulae, hips, posterior superior iliac spine, gluteal fold, posterior knee creases, and medial malleoli should appear level left to right. The scapulae should lie against the rib cage between the second and seventh ribs and about 5 cm (2 in.) from the spinous processes. The calcaneus should be straight with a line bisecting its vertical alignment perpendicular to the floor. Trunk muscles should appear balanced with symmetrical development. The shoulders should be relaxed with the gap between the elbows and lateral trunk equal left to right. Body weight should appear equally distributed over the two feet.

Lateral View

From a lateral or side view, the patient stands with the plumb line slightly anterior to the lateral malleolus (figure 11.3). When the patient is positioned with the plumb line referenced at the ankle, observe the lateral alignment from the head down. The plumb line should pass through the external auditory meatus, the earlobe, the bodies of the cervical vertebrae, the center of the shoulder joint, and the greater trochanter. The plumb line should run midway between the back and chest and the back and abdomen, just posterior to the hip joint, and slightly anterior to the center of the knee just behind the patella. A horizontal line should connect the anterior superior iliac spine (ASIS) and posterior superior iliac spine (PSIS). The patient should remain relaxed with the body's weight balanced between the heel and the forefoot. The knees are straight but not locked. The chin is slightly tucked, and the chest is held slightly up and forward. There is a mild curve inward in the low-back and neck regions.

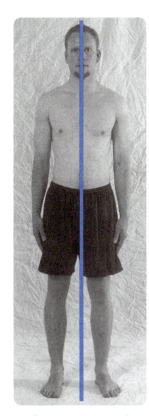

▶ **Figure 11.1** Frontal posture view.

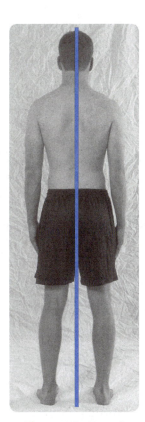

▶ **Figure 11.2** Posterior posture view.

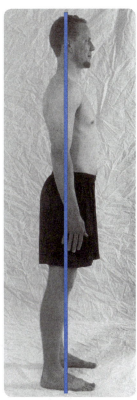

▶ **Figure 11.3** Lateral posture view.

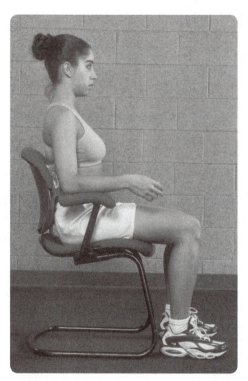

▶ **Figure 11.4** Correct sitting posture with lumbar-roll support.

Correct Sitting Alignment

As in standing, correct sitting posture places the minimum amount of stress on the body. Students in high school and college and many individuals in the work force spend much of their day in chairs. Incorrect sitting posture can aggravate an existing injury, and prolonged sitting with poor posture can lead to injury.

In a correct alignment, the chair seat height must allow the individual's feet to rest comfortably on the floor with the knees and hips at 90°. The chair seat depth should be such that the edge of the seat does not press against the back of the individual's knees. The chair back should support the lumbar and thoracic spine and be high enough to reach the inferior scapular border. A lumbar roll will contour to the curve of the lumbar spine and can provide additional low-back support. Higher-backed executive chairs should provide full thoracic support and permit the person to lean back comfortably. If the chair has arms, they should be at a level that provides for shoulder relaxation and permits the forearms to rest comfortably with the elbows at 90° (figure 11.4).

If the person is sitting at a desk, the chair height should be such that the person's forearms rest comfortably on the desk without hunching the shoulders up or down. If the chair height must be increased to achieve a correct position, a footrest may be necessary to maintain 90° knee and hip positions and still keep the feet flat on the floor. When the individual is using a computer keyboard, the forearms are at 90° or slightly less (0° is full extension), and the wrists are in a neutral position with the fingers resting on the keyboard.

All sitting postures should provide good spinal alignment and normal spinal curves. The head should not be forward nor the shoulders rounded forward.

Pathological Alignment

Unfortunately, most people develop bad posture habits as they age. The best posture can be observed in young children. Toddlers who are learning to stand and walk have good body alignment and move with straight posture. By the time we enter the primary-school years, we develop bad habits that eventually lead to poor posture.

Good posture allows the individual to use his or her body efficiently and effectively. Bad posture, however, places abnormal stresses on the body and increases the demands during performance (Kendall, McCreary, & Provance, 1993). Over time, bad posture habits develop, causing shortening of some structures and lengthening of opposing structures with secondary weakness of both shortened and lengthened structures. This change in strength with a change in relative muscle length is discussed in chapter 7 within the context of length-tension relationships. These changes can impair the individual's efficiency of movement. Inefficient movement burdens an already stressed area during performance and, over time, can cause pain or injury (Sahrmann, 2002). For this reason, the rehabilitation clinician should be aware of the common pathological postures. This knowledge can help the rehabilitation clinician develop an appropriate corrective therapeutic exercise program.

Abnormal alignment is usually recorded in terms of relativity. Rather than precise measurement, terms such as "mild," "moderate," and "severe" identify and grade abnormal alignment. For example, a swimmer may have a mild forward-head posture, or a gymnast may have a severe lumbar lordosis.

Pelvis and Lumbar Area

Common posture faults in the pelvis and lumbar area include excessive lumbar lordosis, flat lumbar spine, and scoliosis. Scoliosis is discussed in the section "Thoracic Area." Often associated with a lumbar lordosis and flat lumbar spine are anterior pelvic tilt and posterior pelvic tilt, respectively.

A normal lumbar curve is slightly lordotic, but an excessive lumbar curve places undue stress on the lumbar spine and other segments (figure 11.5). An excessive lumbar **lordosis,** also referred to as "swayback," is accompanied by an anterior pelvic tilt in which the ASIS is rotated down in relation to the PSIS. It can be caused by tight hip flexors with tight low back extensors pulling on the lumbar spine and by weak abdominal muscles, especially lower abdominals, and weak gluteals. Over time, this abnormal postural alignment can result in tightness of lumbar fascia, increased stress to the anterior longitudinal ligament of the spine, narrowing of the vertebral disk spaces that will cause a narrowing of the intervertebral foramen, and approximation of the vertebral articular facets. These changes can result in nerve root compression, sciatica, joint inflammation, degenerative disk, and vertebral changes.

In a flat lumbar spine, lumbar lordosis is reduced and there is a posterior pelvic tilt so that the PSIS are lower than the ASIS (figure 11.6). Abnormal hip extensor and rectus abdominis tightness is counterbalanced by weak hip flexors and lumbar extensor muscles. This posture reduces the lumbar spine's ability to absorb impact forces and increases the stress of the spine's posterior longitudinal ligament.

Thoracic Area

When you align building blocks, you find that if one block is not placed directly on top of the one below, the next block must be placed askew to compensate for the one adjacent to it that was poorly placed (figure 11.7). The body likewise compensates for malalignments by adjusting positions of adjacent structures in an attempt to keep the body balanced.

Therefore, in the thoracic region, the area can be excessively rounded or excessively flat, depending on the positions of the lumbar or cervical segments. A mild kyphosis in the thoracic spine is normal, but an excessive **thoracic kyphosis,** or excessive rounding of the thoracic area (figure 11.8), in response to a lumbar or cervical lordosis, is pathological. Chest muscles, including the intercostals and pectoralis major and minor are usually tight and are counterbalanced by weak thoracic erector spinae, rhomboids, and trapezius muscles in an excessive thoracic kyphosis. An exaggerated thoracic kyphosis is typically associated with a round-shoulder posture. The scapulae will also be more than the normal 5 cm (2 in.) from the vertebral spinous processes.

A kyphotic posture can lead to **thoracic outlet syndrome,** which is discussed in chapter 16. Secondary cervical problems can result from excessive pressure placed on the cervical area by malalignment of the thoracic spine. People such as swimmers who place high demands on rhomboid and trapezius muscle groups can experience fatigue in these groups because of these muscles' lengthened and weakened status.

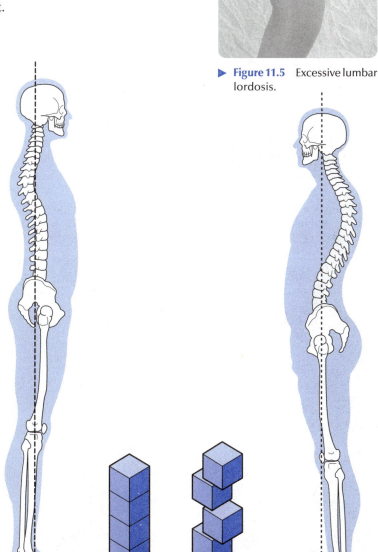

▶ **Figure 11.5** Excessive lumbar lordosis.

▶ **Figure 11.6** Flat lumbar spine.

▶ **Figure 11.7** Building-block alignment.

▶ **Figure 11.8** Kyphosis.

A flattening of the upper back, or a reduction of the thoracic curve, is not as common as a kyphotic posture. This flattening is characterized by an exaggerated attention posture that includes depressed scapulae and flat neck; it results in tightness in the thoracic erector spinae and scapular retractors with secondary weakness of the scapular protractors and anterior thoracic muscles. This posture can also lead to thoracic outlet syndrome because of the increased compression it produces between the first rib and clavicle.

Scoliosis is usually seen in the thoracic or lumbar spine or in both areas. **Scoliosis** is a lateral curve of the normally straight spine and is classified as either a C-curve or an S-curve. A C-curve is indicated as either right or left C-curve according to its direction of convexity. A C-curve with a compensating secondary curve is called an S-curve (figure 11.9). In an attempt to keep the head level, the body compensates for a C-curve by developing a counterbalancing lesser lateral curve that results in an S-curve configuration of the spine. Scoliosis usually also includes a rotation of the vertebrae. If this occurs in the thoracic spine, an asymmetry of rib position is observed from an anterior or posterior view, with one side of the rib cage more anterior than the contralateral side. If leg-length differences are the source of the scoliosis, the pelvic landmarks are not level. Shoulders are often not level in scoliosis as well.

Common causes for scoliosis include congenital deformities of the spine, leg-length differences, and long-term unilateral activities. Tennis players, among others involved in physical activity, may develop a scoliosis because of their participation in a unilaterally demanding sport. Tight soft tissue structures occur on the side of the concavity, while lengthened structures are on the convex side of the scoliosis curve.

Scoliosis can cause muscle fatigue and increased ligamentous stress on the convex side because of weakness of those structures. Impingement of nerve roots with secondary nerve root pain occurs on the concave side. If the scoliosis is caused by a leg-length discrepancy, the longer leg has a lower longitudinal arch to compensate for the leg-length difference.

A scoliosis should not be confused with a lateral shift of the thoracic or lumbar spine. A shift is present when the pelvis and shoulders do not lie in the same frontal plane. Either the pelvis or the shoulders are shifted to the left or right of the midline of the body (figure 11.10). This shift is caused by muscle spasm or pain from an impinged nerve root as the body attempts to move away from the source of pain. It is usually a temporary condition that is relieved when the cause is eliminated.

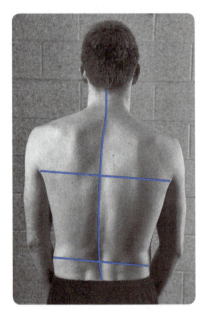

▶ **Figure 11.9** Mild scoliosis. Notice the uneven hips, unequal arm hang, and unequal shoulder and scapula heights.

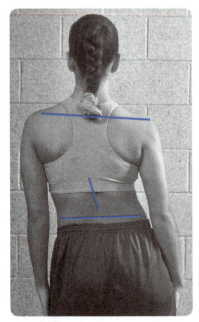

▶ **Figure 11.10** Lateral shift. Notice the uneven hips with a shift of the trunk to the left. Hips and shoulders are not in alignment.

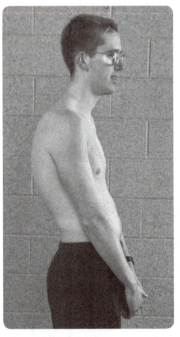

▶ **Figure 11.11** Cervical lordosis, thoracic kyphosis, and lumbar lordosis.

Head and Cervical Area

In response to the abnormal lumbar and thoracic alignment, the cervical spine develops a compensatory alignment. The cervical spine can also develop abnormal alignment with chronically poor posture. For example, sitting with the chin resting on a hand supported by the elbow on a desk or table or keeping the head forward of the body while at a computer will both tend to create exaggerated cervical curves. When the head is positioned forward of the rest of the spine, the lower cervical spine flattens and the upper cervical spine has an exaggerated lordosis. Therefore, cervical **lordosis** refers to an increased flexion of the lower cervical and an increased extension of the upper cervical spine (figure 11.11).

Weakness in the lower cervical and upper thoracic erector spinae and anterior neck muscles is overpowered by tightness in upper cervical muscles including the levator scapulae, sternocleidomastoid, scalenes, suboccipitals, and upper trapezii. This imbalance encourages and perpetuates the abnormal cervical posture.

Many problems can result from prolonged poor cervical posture. Both the weak and the tight muscles experience fatigue. The exaggerated cervical position also increases cervical disc pressure, adds irritation to cervical facet joints, increases nerve root pressure, and impinges on neurovascular bundles to increase the risk of thoracic outlet syndrome. Prolonged abnormal positioning also increases the stresses applied to the cervical spine's posterior and anterior longitudinal ligaments. Scholastic and collegiate athletes who spend their days in the classroom often sit with their elbows on the desk and their chins in their hands, and people in the work force spend their days at a computer sitting in a rounded-back and forward-head position, the most common positions that place increased stress on the cervical spine. Long-term posterior longitudinal ligament stress creates a "dowager's hump" at the base of the cervical spine in persons with chronic forward-head posture. In addition, temporomandibular joint stress can be exaggerated by abnormal cervical posture, leading to temporomandibular joint disorders.

Lower Extremities

Lower-extremity malalignment can begin in the feet, knees, or hips and often affects other structures along the closed kinetic chain. Common postural faults in the lower extremities include excessive flexion or extension, excessive abduction or adduction, and excessive medial or lateral rotation. The normal angle between the femoral neck and the femoral shaft in adults is 120° to 125° (figure 11.12). This angle is larger in infants and children, decreasing from 150° in a newborn to 133° in a teenager until it reaches 120° to 125° in the adult years. An abnormally larger angle is referred to as **coxa valga,** and a smaller than normal angle is called **coxa vara.** As the neck-shaft angle increases with a coxa valga, there is an apparent lengthening of the limb. The opposite is true with a coxa vara, in which the limb shortens as the neck-shaft angle decreases. People with coxa valga have a higher propensity for eventual hip joint arthritis, whereas those with coxa vara are more prone to femoral neck fractures.

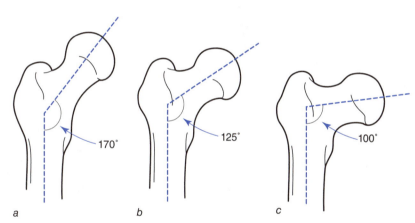

▶ **Figure 11.12** Femoral neck-shaft angles: *(a)* coxa valga causes increased femoral-joint pressure, *(b)* normal position, *(c)* coxa vara produces increased stress on femoral neck.

In the transverse plane of the femur, there is a normal relative forward projection of the femoral neck relative to the femoral condyles. This angle decreases with age during developmental years. A newborn's femoral neck-condyle angle is around 30° whereas in adults it is 8° to 15° (figure 11.13). **Anteversion,** an increased angle, results in greater hip medial rotation and causes squinting patellae and toeing-in during standing. A decreased angle, called **retroversion,** produces greater hip lateral rotation, and in standing, the feet rotate outward. Anteversion decreases hip stability and places the hip at risk for dislocation, whereas retroversion increases the joint's stability.

The normal sagittal alignment of the femur and tibia at the knee is straight; an angling of the knees toward each another is **genu valgus** or **genu valgum.** A bowing outward of the knees is **genu varus** or **genu**

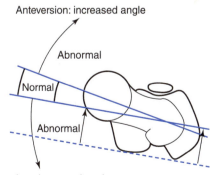

▶ **Figure 11.13** Relative position of the femoral neck and femoral condyles. Normal anteversion in an adult is 8° to 15°.

varum (figure 11.14). These malalignments have a variety of causes. If they occur on one side, leg-length discrepancy is likely the cause. Quadriceps weakness can produce genu valgus. Genu valgus deformities can be the source of excessive foot pronation, and varus deformities can be related to high arches.

In normal standing, the patellae face forward with the feet positioned forward or slightly outward. The condition in which the patellae face toward each other is referred to as **squinting patellae** and may be related to medial hip rotation, hip anteversion, medial tibial rotation, or adduction of the feet (figure 11.15). The condition in which the patellae angle away from each other is referred to as **frog's eye** or **grasshopper eye.** This condition is often the result of lateral hip rotation or tibial rotation, and the feet positioned in abduction.

In a side view, the knee is straight but not locked in a proper alignment. If the line of gravity falls in front of the knee, the knee is hyperextended, a condition referred to as **genu recurvatum** (figure 11.16). Excessive stress is placed on the knee's ligamentous structures in this position. Genu recurvatum is commonly accompanied by excessive lumbar lordosis and anterior pelvic rotation.

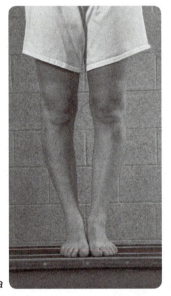
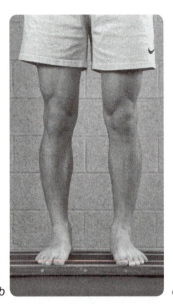
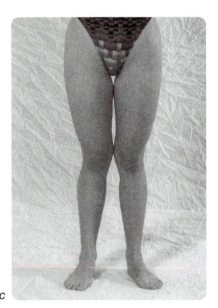

a   *b*   *c*

▶ **Figure 11.14** Knee alignment in the sagittal plane: *(a)* genu varus, *(b)* normal, *(c)* genu valgus.

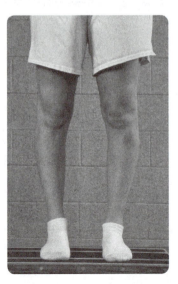
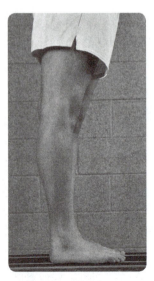

▶ **Figure 11.15** Left squinting patella.

▶ **Figure 11.16** Genu recurvatum.

Tibial torsion is present when the leg appears rotated in relation to the thigh. This is most evident when looking at the positions of the patellae relative to the positions of the feet. In an adult, the feet normally face approximately 12° to 18° from the sagittal axis of the body. In youth, this angle can be as small as 5° (figure 11.17). Excessive tibial torsion is usually a lateral torsion and is correlated with feet facing laterally when the knees face forward; when the feet point forward, the knees are medially rotated. To measure tibial torsion, place the patient in supine with the patellae facing directly upward. A line bisecting the medial and lateral malleoli creates an angle with the plane of the tabletop; this is the tibial torsion measurement (figure 11.18). Normal values are less than 20° to 25° (Sahrmann, 2002). Excessive lateral tibial torsion can increase patellofemoral stresses and lead to instability and fat-pad entrapment.

Medial tibial torsion is associated with genu varum, and lateral tibial torsion is associated with genu valgum. These conditions can become apparent with habitual use of poor sitting postures, especially in children, as seen in figure 11.19.

Foot position can influence knee and hip positions, and the converse is true as well. One determines medial longitudinal arch height by drawing a line from the distal aspect of the medial malleolus to the weight-bearing surface of the first metatarsophalangeal joint. In both weight bearing and non-weight bearing, the navicular tuberosity should be on the line (figure 11.20). If the navicular tuberosity falls below the line, the arch is abnormally low; and if it falls above the line, the arch is abnormally high. A high arch is **pes cavus.** A low arch, **pes planus,** can be associated with excessive foot pronation and calcaneal eversion and accompanied by genu valgum and/or femoral anteversion. A pes planus is usually hypermobile, allowing for excessive rearfoot and forefoot motion during gait. This type of foot structure may not have the stability to create a strong platform for propulsion, and it places excessive stresses on soft-tissue structures and adjacent joints as the patient attempts to perform power and agility activities. The greater the foot's hypermobility, the greater the loss of its stability. Increased stress on foot and ankle structures can lead to injuries such as plantar fasciitis and Achilles tendinopathy.

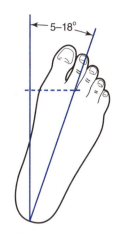

▶ **Figure 11.17** Normal adult foot position in weight bearing.

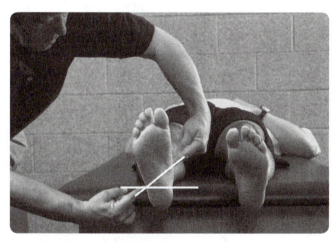

▶ **Figure 11.18** With the patella facing the ceiling, a line between the medial and lateral malleolus forms an angle with a line parallel to the tabletop for identifying the individual's tibial torsion.

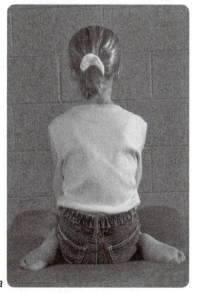

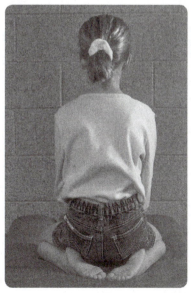

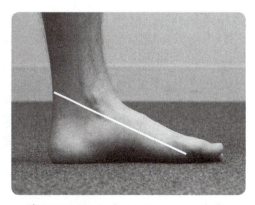

▶ **Figure 11.19** Poor sitting posture for knees: *(a)* encourages lateral tibial torsion; *(b)* encourages medial tibial torsion.

▶ **Figure 11.20** Arch position: normal alignment.

Posture, or the relative alignment of various body segments, includes standing alignment and sitting alignment. Anterior, posterior, and lateral views show whether alignment of the various segments of the body is normal.

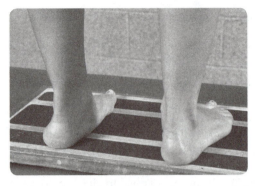

▶ **Figure 11.21** Pronation. Notice the everted position of the left calcaneus.

Calcaneal eversion with increased forefoot pronation is observed from a posterior view of the ankle. In this position, the Achilles tendon appears to be at less than a 90° angle to the floor, and the calcaneus is everted (figure 11.21).

Pes cavus, a higher-than-normal arch, is associated with a more rigid foot structure and produces less mobility of the joints of the rearfoot and forefoot. This type of foot has a reduced ability to absorb stress and is more prone to stress fractures. With reduced flexibility and associated diminution of stress-absorption capacity, increased stress is imposed on the joints of the foot. A high arch is often associated with hammertoes or claw toes and can be related to femoral retroversion.

Toes are normally straight. A positioning of the great toe laterally toward the other toes is called **hallux valgus.** A common cause is hypermobility of the foot. Over time, this additional stress on the first metatarsophalangeal joint during terminal gait causes it to become deformed (figure 11.22).

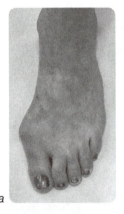

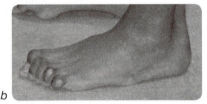

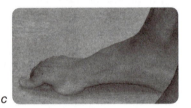

▶ **Figure 11.22** Toe deformities: *(a)* hallux valgus, *(b)* claw toes, *(c)* hammer toes.

© Peggy Houglum

a   b   c

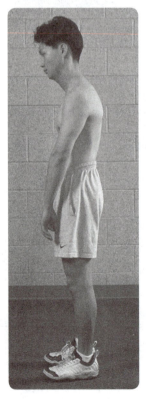

▶ **Figure 11.23** Upper-extremity posture deviation.

Toes that become flexed or extended at the metatarsophalangeal joints or the interphalangeal joints are known as claw toes or hammertoes. **Claw toes** are hyperextended at the metatarsophalangeal joints and flexed at the proximal interphalangeal joints; **hammertoes** are hyperextended at the metatarsophalangeal joints, flexed at the proximal interphalangeal joint, and hyperextended at the distal interphalangeal joint. These conditions are usually accompanied by a high longitudinal arch and a rigid foot. Corns and calluses on the toes develop secondary to abnormal pressures as the elevated portion of the toes rubs against the inside of the shoe.

Upper Extremities

The primary area affected by bad posture in the upper extremity is the shoulders. If a person has a poor thoracic posture with rounded shoulders, the scapulae protract forward and rotate downward and anteriorly on the rib cage. This positioning presents itself as an anterior rounding of the glenohumeral joint, and the dorsal hands will face forward, positioned in front of the anterior thigh rather than at the lateral thigh as they should (figure 11.23). This can lead to glenohumeral impingement, weakness of the scapular rotators, and tightness of anterior shoulder girdle muscles. These soft-tissue changes can cause inefficient use of the shoulder during upper-extremity activities and place the individual at risk for upper-extremity injuries.

MUSCLE IMBALANCES

Muscle imbalances often affect posture. To correct posture, the rehabilitation clinician must be able to identify the muscle imbalances that perpetuate the patient's improper posture.

Causes

Poor posture results from an abnormal relationship between the forces that act on an area. Normal posture occurs when there is a balance of forces acting on bones and joints. Normal posture permits an efficient and effective use of the body to produce the desired motions.

When a body is in bad posture, the joints and muscles are already under stress, and activity increases that level of stress. In bad posture, muscles must work harder to produce desired motions and are not as efficient or as effective. Bad posture can also restrict muscles from performing optimally. For example, a freestyle swimmer with rounded shoulders has difficulty getting enough lateral rotation and abduction on the recovery phase of the stroke, so either hand entry into the water is premature or the swimmer has to compensate with an exaggerated body roll. The swimmer will also suffer an impingement injury of the shoulder because the scapula does not upwardly rotate and retract, as it should. If this swimmer were to come to you with a rotator-cuff tendinopathy and you did not correct the posture and muscle imbalances, your treatment success would be short-lived, for the injury would recur.

Sometimes pain in an area is the result of poor posture or muscle imbalances in another area. The site of pain is not always the source of the problem. For example, a gymnast who complains of back pain and has a lumbar lordosis may in fact be having back pain because of hip-flexor tightness, not a back injury. The hip flexors place abnormal stress on the lumbar vertebrae because tight hip flexors pull on the lumbar vertebrae, increasing low-back stress and making the area more susceptible to injury. The gymnast's back pain could also be related to hyperextended knees, which will pull the anterior pelvis forward, increasing lumbar lordosis.

Commonly, the source of muscle imbalance is a loss of motion or flexibility in a muscle or muscle group and lengthening and weakness from prolonged or sustained stretch of the opposing muscle or muscle group. If a muscle actively shortens, its opposing muscle is lengthened via the neurological reciprocal innervation system. It is this reciprocal activity that allows us to feed ourselves, walk, and perform most activities. For example, when you perform a biceps curl, the biceps shorten and the triceps lengthen; or when you bend your knee, the hamstrings shorten and the quadriceps lengthen.

There is, however, a significant difference between neurological length changes during normal activity and prolonged length changes in a muscle's resting length. Sustained shortening of one muscle from poor posture or prolonged positioning causes a loss of flexibility and strength in that muscle, and the sustained lengthening of the opposite muscle causes a loss of strength and tone in its opposing muscle. Remember from chapter 5, as a muscle either shortens or lengthens from its optimal length, strength declines (length-strength principle).

Additionally, changes in fascia length accompany muscle tissue length changes when the changes occur over time. One can compare the results of sustained lengthening to what occurs when a weight is hung on the end of a rubber band for a length of time. When the weight is removed, the rubber band has less tone than before, and less spring. So, too, a muscle that is positionally lengthened loses its spring and becomes weaker. If a patient performed only flexibility exercises to restore balance, the imbalance, caused by tightness of one muscle and weakness of its opposing muscle, would overpower the effects of stretching and would continue to encourage the imbalanced posture.

Some activities are more likely to cause postural deviations than others are. For example, participants in sports that emphasize muscle activity on anterior more than on posterior body regions, such as swimming and boxing, are more likely to develop postural deviations. Unilateral activities such as racket sports encourage muscle imbalance from left to right and can cause such postural deviations such as scoliosis.

As the body ages, postural deviations become more pronounced. A mild forward-head posture in a young adult becomes a moderate forward-head posture in the middle-aged adult and becomes even more severe as the individual ages. As the muscle naturally weakens with age, it has increasing difficulty opposing tight structures, so pathological postures become even more apparent with aging—further increasing joint and muscle stresses.

Muscle imbalance can also result from joint abnormalities. These abnormalities run the spectrum from hypermobility to hypomobility. When joints are hypermobile, displaying an excessive amount of motion, the muscles must work harder to provide joint stability. This is true for a joint that is uniplanar or multiplanar. Joints that lack normal mobility—hypomobile joints—have less-than-normal motion and place additional stresses on muscles and joints. These conditions can also add stresses to other body segments. For example, the individual who has foot-joint hypermobility with excessive pronation may develop patellar tendinopathy. This may be secondary to additional stresses on the patellar tendon when its insertion rotates medially during prolonged pronation in gait.

Injuries can also cause muscle imbalances. Scar-tissue adhesions following a ligament injury can cause the joint to become hypomobile, especially if the joint was immobilized immediately after the injury. The deleterious effects of immobilization are discussed in chapter 2.

Another cause of imbalances is muscle strains. If the injured muscle is not properly rehabilitated and unwanted adhesions within the muscle occur, the site can become tight, limiting flexibility and causing increased stress to the site or adjacent areas.

Treatment

It becomes important in any injury examination to assess the patient's posture and look for muscle imbalances that either may have contributed to the injury or may result from the injury. You should also look at the total body, not merely the injured site, because postural deviations from other locations may have contributed to the pain or injury.

It is important to correct postural deviations, not only to address the patient's current injury, but also to prevent recurrence. As has been mentioned, if a postural deviation is either the source of an injury or a contributing factor, you must correct the postural deviation as part of the rehabilitation program in order to prevent recurrence of the injury. If you do not, in all likelihood, the injury will recur.

In correcting postural deviations, the rehabilitation clinician must first identify the structure that has become tight and the opposing structure that has become overstretched. He or she can then give the patient exercises to correct the muscle imbalance—that is, to lengthen the short or tight structures and improve stiffness (strength) of the opposing lengthened (weak) structures. For example, if the freestyle swimmer's posture is a rounded-shoulder position, examination will show that the anterior chest muscles are tight; the downward scapular rotators are tight; and the upper back muscles, scapular retractors, and upward scapular rotator groups are lengthened with less tone and stiffness. The treatment program should include lengthening exercises for the pectoralis minor, anterior deltoid, and pectoralis major and strengthening activities for the lower trapezius, middle trapezius, rhomboids, and posterior deltoid. It should also include activities that will recruit and retrain muscles to produce the desired activity correctly. It is useful to provide reminders that will facilitate correct postural alignment—for example, a visual cue such as a colored dot on the face of the patient's watch or on a fingernail can be used to remind the patient to think about and correct his or her posture. An example of a more direct reminder is tape applied between the shoulder blades to help the patient remember to keep the shoulders in correct alignment (figure 11.24).

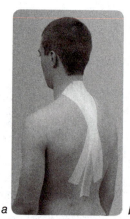
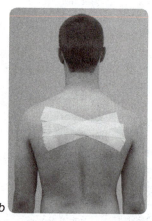

a   b

▶ **Figure 11.24** Stretch pre-tape provides feedback if patient strays from a properly aligned postural position. The tape provides the patient with feedback when he moves out of proper posture. The tape may be worn for 24 hours, if tolerated. If muscle fatigue occurs, the tape should be removed earlier. *(a)* For proper cervical posture, tape is applied to the neck and thoracic back while the patient stands in proper posture. *(b)* For correction of rounded shoulders, the patient retracts the shoulders into proper alignment and stretch pre-tape such as Cover-Roll (BSN Medical, Hamburg, Germany) is applied between the scapulae.

Conscious correction of posture is necessary for bad posture to improve. The patient must become aware of the abnormal posture and then make a deliberate effort to alter the habitual posture; otherwise, posture does not change. As the patient continues to improve muscle balance through proper exercises and to correct bad postural position, and maintains a proper posture more and more frequently, the posture eventually will improve.

It is more difficult in the initial stages than it will be later for the patient to change posture, for two primary reasons. The first one is habit. Habit, whether good or bad, is easy and comfortable and thus difficult for anyone to change. The second reason is the relationship between the lengthened and tight muscles. The tight muscles overpower the lengthened muscles, making it difficult for the patient to maintain a proper posture when attempting correction. But as the muscle imbalance reduces, the task becomes easier. Conscious effort by the patient must occur to achieve the ultimate goal of improved postural alignment.

Posture- and Muscle Imbalance-Related Injuries

To make it easier to understand the muscle imbalance and postural change process, let's look at a couple of examples of injuries and the relationship between improper posture and muscle imbalance.

Lower Extremity

Iliotibial band (ITB) friction syndrome frequently occurs in athletes, particularly in runners. The pain occurs along the ITB and is typically located along the superior-lateral aspect of the knee or toward the hip. The patient reports that the pain worsens with hill running. The examination reveals a tight ITB, and the patient stands with the leg in more medial rotation than normal. Muscle testing demonstrates weakness of the quadriceps and hip lateral rotators, and probably weakness of the gluteus maximus as well. Examination of the soft tissue along the ITB reveals tenderness in areas of soft-tissue thickness.

Treatment includes softening the ITB-restrictive areas with deep friction massage techniques, along with lengthening the tight ITB and strengthening the lengthened, weak gluteus maximus, hip lateral rotators, and quadriceps muscles. Instructions to the patient include conscious positional correction: keeping the leg in only slight lateral rotation alignment when standing or walking. The use of a modality, such as heat, prior to friction massage allows for better massage results by making the soft tissue more pliable.

Upper Extremity

A common upper-extremity problem in patients who participate in upper-extremity sports such as tennis, golf, swimming, and gymnastics is shoulder impingement. This often appears as rotator-cuff tendinopathy, and the patient complains of pain with movements such as shoulder elevation, putting the hand behind the back, and resisted activities. He or she experiences pain through the middle arc of shoulder range of motion, and the impingement tests produce a positive sign. The rotator-cuff tendons are tender to palpation at their insertion on the greater tubercle. Examination of muscles reveals tightness of the pectoralis minor, anterior deltoid, latissimus, and pectoralis major. The rhomboids and levator scapulae may also be tight. Weakness is apparent in the lower and middle trapezii, serratus anterior, infraspinatus, and teres minor. The capsule may have areas of restriction. The scapula may not rotate fully into an upward and retracted position because of weakness of the upward rotators and tightness of the downward rotators.

Effective treatment of this condition must include correcting the faulty posture, strengthening weak muscles, and stretching tight muscles. Optimal balance between muscle length and strength of opposing muscle groups is the goal that will lead to reduced impingement in the shoulder. It is important to make the patient aware of the proper posture of the shoulder and cervical and thoracic spine so that he or she can work at improving posture and alignment. Exercises should include stretching of the anterior capsule, pectoralis minor, pectoralis major, and latissimus. Strengthening exercises should include appropriate exercises for the serratus

Improper posture is often perpetuated by muscle imbalances. Causes of muscle imbalance include overuse, loss of motion or flexibility in a muscle or muscle group, postural deviations, and injuries. It is necessary to determine the muscle imbalances involved before correcting postural deviations.

anterior, lower and middle trapezius, infraspinatus, and teres minor. Restoring the balance between scapular upward and downward rotators, protractors and retractors, and elevators and depressors must be part of the rehabilitation program for resolution of postural defects and muscle imbalances to occur. Because weakness of the lengthened posterior muscles is one of the sources of shoulder impingement, retraining the depressors, retractors, and upward rotators to provide the appropriate movement of the scapula during shoulder movement is vital to reducing impingement of the rotator cuff.

A Challenging Example

Let's look at one more example so you can outline an appropriate program. A basketball player comes to you with complaints of pain around the patella, especially when jumping for a rebound. He also has pain going down stairs, and in the weight room he has pain on the leg extension and squat machines. When he stands in front of you, the patellae face forward and the feet are in a laterally rotated position. In weight bearing, the longitudinal arches are low. When he performs a step-down exercise, you notice that he lacks full control of the knee and that there is a slight knee wobble medially-to-laterally as he lowers himself. Range-of-motion testing shows tightness of the ITB, but range of motion of the knee is normal. Strength testing indicates weakness of the vastus medialis oblique (VMO), and you can see some atrophy of the VMO compared to that in the contralateral knee. There is also weakness present in the gluteus maximus and gluteus medius. With the patient in long sitting, the patella is positioned with its medial side higher than the lateral side. When he contracts the quadriceps, you observe that the patella tracks primarily laterally. What is the cause of this individual's pain, and what treatment plan would you provide for him? Think for a moment before you read on, and identify the types of corrective exercises and the progression you would recommend to resolve this problem.

The cause of the patient's pain is a malalignment and maltracking of the patella. This in turn is caused by a combination of weakness of the VMO, tightness of the ITB, and malalignment of the feet. Lower-than-normal arches can result in a tibial torsion to increase stresses on the patella. Weakness in his glutes causes the thigh to wobble when he lowers himself on a step; this will cause more stress to the patellofemoral joint. You should check hip rotation to eliminate tightness of the lateral rotators. The patella is not tracking normally because of weakness of the VMO and tightness of the ITB overpowering the VMO pull. There may also be an imbalance between the vastus lateralis and the VMO that would add to the lateral tracking. Tightness of the ITB can also be responsible for the lateral tilt of the patella.

Treatment for this patient should include stretching exercises for the hip and ITB and progressive strengthening exercises for the VMO, such as terminal knee-extension exercises, squats, step exercises, and lunges; these exercises should be pain free and should increase in intensity, repetitions, and number of sets as the patient's strength increases. Strengthening the gluteus maximus and gluteus medius is also necessary. For example, exercises may include hip extension, hip abduction, clam exercises, and sidelying bridges. Taping the patella may also reduce the pain. If inspection of the feet reveals excessive pronation, taping the arch and limiting rearfoot motion may be beneficial.

The exercises you select should be designed to increase flexibility of the tight muscles and increase strength of the weak muscles to provide for a restoration of balance between muscles. If modalities are the only treatment technique used or if flexibility is the only type of exercise included, the rehabilitation program will not succeed in relieving the patient's complaints and permitting a full and successful return to sport participation and normal activity.

BODY MECHANICS

Body mechanics is related to posture in that use of proper body mechanics is easier with good posture. **Body mechanics** refers to the way the body is positioned and used during activity. Incorrect body mechanics increases stresses placed on various body segments, but correct body mechanics makes the most effective use of the body's forces and lever systems. Body mechanics is briefly discussed here because an awareness of good body mechanics is important to the rehabilitation clinician from both a personal and a treatment perspective. From a personal perspective, use of proper body mechanics makes you more efficient in the application of manual therapy and exercises. It conserves your energy and makes the most effective use of your body.

From a treatment perspective, knowledge of correct body mechanics in the execution of specific sport activities allows you as a rehabilitation clinician to provide the patient with proper exercises. Such exercises will enhance the patient's performance and include corrective techniques to further prepare the individual for returning to competition.

Basic Principles

A few basic concepts are important to remember regardless of the activity that is being performed. The first principle is that the spine should remain straight. A "straight spine" is one that has the natural curves with the pelvis in neutral. A straight spine has slight lumbar lordosis, thoracic kyphosis, and cervical lordosis. In this position, each vertebra is in correct alignment with the adjacent vertebrae (figure 11.25). Pelvic neutral is present when the pelvis is in a mid-position between an anterior and a posterior pelvic tilt. In this position the stress on the pelvis is minimal, and the vertebrae should be balanced. This position is also called a **neutral spine** or **pelvic neutral.**

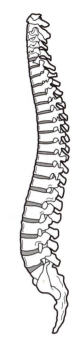

▶ **Figure 11.25** Proper spinal alignment is a "straight spine."

Maintaining a neutral spine is important so forces from the lower extremities are properly transmitted to the trunk and upper extremities. It is easier to understand this concept if you think of the legs, trunk, and arms as three sections connected in series. When the sections are all rigid, forces transfer easily from one section to another; but if the middle section, the spine, is a spring rather than a rigid structure, it is more difficult to transfer forces from one section to another. When the middle segment is not rigid, the forces produced in the lower segment dissipate and are absorbed by the spring and the upper bar, the arms, must develop their own forces—a far more difficult and strenuous method of delivering force for desired activity.

For this reason, it is important for athletes to have a "straight back" during activities, especially those activities that require force transmission. For example, a football lineman squats with the back straight to utilize the driving force from the legs; the warehouse worker keeps the back straight in a squat to transfer the lifting force from the legs to the arms; and the golfer's back is straight so that the summation of forces from the legs and trunk can drive the ball down the fairway. The rehabilitation clinician must also maintain a straight back so the power of the legs, not the arms, is the primary source to deliver manual resistance forces for therapeutic exercises.

If the back is not straight, transfer of forces from the lower extremities to the trunk and upper extremities is not possible. To illustrate the significance of this, have a friend bend over from the waist so that his or her back is not straight, and then push on your friend's shoulders to move the person off balance. Now have your friend bend at the hips but keep the back straight as you again push his or her body off balance. You will find that with the back straight, the power of the legs will provide increased stability and better resistance to outside forces.

When lowering the body to sit or to lift an object, the back should remain straight so less stress occurs in the spine. It is not enough just to bend the knees. The knees must bend, but the hips are also pushed back while the chest is kept up. If the hips are not pushed back, the bend occurs at the waist, not the hips, and the lower back will round, losing the back's proper alignment. If the chest is lowered, the spine will round and lose its proper straight position (figure 11.26b).

Lowering the center of gravity increases the body's stability. This is important to resist outside forces. For example, if you push your friend while he or she is standing fully upright, it will be easier for you to move the person than if he or she squats down to reduce the body's center of gravity. This is one reason linemen in football and rugby get into a squat position.

Broadening the base of support is another method of providing increased stability. If your friend stands with feet together, it is much easier to push him or her off balance than if the

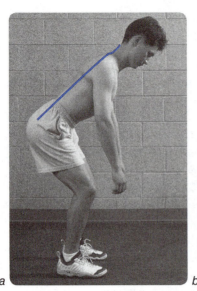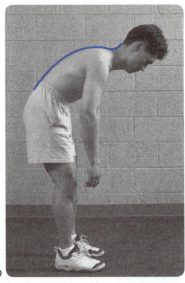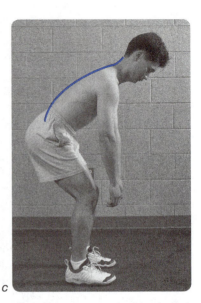

a   b   c

▶ **Figure 11.26** Keeping back straight when bending: *(a)* Knees and hips are flexed, hips are pushed backward, and lumbar curve is maintained, chest is held up. *(b)* Leg and lower back positions are maintained properly, but the head and chest are lowered. *(c)* Leg and chest positions are maintained, but lumbar curve is lost and hips are not pushed backward.

feet are apart. A broader base of support produces a larger area for the center of gravity to move within before balance is lost. When you move an object, a broad base of support will increase your stability.

Another principle of good body mechanics is to stand in the direction of force application. This allows the use of force transfer from the legs. For example, when you throw a ball forward, your feet should be in a backward-forward straddle. This permits transfer of forces from the back leg to the front leg as your trunk rotates and your arm follows through the throwing motion. To see this concept, throw a ball with your feet in a side-by-side stance and then with your feet in a backward-forward straddle stance. You will find that the ball goes farther with the straddle stance. If it is necessary to transfer an object or exert a force from one side of the body to the other, the best stance is a side-by-side stance with the feet in line with the shoulders. For example, if you are resisting a patient's straight-leg raise with the patient supine on the table, your stance should be side by side, as you face the table. This way, as the patient raises his or her leg, your weight can transfer from the leg you have positioned next to the patient's foot (lower) to the one you have positioned next to the patient's hip (upper). You will be able to use a body-weight shift from your lower-positioned leg to your upper-positioned leg as the patient's leg moves.

Abdominal strength is important for force transfer from the lower to the upper extremities. Strong abdominals provide the support needed to keep the back straight, help to diffuse the forces applied to the back, and assist in the transfer of forces from the legs to the arms. Arm and leg movement assisted by stabilization of the spine for the arms and legs will produce the desired activity. You can see this if you have someone resist your shoulder flexion-to-extension movement. You should feel your abdominals tighten as you extend the arm against his or her resistance. You should also feel the abdominals tighten when you resist hip flexion. For these reasons, an injured individual's therapeutic exercise program should include abdominal strengthening exercises.

The Patient's Daily Activities

Performing daily activities using correct body mechanics is important because it conserves energy, makes for efficient and effective use of the body, and reduces stress on the back and other segments. Knowledge of these techniques enables you to instruct patients, especially those with back injuries, to minimize stress to the injured area.

Patients routinely lift and carry objects such as book bags, backpacks, boxes, athletic gear, and gym bags. The way an object is lifted depends on its size and weight. It is important to test the weight of the object before it is lifted. If an object is heavy, the proper way to lift it is to approach it front on. This means facing the object, standing as close to the object as possible and standing so that when the back is straight and the person flexes at the hips and knees, and the arms fall directly over the object. As the individual bends the knees to lift the object, the knees should never be higher than the hips. Positioning the knees greater than 90° imposes a great deal of stress on the knee's meniscus. Additional lowering of the body occurs by pushing the hips backward, bending the knees as far as possible but bending the knees to no more than

90°, and keeping the chest and head up and the back straight. With the abdominals tightened, the person lifts the object by straightening the legs while moving into a standing position (figure 11.27). The object is kept close to the body to reduce its force (force equals weight × distance). The farther away from the body the object is, the more force is required to lift it.

To push or pull an object, the individual places his or her legs in the direction of movement (side-by-side if the object is being moved left to right; backward-forward if the object is to be moved toward or away from the person). The person then moves the object by transferring the body's weight from one leg to the other. If the object is to be moved from the right side of the body to the left, the individual

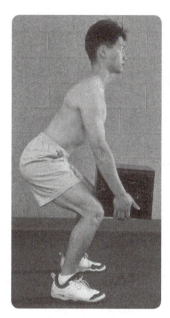 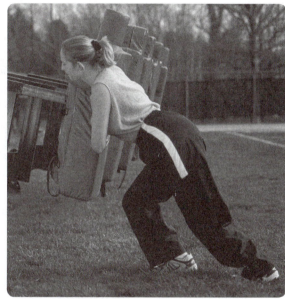

▶ **Figure 11.27** Proper lifting technique.   ▶ **Figure 11.28** Proper pushing technique.

positions the legs in a side-by-side stance, grasps the object, and moves the body weight from the right to the left leg. If the object is to be moved from a position in front of the person to one farther away, the individual begins in a backward-forward stance, grasps the object and moves the body weight from the back leg to the front leg to move the object. The legs, not the arms, provide the force to move the object.

While carrying objects in only one hand, it is best to shift the object periodically from one side to the other, especially when carrying an object for more than a short time. The load is minimized when the object is kept close to the body and no higher than waist level.

The easiest way to push or pull objects is to keep the back straight, lower the center of gravity, and use a wide forward-backward stance position. Keeping the center of gravity low will assist in using the lower-extremity forces to move the object (figure 11.28). Pushing is easier than pulling because better use of the body's weight is made in pushing.

Rising from a chair is performed according to the same principles as bending. As figure 11.29 shows, the back is kept straight; the bend occurs at the hips and knees; and the chest is kept up.

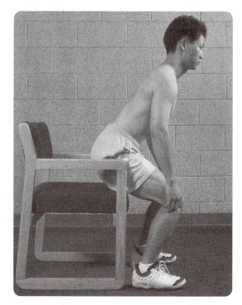

▶ **Figure 11.29** Proper sit-to-stand position.

The proper technique for getting down on the floor is to go down first on one knee then the other before placing the hands on the floor in a quadruped position. From there, the person walks the hands out to get into a prone position, and then rolls into either a sidelying or a supine position. The technique occurs in reverse to return to a standing position.

Athletic Events

Athletic activities, like daily activities, demand a straight back for the optimal transmission of forces from the lower extremities to the upper extremities. Abdominal strength is also important for transmitting these forces. Maintenance of pelvic neutral and straight back is important for force production, injury prevention, and efficiency of movement.

It is beyond the scope of this text to describe proper body mechanics for execution of all activities. However, on the basis of the information presented regarding body mechanics, the rehabilitation clinician should have a concept of the proper posture and position for the execution of many activities. For example, a canoeist must have a straight spine with pelvic neutral to transmit forces from the legs to the arms and move the canoe quickly and forcefully (figure 11.30); a gymnast must be in pelvic neutral as she goes into a kip on the uneven bars; a weightlifter's back must be straight as he lifts the weight overhead (figure 11.31); and a shot-putter must transfer the lower-extremity forces to the upper extremity by keeping the back straight to propel the shot for the desired distance.

The Rehabilitation Clinician's Daily Activities

Just as the patient needs to use the body efficiently and effectively, the rehabilitation clinician must use his or her body correctly in order to be effective, competent, and proficient in the application of rehabilitation techniques.

This means that the rehabilitation clinician must use good body mechanics. It is important that your body weight be equally distributed over both feet, that your feet be

Proper body mechanics is fundamental to proper posture. Important principles include keeping the spine straight, lowering the center of gravity, and keeping the base of support broad. Patients need to perform daily activities using correct body mechanics, and the rehabilitation clinician must also pay attention to his or her own body mechanics.

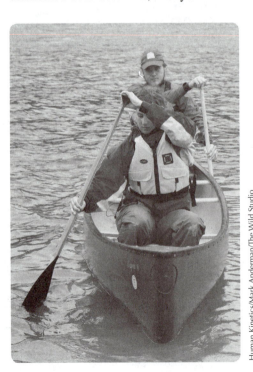

▶ **Figure 11.30** Canoeists with proper technique.

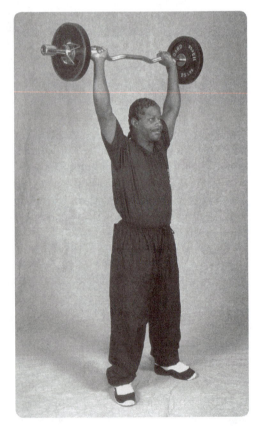

▶ **Figure 11.31** Weightlifter using proper mechanics.

Human Kinetics/Mark Anderman/The Wild Studio

positioned in a correct alignment depending on the direction of the forces you are applying to the patient, and that the force you use is from the legs rather than the arms. Remember to keep the back straight so leg strength rather than arm strength is used. Moving from right to left foot and back again as you move or resist the patient's extremities through a range of motion reduces the demands on your body and conserves energy. Keeping the upper extremities relaxed but in proper alignment makes it easier for you to achieve the transfer of forces from the lower to upper extremities. Figure 11.32 demonstrates using proper body mechanics when working with patients.

Proper body mechanics includes keeping the spine in a neutral position so that you can use your body as effectively and efficiently as possible; a neutral spine allows the powerful lower-extremity muscles to be used as the source of strength. Keeping the back straight, bending the knees, and transferring body weight with movement help to minimize risk of injury and maximize body forces. This is true for the athlete during sport participation, for the rehabilitation clinician during execution of therapeutic exercises, and for employees in daily work activities.

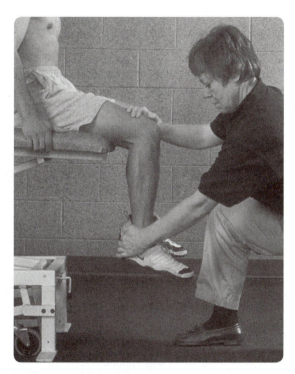

▶ **Figure 11.32** Rehabilitation clinician with proper body mechanics.

BODY-AWARENESS PROGRAMS

Over the years, many programs have been developed to improve body awareness through body movement. Three of these programs are introduced here. The intent is to familiarize you with the various kinds of approaches that body-awareness programs use. The two basic premises common to all these programs is that the techniques produce self-improvement through increased body awareness and that a strong body-mind interaction exists that determines an individual's movement patterns and abilities. The whole body, not just the area of pain or dysfunction, is addressed. Some athletes use these programs to enhance their athletic skill and performance. Others find the programs useful in treating injuries that impede normal body function.

Feldenkrais Method

Moshe Feldenkrais (1904–1984) was a Russian-born Israeli who obtained a doctorate in physics from the Sorbonne in Paris. He held a black belt in judo and was a recognized judo instructor. An old soccer injury of the knee became painful and crippling in Feldenkrais's later years. Physicians were unable to provide a satisfactory medical treatment, so he taught himself medicine, anatomy, therapeutic exercise, and body mechanics. His mechanical and electrical engineering background was an asset as he developed what became known as the Feldenkrais Method. He taught himself to walk pain free using this method. By the 1950s, he gave up his career as a research scientist and devoted his work to teaching and using the Feldenkrais Method.

Dr. Feldenkrais believed that an individual develops inefficient movement patterns for a variety of reasons—that cultural influences, illness, injury, and other factors can cause limited movement leading to inhibition of normal movement ability. In the Feldenkrais Method, movement patterns and habits are assessed before a treatment program is initiated. Feldenkrais believed that a person's unconscious pattern of movement is influenced by several factors, including the unconscious sensorimotor relationship that affects muscles and joints and their associated motor skills and abilities; the individual's perception of balance, space, and gravity; self-image; and kinesthetic awareness. His approach for changing these components to improve movement involves engaging the whole person in the treatment regimen, promoting self-esteem, and improving learning skills.

Pain is avoided in the Feldenkrais Method. Pain encourages the unfavorable muscle movement patterns that the person has established. Movement is usually performed slowly through an easy direction of motion. Slow and easy movement allows the individual to become sensitive to motions and positions, allows muscle relaxation, and permits a change of position through a new and more correct movement pattern.

As the individual progresses, the movements become more advanced in their complexity, speed, size, and trajectory of motion. This process permits an increased awareness of kinesthesia and coordination and causes a decrease in pain.

The Feldenkrais Method encompasses two approaches to this somatically based reeducation. One is "Awareness Through Movement" and the other is "Functional Integration." Awareness Through Movement includes the use of active motion either with the individual or with a group. In 45- to 60-min sessions the instructor guides patients through a series of active movements using imagery and focused attention. Through the guidance, the patients become aware of their somatic reception and the influence it has on their movement. Imagery and visualization help them to develop this awareness and movement perception. The goal is for patients to become aware of their bodies and how their bodies move, the relationship between one segment and another during movement, and influences that affect their movement.

The lessons often include developmental movements such as rolling, crawling, and standing up. They also include somatic awareness, visualization, and imagery for functions such as posture, breathing, and simple movements. The exercises are not vigorous but rather are explorations of the somato-psychic connections that increase self-awareness and facilitate an assessment of sensory-based movement. The movements often start as very small motions with emphasis on ease of movement, comfort, and development of an awareness of the way the muscles and bones are integrated with the individual's somatosensory system and personality.

■ An Example of the Feldenkrais Method

As an example of the Feldenkrais Method, a simple 2-min activity experiment from Alon (Alon, 1990), is reprinted here. It is designed to improve and refine an individual's ability to look up. Take a couple of minutes to go through it and note any changes you experience. To perform the activity, go through the following steps:

In a sitting position, raise your head upward and try to see the ceiling. Make a note how this movement works for you. At what point in your reach do you have a feeling of difficulty? What happens to your breathing? Now, shift your attention to the feet. Take off one shoe and extend that foot forward, as far as you can; the sole stays flat on the floor. Begin to slowly flex your toes downward, dragging them along the floor closer to your heel. In this position, lift the ball of the foot from the floor and decrease the angle of bending in the ankle. All this time, the heel is still anchored to the floor. This is an unusual combination of movements involving the foot. Allow the foot to return to its comfortable place on the floor, and repeat the whole sequence several times.

In the next step, place your foot in full contact with the floor again, but this time, bend the toes upward, raising them into the air while the ball of the foot stays on the ground. Alternate several times between the two movements, from bent ankle to outstretched ankle, with the heel planted all the time on the floor. The toes point to the floor when the foot comes up, and they are turned to the ceiling when the ball of the foot rests on the floor. See if you can reduce the amount of effort you invest in bending the ankle and the toes. Notice that to design a strange arrangement that is perhaps totally new to you, you have to use a device other than direct physical power. Identify within yourself this quality of listening and clarification—it is this quality which makes the difference between exercise and learning.

Now, bring the foot back to its usual place, and again lift your head so as to look at the ceiling. Has your scan of the ceiling now been made a bit easier than it was earlier?

From R. Alon, 1990, "An Example of the Feldenkrais Method" from *Mindful Spontaneity: Lessons in the Feldenkrais Method.*

Small movements progress to more complex, larger, and faster ones until the movements are functional and can be put to daily use. Imagery and verbal suggestion guide the patient toward incorporating the new movement patterns into daily activity.

Functional Integration uses individualized sessions designed to meet the person's specific needs to improve movement. As with Awareness through Movement, Functional Integration is a learning-based method of improving movement efficiency, coordination, awareness, and self-control. Movement awareness and response are facilitated through touch, imagery, repetition, and guidance. A new awareness and perception of movement are created and integrated into the individual's motions through the instructor's guidance, like one dance partner being guided by the other, until the new neuromuscular patterns become ingrained and translate into a change in the patient's active performance.

The Feldenkrais Method is a complex system that takes time to learn. There are several classifications of Feldenkrais-trained professionals. Awareness-through-movement Feldenkrais teachers must have a minimum of 2 years of instruction; Feldenkrais practitioners have a minimum of 4 years of instruction; assistant trainers have a minimum of 7 years of activity; and trainers must have at least 11 years in the area. The Feldenkrais Guild in Albany, Oregon, is the accrediting body for the Feldenkrais Method. For more information about the Feldenkrais method, see the Feldenkrais Guild of North America's Web site at www.feldenkrais.com.

Alexander Technique

Frederick M. Alexander (1869–1955) was an Australian-born actor who owned his own theater company and performed readings of Shakespeare. Before the invention of microphones, voice projection was vital to an actor's livelihood. After many fruitless attempts by physicians to cure the projection difficulty Alexander had, he discovered that his problem lay in his body posture and movement. He discovered how faulty posture, incorrect movement patterns, and inefficient movement could affect health, movement, and body function. He eventually abandoned his theatrical career and studied the human body and techniques to improve its efficiency of movement. In the early 1900s, he moved from Australia to England, where he taught his techniques.

Alexander discovered that posture is complex and that it involves not just sitting or standing straight, but also supporting and balancing against gravity during all daily activities. Children, he noticed, have good posture and good mechanics; but as people become older, the stresses and strains of life increase muscle tension and affect posture, as well as the way they use the body. Alexander believed that daily stresses over time produce increased muscle tension. This increased tension causes people to use their bodies inefficiently and ineffectively, eventually leading to injury and poor performance. For this reason, Alexander advocated unlearning, rather than learning. He felt that once we discarded the old, incorrect way of performing activities, the body would move naturally and easily.

The Alexander Technique involves the self-examination of functions such as posture, breathing, balance, and coordination. It is an educational process that includes an increased perception of kinesthesia and balance, self-awareness, and natural, stress-free movement. The Alexander Technique is also used to improve functional activities for fine-arts performers and athletes. As an individual's awareness, kinesthesia, and performance improve, pain is relieved and movement becomes more efficient.

The Alexander Technique includes first becoming aware of and releasing the tension that has become habitual over many years of improper movement; it then focuses on re-education to new ways of standing, sitting, and moving that are easier, more efficient, and less stressful to the body. The final phase of the technique includes development of new ways of handling the stresses encountered in daily living so that unnecessary muscle tension does not return. Changing behavior is vital to creating an effective and permanent alteration in body movement. Alexander's method of body awareness, re-education, and self-awareness allow the individual to make choices that ultimately influence movement. His intent was to create a re-education process that provides a stronger awareness of inner and outer self.

Alexander discovered that the body works as a whole, not in parts. He saw that a painful body part may be influenced by another area that may be the actual site of the pain or dysfunction. He also discovered that an individual produces the same reaction repeatedly until the abnormal motion becomes habitual and feels natural, even though it is abnormal. To correct these problems, he inhibited old motions, encouraged new and more correct motions, and had the individual repeat the corrected motions until the new task became natural. He would use light touch, verbal cueing, and self-awareness techniques until the individual did not need the touch and verbal cueing to perform the task correctly.

Alexander Technique sessions usually last 30 to 60 min and involve group classes or individual lessons. These lessons are a cooperative effort between the participant and the instructor. As the participant receives feedback, he or she gradually feels a lightening sensation. Normally, no more than about eight sessions are needed.

Alexander thought that there were two levels of control or "direction," primary and secondary. The primary control, according to Alexander, stems from the core of the body—the head, neck, and back. If freedom of this primary direction is not managed first, secondary control is not possible. Alexander's primary directions include release of neck, head, and back tension. Releasing the neck is necessary before releasing the tension in the head, and both those sites must be released before the back tension can be released.

Once the primary directions have been applied, the secondary directions can follow. These directions are more numerous and involve the extremities. Depending on where tension is, the secondary release areas may include the shoulders, hips, hands, knees, or other sites. For example, to release tension in the feet, the individual may be instructed to think of the feet spreading onto the ground as the toes lengthen. To release the tension in the upper chest, the person may be instructed to allow the shoulders to release away from one another.

The Alexander Technique is one of thought rather than of action. It emphasizes the individual's thinking of the release rather than actually performing the activity. Alexander believed that attempts to produce the action increases muscle tension instead of relieving it. The individual must practice following the directions several times so that he or she becomes very familiar with them and can feel a change in control. Awareness of actions and performance makes one better able to control those actions and change performance.

Alexander Technique instructors must obtain a minimum of 1,600 hours, or three years, of experience and education before they can become certified. The American Center for the Alexander Technique is headquartered in New York City.

It will be helpful to consider a couple of athletic activities and incorporate into them the Alexander Technique of improved awareness and conscious correction with assistance. The common activity of running requires an inefficient expenditure of energy if it is not performed correctly. The Alexander Technique teacher uses gentle touch and verbal instructions to correct the runner's movements until the runner is able to perform the technique using self-awareness and self-correction.

Used in soccer, the Alexander Technique can also be used to improve kicking technique. The Alexander Technique teacher can provide instruction to permit the soccer player to release unwanted muscle tension, become aware of muscle activity, and correct the kicking technique to permit a more effective and efficient movement.

For more information about the Alexander Technique, see http://alexandertechnique.com, www.life.uiuc.edu/jeff/alextech.html, or www.ati-net.com.

Pilates Method

Joseph H. Pilates (1880-1968) was born in Germany. He was a sickly child, suffering from asthma, rickets, and rheumatic fever. Determined to overcome his illnesses, he underwent self-study and practice in a combination of yoga, Zen, and ancient Greek and Roman physical conditioning regimens. Prior to World War I he was living in England and working as a performer and boxer. During the war, he was interned with other German nationals in a camp where he began instructing his fellow camp members in his exercise routines. From England, he moved to New York City where he opened a studio and used his techniques with dancers.

Pilates called his exercise regimen "Contrology." He defined it as the art of control. He believed that our will should control our muscles. He was a firm believer that movement starts from our core: the abdominal, lower back, buttock, and hip muscles. The body's balance and stability originated in these muscles. He called these muscles the "powerhouse" of our bodies.

His method was based on a philosophy that integrated body awareness with conditioning. The goal was to improve flexibility, coordination, strength, tone, muscle control, and mental conditioning to improve the whole person. Pilates was also concerned with the process, so he advocated continuous movement through a natural evolution: moving from one exercise to the next to ultimately build strength from the inside out and rebalance the body. He believed that balance was the factor to seek, and since everyone is different, each person's program must be individually designed. Because of this belief, he often did not teach the same exercise from one day to the next but rather adjusted to meet the individual's needs.

Although different pieces of equipment have been designed for the Pilates Method, it is not necessary to use equipment to perform Pilates exercises. During his life, Joseph Pilates designed 500 exercises. This is probably because he designed programs to meet the needs of the individual. He did not organize or form an association to carry on his techniques and methods; for this reason, there are many different instructors, companies, and businesses today that have created programs based on the Pilates Method and various versions of it. Pilates classes can be found around the country in workshops, private sessions, health clubs, hospitals, clinics, and gyms.

The Pilates Method revolves around a few basic principles. Most advocates list eight to nine principles. The first principle is *relaxation*. Relaxation allows the body to release tension and stress and provides a nice balance for body and mind. Many people use relaxation at the beginning of their Pilates workout to rid themselves of the day's stress and allow themselves to concentrate better on the session. Relaxation enhances correct firing patterns to improve posture and breathing. The next principle is *concentration*. Since the mind is used to reeducate the muscles, Pilates exercises should be performed in an environment without distractions to achieve the necessary level of concentration. Focusing your mind on your movements enhances the sense of where your body is in space. *Control* is learned using concentration and practice of each exercise. Exercises start simple and become more complex as control improves. Another principle is *breathing*. Using the diaphragm and other respiratory muscles encourages both flexibility and strength of the rib cage and its muscles. This allows for optimal use of breathing during exercises to both prepare for movement and aid in the exercise and recovery. *Centering* is the fifth principle and deals with the idea that motion and energy begin in the center or the core and branch outward to the periphery. Using the core muscles as stabilizers produces effective and safe body movements. *Postural alignment* is important for safety during exercises and correcting muscle imbalances. A correct posture will encourage proper muscle activation and coordination. *Fluidity of movement* means moving slowly and gracefully with control. Slow movements allow you to monitor your posture and muscle activity to assure correct activation patterns. The exercises are performed with the individual moving from one exercise to the next, flowing gracefully through the exercise routine. Since Pilates movements are executed with precision, motions should be slow to more accurately assess them as you perform them. Finally, *stamina* is achieved as you progress in the program. As motion becomes more efficient, endurance improves. Your body becomes less tired with activities you found previously exhausting because your body moves with less stress and more energy conservation.

Body-awareness programs, which focus on self-improvement through awareness of movement patterns and abilities, include the Feldenkrais Method, the Alexander Technique, and the Pilates Method.

■ A Pilates Method Example

The following example of a progression of the Pilates Method is based on a program outlined in *The Pilates Body* (Siler, 2000). Outlined below is a description of sequential exercises for beginners; each exercise is performed 3 to 5 times:

1. Lie down on a floor mat on your back with your hips and knees flexed and feet comfortably on the floor; the arms are extended along the sides. Tighten your buttocks, squeeze the knees together, pull your navel to your spine, inhale, and roll up slowly, starting with moving your chin to your chest and moving your shoulders and trunk up and forward. As your body comes up into a sitting position, you exhale and the legs are simultaneously stretched forward into extension. As you move sequentially through this motion, imagine a progression of lifting from the beginning with your chin lifted to your chest, your chest lifted over your ribs, your ribs lifted over your abdomen, and your abdomen lifted over your hips. To return to the starting position, breathe in, squeeze the buttocks, tuck your coccyx, and pull your navel to your spine as you start to flex your knees. Reverse the roll-up sequence, and exhale as you feel your back begin to unroll onto the mat. By the end, your head and arms should be resting on the mat.

2. Begin in the starting position of the first exercise. Pull your navel to your spine and extend one leg to the ceiling with the hip in lateral rotation. Maintain the navel-to-the-spine position and perform a hip circle, inhaling and beginning the movement in an adducted position, circling down, around, and breathe in as you move the leg up to the start position; the circle should be large enough to maintain control and prevent the leg from wobbling and not permit the buttocks to lift off the mat. Once you have completed the 3 to 5 repetitions, perform the exercise in the opposite direction, and then repeat the exercise with the other leg. Return to the starting position.

3. In a sitting position with the hips and knees flexed, placed a hand under each distal thigh and lift the feet off the floor until you are balancing on your coccyx. Become round like a ball by tucking your chin to your chest and moving your elbows away from your sides. Pull your navel to your spine, inhale, and roll backward, maintaining your arm and leg positions relative to each other and to your chest. Exhale as you return to the starting position but do not touch the feet to the floor. Create the movement from your abdominals, not your neck, shoulders, or legs.

4. Lie on your back with your knees pulled toward your chest. Grab one shin with your hands and extend the other leg to the ceiling. Place the outside hand on the flexed leg's ankle and the other hand on the flexed leg's knee; both shoulders should remain depressed throughout the exercise. Pull your navel to your spine and lift your head and neck to reach your chin toward your abdomen. Exhale and hold the position. Keeping your navel to your spine, inhale and switch arm and leg positions, maintaining a flat back to the mat. Squeeze the buttocks as you switch leg positions.

5. Sit in a long-sitting position with your knees flexed slightly and your feet separated wider than your hips. Flex the shoulders to 90° with the elbows extended in front of you and your scapula depressed. In this position, flex your ankles and inhale to extend your trunk longitudinally. As you bring your chin to your chest, roll downward and bring your navel to your spine. Keeping your hips stable, exhale and move your upper body forward while resisting the stretch forward by pulling back with your abdominals. Now inhale and reverse back to the chin-tucked position. Then exhale as you return to the tall seated starting position. At the very end you should be sitting tall with your back flat and your scapulae depressed.

The advantage of Pilates is that anyone at any level of fitness may begin the program. It is not meant to increase bulk, but its goal is to create total body awareness and control through a coordinated effort between the mind and body. The exercises should be pain free. The method can be used for general health, rehabilitation, and sport-specific training. For more information about the Pilates Method, see www.pilates.com or www.pilates.net.

SUMMARY

Since poor posture can have an impact on injury and injury recovery, patient posture is evaluated as part of the rehabilitation evaluation. Posture assessment includes evaluation of posture from anterior, posterior, and lateral views, and looking for abnormalities in alignment from the head down to the toes. Muscle imbalances account for many postural deviations and must be corrected if a rehabilitation program is to have a lasting positive outcome. Instructions in proper body mechanics are incorporated early in a rehabilitation program. Proper body mechanics allows the body to be used more efficiently and effectively, and it reduces the risk of injury.

KEY CONCEPTS AND REVIEW

1. Identify the primary elements of proper alignment in standing from an anterior, posterior, and side view.

In an anterior position, a plumb line should bisect the nose and mouth and should run through the central portion of the sternum, umbilicus, and pubic bones. The earlobes should be level with one another, as should the shoulders, fingertip ends, nipples, iliac crests, patellae, and medial malleoli. The patellae should point straight ahead, with the feet straight or turned slightly outward. The knees and ankles are in line with each other with the knees angled neither inward nor outward in relation to each other.

From a side view, the plumb line should pass through the external auditory meatus, the earlobe, the bodies of the cervical vertebrae, the center of the shoulder joint, and the greater trochanter. The plumb line should run midway between the back and chest and between the back and abdomen, slightly posterior to the hip joint, and slightly anterior to the center of the knee just behind the patella. A horizontal line should connect the ASIS and PSIS. The patient should remain relaxed with the body's weight balanced between the heel and the forefoot. The knees are straight but not locked. The chin is slightly tucked and the chest is held slightly up and forward. There is a mild curve inward of the low back and neck regions.

In the posterior view, a plumb line should bisect the head and should follow the spinous processes from the cervical through the lumbar spine. The earlobes, shoulders, scapulae, hips, PSIS, gluteal fold, posterior knee creases, and medial malleoli should appear level left to right. The scapulae should lie against the rib cage between the second and seventh ribs and about 5 cm (2 in.) from the spinous processes. The calcaneus should be straight, and the calcaneal tendon should be perpendicular to the floor. Trunk muscles should appear balanced, with symmetrical development. The shoulders should be positioned down and relaxed. Body weight should appear equally distributed over both feet.

2. Discuss common postural faults and describe their causes.

A muscle strength imbalance or shortening of a muscle or group can cause common postural faults. These changes usually occur over time and can cause any number of postural changes, depending on the specific area. Some examples of common postural faults include anterior-posterior or lateral spinal deformities such as scoliosis, lordosis, and kyphosis; hip anteversion and retroversion; winking or frog-eye patellae, genu recurvatum; genu and ankle varus and valgus; pes cavus and pes planus; and hammertoes, claw toes, and bunions.

3. Outline corrective exercises for common postural faults.

Once the cause of the fault has been determined, corrective exercises are used to reduce or relieve the fault. In many instances, strengthening of weak muscles combined with stretching of tight structures is fundamental and vital to correction, especially the strengthening of the weak muscles. In addition, the individual must make a conscious effort to correct postural faults in order to stop poor habits and establish new, correct ones.

4. Explain the importance of good posture and proper body mechanics in athletics.

Good posture is vital to good execution of sport activity because it improves efficiency and reduces the risk of injury. Imbalances that occur because of poor posture and mechanics place the body at risk of injury because of already increased stresses on structures. One area must compensate for the deficiencies in another area, causing the body to perform less efficiently and effectively.

5. List the basic principles of good body mechanics.

Maintain a "straight" spine so that forces from the legs can be transferred upward; reduce the height of the center of gravity for increased stability; widen the base of support for more stability; stand in the direction of movement or force application; and maintain good strength in the abdominals and lower-extremity muscles.

6. Discuss an example of the use of proper body mechanics by the rehabilitation clinician during a treatment program.

When providing manual resistance, the rehabilitation clinician stands close to the patient, uses leg strength to deliver the manual resistance, keeps the back straight, and stands with the feet in the direction of the resisted movement.

7. Explain the differences and similarities between the Feldenkrais Method, the Pilates Method, and the Alexander Technique.

All methods are based on correction of the dysfunctional somatic feedback system and use of self-awareness, reeducation, and repetition as part of the correction process. The Feldenkrais Method improves movement through changing awareness of movement; it engages the entire person in the treatment program by promoting self-esteem and improving learning skills. The Pilates Method controls body movement through a balance between mind and body. The core muscles serve as the "powerhouse" from which movement is initiated, and movement follows a smooth flow from one motion to the next. The Alexander Technique emphasizes the unlearning of old and improper habits and establishing new habits based on self-evaluation and increased perception of kinesthesia and natural movement.

CRITICAL THINKING QUESTIONS

1. You are working in an industrial clinic where back injuries are frequently treated. In an effort to be more efficient, you design a handout for these back patients that will include instructions for proper lifting and sitting. What items will you include in the handout? Will you include any precautions? What about general information on back anatomy and mechanics? Why would you or would you not include this information?

2. A shoulder patient you are treating has poor upper-back and cervical posture. You feel that this is complicating the shoulder injury and that you must correct the patient's posture before you can effectively impact the shoulder. How can the thoracic and cervical posture affect the shoulder? What will you do to improve this posture? What cues and instructions will you provide the patient?

3. The secretary for your department spends most of her day at the computer and on the phone. She is complaining about upper back and neck pain and has asked you to help her. On what areas will your examination be focused? What is the probable cause for her complaints, and what can she do to alleviate the problem?

4. A patient with plantar fasciitis has some postural deviations in the lower extremities. In addition to excessively pronated feet, she also has tibial torsion and squinting patellae. What other deviations in the hips would you expect, given these abnormalities?

5. Based on the opening scenario for this chapter, what instructions would you give Dee on proper lifting mechanics? What precise lifting instructions would you give her? What types of lifting activities would you include in her program?

6. When you are providing lower-extremity proprioceptive neuromuscular facilitation (PNF) to a patient who is lying on the table, what correct body mechanics would you use? What would be the position for your base of support? How would you transfer your body weight? Where would your body be positioned to offer the best resistance on hip extension? On hip flexion?

LAB ACTIVITIES

1. Perform a posture analysis on a lab partner. Identify all areas of malalignment or deviations from normal. Evaluate his/her posture from all three angles. Identify if there are any corrective causes for these postural deviations. What exercises would you provide to correct or reduce these deviations?

2. If you have a digital camera, take photos of your friends of family members who have postural deviations. Identify which deviations each has and if the deviation is mild, moderate, or severe.

3. In a group of three or four classmates, go around campus and take digital photos of as many postural deviations as you can find. After a specific time established by your instructor, report (along with the other teams) the types and numbers of postural deviations you have captured. The team with the greatest number or types of postural deviations and that correctly identifies them is the winner.

4. Have your lab partner lie supine on the treatment table. If you are going to provide manual resistance to your lab partner's hip flexion and hip extension motions, how are you going to stand and move as he moves the hip through the range of motion? What is the best position for your body? Where is the best placement of your hands on your partner's leg for your mechanical advantage? How do you move your body to allow the resistance to be easier for you? Where is your arm offering the resistance in comparison to where your body is throughout the exercises? What have you learned from this activity?

5. Have your lab partner sit on the end of a treatment table. Offer him/her manual resistance to knee extension. How are you going to position your body to make the activity easiest for you? Where is your body in relation to your lab partner's leg? How does your body movement change as the leg goes through its range of motion? What must you do to continue to make the manual resistance exercise an easy activity for you? What have you learned from this activity?

6. Have your lab partner perform an athletic activity such as a tennis serve, basketball free-throw or layup, soccer kick, volleyball serve or net block, football pass or front line block, or baseball toss. What instructions are you going to provide that will allow your partner to perform the athletic activity using good body mechanics? Have him/her repeat the performance using your instructions; how was the performance this time? What additional tips and instructional points do you need to provide for your partner to perform with better body mechanics? What are the basic principles that your lab partner must remember to perform the activity correctly? Once your partner is able to perform the activity using good body mechanics, how did the actual performance change (in terms of distance thrown or kicked, force produced, or speed of delivery)? Why?

ADDITIONAL SOURCE

Hislop, H.J. and J. Montgomery. 2002. *Daniels and Worthingham's muscle testing. Techniques of manual examination*. Philadelphia: WB Saunders.

Ambulation and Ambulation Aids

OBJECTIVES

After completing this chapter, you should be able to do the following:

1. Discuss the general concepts of gait.
2. Identify the range-of-motion changes during the gait cycle.
3. Explain the muscle activity involved in ambulation.
4. Describe the general mechanical differences between walking and running.
5. Discuss one abnormal gait commonly seen following a musculoskeletal injury.
6. Outline the various types of gait with assistive devices.
7. Explain the technique involved in stair climbing with assistive devices.
8. Identify the safety measures involved in ambulating with assistive devices.

▶ When Michelle, a 38-year-old competitive soccer player, first injured her ankle, she was unable to walk on it. Her second-degree sprain was conservatively treated with a cast for two weeks and then placed in a splint for four weeks. By the time Drew Williams, certified athletic trainer, saw Michelle, she was out of the splint and off crutches but was still not able to walk normally. Drew analyzed her gait to evaluate for deficiencies in range of motion and strength before performing specific motion and strength tests. He did not have her run because she was not walking normally, but he knew that one day he would analyze her running gait as well.

Since Michelle was still limping severely, he instructed her in how to walk with a cane. She didn't want to use crutches any longer, but saw the cane as a compromise until she could walk normally without it. Drew was careful to provide her with precautions about using the cane and would not allow her to use it on her own until she demonstrated proper use on the floor, carpet, and stairs.

Walking is the best possible exercise.
Habituate yourself to walk very far.

THOMAS JEFFERSON, (1743-1826), third president of the United States (1801-1809);
author of the Declaration of Independence

People have been walking long before Mr. Jefferson advocated it as exercise. Watching how a patient moves during ambulation, from the feet all the way up to the head, can yield important information to the rehabilitation clinician. To know whether a patient ambulates normally, you must understand what normal gait is. Before you can instruct a patient in how to use assistive devices during ambulation, you must first understand the mechanics of those assistive devices and the desired gait with the devices.

Ambulation is a normal activity that most of us perform every day without thinking about it, about what it involves, or about how we do it. We just do it. When an injury prevents normal ambulation, walking suddenly becomes difficult and energy consuming. It no longer is something we take for granted, and it no longer is automatic.

This chapter introduces the mechanics of walking and introduces differences between walking and running. We will consider normal ambulation, common pathological gaits, and ambulation with assistive devices. Topics include the mechanics of assistive device applications, various gaits with different types of assistive devices on different surfaces, and methods of selecting assistive devices for the patient.

NORMAL GAIT

Ambulation, or walking, is the locomotion method we use to move our body from one place to another. The way we walk is called *gait*. Although each person's gait is slightly different from everyone else's, all normal gaits have basic similarities. In fact, considering how many body types and sizes there are among human beings, it is surprising how little normal gait differs from one person to the next. Major differences commonly result from postural variations, weaknesses, structural abnormalities, and soft-tissue length alterations, some of which are discussed in chapter 11. Knowledge of normal gait is essential to the rehabilitation clinician so that he or she can correct abnormal gait following injury and understand the use of assistive devices.

Gait Cycle

One **gait cycle** is the time from the point at which the heel of one foot touches the ground to the time it touches the ground again. A gait cycle is divided into two phases, the stance phase and the swing phase. The **stance phase** occurs when the foot is in contact with the floor and the extremity is bearing partial or total body weight. The stance phase is subdivided into three parts. **Heel strike,** or **foot strike,** occurs when the heel or foot first comes in contact with the floor. **Foot flat,** as the term implies, occurs when the foot is flat on the floor. Just as the heel may not be the first part of the foot to strike the ground in runners and some pathological gaits so that "foot strike" is more appropriate than "heel strike," some believe that the term "foot flat" should be replaced with the term "reversal of fore shear to aft shear" since the foot may not achieve a flat position in some pathological gaits (Chambers & Sutherland, 2002). The **midstance** phase occurs when the foot is directly under the body's weight and the entire foot is in contact with the floor. Because the body weight is transferred entirely to the one supporting leg and the other leg is in the middle of its swing phase, this is also referred to as **single-leg support. Heel-off** occurs when the weight begins to transfer to the front of the foot, and the heel lifts off the floor. Partial weight remains on the extremity as the contralateral extremity is now in contact with the floor again. **Toe-off** occurs when the foot comes off the floor. From that point, the swing phase begins. This phase is also referred to as *push-off,* since the extremity now propels the body forward and the leg continues into the second phase of gait.

The second gait phase, **swing phase,** occurs when the foot is not in contact with the floor and no weight is borne on the extremity. The swing phase begins immediately after toe-off and is divided into early-, mid-, and late-swing phases. Immediately after toe-off, the leg begins its early swing, or **acceleration phase,** as momentum increases from the thrust obtained at toe-off and propels the extremity forward. The mid-swing of the swing phase is also called **swing-through.** The leg continues its swing-through until just before heel strike when it goes through the late swing, or **deceleration phase,** to slow its forward propulsion, make a smooth contact with the floor, and begin a new gait cycle. Alternative terminology can also be used and is often seen in research reports on gait. With this nomenclature, the initial heel (foot) strike with the floor is termed **initial contact,** and as the foot progresses to increased weight bearing, it goes from initial contact to **loading response** (foot flat), then **midstance** (single-leg support). In this terminology, heel-off is **terminal stance** and progresses to **preswing** (toe-off). The swing phase begins after preswing and is divided into **initial swing** (early swing/acceleration), **midswing** (swing-through), and **terminal swing** (late swing/deceleration). Some researchers and clinicians prefer this terminology because the terms provide for greater consistency and descriptor accuracy in reporting analysis and results.

Clinicians vary in the terminology they use. Clinicians' choice of terminology for gait analysis most often depends on the method they were taught and on what is most intuitive for them. Both groups of terms are presented here so you can become familiar with each. These alternative terms are used interchangeably throughout this text.

One gait cycle from the beginning of stance phase to the end of swing phase is 100%, and stance phase is 62% (usually rounded off to 60%) of the gait cycle. Within the stance, heel strike to foot flat covers 0% to 12% of the gait cycle; midstance occurs over the next 12% to 30%; heel-off begins at 30% and continues until toe-off at the start of the swing cycle (figure 12.1). The remaining 38% (usually rounded off to 40%) of the gait cycle occurs during the swing phase. As speed of the gait increases, the percentages between the stance and swing phases become more equal. In running, the percentage becomes greater for the swing phase than for the stance phase.

During the first and last 10% of stance in walking, the body is supported by both lower extremities (Ounpuu, 1994). This occurs at the beginning of the stance phase during heel strike for one leg and at the end of the stance phase, just before toe-off, for the other. This part of stance is referred to as **double-limb support.**

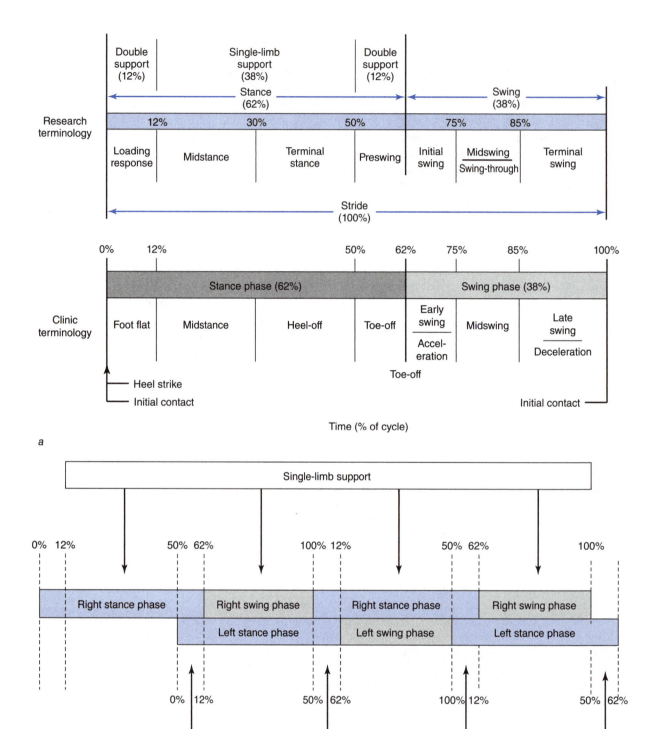

▶ **Figure 12.1**   (*a*) Single-leg gait cycle, (*b*) double-leg gait cycle.

Center-of-Gravity Pathway

The body's center of gravity propels forward during ambulation. Its relative position also changes because of the associated changes in position of the joints and extremities during ambulation. Before we can understand the changes that occur and their importance, we must clarify some terms.

Stride length is the distance from heel strike of one foot to heel strike of the same foot in one gait cycle. **Step length** is the distance from heel strike of one foot to heel strike of the other foot in one gait cycle. Although stride length depends on the individual's height, an average stride length is 156 cm (61 in.) (Lehmann, 1990).

The body's side-to-side movement as weight shifts from one lower extremity to the other is **stride width** (figure 12.2). It is the distance between the midline of one foot at midstance and the midline of the other foot at midstance. Stride width also has individual determining factors such as body size and weight, but the average stride width ranges from 5 cm (about 2 in.) (Chambers & Sutherland, 2002) to 8 cm (about 3 in.) ± 3.5 (Lehmann, 1990).

There is large variation in the rate at which individuals walk. Reports of what is normal walking speed vary. The range is from just under 60 strides per minute (Lehmann, 1990; Murray, Drought, & Kory, 1964) to 101 to 122 steps per minute (Winter, 1987). Stance and swing phases are directly influenced as cadence increases to jogging, running, and sprinting speeds. We will consider the mechanics of running in the section "Normal Running Gait" later in this chapter.

As the body is propelled forward, it attempts to create motion that is as efficient as possible. Keeping the center-of-gravity movement to a minimum is how we achieve efficiency of movement. Short of the lower extremities being wheels instead of legs, a multijoint system is the best way to propel the body forward efficiently. Although a wheel system would move the body very efficiently over flat surfaces, movement over uneven surfaces would become quite difficult. Using a number of joints from the pelvis to the foot, the body minimizes center-of-gravity pathway changes by changing the position of the joints as the body moves, and simultaneously allows for adjustment to varying types of surfaces and terrain.

In order for propulsion of the body to be smooth and efficient, the body must produce enough force to move forward but also control the movement and momentum so that the body remains stable as its positions change. It must also absorb the impact shock of moving weight from one leg to the other. All these capabilities must be present and must be controlled if movement is to be efficient and effective. Loss of one of the contributing factors can result in poor quality of movement, high-energy requirements, or injury.

Since the body does not move on wheels, its bipedal system causes an efficient sinusoidal motion of the body's center of gravity that rises and falls an average of about 4 cm (1.6 inches) (Chambers & Sutherland, 2002). Moving the body's center of gravity in a wavelike fashion conserves energy and reduces impact forces (figure 12.3).

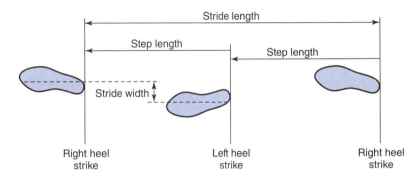

▶ **Figure 12.2** Stride length and stride width.

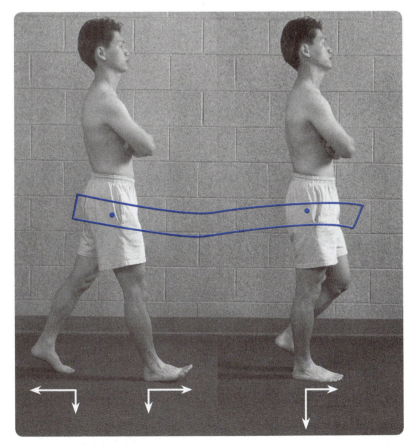

▶ **Figure 12.3** Sinusoidal motion.

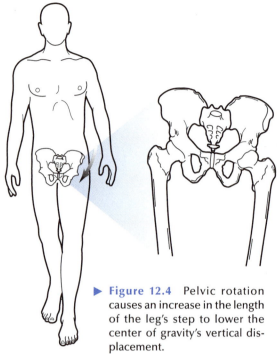

▶ **Figure 12.4** Pelvic rotation causes an increase in the length of the leg's step to lower the center of gravity's vertical displacement.

Determinants of Gait

The body's center of gravity moves through a sinusoidal movement in both vertical and horizontal directions during locomotion. This sinusoidal movement was originally thought to be produced through what Saunders and colleagues (Saunders, Inman, & Eberhart, 1953) identified as six determinants of gait. Their theory stated that energy expenditure requirements during gait were minimized by minimal changes in the body's center of gravity. Although more recent investigations have disproved their theory, the concepts presented in their original theory help to identify how the cooperative efforts of the trunk, pelvis, and extremities provide an efficient system of gait (Childress and Gard, 1997; Gard and Childress, 1999). For this reason, these concepts are presented here.

Pelvic Rotation

Pelvic rotation occurs around a vertical axis in the transverse plane. As one leg swings forward, the pelvis rotates forward to increase the length of the leg's step. The pelvis attains its maximum rotation on one side, 4°, at the point of double-leg support. With lengthening of the leg, the center of gravity is prevented from dropping lower than it otherwise would (figure 12.4). The pelvis rotates 4° on the opposite side as that leg rotates forward during the same process. The total pelvic rotation is 8°, or 4° on each side.

Pelvic Tilt

During midstance, the pelvis tilts downward on an anterior-posterior axis from the stance leg so that the hip on the swing-leg side is lower than that on the stance-leg side (figure 12.5). The hip abductors of the stance leg control this movement. Because the body's center of gravity is midway between the hips, it moves downward when the swing leg is lowered. This movement lowers the center of gravity during midstance by five degrees and reduces the vertical displacement of the center of gravity by 3/16 inch.

Knee Flexion at Midstance

At heel strike, the knee is in extension, but immediately afterward, it begins to flex until it flexes to 15° by midstance (figure 12.6). This knee flexion lowers the center of gravity when it is at its highest point of the sinusoidal motion curve.

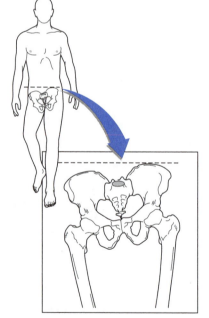

▶ **Figure 12.5** Pelvic tilt decreases vertical displacement of the center of gravity.

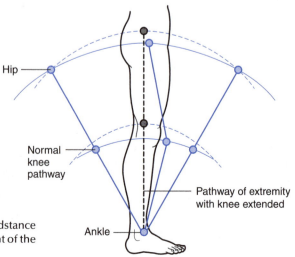

Hip

Normal knee pathway

Pathway of extremity with knee extended

Ankle

▶ **Figure 12.6** Knee flexion at midstance decreases vertical displacement of the center of gravity at midstance.

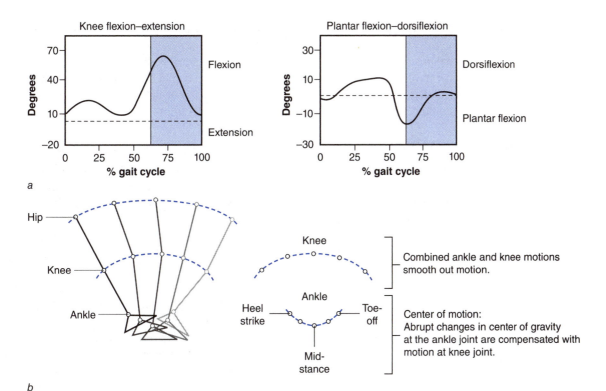

▶ **Figure 12.7** Knee and ankle motions in gait. The opposite motions occurring at the ankle and knee reduce vertical excursion of the center of gravity.

Ankle Motion

The center of gravity of the ankle joint is highest at heel strike and toe-off and lowest at midstance. This is the opposite of what happens with the knee joint, as seen in figure 12.7. These combined motions help to reduce the vertical excursion of the center of gravity and smooth out its sinusoidal curve.

The combined effects of pelvic rotation, pelvic tilt, and knee and ankle motions during stance minimize the overall vertical displacement to less than 5 cm.

Lateral Motion of Pelvis

In order for a person to stand with stability, the center of gravity must be over the base of support, the feet. When we stand on two feet, the center of gravity falls between the feet. To stand on one leg, the center of gravity must shift so that it is over the supporting leg. If the thighs were arranged in a parallel fashion, a maximum shift of 15 cm (6 in.) of the pelvis would be needed to transfer the center of gravity from one supporting leg to the other during single-limb support (figure 12.8). Because the femurs are not straight but angled medially to place the knees in a slight valgus position, the lateral shift required of the pelvis to move from one leg to the other is only 4.3 cm (1.7 in.) for an adult. This lateral sway of less than 5

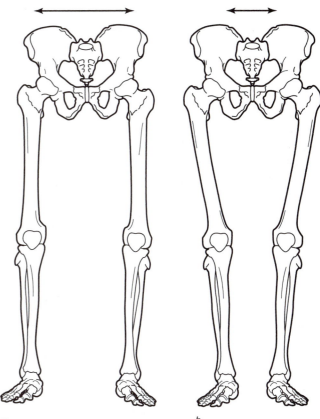

▶ **Figure 12.8** Hip and knee alignment in lateral pelvic shift. Adducted thigh alignment reduces lateral sway during gait. *(a)* If thighs were parallel, it would require a lateral movement of 15 cm during ambulation. *(b)* Normal hip angulation minimizes lateral pelvic motion during ambulation to less than 5 cm.

cm (2 in.) is also a sinusoidal curve, making the movement from one leg to the other during gait smooth.

The maximal position of the left-to-right sinusoidal curve occurs during midstance of each leg and is at the midline during double-limb support. The maximal height of the sinusoidal curve in vertical displacement also occurs during midstance of each leg and is at its lowest point during double-limb support.

Gait Kinematics

The sinusoidal curves of motion that occur during ambulation are caused by changes in the joints' ranges of motion. Some of these changes are not large but are important for smooth motion. Movement occurs in the sagittal, frontal, and transverse planes. If movement in one plane is restricted, smooth gait will not occur. Therefore, the clinician needs to understand the sequence, degree, and timing of joint motion so that when deficiencies exist, he or she can correct them.

Trunk and Upper Extremities

Throughout all cycles of normal gait, the trunk is in an erect and neutral position. This is necessary to maintain the center of gravity over the base of support. Trunk movement is coordinated with pelvic movement so that as the pelvis rotates in one direction, the trunk rotates in the opposite direction (figure 12.9). The swing momentum of the arms assists the trunk in its rotation, so trunk movement is less. This coordinated movement between the pelvis and trunk aids in making the gait smooth and stable.

Pelvis

Pelvis movement is defined in terms of iliac crest movement. Forward motion of the iliac crest produces an anterior pelvic tilt, and backward motion produces a posterior pelvic tilt. Pelvis motion in the frontal, sagittal, and transverse planes is seen in the graphs in figure 12.10.

Heel Strike to Midstance   As the heel hits the ground at heel strike, the pelvis remains level and is in a 5° forwardly rotated position in the sagittal plane; as the body progresses toward midstance, the pelvis reduces its anterior tilt. In the frontal plane, it is elevated 4° at heel strike and begins to drop after initial contact has been made. As the leg goes from heel strike to midstance, the pelvis medially rotates 4°.

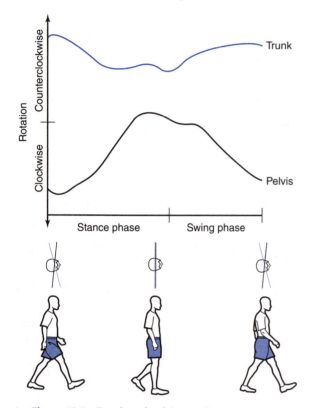

▶ **Figure 12.9**   Trunk and pelvic rotation.

Adapted from M.P. Murray, A.B. Drought, and R.C. Kory, 1964, "Walking patterns of normal men," *Journal of Bone and Joint Surgery* 46-A: 335-360, fig. 10.

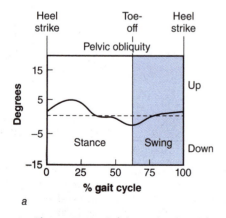

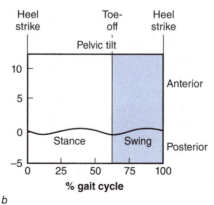

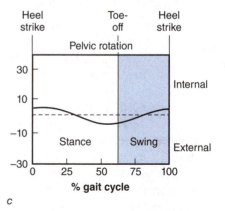

▶ **Figure 12.10**   Pelvic motion in *(a)* frontal plane, *(b)* sagittal plane, *(c)* transverse plane. Pelvic motion is a triplanar event.

Midstance to Toe-Off By the time the leg reaches the end of stance phase, the pelvis has moved into a posterior rotation position of about 5°. In a frontal plane during midstance to toe-off, the pelvis continues to drop until it reaches a total of 8° of lateral movement. During the final moments of stance phase, the pelvis rotates laterally, 8° from the initial position of 4° medial rotation to an ending stance position of 4° lateral rotation.

Early Swing In early swing, the pelvis is level and in a posterior rotation of 5° moving toward anterior rotation. In the frontal plane, it begins to move from a downward to an elevated position. Rotation in the transverse plane is gradual from 4° of lateral rotation to 4° of medial rotation by late swing.

Late Swing The pelvis continues to be level throughout the gait cycle, moving in the sagittal plane from an anterior position at the middle of the swing phase to a posterior position by the end of late swing. Frontal plane movement continues from its maximum downward position during early swing on its way toward an elevated position such that it is slightly elevated by the end of swing. Rotation also continues to progress in a medial direction as swing phase is terminated.

Total motions of the pelvis during a gait cycle are 4° of anterior-posterior tilt, 8° of lateral tilt, and 8° of rotation.

Hip

Hip motion also occurs in three planes of movement: the frontal, sagittal, and transverse planes (figure 12.11).

Heel Strike to Midstance At heel strike the hip is in 30° of flexion, slight adduction of 2° to 6°, and near-neutral rotation at 5°. As the leg advances in the stance phase, the hip becomes less flexed, becomes less adducted, and goes from slight medial rotation to slight lateral rotation.

Midstance to Toe-Off In the last half of the stance phase, the hip goes from 10° of extension at heel-off to ~5° to 0° extension at the time of toe-off. The hip is at neutral in the frontal plane at heel-off and goes into 4° of abduction at toe-off. After midstance, the hip moves from medial rotation to neutral at heel-off until it reaches 4° of lateral rotation at toe-off. Part of the apparent hip extension that occurs from midstance to toe-off is actually the result of a posterior rotation and downward tilt of the pelvis.

Early Swing In its initial swing, the hip continues to flex to 15° to 20°, reaches its maximum abduction of an average of 5°, and continues to have slight lateral rotation.

Late Swing Sagittal plane movement continues to advance to ~30° just before the end of swing. Frontal plane movement continues to advance from maximal abduction just after the start of early swing toward the midline until a neutral position occurs just before heel strike. Transverse plane movement oscillates throughout swing from medial to neutral to lateral rotation then back to slight medial rotation just before heel strike.

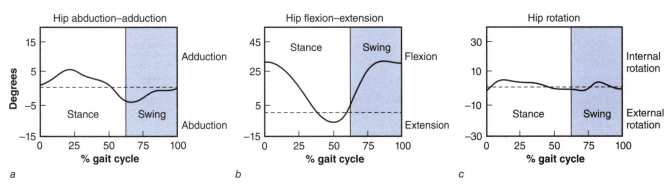

▶ **Figure 12.11** Hip motion in the *(a)* frontal plane, *(b)* sagittal plane, *(c)* transverse plane. Hip motion is triplanar with the greatest movement occurring in the sagittal plane and the least occurring in the transverse plane.

Total hip motions occurring during the gait cycle include 43° in the sagittal plane from flexion to extension, 13° of abduction-adduction in the frontal plane, and 8° of rotation in the transverse plane.

Knee

The knee performs the greatest amount of motion during the swing phase of the gait cycle. Rotation of the knee occurs throughout the gait cycle. Knee rotation is most likely affected by a combination of tibial rotation and hip rotation occurring synchronously.

Heel Strike to Midstance   At heel strike, the knee is in or close to full extension. The tibia is laterally rotated 8° to 10°. As weight acceptance on the leg increases, the knee flexes to 15° and tibial rotation begins to occur in a medial direction (figure 12.12).

Midstance to Toe-Off   By the time the extremity reaches midstance, the knee has achieved its maximum degree of flexion in the stance phase and begins to move into full extension at heel-off. After achievement of maximal tibial medial rotation just before midstance, a return to lateral rotation occurs during the later half of stance until maximal lateral rotation occurs immediately before toe-off. Immediately before toe-off, the knee is passively flexed to 35° by the active movement of the ankle as it goes into plantar flexion and forces the weight-bearing knee to flex.

Early Swing   The knee continues to progress to a maximum of 60° of flexion; this occurs so that the foot clears the ground during the swing phase. In the body's attempt to conserve energy, foot clearance from the floor during swing is only a mere 0.87 cm (.3 in.) (Rodgers, 1988). That small clearance leaves little room for error. It is no wonder that fatigue or restricted

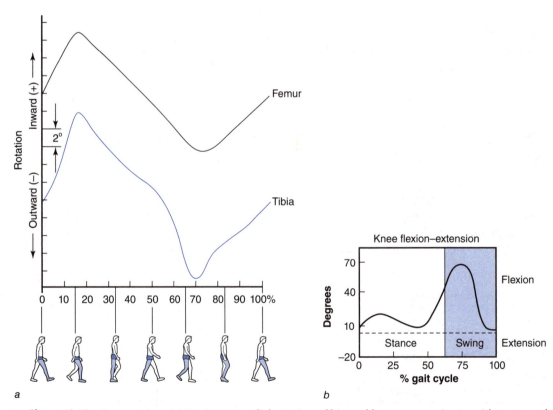

▶ **Figure 12.12**   Knee motion: *(a)* Maximum medial rotation of hip and knee occur prior to midstance, and maximum lateral rotation occurs at the end of stance and into early swing phase. *(b)* Maximum knee extension occurs after midstance, whereas maximum knee flexion occurs in swing phase.

knee motion will increase the likelihood of stubbing the toe when the foot is moving off the ground. The tibia begins moving from the maximum laterally rotated position that it was in at toe-off toward inward rotation, although it continues to maintain some degree of lateral rotation throughout swing.

Late Swing   After achieving 60° of flexion in the first half of swing, the knee moves progressively and steadily toward extension until it is at 0° just before heel strike. Total knee range of motion in the sagittal plane is 60°, and tibial rotation is 18°. Maximum knee flexion during the stance phase occurs during midstance, and maximum knee flexion during the swing phase occurs during midswing. Maximum knee medial rotation occurs between heel strike and midstance in what researchers call the loading response, and maximum lateral rotation occurs at toe-off.

Ankle

The ankle and foot work together during gait and provide balance that is needed as the body moves over uneven ground. The ankle joint is responsible for forward motion and stability, and the foot joints are responsible for medial and lateral adjustments. The foot and ankle are complex structures and demonstrate highly variable structure and function from one individual to the next. As with other measurements indicated here, the values given are averages.

Heel Strike to Midstance   At heel strike, the ankle and toes are in neutral (figure 12.13). The ankle moves into 15° of plantar flexion before midstance as more weight is borne by the extremity. The subtalar joint moves into pronation to accept the impact forces of weight bearing. The toes remain in a neutral position through midstance.

Once the leg moves into midstance, the ankle moves into 10° of dorsiflexion. This 10° permits a smooth glide of the limb as the body moves over its support. A lesser amount of motion causes the body to lurch as it moves into midstance. Once heel strike occurs, the calcaneus everts to cause subtalar pronation. This pronation permits the midtarsal area to remain flexible and to adapt to varying terrains. Pronation also allows the foot to act as a shock absorber. The subtalar joint remains in pronation until just before midstance when it begins to supinate. The longitudinal arch passively lengthens from heel strike until it reaches its maximum length at midstance. At heel strike, the foot makes contact with the ground on the posterior aspect of the heel, slightly lateral to the midline. As the body moves forward and more weight is borne on the extremity, the weight is transmitted distal to the heel to the midtarsal foot.

Midstance to Toe-Off   Following midstance, the ankle moves quickly from 10° of dorsiflexion to about 20° of plantar flexion by the time of toe-off. The calcaneus inverts and causes the subtalar joint to move into supination so the foot will become stable for propulsion at toe-off. The longitudinal arch begins to shorten, and the metatarsophalangeal joints extend to 30° after midstance until reaching maximum extension of about 60° at toe-off. The interphalangeal joints remain in neutral throughout the stance and swing phases of gait. As stance progresses, the body's weight is advanced forward on the foot (figure 12.14). At midstance, it is located just behind the metatarsal heads, and at toe-off the weight is primarily over the first and second metatarsophalangeal joints.

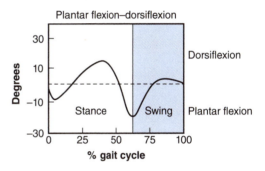

▶ **Figure 12.13**   Ankle motion.

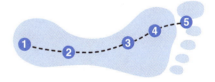

Key

1 = Initial contact (heel strike)

2 = Loading response (foot flat)

3 = Midstance

4 = Terminal stance (heel-off)

5 = Preswing (toe-off)

▶ **Figure 12.14**   Weight transmission during walking: Initial contact at heel strike occurs in the posterior-lateral heel and advances forward on the foot through the stance phase. At midstance the body's weight is just behind the metatarsal heads and at toe-off the weight is primarily over the first and second metatarsal heads.

Early Swing   Once toe-off occurs, the ankle begins movement toward dorsiflexion until it reaches a neutral position. By the time of middle swing, the ankle and toes are in a neutral position.

Late Swing   The ankle and toes remain close to neutral throughout the remaining part of the swing phase. The subtalar joint remains in pronation through the swing phase.

Total movement from plantar flexion to dorsiflexion in the sagittal plane is 30°. A great deal of motion in the lower extremities occurs during one stride. Figure 12.15 presents a summary of the joints' motions during ambulation. The motion is usually rapid, and some motions are difficult to detect visually without a video camera or similar device that can slow the motion so visual detection is possible. If visual recording devices are not available, it is useful to have the patient walk on a treadmill at a comfortable pace while you observe the gait from anterior, lateral, and posterior views. It is best to take an overall perspective first and notice any gross abnormalities in stride-length differences, stride width, and cadence. The next focus is on individual segments, investigating one at a time to discover any abnormalities in each of the joint's movements. These may include pelvic obliquity, premature heel-off or toe-off, knee position during various phases of gait, and calcaneal position during weight bearing. It makes little difference if your segmental observations begin proximally or distally, but whatever routine you select, perform it in the same manner consistently so you don't overlook any segment.

Gait Kinetics

Movements that occur during ambulation are the result of forces acting on the body. These forces include primarily those produced by the muscles, ground reaction forces, gravity, and momentum.

Muscles

The muscles function in gait to produce acceleration, deceleration and shock absorption, and stabilization. Acceleration propels the body or segment forward to produce motion. Acceleration is generally the result of the muscle's concentric activity. Deceleration slows down momentum of the segment or body to produce a smooth and controlled motion during ambulation. Deceleration occurs with eccentric activity. Like deceleration, shock absorption is primarily an eccentric muscle activity. Shock absorbers reduce impact forces on the body when the extremity first contacts the ground. Muscles that act as stabilizers are used as guy wires to hold a segment stable during movement. Isometric activity frequently produces stabilization. Some muscles act at times during gait as accelerators and at other times as decelerators. Other muscles are primarily stabilizers of the body or segment.

Obviously, not all muscles are active all the time during gait. The cyclic activity of a muscle in gait provides periods of rest for a muscle. Brief periods of peak muscle activity followed by less activity or periods of rest give the muscle enough recovery time so that an activity such as walking can continue for extended durations, if necessary. Because walking is the means by which we move our body from one location to another, it matters quite a bit that locomotion does not require continuous muscle activity.

The greatest energy requirement of muscles is present during the stance phase; less energy is required during the swing phase. The times of the greatest amount of muscle activity are in the first 10% of the stance phase and the last 10% of the swing phase. Periods of relative inactivity occur during midstance and the swing phase. The times of greatest muscle activity are during periods of acceleration and deceleration. The swing phase is a relatively quiet time of muscle activity because the momentum produced during the final stages of stance carries the lower extremity forward. As muscles prepare the extremity for heel strike during the final stages of swing and propulsion during preparation for swing in the final stages of stance, their activity increases.

Normal Gait

	Stance 60%					Swing 40%		
	Heel strike (initial contact)	Foot flat (loading response)	Midstance	Heel-off (terminal stance)	Toe-off (preswing)	Early swing (initial)	Midswing	Late swing (terminal)
	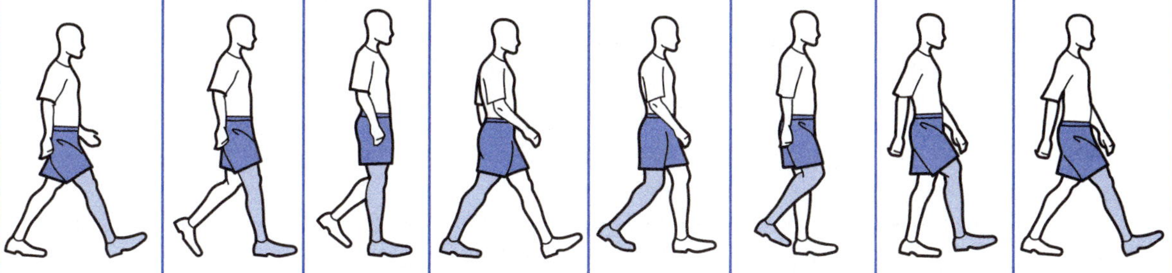							
Trunk	Erect Neutral	Erect Neutral	Erect Neutral	Erect Neutral	Erect Neutral	Erect Neutral	Erect Neutral	Erect Neutral
Pelvis	Level Forward rotation	Level 5° forward rotation Upward lateral rotation	Level Neutral rotation	Level 5° posterior rotation Downward lateral rotation	Level Posterior rotation Downward lateral rotation	Level Posterior rotation moving forward Lateral position is down	Level Neutral lateral rotation moving up	Level 5° forward rotation
Hip	30° flexion Slight adduction Near-neutral rotation	30° flexion Slight adduction Slight rotation	Extends Slight adduction Slight medial rotation	10° hyper-extension Slight abduction	5° neutral Extension Slight medial rotation 4° abduction	20° flexion Slight lateral rotation 5° abduction	Flexing Lateral rotation	30° flexion Mild lateral rotation going to medial rotation
Knee	Full extension Tibia in lateral rotation	15° flexion Tibia in medial rotation	Moves toward extension	Full extension	35° flexion	Cont. to 60° flexion Tibial lateral rotation	Begin to move to 30° flexion Tibial lateral rotation	Cont. to extend
Ankle	Neutral	15° plantar flexion Pronation	10° dorsi-flexion Starts to supinate	Moving into plantar flexion Supinating	20° plantar flexion	Moving to neutral	Neutral	Neutral
Toes	Neutral	Neutral	Neutral	MTP: 30° extension IP: Neutral	MTP: 60° extension IP: Neutral	Neutral	Neutral	Neutral

▶ **Figure 12.15** Summary of kinetics and kinematics for the hip, knee, and ankle in the sagittal plane through the gait cycle. Movement is a smoothly flowing change of range of motion in each joint throughout the gait cycle.

Hip

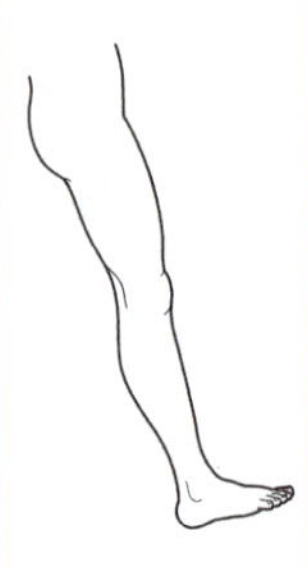 Initial contact/ Heel strike	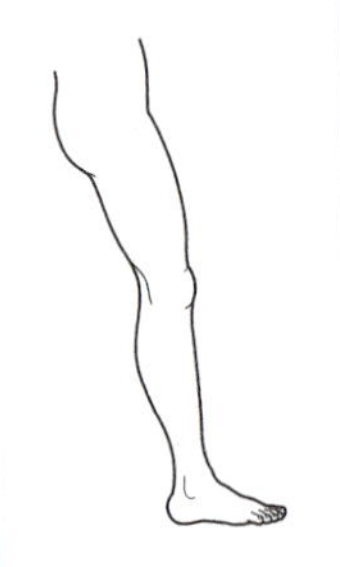 Loading response/ Foot flat	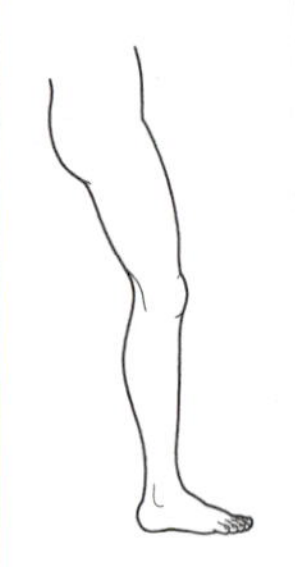 Midstance/ Single-leg support	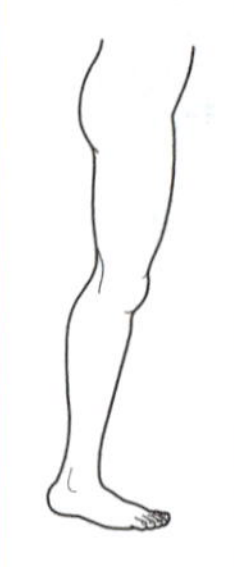 Terminal stance/ Heel-off	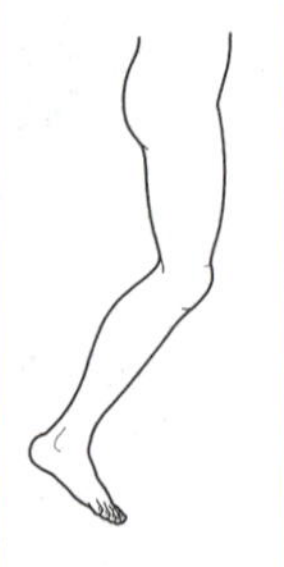 Preswing/ Toe-off	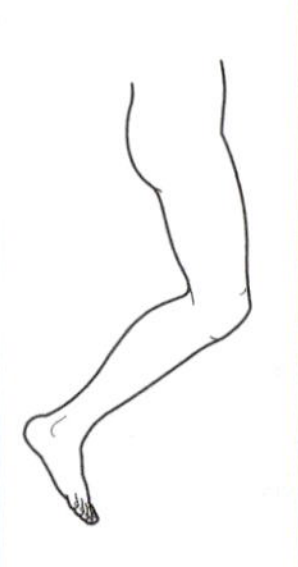 Initial/ Early swing	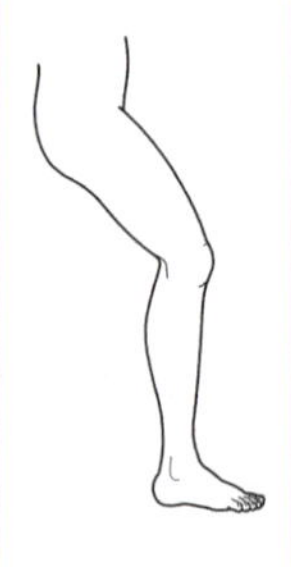 Midswing/ Swing-through	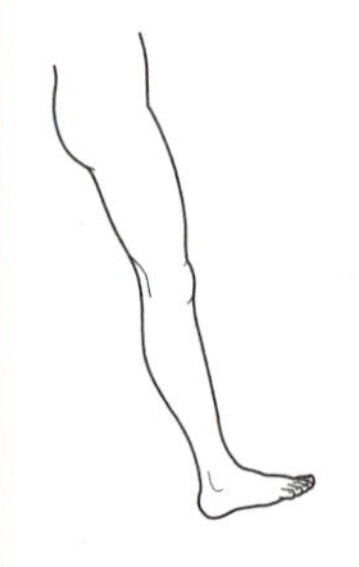 Terminal/ Late swing
0%	0–15%	15–40%	40–50%	50–60%	60–75%	75–85%	85–100%
ROM Flexion 30° neutral abduction, adduction rotation	30° flexion	Full extension	10° hyper-extension	Neutral extension	20° flexion	Flexion from 20° to 30°	30° flexion
Muscle activity Gluteus maximus, medius, tensor fascia lata, and hamstrings	Gluteus maximus, gluteus medius, tensor fascia lata, and hamstrings	Gluteus medius, tensor fascia lata	Hip flexors to prevent further extension	Hip flexors to initiate swing	Hip flexors	Hip flexors	Hamstrings to decelerate hip

Knee

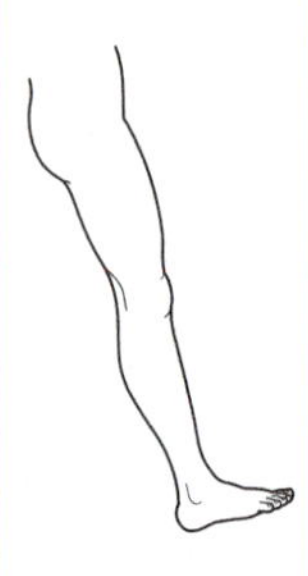 Initial contact/ Heel strike	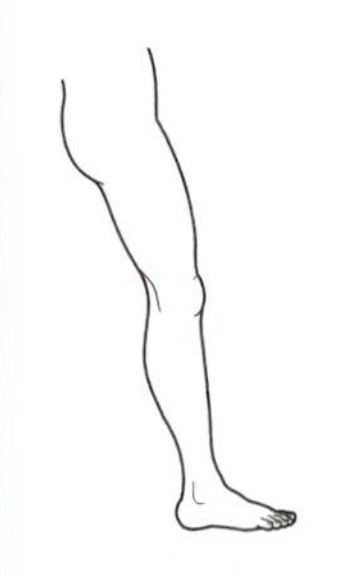 Loading response/ Foot flat	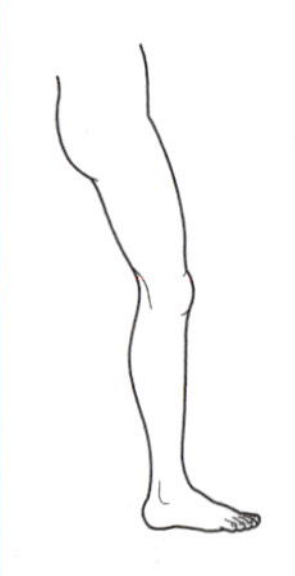 Midstance/ Single-leg support	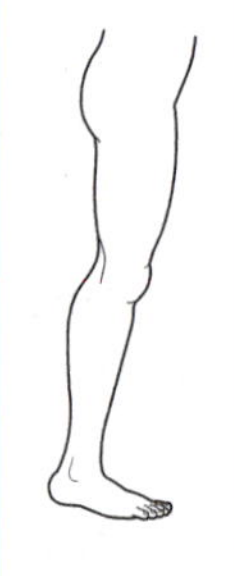 Terminal stance/ Heel-off	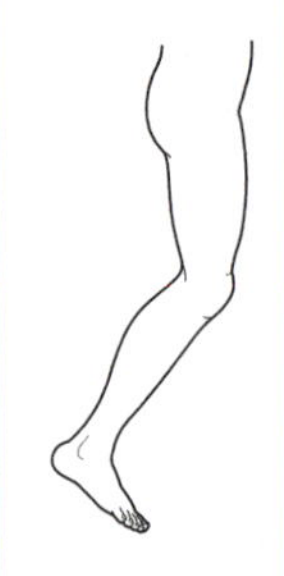 Preswing/ Toe-off	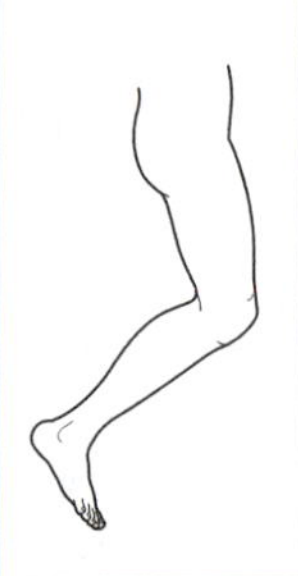 Initial/ Early swing	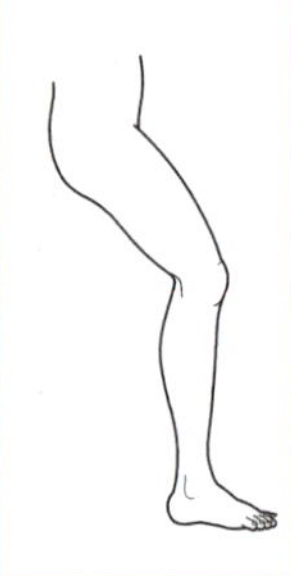 Midswing/ Swing-through	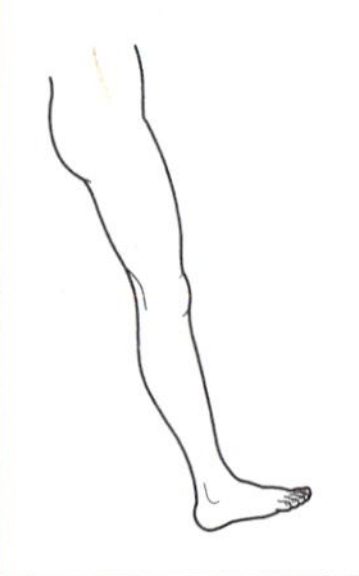 Terminal/ Late swing
0%	0–15%	15–40%	40–50%	50–60%	60–75%	75–85%	85–100%
ROM Full extension	15° flexion	Moving toward full extension	Full extension	35° flexion	60° flexion	From 60° to 30° flexion	Extension to 0°
Muscle activity Quadriceps	Highest point of quadriceps activity Hamstrings active as hip extensors	Quadriceps first half of midstance Once knee is extended, quadriceps silent	None	None	Short head of biceps, sartorius, gracilis	None	Quadriceps and hamstrings decelerate the lower extremity

▶ **Figure 12.15** *(continued)*

362 ■

Ankle

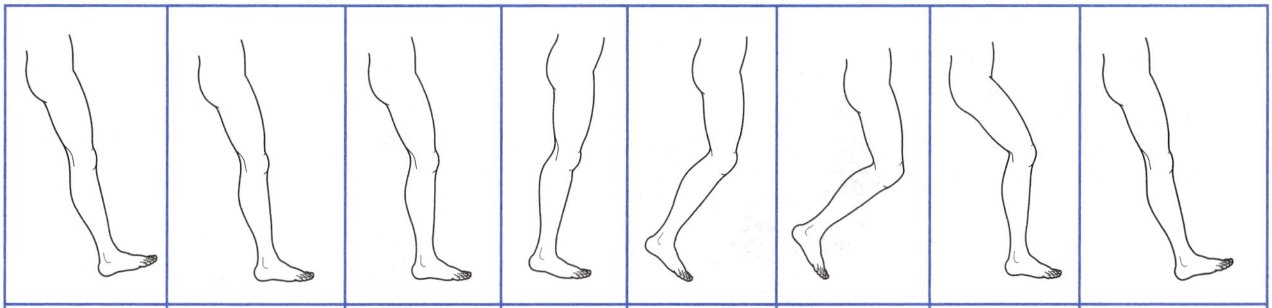

Initial contact/ Heel strike	Loading response/ Foot flat	Midstance/ Single-leg support	Terminal stance/ Heel-off	Preswing/ Toe-off	Initial/ Early swing	Midswing/ Swing-through	Terminal/ Late swing
0%	0–15%	15–40%	40–50%	50–60%	60–75%	75–85%	85–100%
ROM Neutral	15° plantar flexion	Neutral to 10° dorsi-flexion	Heel-off Prior to heel contact, opposite foot Moving into plantar flexion	20° plantar flexion	10° plantar flexion moving to neutral	Neutral	Neutral
Muscle activity Dorsiflexors maintain neutral position	Dorsiflexors control amount of plantar flexion, prevent foot slap	Plantar flexors control advance of tibia	Plantar flexors control tibia, restrict dorsiflexion	Dorsiflexors begin activity	Dorsiflexors active for toe clearance	Dorsiflexors maintain neutral position	Dorsiflexors maintain neutral position

▶ **Figure 12.15** *(continued)*

Let's take a brief look at the specific muscles that produce ambulation. Once you know what muscles are important for gait, it becomes easier to instruct in corrective gait training and provide therapeutic exercises to correct gait deficiencies.

An easy way to look at gait muscles is to divide them into categories according to their function. These categories include shock absorbers, stabilizers, accelerators, and decelerators. Some categories overlap because, for example, shock absorption requires deceleration. It is helpful to further divide categories according to the various body segments the muscles influence. Refer to figure 12.16 for a summary of the muscle activity described in the following sections.

Shock Absorbers During the first 15% of stance from initial contact to loading response, the quadriceps work as shock absorbers to reduce impact forces. These forces are based on the impact of the body contacting the ground, and the ground pushing back as a reaction of the body's impact (ground reaction force, or GRF). This principle is based on Newton's 3rd Law of Motion (see chapter 3) regarding action-reaction. Depending on the speed of locomotion, the ground reaction force can be anywhere from 110% at normal walking speed (Perry, 1992) to well over 700% of the body's weight (Williams, 1985). Muscles absorb these forces by eccentrically moving the lower extremity joints. At initial contact, the foot extensors also work as shock absorbers to prevent the foot from slapping onto the ground.

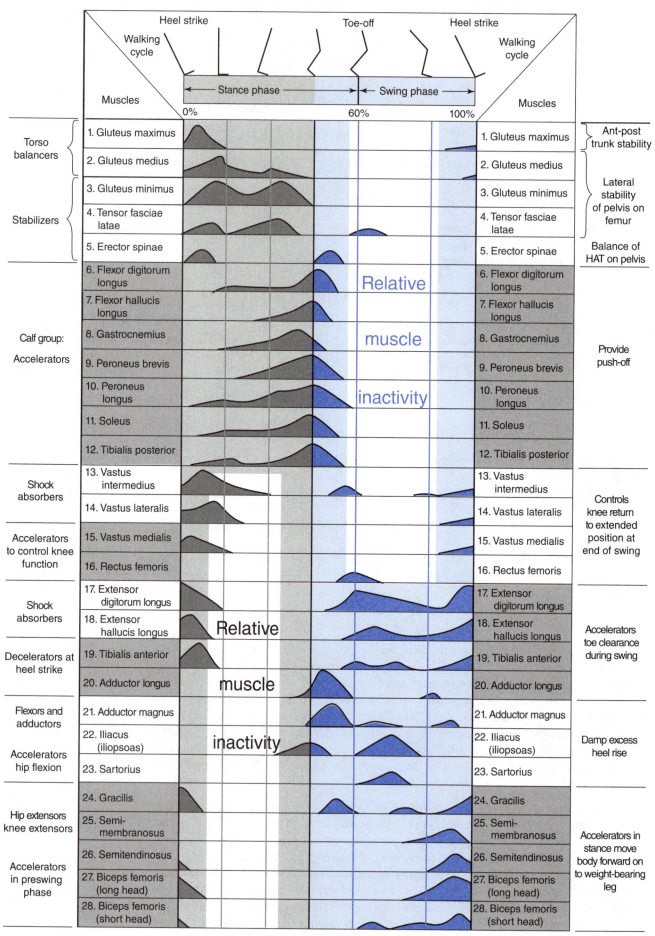

▶ **Figure 12.16** Muscle activity during gait. Peaks indicate periods of highest activity on each graph.

Adapted from J. Perry, 1992, *Gait analysis: Normal and pathological function* (Thorofore, NJ: SLACK Incorporated).

The quadriceps group decelerates knee flexion and controls the amount of knee flexion that occurs during the first 15% of the gait cycle. At the instant the heel makes contact with the floor, the foot dorsiflexors are at their peak output as they work first isometrically to keep the forefoot off the floor; they then immediately act eccentrically to control the lowering of the foot to the floor, functioning as a decelerator and shock absorber so that the movement is smooth.

Stabilizers   The hip extensors and torso muscles act as stabilizers to maintain the trunk in an erect position as the weight transfers from one leg to the other, preventing excessive side tilting of the pelvis or trunk. The gluteus maximus stabilizes the spine to prevent a forward lean of the trunk during weight bearing and during weight transfer from left to right; the gluteus medius, gluteus minimus, and tensor fascia lata stabilize the pelvis laterally on the femur; and the erector spinae muscles balance the head, arms, and trunk on the pelvis. These groups reach their peak levels of activity during the beginning and late stages of stance when weight is transferred from one leg to the other. The tensor fascia lata also works during initial swing phase to stabilize the pelvis to prevent lateral tilt.

Accelerators   Accelerators in the leg and thigh have peak outputs at various times during gait. The posterior calf accelerators exhibit peak activity during the end of stance phase as they propel the leg forward, providing for a push-off to produce an accelerated passive momentum of the extremity forward during swing phase. The posterior calf muscles begin activity during the middle portion of the weight-bearing phase as they provide control and balance during weight bearing. This is especially true of the lateral leg muscles, the ankle inverters and everters. Since the peroneals and tibialis posterior work through the majority of the weight bearing phase, it is easy to appreciate how tendinopathy may develop when their workload is increased because of poor foot mechanics, as seen in an excessive pronator.

During swing, the foot and toe dorsiflexors are working to lift the foot and toes to clear the floor and prepare the foot for the right position at heel strike.

The thigh accelerators work primarily in the early and middle stages of swing to increase hip flexion to clear the foot from the ground. They also adduct the thigh to keep it close to the support leg to reduce the energy requirements for holding the trunk erect during single-leg stance on the opposite leg.

Decelerators   During swing phase, the hamstrings work as decelerators of the knee to slow the swing of the leg so that initial contact occurs smoothly. The hamstrings also act as accelerators in the very early portion of stance phase to bring the body forward onto the weight-bearing leg.

It is worthwhile to note that the shock-absorbing activity of the quadriceps group, mentioned earlier, may also be categorized as a decelerating activity. Shock absorption is provided through muscle deceleration. Therefore, this is also true for the dorsiflexors during the early portion of stance phase.

Ground Reaction Forces

Ground reaction forces are the forces exerted between the body and the ground during ambulation. Since the foot hits the ground at an angle with the body moving in a direction, the ground produces reaction forces in more than one plane. One is a shearing force that is parallel to the ground, and the other is an impact force that is perpendicular to the ground. Shear forces occur in both fore-aft and lateral-medial directions. At initial contact, the fore-aft shear force is a forward force, and during preswing, it is a backward force. If you step on ice and lose your footing at initial contact, the forward force causes your extremity to slip forward. The reverse is true if you lose your footing during preswing; your foot slips backward.

Shortening stride length reduces fore-aft shear forces but increases vertical forces (figure 12.17). This is why it is safer to walk on ice with a shortened stride length: There is less forward force to slip the foot forward at initial contact and less backward force to slip the foot backward during preswing. Additionally, with a shortened stride, there is a larger foot surface in contact at both the start and end of stance.

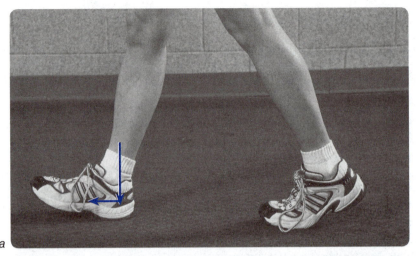

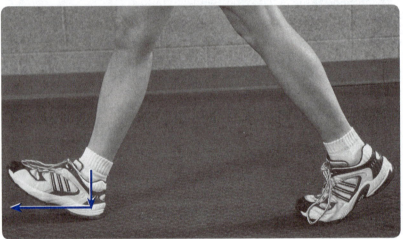

▶ **Figure 12.17** Shortened stride reduces fore-aft shear force. *(a)* Shortened stride produces a greater perpendicular force vector than fore-aft force vector. *(b)* A longer stride produces a greater fore-aft force vector than perpendicular force vector.

Elements of gait include the gait cycle, the center-of-gravity pathway, gait kinematics, and ground reaction forces. Lower-extremity injuries can lead to abnormalities of these elements and are reflected in the patient's pathological gait.

Fore-aft, or anteroposterior, forces are indicative of the deceleration forces that slow the body during initial contact and the acceleration forces that speed up the body before preswing. The medial-lateral shear force is predominantly a medial shear force through initial contact; it moves to a lateral shear force as weight transfers to the front of the foot. The medial-lateral shear forces coincide with how the body weight transfers from side to side during gait.

Vertical forces applied to the foot during stance are the effects of the body's weight. The amount of vertical force varies through the gait cycle and reflects the altering forces of shock absorption and deceleration during heel strike and acceleration as the extremity prepares to propel forward and move into the swing phase. The greatest vertical force occurs during push-off as acceleration for forward propulsion occurs. Vertical forces are at minimal levels when the body weight is shared with the other lower extremity during double-limb support (figure 12.18).

Awareness of ground reaction forces is important in examination of gait and musculoskeletal injury. Some of the greatest forces applied to the foot occur during acceleration. This can be crucial information when you are treating a patient who is a runner or participates in any activity in which ground reaction forces affect performance. For example, a pitcher who is experiencing first metatarsophalangeal joint pain will have difficulty during ball release

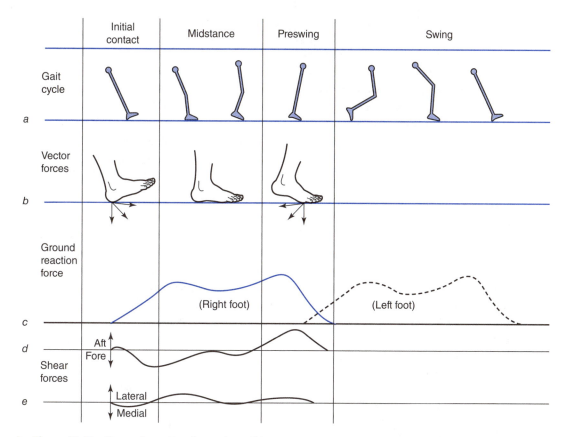

▶ **Figure 12.18** Ground reaction forces in walking.

Adapted from D.E. Klopsteg and P.D. Wilson, 1954, *Human limbs and their substitutes* (Washington, DC: National Academy of Sciences).

and will require treatment of the great toe, since ground reaction forces applied to the painful joint significantly affect the follow-through.

GAIT ANALYSIS

Now that you know the muscle and joint activity during gait, investigating a patient's gait is a matter of comparing these factors with the patient's presentation. To avoid forgetting something during the examination, it is best to establish a routine for yourself. Have the patient walk with and without shoes since shoes could mask some deviations you might otherwise not notice. Also, have the patient in shorts and female patients in a sports bra or male patients shirtless so you are able to observe the entire body during gait analysis.

An overall view of a patient's gait occurs first in gait assessment. Listen to the cadence. Is it even and rhythmical or is there disparity between the left and right foot sounds?

Next, look at gross movements. See how the body is carried and how it moves. Does the gait appear smooth or is it halting? Do the shoulders rotate in opposite direction to the hips, and do both segments rotate through an appropriate degree of motion and equally, left to right? Uneven or restricted motion could indicate back problems. Are the strides even? An unequal stride may be from an unequal leg length or soft tissue restrictions on one side. Is the arm swing relaxed and equal? Does the arm swing come from the shoulders or the elbows? If it comes from the elbows, this could indicate a shoulder problem. Do the trunk and neck sit erect on top of the pelvis? If the trunk is forward of the pelvis, either weakness in the gluteals or tightness in hip flexors may be the cause. If the head is forward of the trunk, tightness in the anterior shoulder girdle and/or cervical muscles along with weakness in the posterior shoulder girdle and neck may be present. Are the feet no more than about two inches apart during gait? If they are farther apart, balance, confidence in balance, or tight lateral hip muscles may be a problem.

After making an overall assessment, begin a joint-by-joint examination while the patient continues walking. Look from an anterior, posterior, and lateral view to obtain the best information. You may start from either the feet or the trunk but stay with whichever you choose so you do not overlook any segment. You may also look at each segment from a posterior, anterior, and lateral view, or if you find it easier, you may choose to look at a segment from all views then go on to the other segments in the same manner. If the patient's endurance is limited, it may be better to obtain all information from one view before moving to another view since it will take less time to approach the examination in this manner.

Head position, shoulder position, shoulder movement relative to pelvis movement, knee alignment, and foot and heel positions during stance are examined from anterior and posterior views. A posterior view of the ankle includes noticing the number of toes you can observe on each foot; the number should be equal; if one extremity reveals more than the other, that extremity has either tibial torsion or hip lateral rotation greater than its contralateral extremity. See if you can see the same amount of the plantar foot when the foot moves from heel-off to right after toe-off. Less on one side than the other may indicate either a shortened or prolonged stride length or tightness in the Achilles. Does the calcaneus move immediately into pronation at heel strike then rotate into inversion during midstance, or does it stay in pronation throughout the stance phase? Prolonged pronation may indicate an excessively flexible foot that requires extraneous support. Does the heel hit the ground on the lateral aspect, or does it contact the floor in the middle or medial heel? More pronation than usual may be the cause of this foot position. Does the heel hit the floor and allow the foot to roll into pronation, or does the weight stay on the lateral foot? This action may be indicative of a restricted rearfoot with high arches. Does the foot hit the floor in the midfoot, not the rearfoot? If the foot lands more distal than the heel, the stride length is shortened. Does the heel come off the ground before it should? If this is the case, either weakness of the quadriceps or tightness of the Achilles may be a problem. Do the posterior legs appear the same or is one smaller or less defined than the other one? Size or definition differences may reflect a difference in strength.

Moving up to the knee from a posterior perspective, compare left to right to see if the posterior knees are the same, or does one expose more of the medial knee than the other? If the latter is the case, there may be tibial torsion or excessive medial hip rotation. As the foot moves into heel off, do both knees remain in a forward position, or does one start to rotate laterally or medially? Excessive rotation of the knee during latter stance may indicate tightness or weakness in the extremity. Check the relative alignment of the knee with the ankle and hip to note any valgus or varus condition. Observe for any size and definition distinctions between the right and left thighs.

Continuing to move more proximally from a posterior view, observe for muscle size and definition of the gluteus maximus on each side. Do the hips stay level throughout the gait or does one drop significantly during swing? The opposite gluteus medius is weak if this drop is observed. Does one leg swing out in a circumduction pattern during swing or do they both swing through in the proper manner? If it swings out, there may be weakness in the hip flexors or reduced flexibility in the knee.

Skin creases in the thoracolumbar spine should mirror each other as the hips and shoulders rotate opposite to one another. If there is less motion or skin mobility on one side, it may indicate low back restriction or a history of pain in that area. Do the contralateral paraspinals contract with the weight bearing extremity? Are they easily observed or do they lack muscle bulk? Lack of muscle definition in the lumbar paraspinals along with atrophy of the gluteals may indicate low back problems.

From an anterior perspective and starting from the same joint as in the posterior view, make a lot of the same observations to reconfirm your posterior observations. Since you are unable to observe the heels, look at the toes. Do they look the same left to right when the foot lands? Is each foot's rotation the same? Are the toes dorsiflexed the same amount? Do you see differences between the longitudinal arches during weight bearing? Is there atrophy in the anterior tibialis on one leg or are they the same? Do the patellae face forward when the foot is on the ground? If the patella moves to a squinting position, the individual may have excessive pronation, tibial rotation, or patellofemoral problems. Is the knee straight or in valgus or varus? If it is in valgus, the quadriceps may be weak. Do the hips remain level from an anterior perspective as they did from the posterior view? Does the navel maintain a forward position, or does it rotate or shift to one side?

The lateral view offers additional insight into pathologies you have already discovered, or it may reveal other new ones. Lateral-view examination includes observations of knee position at heel strike, midstance, and heel-off; head, trunk, and hip alignment; swing-through motion of the lower extremity; arm swing; pelvis motion; and timing of heel strike, heel-off, and toe-off. Again, starting at the ankle, it should be observed that each heel hits the ground at the same distance in front of the body. Each heel should lift off the ground and each foot should come off the ground at the same point in stance. If this does not occur, a leg length discrepancy, unilateral tightness in hip extensors or flexors, or weakness in the hip or knee may be present. When the heel hits the ground, is the ankle in neutral? Does the ankle remain at neutral throughout swing?

Moving to the more proximal joint from a side view, we continue to observe for gait characteristics. When the heel hits the ground, is the knee in extension, but does it move immediately into some flexion as the body's weight is borne on that extremity? If the knee remains in extension, it may be that the quadriceps is weak or the knee lacks normal motion. As the limb moves behind the body's center of gravity, does the knee start to move into flexion as the heel lifts off the ground? During swing, does it move freely into about 60° of flexion? If it fails to achieve this much motion, it may be restricted in flexion motion.

Since the hip has its greatest flexion motion during swing, does it move smoothly and fully during mid-swing as it should? It has its greatest extension motion during stance just before heel off. Is it able to be in extension at that time, or does it remain in some degree of flexion? If it stays in flexion, it may be either tight in its hip flexors or weak in its hip extensors. Does the pelvis remain level throughout gait or is the anterior pelvis tilted more forward? If this is the case, tight hip flexors may be present.

From a lateral view, the head, shoulders and pelvis should remain level throughout the gait cycle. The head remains directly over the shoulders, and the shoulders remain directly over the hips and pelvis. If either is forward of its more proximal segment, tightness of the anterior structures and weakness of the posterior structures is likely present.

Once the gait examination is completed, any deviations discovered are confirmed by an investigation of the structure. For example, if the patient displayed a forward trunk lean during gait, a strength assessment of the hip extensors and a flexibility assessment of the hip flexors are performed to locate the source of the gait deviation. Once the cause of the deviation is identified, exercises are then incorporated into the therapeutic exercise program to correct the problem.

PATHOLOGICAL GAIT

Pathological gait results when injury, weakness, loss of flexibility, pain, or bad habit prevents a segment from moving as it should during ambulation. The body continues to ambulate, but it must make adjustments to accommodate for the loss of normal function. This places stress on other segments and promotes weakness, and if the situation continues, it can cause additional injury. Here we consider a few typical pathological gaits that result from musculoskeletal injuries.

Gluteus Medius Gait

If an individual sustains an injury that necessitates prolonged non-weight bearing on an extremity, or if he or she directly injures the hip, the gluteus medius can become weak. Once the patient resumes full weight bearing, the gluteus medius is too weak to maintain a level pelvis during single-leg stance. A drop of the pelvis occurs on the uninvolved side. This drop occurs from initial contact on the involved side through to initial contact on the uninvolved side. This is known as a **Trendelenburg,** or **gluteus medius, gait.**

When the gluteus medius is weak, the pelvis drops on the contralateral, non-weight-bearing side because the strength of the weight-bearing gluteus medius is insufficient to hold the pelvis level. Consequently, the weight of the pelvis overcomes the strength of the gluteus medius so the pelvis drops downward on the opposite side. To compensate for this, a patient may move the trunk laterally over the weak hip. This movement forces the erector spinae and quadratus lumborum of the opposite side to contract and lift the pelvis. This compensation reduces the gluteus medius' strength requirements by shortening the pelvis's lever arm length.

Quadriceps Gait

Surgery or severe injury to the knee or quadriceps can leave the quadriceps very weak and unable to function properly during ambulation. Even after strengthening the quadriceps, the patient can continue to ambulate with a pathological gait because of bad habits established during ambulation when the muscle was too weak to be used properly. With a quadriceps gait, the patient keeps the knee extended at heel strike and through the stance phase. If the quadriceps is very weak, a lurch immediately after heel strike can occur as the individual forces the femur backward and the trunk forward to passively lock the knee by keeping the body's center of gravity in front of the knee. The hip extensors then stabilize the knee to keep it locked after heel strike.

Ankle Tightness

If an individual sustains an ankle sprain and subsequently suffers a loss of dorsiflexion motion, a pathological gait develops. During midstance when the ankle should move suddenly from plantar flexion to dorsiflexion, the person lurches forward over the foot, experiences increased knee extension, and moves quickly toward heel-off in an attempt to shorten the time requirement for dorsiflexion. There will be a rapid movement from initial contact to loading response if the ankle does not have dorsiflexion to 0°, and the patient may either hike the involved hip upward or increase knee and hip flexion to clear the toes from the floor during the swing phase.

Antalgic Gait

When an individual suffers an injury or inflammation and ambulates with pain in any joint, muscle or tendon, you can observe a typical, obvious pathological gait. The patient reduces the time spent on the painful extremity to minimize the stresses placed on it during gait. Therefore, the stride length is altered and the cadence is asymmetrical; initial contact is not "heel strike" but occurs in the middle to distal foot to minimize impact stress. If the knee is the painful region, knee flexion during midstance may be exaggerated if the knee has increased edema; and knee motion is minimized during the swing phase. To compensate for the lack of motion during the swing phase the patient hikes the hip, goes up on the toes of the uninvolved leg during midstance, or uses a circumduction swing to clear the foot from the floor. If the hip is the site of pain, the hip is usually kept in about 30° of flexion since the joint is least irritated by weight-bearing pressures in this position. The ankle is placed in 10-15° of plantar flexion with weight bearing on the forefoot to relieve joint pressures at the ankle during ambulation.

NORMAL RUNNING GAIT

Running and walking differ, just as running differs at different speeds. Running differs from walking in that the stance phase is shortened, the swing phase is lengthened, there is no

Pathological gait is a reflection of injury, weakness, loss of flexibility, pain, or bad habits. As with normal gait, observation of pathological gait begins with an overview assessment and proceeds with segmental assessment.

time of double support, and there is a nonsupport phase in which neither leg is weight bearing. The nonsupport phase in running, also referred to as the **double float** phase, occurs during the early-initial swing phase of one leg and the end of terminal swing for the other leg (figure 12.19). Since gait characteristics also change with a change in running speed, categories of running must be defined.

A variety of factors affect running mechanics, including speed, age, somatotype, fatigue, surface, footwear, and skill level. Researchers who compare running speeds vary considerably in their categorizations. In one study, for example, slow runners are defined as those who run 4 m/s (4.4 yd/s), or are able to run a mile in 6:42

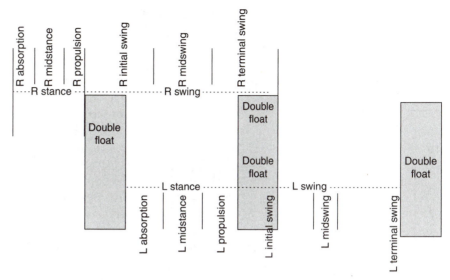

▶ **Figure 12.19** Model of one running stride: Double float is unique to running and occurs when there is nonsupport of either extremity.

Adapted from S. Ounpuu, 1994, "The biomechanics of walking and running," *Clinics in Sports Medicine* 13: 843-862.

(6 min, 42 s). A fast runner is defined as one who runs 8 m/s (8.7 yd/s) or 91 m (100 yd) in 11.4 s. A sprinter is able to run 10 m/s or 100 yd in 9.1 s (Dillman, 1975). In another study, a runner is defined as someone moving at 19.3 kph (12 mph; slightly less than a 5-min mile), and a sprinter is one who is able to run 27.6 kph (17.1 mph; 109 m in 12.2 s) (R. A. Mann & Hagy, 1980). Whereas the average walking speed is approximately 1.4 m/s (1.5 yd/s), ranges in running speeds vary from 2 to 5.5 times the speed of walking (Perry, 1990). These variations make analysis and comparison of results difficult at best.

In most instances, terminology used for running is the same as for walking. A few additional terms are used for running, however. A running stride is from toe-off of one foot to toe-off of the opposite foot, and one **running cycle** includes two running strides. Because runners do not always impact the ground at the heel, initial contact is called **foot strike** rather than heel strike. **Cycle time,** or stride time, is the amount of time it takes to perform one step length. **Stride rate** is the inverse of stride time. As mentioned previously, the nonsupport phase is the time when there is no weight bearing. The stance phase is sometimes referred to as the *support phase* for consistency with the term "nonsupport phase."

Stride Length and Stride Rate

Although researchers differ in their definitions of running speeds, the information available on running yields several basic observations. Stride length and cadence increase with an increase in velocity. Cycle time decreases with an increase in speed. After about 7 m/s (7.6 yd/s), stride length does not increase remarkably, but stride rate does (figure 12.20).

Joint Motions

Generally, as speed increases, the body tends to move its center of gravity lower by increasing the degree of hip flexion, knee flexion, and ankle dorsiflexion during the early stages of the stance phase.

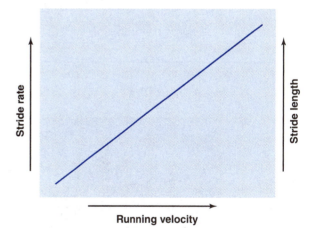

▶ **Figure 12.20** Relationships between stride length, stride rate, and running speed. As speed increases, stride length and stride rate increase.

The hip increases its flexion during midswing with increases in speed, but hip position changes little with speed variations during weight bearing except in sprinting when the hip never reaches full extension. Generally, hip motion increases as speed increases (figure 12.21).

The knee motion also changes with changes in speed. Like the hip, there are greater degrees of knee flexion and there is less extension with greater speeds. During sprinting, the knee does not extend; it continues through the gait cycle in varying degrees of flexion. Some evidence indicates that at higher speeds the trend is toward extension at toe-off, although full extension is not achieved (Williams, 1985). During the swing phase, knee flexion has been recorded at more than 120° (Williams, 1985). Increased knee flexion provides for additional shock absorption, but it also requires greater quadriceps output. This topic is discussed later in the section "Kinetics."

Ankle plantar flexion at toe-off has been recorded in ranges between 59° and 75° (Williams, 1985). Which part of the foot makes initial contact with the ground depends on the angles of the hip, knee, and ankle. Runners most often land on the midfoot. As a rule, faster runners tend to land at the midfoot, and slower runners land at the rearfoot (Williams, 1985).

Although an erect trunk is thought to be the best position for running form, most reports indicate that runners use a forward trunk lean throughout the running cycle (Williams, 1985). The amount of trunk lean increases from 4° to 7° in runners at speeds up to 7 m/s (7.7 yd/s) and to 11.6° in sprinters running at 9.2 m/s (10.06 yd/s) (Williams, 1985).

Ground Reaction Forces

As speeds increase, ground reaction forces also increase. In running and walking, ground reaction forces reach two peaks. The first is at impact during initial contact. This peak, which occurs very quickly with running impact, is referred to as the impact peak. The second peak occurs during the last half of support and is referred to as an action peak because of muscles' influences on it during acceleration prior to toe-off (figure 12.22).

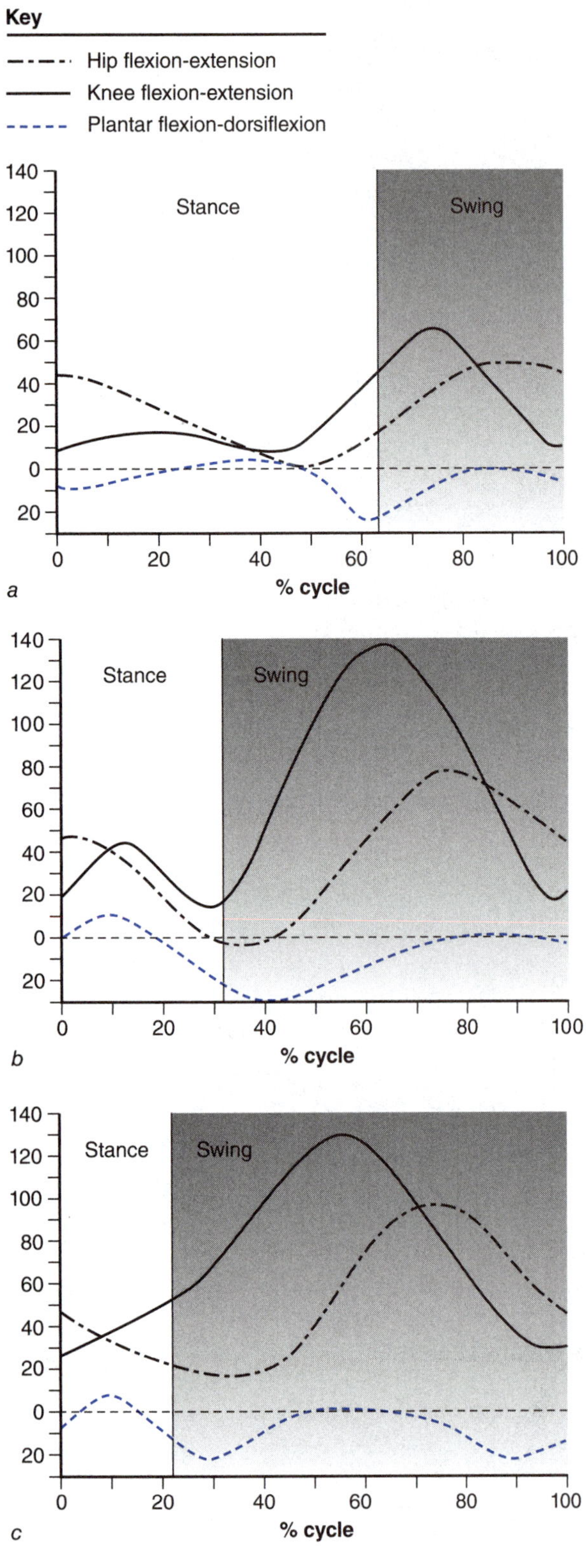

Key

- –·–·– Hip flexion-extension
- ——— Knee flexion-extension
- – – – Plantar flexion-dorsiflexion

▶ **Figure 12.21** Sagittal plane ranges of motion during gait when *(a)* walking, *(b)* running, and *(c)* sprinting. As speed increases, the swing phase (nonsupport phase) time increases, and joint ranges of motion change.

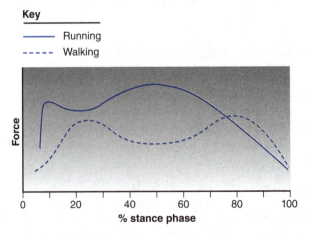

Key

- ——— Running
- – – – Walking

▶ **Figure 12.22** Ground reaction forces in running and walking. The impact ground reaction force in running occurs very quickly.

Based on data from Ounpuu, 1994.

Vertical impact forces encountered during running are mathematically combined with joint positions to determine joint moments. Joint moments are the stresses applied to the joints. During running, the knee encounters flexor moments 7.7 times greater than those encountered during walking (Williams, 1985). The hip and ankle flexion demands during running are double those during walking (Perry, 1990).

Body weight, surfaces, shoes, speed, and where on the foot the runner lands all influence the impact peak forces. Softer surfaces can eliminate the impact peak. A good running shoe has a lower impact peak than a poorly constructed shoe. Runners who land on the midfoot or forefoot have a significantly reduced impact peak compared to those landing on the rearfoot; and runners landing on the rearfoot have a single peak whereas runners landing on the midfoot have a biphasic peak impact. Faster runners have greater ground reaction forces than slower runners.

Kinetics

Specific activity varies greatly, depending on running speeds and on the investigation, but a general conclusion is that muscle activity increases with increased running speeds, as seen in figure 12.23.

Hip

There is an increase in hamstring activity from heel strike and throughout stance as the hamstring assists concentrically in hip extension. The semimembranosus is at a particular advantage to provide hip extensor force since it is 1.4 times larger than the biceps femoris (Perry 1990). The hamstrings also play a concentric and stabilizing role during trunk lean.

The rectus femoris is more active at foot strike, but this activity diminishes by the end of support. The rectus femoris is active concentrically during hip flexion in the early swing phase to lift the extremity for swing. The hamstrings and hip extensors in the late-swing leg act eccentrically to slow hip flexion and prepare the leg for the support phase.

Knee

The quadriceps, especially the vastus lateralis and vastus medialis, are extremely active at foot strike; they continue to be active along with the rectus femoris during the early portion of support. High demands are placed on the quadriceps muscles during most of the stance phase. Their activity diminishes as the leg continues to the end of support, but increases again just

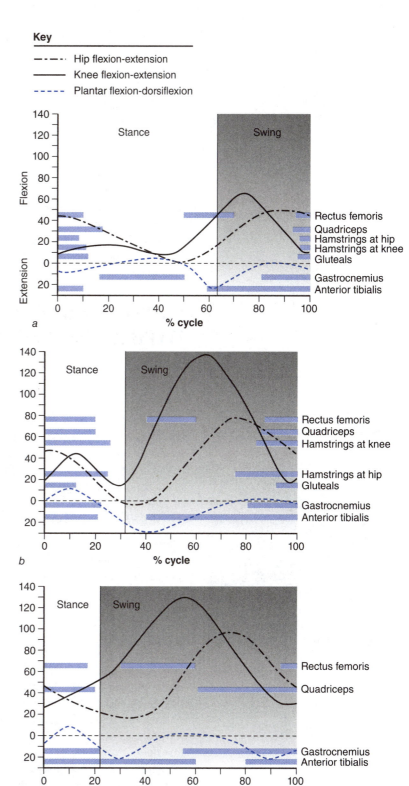

▶ **Figure 12.23** Muscle activity with sagittal plane range of motion during *(a)* walk, *(b)* run, and *(c)* sprint.

Based on data from Mann & Inman, 1964.

Running gait differs from walking gait in several major ways—stride length and rate, joint motions, ground reaction forces, and kinetics.

prior to foot strike in preparation for its impact-loading response. As running speeds increase, the amount of time the quadriceps are active in both the stance and swing phases increases.

The hamstrings begin their aggressive activity in the last half of swing phase to prepare the knee to land in the stance phase. The hamstrings continue their activity halfway through stance and may be an active restraint against anterior tibial shear. During the last half of stance, the hamstrings and quadriceps co-contract, presumably for additional knee support.

Ankle

At foot strike, the tibialis anterior and triceps surae group co-contract to stabilize the foot at impact. The contraction of the posterior muscle group through most of the stance phase may provide tibial stability for improved quadriceps function. If the runner's foot strike occurs at the heel, the tibialis anterior immediately eccentrically contracts to control foot pronation. The triceps surae concentrically contracts to provide thrust for propulsion of the body into the nonsupport phase. This is especially true for faster speeds (Williams, 1985).

MECHANICS OF AMBULATION WITH ASSISTIVE DEVICES

Now that you have an understanding of normal gait mechanics, you will more easily appreciate the intricacies of ambulation with assistive devices. Assistive devices are used either to provide additional stability during ambulation or to reduce or eliminate weight bearing on a lower extremity. They can permit the patient to walk safely and unassisted by others. As a rule, assistive devices are used in gait if the patient is unable to walk normally. Assistive devices are used in this instance to prevent the added stresses of abnormal gait from causing additional injury and avoid establishment of poor gait habits.

Types of Assistive Devices

There are several different types of assistive devices used in ambulation. The type selected is dependent upon several factors such as the patient's age, physical ability and agility, patient size, balance, injury, weight-bearing status, and comfort level. Table 12.1 includes a list of the various assistive devices commonly used in rehabilitation.

Fitting

Before a patient can use any assistive device, the device must be properly fitted to the individual's height. Axillary, or underarm, crutches are measured with the crutch tips flat on the ground and approximately 15 cm (6 in.) lateral to and 15 cm in front of the foot (figure 12.24). There should be a two- to three-finger space between the top of the axillary pad and the patient's axilla. The handgrip should be at a level such that there is a 20° to 30° bend in the elbow with the crutch at the correct length as the patient stands with the crutches 15 cm laterally and 15 cm anterior to the feet.

Forearm (Loftstrand) crutches are adjusted so that the handgrip is at the level of the greater trochanter and the forearm cuff is just distal to the elbow. This should provide for about a 30° elbow bend during weight bearing. Cane measurements are made with the arm in a relaxed resting position at the side and the cane next to the leg. The top of the cane handle should be at wrist or greater trochanter level.

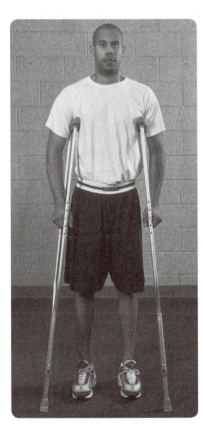

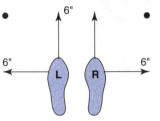

▶ **Figure 12.24** With the crutches 15 cm (6 in.) lateral and anterior to the feet, and the shoulders relaxed, proper crutch height should allow two to three fingers between the axilla and axillary pad. Elbows should be flexed 20° to 30°.

TABLE 12.1   Assistive Devices Used in Gait

Assistive device	Types available	WB status	Selection criteria	Correct fitting	Notes
Walker	1. Pick-up 2. Front-wheeled 3. Four-wheeled	PWB NWB extremity FWB or PWB	Needs balance assistance Poor proprioception Older patient	Height is at patient's greater trochanter in standing	Unless an athlete has multiple injuries, walkers are not usually used with this group. Stairs can be difficult with a walker, but a walker provides the greatest stability of any assistive device.
Cane	1. Walker cane 2. Large-base quad cane 3. Small-base quad cane 4. Single-ended cane (straight or curved)	PWB	A cane can increase balance by expanding the base of support. It also reduces pain during gait. The walker cane may be used by a hemiplegic patient without use of one UE. The 4-prong canes (large/small base) offer greater balance and may be used for more weight bearing reliance.	Used in the contralateral hand, the top of the cane should be at the level of the greater trochanter so there is a 20-30 degree bend at the elbow. Another way to measure it is to have the patient stand with arms at sides; top of the cane is at the break in the wrist.	Used in the contralateral hand, the cane reduces weight bearing stress on a weak gluteus medius. A cane reduces forces on the involved LE by up to 25% (Kumar, Roe et al. 1995). Patients may progress from crutches to a cane as balance, strength, and WB status improves.
Crutches	1. Underarm 2. Loftstrand or forearm	NWB PWB	Underarm crutches are used by patients who have good balance. Loftstrand (forearm) crutches are used by patients who must remain on crutches throughout their lives or for extended times.	There is 2-3 finger-width between the top of the crutch and the patient's axilla. The hand grip is measured the same as for other assistive devices. The forearm band of Loftstrand crutches is distal to the elbow.	Crutches offer more mobility than a walker. They can be used on stairs, ramps, and inclines more easily than a walker. Patients are able to ambulate faster than with a walker. They can be treacherous in ice, snow, rain. Crutches are used most often with younger and agile patients. Loftstrand crutches allow the patient's hands to be free but not let go of the crutches while standing.

Gait Patterns With Crutches

A basic concept in the use of assistive devices is to keep the center of balance within the base of support. A person is more stable when using assistive devices because the base of support is increased (figure 12.25). Gait patterns are designated according to the number of support points in contact with the floor. These contacts include the assistive devices and the feet.

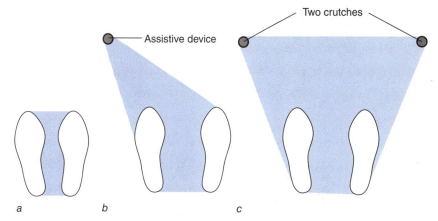

▶ **Figure 12.25** Base of support with (a) no assistive devices, (b) one cane or crutch, (c) two crutches. The base of support area is increased when assistive devices are used. As long as the patient's center of gravity falls within the base of support, the patient is stable.

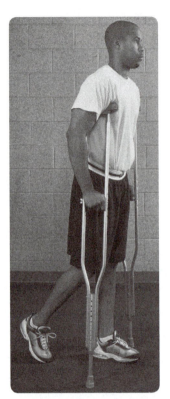

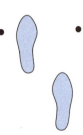

Two-Point Gait

A two-point gait is used when partial weight bearing (PWB) is allowed on the involved extremity. This gait is so named because of the fact that both lower extremities are in contact with the ground, but one requires two assistive devices, one on each side of the body. In this gait, the injured leg moves forward with the crutches, and some body weight is placed on the injured extremity. The amount of weight permitted is dictated by the patient's pain or the physician's prescription. In this gait, the crutches and involved leg advance simultaneously. Partial body weight is placed on the extremity, and the remaining weight is placed on the hands (figure 12.26). The uninvolved leg then advances forward in a normal stride, passing the opposite leg as it swings through.

Three-Point Gait

A three-point gait is so termed because there are three points of contact with the floor—two made by the assistive device and one made by the uninvolved extremity's foot. This gait is used when the patient is unable to bear weight on one extremity. It is also called a right (or left) non-weight-bearing (NWB) gait. For young, healthy individuals who have been injured, underarm crutches are the most frequently used assistive devices. Forearm crutches or a walker can also be used in a three-point gait.

In a three-point gait, while remaining non-weight bearing (NWB) on one LE, the patient advances the crutches simultaneously in front of the body along with the NWB extremity; he or she then bears weight on the crutch handles and lifts the weight-bearing leg by pushing down on the crutch hand grips to move the weight bearing extremity either up to or past the crutches (figure 12.27).

▶ **Figure 12.26** A two-point gait is used when partial weight bearing is permitted. The crutches move with the involved extremity with partial weight on the crutches and partial weight on the lower extremity.

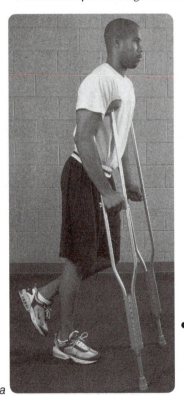

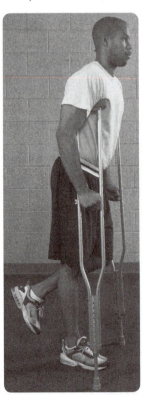

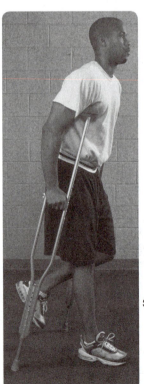

Swing-to

Swing-through

▶ **Figure 12.27** In a three-point gait, the patient places the crutches in front of the body *(a)* and advances the weight-bearing leg either to the crutches *(b)* or in front of the crutches *(c)*. Weight is borne entirely by the hands during the swing-to or swing-through phase of this gait.

A gait in which the individual swings the weight-bearing leg to the crutches is called a **swing-to gait.** If the weight-bearing leg is advanced far enough to land in front of the crutches, the gait is a swing-through gait. The **swing-through gait** is more difficult and requires more self-confidence than the swing-to gait does. A patient who is hesitant about using the crutches uses a swing-to gait initially; as the individual gains confidence and it is safe to do so, he or she advances to a swing-through gait. The swing-through gait is faster than the swing-to gait, but requires more balance and control.

Four-Point Gait

A four-point gait is used by individuals who have bilateral lower-extremity involvement. This gait involves using one crutch with each contralateral lower extremity. For example, the left crutch advances with the right leg and the right crutch moves with the left leg. This type of gait is not used if only one extremity is involved.

Single Support

When a single device, either a cane or a crutch, is used, it is placed in the hand contralateral to the leg injury. Single devices are used primarily for stability, not weight-bearing support, because only about 25% of the body's weight can be borne on a cane or on one crutch (Kumar, Roe, & Scremin, 1995; Lehmann, 1990).

Single support is essentially a second-class lever system. It is designed to be efficient so minimal force from the upper extremity is required to produce the desired effect of support for the involved leg. The injured lower extremity's hip is the fulcrum from which the cane or crutch leverage is applied. The head, arms, and trunk (HAT) are the resistance force that is positioned between the fulcrum and the cane or crutch (figure 12.28). If the cane or crutch were placed in the hand on the same side as the injured leg, it would not provide the intended assistance for reduced weight on the involved extremity, and the patient would have to lurch over the outside of the involved leg to place the HAT weight between the cane and the injured leg.

In a single-support gait, the cane or crutch moves with the injured leg so the two advance together. As the patient bears weight on the injured leg and swings the uninvolved leg forward, some weight is also applied to the single-support device. This gait is used when minimal support for balance is required or when the patient is able to bear weight on the extremity but displays an abnormal gait because of pain, loss of motion, or weakness. A gluteus medius gait is relieved with a cane used in the contralateral hand during ambulation.

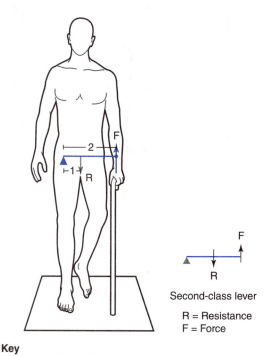

Key
1 = Lever-arm length of body weight
2 = Lever-arm length of cane support

▶ **Figure 12.28** Ambulation with single support allows reduced force application to the involved lower extremity.

Assistive Devices on Various Surfaces

The patient will be ambulating with assistive devices on varying surfaces such as stairs and ramps, so he or she needs to receive instruction before he or she is able to safely use the assistive devices without supervision. Risk of injury and falling is significant until the patient is safe on all surface types.

Stairs

When maneuvering stairs with a railing, the patient should use the handrail. A railing provides greater safety since it is more stable than crutches on stairs. If the person is using two crutches, both are placed in the same hand, the one away from the railing. If the stairs have a handrail on each side, it is easiest if the patient places the hand of the uninvolved side on the railing when going up or down the stairs.

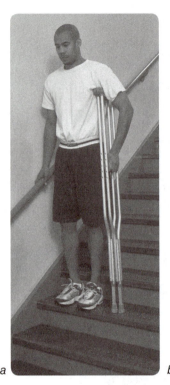 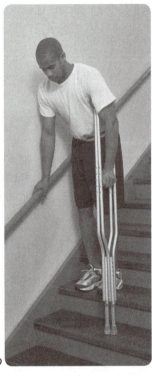 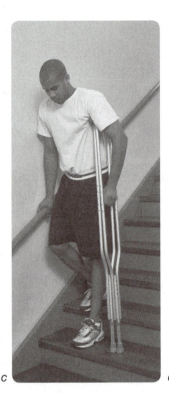 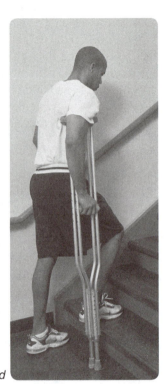

a   *b*   *c*   *d*

▶ **Figure 12.29** How to ambulate on stairs with crutches: *(a)* Use the rail if one is present and place both crutches in ipsilateral hand to the involved LE. *(b)* Advance the crutches to the lower step and move the rail hand to keep the hands even. *(c)* Lower the body to the step, bearing weight on the hands as the involved leg is lowered before the uninvolved leg. *(d)* When going up stairs, the uninvolved leg leads, and the crutches remain on the lower step with the involved leg until the uninvolved leg is secure on the higher step.

Stair climbing involves two important factors to remember. One is that the uninvolved leg advances up the stairs first and the involved leg advances down the stairs first. This can be confusing, so you can use a simple reminder. "The good go up to heaven and the bad go down to hell," is a reminder that most patients find easy to recall.

The second concept is that the assistive device always goes with the involved leg. In other words, the crutches go on the same step as the injured extremity. For example, when descending stairs, the patient grasps the railing with one hand and holds both crutches in the opposite hand (figure 12.29a). The crutches advance down a stair step (figure 12.29b); then the involved extremity is lowered to the same stair step (figure 12.29c). The patient bears weight on the arms and involved leg, if weight bearing is permitted, and then lowers the uninvolved leg to the same stair step. For ascending stairs, the process is the reverse; the uninvolved leg is advanced up the stairs first (figure 12.29d), and then the crutches and involved leg are raised to the same stair step.

If the stairs do not have a railing, the patient must use the crutches in each hand in lieu of a railing. This is less safe and requires more concentration, especially in the first few attempts; but navigation is feasible according to the same concepts as with a railing. Curbs are essentially stairs without railings and are managed the same way.

Ramps

Ramps may have varying degrees of incline, but the principle for ambulating on them with assistive devices is the same in any case. The most important concept on ramps is that, as with stairs, the crutches and involved leg move together. The other important additional concept is that the individual must take shorter steps going up and down a ramp. The tendency is to take larger steps going down a ramp, but this can be dangerous and lead to falls. The patient should also remember to maintain an upright posture going down ramps since the natural pattern is to lean forward. This can lead to falling, but a reminder to take shorter steps can reduce this risk.

Transfers

Getting up and down from a chair when a patient is using assistive devices can be treacherous. Using the correct technique will ensure greater safety. If using crutches, the individual places both crutches in the hand on the involved side. The patient grasps the handgrips with the hand and places the crutches in a vertical position near the chair but in front of it and to its side. The other hand is placed on the arm of the chair or on the seat if there are no chair arms. The patient pushes from the crutch handgrips and chair simultaneously to gain assistance in standing. He or she then places a crutch under each arm before proceeding. This technique is used with two crutches, one crutch, or a cane. The steps are reversed to move from standing to sitting.

Safety Instructions and Precautions

Walking with assistive devices can be energy consuming and poses a risk of falling, especially if the activity is performed incorrectly or with faulty equipment. Precautions should be taken at the outset to minimize these factors.

Equipment

Crutch tips, handgrips, and axillary pads should be inspected to make sure that they are not worn or damaged. Lack of tread on a crutch or cane tip can cause the assistive device to slip when weight is applied to it. Cracked or damaged handgrips and axillary pads can cause the pads to become loosened during use and put the patient at risk of falling.

If the crutches are adjusted with screws, the screws should be secured and in working order. Wing nuts should be firmly in place.

Environmental Factors

Throw rugs are among the environmental factors that pose a risk to people using assistive devices. The patient must take care not to trip when walking on rugs of this type. Removing them until the person is able to ambulate without the assistive device may be the safest thing to do.

Extra caution must be taken in rain, ice, or snow. A slippery surface increases the patient's risk for falling. Instructions to ambulate more slowly and use smaller steps should be given. If the crutches are advanced too far forward, the fore-aft shear force, discussed earlier, has a greater forward than downward component, causing the crutch to slip forward and putting the person at risk for falling.

To avoid someone accidentally tripping over or kicking the assistive device, the patient should keep the crutches or cane to his or her side rather than in front, but not so far out as to present an obstacle for another person. An exaggerated outward position also places too much pressure on the patient's sides if axillary crutches are being used. The devices should be advanced far enough forward to provide for an economical gait but not so far as to endanger the patient's balance and increase the risk of falling.

Axillary Crutches

The patient should be instructed in proper use of axillary crutches. The purpose of the axillary pad is not to allow the patient to rest the axilla but rather to serve as a cushion against the lateral chest wall so that the crutch does not slip out from under the arm. Resting the axillae on these pads poses a risk of radial nerve damage from pressure on the nerve as it runs through the axillae. The patient's weight should be borne through the hands, not the axillae.

The rehabilitation clinician should understand several issues regarding the use of assistive devices for ambulation. These include proper fitting, correct gait patterns, proper use on various types of surfaces, and safety instructions and precautions.

SUMMARY

Before we can assess pathological gait, we must understand normal gait. There are two phases of gait, stance (62%) and swing phases (38%). Each of these phases is further divided to allow us to analyze gait. The stance phase is divided into initial contact or heel strike, foot flat or loading response, midstance, terminal stance or heel-off, and pre-swing or toe-off. The swing phase is divided into early swing or acceleration, mid-swing, and late swing or deceleration. Determinants of gait provide for a less dramatic sinusoidal motion of the body to make ambulation more economical. Each joint moves through specific ranges of motion during a normal gait speed. As the gait speed increases, the joint angles also increase. Muscles providing force for ambulation act as accelerators, decelerators, or stabilizers. Ground reaction force occurs because of the impact of the foot on the ground at initial contact and the foot pushing away from the ground at pre-swing. Depending upon the size of the stride, the forces applied downward, as opposed to forward or backward, will vary. There is a brief period of double stance during normal walking, but running has no such period. Running has only stance phase and float phase when neither foot is in contact with the ground. Ambulation with assistive devices is necessary when the injured extremity must be protected from full weight bearing. Depending on the weight bearing restriction, partial or no weight bearing on the extremity may be indicated. In the case of non-weight bearing, crutches or a walker are used for ambulation. In the case of partial weight bearing, one crutch or a cane may be used. Specific sequences are used for the various devices and weight bearing requirements for ambulation on a flat surface, stairs, and hills or ramps. The patient should be measured to ensure the assistive device is at the correct height for the patient, and the patient should be instructed in proper ambulation using these devices before independent use is allowed.

KEY CONCEPTS AND REVIEW

1. Discuss the general concepts of gait.

The gait cycle is divided into two phases, stance and swing. The stance phase is divided into initial contact, or heel strike; loading response or foot flat; midstance; heel-off, or terminal stance; and preswing, or toe-off. The swing phase is divided into initial, or early swing; mid-swing; and terminal swing. In normal walking, the stance phase constitutes about 60% of the gait cycle. Double support occurs during loading response and preswing.

2. Identify the range-of-motion changes during the gait cycle.

At initial contact, the hip is at 30° flexion, the knee is at full extension, and the ankle is in neutral. By midstance the hip is extending, the knee has moved from 15° flexion toward extension, and the ankle has moved from 15° plantar flexion to 10° dorsiflexion. At toe-off the hip has moved from 10° extension to neutral, the knee is in 35° flexion, and the ankle is in 20° plantar flexion. During swing, the hip moves from 20° to 30° flexion, the knee moves into 60° flexion and progresses to full extension, and the ankle remains in neutral.

3. Explain the muscle activity involved in ambulation.

Muscles are divided into groups: accelerators, decelerators and shock absorbers, and stabilizers. Muscles act in cyclic fashion, with the greatest activity occurring during early and late stance and early and late swing as muscles prepare to change activity.

4. Describe the general mechanical differences between walking and running.

In running, there is a double-float portion in the gait cycle during which the body is not supported by either lower extremity. The stance phase is divided into initial contact, midstance, and toe-off. The swing phase becomes longer than the stance phase, the stride length increases in a curvilinear (nearly linear) fashion in relation to running speed, and ranges of motion for all joints increase with increased running speeds.

5. Discuss one abnormal gait commonly seen following a musculoskeletal injury.

Prolonged knee extension is an example of a common gait following knee injury and subsequent quadriceps weakness. It occurs because the quadriceps lack control of the knee, and keeping the knee locked prevents the knee from buckling during weight bearing.

6. Outline the various types of gait with assistive devices.

A four-point gait is used when both lower extremities require an assistive device during ambulation. A three-point gait is used with two crutches when weight bearing on the involved extremity is prohibited. A swing-to or swing-through gait can be used with a three-point gait. A two-point gait is used when partial weight bearing on the involved extremity is permitted. The involved extremity is placed between two crutches; some weight is borne by the crutches and some by the extremity. When a cane or single crutch is used, it is placed in the hand opposite the involved extremity, and weight is simultaneously borne by the involved extremity and the cane.

7. Explain the technique involved in stair climbing with assistive devices.

When going up stairs, the patient places the uninvolved extremity on the upper stair, places weight on the crutches or the crutches (on the lower stair step) and handrail, and hops up. The crutches and involved extremity then are raised to the stair step. Going down stairs, the individual places the involved extremity and crutches on the lower stair before lowering the uninvolved leg.

8. Identify the safety measures involved in ambulating with assistive devices.

The assistive device should be adjusted for proper fit; crutch tips, pads, and grips should be inspected for wear before use. Proper instruction in the use of assistive devices on various surfaces and in proper transfer techniques should be provided before the patient is permitted independent use. Instructions should cover use on slippery surfaces, avoiding axillary pressure with crutches, and proper weight bearing on the involved extremity. Scatter rugs should be removed from the patient's environment, and the person should receive instruction about keeping the assistive device close to the body to avoid tripping or falling.

CRITICAL THINKING QUESTIONS

1. If the patient you are treating has limited range of motion in dorsiflexion and plantar flexion, what kind of gait deviation would you expect to see? How would it alter the timing of the knee and ankle motions? Would the patient have normal knee motion during weight bearing? If not, why not? What possible substitutions might the patient use to compensate for the loss of ankle motion?

2. If a patient has weak quads, there will be full knee extension during midstance. Why will this occur? What must be done before normal knee flexion during midstance occurs?

3. If hip flexors are tight, what changes in gait will occur? What changes in pelvic rotation can occur? Will tight hip flexors cause an apparent short-leg syndrome? Why?

4. If the hip abductors are weak, what type of abnormal gait would you expect to see? Identify what can be used to correct this type of gait, and explain the mechanics of how the correction works.

5. You are developing a handout for instructions on gait with crutches. Assuming that the instructions will be for conditions that are non-weight bearing on one extremity, what

instructions will you include? What precautions will you include? What surfaces will you deal with in your instructions?

6. Based on the chapter's opening scenario, what instructions should Drew give Michelle for ambulation with a cane? What precautions should he also include? What criteria should he use to determine when Michelle can begin running?

LAB ACTIVITIES

1. In groups made up of three or four students, evaluate each person's gait. Evaluate gait from anterior, lateral, and posterior views. Identify any gait deviations for each person. List the deficiencies that are causing the gait deviations and identify corrective exercises for each one.

2. In your same group, go to the campus mall or student union and watch people walking. How many gait deviations can you identify? Is there a common one or are there many various gait abnormalities? Can you identify the source of the gait deviation? How did findings of other members in your group compare to yours?

3. Measure your lab partner for axillary crutches. Measure your partner for a cane. Instruct him or her in a gait with the crutches with NWB on one leg. Instruct him or her in a gait using PWB on one leg. Practice rising from and lowering to a chair, ambulation on a flat surface, up and down ramps, and up and down stairs.

4. Using a three-point gait, walk around campus with crutches. What were the most difficult aspects of walking around campus with crutches? What surprised you the most? How did you find people around you responding to your crutches? What precautions did you take or fears did you find yourself feeling?

ADDITIONAL SOURCES

Childress, D.S., and S.A. Gard. 1997. Investigation of vertical motion of the human body during normal walking. *Gait and Posture* 5:161.

Gard, S.A., and D.S. Childress. 1999. The influence of stance-phase knee flexion on the vertical displacement of the trunk during normal walking. *Arch Phys Med Rehabil* 90:26.

13

Aquatic Therapeutic Exercise

OBJECTIVES

After completing this chapter, you should be able to do the following:

1. Identify and discuss the physical properties of water that affect the ability to exercise in water.

2. Define and explain the difference between assistive and resistive aquatic equipment and give examples of each.

3. List precautions and contraindications for aquatic exercise.

4. Identify three advantages of aquatic therapeutic exercise.

5. List three aquatic exercises for each body segment and identify their purposes.

▶ Before Casey Marran became a certified athletic trainer she had been a swimming instructor at the local beaches during the summer. She was well aware of the physical properties of water and of ways it can be used to either assist a body in water or resist it. In her current job as aquatic rehabilitation clinician at the city's largest sports medicine facility, she felt her position was a perfect match for her since it combined her sports medicine knowledge with her love for the water.

Casey's patients have various kinds of injuries and are at different levels within their rehabilitation programs. Casey enjoys this situation because it allows her to make use of the various pieces of exercise equipment and water's various properties. With some patients she uses the water to eliminate weight bearing for ease of lower-extremity activities. With others she uses the water to resist movement in strengthening activities. Still other people are in the water to stress their cardiovascular systems. Some weight-bearing patients are in shallow water so that they encounter greater weight-bearing forces, while others are in the deeper end for activities that allow less weight bearing. Some patients use water dumbbells for resistance activities, whereas others are challenged simply by the water's drag and viscosity. Several of the patients are just beginning their rehabilitation work and use the water to gain motion, while others are in the final phases, letting the water provide them with an aggressive exercise program.

We can't solve problems by using the same kind of thinking
we used when we created them.

ALBERT EINSTEIN, physicist, 1879-1955

Thinking outside the box can be challenging, but it can also be fun. When we create therapeutic exercise programs for our patients, it is important to be creative with our programs. Many rehabilitation clinicians have a swimming pool available to them but do not make use of it. There are often times that the best exercises we can create for our patients will be aquatic exercises.

This chapter includes information that you may apply using your newly gained knowledge of exercise from previous chapters. General concepts and principles of aquatic exercise are introduced first. Examples of exercises for the trunk, lower extremities, and upper extremities are then presented.

Water-based treatment has been in existence for a long time. The ancient Greeks and Romans used water therapeutically. The development of whirlpools and Hubbard tanks promoted the use of water in the early 1900s. Recently there has been a resurgence of interest in aquatic therapy, emphasizing its use in exercise rather than its more traditional effects. This chapter addresses the therapeutic exercise use of water rather than its use as a thermal modality.

Aquatic therapeutic exercise is the application of therapeutic exercise that takes place in water. Exercise in water is advantageous when the patient is unable to perform land-based exercises, allowing the individual to begin exercises sooner than would otherwise be possible. It also provides a means of exercise while the patient is non-weight bearing on an injured lower extremity. Aquatic therapeutic exercise (aquatic therex) can offer the patient a total exercise program that includes activities for cardiovascular conditioning, flexibility, strength, and muscle endurance. It can be instituted early in a rehabilitation program and can continue past the time when the patient is able to perform land-based exercises.

PHYSICAL PROPERTIES AND PRINCIPLES OF WATER

An understanding of how water affects the body's ability to move and exercise is necessary before one can apply water exercises. Although some of these properties can be specifically determined by formulas, we will not focus on the precise mathematical applications here. It is important only to appreciate that one can acquire an understanding of the impact of these properties on the body exercising in water by gaining a thorough knowledge of these mathematical formulas.

Specific Gravity

Specific gravity is also called **relative density.** It refers to the density of an object relative to that of water. It is, then, a ratio of an object's weight to the weight of an equal volume of water. The specific gravity of water is 1. If an object has a specific gravity greater than 1, it will sink in water since its relative weight per volume is more than that of water. If an object has a specific gravity of less than 1, it will float in water. If the object's specific gravity is 1, it will float just below the water's surface.

Specific gravity for the human body varies from one individual to another and from one body segment to another within the same individual. The individual's specific gravity depends on the body's composition of lean and fat mass and the distribution of body fat. The specific gravity of fat is 0.8, bone is 1.5 to 2.0, and lean muscle is 1.0 (Hay, 1993). The average range of specific gravity for the human body is 0.95 to 0.97 (Davis & Harrison, 1988). Since the specific gravity of the average human body is less than 1, people will most often float. Women usually have more body fat than men, so women float better than men. A lean, muscular person may have a specific gravity of 1.10; an obese individual may have a specific gravity of 0.93 (Edlich et al., 1987). These wide variations in individual specific gravities lead to a wide range of abilities to float. Patients who are more muscular and have less fat mass may have a difficult time floating and may require flotation devices during aquatic exercise programs.

Buoyancy

Archimedes' principle of buoyancy states that a body partially or fully immersed in a fluid will experience an upward thrust of that fluid that is equal to the weight of the fluid the body displaces. Buoyancy and specific gravity are closely related in that a body with a specific gravity of less than 1 will float because the weight of the water it displaces is more than the weight of the full body. For example, if a person has a specific gravity of 0.95, 95% of the body is submerged and 5% of the body floats above the water's surface. The amount of water displaced is 95% of the body weight. Specific-gravity values, in essence, indicate the amount of the body that floats and the amount that is submerged; and the weight of the body or part of the body submerged is equal to the weight of the water it displaces.

Center of Buoyancy

Center of buoyancy is the center of gravity of the displaced fluid and the point at which the buoyant force acts on the body. In water, two opposing forces act on the body. Buoyancy is the upward force, and gravity is the downward force. Each has a center point of balance. When a floating body is in equilibrium, the center of buoyancy and the center of gravity are in vertical alignment with each other (figure 13.1). In this position, the body is balanced. If the center of buoyancy and the center of gravity are not in vertical alignment with each other, the body is out of equilibrium and will tend to roll or turn. For example, if you place a kickboard between your knees, the center of buoyancy will cause your lower extremities to float upward.

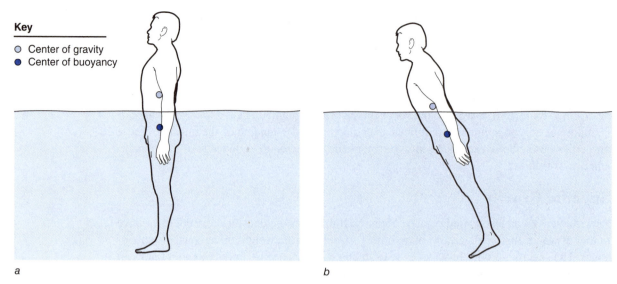

▶ **Figure 13.1** When the center of buoyancy and the center of gravity are not in vertical alignment, a person must actively work to keep from rolling in the water. *(a)* The body is in equilibrium; the centers of gravity and buoyancy are aligned vertically. *(b)* The body is not in equilibrium; the centers of gravity and buoyancy are not aligned vertically.

Hydrodynamics

The fluid's resistance to movement, the size and shape of the object moving, and the speed of the object govern movement through water. Some of the factors that impact a body's movement through fluid are interrelated.

Viscosity

Viscosity is the resistance to movement within a fluid and is caused by the friction of the fluid's molecules. Additional factors include physical properties such as cohesion (the attraction of water molecules to adjacent water molecules), adhesion (the attraction of water molecules to the individual's body), and surface tension (the attraction of water molecules on the surface to each other). Movement within the water is resisted by the adhesion and cohesion of water molecules to the person in the water and to other water molecules, respectively. Surface tension provides a resistance when an individual attempts to break the water's surface with the body or a body segment.

Drag

Drag is the water's resistance to a body that is moving through it. There are three types of drag: form drag, wave drag, and frictional drag (Koury, 1996).

Form Drag Form drag is the resistance that an object encounters in a fluid and is determined by the object's size and shape. A larger object has more drag than a smaller object. A broad object has more drag than a streamlined object. Form drag is directly related to turbulence. The greater the form drag, the greater the turbulence. Turbulence produces a low-pressure area behind the object that tends to pull the object backward (figure 13.2).

A streamlined object moving through water produces a laminar flow—a smooth movement of water that causes a minimal amount of resistance to movement. There is less form drag because of less turbulence. The water molecules all travel at the same speed past the body. Friction of the fluid is minimal because the water molecules separate easily, moving smoothly behind the object.

On the other hand, a broad object produces a turbulent flow as it moves through the water. The object has more form drag because of the greater turbulence created behind it. The layers of the water move irregularly as they run into the object and rush to

Streamlined object

a

Broad-shaped object

b

▶ **Figure 13.2** Form drag: *(a)* laminar flow, *(b)* turbulent flow. Form drag is caused by turbulence behind an object moving through a fluid.

move past and behind it. This causes a circular movement of the water layers as they rejoin behind the object. This circular motion of water layers pulling against the moving object is called an **eddy.** Because of the disturbance caused by the eddy, a wake or trail is left in the water (seen as either bubbles behind the body or white water, depending on the amount of turbulence created).

Form drag can be used in an aquatic therex program as a means of altering resistance to exercises. A change in the position of the body or body segment can increase or decrease form drag. For example, moving the arm horizontally in the water with the palm down causes less form drag than with the hand in a vertical position. Shortening or lengthening the body's extremity decreases or increases the form drag, respectively, since the longer lever arm pushes more water than a shorter one. Adding equipment such as hand paddles increases the surface area of the hand, and other equipment such as long paddles increases the lever-arm length; both provide additional form drag to increase the resistance of an exercise.

Wave Drag   Wave drag is the water's resistance because of turbulence. The greater the speed of an object, the greater the wave drag. Wave drag is reduced if movement remains under water. The amount of water wake is an indication of wave drag. Swimming pools often have a splash gutter around the periphery to reduce wave drag for swimmers.

Exercises performed in calm water produce less resistance than those performed in turbulent water. The individual can create wave drag during an exercise by changing positions frequently and rapidly. Increasing the speed of an exercise also increases the wave drag that the exercise causes. For example, walking in water provides the body with 5 to 6 times the resistance that walking in air does. Running water, however, increases the resistance to more than 40 times that of air (McWaters, 1988).

Frictional Drag   Frictional drag is the result of water's surface tension. This is not a factor in therapeutic exercise, but it becomes an important element for the competitive swimmer. Frictional drag can add crucial milliseconds to a race time, and swimmers can reduce it by shaving body hair before competition. Recently, custom-made bodysuits constructed from unique new fibers reduce frictional drag.

Hydrostatic Pressure

Pascal's law states that pressure from a fluid is exerted equally on all surfaces of an immersed object at any given depth (figure 13.3). The more deeply the object is immersed, the greater

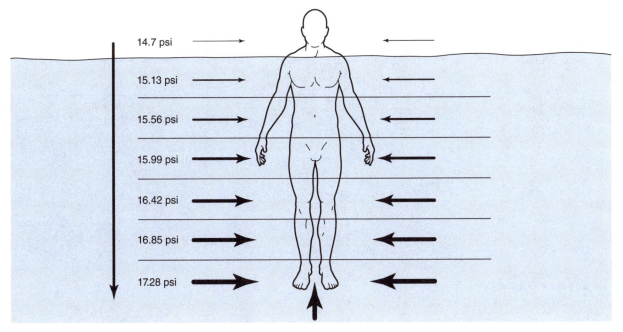

14.7 psi

15.13 psi

15.56 psi

15.99 psi

16.42 psi

16.85 psi

17.28 psi

▶ **Figure 13.3**   Pascal's law.

Several major physical properties of water, including specific gravity, buoyancy, center of buoyancy, and hydrodynamics, affect the way people exercise in water.

the pressure it encounters. Atmospheric pressure at the surface is 14.7 psi (pounds per square inch). For every foot of submersion, water pressure increases by 0.43 psi (Edlich et al., 1987). Hydrostatic pressure can positively affect edema both by reducing post-injury edema and by allowing exercise without the risk of increasing edema.

Weight Bearing in Water

Since buoyancy and gravity are opposing forces on a body in water, the more deeply the body submerges in water, the less weight is borne by the lower extremities (figure 13.4). Because a male's center of gravity is higher than a female's, the specific percentage of body weight borne at different depths varies slightly from female to male. For example, with the body immersed to the xyphoid process, females bear 28% of their weight whereas males bear 35% of their weight (Thein & Brody, 1998).

These percentages are useful information, especially in the early stages of rehabilitation. For example, an injured basketball player who is partial weight bearing to 50% on the left lower extremity can perform therapeutic exercises for the left leg in water that is at hip level. As the patient is permitted to bear more weight on the leg, he or she can perform the exercises in shallower water.

Changing walking speed in the water will change the weight-bearing forces in the water (Harrison, Hillman, & Bulstrode, 1992). Generally, the faster a person walks in the water, the higher the weight-bearing percentages. For example, if you walk at a slow pace, you must walk in water that is at a level below the axilla in order to be 50% weight bearing. If you walk at a fast rate, 50% weight bearing occurs in water above the axilla level.

EQUIPMENT

In recent years, more and more manufacturers have produced more types and varieties of aquatic exercise equipment. Aquatic equipment can be divided into safety equipment and exercise equipment. Exercise equipment is used and classified as assistive or resistive.

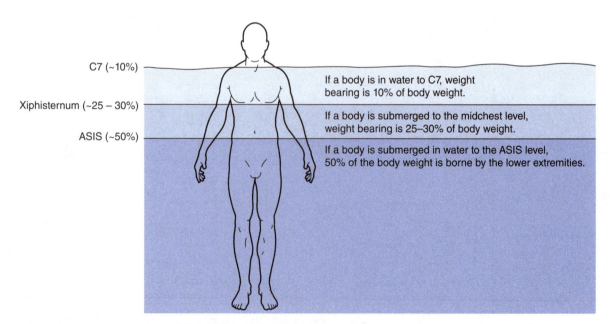

▶ **Figure 13.4** Weight bearing in water.

Safety Equipment

The specific safety equipment required at a pool depends on the size of the pool and on state regulations. Safety equipment includes various rescue equipment such as ring buoys, the shepherd's crook, and rescue tubes. Ring buoys are useful in towing and in-water rescues; the shepherd's crook is used for rescue of victims from the side of the pool. A rescue tube has an attached towrope and can support one or more persons. It is flexible enough to wrap around a body.

Spine boards should be among the items of safety equipment at a pool (figure 13.5). These are made of wood, plastic, or fiberglass and have neck and head straps and/or supports. Transport litters or stretchers should be readily available.

Secondary safety equipment should include a basic first-aid kit. In addition to the routine first-aid items, the kit should contain items such as rubber gloves, earplugs, nose plugs, and waterproof bandages.

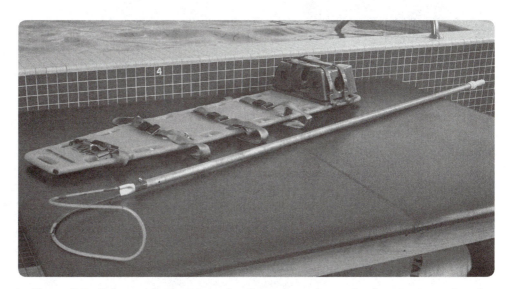

▶ **Figure 13.5** Safety equipment. A shepherd's crook or other retrieval equipment and a spine board should be readily available.

Exercise Equipment

Exercise equipment most often comprises items that are portable but may also include installed or fixed equipment. Rails and benches are examples of fixed equipment. Portable items may range from simple kickboards to elaborate in-water gym equipment. The selection of specific items depends on the budget and on the sophistication of the pool exercises incorporated into a rehabilitation routine.

Assistive Devices

Assistive exercise equipment helps to stabilize or support the patient in a desired position while in the water; this may be upright, supine, or prone. Flotation devices are used to maintain buoyancy in these positions. They can also serve to assist in the motion of an exercise and often are used to provide additional motion of a joint. The following sections deal with some of the more commonly used devices.

Flotation Cuffs Flotation cuffs are worn on the upper arms or on the ankles to provide buoyancy for the arms or legs (figure 13.6). When used on the ankles, they can facilitate gait activities or provide buoyancy for range-of-motion activities.

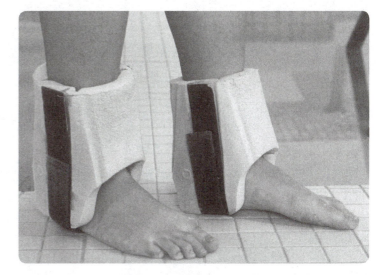

▶ **Figure 13.6** Flotation cuffs.

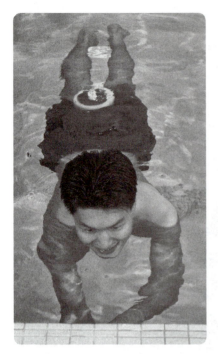

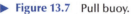

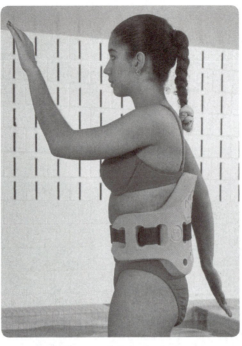

▶ **Figure 13.7** Pull buoy.

▶ **Figure 13.8** Flotation belt.

Pull Buoys Pull buoys are usually Styrofoam devices that are held between the thighs to provide flotation for the legs and lower body during arm exercises (figure 13.7).

Vests and Belts Vests and belts are used to maintain buoyancy for the trunk during deep-water arm or leg exercises. They are also used for deep-water running and prone- or supine-position exercises (figure 13.8). They should fit comfortably and snugly so they do not ride up. They should also fit well enough not to impede arm or leg movement.

Kickboards Kickboards provide buoyancy for the arms, legs, head, or trunk. They are available in soft or hard materials and can be used in a vertical, supine, or prone position. They can be used on the water's surface or under the water (figure 13.9). A disadvantage of using kickboards with the arms is that prolonged positioning can cause shoulder fatigue.

Water Dumbbells Water dumbbells resemble regular dumbbells, but they are made of Styrofoam, and the bar is padded (figure 13.10). The dumbbell can be placed under the axillae or under the knees to provide buoyancy. Dumbbells offer buoyancy to the arms without adding to the stress of the shoulders the way kickboards can. The bars come in different lengths: The shorter lengths are used under the axilla or held in each hand, and the longer lengths are used under the knees or held with both hands.

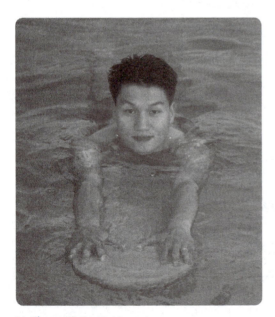

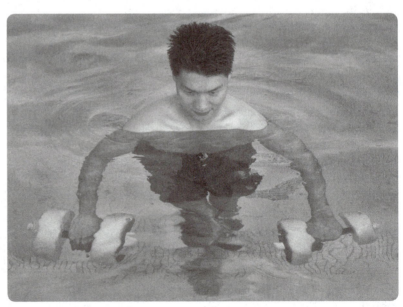

▶ **Figure 13.9** Kickboard.

▶ **Figure 13.10** Water dumbbells.

Other Buoyancy Equipment Other buoyancy equipment encompasses items such as inner tubes, water mattresses, ski belts, and cervical float collars. Facilities with restricted budgets may use empty plastic gallon containers as flotation devices.

Resistive Devices

Resistive devices can advance the difficulty of an exercise to increase muscle strength or endurance. They increase exercise difficulty by increasing a body segment's surface area, requiring increased speed of movement, or adding buoyancy or weight.

Lower Extremity Lower-extremity resistive devices are designed to increase resistance to lower-extremity movement. They do this by either increasing the friction during ambulation in the water or increasing the form or wave drag of the lower extremity.

Water shoes are used when the patient is in shallow water and able to touch the bottom of the pool. They are not used during swimming or kicking. They increase the weight of the lower extremity and increase the leg's drag in the water. Their rubberized soles make them good for providing traction during walking, running, or jumping activities. The surface of the sole results in an increase in friction to increase resistance as well as providing stability during these activities.

Fins, which come in a variety of styles and lengths, increase resistance because of the increase in drag they produce. The shorter fins are more appropriate for patients with limited ankle range of motion. Shorter fins are more manageable in the water, offer less resistance than longer fins, and allow the patient to perform a more normal kick while swimming. Any fin that is used should fit the patient well and not pinch, as pinching can cause blisters or cramping.

Boots covering the feet and ankles increase form and/or wave drag during the exercise (figure 13.11). Extension panels on the front or sides of the boot cause turbulence of the water during movement to increase the extremity's form and wave drag. Boots can be used during exercises or walking and running activities to increase difficulty of the activity.

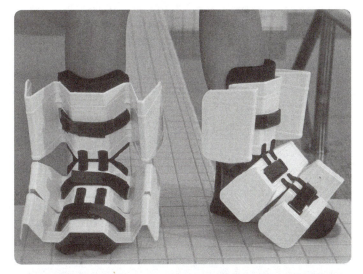

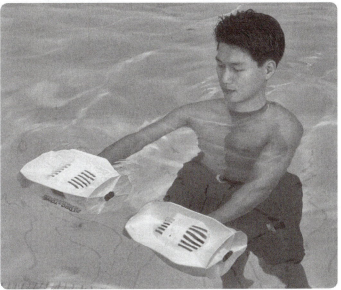

▶ **Figure 13.11** Boots and bells.

Upper Extremity Upper-extremity resistive devices, like those for the lower extremity, are designed to increase extremity resistance by increasing form or wave drag or turbulence.

Webbed gloves are the least-resistive devices for the arms. They can be used earlier in the aquatic exercise program than some of the other devices. The gloves are made of Lycra, nylon, or neoprene, so they are soft and pliable. They thus permit the patient to close or open the hand to reduce or increase the water resistance during an exercise.

Paddles either are handheld or are attached to the hand with straps. They come in a variety of sizes and shapes. The larger the size, the more resistance the paddles produce by increasing form and wave drag. Some paddles look like dumbbells except that they are flat and their disks can be open-vented or close-vented to reduce or increase resistance. Typically made of rigid plastic, paddles offer more resistance than gloves.

Major categories of aquatic equipment include safety equipment and exercise equipment. Equipment for exercising in the water comprises many types of assistive devices, which help to stabilize or support the patient in the pool, and resistive devices that increase the difficulty of an exercise.

Bells provide greater resistance to the arms than the other devices and so are appropriate in the later stages of an aquatic exercise program. Like the boots, they offer resistance by providing turbulence and form and wave drag. They are similar in structure to the boots (figure 13.11) and have either side panels or hollow cores.

Cardiovascular Devices Cardiovascular devices are available either as separate aquatic containers or as special treadmills that are immersed in swimming pools. The separate containers offer resistance by providing turbulence against an individual who is walking. These devices are costly, but they may be an aquatic exercise solution for facilities without swimming pools. They do require substantial space and some maintenance but obviously not as much as a regular swimming pool.

INDICATIONS, ADVANTAGES, PRECAUTIONS, AND CONTRAINDICATIONS

Although aquatic exercise has the advantage that it can begin early in a rehabilitation program when other forms of exercises are contraindicated, aquatic exercise is not for everyone. Before deciding to use an aquatic therapeutic exercise program, the rehabilitation clinician must be aware of the indications, as well as the limitations and dangers, of this type of system.

Indications

An aquatic therapeutic exercise program is indicated when the patient has many of the typical signs and symptoms associated with musculoskeletal injuries. These include pain, edema, muscle spasm, loss of motion, weakness, limited endurance, or restricted weight-bearing status. Aquatic exercise can also serve as a method of maintaining cardiovascular conditioning or normal status of the uninvolved extremities.

Advantages

The indications lead naturally to advantages of the use of aquatic exercises. Aquatic exercise can be particularly beneficial when the patient is non-weight bearing on the injured extremity. While the patient may be restricted in activities on dry land, he or she may perform a wide range of activities in the water. The warmth of the water causes a relaxation of muscles. The buoyancy reduces joint compressive forces to allow movement and positioning with reduced pain. The warmth of the water also reduces pain sensation by bombarding the sensory system with temperature input and decreasing the painful noxious input that travels the same pathways. This relief of spasm and reduction of pain assists in breaking down the pain-spasm injury cycle discussed in chapter 2.

Reduction of joint compressive forces and relaxation of muscles permit better movement of the injured area. Buoyancy equipment can help even further to reduce stress of area muscles and permit greater ease of movement. Reduction of gravitational forces on the body allows activity when weight bearing on land is not permissible. Walking in water with reduced weight bearing makes it possible for muscles to function properly for the gait sequence. This encourages the maintenance of muscle tone and balance. Weight bearing can be progressive if the patient walks in water of decreasing depths: The lower the water level, the greater the weight bearing.

Instituting exercises early helps the patient maintain or develop a healthy attitude, promotes body awareness and balance, and stresses newly forming tissue without overstressing it. The healing process is advanced because of the greater exchange of nutrients and metabolites that occur with improved circulation in the injured site. Movement in water can often relieve or reduce pain due to immobilization or edema. If pain and edema are reduced to positively affect the pain-injury cycle, the healing rate may be accelerated so that recovery occurs more readily.

The patient's ability to begin exercises sooner also helps to prevent the deconditioning that can play a part in delaying the return to full participation.

Precautions

As with any exercise, the rehabilitation clinician must be aware of precautions and must take special care to administer the aquatic rehabilitation program with these in mind. In the presence of any doubt or question about the patient's ability to perform an aquatic program, it is essential to consult the physician in advance.

Fear of the Water

A patient's fear of water often calls for encouragement and patience. It is advisable to use a vest, even in shallow water, for reassurance. The patient should begin in shallower water if the injury permits. As a rehabilitation clinician, you may have to give the patient assistance and physical support through a hands-on approach until he or she becomes more comfortable in the water. Any patient who experiences an excessive fear of the water should not be forced into an aquatic exercise program.

Medications

Some medications that affect heart rate, blood pressure, or respiration, or any other medication that may alter cardiorespiratory function, may impact the patient's ability to exercise in the water. The rehabilitation clinician should check with the patient's physician or pharmacist before permitting the individual in the water.

Ear Infections

If the patient has a tendency toward chronic ear infections, he or she should apply proper protective ear devices before entering the water. Exercises should be designed so the patient's head is kept above the water to reduce the risk of an infection.

Specific Conditions

Patients with certain systemic or compromising diseases such as diabetes, cardiovascular disease, or seizure disorders should be carefully monitored while in the water. If the person is sensitive to the pool chemicals, it is essential to observe for unwanted side effects.

No patient should ever be in the pool alone, even if he or she is a good swimmer. Someone should always accompany patients during aquatic exercise.

Contraindications

Under certain conditions or in certain situations, patients should not be allowed in the pool for aquatic therapeutic exercises. These are absolute contraindications that, if ignored, could lead to serious consequences.

Illness

A patient who has a contagious infection and is at risk of transmitting the infection to others should not be allowed in the water.

A severe cold or the flu warrants keeping the patient out of the water until he or she has recovered. Any urinary tract infection should be resolved before the patient is allowed in the water. If the patient has a temperature of 100 °F, aquatic exercise must be postponed. Not only is a fever a problem in that it indicates an illness; it may rise further because of the temperature of the water and the exercise.

One major advantage of aquatic therex, among others, is that exercise in the water is feasible for patients who are not yet weight bearing. Precautions and contraindications relate to the use of medications, various medical conditions, and illness.

Open Wounds

Open wounds should be healed before a patient is allowed into the pool. After surgery, the healing time is usually about seven days. However, if any portion of the surgical scar is open, the patient should remain out of the water.

Other Medical Conditions

Some conditions are not usually found in the young population but need to be mentioned as a point of information. Conditions that are absolute contraindications for an individual's participation in an aquatic exercise program include tracheostomy, severe kidney disease, presence of a nasogastric tube, fecal incontinence, radiation treatments within the past three months, and a history of uncontrolled seizures.

AQUATIC THERAPEUTIC EXERCISE PRINCIPLES AND GUIDELINES

As with therapeutic exercises on land, aquatic therapeutic exercises follow a progression. They begin with range-of-motion and flexibility exercises, progress to strength and endurance exercises, and then advance to coordination and agility activities before the patient begins doing functional and performance-specific activities. An exercise session should begin with a warm-up and end with a cool-down.

The length of the warm-up depends on the temperature of the water. Therapeutic pools used exclusively for exercise are often set at 92° to 98 °F (33°-37 °C). Swimming pools are set at a lower temperature, 80° to 85 °F (27°-30 °C). The cooler the pool temperature, the longer the warm-up should be.

A cool-down is particularly important if the exercise session has included cardiovascular activities. Cool-down activities can include walking, easy treading water, or sculling in deep or shallow water. It is important to remind the patient to rehydrate following exercises in the pool. Because of the warm water temperature, the patient will perspire and not realize it.

Principles Related to Water Properties

The rehabilitation clinician determines the essential exercises of the aquatic exercise session on the basis of specific findings and gears the session toward correcting the deficiencies observed. The same progression principles are used for aquatic exercises as for dry-land exercises.

Additionally, because of the properties of water discussed earlier, other factors enter into the selection of specific exercises. These factors include hydrostatic pressure, drag and turbulence, and buoyancy.

Hydrostatic pressure can affect the edema of a segment. It is more advantageous to exercise a swollen extremity in deep water than in shallower water because of the greater hydrostatic pressure at greater depths.

A longer lever arm increases form drag. The straighter the arm, the greater the resistance. It is best to start with a shorter lever arm and progress to longer ones as strength improves. You can make additional changes in lever-arm length by changing the position of the resistive equipment. The farther away from the body's core the resistance is, the greater it is.

Resistance can be provided for a body segment using the properties of water. Increasing the speed of the activity causes increased resistance to movement. Moving objects toward the surface of the water, increasing resistive surface area by using the equipment discussed earlier, and using floats can all increase water resistance to provide for additional strength gains. Exercising in differing depths of water will also change the weight bearing and resistance.

Buoyancy can make an exercise easier or more difficult, depending on the relative position of the center of buoyancy and center of gravity. Buoyancy becomes a greater factor for the body in deeper water.

Aquatic Exercise Progression

Although we have noted that an aquatic therex program can serve to maintain cardiovascular conditioning and status of the uninvolved extremities, we will not consider such exercises in detail. The emphasis here is on the injured segment. Keep in mind that cardiovascular activities are usually performed in the deep water unless in-water treadmills are available. Deep-water cardiovascular exercises include activities such as running, treading water, and swimming. If it is desirable to exercise the uninjured extremities, the more advanced exercises presented later in this chapter can be used.

Early-Phase Exercises

The early portion of an aquatic therex program includes gait-training activities in appropriate-depth water, range-of-motion exercises, and perhaps early strengthening activities, if these are indicated and tolerated. Gait training emphasizes the correct manner of ambulation, proper posture, and good balance. The rehabilitation clinician should rely on knowledge of proper posture and proper gait timing and sequencing, as discussed in chapters 11 and 12, to assist and instruct the patient in correct posture and gait techniques. The goals in this phase are to achieve normal gait in water and restore normal range of motion.

It is beneficial to use buoyancy equipment in range-of-motion exercises. Buoyancy equipment allows the extremity to come to the water's surface, where range-of-motion gains are easiest to achieve. At the surface, the drag is at a minimum, so movement is made with less effort. Resistance exercises in the beginning are low level and are provided without resistive devices. Use of the body segment's own drag in the water is sufficient in the early stage of strengthening activities. Speed of movement is kept slow initially so that less resistance is offered by the water. Koury (Koury, 1996) recommends limiting initial bouts of resistance exercises to one to two sets of 10 to 15 repetitions, but the specific numbers of sets and repetitions are individually determined and based on the patient's level of fitness, tolerance, and ability and on the program goals. Increasing the repetitions or increasing the sets makes the exercise progressive. The method selected to provide progression specifically determined by the individual's tolerance, normal activity demands, rate of healing, and fitness level.

Middle-Phase Exercises

As the patient progresses, restoration of muscle strength and endurance—the goal of the middle phase—receives more emphasis.

Viscosity-producing drag and buoyancy-permitting motion are now used to provide resistance to increase strength. Speed of motion and lever-arm length are other variables that change the resistance. Deeper water offers additional resistance because it increases pressure on the extremity and increases stability requirements.

Progression with resistive equipment includes starting with short objects and progressing to longer objects. Using lower-profile objects is less difficult than exercising with higher-profile objects. The more drag an object provides, either because it increases the water's resistance or because its profile is made larger, the greater the resistance. The more turbulence the object produces, the greater the resistance. The farther along the extremity the object is placed, the greater the resistance it offers. Each of these ways of increasing resistance creates an additional level of difficulty.

As was done in the early-phase exercises, you can increase the intensity of an exercise by increasing the repetitions or sets. This will help improve endurance more than strength, but there will also be strength gains at a lower rate. This principle is discussed in chapter 7.

Advanced-Phase Exercises

The later stages of the aquatic therex program present a progression toward achieving the goal, normal restoration of the ABCs of proprioception—agility, balance, and coordination. This prepares the patient to withstand the stresses that will be applied during land-based activities.

Gait-training activities can now include walking at a faster pace or running, side-stepping, cariocas, and retrograde walking. Hopping, jumping, squatting, and other sudden changes in direction are also appropriate in this phase. Coordination exercises with eyes open and eyes closed can be included as well.

Strength activities can continue to increase in intensity if the rehabilitation clinician uses more aggressively resistive equipment, increases the speed, requires more than one activity simultaneously, increases repetitions and sets, or changes the shape or size of the resistive equipment.

Land-based exercises may have started during this phase or during the middle stage. Whether or not the aquatic therex program continues depends on the patient's interest in the program, the rehabilitation clinician's preference, rehabilitation goals, and equipment and pool availability.

End-Phase Exercises

If a patient continues in the pool for therapeutic exercises, this is the final stage of aquatic-based exercises. Because of advancement to land exercises, aquatic exercises either constitute a fraction of the time of the total therapeutic exercise program or are discontinued; however, some patients may prefer to continue in the water because of satisfaction they receive from their workouts. The goal in this phase is to prepare the patient for the specific demands of his or her activity.

Exercises during this phase mimic the skill demands of the patient's sport; include aggressive coordination, agility, and speed activities; and reinforce performance of specific skills using proper posture. High-demand activities can include plyometrics such as box jumping drills and bench stepping in the water. Activity-specific activities can include the use of equipment such as a golf club, tennis racket, or baseball bat in the water.

Progression Guidelines

Progression requires close observation by the rehabilitation clinician and accurate reporting by the patient to the clinician. You should observe the patient's response to the exercise program and the quality of performance. If the patient is able to perform the required exercises correctly, swiftly, and without difficulty, he or she advances to the next level of difficulty. You must also examine the patient's range of motion, strength, and balance and record improvements or changes.

The patient must communicate to the rehabilitation clinician any increases in pain or swelling or other symptoms following an exercise session. In the absence of any injury aggravation, he or she continues to progress in the program. It is essential to advance the patient at a rate that will provide for a continued overload, but not so quickly that his or her body is unable to adapt to the stresses and or suffers a re-injury.

DEEP-WATER EXERCISE

Even patients who are unable to swim can exercise in deep water. Because of its advantages, deep-water exercise warrants special attention in this chapter. We will look briefly at the benefits of this type of exercise.

The most obvious benefit of deep-water exercise is that it involves no weight bearing and no impact forces on the body. This is particularly important if the patient wants to exercise but either is unable to tolerate impact forces or needs to remain completely non-weight bearing. For example, a basketball player with patellar tendinopathy that causes sufficient pain to restrict ground running may be able to tolerate running in deep water. Deep water running can help keep the individual's cardiovascular fitness level and strength intact during the rehabilitation process. A runner with a stress fracture is another example of a patient who can benefit from deep-water running.

Since gravity is opposed by buoyancy in deep water, the forces of gravity on a submersed body are minimal. If weights are applied to the ankles, a slight traction force is produced by the force of gravity and the counterbalance force of buoyancy. This can be important for a patient who has low-back pain secondary to either facet irritation or intervertebral disk compression.

Deep-water exercises are essentially concentric. Trauma to acutely injured tendons, muscles, or bones is reduced without eccentric activity, yet good strengthening can be provided with deep-water exercises.

Important benefits of exercise in deep water include the absence of weight bearing and the lack of impact forces on the body of the patient.

■ Some Recommendations for Optimal Benefits

During deep-water exercises, the body should remain in good alignment to keep stresses reduced and to use muscles effectively. The head should be out of the water and in proper alignment with the rest of the body. There should be no forward positioning of the neck or upward positioning of the chin to produce an excessive cervical lordosis. The lumbar and thoracic spine should be in correct alignment as discussed in chapter 11 in relation to proper standing posture (figure 13.12). Buoyancy vests or belts help the patient maintain a good postural alignment in deep water. If the spine is not in a neutral position, the center of gravity and the center of buoyancy will not be in a vertical alignment. It becomes more difficult for the patient to maintain a vertical position in deep water when the spine is not in good alignment.

To keep the spine in a good alignment, the patient should attempt to keep the chest lifted and to maintain some tension in the abdominals and gluteals. This preserves good spinal alignment in the water just as it does on land.

Arm activity during deep-water exercises should occur from the shoulders, not the elbows. The arms, as in land running, are used in a pumping activity, with initiation of the activity occurring at the shoulders.

As in ground running, hip flexion and extension coincide with knee flexion and extension. The ankle goes into plantar flexion during leg extension motion and into dorsiflexion as the hip moves into flexion.

Throughout deep-water running, the spine remains in neutral with a slight forward inclination (figure 13.13). The movement through the water is produced by the extremities, not the trunk. It is necessary for the trunk muscles, the abdominals and the back extensors, to act as stabilizers of the trunk as the body is propelled through the water by the arms and legs.

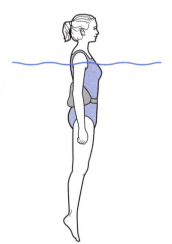

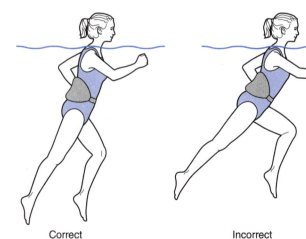

Correct   Incorrect

▶ **Figure 13.12**   Correct vertical alignment.   ▶ **Figure 13.13**   Position for deep-water running.

AQUATIC THERAPEUTIC EXERCISES

The sections that follow present a variety of aquatic exercises for the spine, the lower extremities, and the upper extremities. First, though, a few special points relevant to water-based exercise deserve mention. The first point concerns refraction in water and its effect on observation. When light rays move from the air through water, they bend as a result of the lower density of water compared to that of the air. This bending of the light rays makes the bottom of the pool appear closer to the surface than it actually is. It also makes the submerged portion of the patient's body appear distorted (figure 13.14). The submerged body segments appear to be flexed at a different angle than the body segments that are not in the water. This can make it difficult for someone standing at poolside to accurately judge the position of the body or body segment. At times it may be necessary for the rehabilitation clinician to get into the water with the patient to make sure the positioning is correct, especially if the patient has difficulty with proprioception and is unable to align him- or herself correctly without tactile guidance.

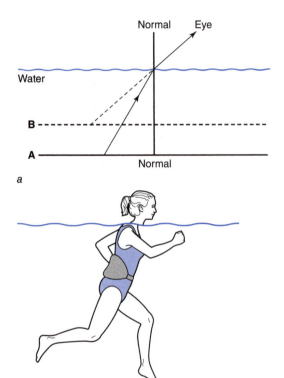

a

b

▶ **Figure 13.14** *(a)* Refraction of light causes rays reflected from the true bottom of the pool A to appear at a false bottom B. *(b)* Refraction can create illusions in alignment of body segments.

The patient should wear a vest or ski belt while performing deep-water exercises. The use of fins can make deep-water exercises more difficult, so goals of the exercise should be determined before the decision to use them is made.

Another point relates to exercises in shallow water. It is advisable for a patient exercising with the feet on the bottom of the pool to wear aquatic shoes. These will enhance balance and provide friction resistance, as well as protecting the patient's feet from abrasions.

The exercises described here are intended only as suggestions and are presented in a progressive series. The exercises are far from all-inclusive. Indeed, the range of possible exercises is limited only by the patient's abilities and your imagination and knowledge. If you know the goals of the therex program, understand the injury limitations, know the patient's abilities, and have an appreciation of the water's physical properties, you can incorporate any appropriate exercise into the aquatic therex program that your ingenuity allows.

A final point is that you should determine the depth of the water for the exercise according to the patient's confidence in the water, weight-bearing status, and the goals for the treatment session.

Some of the exercises are presented, along with their purposes, in the following sections. For many of the strengthening exercises, however, the discussion does not specify which muscles the activity is designed to strengthen. Using your knowledge of kinetics and aquatic principles, attempt to identify the muscles for which each exercise is intended.

Exercises for the Spine

An important concept to remember about aquatic spine exercises is that the patient should maintain a neutral spine during all activities. This keeps the vertebrae in good alignment, places minimal stress on the spine, and uses the spine and trunk most efficiently, effectively, and correctly. If the patient is unable to maintain a proper spinal alignment during an exercise, the intensity, complexity, or demand level should be decreased and the patient should concentrate on a lower-level exercise until he or she has mastered spinal alignment at that level. If an individual has difficulty identifying correct spinal alignment with even the basic exercises, it may be necessary for the rehabilitation clinician to get into the pool and use tactile stimulation to provide sensory feedback. This feedback will help the patient identify and learn correct neutral spine alignment.

You will see that many of the exercises described here are similar to land exercises. When patients perform them in warm water, the activity is often easier and more comfortable.

Spine Exercises in Shallow Water

The following sections describe only a few of many exercises that could be suggested for the spine. They begin with the cervical spine and move to the pelvis and advance from easiest to most difficult.

■ **Neck Stretches.** To stretch the lateral neck, the patient holds the right arm down and across the front of the body and then side-bends the neck to the left, as seen in figure 13.15a. Reverse neck and arm position to stretch the left lateral neck. Figure 13.15b shows an alternative stretch in which the left hand is over the head. In this position, the patient provides a gentle stretch with the left arm while keeping the opposite arm behind the back. Substitutions for these exercises should be corrected. Most common substitutions include flexing the neck forward or rotating it to the stretch side or flexing the trunk rather than the neck. In the neck flexion stretch in figure 13.15c, the patient places both hands on the back of the head and performs a gentle pull of the head forward and downward with the hands as the chin is tucked

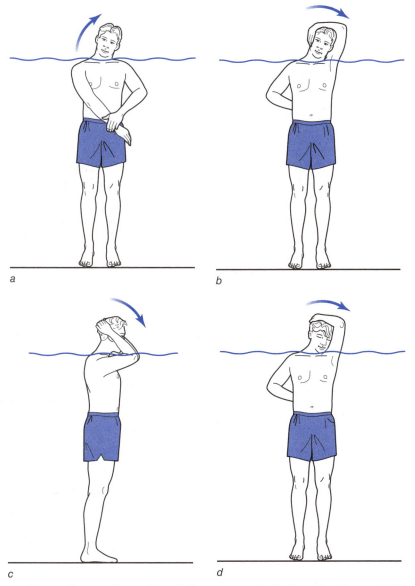

a

b

c

d

▶ **Figure 13.15** Neck stretches, shallow water: *(a)* active lateral neck stretch, *(b)* stretch to right lateral neck with assistance of left arm, *(c)* stretch to posterior neck muscles using weight of both arms to assist, *(d)* right levator scapula stretch.

toward the chest. It is important to instruct the patient to only use the weight of the arms and not add additional force in the stretch. The levator scapula stretch (13.15d) is similar to that seen in figure 13.15b except that the neck is rotated slightly to face toward the axilla. Substitutions to watch for include rotating the neck too far, side bending the trunk, and trunk flexion.

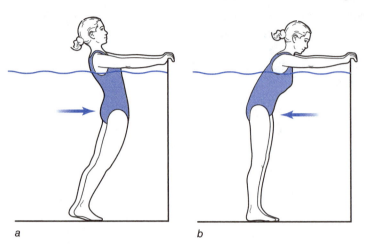

▶ **Figure 13.16**   Spine: *(a)* extension, *(b)* flexion.

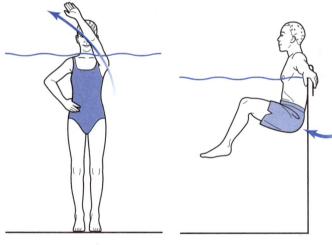

▶ **Figure 13.17**   Lateral trunk stretch.

▶ **Figure 13.18**   Pelvic roll.

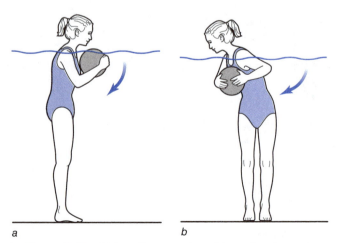

▶ **Figure 13.19**   *(a)* Standing crunches, *(b)* rotational crunches.

■ **Spine Extension-Flexion.** Standing with hands on the pool wall and feet shoulder-width apart, the patient keeps the arms straight throughout the exercise (figure 13.16). The hips are pressed forward toward the wall, then backward. During the move forward, the chest is lifted upward; when moving backward, the patient attempts to make the spine rounded. A common substitution is rocking on the feet rather than stretching the spine or pushing and pulling with the hands on the wall.

■ **Lateral Stretch.** With the feet shoulder-width apart, the patient raises one arm overhead and reaches upward and across the body (figure 13.17) feeling a stretch on the arm-elevated lateral trunk side. Substitutions include leaning to the side from the hips and rotating the trunk.

■ **Pelvic Roll.** With the back against the pool wall, the patient supports himself or herself by holding on to the edge of the pool as seen in figure 13.18. With the lumbar spine kept flat against the pool wall and the abdominals tensed (pulling the naval to the spine), the legs are lifted until the knees and hips are at 90°. In this position, the patient slowly lifts the pelvis off the wall by increasing the tension of the lower abdominals. The pelvis is rolled back to the wall before the legs are lowered. If pain is reported during this exercise, the patient is likely substituting with hip flexors and arching the back. Instruct the patient to maintain the lower back in contact with the pool wall. If the correct position cannot be maintained, instruct the patient to lift only one leg at a time and alternate them in the exercise until sufficient strength is acquired to perform the exercise properly. Another substitution is pushing off the pool floor with the feet rather than lifting the legs.

■ **Standing Crunch.** The patient stands with a flotation device or a ball against the chest (figure 13.19). The abdominals are contracted to flex the spine, and the position is held for at least 5 to 10 s. A pelvic tilt should be maintained throughout the exercise. This exercise can be modified to include rotational crunches as seen in figure 13.19b. The trunk is rotated about 10° to one side before the crunch is performed. The motion is repeated to the opposite side. Substitutions include pushing the ball down with the arms, not maintaining pelvic neutral, and using the hips to rotate rather than the abdominals.

■ **Trunk Rotation.** In a neutral standing position with the abdominals tightened, the patient rests the arms on a kickboard that is floating in the water. Slowly and in a controlled manner, he or she rotates the trunk to one side and then to the other maintaining tension in the abdominals throughout the movement (figure 13.20). The motion should not cause any pain. If pain is present, the motion should be restricted to a pain-free range. The exercise can be advanced through increasing the surface area of the resistance device. Substitutions include rotating with the hips and knees rather than the abdominal muscles and pushing the board with the arms rather than maintaining the board and arms in the same position throughout the range of motion.

■ **Wall Push-Offs.** The wall push-off strengthens the thoracic spine. Standing away from and facing the pool wall, the patient keeps the spine straight and does not bend at the hips or the back during the exercise (figure 13.21). The feet are kept in the same position throughout the exercise. The patient begins the exercise with the hands on the pool wall and the arms straight. He or she then leans forward by dorsiflexing the ankles and bends the arms until the chest comes close to the pool wall, and finally pushes away from the wall until the arms are straight. Substitutions include not keeping the spine straight and leading with the hips.

■ **Pull-Downs.** With the feet shoulder-width apart, the knees slightly flexed to relieve low back stress, and the spine in neutral, the patient moves arm bells from in front of the body downward toward the sides (figure 13.22). The elbows maintain a partially flexed position and the spine in neutral throughout the motion. As strength improves, the elbows maintain an extended position throughout the exercise. A common substitution includes trunk flexion to move the dumbbells.

Spine Exercises in Deep Water

The patient must have good trunk control in order to perform the spine exercises. An individual who has difficulty with the exercise should perform it in waist-high or chest-high water first.

■ **Double-Leg Lift.** With flotation devices in the hands or under the arms, the patient maintains a neutral spine as he or she lifts the legs to a 90° hip flexion position with the knees extended (figure 13.23). The abdominals must remain contracted throughout the exercise. If a neutral spine position cannot be maintained during this exercise, have the patient either begin with a single-leg lift or flex the knees so the hips and knees are at 90° at the top of the motion. If the patient substitutes by arching the back, spinal neutral is lost. Another substitution is flexing the knees to shorten the lower extremity's lever arm length.

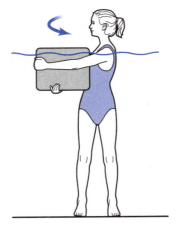

▶ **Figure 13.20** Trunk rotation.

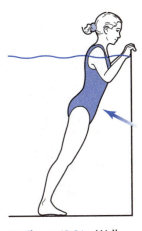

▶ **Figure 13.21** Wall push-off.

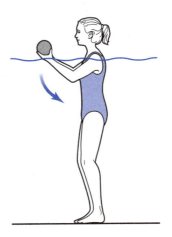

▶ **Figure 13.22** Pull-down.

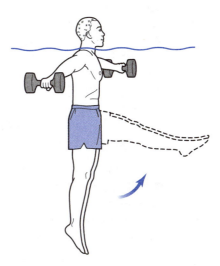

▶ **Figure 13.23** Double-leg lift.

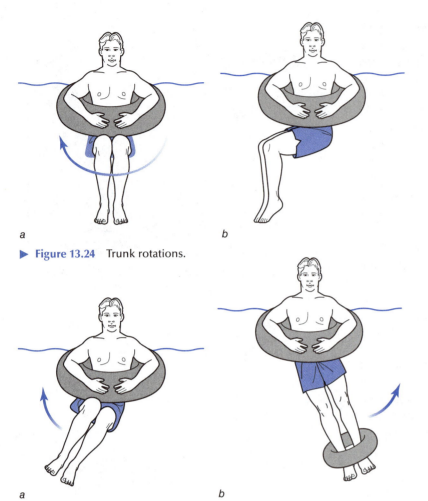

▶ **Figure 13.24**   Trunk rotations.

▶ **Figure 13.25**   *(a)* Lateral flexion and *(b)* added resistance with flotation device at feet.

■ **Trunk Rotations.** Using a flotation tube, the patient maintains a vertical position in the water (figure 13.24). The hips and knees are flexed, and the oblique muscles are used to rotate the hips first in one direction and then to the opposite side. The exercise is more demanding if the knees are fully extended. Substitutions include initiating the exercise with the hips or the shoulders rather than the abdominal obliques

■ **Lateral Flexion.** Using a flotation tube or other flotation device, the patient flexes the hips and knees to 90° (figure 13.25a). He or she maintains this position while lifting both hips laterally toward the left ribs, returning to the start position, and then lifting both hips laterally toward the right ribs. The back should not twist or arch during this exercise. You can make this exercise more difficult by having the patient supine in the water with a flotation device at the waist and a small flotation tube or bells at the feet (13.25b). A common substitution is arching the back and moving the legs in an arc around to the other side rather than moving back to the start position before lifting to the opposite side.

Exercises for the Lower Extremities

Exercises in this section begin with the simpler exercises in shallow water and advance to deep-water exercises. Keep in mind that the patient may progress to some deep-water activities while still needing to continue with some shallow-water activities. A patient moves from shallow to deep water exercises when the short-term goals are achieved and the patient is comfortable moving to deep water.

Ambulation and Balance Activities in Shallow Water

The following are examples of shallow-water exercises. You can increase difficulty by increasing the depth of the water in which the patient performs the activity. As previously discussed, the patient should maintain body control throughout each exercise.

■ **Forward walking.** This is useful as a gait-training exercise. Encourage the patient to maintain a correct gait pattern, as outlined in chapter 12, while in the water. Look for correct trunk stability. If necessary, the patient may use buoy lines or may walk along the side of the pool, holding on for balance in the beginning. Substitutions include any gait deviations that may be expected during land walking. The patient's specific substitution may relate to the specific injury. For example, if the knee is injured, the patient may not be willing to flex it sufficiently during swing phase and opt to raise up on the contralateral toes to clear the involved extremity's foot.

■ **Backward walking.** This exercise works particularly on the extensor muscles of the trunk and legs. It is good for balance and coordination as well. Emphasize normal stride backward with a good toe-to-heel pattern, normal and equal stride length, and proper weight shifting. The patient should maintain proper trunk alignment. The most common substitution is a forward trunk lean.

■ **Toe walking.** The patient walks on his or her toes. This exercise is good for strength and proprioception. Substitutions to watch for include not raising up as high as possible on the toes and letting the heel touch the floor during contralateral swing.

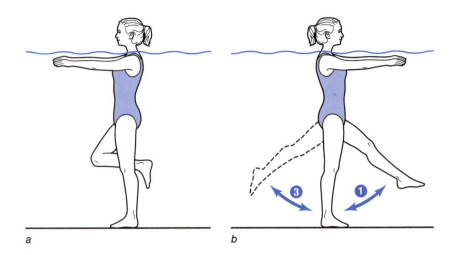
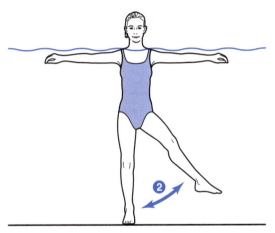

■ **Heel walking.** The patient walks on the heels. This is a strengthening exercise for the dorsiflexors and is a proprioceptive exercise as well. Substitutions include hip flexion, not maintaining a high toe lift, and allowing the toes to touch the floor after mid-stance.

■ **Single-leg balance.** The patient stands on the involved leg, moves the contralateral leg forward, and holds that position for 30 s (figure 13.26). To advance this exercise, you can have the patient stand on the involved leg while moving the uninvolved leg forward and backward or sideways. This exercise focuses on static balance improvement. Substitutions include using the trunk to move the extremity, flexing the weight bearing or non-weight bearing knee, and trunk lean.

▶ **Figure 13.26** Single-leg balance: *(a)* Static, *(b)* with contralateral leg movement. The trunk should remain stable and erect throughout the exercise, with tension maintained in abdominal and gluteal muscles.

■ **Lunges.** The patient performs a forward lunge by taking a large step forward and then bringing the back leg up to meet the front leg. This activity is good for increasing strength and range of motion of the hip and knee. Good trunk alignment is necessary throughout the exercise. The patient can also do backward lunges and side lunges to increase hip extension and hip abduction, respectively. These exercises are good for balance and strength as well. Substitutions include trunk lean, not using proper weight transfer, and not flexing the knee sufficiently.

■ **Grapevine.** The grapevine is also referred to as a carioca or braid step. The patient first steps to the side with the first leg, then in back (crossing behind the first leg) with the second leg, out to the side again with the first leg, then in front (crossing in front of the first leg) with the second leg. This exercise is good for improving proprioception through improving coordination and balance. Substitution includes rotating the trunk rather than facing the same direction as the patient moves in the water.

■ **Running.** Analogously to walking in the water, water running should imitate the technique of land running as much as possible. The patient should use the arms to keep an upright posture and should avoid the tendency to lean forward. Running forward, running backward, and cutting can all be performed in shallow water as a prelude to land running. The primary substitution includes using the trunk rather than the legs to obtain sufficient speed and motion.

Hip Exercises in Shallow Water

Good trunk stability is important during all of the following hip exercises. You should instruct the patient to maintain vertical trunk alignment and to maintain tension in the abdominals to assist in this activity. If the patient is unable to demonstrate good trunk alignment, it may be necessary to work on the previously presented trunk activities in addition to the lower-extremity exercises here.

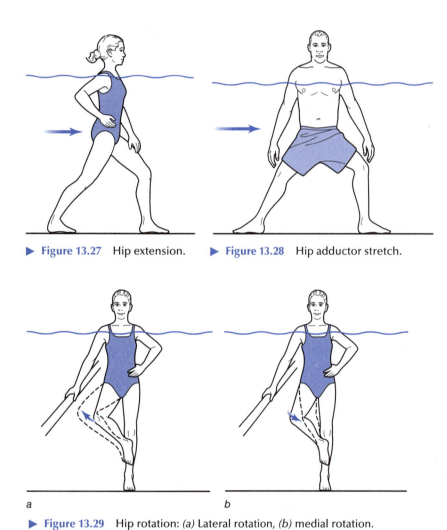

▶ **Figure 13.27**   Hip extension.

▶ **Figure 13.28**   Hip adductor stretch.

a

b

▶ **Figure 13.29**   Hip rotation: *(a)* Lateral rotation, *(b)* medial rotation.

■ **Hip extension.** This activity can be used to stretch the hip flexors and strengthen the hip extensors (figure 13.27). The patient stands in a backward-forward straddle position with the involved leg behind. The spine is maintained in neutral throughout the exercise. Keeping the abdominals tense will help ensure a correct spinal alignment. The involved knee remains extended and the hip is pushed forward while the heel stays on the floor. The gluteals are tightened during the exercise. Substitutions include arching the back, lifting the heel off the floor and flexing the knee.

■ **Hip adductor stretch.** In this activity for stretching the hip adductors, the patient stands in a side-straddle position (figure 13.28). The uninvolved knee is flexed as the weight is shifted to that side. The involved knee is kept extended, and the trunk is maintained in an upright position. Substitutions include lateral trunk flexion or rotation, hip flexion on the involved side, or hip lateral rotation.

■ **Hip medial-lateral rotation.** These exercises can be used to stretch one group as they strengthen the opposing muscle group. The patient may need to hold on to the pool wall or rail. The knee and hip of the involved extremity are flexed, with the sole of the foot on the shin of the opposite leg (figure 13.29). The knee of the involved leg then rotates outward as far as possible to stretch the medial rotators. To stretch the lateral rotators, the knee moves inward toward the opposite leg. The trunk should remain in neutral throughout the exercise, and the pelvis and back should not rotate. Substitutions include rotating the pelvis or trunk or rotating the entire body on the standing extremity.

■ **Figure-8s.** This alternative to the rotation exercise just described offers resistance more than it increases in range of motion. The patient draws figure-8s in the water with the entire leg, initiating the movement from the hip, not the knee or ankle. Progressions from this exercise can include proprioceptive neuromuscular facilitation patterns in the water and breaststroke kicking. The common substitutions for this exercise are rotating the pelvis and rotating from the knee or ankle.

Knee Exercises in Shallow Water

The first two knee exercises that follow are flexibility exercises; the others are strengthening exercises. The initial strengthening exercises should use only the limb as the source of resistance. As the patient's strength and control improve, you can add drag equipment to the activity or can have the patient perform the exercise faster as long as he or she maintains control of the limb.

- **Quadriceps stretch.** This stretch is similar to the land exercise in which the patient grasps the ankle of the involved leg, which is positioned behind, and attempts to pull the foot toward the buttock. The knee should remain pointing downward, and the trunk should remain in a neutral position. Substitutions include flexing the hip, flexing the trunk, and grasping the foot on the side of the hip rather than behind it.

- **Hamstring stretch.** The patient places the involved foot on the pool wall or on a step. The knee is slightly flexed, and as the stretch is applied, the knee is extended (figure 13.30). Good trunk alignment is maintained throughout the exercise with trunk forward lean coming from the hip, not the back. Substitutions include posterior rotation of the pelvis and extending the hip.

- **Single-leg bicycle.** The patient flexes and extends the involved hip and knee in a cycling pattern while holding on to the side of the pool (figure 13.31). The trunk remains in neutral and does not move. This exercise is more difficult if the patient performs it without holding on to the side of the pool. Substitutions include using the trunk to move the lower extremity and using the arms for force transfer rather than using lower extremity strength. Also, hip abduction or rotation may be observed, but should be corrected so the hip, knee, and ankle maintain vertical alignment with each other.

- **Squats.** With the feet shoulder-width apart, the patient slowly bends the knees until the thighs are almost parallel to the pool floor. The spine should remain in a neutral position throughout the exercise. You can make this exercise more difficult by having the patient perform it without holding on to the side of the pool or perform it only on the involved leg. In a further progression, the patient performs a jump squat so that he or she lifts off the pool floor. Hip flexion, hip hiking, hip abduction, and weight transfer to the uninvolved extremity are all substitutions to watch for and correct in this exercise.

- **Step-ups.** The involved leg is placed on the top of a box, stair, or platform. The patient steps onto the box by lifting his or her body upward, using the knee and hip muscles (figure 13.32). The trunk remains in a neutral position throughout. This exercise can be performed with the patient standing in front of, behind, or at the side of the box for forward step-ups, reverse step-ups, or lateral step-ups, respectively. The patient should avoid trunk lean or hip hike, all common substitutions in this exercise.

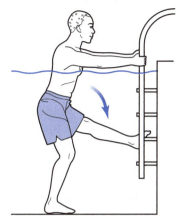

▶ **Figure 13.30** Hamstring stretch.

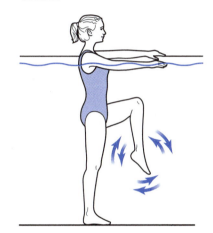

▶ **Figure 13.31** Single-leg bicycle.

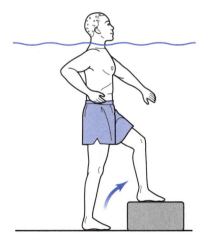

▶ **Figure 13.32** Step-up.

Ankle Exercises in Shallow Water

The ankle exercises outlined here are similar to those frequently performed on land, but the water is an ideal place to begin these exercises when weight bearing on the extremity is limited. In these situations, the patient begins in deeper water and progresses to shallower water as more weight bearing is permitted.

■ **Gastrocnemius-soleus stretch.** The patient stands facing the pool wall and places the involved leg behind him or her and the uninvolved leg in front. The heel of the involved leg is kept in contact with the pool floor, the knee is kept extended, and the body weight is moved forward onto the hands and front leg. This stretches the gastrocnemius. For stretching the soleus, the leg is brought forward slightly; the involved knee is bent; and the heel is kept on the pool floor as the weight is moved forward. Substitutions seen with this stretch include flexing the hips, raising the heel off the pool floor, flexing the knee, and laterally rotating the extremity.

■ **Heel raises.** To perform this activity the patient may need initially to hold on to the side of the pool for stability. The patient slowly rises up onto the toes while the knees remain straight. The body should not lean or move forward. This exercise becomes more difficult if the patient does not hold on to the side of the pool. It is also more difficult if he or she stands only on the involved leg or moves to shallower water. Substitutions include rocking the body forward rather than moving the body directly upward with the heel raise, flexing the knee, and transferring weight to the uninvolved extremity.

■ **Ankle walking.** The patient walks the length or width of the pool, first on the toes, then on the heels, then on the lateral side of the feet, finally and on the medial side of the feet. Progressions include increasing the stride length, increasing the speed, moving to shallower water, and using resistive equipment. Substitutions seen may include knee valgus or varus positioning, hip rotation, and body lean.

■ **Hopping.** The patient jumps forward, using the arms to assist while maintaining the spine in neutral (figure 13.33). The knees flex to absorb the impact-landing forces. Progression of this exercise includes advancing from double-leg to one-leg hops, moving to shallower water, increasing the repetitions or sets, and increasing the speed. Substitutions to avoid include flexing the trunk to lose spinal neutral and not landing vertically.

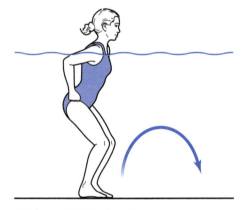

▶ **Figure 13.33** Hopping.

Ambulation Activities in Deep Water

The following activities are appropriate when weight bearing is restricted. Cycling and running in deep water can also serve as both cardiovascular activities and lower-extremity exercises. The most common substitution for any exercise in this group is using the trunk or arms rather than the lower extremities for power and motion.

■ **Stride walking.** Stride walking is the use of exaggerated strides that are initiated from the hips. The spine should remain in neutral during the exercise.

■ **Cycling.** Cycling is performed with the patient in a vertical position. The patient mimics a bicycle motion with exaggerated hip and knee movement. The motion can be either forward or backward.

■ **Running.** Running in deep water, as with walking activities, is a good exercise for patients who must remain non-weight bearing. Running in deep water can include jogging or sprinting. The form is as close to land running as possible. The trunk should remain in neutral throughout the running phase.

■ **Cross-country skiing.** The patient performs a reciprocal motion of the arms and legs, similar to the cross-country skiing action, while maintaining a neutral spine position as seen in figure 13.34.

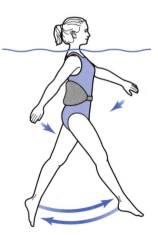

▶ **Figure 13.34** Cross-country skiing.

Hip Exercises in Deep Water

Deep-water exercises are more difficult than shallow-water exercises because in addition to staying afloat, the patient must also work to maintain an upright posture and stable trunk during the exercise. Instructions to keep abdominal muscles tense and the chest elevated can be useful cues. Use of a flotation belt can assist the patient in the early phases of deep-water exercise. Substitutions in these exercises will be most notable in trunk movement; trunk movement is indicative of poor trunk and spine control that becomes readily apparent when the body is not stabilized by contact with the ground. If the patient is unable to maintain trunk stability in any of these exercises, the patient either may not be concentrating on the activity or does not have the strength required for the exercise. If the latter is the reason, instruct the patient to perform the exercise in shallower water before advancing it to deep water.

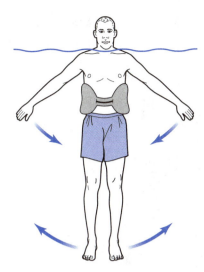

▶ **Figure 13.35** Jumping jacks.

■ **Jumping jacks.** The elbows and knees are kept straight, and the spine is in neutral (figure 13.35). The arms begin in an abducted position. As the hips are abducted, the arms are adducted, and vice versa.

■ **Double-knee lift.** The patient lifts both legs together, bringing the knees toward the chest while the spine remains in neutral (figure 13.36).

■ **Flexion with lateral rotation.** The patient is in a vertical position with the spine in neutral (figure 13.37). The legs move together, simultaneously into hip flexion and lateral rotation, and then return to the starting position.

■ **Hip abduction.** In a vertical position, the patient keeps the knees extended and the spine in neutral. The hips are both abducted simultaneously and then returned to the starting position. This exercise is more difficult if the patient performs abduction with the hips in a 90° flexion position, as seen in figure 13.38.

■ **Flutter kicking.** Flutter kicking prone or supine, with two legs or with one, is useful for the hip. A substitution for this exercise is initiating the movement from the hip rather than the knee.

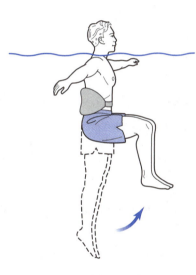

▶ **Figure 13.36** Double-knee lift.

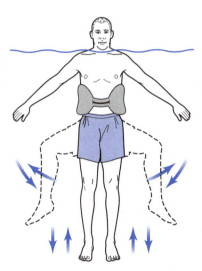

▶ **Figure 13.37** Hip flexion with lateral rotation.

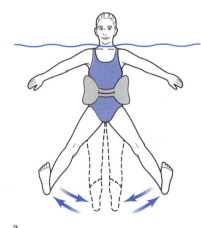

a

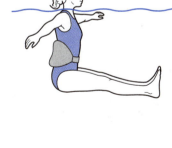

b

▶ **Figure 13.38** Hip abduction in 90° hip flexion: *(a)* front view, *(b)* side view.

Knee Exercises in Deep Water

The knee exercises suggested here become more difficult if the patient performs them with both legs simultaneously or with resistance attached to the feet. Trunk and hip control should be maintained throughout the exercises.

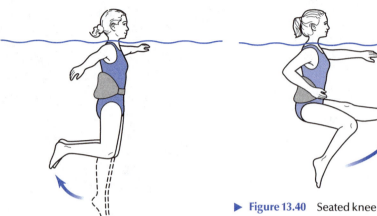

▶ **Figure 13.39**   Double-knee bend.

▶ **Figure 13.40**   Seated knee extension.

■ **Double-knee bend.** In a vertical position with the spine in neutral, the patient simultaneously flexes both knees while keeping them pointing directly downward (figure 13.39). The substitution for this exercise is flexing the hips.

■ **Seated knee extensions.** With the hips flexed to 90° and the thighs together, the patient extends the involved knee to full extension (figure 13.40). A vertical position is maintained throughout the exercise. To make this exercise more difficult, have the patient extend both knees simultaneously. The common substitution is extending the hips. The trunk may also flex if the patient does not have good trunk control.

Exercises for the Upper Extremities

Keep in mind that just as with the lower-extremity exercises, the following exercises for the upper extremities do not constitute a complete list but are merely some suggested activities for use in therapeutic exercise. Although weight bearing is not the issue for the upper extremity that it is for the lower extremity, aquatic exercises can provide the patient with another way of rehabilitating the extremity. Diversification of activities can help to maintain the patient's interest in the therapeutic exercise program, and the variety can be enjoyable for the rehabilitation clinician as well.

Shoulder Exercises in Shallow Water

Presentation of upper-extremity exercises will start with the shoulder and progress through the upper extremity, beginning with stretches and advancing to strengthening exercises.

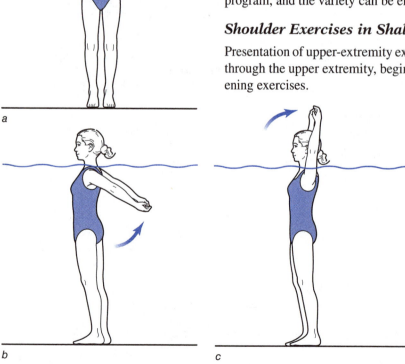

▶ **Figure 13.41**   Capsule stretches: *(a)* Posterior, *(b)* anterior, *(c)* inferior.

■ **Pectoralis stretch.** In water above shoulder level, and with the arms elevated to shoulder level with elbows extended, the patient horizontally abducts the arms, squeezing the shoulder blades together. The palms should be facing upward. A common substitution is shoulder shrugging.

■ **Capsule stretch.** With the involved arm at shoulder level, the patient grasps the elbow of the involved arm with the uninvolved hand and pulls the involved arm across the chest to stretch the posterior capsule (figure 13.41a). To stretch the anterior capsule, the patient grasps the hands behind the back and attempts to lift the hands upward (figure 13.41b). Figure 13.41c demonstrates the inferior-capsule stretch with the patient's hands overhead. Arching the back or flexing the trunk are substitutions in this exercise.

■ **Lateral rotator stretch.** For this stretch of the lateral rotators, the patient places the involved hand on the low back (figure 13.42a). Keeping a neutral spine and erect posture, the patient flexes the elbow and reaches upward as high as possible on the back with the hand. In an alternative stretch, the patient grasps a bar or stair rung behind the back and attempts to bend the knees (figure 13.42b). Forward trunk flexion and wrist extension are substitutions in this exercise.

■ **Medial rotator stretch.** The patient stands with the involved side near the pool wall. The elbow is at the side and flexed to 90° with the palm on the wall (figure 13.43). The patient rotates the trunk away from the wall while keeping the hand in contact with the wall surface and the elbow at his or her side. This exercise stretches the medial rotators. Substitutions include extending the elbow, rotating the pelvis rather than the trunk and stepping away from the wall.

■ **Shoulder press-down.** This is a shoulder-strengthening exercise. Using dumbbells or another flotation device, the patient allows the arms to elevate under the water as the elbows flex until the upper arms are at shoulder level and in an abducted position (figure 13.44). The patient then pushes the dumbbells downward until the elbows are extended. Using the trunk to push down by flexing the trunk forward is a common substitution.

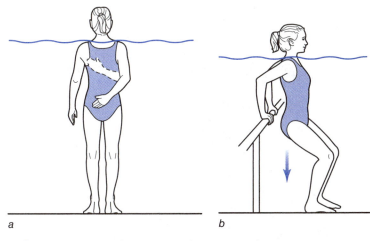

▶ **Figure 13.42** Lateral rotator stretch, *(a)* active, *(b)* passive.

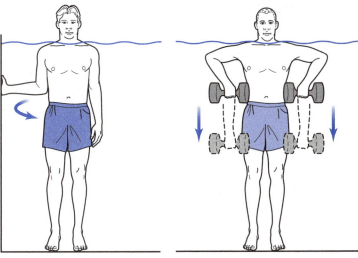

▶ **Figure 13.43** Medial rotator stretch.

▶ **Figure 13.44** Shoulder press-down.

■ **Shoulder abduction-adduction.** Using resistive devices and keeping the elbows extended, the patient abducts the arms until the hands are at shoulder level and then returns to the starting position. The trunk remains in a neutral position. Trunk flexion is the most common substitution.

■ **Shoulder flexion-extension.** This exercise is similar to the preceding one, but the arm moves from flexion at shoulder level to hyperextension with the hand moving past the hips (figure 13.45). Trunk flexion is the most common substitution.

■ **Horizontal abduction-adduction.** In this exercise the patient keeps the arms at shoulder level and the elbows straight. The spine is kept in neutral. With resistive devices in the hands, the patient moves the arms through horizontal abduction and horizontal adduction. Arching and flexing the back is the substitution pattern for these movements.

■ **Medial rotation-lateral rotation.** With the elbow at the side, the spine in neutral, and a resistive device attached to the hand, the patient moves the arm into lateral rotation and then medial rotation. If only one direction is desired, on the return to the starting position the hand is rotated so that the hand's profile in the water is reduced. Substitutions include shoulder abduction or adduction.

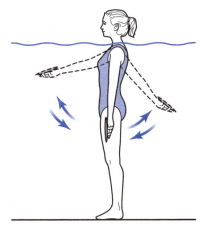

▶ **Figure 13.45** Shoulder flexion-extension.

Elbow Exercises in Shallow Water

Stretching exercises are often more comfortable when performed in water. The elbow is particularly uncomfortable to stretching and may be stretched more effectively in the pool than on land. Strength exercises can also be useful when performed in the pool. Consider the following activities:

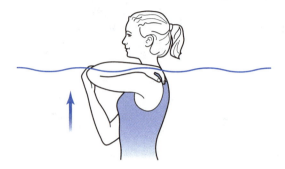

▶ **Figure 13.46** Elbow extensor stretch.

- **Elbow extensor stretch.** To increase elbow flexion range of motion, the patient flexes the elbow as far as possible, and then applies additional force by using the contralateral hand to push the hand toward the humerus (figure 13.46). A common substitution is shoulder flexion.

- **Forearm curl.** Using a resistive device to strengthen the elbow flexors, the patient flexes the elbow as the shoulder is abducted and the hand is moved toward the water's surface. The shoulder and trunk are maintained in a stable position throughout the exercise. Trunk extension is a common substitution.

- **Supination-pronation.** With the elbow maintained at the side at 90° of flexion, the patient grasps a resistive device in the hand. The forearm is slowly moved from a palm-up position through a full range of motion to a palm-down position, and then to the starting position. To avoid substitutions, the trunk and shoulder are maintained in stable positions throughout the exercise.

- **Elbow extension.** With the elbow held at the side and a resistive device in the hand, the patient moves the elbow from a fully flexed to a fully extended position. The hand should remain in a palm-down position. Substitutions include trunk flexion and shoulder extension.

Upper-Extremity Exercises in Deep Water

Because so many of the deep-water exercises for one upper-extremity joint simultaneously engage the other upper-extremity joints, we will consider all the deep-water upper-extremity exercises together.

▶ **Figure 13.47** Bent-arm pull.

- **Bent-arm pull.** With the body maintained in a vertical position, the patient keeps the arms at approximately shoulder level (figure 13.47). As one shoulder moves into hyperextension with the elbow flexed, the contralateral shoulder moves to 90° flexion, with its elbow moving from flexion to full extension. The upper extremities then reverse their positions. The trunk should not rotate during this exercise.

- **Straight-arm pull.** With the body in a vertical position, the elbows extended, and the trunk stable and erect, the patient alternately swings the shoulders forward into flexion and then backward into hyperextension (figure 13.48). As the shoulder flexes, the hand faces upward; as the shoulder extends, the hand faces downward. Substitutions include flexing the elbow, using the trunk rather than the shoulder to provide the motion with trunk flexion during shoulder extension and trunk extension during shoulder flexion, and abducting the shoulder.

- **Arm circles.** In a vertical position, the patient places the arms at shoulder level (figure 13.49). With the elbows in exten-

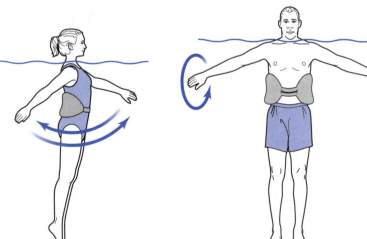

▶ **Figure 13.48** Straight-arm pull.

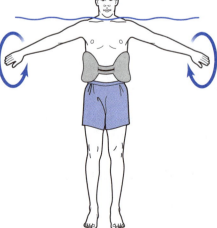

▶ **Figure 13.49** Arm circles.

sion, the arms are moved in circles, clockwise and counterclockwise. Changing the size of the circles, changing the speed of movement, or attaching resistive devices to the hands can alter the resistance. Flexing the elbows is the most common substitution.

■ **Breaststroke.** With the body in a vertical position, the patient keeps the arms at shoulder level. Shoulders begin in horizontal adduction and move through a full range of motion to end in horizontal abduction, as during a breaststroke. Substitutions include moving the trunk into flexion, dropping the arms downward, and not moving the shoulders through an entire range of motion.

■ **Shoulder press.** In a vertical position, the patient pushes both upper extremities forward at shoulder level from the chest as in a bench-press exercise with weights (figure 13.50). To increase the resistance of this exercise, you can add resistive devices, increase speed, or increase the number of repetitions. Losing pelvic neutral is a substitution, especially when resistance is added.

■ **Elbow press.** In a vertical position, the patient flexes and extends one elbow and shoulder, alternating the motion with the contralateral extremity (figure 13.51). The movement occurs in an up-and-down motion in front of the body. Substitutions include not moving the extremities through a full range of motion and moving the arms to the sides of the body.

■ **Wave.** In a vertical position, the patient places the upper extremities at shoulder level in abduction. With the elbows in extension, the wrists are alternately flexed and extended through their full range of motion. Substitutions include flexing the elbows, dropping the arms towards the sides, and not moving the wrists through the full motion.

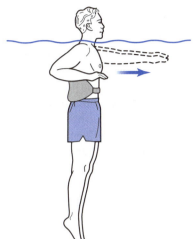

▶ **Figure 13.50** Shoulder press.

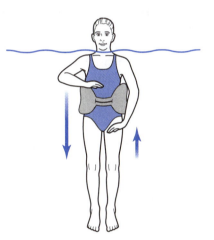

▶ **Figure 13.51** Elbow press.

Many water-based therapeutic exercises are similar to exercises that patients do on dry land. As with dryland exercise, most aquatic exercises for the spine and the lower and upper extremities can be made more demanding to provide a progression.

SUMMARY

Specific gravity is the density of an object relative to that of water. The specific gravity of water is 1, so anything with specific gravity greater than 1 will sink and anything with specific gravity less than 1 will float. The specific gravity of the average body is 0.95 to 0.97. Moving the body in water causes resistance in the water; this is drag. The more drag a body has, the more resistance the water creates. Drag can be used as a resistive force just as buoyancy can be used as an assistive force for the body in water. Water exercises may be used early in a rehabilitation program if the body segment is unable to bear weight or if it is too weak to withstand resistive forces. The deeper in the water a patient's body is placed, the less weight is borne by the lower extremities. Devices are available to assist with floatation in water and other devices are available to provide additional drag, or resistance. As with any therapeutic exercise, there are advantages, disadvantages, and contraindications for aquatic exercise; the clinician must be aware of these factors before including aquatic exercise in a rehabilitation program.

KEY CONCEPTS AND REVIEW

1. Identify and discuss the physical properties of water that affect the ability to exercise in water.

The physical properties of water, including specific gravity, buoyancy, center of buoyancy, and hydrodynamics, influence the way a patient is able to exercise in water. Water has a specific gravity of 1. If a body's specific gravity is less than 1, the body will float; but if the specific gravity is more than 1, the body will sink. Buoyancy occurs when the specific gravity is less than 1. In order for a body to remain upright while floating, the center of buoyancy must be in line with the center of gravity; otherwise, the patient must work to maintain an upright position. Drag is the resistance to movement in water; the greater the drag, the more resistance there is. We can influence drag by increasing the speed of movement, turbulence, surface area being moved, and depth of the water.

2. Define and explain the difference between assistive and resistive aquatic equipment and give examples of each.

Assistive devices in the water provide the body support to aid in buoyancy; examples are the kickboard and the flotation belt. Resistive equipment in the water increases the drag and makes it more difficult for a body to move; examples are paddles and boots.

3. List precautions and contraindications for aquatic exercise.

The most common precaution relates to the patient's fear. Other precautions relate to certain medications that can compromise the patient's situation, to ear infections, and to certain medical conditions. A patient who has epilepsy, for example, may be endangered in a pool and must be closely observed. Contraindications include illness, open wounds, and medical conditions that may be dangerous for either the patient or others in the pool; in these cases, the individual must not be allowed in the pool.

4. Identify three advantages of aquatic therapeutic exercise.

Aquatic exercise can begin early in the therapeutic exercise program. Patients with non-weight-bearing conditions can begin water exercises before land exercises. Aquatic therex can relax muscle spasm and pain, and provides for diversity and variety in the patient's rehabilitation program.

5. List an aquatic exercise for each body segment and identify its purpose.

An example of a trunk exercise is the lateral stretch in shallow water, used to improve flexibility. An example of a lower-extremity exercise is step-ups in shallow water, which increases strength of the knee muscles, especially the quadriceps. An upper-extremity exercise is the shoulder press-down with water dumbbells, used to strengthen the shoulder depressors.

CRITICAL THINKING QUESTIONS

1. Why is it that some of the patients you place in the pool have no trouble floating while others must work to keep their heads above water? What principle does this phenomenon involve?

2. If the patient you are rehabilitating is non-weight bearing on an injured ankle but wants to perform cardiovascular activities in the pool, what program will you design for him? What water depth should he be in for resistive exercises?

3. The softball player with whom you have been working to rehabilitate her shoulder is fearful of going into the water. You would like to have her in the pool, since water activity would help increase her shoulder motion and strength. What would you do to encourage her to get into the pool and relieve her fears? What would be your initial exercises with her, and at what water depth would you place her?

4. You are using the pool to rehabilitate a gymnast with a hip strain until she has less pain with land activities. Her motion is good, but her strength is limited in all hip motions, especially abduction. List resistive exercises that you will include in her pool program, and provide a progression for each one.

5. Identify a simple core stabilization exercise that you would use for a patient with a recent back injury, and include a four-step progression for the exercise. What would your criteria be for advancement from one level to the next?

LAB ACTIVITIES

1. While standing in waist-deep water, move your hand through the water in the following manners:
   a. With the fingers together and the hand parallel to the water surface
   b. With the fingers together and the hand perpendicular to the water surface
   c. With the fingers apart and the hand perpendicular to the water surface
   d. With the hand grasping a paddle and perpendicular to the water surface

   Rate the movements from easiest to perform to most difficult. Which one was easiest and which one was most difficult and why?

2. Walk across the pool in waist-high water. Walk across the pool in chest-high water. Walk across the pool in neck-deep water. Which depth was the most difficult to walk in? Why? At which depth did you feel the most weight applied through your feet? Why?

3. Now run across the pool at the same depths in question 2. Which depth was the most difficult? Why?

4. While maintaining pelvic neutral in chest deep water, perform a single knee to chest exercise, alternating legs. Now repeat the activity in deep water. Which was the more difficult exercise and why?

5. While maintaining pelvic neutral in chest-deep water, perform a shoulder flexion-extension exercise, alternating arms. Now repeat the activity in deep water. Which was the more difficult exercise and why? What do the results of this activity and the one in question 4 teach you in terms of rehabilitation exercises in the pool?

6. Create an aquatic program for a lower-extremity injury beginning with NWB and progressing to partial then full weight-bearing activities. Don't forget to design exercises to include pelvic stabilization during lower-extremity exercises.

7. Create an aquatic program for an upper extremity injury. Don't forget to design exercises to include pelvic stabilization during lower extremity exercises.

Swiss Balls and Foam Rollers

OBJECTIVES

After completing this chapter, you should be able to do the following:

1. Explain how Swiss balls and foam rollers can increase the challenge of a traditional exercise.

2. Identify which rehabilitation parameters improve by the use of Swiss balls or foam rollers.

3. Discuss safety factors, precautions, and contraindications relating to the use of Swiss balls and foam rollers.

4. Explain how to properly fit a Swiss ball.

5. List one exercise each for the trunk, upper extremity, and lower extremity using a Swiss ball, and identify its purpose.

6. List one exercise each for the trunk, upper extremity, and lower extremity using foam rollers, and identify its purpose.

▶ Of all the exercise equipment in the sports medicine facility where Owain Turngher worked, he enjoyed the Swiss balls and foam rollers the most. He believed that these items could provide a challenging and interesting rehabilitation program for any of his patients. In his opinion, no other piece of equipment challenged the trunk muscles as well as the foam roller. Owain routinely placed all his patients on it, since not only back injuries but also upper- and lower-extremity injuries could benefit from the challenge of the foam roller.

As much as he liked foam-roller rehabilitation, Owain also liked the Swiss ball for its versatility in upper- and lower-extremity and trunk rehabilitation. Whenever possible, he liked to include both the Swiss ball and foam roller in a patient's program. When patients were ready to advance to a home program, he would often provide patients with a Swiss ball and foam roller so they could perform exercises at home.

Today, Mike Xaviar, a patient Owain has seen for the past week is ready for a home exercise program. Owain plans to give Mike a group of fun yet challenging home exercises that he knows Mike will enjoy performing on the Swiss ball. During his first appointment, Mike mentioned that he had a Swiss ball at home. Owain assured him at that time that he would be using it for home exercises soon since Swiss balls can be used for many various exercises.

Games lubricate the body and the mind.

BENJAMIN FRANKLIN, 1706-1790, author, scientist, inventor, American diplomat

Rehabilitation and the treatment of musculoskeletal injuries have changed over the years. Many techniques we use today were unknown 20 years ago. Among the changes in therapeutic exercise techniques is the use of Swiss balls and foam rollers. These are both relatively new items in the orthopedic and rehabilitation arena that are commonly used in therapeutic exercise programs today. They are used to create exercises that achieve desired goals and inject an element of fun into an exercise.

This chapter presents information about how to introduce Swiss balls and foam rollers into the rehabilitation program, techniques to use, and examples of exercises that patients can perform with them. We also consider indications, precautions, and contraindications that represent crucial guidelines for the use of Swiss balls and foam rollers in therapeutic exercise programs.

There is a large void in research demonstrating the efficacy of exercises using either Swiss balls or foam rollers. Although clinicians lack the empirical evidence, using unstable surfaces such as Swiss balls and foam rollers makes intuitive sense when the goal is to require additional muscle group activity, challenge the patient's stability, or add variety to a program. One of the few investigations regarded muscle recruitment differences between low-level Swiss ball exercises and other early stabilization exercises for the spine; the study did not show any additional output in the muscles tested (Drake, Fischer, et al., 2006), but the study looked only at prime movers and not synergists or other regional muscles. Unfortunately, Drake et al. used healthy individuals, not patients, and even they concluded in their discussion that using patients or more aggressive exercises may change the results (Drake, Fischer, et al., 2006). It is clear that research of Swiss ball and foam roller exercises is in its infancy. Until evidence proves or disproves the theories of Swiss ball and foam roller use, clinicians will rely on their clinical experiences and patient outcomes to guide their choices.

SWISS BALLS

The Swiss ball, a large vinyl ball, was developed by an Italian toy manufacturer and first produced in 1963 under the name Gymnastik, and later, Gymnic. Using the Bobath method,

Dr. Elsbeth Kšng, a Swiss pediatrician, and Mary Quinton, an English physiotherapist, developed pediatric neurological rehabilitation programs using Swiss balls. In the 1960s, Dr. Susan Klein-Vogelbach, a physical therapist in Switzerland, began using the Swiss balls as an instructional tool in classes for adult orthopedic and other medical problems.

The term **Swiss ball** derives from the fact that U.S. physical therapists who introduced the balls in this country first saw them used in clinics in Switzerland (Posner-Mayer, 1995). Although Swiss balls were introduced in the United States during the early 1970s, they did not begin to catch on until the late 1980s. Today, many facilities use them for a wide range of orthopedic activities, including spinal stabilization, upper- and lower-extremity strengthening and flexibility, balance and coordination, and body awareness.

Swiss-Ball Challenges

Most patients enjoy exercising with balls. Balls provide a diversion from boring exercises. Swiss-ball activities can also be more challenging than regular exercises. Swiss balls used in therapeutic exercises can stimulate interest, offer activity complexity, and motivate the patient to perform more diligently.

The Swiss ball can provide challenges within a variety of rehabilitation parameters. Swiss-ball exercises increase flexibility, strength, muscle endurance, balance, coordination, and joint- and body-position awareness (Naughton, Adams, et al., 2005). They are used in open and closed chain activities. They can provide for a progression of difficulty so the patient is continually challenged as parameters improve. Swiss balls can also offer the patient a number of stimulating activities.

A simple activity becomes more complex and challenging when it incorporates additional elements. For example, standing on the ground is a relatively simple activity for a patient, but standing on a boat that is moving through water, or standing on skis while moving downhill, is more challenging. Sitting on a chair at a desk requires little balance; sitting on a Swiss ball requires more balance. Lying on a table is no challenge, but lying prone on a Swiss ball with only one hand in contact with the ground requires effort.

Activity on a Swiss ball requires more effort because the surface is unstable—the instability challenges balance. Coordination is more difficult on a Swiss ball because more than one body segment and more than one system must participate simultaneously to maintain position or balance during an activity. Coordination is additionally tested if the patient is required to perform more than one activity while on the Swiss ball.

Body weight can be used in a variety of positions to offer resistance during activity. Using weights during exercises on the Swiss ball makes the exercise more stressful. The unstable surface requires a greater effort by the exercising muscles, as well as effort by a greater number of muscles, to perform the exercise. Increasing repetitions, sets, and difficulty of the exercises on the Swiss ball can each improve muscle endurance or strength.

Other Swiss ball exercises improve flexibility. Many people find the ball a comfortable surface on which to perform stretching exercises. The Swiss ball can also provide a comfortable and relaxing gravity-assisted method of stretching (figure 14.1).

When an individual performs an activity, the body receives feedback on the accuracy and quality of the performance in the form of sensory information from visual, auditory, vestibular, and

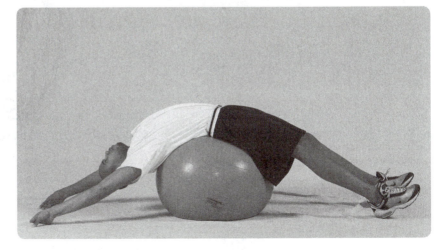

▶ **Figure 14.1** Gravity-assisted Swiss-ball stretch.

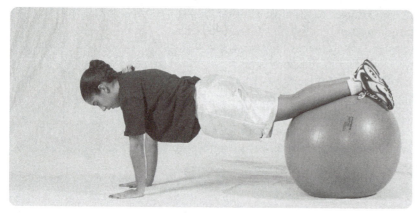

a

b

▶ **Figure 14.2** Reduced base of support from two arms *(a)* to one arm *(b)* on Swiss ball increases the activity's difficulty.

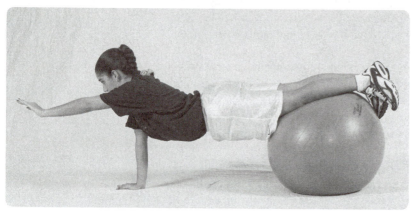

a

▶ **Figure 14.3** Increased lever-arm length on Swiss ball increases the activity's difficulty. Ball is moved from the thighs *(a)* to the distal legs *(b)*.

b

somatosensory systems. Adjustments in performance occur based on the feedback received and interpreted at various neural levels as discussed in chapter 8. Swiss-ball exercises facilitate joint- and body-position awareness because there is a continual change of position, and the body must adjust and adapt to those changes appropriately, while performing the activities correctly.

Increasing Swiss-Ball Challenges

Regardless of the parameter you are challenging, you can provide exercise progressions on the Swiss ball. The obvious modification is the addition of resistance equipment such as weights, rubber tubing/bands, pulleys, or the use of manual resistance to increase strength gains.

Other modifications include decreasing the base of support. For example, if a patient is balancing on the ball with both hands on the floor, a narrower placement of the hands will make the activity more difficult. This activity becomes even more difficult if you have the patient perform it with only one hand on the ground, or perform movement on the ball while supporting the body with one hand on the floor (figure 14.2).

Based on information from chapter 3, increasing the lever-arm length makes the activity more difficult. For example, a push-up performed on the Swiss ball will increase in difficulty if the ball is moved from under the thighs to under the shins (figure 14.3).

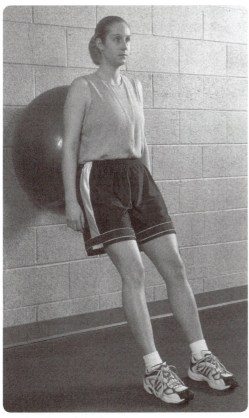
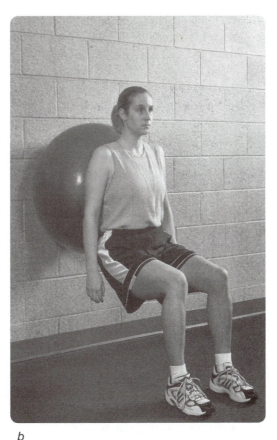

a   b

▶ **Figure 14.4** Moving through a greater ROM on the Swiss ball requires greater muscle activity. *(a)* Slight squat motion, *(b)* full squat.

Increasing the distance traveled is another way to make the exercise more difficult. Going through a greater range of motion requires recruitment of more muscle fibers, so the muscle must work harder. For example, the difficulty of a squat exercise with the Swiss ball is increased if the range of motion of the squat is increased (figure 14.4).

As with many other exercises, increasing the speed of movement and requiring the same amount of control as with the slower speed will increase the difficulty of the exercise on a Swiss ball.

Equipment and Exercise Area

There are currently several manufacturers of vinyl Swiss balls. Gymnic and Physioball are well-known Swiss-ball names. These balls are durable enough to withstand an individual's weight. The Gymnic ball will hold 454 kg (1,000 lb), while the Physioball resists loads up to 299 kg (660 lb).

Swiss balls come in various sizes. Each company makes balls in different colors corresponding to different sizes, but because the colors vary among the companies, you should select balls according to size, not color. Ball size is indicated by diameter. The size to select for a particular patient is determined by the patient's height and hip & knee position in sitting. Table 14.1 lists appropriate Swiss-ball sizes for individuals of varying heights.

TABLE 14.1 **Swiss Ball Sizes**

Patient's height	Circumference (cm)	Diameter (in.)
Under 5 ft	45	18
5 ft to 5 ft 7 in.	55	21 Aw
5 ft. 8 in. to 6 ft. 2 in.	65	25
6 ft 3 in. to 6 ft. 10 in.	75	29 Aw
Over 6 ft 10 in.	85	33 Aw

When the patient is sitting on the ball, the hips and knees should be at 90°. If the patient's height is between the heights listed in table 14.1, use the larger-sized ball and under-inflate it to fit the patient.

The floor surface should be firm and smooth but not slippery. Firm mats, linoleum, hardwood, and low-pile carpet are good surfaces. Surfaces should not be rough or uneven. Swiss balls should not be used outdoors because of the unevenness of the surface and because objects on the ground, such as pebbles or debris, can puncture them. The area where a patient exercises with a Swiss ball should be spacious enough to allow moving and rolling without danger of hitting furniture or other objects that could cause injury.

Safety Factors

The rehabilitation clinician should keep some safety factors in mind when beginning an exercise session that uses a Swiss ball. The patient's clothing should be free of objects such as belt buckles that may puncture the ball. The patient should wear rubber-soled shoes that provide traction. If the shoes are worn outdoors, the soles should be inspected for pebbles that could fall off and puncture the ball.

The patient's clothing should be proper athletic wear that allows freedom of movement. If the individual will be on the floor on the knees, he or she should wear sweatpants or warm-up pants that will protect the skin from abrasions. Pants of these types will also prevent the skin from sticking to the ball and reduce restriction of movement or skin discomfort.

When performing exercises on the Swiss ball, patients should not combine bouncing on the ball with bending and twisting or rotating the spine. This can cause injury to the spine. The exercises should be performed with control and not so quickly that the motions are incorrect.

The patient's hair should be restrained if necessary, so that it does not impede the exercise, hamper vision, or get in the way.

Contraindications

Although contraindications are not commonly seen in the young population, the rehabilitation clinician should be aware of them since they may occur in adults. An individual who has a fear of using or falling off the ball, and who cannot be reassured, should not use the Swiss ball. Increased pain, dizziness, or any other undesirable symptom is an indication to stop the exercises. Any disease or injury that is contraindicated for specific exercises should be avoided. For example, a patient who is non-weight bearing should not use the feet to stabilize while sitting on the ball.

Swiss balls can be used in a progression of exercises to challenge flexibility, strength, muscle endurance, balance, coordination, and joint- and body-position awareness. Ball size is chosen according to the patient's height and hip and knee position in sitting. Safety factors include avoidance of bouncing in combination with spine movements and being aware of several contraindications.

■ Swiss-Ball Care

As mentioned earlier, the Swiss ball should not be used outdoors. A Swiss ball can be easily damaged by pebbles or other sharp or hard objects on the ground. The balls should be kept away from excessive or prolonged heat sources such as lamps, heat ducts, and direct sunlight.

Swiss balls should be inflated when at room temperature. They can be inflated with an air compressor, air-mattress pump, or gas-station air compressor or pump with a trigger nozzle attachment. A bicycle pump will not work well because of the large volume of air the ball requires—using a bicycle pump will simply take too long. A ball is maximally inflated when it is firm; but as already indicated, less-than-maximal inflation is appropriate when a patient's height requires a slightly smaller ball.

Warm, soapy water and a cloth are used to clean the ball. Abrasive or chemical cleaners may cause damage and should be avoided.

SWISS-BALL EXERCISES

Many Swiss-ball exercises are used for trunk stabilization, but a number of these can be used to strengthen the upper and lower extremities as well. The activities described here by no means represent all Swiss-ball exercises and are examples only. As with many other therapeutic exercises, specific Swiss-ball activities are limited only by the patient's restrictions and the rehabilitation clinician's knowledge and imagination.

Trunk Exercises

For all Swiss-ball exercises, the patient is instructed to maintain a pelvic-neutral posture throughout the activity. To maintain this position, the patient must know where his or her pelvic neutral is located and keep some tension in the muscles controlling the position, especially the abdominals.

Bounce and Kick

This is a stabilization exercise. The patient sits on the ball in pelvic neutral. Without rotating the spine or hips, the patient bounces on the ball. While bouncing, he or she alternates kicking out one leg and then the other, one kick for each bounce (figure 14.5). This becomes more difficult if the patient simultaneously raises the opposite arm.

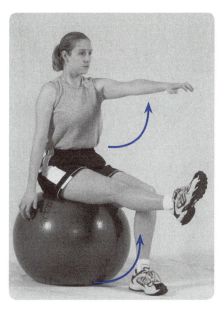

▶ **Figure 14.5** Bounce and kick.

Side Foot Reach

This is also a stabilization exercise. The patient sits on the ball in pelvic neutral. The arms are crossed (figure 14.6). As the patient bounces on the ball, he or she extends one leg out to the side and then brings it back to the starting position. Movements should coincide with the bounces. The opposite leg is then moved to the other side in similar fashion. This exercise is more challenging if arm movements are added, with the same-side arm extending sideways simultaneously with the leg.

Lateral Glide

The lateral glide is for pelvic flexibility. The patient sits on the ball in pelvic neutral (figure 14.7). The pelvis is rolled out to one side and then the other, the patient then returns to pelvic neutral. The patient uses the trunk muscles to perform the exercise, not the legs.

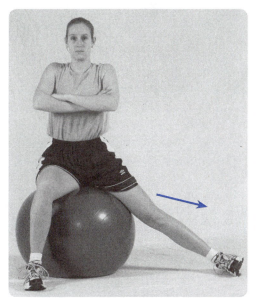

▶ **Figure 14.6** Side foot reach.

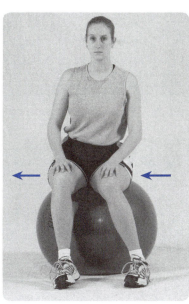

▶ **Figure 14.7** Lateral glide to the right.

Pelvic Circles

This exercise is for pelvic flexibility. The patient sits on the ball in pelvic neutral and rotates the pelvis first clockwise and then counterclockwise (figure 14.8). The pelvic and trunk muscles are used to produce the motion, not the legs. The legs and shoulders should move minimally.

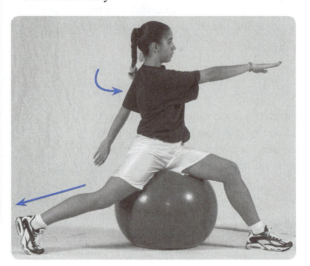

Figure 14.8 Clockwise pelvic circles.

Figure 14.9 Trunk rotation in sitting.

Trunk Rotation in Sitting

This exercise is for trunk flexibility. The patient sits on the ball in pelvic neutral with the arms abducted to 90°. The trunk is rotated to the left, and the right arm reaches in the direction of the trunk rotation as the right leg is extended behind the person (figure 14.9). The patient returns to the starting position and repeats the motion to the right.

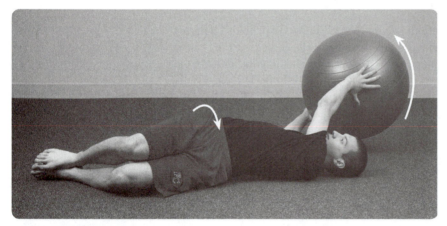

Figure 14.10 Trunk rotation in supine.

Trunk Rotation in Supine

This is a variation of the exercise just described. The patient lies supine on the floor with the knees and hips flexed, holding the ball in the hands with the arms straight and directly overhead. Keeping the abdominals tight to stabilize the spine, the individual moves the ball to the right as the hips are rotated to the left (figure 14.10). The hip movement is initiated from the low-back and oblique abdominal muscles, not the hips or legs.

Stretch in Kneeling

This stretch for the back can also be used for the shoulders. The patient kneels on the floor with his or her hands on the ball, which is in front of the person. The patient bows forward and lets the ball roll out (figure 14.11). The elbows are extended as the patient attempts to lower the upper trunk toward the floor.

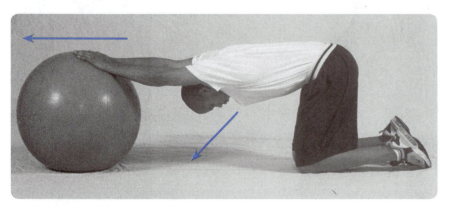

Figure 14.11 Stretch in kneeling.

Lateral Stretch

This stretch is for the lateral trunk. The patient kneels beside the ball and lies sideways over the ball to touch the lower hand to the floor (figure 14.12). The upper arm is extended overhead as the patient lies in sidelying across the top of the ball.

Thoracic Stretch

The patient sits on the ball with the feet about shoulder-width apart. He or she then lies back on the ball as it rolls up the back until the buttocks are toward the floor and the shoulder blades are on the ball (figure 14.1, p. 417). The patient then raises the arms overhead and moves the ball position so the head moves closer to the floor and the knees are straight with the ball supporting the back and hips.

Supine Leg Lift

This exercise strengthens the back extensors. The patient sits on the ball then lies back as he or she walks out until the head and shoulders are supported on the ball (figure 14.13). While the individual maintains pelvic neutral, he or she alternately lifts the legs off the floor in a marching sequence. There should be no rolling of the trunk or hips, and the pelvis should not drop. This exercise becomes more difficult if performed with the arms overhead.

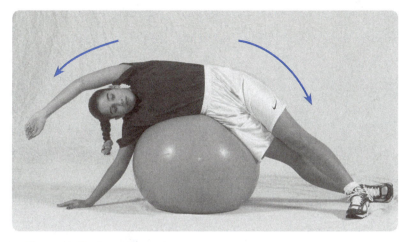

▶ **Figure 14.12** Lateral stretch.

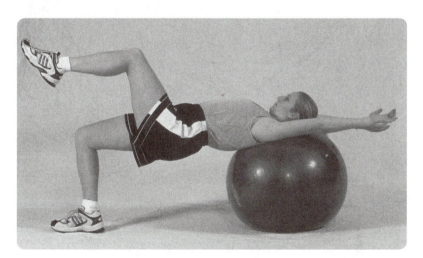

▶ **Figure 14.13** Supine leg lift.

Hip Rotation

The abdominal oblique muscles are strengthened with this exercise. The patient lies supine on the floor, with the legs on the ball and arms at the sides (figure 14.14). The individual rolls the knees from side to side as far as possible without falling off the ball. The abdominals, kept tightened, initiate the movement of the hips. The back should not arch, and the shoulders should remain on the floor throughout the exercise.

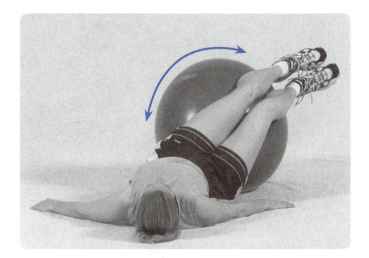

▶ **Figure 14.14** Hip rotation.

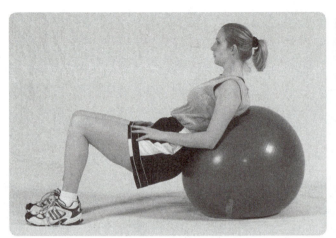

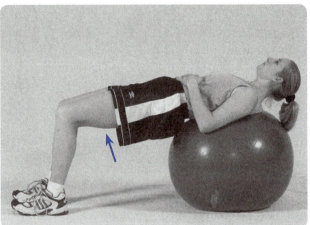

a

b

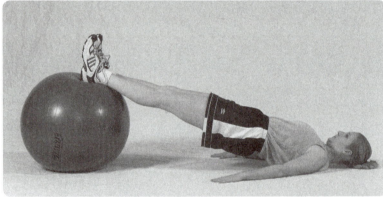

c

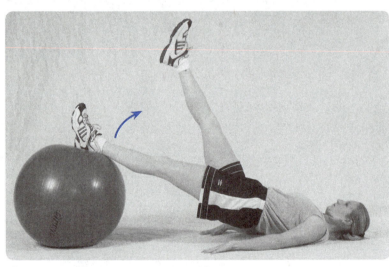

d

▶ **Figure 14.15** Bridging: *(a)* beginning position, *(b)* end position, *(c)* variation—isometric hold with feet on ball, *(d)* variation—alternate leg raise while maintaining pelvic neutral position.

Bridging

This exercise, which strengthens the back extensors, can be performed in two positions. In one variation, the patient is supine on the ball so the scapulae are on the ball, the hips and legs are off the ball, and the feet are on the floor about shoulder-width apart (figure 14.15, a and b). The pelvis is in neutral and the abdominals are tight as the patient lifts the buttocks and extends the hips. Hip elevation motion occurs at the buttocks, not the feet or knees, and the pelvis is kept in neutral throughout the activity. This exercise is more challenging if the patient marches in place while maintaining pelvic neutral.

The other variation of this bridging exercise is with the patient lying supine on the floor and the feet on the Swiss ball. Keeping pelvic neutral, the individual lifts the hips off the floor as the buttocks and abdominals are tightened (figure 14.15c). You can make this exercise more difficult by having the patient alternate leg lifts off the ball (figure 14.15d). The exercise also becomes more challenging if you have the patient change the arm positions, from arms extended away from the hips, to arms across the chest, to hands behind or above the head.

Back Extension in Prone

This exercise strengthens the back extensors. The patient lies prone on the ball; the ball is under the lower abdomen and pelvis, and the balls of the patient's feet are on the floor. The trunk is flexed forward with the pelvis in neutral (figure 14.16a). The patient lifts the trunk by squeezing the gluteals and the lower back paraspinal muscles. The arm positions change to increase the difficulty of the exercise, beginning with the hands behind the back and progressing so that the hands are out to the sides (figure 14.16b) and then overhead (figure 14.16c). To create an additional level of difficulty, the patient places his or her feet on a chair as seen in figure 14.16, d through f.

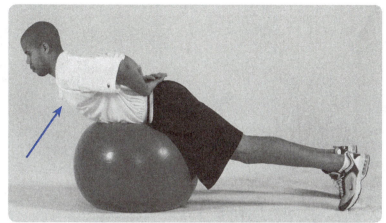

a

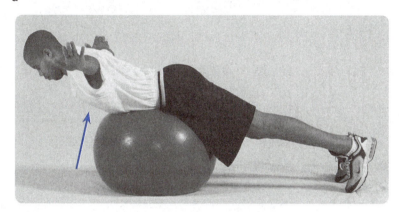

b

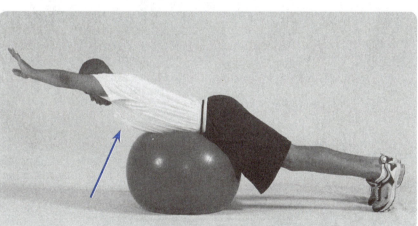

c

▶ **Figure 14.16** Back-extension progression. Changes in arm placement change the exercise's difficulty by moving the center of gravity. Additional levels of difficulty of the back-extension progression are shown in parts d through f. *(continued)* ▶

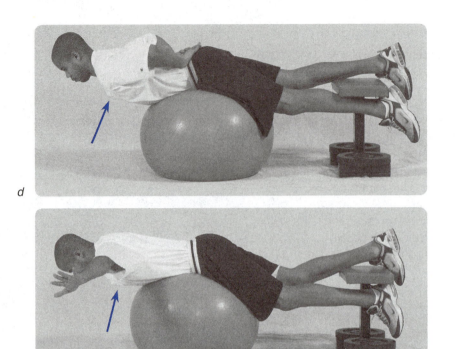

d

e

f

▶ **Figure 14.16** *(continued)*

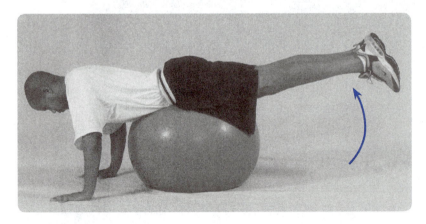

▶ **Figure 14.17** Prone leg lift.

Prone Leg Lift

This leg lift strengthens the trunk extensors. The patient lies prone on the ball with the hands and the balls of the feet on the floor. The Swiss ball is under the lower abdomen and pelvis. The patient squeezes the buttocks to raise the legs, keeping the pelvis in neutral and the knees straight (figure 14.17).

Swimming

This exercise strengthens the midback region. In prone with the ball placed under the patient's abdomen and both knees extended, with only the balls of the feet on the floor, the patient places one arm overhead in full shoulder flexion in front and the other behind in shoulder extension (figure 14.18a). The patient maintains a neutral spine as the arms reverse positions (figure 14.18b). The trunk should not rotate as the arms move. Weights can be added to increase the difficulty of the exercise.

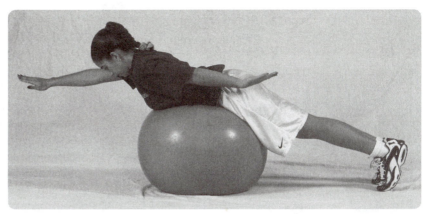

a

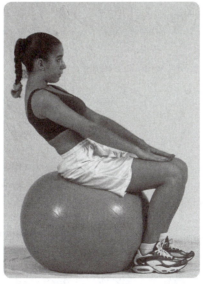

b

▶ **Figure 14.18** Swimming.

Seated Abdominal Strengthening

The patient sits on the Swiss ball in pelvic neutral. The feet are shoulder-width apart. Maintaining pelvic neutral, the person leans back on the ball, moving from the hips, not the spine (figure 14.19a). Changing the arm positions changes the difficulty of the exercise. The least-difficult variation is with the arms outstretched in front of the hips. As the arms move upward toward the head, the exercise difficulty increases. This activity can stress the oblique muscles if the patient places the arms overhead and alternately lowers each arm to the opposite knee as seen in figure 14.19b.

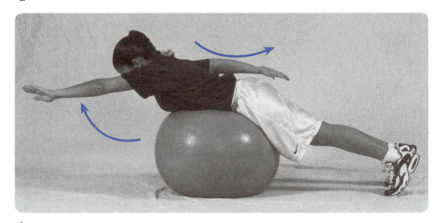

a   *b*

▶ **Figure 14.19** Seated abdominal strengthening: *(a)* with arms forward, *(b)* more difficult with alternating arms overhead while reaching toward the opposite knee, which will stress oblique muscles.

Ball Lift

The purpose of this exercise is to strengthen the lower abdominals. The patient lies supine on the floor and maintains pelvic neutral. The ball is picked up between the ankles, and the hips are maintained at 90° flexion (figure 14.20a). With the lower abdominals kept tight, the knees are flexed and extended at 90°. The progression for this exercise is advancing from flexing and extending the knees with the hip position maintained in flexion to extending the hips and simultaneously extending the knees as the lower extremities are lowered to the floor (figure 14.20b). It is important that the lower abdominals remain tense throughout this exercise and the lower back maintains contact with the floor.

To increase the difficulty, the patient rotates the legs, bringing one in front of the other and then reversing positions. Again, the pelvis should remain in neutral, and the lower spine maintains contact with the floor, as seen in figure 14.20c.

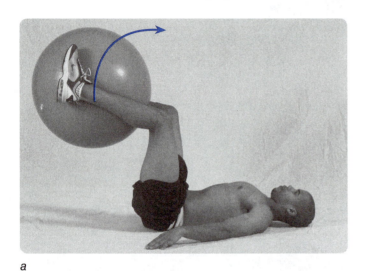

a

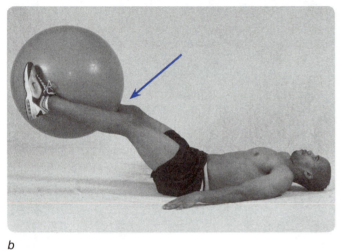

b

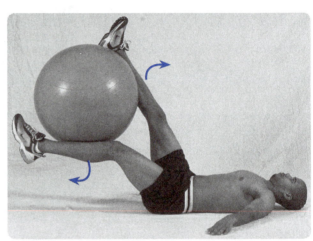

c

▶ **Figure 14.20** Ball lift: *(a)* Hips are at 90° and knees are extended, *(b)* legs are lowered while back remains flat, *(c)* legs are rotated with spine in neutral.

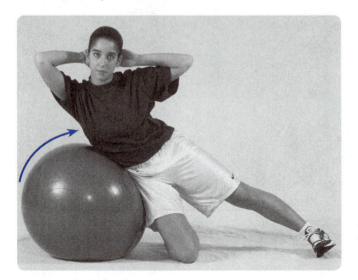

▶ **Figure 14.21** Side sit-up.

Side Sit-Ups

This sit-up strengthens the obliques. The patient kneels on the floor beside the ball. The individual then lies sideways on the ball, with the lateral hip and trunk in contact with the ball and the outer knee extended laterally away from the ball and to the side in abduction (figure 14.21). The patient then lifts the trunk sideways off the ball while maintaining contact on the ball with the hip. Progression of this exercise includes moving the knee closest to the ball off the floor and having only the feet in contact with the floor while the lateral trunk is in contact with the ball.

Prone Walk-Out

This exercise strengthens the abdominals. The patient walks forward until the ball is at the shins and the arms support the weight of the trunk in a push-up position as shown in figure 14.22a. Pelvic neutral is maintained while this position is held on a timed basis.

A variation of this exercise is to have the patient maintain pelvic neutral while bringing the knees up toward the chest (figure 14.22b). You can add difficulty by having the patient roll the ball to one side and then to the other so that the side of the thigh comes in contact with the ball while the legs remain in the position seen in figure 14.22b. This variation also exercises the oblique muscles.

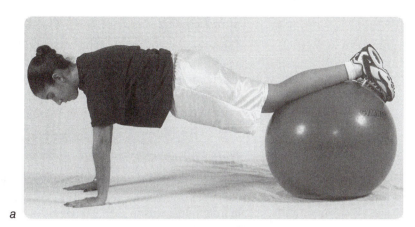

a

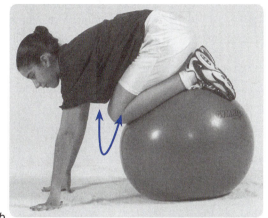

b

▶ **Figure 14.22** Prone walk-out: *(a)* beginning position, *(b)* ending position. The ball can be rolled from side to side for an additional level of this exercise (see arrow).

Lower-Extremity Exercises

Some of the trunk exercises also can be used for the lower extremities. It should not be difficult for you to identify which trunk exercises also exercise the lower extremities. A few additional exercises for the lower extremities are described here.

Reverse Squats

This squat strengthens quadriceps, calf, and gluteal muscles. The patient places the ball on the wall and leans prone on the ball with the ball at waist level (figure 14.23a). The patient remains on his or her toes throughout the exercise, and the feet are shoulder-width apart. The individual squats down to a comfortable level and returns to the start position (figure 14.23b). This exercise is substantially more difficult when performed in a unilateral leg stance position.

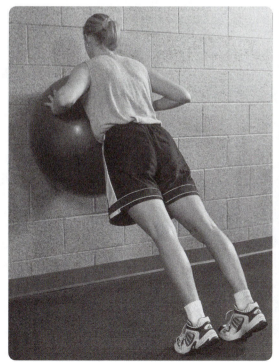

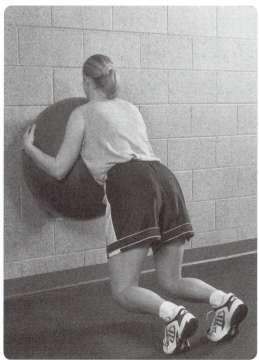

▶ **Figure 14.23** Reverse squats: *(a)* start position, *(b)* end position.

a

b

Side Leg Lift

This exercise strengthens hip abductors. The patient kneels and lies sideways on the ball in a position similar to the side sit-up position shown in figure 14.21. The top leg rises toward the ceiling with the knee extended and the leg in line with the trunk. The raised leg should not move in the sagittal plane. If the patient is performing the exercise correctly, it will feel as if the hip is in hyperextension. Do not allow hip flexion or rotation, knee flexion, or trunk rotation during the exercise.

Half Squat

This exercise strengthens the quadriceps. The patient stands with the ball on the wall and in the patient's low back region. The feet are positioned shoulder-width apart, and far enough in front of the person so that when he or she squats, the knees do not flex more than 90° (see figure 14.4, p. 419). Additional knee flexion places too much stress on the patellofemoral joint. A patient who has knee pain during this exercise should place the feet farther forward or reduce the depth of the squat.

Hamstring Curl

This exercise strengthens the hamstrings. The patient lies supine on the floor with his or her feet on the Swiss ball. The hips remain off the floor so the trunk and legs form a straight line, as illustrated in figure 14.15a. While keeping the hips elevated, the patient flexes the knees to move the ball closer to the hips, and then extends the knees to the starting position. A progression includes starting with the arms on the floor near the hips and then moving them to the chest and overhead. In another progression, the patient first uses both legs, then crosses the uninvolved over the involved leg on the ball, and finally maintains only the involved leg on the ball.

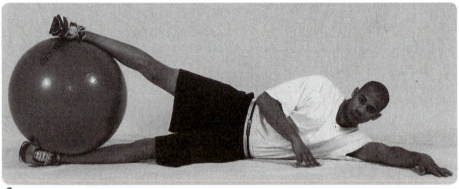

a

Sidelying Ball Lift

This exercise strengthens the hip and trunk muscles. The patient is sidelying with the knees and hips extended; the floor arm is overhead, and the top hand is on the floor for stabilization as shown in figure 14.24a. The ball is grasped between the feet and legs, and the pelvis is maintained in neutral. Both legs are lifted off the floor as high as possible, with the legs and spine kept straight (figure 14.24b).

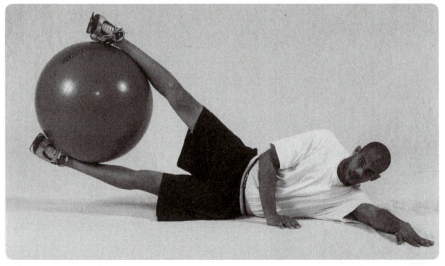

b

▶ **Figure 14.24** Sidelying ball lift: *(a)* start position, *(b)* upward lateral movement of the legs.

Ankle Motion Exercise

This is a balance exercise for the lower extremity. The patient stands in pelvic neutral with the uninjured foot on top of the ball; he or she then writes the alphabet with the uninjured foot, using the ball as a base of support (figure 14.25).

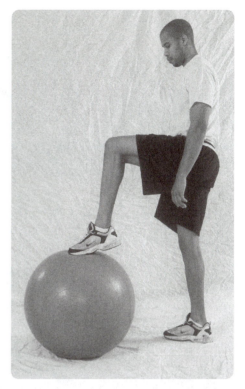

▶ **Figure 14.25** Ankle motion exercise.

Upper-Extremity Exercises

Some of the trunk exercises, and even the lower-extremity exercises, can also be used for the upper extremities. Although they are not mentioned here, many upper-extremity exercises using rubber tubing and rubber bands, as well as medicine-ball exercises, become more difficult when performed on the Swiss ball.

Prone Fly

This exercise strengthens scapular retractors. The patient lies prone on the Swiss ball with the ball under the lower abdomen or upper thighs. The legs are straight, with the toes in contact with the floor. The patient's arms are anterior to the chest and resting on the floor, and elbows are flexed (figure 14.26). The patient lifts the elbows toward the ceiling while keeping the shoulders elevated to about 90° and squeezes the scapulae together. Weight is used to provide resistance.

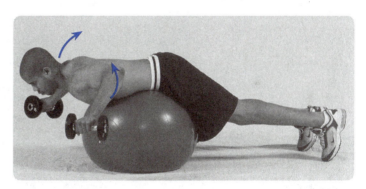

▶ **Figure 14.26** Prone flys.

Triceps Extension

The patient is reclined with the ball supporting the low back or midback as illustrated in figure 14.15a or seated on the ball. Abdominal tension maintains pelvic neutral. The arms are elevated overhead with the elbows flexed and hands behind the shoulders. Keeping the arms above the head, the patient extends the elbows.

Swiss-ball exercises can improve trunk stabilization, flexibility, and strength; there are also many Swiss-ball exercises for strengthening the upper and lower extremities. The upper-extremity exercises become more challenging if the Swiss ball is used in combination with such devices as rubber bands or tubing and weights.

Push-Ups

The patient lies prone on the ball with hands on the floor and feet elevated. The ball is under the lower abdomen or pelvis (figure 14.27a). With the hands positioned as close together as possible and still complete the exercise, the patient performs a push-up, keeping good spinal alignment throughout the motion (figure 14.27b). Progressions of this exercise include moving the ball under the thighs, placing the ball under the legs (figure 14.27c), and reversing the body position so the hands are on the ball and the feet are on the floor (figure 14.27d).

Scapular Retraction

This exercise uses the Swiss ball with rubber bands or tubing. The patient sits on the ball, with the feet on a foam roller for a more difficult exercise or on the floor for a less difficult exercise. The patient pulls the bands and squeezes the scapulae together while maintaining balance on the Swiss ball and the elbows below shoulder level (figure 14.28). Upper-extremity exercises using rubber tubing, medicine balls, and other equipment become more challenging with the patient on a Swiss ball.

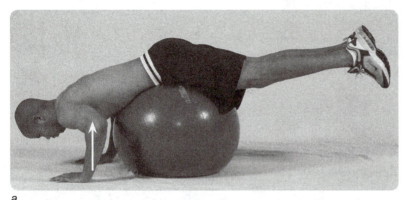

a

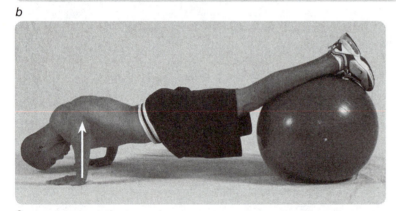

b

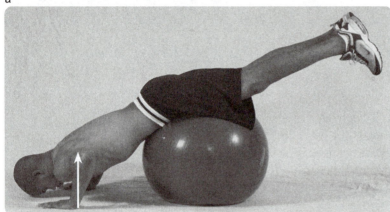

c

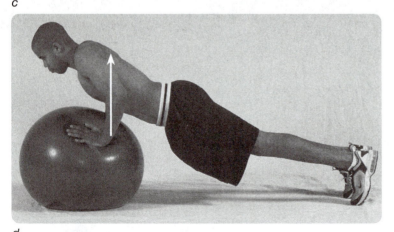

d

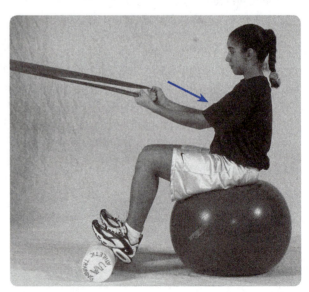

▶ **Figure 14.27** Push-up progression: *(a-c)* Progression is provided by increasing the lever-arm length; *(d)* progression is provided by using an unstable base for the arms.

▶ **Figure 14.28** Scapular retraction.

FOAM ROLLERS

Moshe Feldenkrais was one of the first to use rollers as a therapeutic tool. He used rollers in his Feldenkrais Method, discussed earlier in this text (chapter 11). Feldenkrais used wooden rollers until 1972, when he was introduced to **foam rollers** while in the United States.

In recent years, the use of foam rollers has become commonplace for rehabilitation in neurological, orthopedic, and sports medicine facilities. Several annual professional workshops and seminars in foam roller use take place across the country.

Use of foam rollers in therapeutic exercise improves body awareness and joint-position sense, enhances balance and proprioception, aids in muscle reeducation, and promotes flexibility and strength. Because of its cylindrical shape, the foam roller provides little contact with the floor and moves quickly and easily; standing on the roller challenges the patient's balance reaction. As with the Swiss ball, the roller presents an unstable surface and, thus, a more challenging platform for performing what are otherwise easily managed activities. The use of foam rollers offers the patient a diversion from routine exercises and still accomplishes many of the same goals that more traditional exercises do. Rollers are relatively inexpensive and can be used in the treatment facility and at home.

Foam-Roller Design

Most foam rollers are made of Ethafoam, which is a polyethylene product; others are made of polyurethane. They all are cylindrical and come in a variety of lengths, circumferences, and densities. Diameters include 7.6, 10.0, and 15.2 cm (3, 4, and 6 in.). The lengths vary from 30 cm to about 180 cm (1-6 ft). Half-rollers may be purchased, or rollers can also be cut in half longitudinally with a bread knife to form a half roll so one side is flat and the other is a half circle.

The Ethafoam rollers are dense rolls that can support up to 159 kg (350 lb). Because of their buoyancy, patients can also use them in aquatic therex programs. Their density makes them effective for use in soft-tissue and joint mobilizations, and they are firm enough for muscle strengthening. The Ethafoam rollers can also be used to improve proprioception. The softer polyurethane rolls offer more stability. They can be more comfortable to lie on than the Ethafoam rollers, but they tend to lose their shape more quickly and become difficult to roll with repeated use.

Precautions and Contraindications

Before the rehabilitation clinician uses a foam roller, he or she must observe several precautions and must examine the patient for existing contraindications. If an individual has contusions, acne, or other skin disturbances, the rehabilitation clinician should observe for responses that aggravate the condition.

Patients experiencing temporary conditions of vertigo brought on by ear infections or other disorders should either postpone using a foam roller or should use the roller under careful supervision and be sure to perform slow, controlled, and adequately supported movements.

Hypermobility of joints, postpartum hypermobility, and acute fractures are conditions that require caution in the use of foam rolls. Performing some activities on a foam roller can aggravate these types of hypermobility.

A patient showing signs of nausea, light-headedness, pallor, or shortness of breath should be taken off the foam roller. The few outright contraindications for the use of foam rollers are common sense ones. Any symptoms of increased pain, dizziness, nausea, or tinnitus are contraindications, as are any full-weight-bearing restrictions. Other contraindications not commonly seen in young adults but that may occur in older patients include osteoporosis, connective-tissue disorders such as fibromyalgia and rheumatoid arthritis that are in a flare-up condition, current use of anticoagulant medication, and tumors.

Foam rollers help to improve joint- and body-position awareness, balance, proprioception, flexibility, and strength. Precautions relate to various skin conditions and various types of hypermobility, and the rehabilitation clinician should keep in mind several contraindications.

FOAM-ROLLER EXERCISES

As with the Swiss-ball exercises, the foam-roller exercises described here do not represent an entire program but serve only as examples. The exercises suggested may give you ideas for others. You can use foam rollers in conjunction with equipment such as the Swiss ball, rubber tubing and bands, and other exercise equipment. The following exercises are presented according to body segments.

Trunk Exercises

Some of the exercises described here for the trunk may also be used for upper and lower extremities. Some are stretching exercises, some are for strengthening, and others are self-massage techniques. The massage techniques are presented first.

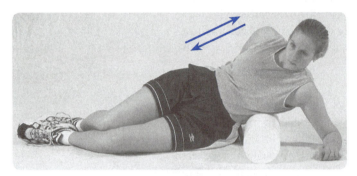

▶ **Figure 14.29** Quadratus massage.

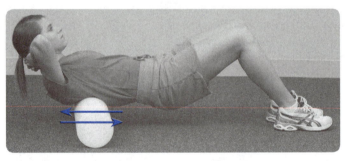

▶ **Figure 14.30** Thoracic massage.

Quadratus Massage

This exercise relaxes the quadratus lumborum to increase range of motion. The patient positions the foam roller under the quadratus lumborum in a semi-reclined, three-quarter position with the foam roller as seen in figure 14.29. The individual leans back on the roller and gently rolls up and down over the foam roller to relax the quadratus.

Thoracic Massage

This exercise massages the thoracic area to relax muscles and improve range of motion. The patient lies supine on a foam roller positioned perpendicular to the line of the body. The roller is placed under the thoracic region (figure 14.30). The patient supports his or her head in both hands and keeps the buttocks lifted off the floor and the feet flat on the floor. He or she rolls gently up and down from the lower ribs upward to the shoulders.

Low-Back Mobilization

The purpose of this exercise is to improve low-back flexibility. The patient stands with feet shoulder-width apart; the foam roller is hooked under the elbows and across the low back. The patient arches the back into the roller.

Cat Stretch

This is a back-flexibility exercise using two foam rollers. The patient is in a kneeling quadruped position, with both knees on one roller and both hands on another roller. The patient arches the back up as high as possible by tightening the abdominals and then sags the back toward the floor.

Quadruped Balance

This exercise develops balance and pelvic stabilization. The patient kneels on one roller and places the hands on a second roller, as in the cat stretch just described. Keeping pelvic neutral throughout the exercise, the patient first lifts one leg and the opposite arm and then reverses the extremity positions (figure 14.31).

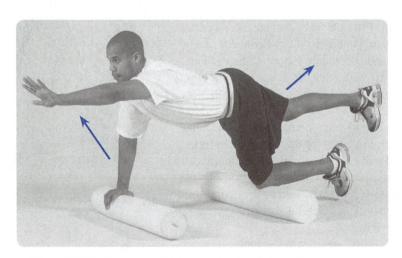

▶ **Figure 14.31** Quadruped balance using two foam rollers.

Supine Lower Abdominal Exercise

This exercise strengthens the lower abdominal muscles. The patient lies supine with the knees flexed. The roller is placed between the knees (figure 14.32). The patient tightens the lower abdominals and lifts the knees toward the chest, keeping the back flat on the floor. The back should not arch at any time during this exercise.

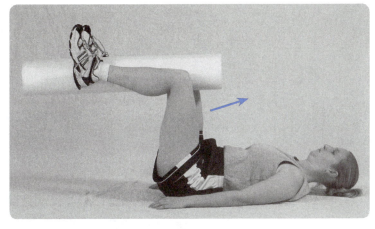

▶ **Figure 14.32** Supine lower abdominal exercise.

Supine Oblique Exercise

This exercise strengthens the obliques. The patient lies supine on the foam roller and places the feet on a Swiss ball (figure 14.33). While keeping the knees extended, the patient rolls the ball from side to side. The back should not arch.

Abdominal Crunch

This exercise strengthens the abdominals. The patient assumes a kneeling position; the roller is under both knees, and the hands are flat on the floor. The patient pulls the knees up toward the chest as the foam roller moves down the legs. This exercise becomes more difficult if the patient begins the exercise in a prone position (figure 14.34a) and moves to the same end position as in the easier exercise (figure 14.34b).

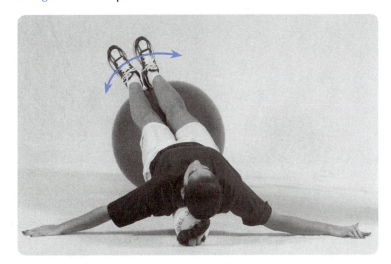

▶ **Figure 14.33** Oblique exercise.

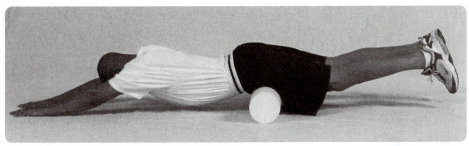

a

▶ **Figure 14.34** Abdominal crunch: (a) start position, (b) end position.

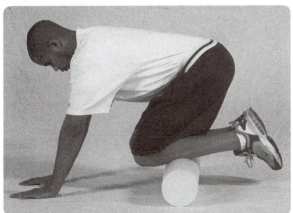

b

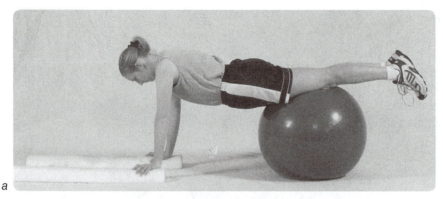

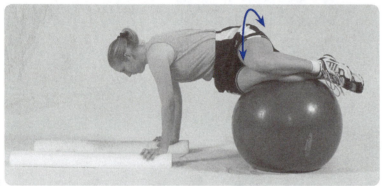

▶ **Figure 14.35** Rotational crunch: *(a)* start position, *(b)* with knees up, patient rolls side to side from one hip to the other.

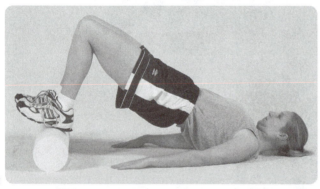

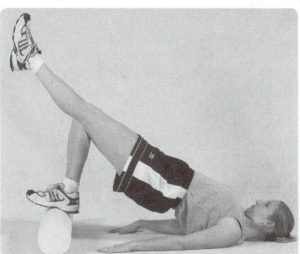

▶ **Figure 14.36** Bridging: *(a)* start position, *(b)* end position.

Rotational Crunch

This exercise strengthens the obliques. The patient lies prone on a Swiss ball with the thighs on the ball and each hand on a half roller, flat side down (figure 14.35a). The patient brings the knees toward the chest and then rotates the hips, first to one side and then to the other, so that the bottom lateral thigh rests on the ball (figure 14.35b). A pelvic neutral position is maintained throughout the exercise. This exercise becomes more difficult with the half rollers placed flat side up.

Bridging

This exercise strengthens hamstrings, hip extensors, and back extensors. The patient lies supine on the floor with the feet placed on a horizontally positioned foam roller (figure 14.36a). The patient lifts the hips upward and rolls the roller toward the buttocks. This activity becomes more difficult if the individual performs it with only one leg at a time (figure 14.36b). A pelvic neutral position is maintained throughout.

Quadratus Lumborum Strengthening

The patient lies supine longitudinally on the foam roller. The knees are flexed and the feet flat on the floor. The shoulders and elbows are at 90° in a goalpost position. The patient brings the right elbow and the right rear pocket toward each other without changing the arm position and then repeats the movement to the opposite side (figure 14.37).

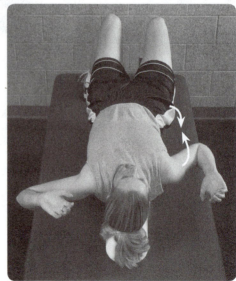

▶ **Figure 14.37** Quadratus lumborum strengthening.

Lower-Extremity Exercises

Foam-roller activities for the lower extremities can include techniques for massage, flexibility, strengthening, and proprioception.

Iliotibial-Band Massage

This exercise massages the iliotibial band (ITB) to increase flexibility. The patient lies on his or her left side with the left elbow flexed. The roller is placed under the left thigh, and the left leg is positioned under and in front of the right leg (figure 14.38). The patient gently moves the roller over small sections at a time from the knee to the hip, concentrating on those areas of greater tenderness. Reverse position to massage the right ITB. Areas of tenderness will be areas of soft-tissue restriction. This massage causes no discomfort in non-restricted areas.

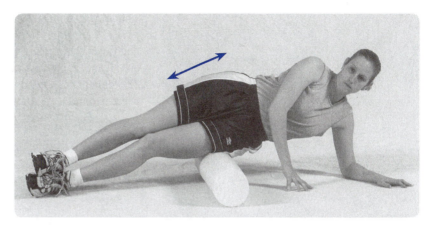

▶ **Figure 14.38** Iliotibial-band massage.

Quadriceps Massage

This exercise massages the quadriceps to increase flexibility. The patient lies prone on the floor with the roller in a horizontal position under and across the thighs. The individual then places his or her upper-body weight on the hands and pulls the body back and forth with the arms, allowing the roller to move up and down the anterior thighs.

Standing Balance

This exercise improves balance. The patient stands with both feet on a horizontally positioned foam roller (figure 14.39). To prevent falling, the patient needs to mount the roller using both hands to grasp a support structure, such as a table, handrail, or spotters. To prevent the roller from moving forward and forcing the patient in a backward fall, the patient must be instructed to place his or her center of gravity over the foot on the roller before stepping onto the roller. The patient's balance must be secure before letting go of the support. It may be necessary for the clinician to assist with additional manual support during the initial trials of this activity. If this exercise is too difficult, the patient can begin by standing with both feet on a single half roller or each foot on separate half rollers with the flat side up. You can make this exercise more difficult by having the patient stand only on one leg. Standing in a forward-backward (heel-to-toe) tandem position on the roller is also more advanced.

Anterior Tibialis Stretch

The patient kneels on the floor. The foam roller is on the ground behind the body and crosswise to the body. The dorsa of the distal feet are placed on top of the roller. The patient then leans back to sit on his or her heels while keeping the distal feet on the roller.

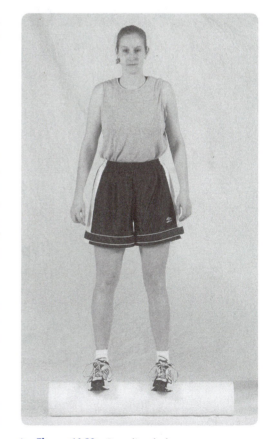

▶ **Figure 14.39** Standing balance.

Gastrocnemius Stretch

The patient stands on the flat portion of a half roller, with the balls of the feet on the roller and the heels on the floor. The knees are extended but not locked, and the body leans forward slightly while the patient places the hands on the wall or other structure for balance and support.

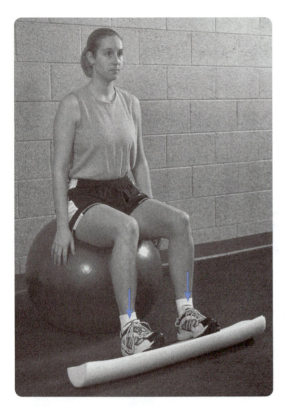

▶ **Figure 14.40** Sitting soleus stretch.

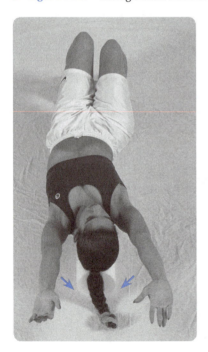

▶ **Figure 14.42** Arm stretches.

Soleus Stretch

The patient sits in a chair and places the balls of the feet on a half roller, flat side up (figure 14.40). He or she then pushes the heels to the floor.

Squats

The patient stands on a full foam roller, with the roller in a horizontal position and the feet about shoulder-width apart. The patient squats and raises the arms in front to maintain balance (figure 14.41). This is an advanced exercise that requires good balance and postural control. The patient may need stabilizing assistance from a spotter or need to use one hand on a stable object until balance is maintained.

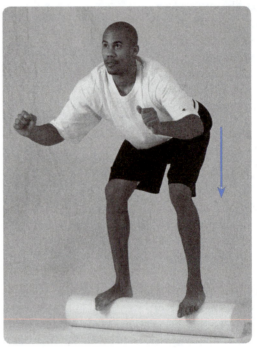

▶ **Figure 14.41** Squats.

Upper-Extremity Exercises

Upper-extremity exercises on the foam roller can begin early in a therapeutic exercise program in the form of flexibility exercises and then progress to open and closed kinetic chain activities as the patient improves.

Arm Stretches

The patient lies supine longitudinally on the roller with the hips & knees flexed and feet flat on the floor about shoulder width apart. The patient then moves the arms into 90° abduction, then 135°, and then overhead (figure 14.42). During each of these movements, he or she attempts to pull the elbows and forearms to the floor.

Push-Ups

The patient kneels on the floor, places the hands shoulder-width apart on the roller, and then performs a push-up. With the hands on the roller, the progression for this exercise is from the modified position on the knees, to the regular position, to a position in which another roller is placed under the knees, and finally to a position in which either an additional roller is placed under the shins or the legs are placed on a Swiss ball.

Resistance-Band Exercises in Standing

Isolated or combined movement patterns using rubber tubing or bands can be performed on foam rollers. The beginning-level exercise is performed on half foam rollers, flat side up (figure 14.43), and the more advanced exercise is performed with the patient standing on a full foam roller.

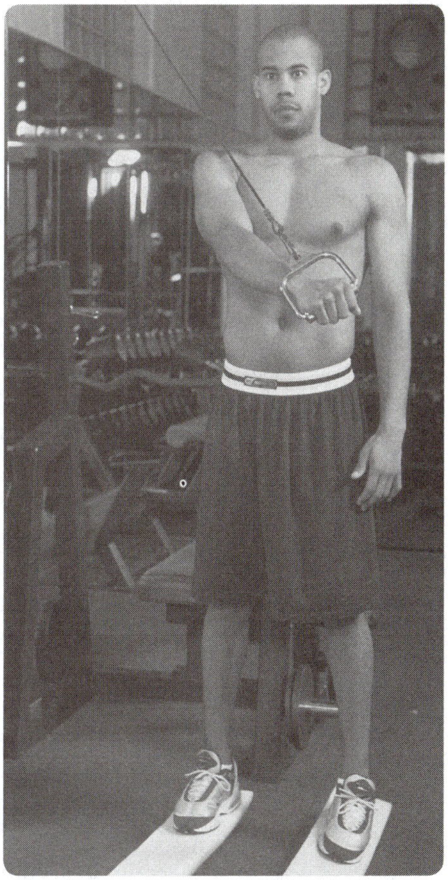

Resistance-Band Bench Press in Supine

The patient lies in a supine hook-lying position with the hips and knees flexed and the feet flat on the floor. The resistance band is secured under the roller at chest level. The patient grasps the band in each hand pushes the hands toward the ceiling until the elbow is in full extension. This exercise can be performed with either one arm or both (figure 14.44). Doubling the band will increase resistance.

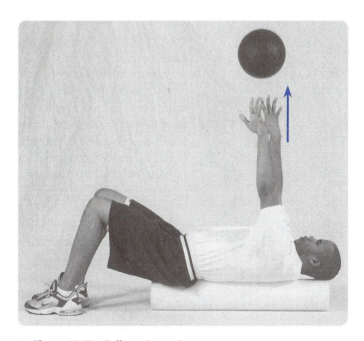

▶ **Figure 14.43** Resistance-band exercise in standing.

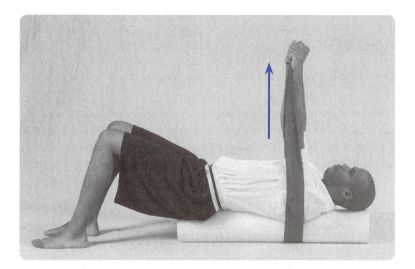

▶ **Figure 14.44** Resistance-band bench press in supine.

Ball Toss in Supine

The patient lies in a supine hook-lying position on the roller with the hips and knees flexed and feet flat on the floor. He or she then tosses either a Swiss ball or a medicine ball toward the ceiling (figure 14.45). The way the patient catches the ball depends on the purpose of the exercise. If the shoulders are emphasized, then the shoulders horizontally flex to catch the ball and horizontally extend to toss the ball. If the elbows are the reason for the exercise, the shoulders are kept relatively stable and elbow flexion and extension is performed to catch and release the ball, respectively. Wrist exercises in this position will maintain the elbows and shoulders in a relatively stable position while the wrists move from extension and radial deviation to flexion and ulnar deviation during catching and tossing the ball, respectively.

▶ **Figure 14.45** Ball toss in supine.

Patients can perform foam-roller exercises for the trunk, lower extremity, and upper extremity with or without other equipment, such as Swiss balls and rubber tubing and bands.

Triceps Press

The patient sits on the floor with the knees extended out in front of the body. One roller is under the ankles, and a short roller is at each side of the body near the hips. The patient places his or her hands on the rollers next to the hips and presses down to extend the elbows and shoulders and lift the buttocks off the floor. The scapulae should depress as much as possible.

SUMMARY

Swiss balls and foam rollers are inexpensive equipment that can make rehabilitation more interesting and challenging for the patient. These items may be used for upper and lower extremities and the trunk. They can be used for both flexibility and strength exercises. Some exercises can also combine the use of both pieces of equipment at the same time. Contraindications must be respected, and the patient must be properly instructed and spotted by the clinician before the patient is allowed independent use of these items.

KEY CONCEPTS AND REVIEW

1. Explain how Swiss balls and foam rollers can increase the challenge of a traditional exercise.

Swiss balls and foam rollers provide an unstable surface for an exercise. They can be used for open and closed chain activities. They can provide a progression of difficulty to continually challenge the patient as parameters such as flexibility, strength, and balance improve. Swiss balls can be used throughout a therapeutic exercise program to offer a number of stimulating challenges to the patient.

2. Identify the rehabilitation parameters that are benefited by the use of Swiss balls or foam rollers.

Flexibility, strength, muscle endurance, balance, coordination, and joint- and body-position awareness may each be stressed with Swiss ball and foam roller activities.

3. Discuss safety factors, precautions, and contraindications relating to the use of Swiss balls and foam rollers.

For safety, the patient's clothing should be proper athletic wear to allow freedom of movement and should be free of objects such as belt buckles; shoes should have rubber soles to provide traction; bouncing on the ball should not be combined with bending and twisting or rotating of the spine; long hair should be restrained; and exercises should be performed with control and not too quickly. Precautions for the rehabilitation clinician to observe include carefully explaining and demonstrating the exercise before having the patient attempt it, taking proper care of the equipment, fitting the ball correctly, and not using the equipment if you have any doubt about an patient's ability to handle it. Contraindications include fear of falling off the ball or roller, use of any medication that poses a danger, and complaints of dizziness or increased pain.

4. Explain how to properly fit a Swiss ball.

With the patient sitting on the ball and the feet flat on the floor, the hips and knees should be at 90°.

5. List one exercise each for the trunk, upper extremity, and lower extremity using a Swiss ball, and identify its purpose.

A bridge is an exercise for strengthening the back extensors; hip rotations in supine are used to gain flexibility and strength of the hip muscles; and a push-up with the pelvis on the ball can serve as an early upper-extremity strengthening exercise.

6. List one exercise each for the trunk, upper extremity, and lower extremity using foam rollers, and identify its purpose.

Lying on the foam roller and lowering the knees from the chest is a lower-abdominal strengthening exercise; lying sideways on the roller and rolling the lateral thigh along the foam roller is a massage technique for the ITB; and lying with the foam roller down the spine with the arms out to the side is a stretch for the anterior shoulder.

CRITICAL THINKING QUESTIONS

1. Because the Swiss ball can be used early in rehabilitation, you decide to use it in stabilization exercises for weak scapular muscles. Identify three low-level stabilization exercises that would incorporate the Swiss ball. What would be a more rigorous Swiss-ball scapular exercise? Identify an upper-extremity Swiss-ball exercise that can also be used for the trunk.

2. You have decided to give a Swiss ball to a patient with a back injury. You feel that she is now ready to continue the Swiss-ball exercises on her own at home. You want to limit the total number of Swiss ball exercises to 10 so that the patient will be more likely to perform all of them. Identify no more than 10 exercises that you would give this patient, and justify each one.

3. A patient wants to buy a Swiss ball to use at home during the semester break but does not know what size to buy. What guidance would you give him?

4. A patient with weak abdominals is going home for the summer and wants to take with her either a Swiss ball or foam roller, but not both. Which one would you advise her to take with her and why? List four exercises on the piece of equipment you have selected.

LAB ACTIVITIES

1. Measure your lab partner to select a Swiss ball that is the correct size for her.

2. Of the following Swiss ball exercises, select five trunk exercises to teach your lab partner. Be sure to have your "patient" maintain pelvic neutral throughout each exercise. As your partner is performing each exercise, use verbal cues to correct for any errors in his or her performance. Identify the purpose of each exercise.

    a. Bounce and kick
    b. Side foot reach
    c. Lateral glide
    d. Pelvic curls
    e. Trunk rotation in sitting
    f. Trunk rotation in supine
    g. Stretch in kneeling
    h. Lateral stretch
    i. Thoracic stretch
    j. Back extension in prone
    k. Supine leg lift
    l. Hip rotation
    m. Bridging
    n. Prone leg lift
    o. Swimming with 5 lb weights
    p. Seated abdominal strengthening
    q. Ball lift
    r. Side sit-ups
    s. Prone walk-out

3. Of the following Swiss ball exercises, select three lower extremity exercises to teach your lab partner. Be sure to have your "patient" maintain pelvic neutral throughout each exercise. As your partner is performing each exercise, use verbal cues to correct for any errors in his performance. Identify the purpose of each exercise.

   a. Side leg lift
   b. Half squat
   c. Reverse squat
   d. Hamstring curl
   e. Sidelying ball lift
   f. Ankle motion exercises

4. Of the following Swiss ball exercises, select three upper extremity exercises to teach your lab partner. Be sure to have your "patient" maintain pelvic neutral throughout each exercise. As your partner is performing each exercise, use verbal cues to correct for any errors in his performance. Identify the purpose of each exercise.

   a. Prone flys
   b. Triceps extension
   c. Push-ups
   d. Scapular retraction

5. Create an original Swiss ball exercise for the trunk, upper, and lower extremities that is not included in your text. Identify the purpose of each exercise.

6. Of the following foam roller exercises, select five trunk activities to teach your lab partner. Be sure to have your "patient" maintain pelvic neutral throughout each exercise. As your partner is performing each exercise, use verbal cues to correct for any errors in her performance. Identify the purpose of each exercise.

   a. Quadratus massage
   b. Thoracic massage
   c. Low-back mobilization
   d. Cat stretch
   e. Quadruped balance
   f. Supine lower abdominal exercise
   g. Supine oblique exercise
   h. Abdominal crunch
   i. Rotational crunch
   j. Bridging
   k. Quadratus lumborum strengthening

7. Of the following foam roller exercises, select three lower extremity activities to teach your lab partner. Be sure to have your "patient" maintain pelvic neutral throughout each exercise. As your partner is performing each exercise, use verbal cues to correct for any errors in his performance. Identify the purpose of each exercise. You may use either half rollers or full rollers for the exercises.

   a. Iliotibial band massage
   b. Quadratus massage
   c. Standing balance
   d. Anterior tibialis stretch
   e. Gastrocnemius stretch
   f. Soleus stretch
   g. Piriformis stretch
   h. Squats

8. Of the following foam roller exercises, select three upper extremity activities to teach your lab partner. Be sure to have your "patient" maintain pelvic neutral throughout each exercise. As your partner is performing each exercise, use verbal cues to correct for any errors in his or her performance. Identify the purpose of each exercise.

    a. Arm stretches

    b. Push-ups

    c. Resistance-band exercises in standing

    d. Resistance-band exercises in supine

    e. Ball toss in supine

    f. Triceps pass

9. Design an exercise for the trunk, lower extremities, and upper extremities using a combination of the Swiss ball and foam roller. Indicate the purpose of each exercise and the muscle(s) it is working.

ADDITIONAL SOURCES

Craeger, C.C. 1996. *Therapeutic exercises using foam rollers.* Berthoud, CO: Executive Physical Therapy.

Institute of Physical Art. 1991. *Integrating function: The foam roller approach.* Steamboat Springs, CO: Institute of Physical Art.

Therapeutic Exercise for Tendinopathy

▶ During her career, Ella Bella has seen many athletes with tendinopathy. As much as she urges athletes to report early onsets of tendinopathy, it seems that they consistently wait until the problem becomes much more difficult to treat than it would have been if the athlete had been seen in the early stages of the condition.

Ella knows that tendinopathy cannot be treated like acute injuries, especially during the initial stage of care. She enjoys the challenge of treating cases of tendinopathy because she has to be a detective to discover its causes and reduce the risk of the tendinopathy returning later. Now she is confronted with managing and treating one of the runners on the high school's 4 × 200 meter relay team. The team is expected to take first place in the state track meet, but she knows they won't if she doesn't effectively treat Tyler before the track meet. Before she determines the best treatment outcomes for Tyler, she must play detective to identify the reasons he has developed Achilles tendinopathy and determine how involved it is.

Act as if what you do makes a difference. It does.

WILLIAM JAMES, 1842-1910, American philosopher and psychologist

Although tendinopathy can affect many body segments, it is worthwhile to discuss this condition in a separate chapter rather than including it in each of the chapters on specific body segments. Looking at tendinopathy separately makes sense because treatment of tendinopathy differs from treatment of acute conditions, yet treatment of tendinopathy is essentially similar for all body segments.

TERMINOLOGY

By the very nature of tendon function during force transmission and tendons' positions between muscle and bone, they undergo tremendous stress and strain during work and athletic activities. Although we do not understand the evolution of pathology that occurs within tendons, we do realize that injury occurs frequently within the tendon's structure. Some of the confusion in discussing tendon pathology occurs with the myriad terms used to describe tendon conditions. These terms relate to the specific tissue involved. **Tenosynovitis** is an inflammation of the synovial sheath that surrounds a tendon. **Paratendinitis** is an inflammation and thickening of the paratenon sheath of tendons that do not have synovial sheaths. **Tendinitis,** also spelled *tendonitis,* is the global term used to identify an inflammation of a tendon. **Tendinosis** is a non-inflammatory condition that involves microscopic tears of the tendon caused by repeated trauma. Since each of these terms can only be accurately applied after biopsy (Maffulli, Khan, & Puddu, 1998; Wang, Iosifidis, & Fu, 2006) and biopsy is not usually performed on patients, these terms are no longer used to describe inflammatory conditions of tendons. These terms are often used interchangeably, but incorrectly, so current best-practices discourage their use. It has been suggested that the term **tendinopathy** be used to discuss and identify conditions of a tendon that demonstrates signs and symptoms of pain, swelling, and reduced function (Maffulli et al., 1998). Hence, *tendinopathy* is the term used in this text.

TENDON STRUCTURE

To develop an appreciation of tendinopathy and its treatment, you must first understand the structure and function of a tendon. The specific structure varies somewhat from one tendon to another, but all tendons contain certain basic components. Normal tendon is composed of

Tendinopathy is the term used to identify a tendon that presents with pain, swelling, and impaired function.

collagen bundles that contain fibroblasts and an extracellular matrix. The extracellular matrix is composed primarily of water, Type I collagen, and ground substance. Type I collagen is a tendon's primary fiber component. Tendons are viscoelastic because of glycosaminoglycans, glycoproteins, and other substances in the ground substance that form a gel-like structure that supports the extracellular matrix. Because tendons are viscoelastic, they take on all the properties of viscoelastic tissue discussed in chapter 5. The tendon's blood vessels and nerves are contained in the **epitenon,** the loose areolar tissue that surrounds the tendon. The epitenon is intimate with the **endotenon** which extends itself between the collagen bundles. **Synovial sheaths** surround tendons that are subjected to greater than normal friction stresses, such as the Achilles and biceps tendons. If a sheath is present, it contains the primary blood supply for the tendon. Sheaths have two layers, an outer fibrotic and a thin inner layer. Between these two layers is a very small amount of **synovial fluid** to reduce friction in these high-stress areas.

The tendon connects to the muscle at the myotendinous junction and to the bone at the osteotendinous junction. Both sites are highly specialized in the cellular make up and provide secure attachments for the tendon to the respective structures. These locations are rarely sites of tendinopathy.

In normal resting, a tendon has a crimped or wavy appearance, but as a load is applied to the tendon it becomes stiffer and is subject to the stress-strain principles discussed in chapter 5. A tendon's tensile strength is determined by how well it resists the stress applied to it. One estimate is that a tendon's tensile strength is about four times the maximal force produced by its muscle (Elliot, 1965). Because a tendon's tensile strength is so much greater than its muscle's force generation, there must be factors other than tensile strength that enter into tendinopathy injuries. Exactly what these additional factors are has yet to be determined.

The basic structure of a tendon consists of collagen bundles containing fibroblasts and extracellular matrix. When a load is applied to a tendon it becomes stiffer and is subjected to stress-strain principles.

ETIOLOGY

Causes of tendinopathy are not yet clear. Different theories have evolved regarding the source of this malady. Three different theories are prevalent, yet none is without its unanswered questions. One theory is based on mechanical stressors that repeatedly stress the tendon within its normal stress ranges but then cause fatigue that ultimately results in failure of the tendon (Rees, Wilson, & Wolman, 2006). If it is assumed that repetitive stress is the cause of damage, it is realized that fibroblasts entering the area will produce scar tissue and weaken the structure. This theory supports scar tissue formation, but it does not explain how stress applied at a submaximal level causes the problem.

A second theory is based on vascular supply. Tendons lack good vascular supply and are, therefore, susceptible to compromised perfusion. The greatest blood vessels are located at the junctions between the tendon and the muscle and the tendon and the bone, not sites of tendinopathy. Tendons that are recognized for their reduced vascularity include the Achilles, patellar, posterior tibial, biceps, and supraspinatus tendons (Fenwick, Hazleman, & Riley, 2002). These are the tendons that are most often affected by tendinopathy, and they are most often affected at their sites of hypovascularity (Fenwick et al., 2002). Once tendinopathy occurs, there is hypervascularity at the site; however, increasing blood supply to the area does not aid in repairing the site and actually seems to promote the pain and chronicity of the condition (Fenwick et al., 2002). Why this counterintuitive promotion of tendinopathy occurs in the presence of increased vascularity is unknown but provides an argument against support of reduced vascularity as a theory of tendinopathy etiology.

A third theory is a neurally-based theory that is based on findings of various researchers. Substance P, a pain neurotransmitter, has been found in some tendinopathy sites, and since there is a close association within tendons of nerve cell endings and mast cells, chronic tendon overuse could lead to disproportionate neural facilitation to promote mast cell activity (Rees et al., 2006). Remember from chapter 2 that mast cells increase localized blood flow and fibroblast production, both important elements in tendinopathy. Unfortunately, the neural theory is not yet fully substantiated and needs additional research before it is confirmed.

It is plausible that tendinopathy involves a combination of these theories (Rees et al., 2006). Regardless of the theory behind the condition, the consequence is the same: pain, swelling, and reduced function result. If excessive stress is involved, it may take the form of cumulative trauma or acute trauma, such as a direct blow. Most cases of tendinopathy are considered overuse injuries. In overuse injuries, cumulative trauma is thought to be the cause. In traumatic tendinopathy, the tendon suffers a sudden severe injury and does not have sufficient time to recover before additional loads are applied to it, so breakdown occurs. Pain, swelling, and reduced function are the clinical manifestations of tendinopathy.

It is likely that tendinopathy is a multifactorial condition. If this were not true, then all individuals who overstress their tendons would develop tendinopathy, but this is not the case. Therefore, the clinician must investigate and identify all of the possible causative factors relevant for an individual with tendinopathy.

There are factors that must be examined in any patient who has tendinopathy since they may have an influence in both the onset and the propagation of tendinopathy. These factors are divided into two categories, extrinsic and intrinsic factors. Extrinsic factors can include an excessive or overly frequent load application, inappropriate equipment or footwear, training errors, and occupations (Rees et al., 2006). Common intrinsic factors include age, gender, pathomechanics, and either genetic or acquired systemic diseases such as Marfan's or diabetes mellitus (Rees et al., 2006).

In the area of extrinsic factors, loading errors include excessive increases in the progressive overload, excessive durations or distances, and excessive increases in speed. Examples are increasing hill-running workouts in speed, distance, or incline; increasing the intensity of jump workouts; throwing too far, too hard, too fast, or for too many repetitions; and typing at a computer too long without a break. Any type of loading error can be the problem, but they all essentially increase the workload to a level greater than the tendon is able to tolerate. As a rule of thumb, an increased workload of 10% to 15% a week is usually safe and tolerable.

Technique and execution errors can place additional stress on a tendon. For example, if a tennis player hits a backhand late, extensor tendons on the lateral epicondyle suffer significant increases in stress.

Inappropriate equipment and standing or training surfaces can alter forces placed on the body. For example, if the tennis player's racket grip is too large, the athlete must grip harder to hold onto the racket. This increases the stresses applied to the elbow where the tendons insert. If an athlete ties his or her shoes too tightly, the foot's extensor tendons incur increased pressure and tendinopathy can develop. Playing basketball on a vinyl-covered concrete floor rather than a force-absorbing suspended wood floor can make a player susceptible to patellar tendinopathy. Using a too-short computer desk chair can lead to carpal tunnel syndrome.

Structural abnormalities and muscle imbalances are intrinsic factors that place additional stresses on tendons by altering normal biomechanics. If a patient excessively pronates when running, the medial Achilles and posterior tibialis tendons encounter an excessive stretch while contracting. If the rotator cuff is weak, the humerus does not glide into the inferior aspect of the glenoid during shoulder motion, so soft tissues become subject to impingement, especially during arm elevation activities. Tendons that are compressed against bone or retinacular pulleys and tendons that are subject to high-friction forces are susceptible to tendinopathy. For example, the biceps tendon's common site of tendinopathy is the point at which the transverse ligament holds the tendon in the bicipital groove.

Stresses applied to a tendon may cause the tendon to alter its behavior as it attempts to adapt to them. As with muscle, bone, and other structures, tendons respond to overload stresses by hypertrophying and remodeling. How much stress is enough to cause hypertrophy of the tendon, without overloading it to cause breakdown, becomes the question—a question that researchers have not yet answered.

From a clinical standpoint, the best answer in the absence of definitive research conclusions must come from the observational skills of the clinician. Monitoring the patient's tendon

Tendinopathy involves changes within a tendon such as thickening of the tendon's sheath, areas of fibrosis and tissue thickening, and formation of nodules.

responses to stress and adapting the therapeutic exercise program accordingly is the best method, at present, for determining appropriate load applications. Increase in pain, crepitus, or edema are clinical signs that overload has been excessive.

TENDON RESPONSE

When a tendinopathy occurs, we know that pain, swelling, and reduced function occur. There are also other changes that have been documented. At the macroscopic level, the tendon's sheath is thickened. Additionally, areas of fibrosis and connective tissue thickening can often be palpated. Nodules and adhesions can be palpated on superficial tendons. Tendons do not appear to be inflamed but do have collagen degradation (Tasto et al., 2004). Additionally, there are normal levels of prostaglandins, cells that mediate inflammation (Alfredson, 2006) and evidence of nervous system pain modulators (Alfredson & Cook, 2007), in affected tendons. Therefore, rather than a prostaglandin-mediated condition, tendinopathy may be a neurogenic-mediated condition (Alfredson, 2005). The process of increased vascularity with tendinopathy is actually an increase in neurovascularity, so neural input in the form of pain amplifies along with the vascular supply. Since tendinopathy is not a prostaglandin-mediated inflammation, the use of NSAIDs in treating tendinopathy does not appear warranted (Alfredson, 2006).

How a tendon responds to threats of tendinopathy depends on its ability to withstand those threats, the etiology factors we have discussed previously. Healthy tendons may adapt to those threats through matrix adaptations. Depending on existing intrinsic and extrinsic factors, however, a tendon may be unable to withstand the threats (figure 15.1), and symptoms occur. Rehabilitation intervention then becomes necessary for the tendon's recovery and ability to restore normal function.

GENERAL TREATMENT

Treatment of tendinopathy includes the identification and modification of those internal and external factors causing the patient's tendinopathy. This aspect cannot be overemphasized. If the rehabilitation clinician does not alter these contributing factors, the patient will be plagued with recurrent episodes of tendinopathy and ultimately develop a chronic condition that will be frustrating for both the patient and clinician.

> The fundamental cause of any form of tendinopathy, including conditions resulting from repetitive stress and those resulting from acute trauma, is excessive stress on the tendon.

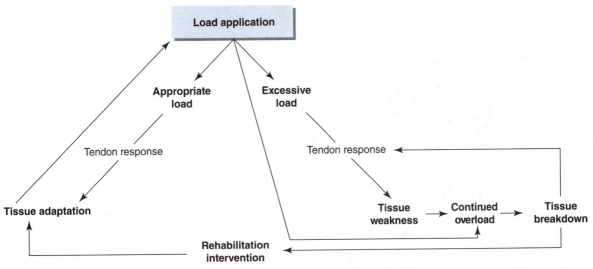

▶ **Figure 15.1** Load application and tendon response: When applied tendon loads are excessive without sufficient recovery time, tissue breakdown may occur. It is thought that tendon health is maintained when load applications permit adequate tissue adaptation.

To identify the cause, the rehabilitation clinician must take a thorough history; rely on the patient, coach, or supervisor for information about load changes and poor technique; personally observe the patient's execution; investigate equipment use and play or work surfaces; and evaluate for muscle imbalances and structural abnormalities. To prevent the tendinopathy from recurring, each causative factor must be changed before the patient can be safely returned to full participation.

One of the most difficult problems for the rehabilitation clinician in dealing with tendinopathy is identifying where the tendon is in the healing process. The injured individual's symptoms and response to the first treatment may be the best means of identifying the healing stage for overuse tendinopathy. An injury's healing stage is important to pinpoint because this is what determines the treatment course, as outlined later in this chapter. Therefore, initial treatment decisions are the most difficult. The goal is to help the patient progress without aggravating the injury. Lacking knowledge of where in the healing process the tendon is makes accomplishing this goal challenging. Before therapeutic exercises begin, the tendinopathy pain must be brought under control. The intensity of the symptoms can guide you in determining early treatments. If you are unsure of how aggressive a treatment should be, it is better to err on the side of caution and do less aggressive treatment than to provide more aggressive treatment and increase pain and swelling. The accuracy of your trial-and-error results during the initial treatment session depends on your knowledge of the patient's injury responses and tissue healing phases, skill in observation and history taking, and good judgment. If the tendon becomes more irritable because of your treatment, you know that the tendinopathy is now easily irritated, and you can gear future treatment accordingly. If the first treatment either improves the symptoms or has no effect, treatment can advance to the next level.

Since tendinopathy is essentially a diagnosis based on symptoms, the symptoms serve as the primary guidelines for determining the intensity of the treatment: The more intense and prolonged the symptoms, the less aggressive the treatment. General guidelines based on work by Stanish et al. (2000) can help you ascertain the intensity of the tendon's condition and select an appropriate initial treatment (table 15.1). For example, if the patient has Achilles tendon pain while walking to class, you know the tendinopathy is irritable and the patient will be able to tolerate little exercise. On the other hand, if the individual has Achilles pain only while running, the initial treatment can include therapeutic exercises.

It is important to continually monitor the tendon's response to treatment throughout the rehabilitation program. Pain and swelling are key signs that should be respected and regarded with care. Any increase in symptoms indicates the treatment is too aggressive. Thermal or electrical modalities and medication, as well as a reduction in activity, can be used to relieve symptom exacerbations.

TABLE 15.1 Classifications of Tendinopathy*

Classification	Level 1	Level 2	Level 3	Level 4	Level 5	Level 6
Intensity	Mild	Mild	Moderate	Moderate	Severe	Severe
Pain	No pain	Pain only with extreme exertion but stops when activity stops	Pain with extreme exertion lasting 1-2 hours post-activity	Pain with moderate activity lasting 4-6 hours post-activity	Rapidly increasing pain with any exertion lasting up to 24 hours post-activity	Pain during activities of daily living
Performance limitations from pain	None	None	No change in normal workouts but limits extreme exertion	Unable to perform normal workout activities	Unable to participate in any sport or work activity	As with level 5 and difficulty with some activities of daily living

*Modification of categories based on work by Stanish et al., 2000.

Therapeutic exercises are a critical aspect of tendinopathy treatment, but they must be provided only when appropriate; otherwise they can aggravate the condition. When exercises are used, flexibility exercises are usually a chief component. Concentric and eccentric strengthening exercises stress the tendon and play a vital role in preparing the tendon for normal functional activities. Of these, eccentric exercises play a particularly important role in treatment of tendinopathy (Eriksson, 2006; Jonsson & Alfredson, 2007; LaStayo et al., 2003; Woodley, Newsham-West, & Baxter, 2007). There is evidence that eccentric exercises promote tendon health and reduce the signs and symptoms of tendinopathy by reversing neovascularization, via a mechanism that is not yet understood (Ohberg, Lorentzon, & Alfredson, 2004). The end result regardless of the mechanism, however, is reduced pain, improved strength, and an optimal return to normal function. Once signs and symptoms of tendinopathy are resolved, the patient is guided through concentric, plyometric, and agility activities prior to return to functional activities.

Eccentric exercises should be a part of any therapeutic exercise program in the treatment of tendinopathy. Regardless of the body segment involved, eccentric exercises play a key role in resolution of tendinopathy. Beginning these exercises as soon as is reasonably possible provides for the best management of tendinopathy. The following section provides a progressive treatment outline and rationale for the steps. Eccentric exercises and other treatment considerations and progressions are included.

> Guidelines for treatment that relate to all forms of tendinopathy include two critical components: identifying the cause of the condition and modifying the causative factor. Selection of treatment depends on the irritability of the condition.

SPECIFIC TREATMENT

A tendinopathy rehabilitation program follows a logical progression that is carefully designed to allow the patient to advance to full participation and normal activity. Figure 15.2 depicts this rehabilitation progression for tendinopathy. The progression consists of six phases that are determined by the tendon's healing stage and its response to the treatment parameters within each phase. Despite this outline of phases, each patient's progression from one phase to another must be individually decided. At no time do you want an exacerbation of symptoms from one treatment session to the next. If this happens, it is essential that you return

Phase	Maintain CV and uninvolved segments	Pain control	Eccentric exercises	ROM exercises	Strength and endurance	Agility	Functional activities and activity-specific exercises
1. Tendinopathy classification levels 5, 6	■	■					
2. Tendinopathy classification levels 3, 4	■	■	■				
3. Tendinopathy classification levels 2, 3	■	■	■	■	■		
4. Tendinopathy classification levels 2, 3	■	■	■	■	■	■	
5. Tendinopathy classification levels 1, 2	■	■	■	■	■	■	■

▶ **Figure 15.2** Tendinopathy treatment phases and rehabilitation: Emphasis in phase I is on reducing pain during activities of daily living (ADLs). Phase II begins with eccentric and flexibility exercises once the pain during activities of daily living subsides. As the patient's injury improves, phase III includes additional strength exercises. Phase IV begins with agility activities and eventually progresses to phase V, where functional activities are added in preparation for return to full participation.

the patient to the previous level and allow the tendon time to adapt to that stress level before advancing the person to the next level.

Early tendinopathy rehabilitation is similar to early rehabilitation of other injuries. In addition to maintaining the patient's cardiovascular conditioning level and the parameters of the uninvolved segments and extremities, the rehabilitation clinician uses techniques to relieve the pain and dysfunction. Modalities that are effective to relieve pain include laser, ultrasound, cryotherapy, and transverse friction massage (Rees et al., 2006).

Cross-friction massage, described in chapter 6, helps to release adhesions between newly formed collagen and adjacent structures. These adhesions can cause continued discomfort by preventing normal tissue mobility and irritating the local tissue when movement is attempted. The cross-friction massage can also exert tensile force on the tendon by causing a bowstring effect (Gross, 1992).

Eccentric exercises are initiated early in a rehabilitation program before pain is resolved with modalities. If a patient has tendinopathy pain that interferes with activities of daily living, it is wise to wait until pain does not occur with these activities before beginning eccentric exercises. The recommended program of eccentric exercises is consistent among researchers: 3 sets of 15 repetitions performed once to twice daily for 12 weeks (Alfredson, Pietila, Jonsson, & Lorentzon, 1998; Jonsson, Wahlstrom, & Ohberg, 2006; Young, Cook, Purdam, Kiss, & Alfredson, 2005).

Stanish et al. recommend a progression of eccentric exercises with speed being the changing variable (Stanish, Curwin, & Mandel, 2000). Eccentric exercises begin with a slow speed and increasing every two days until a fast speed is achieved by the end of the week. Other advocates of eccentric exercises do not use speed as the variable but increase resistance as the means of progression (Alfredson et al., 1998; Jonsson et al., 2006; Young et al., 2005). However, they do not indicate any specific goal when a progression should be made. Using a combination of all four programs, table 15.2 outlines a progressive program of eccentric exercises for a tendinopathy program. It is expected that pain will be produced with eccentric exercises (Alfredson, 2006). Clinical experience has indicated that best results occur when the patient experiences little or no pain after the first set. By the last set, however, the patient usually reports pain, especially during the first few weeks of the program. As long as the patient is able to continue the exercise, progression is continued throughout the twelve weeks.

The reason it is important to consider the speed of exercise as a component in the early rehabilitation phase of eccentric exercises has to do with the force-velocity relationship of muscle, discussed in chapter 5; according to this principle, the faster the eccentric activity, the greater the force exerted. The tension on the tendon is increased when the speed of the eccentric movement is increased. This progression allows for a gradual buildup in overload and increases strength output as the tendon's tolerance improves. Once the patient tolerates the increased exercise speed, an increase in resistance is provided.

Loss of flexibility, a contributing factor to tendinopathy, is seen in many cases. Flexibility exercises should be a part of a tendinopathy rehabilitation program. As the tendon adapts to the eccentric exercises, other strengthening exercises can be initiated. These early strengthening exercises include low-load, high-repetition concentric-eccentric exercises. Endurance activities put less stress on the tendon and still permit strength gains, but the patient's response to these activities are carefully monitored. The patient begins strengthening with endurance exercises and he or she can often advance relatively rapidly to exercises that emphasize strength. How quickly this occurs depends on the tendon's response to the activities; pain is the most useful sign to guide the program.

During the last half of Phase III and beginning into Phase IV, when strength is the primary emphasis and the tendon is tolerating eccentric and concentric exercises, the patient progresses to plyometric exercises. These should be low-level and low-impact exercises and should progress as the patient tolerates.

Within this period the patient transitions to Phase IV, agility becomes the primary focus. Strength and flexibility exercises continue, but the activities become more strenuous as the

Components of specific treatment programs for tendinopathy may include relief of pain and dysfunction in addition to exercises in a progression that is consistent with the phases of the condition.

TABLE 15.2 Eccentric Exercise Progression

Day	Speed	Reps	Sets	Notations
1	Slow	15	3	If significant pain occurs with the first repetition at the new speed, the patient resumes the old speed for one more day.
2	Slow	15	3	
3	Moderate	15	3	
4	Moderate	15	3	
5	Fast	15	3	
6	Fast	15	3	
7	Fast	15	3	

Week	Resistance	Reps	Sets	Notations
2	Initial weight UE: 1 lb - 3 lb LE: 5 lb - 10 lb	15	3	All sets are performed at a fast pace starting at week 2. If significant pain occurs with the first set using a new weight, the patient resumes the previous weight level for another three days. Incremental increases are the same as the first day. Not all patients will begin with these recommended weights. Specific weights will be determined by patient size, strength, and response to exercise; the specific muscle being treated; and other individual factors.
3		15	3	
4		15	3	
5		15	3	
6		15	3	
7		15	3	
8		15	3	
9		15	3	
10		15	3	
11		15	3	
12		15	3	

UE = upper extremity; LE = lower extremity.

patient is prepared for the final phase in which functional activities are the primary thrust. It bears repeating here that if symptoms return or become exaggerated during any progression, the patient should remain at the lower level for a couple of days more to allow the tendon additional time for adaptation to stress at that level.

EXAMPLES OF TENDINOPATHY CASES

The best way to demonstrate rehabilitation for tendinopathy injuries is to provide examples. This section presents two examples, one for the lower extremity and one for the upper extremity. For one final example, you will be asked to outline an appropriate rehabilitation program.

Lower-Extremity Case

A 20-year-old collegiate cross country runner, Sally, presented with complaints of right Achilles pain that had begun about three months earlier. She usually ran about 65 km (about 40 miles) a week on varying terrain. At first she had pain only when running hills, but at the time she came to the clinic she was experiencing pain even when walking across campus. She finally sought treatment because the intensity of the pain made it impossible to run.

Examination

On examination, Sally had a mildly antalgic gait. She had prolonged pronation in the stance phase of gait. She was unable to hop on the right leg because of pain. Although Sally said that she performed stretching exercises, her ankle dorsiflexion was 0° when the rearfoot was stabilized in subtalar neutral. Palpation revealed swelling along the Achilles tendon and a painful nodule about 8 cm (3 in.) above the tendon's distal insertion.

Treatment

Sally was instructed to stop running for the time being. She was advised to continue her cardiovascular conditioning either in a pool or by performing stationary cycling using only the left leg. She could continue any weight exercises with the upper extremities, left lower extremity, and trunk, but was instructed not to use the right leg for any exercise.

Sally was given crutches and instructed in partial weight bearing on the right. Right lower-extremity weight bearing was allowed only to the extent that her gait was pain free. Sally's first treatment included the use of phonophoresis, ice, and strapping to reduce her excessive pronation.

On the next day Sally returned, feeling better. The phonophoresis treatment was repeated. Cross-friction massage was used, first in non-tender areas and then on the nodule and in other tender areas as Sally was able to tolerate. The strapping helped to reduce the pain, so Sally was measured for orthotics as a permanent correction for her excessive pronation. Ice was applied as a final treatment.

By her third visit Sally was able to walk around campus without pain, so the use of crutches was discontinued. She was instructed in proper stretching exercises for the gastrocnemius and soleus. She was also started on a progressive eccentric exercise program of 3 sets of 15 repetitions. She was instructed to stand on the edge of a stair step and use only the left lower extremity to raise up on the ball of her foot, then use only the right lower extremity for the eccentric phase of the motion going down. She started out doing the exercise slowly for the first two days then moved to a moderate motion for two days before she was able to do the exercise in a fast motion. She reported that she felt some pain after the second set and more pain after the third set of her exercise, but her rehabilitation clinician informed her that she was having normal reactions to the exercise and to continue them. She was taught how to self-administer cross-friction massage.

By the sixth week she was feeling good, so exercises included concentric activities and were soon advanced to include trampoline jumping activities, lateral-movement exercises, and fast walking. Fast walking progressed to alternately walking and jogging, then jogging, then running on flat surfaces, and finally running hills.

Upper-Extremity Case

Tom, a 24-year-old, right-handed baseball pitcher, was seen because of pain in the right shoulder. He reported that the pain was located over the deltoid tubercle and that it sometimes radiated down the lateral arm to the elbow. He was unable to sleep on his right side. The pain had started about two months before, in the beginning of the season after Tom had pitched seven long innings in a game. He usually had pain during the last two innings that he pitched, especially with curve balls; the pain would last for about 2 or 3 h after he had finished pitching. He was pitching more during the current season than he had the year before. In the off-season, he had fallen while skiing, landing on his right shoulder but did not think at the time that the shoulder was injured. It was just sore for a couple of days, and he did not seek any medical attention. During preseason, the flu kept Tom out of most of the regular preseason conditioning program.

Examination

Active range of motion and overpressure of the neck were normal. Shoulder range of motion was normal for a pitcher, but Tom had pain during the middle arc of shoulder elevation, especially abduction. Weakness was present, and Tom complained of pain with resisted manual muscle tests to lateral rotation and abduction in the scapular plane. He had shoulder tenderness when he put his hand behind his back and raised it upward along his back. There was tenderness to palpation of the greater tubercle. The findings were consistent with a tendinopathy of the supraspinatus. Tom's history indicated that the irritability of the tendon was moderate.

Treatment

Because the injury had moderate irritability, Tom was able to begin exercises on the first treatment. The first treatment included eccentric exercises with the supraspinatus. The clinician would passively elevate the shoulder and have Tom eccentrically resist against gravity to lower the arm to his side. Scapular rotator muscle exercises were also started. Ice application ended the treatment session. Home exercises included three sets of 15 repetitions for eccentric exercises against the supraspinatus. Tom was told that he could also do scapular rotator exercises, such as push-ups, seated push-ups, and flys, as long as they were pain free.

The eccentric exercises progressed to where Tom was able to perform the exercises with weights, starting with 2 lb and progressing steadily in his routine to 8 lb. Agility and plyometric exercises with medicine balls and rubber tubing exercises were soon added as Tom continued to improve.

A throwing progression similar to the one outlined in chapter 10 was given Tom. He began with tosses, progressed to throwing, and increased the speed and distance of the throws as he was able to tolerate.

■ A Challenging Case

Joe, a 19-year-old, right-handed tennis player, complains of right elbow pain. The pain is located over the lateral elbow and sometimes radiates down the dorsal forearm. It began about four months ago, about three weeks after Joe had bought a new tennis racket and started playing in two leagues. He stopped playing for a month until he was pain free, but when he went back to playing, the pain returned. He plays or practices tennis daily. He has noticed that the elbow especially bothers him on his tennis backhand, when he attempts to lift heavy objects, and when he shakes hands.

Examination

The right elbow and forearm have full range of motion in all planes. The neck and shoulder also have normal motion. There is pain to resisted wrist extension. Joe's grip strength on the right is 8 kg (17.6 lb) weaker than that on the left. Palpation of the lateral epicondyle reveals swelling over the epicondyle and tenderness to even light palpation. There is some tenderness to palpation extending into the proximal wrist extensor muscle bellies in the forearm.

Questions for Analysis

1. What will you include in your first treatment session?
2. What instructions will you give Joe about what he should and should not be doing at home?
3. How will you advance him in his program?
4. What will be the progression of your eccentric exercise program?

SUMMARY

Tendinopathy, rather than tendonitis or other myriad terms used in the past, is the current term used to identify tendon conditions that demonstrate signs and symptoms of pain, swelling, and reduced function. There is no inflammatory process going on with tendinopathy, so *tendinitis* is not an accurate term. The condition may affect the tendon itself, its sheath, or the paratenon, but the specific problem is difficult to identify and they are essentially treated the same, so the general term, *tendinopathy,* is used by the medical community to pool these conditions into one.

Three primary theories have been advanced to understand the sources of tendinopathy; none as yet have been verified. Regardless of the source or condition, since most cases of tendiopathy are likely to be multifactorial in origin, the first step is to identify what is causing the signs and symptoms. Once the causes are identified, steps are taken to correct these causes. The most effective rehabilitation exercises for tendinopathy are eccentric exercises. Additionally, flexibility and strength gains may be required to fully recover from the condition, but eccentric exercises are used early and into at least the middle phase to provide effective recovery from tendinopathy. This chapter provides examples of progressive eccentric exercise programs for tendinopathy.

KEY CONCEPTS AND REVIEW

1. Define tendinopathy.

Tendinopathy is an irritation of the tendon that is displayed as pain, swelling, and reduced function. Unless visualized in surgery, the precise structure involved is difficult to determine.

2. Discuss various etiologies of tendinopathy.

Tendinopathy can occur as a traumatic or an overuse condition. The three prevalent theories regarding tendinopathy regard a mechanical theory, a vascular theory, and a neural theory. The mechanical theory indicates the cause based on excessive or repetitive stress: The tendon breaks down because cumulative trauma is applied without an opportunity for the tendon to recover before additional stress is applied. The vascular theory bases the cause of tendinopathy on reduced vascular supply to tendons that result in tissue breakdown, but evidence reveals that pathological tendons have an increased neovascular supply. The neural theory states that neurovascular growth in the pathological area produces neural chemicals that create pain and enhance fibroblastic responses. It is likely that the cause of tendinopathy involves a combination of these theories. Extrinsic and intrinsic factors may also play a contributing part in tendinopathy.

3. Explain the response of tendons to treatment.

Tendinopathy does not show evidence of inflammation from what normally causes inflammation, prostaglandins. Since prostaglandins are not in the area, NSAIDs are not of usual benefit in cases of tendinopathy. Eccentric exercises have been found to be the most effective treatment in resolving tendinopathy. It is thought that the eccentric exercises promote tendon health and reduce the signs and symptoms of tendinopathy by reversing neovascularization through some mechanism that is not yet understood. Researchers have consistently found that a once to twice a day program of eccentric exercises performed as 3 sets of 15 repetitions for 12 weeks provides consistent positive results, regardless of the body segment involved.

4. Outline the progression of a tendinopathy treatment program.

Treatment for tendinopathy is divided into five phases. In addition to correcting the cause and maintaining the conditioning status of unaffected segments, treatments should address restoration of flexibility, muscle endurance, strength, agility, and functional performance. These goals are accomplished by careful progression of the program, beginning with modalities if the tendon is very irritated and interferes with daily activities. Cross-friction massage is also included to break up adhesions and promote pain reduction. Eccentric exercises and flexibility exercises are started as soon as possible. Each of these are instructed to the patient and performed at least daily. Observation by the rehabilitation clinician and reports by the patient regarding the tendon's response to treatment determine the rate of progression. If the tendon responds negatively to the treatment, the rehabilitation clinician should return the patient to the previous exercise stress level and resume modalities as indicated. To reduce the chance of recurrences, it is important that the rehabilitation clinician identify and correct the underlying precipitating factor.

CRITICAL THINKING QUESTIONS

1. A patient with Achilles tendinopathy has advanced nicely over the past three weeks of treatment. He has responded well to all therapeutic exercises. Today, however, he returns for additional treatment, complaining that since yesterday's treatment he has experienced the same pain that he had at first. Yesterday you increased the number of repetitions of the eccentric exercises he had been doing. What will your treatment today include? What will your criteria be for again attempting the program you tried yesterday?

2. A tennis player reports that she has tennis elbow for the second time this season. Last year she experienced the condition toward the end of the season, but with rest it went away. She wants to know what you will do for her, why this problem is recurring, and how it differs from a forearm strain she had two years ago. Explain how you will answer her questions.

3. A basketball player who has been unable to run for the past six weeks because of peroneal tendinopathy has responded well to your rehabilitation program. He is now ready to start running. What will the first day's running program be, and how will you have him progress to normal running activities?

LAB ACTIVITIES

1. Perform the following heel raise exercises on a stair ledge:
   a. Slow-speed drop of the heels from the top of a heel raise, 3 × 15; rest 2 min.
   b. Moderate-speed drop of the heels from the top of a heel raise, 3 × 15; rest 2 min.
   c. Fast-speed drop of the heels from the top of a heel raise, 3 × 15; rest 2 min.
   When during each set of exercises did you begin to feel a burn in your calf? At which speed did the exercise seem the easiest? Why?

2. If you are treating a patient with an Achilles tendinopathy, explain ways you could increase the progression of an eccentric exercise program other than increasing speed.

3. Perform the following wrist extension exercises using a 5 lb or 8 lb weight, 3 × 15, with the wrist hanging over the edge of a table top:
   a. Slow-speed drop into full wrist flexion from full wrist extension
   b. Moderate-speed drop into full wrist flexion from full wrist extension
   c. Fast-speed drop into full wrist flexion from full wrist extension
   Where did you feel the burn occur? Did the repetition at which the burn began vary for each speed? At which speed did the weight seem the lightest? Why?

4. If you are treating a patient with tennis elbow, explain ways you could increase the eccentric program's progression other than increasing speed.

5. Going back to the scenario at the beginning of the chapter, Ella has determined the cause of Tyler's Achilles tendinopathy and corrected those conditions. Without including any modalities, outline only a therapeutic exercise program and the progression you think would be appropriate for Tyler's condition. Include both the eccentric program and other exercises as well.

CHAPTER 16

Therapeutic Exercise for Joint Replacement

OBJECTIVES

After completing this chapter, you should be able to do the following:

1. Know the various terms and abbreviations for total joint replacements.

2. Identify the progression of osteoarthritis and how it leads to joint replacement.

3. Appreciate the secondary factors that add to debilitation when osteoarthritis occurs.

4. Describe the options available to a young person with osteoarthritis of the knee.

5. Identify the precautions involved in treatment and care following total hip joint replacement surgery.

► Floyd Williams has been at his job as an athletic trainer in the town's largest sport clinic for the past two years, ever since he graduated from Cue Creek College where he received his degree in athletic training. Today he has on his schedule a patient he will see for the first time. She is Jan Violet, a total knee replacement patient. According to the chart, Jan is 31 but required a total knee arthroplasty because of a severe knee injury she suffered as an interscholastic field hockey player at Twinsdale High School. Her surgery was six weeks ago. When Floyd examines Jan, he finds that she has a well-healed surgical scar and is able to walk with one crutch, but when she tries to walk without any assistive devices, she has a slight limp. Her active knee motion is 15° to 90°, and her hip strength is 4–/5 in her gluteus medius and 4/5 in her gluteus maximus, just as Floyd would expect. He has worked with total hip joint patients before, but this is his first total knee patient. He is already making mental plans for her rehabilitation program.

A mind once stretched by a new idea
never regains its original dimensions.

AUTHOR UNKNOWN

This chapter on joint replacements is probably a first for an athletic training rehabilitation text, although the topic can hardly be called irrelevant to athletic trainers. As more certified athletic trainers encounter joint replacement patients, it is necessary that they understand the techniques and precautions surrounding these procedures. This chapter presents information about these techniques and precautions. By the end of this chapter, your mind will once again have been expanded with new knowledge and your skills will broaden to include management of these types of patients. As you read this chapter, imagine how you would manage Floyd's patient, Jan, described in the opening scenario. Use the information here to provide a rationale for the program you imagine you will provide her.

Advances in joint replacement surgery within recent years have made the possibility of younger patients undergoing joint arthroplasty more of a reality. Indeed, sometimes this surgery is a necessity that cannot be delayed. Unfortunately, if a relatively young person receives a joint replacement, it is likely that he or she will eventually require revision surgery because the individual's lifetime is greater than the joint's longevity, at least currently. As technological advances continue, it is expected that artificial joints will continue to improve and last longer.

Because more individuals continue to be very active into their retirement years and because nearly half of this country's certified athletic trainers, according to recent data, obtain positions in sport clinic and hospital environments, it has become necessary to include this chapter in the text. Additionally, we have seen professional athletes undergo total joint replacement and sometimes even return to professional sport. For example, National Basketball Association player and, later, referee Leon Wood underwent a total hip replacement and then returned to officiating; Kansas City Royals left fielder Bo Jackson, Professional Golf Association golfer Jack Nicklaus, and 31-year-old Tour de France cyclist Floyd Landis all underwent hip replacement surgery and returned to their respective sports; and tennis professional Jimmy Connors, as well as many other professional sport competitors, underwent total joint replacement surgery after retirement.

It is very likely that certified athletic trainers, as rehabilitation clinicians working in various sport clinic environments, will encounter total joint replacement patients. These patients will often want to return to their sport and leisure activities. It is the responsibility of rehabilitation clinicians to guide these patients through a successful program that will allow them to do just that. In order to provide these patients good rehabilitation programs, a clinician must understand the details and implications of joint replacement surgery, realize precautions, and appreciate physical and physiological impacts. These are the topics explored in this chapter.

HISTORY

Severe and disabling pain secondary to arthritis from either disease or injury has been the primary factor motivating surgeons to find functional substitutions for worn joints. Although procedures involving replacement of half of a joint, either the concave or convex portion, have been around since the late 1800s, it was only in the latter half of the 20th century that total joint replacements became a reality. The physician generally accredited with performing the first total joint replacement was an English surgeon and researcher, John Charnley. In 1958, he replaced both the acetabulum and femoral head of a patient's hip joint and secured the metal ball and Teflon socket with a dental adhesive known as bone cement. These early total hip procedures were successful from the outset.

The first plastic and metal knee replacement was installed and secured with bone cement 10 years later by an orthopedist protégé of John Charnley, Frank Gunston. This knee joint was further refined by John Insall, a surgeon who added a prosthetic patella. Dr. Insall used bone cement as well, but was the first to use specifically designed tools to more accurately cut and prepare the bones for their prosthetic implants.

Total shoulder joint replacements have taken a longer route to their current status than the hip and knee replacements. Shoulder joints have evolved through at least four generations to the most contemporary version. Although many surgeons use a humeral head and glenoid socket, some are finding more success in difficult cases with the *reverse total shoulder arthroplasty* (rTSA) (Nicholson, 2006). This rTSA replacement places the concave joint surface on the humerus and the convex joint surface on the scapula. Total shoulder joint replacement, as well as knee and hip arthroplasty, is discussed in more detail later in this chapter.

Today's joint replacements are made of durable alloys of chromium cobalt and titanium along with polymer materials. The science and technology of metallurgy has advanced in the past several years to provide for lower friction between metallic joint surfaces. These metals are stronger, as well, to allow for more durability and longer life of the joint. The first total joint replacements were expected to last no more than 10 years, but current devices are much better; 90% of them last between 10 and 20 years (Bauman et al., 2007).

Today's materials are biocompatible, which makes it unlikely that they will be rejected by the body. Computer-assisted techniques are now frequently used to ensure an exacting insertion of the joint surfaces to provide optimal postoperative joint function. Many of the body's joints are now replaceable with artificial joints. The most commonly replaced joints are the hips and knees; but shoulders, elbows, ankles, and even the interphalangeal joints of fingers and toes have artificial joint replacements.

INDICATIONS FOR JOINT REPLACEMENT

Joint replacement surgery has many alternative names. It is most commonly referred to as **arthroplasty** or *total joint arthroplasty.* Surgeries for specific joints are designated accordingly; for example, total knee replacement is also known as total knee arthroplasty, TKR, or TKA. Likewise, total hip replacement is also called total hip arthroplasty, THR, or THA. When laypersons hear discussions of total joint replacement, they commonly imagine that the entire end of the given bone is removed and replaced. However, this is not accurate. The part of the joint that is removed and replaced is limited to articular portions of the bone that make up the joint surfaces.

Before we can discuss total joint replacements, however, we must identify why they are required. It is important to recognize certain indications for those individuals who would benefit from such a procedure. This section also covers alternatives for treatment and discusses when such treatments should be performed.

Technological advances will allow younger individuals to receive total joint arthroplasty than in the past. Professional athletes have returned to sport participation following total joint replacement.

Progression of Arthritic Changes

There are several different types of arthritis. The arthritic conditions for which arthroplasties are performed are primarily rheumatoid arthritis and, most commonly, osteoarthritis. Osteoarthritis is often the result of primary or secondary trauma to a joint at an earlier age. As the individual gets older, evidence of fraying and thinning of articular cartilage appears, eventually producing degeneration of the joint's articular surface. Because osteoarthritis is a degenerative condition of the joint, it is also referred to as *degenerative joint disease* or DJD. Once the articular cartilage is worn, the bone itself has no protection. Since articular cartilage has no pain receptors but bone does, the patient begins to experience gradually progressive and worsening episodes of pain with use or weight bearing of the osteoarthritic joint. The degree of pain is sufficient to compromise daily activities, making even walking difficult in the case of lower-extremity joint involvement. Upper-extremity joint osteoarthritis is also debilitating; overhead and functional activities become difficult if not impossible to perform.

Osteoarthritis is a common condition. It affects more than 7 million Americans and more than half of the population over the age of 65 (Weng and Fitzgerald, 2006). A national survey of hospitals showed that over 570,000 patients underwent either hip or knee replacements in 2002 (Weng and Fitzgerald, 2006). This number is expected to rise by significant proportions in the next 20 years. Many individuals who suffer joint injuries today will be patients undergoing joint replacement surgery 20 years from now.

Although osteoarthritis is certainly painful and very disabling, it is not a life-threatening condition. For this reason, arthroplasty is considered an elective surgery, although an individual affected by DJD would probably dispute that classification. One of the greatest risks of arthroplasty surgery is an embolism resulting in death (Brady, Masri, Garbuz, & Duncan, 2000). Why, then, is arthroplasty considered a reasonable treatment for disabling osteoarthritis? The reason is quality of life. If pain interferes with daily activities, making even simple tasks painful and enjoyable activities such as participating in sport impossible, then patients perceive their value of life as significantly diminished.

The change in the quality of life after arthroplasty has consistently demonstrated that the benefits outweigh the risks. With today's preoperative precautions, rehabilitation techniques, and postoperative procedures, the most severe surgical risk of an embolism is diminished. Total joint replacement should always be considered as a last resort treatment, but when pain and disability interfere with quality of life, joint replacement is usually the best option.

Examination and Selection

Prior to total joint surgery, the surgeon must examine and assess the patient. One of the more relevant qualities that ensures success is the patient's self-efficacy and expectations (Hawker, 2006). If the patient has confidence that the surgery will be beneficial and is knowledgeable about the procedures and postoperative expectations, he or she will perform better in the rehabilitation program and is more likely to benefit from the experience.

The rehabilitation clinician is able to contribute to the patient's self-efficacy and expectations by providing preoperative treatments to achieve optimal strength and mobility prior to the surgery. Preoperative instructions in proper gait with assistive devices will also be beneficial. Informing the patient in advance about the procedures that will be performed immediately after surgery, about when he or she will begin exercising and walking, and about the types of exercises and estimated duration of treatment postsurgery will prepare the patient and help him or her to form realistic expectations. Conveying this information is important for allaying patient concerns.

The patient must have confidence in the surgeon and the rehabilitation clinician for a successful outcome. It is likely that the patient will seek recommendations from a number of sources, including the primary care physician, the rehabilitation clinician who is providing preoperative care, friends and relatives who have had the procedure, and coworkers. As an allied health care provider, it is important to provide an honest and professional perspective regarding any physician about whom the patient inquires. If you are asked to recommend a physician, it is unwise to provide only one name; it is better to offer at least three.

Progression of Prearthroplasty Treatment Options

The osteoarthritic process is a long one. It may start as early as the late 20s or early 30s. People in these age groups who have osteoarthritis either experienced a severe injury as a youngster or teenager, have undergone one or more surgeries of the joint, or have suffered injuries to other segments that secondarily affected the joint. For example, if an athlete experienced shoulder instability with rotator cuff tears, osteoarthritis may develop in the glenohumeral joint later in life. If an osteoarthritic patient is young, efforts to delay total joint replacement are the best option, utilizing a number of different procedures. The earliest attempts are usually self-determined and include voluntary and subconscious efforts such as reducing activity, minimizing joint stress, and altering movement patterns. It is when the pain becomes severe or disabling that the patient consults with a physician.

In the very early days of joint pain, many individuals resort to medication for pain relief. Some use over-the-counter or prescription-dose anti-inflammatory medication; however, long-term use of these drugs can be problematic for the liver or kidneys. Some people use an over-the-counter medication, glucosamine chondroitin, to relieve joint pain. As mentioned in chapter 2, articular cartilage is composed of glucosamine aggregates that help to maintain appropriate water levels in the extracellular matrix of the cartilage. Chondroitin is also a part of the articular cartilage extracellular matrix. There is some evidence that use of this medication results in reduced joint pain and improvement in mobility (Brief, Maurer, and DiCesare, 2001). As the osteoarthritis progresses, however, relief with medications does not occur, and patients find themselves resorting to other methods of pain relief.

Some physicians may inject the joint or refer osteoarthritic patients for rehabilitation (or both) before any discussion of surgery. Pain and reduced function secondary to the pain will produce muscle weakness and declining mobility. Muscle weakness and motion loss then become factors in placing more stress on already weakened joints. The cycle continues until the patient seeks medical care. Strengthening and improving joint flexibility reduce stress to the joint. Less stress will reduce pain. In mild cases of osteoarthritis, this intervention may provide enough pain relief to allow the patient to return to activities with the use of medication.

As the arthritic condition advances, steps that are more drastic may be necessary. As discussed in chapter 2, various surgical techniques to encourage articular cartilage regeneration or repair are usually the first procedures used. As you recall, these procedures include abrasion arthroplasty, subchondral drilling, and microfracture. These measures cause bleeding from subchondral bone to allow entrance of stem cells to the articular surface. These stem cells then differentiate into articular cartilage cells. Depending on where the lesion is, how large it is, and the postoperative care provided, the repair may provide good protection for a few years. Osteochondral plugs and autologous chondrocyte transplantation are also discussed in chapter 2 as means of restoring damaged articular cartilage. Patients usually resume full, normal activities after appropriate rehabilitation following these surgical procedures. As mentioned in chapter 2, there is evidence to indicate that young individuals who undergo either regenerative or reparative techniques may have longer lasting results than older adults, provided restriction of jumping and other impact activities is prolonged following the procedure.

Arthroscopic debridement is a short-term pain-relieving technique. This procedure usually relieves pain enough to allow the patient more function, but it is not reparative; it will not make the joint better. It is a temporary measure that provides the patient with temporary relief. "Temporary" may be anything from a few months to a couple of years, depending on the patient's activity level and amount of degeneration prior to the debridement.

The last resort, especially in a patient younger than 70 years old, is an arthroplasty. If the individual undergoing the arthroplasty is 50 years of age or younger, it is likely that a noncement arthroplasty will be performed. Not using cement will allow for an easier arthroplasty replacement when needed, 20 years or so later.

Degenerative Changes and Dysfunction

As already mentioned, pain is the primary disabling factor in osteoarthritis. Pain interferes with all activities. It is not resolved but may be contained with some medications; however, the degeneration will eventually reach a point where pain overrides any activity. Some individuals have a higher pain tolerance than others, so these patients' objective findings may be more significant than those of people with lower pain tolerance levels. But this by no means suggests that persons with less pain tolerance do not have significant degenerative changes. Anyone whose objective tests demonstrate osteoarthritis with clear joint degeneration will have considerable pain. If steps are not taken to assuage the pain, it will continue to reduce the patient's ability to function.

By the time the patient decides to have an arthroplasty, the joint has incurred exceptional damage. An X-ray frequently reveals bone-on-bone wear with a loss of joint spacing and the presence of **osteophytes,** which are bone spurs within the joint. Depending on the joint involved, visible deformity may also be present. For example, in knee osteoarthritis, a common deformity is genu varum; in hip osteoarthritis, it may appear that the leg is shorter than the nonarthritic extremity.

Muscles surrounding the joint are atrophied. Since the patient is reluctant to use the joint because of pain, the muscles become significantly weaker. Muscle weakness compounds joint stresses when attempts are made to use the joint.

Lack of use and weaker muscles also lead to reduced mobility. In addition, the loss of joint structure will make normal motion impossible. The amount of lost motion depends on a number of factors, including the time since disability began and the patient's functional and activity level in spite of the pain. Pain throughout motion and especially at the end of joint motion is common.

If a lower-extremity joint is the affected joint, the gait will be pathological. It is likely the patient will have an antalgic, or painful, gait. The cadence will be asymmetrical with more time spent on the uninvolved extremity. The stride length on the involved extremity will be shorter, and the affected extremity will likely have abnormal initial contact and preswing phases.

Whether an upper- or a lower-extremity joint has osteoarthritis, the entire extremity will be affected. For example, if the elbow is osteoarthritic, the shoulder and wrist will be weak and may even have reduced motion. The same is true in the lower extremity; if the ankle is affected, both the hip and knee will also demonstrate weakness and even loss of normal motion. Therefore, the entire extremity must be examined and treated during rehabilitation.

SURGICAL PROCEDURES

It was once thought that patients younger than 70 years and over 200 lb (91 kg) could not be considered for total joint replacement (Hawker, 2006). Because of new technologies, however, this is no longer true. It is estimated that there are soon to be over 2 million Americans between 45 and 64 years old who will have osteoarthritis (Bauman et al., 2007). We will soon be treating arthroplasty patients who will commonly expect to return to physical activity with their new prosthesis. Before we can design optimal rehabilitation programs, we must understand the surgical procedures involved with arthroplasty.

Overview

The arthroplasty surgeries currently performed are, for the most part, variations of their original procedural predecessors. This section provides general information regarding the main joint replacement surgeries and the ones you are most likely to encounter. These arthroplasty procedures include the hip, knee, and shoulder.

Less frequently used than others is the **hemiarthroplasty** procedure. As the name implies, only half of the joint is replaced. In the shoulder and hip, this usually involves either the convex or the concave surface. In the knee, it can be either the femoral or the tibial segment or the medial or lateral half of the joint. When a joint arthroplasty is restricted to either the medial or the lateral aspect of the joint, it is a *unicompartmental knee replacement;* this is most often performed in the knee. Hemiarthroplasties are not discussed in this chapter.

The surgical procedure for joint replacements is very complex technologically, physically, and biomechanically. The joint surfaces must be aligned properly to ensure good total alignment of the extremity. Poor alignment may result in abnormal rotation of the extremity, limb-length differences, and deficient concave-on-convex congruency. Although computer-assisted technology now provides for more exact positioning of the joint replacement segments, not all surgical facilities have this equipment (figure 16.1). Surgeons at facilities without this technology must rely on their experience and measurements for accuracy in prosthesis sizing, positioning, and alignment. The size of the replacement joint must be appropriate for the size of the individual; the patient's joint size is estimated in advance of the surgery, but prostheses of multiple sizes are sterilized to be available during the surgery so the correct size may be selected after the joint is exposed. The total joint manufacturer's representative is often in attendance during the surgery to assist in determining the most appropriate joint replacement size. Finally, infection is a risk for any surgery. It becomes especially important to avoid infection for a total joint replacement surgery. If an infection occurs in the joint following such a procedure, the joint is at risk of osteomyelitis, a condition that will threaten the joint's survival.

Implantation of the joint surfaces can be performed either using bone cement or not cementing the prosthesis to the bone. Cementless total joints rely on bone ingrowth around the prosthesis to stabilize and secure it. Although there is common consensus among surgeons that a noncemented prosthesis should be used in younger patients who will eventually require resurfacing (Weng and Fitzgerald, 2006), there is no general agreement as to whether cement or no cement is the best option in other patients; the selection is based on individual surgeon preference.

Patients undergoing cemented arthroplasty procedures are usually permitted full weight bearing immediately following surgery. Some surgeons may restrict weight bearing in noncemented arthroplasties, but other surgeons allow full weight bearing for either procedure. When restricted, weight bearing with cementless joint implants is usually toe-touch weight bearing for the first six weeks following total hip arthroplasty. Over the next six weeks, the patient progresses to full weight bearing.

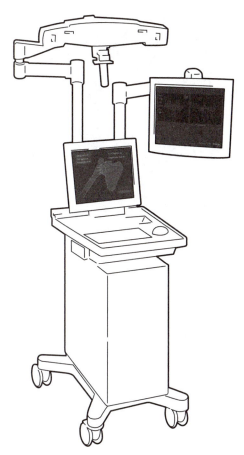

▶ **Figure 16.1** Computer-assisted total joint replacement machine.

Hip Joint Replacement Surgery

Total hip arthroplasty or replacement (THA or THR) is an arthroplasty that may be performed at any age. In addition to the arthritic conditions already mentioned, THA may be required in cases of avascular necrosis where destruction of the femoral head has occurred. Following this surgery and its rehabilitation, patients often wonder why they did not have the procedure sooner, for it gives them much more mobility and restores their function to a level that had been lost often years before.

There are different surgical approaches for THA. The anterior approach places the incision between the sartorius and tensor fasciae latae muscles. This approach misses the hip abductor muscles, but more physicians prefer one of the lateral approaches that require at least some detachment of the hip abductors, a factor that affects postoperative rehabilitation (Brander and Stulberg, 2006). The anterolateral and direct lateral approaches are two of the most often used techniques. Although they both require some release of the hip abductor muscles, they have a lower risk of postoperative dislocation. The posterolateral approach, on the other hand,

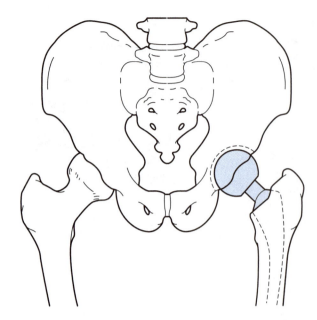

▶ **Figure 16.2**   Total hip arthroplasty (THA).

does not disrupt the gluteus medius, but there is greater risk of dislocation using this procedure (Brander and Stulberg, 2006). The gluteus maximus is split and the small lateral rotators are released in the posterolateral approach.

More recent advances in surgical approaches to hip arthroplasty include the use of minimally invasive THA. Rather than the extensive 8 to 10 in. (20-25 cm) incision, minimally invasive surgery uses one or two small sutures, as small as about 2 in. (5 cm) long (Ulrich et al., 2007). One-incision procedures use either an anterior or an anterolateral approach. If two incisions are used, the second incision is posterior to allow placement of the femoral stem of the ball portion of the THA into the femoral shaft. The goals with minimally invasive surgery are to create less postoperative pain and soft-tissue damage and thereby allow the patient a more rapid postoperative rehabilitation course. Evidence, however, is conflicting on these advantages over those of more traditional THA approaches; some studies show better early postsurgery recovery with the minimally invasive technique while others show no long-term differences between the two techniques (Berry et al., 2003; Brander and Stulberg, 2006; Pagnano et al., 2006; Ulrich et al., 2007).

Regardless of the approach used, once the hip joint is exposed, the joint is dislocated. The humeral head is removed at the femoral neck. The acetabulum is reamed to prepare it to accept the prosthesis. Both replacement ends of the joint are cemented or press fit into their respective bone segments in their proper positions, and the joint is relocated (figure 16.2). The surgeon then closes the wound, layer by layer.

The two greatest postoperative complications include deep vein thrombosis (DVT) and hip dislocation (Brady et al., 2000). Patients wear thromboembolic disease (TED) hose, or stockings, that are applied in the operating room and continue to be worn for a few weeks following surgery. Motions that increase the risk of hip dislocation include hip adduction and flexion, so these motions are restricted for up to two months. The surgical incision is closed with metal staples that are removed about two weeks after surgery. The patient is required to sleep with an abduction pillow between the legs to keep the hip from moving into adduction during sleep; this pillow may be required for up to three months postoperatively. When sitting, the patient is instructed to use an elevated seat for about two months so that the hip is at greater than 90° (about 100°) of flexion; there is increased risk of posterior dislocation if the hip reaches 90° or less. Additional instructions that should be enforced for six to eight weeks include not crossing the legs or moving the leg across the body's midline, avoiding medially rotating the hip beyond 0° (if the posterolateral approach was used), and avoiding extension and lateral rotation (if a lateral or anterolateral approach was used). If the gluteus medius was detached and then reattached during surgery, the patient is to avoid active abduction for up to six weeks post-op to allow the incised muscle to heal before stressing it.

Knee Joint Replacement Surgery

Total knee replacement or arthroplasty (TKR or TKA) is an effective treatment of knee osteoarthritis after other treatment attempts have failed to provide the patient with lasting pain relief. According to the Centers for Disease Control (2008), the year 2002 saw over 380,000 TKA procedures in the United States. These common but complex procedures are being performed more frequently as we find older athletic knees suffering the results of injuries that occurred at earlier ages.

Total knee arthroplasties are not usually performed on young patients. For this reason, most physicians will cement the prosthesis in place. Some surgeons prefer to use a hybrid TKA.

These TKAs have a porous-coated femoral component, encouraging bone ingrowth, rather than being cemented into the medullary canal. Patients undergoing cemented TKAs are permitted full weight bearing immediately following surgery. Some surgeons are also now permitting immediate full weight bearing in patients with cementless TKAs. If full weight bearing is not permitted, toe-touch weight bearing is the limitation for about six weeks postoperatively.

There are three basic components to a total knee prosthesis: the femoral, tibial, and patellar components. The femoral and tibial components are often metal. The tibial platform, which interfaces with the femoral component, has a polyethylene plate to ensure reduced wearing between the two metal surfaces. Some of the new metallic products may eventually lead to metal-on-metal joint surfaces, a design that would last longer than the metal-on-polyethylene design; but for now, the metal-on-polyethylene joint is considered the state-of-the-art model. The patella component is a button-like device. It is a polyethylene structure that is placed on the posterior side of the resurfaced patella bone.

As with THAs, there are different types of TKAs. The primary difference between the various TKAs has to do with posterior cruciate stability. One type retains the person's posterior cruciate ligament (PCL), and the other provides a posterior-stabilized substitution in its design. Both provide for anterior-posterior stability, but the former allows the body's existing PCL to provide stability while the latter creates anterior-posterior stability through the conformity of the two implant segments.

The surgeon may opt to perform a patellar resurfacing or leave the patella alone and not install a patellar button. People who do not undergo a resurfacing are likely to suffer anterior knee pain and joint swelling for several weeks following surgery (Brander and Stulberg, 2006). Patellar resurfacing includes shaving of the posterior patella surface and attachment of a patellar button on the posterior aspect of the patella (figure 16.3).

As with THA, computer-assisted techniques are available for TKA procedures and provide the most accurate bone cuts, sizing, and orientation of the prosthetic segments. Computer-assisted procedures are not yet universally performed with all TKA surgeries. However, since joint replacements that are properly implanted have the greatest survival and longevity rate, it is anticipated that all surgeons will eventually convert to this system of arthroplasty implants. Because of the materials now used and the installation techniques employed, surgeons are currently optimistic that computer-assisted total knee joint implants will last more than 20 years (Brander and Stulberg, 2006).

Surgical approaches for TKAs are anterior. The surgeon's selection of a medial parapatellar approach through the quadriceps tendon, a vastus-splitting approach through the vastus medialis muscle, or a subvastus approach medial to the vastus medialis is based primarily on personal preference. The incision is more than 8 in. (20 cm) long. As with the hip, a minimally invasive technique is also possible for the knee. This technique usually requires an incision from the superior aspect of the patella to the tibial tubercle. Either the traditional incision or the minimally invasive incision is closed with metal staples.

Once the various skin, fascia, and muscle layers are opened in the surgical procedure and the patella is laterally dislocated, the knee joint is exposed. The collateral ligaments, if intact, are maintained. The anterior cruciate ligament is excised, but as mentioned previously, the posterior cruciate may be left intact or removed, depending on the surgeon's preference and condition of the PCL. Precise osteotomies remove the arthritic joint surfaces, and the tibia and femur are prepared to accept the

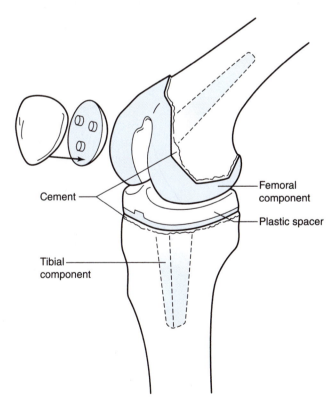

Cement

Femoral component

Plastic spacer

Tibial component

▶ **Figure 16.3** Total knee arthroplasty (TKA).

component parts. Once the sizing and alignment are complete, the joint segments are inserted and cemented in place, and the patella is resurfaced and then restored to its proper position.

As with the hip, risk of DVT necessitates the use of TED hose. These stockings are usually used for six weeks. Although the tibiofemoral joint is not usually at risk of dislocation following this surgery, the patella is at risk for subluxation (Brady et al., 2000). There are no restrictions on sitting as there are with THA. Walking and exercises begin the day following surgery. Depending on the age, agility, and strength of the patient, a walker or crutches are used to initiate gait training.

Shoulder Joint Replacement Surgery

Total shoulder arthroplasty or replacement (TSA or TSR) is a last-resort surgery for people with severe osteoarthritis of the shoulder. Unfortunately, people under the age of 65 are often affected with this condition. For these individuals, the best option may be a resurfacing of the joint or a hemiarthroplasty, a surgical procedure that usually involves replacing the humeral head. The best results, however, have occurred with TSA rather than with the hemiarthroplasty procedure (Dines et al., 2006). Patients who receive TSAs are younger than those who receive either the THA or the TKA (Dines et al., 2006).

Individuals considered good candidates for a TSA have intact rotator cuffs. If a TSA is the only option remaining but the rotator cuff is neither repairable nor viable, an rTSA may be necessary (Nicholson, 2006).

There are two major types of TSA—the traditional one with the humeral head and glenoid fossa (figure 16.4a), and the rTSA, in which the convex portion of the joint is attached to the scapula and the concave portion becomes part of the humerus (figure 16.4b). It has been recommended that the rTSA be reserved for individuals with severely disabled shoulders, because investigations demonstrate a significant reduction in function six years after implantation (Guery et al., 2006). It is unclear, however, whether this occurs because of faulty design of the prosthesis; or because the patients had very deficient shoulders prior to the surgery; or because the rotator cuff's center of rotation is altered, causing increased stresses on the scapular component (Dines and Levinson, 1995). Although the rTSA has been available in Europe since 1994, it has been used in the United States only since 2003 (Nicholson, 2006),

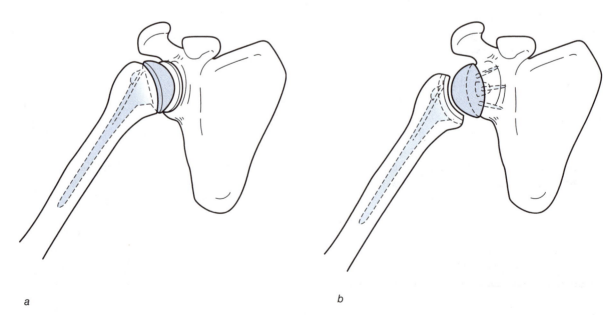

a　　　　　　　　　　　　　　　　　　　　　　　*b*

▶ **Figure 16.4**　Total shoulder arthroplasty (TSA). *(a)* Traditional TSA; *(b)* reverse TSA.

so it remains a relatively new procedure whose long-term benefits and disadvantages are yet to be revealed.

The TSA surgical procedure varies somewhat, but the basic technique involves an anterior incision from a point lateral to the coracoid process and inferiorly toward but not to the axilla. The pectoralis tendon is detached, as is the subscapularis tendon. The humeral head is then excised. The humeral head replacement is either cemented in or placed in the humeral medullar canal without cement. The cementless technique relies on bone ingrowth to secure the prosthesis. The glenoid is then prepared for its prosthesis before the artificial glenoid is cemented in place. The detached tendons are then reattached and the surgical site is closed by layers. Staples or Steri-Strips hold the skin layer in place.

Postoperatively, the patient may have the arm in a sling or an immobilizer with the shoulder positioned in medial rotation, adduction, and some forward flexion. If other procedures such as a rotator cuff repair were also performed during the TSA, other postoperative restrictions may also be indicated. Communication between the surgeon and rehabilitation clinician must occur so that appropriate follow-up rehabilitation can be provided.

Common restrictions following TSA include limits on passive range of motion. Passive range of motion may be limited to 30° of lateral rotation and no abduction beyond 0° for the first four to six weeks. This is to protect the anterior capsule and subscapularis and pectoralis tendons that were reattached during the implant surgery.

Other Joint Replacement Surgeries

As previously mentioned, there are joint replacements for most of the other joints of the body. The hip, knee, and shoulder, however, are the most commonly replaced joints. It is highly likely that you will treat a patient with one of these athroplasties. This chapter deals with only these three joints; the other joint replacement surgeries are beyond the scope of the chapter. Several joint replacement texts and journal articles on these other joint replacement techniques are available. If you have interest in these procedures, it is recommended that you pursue these sources for additional information.

SPECIAL REHABILITATION CONSIDERATIONS

When a total joint replacement occurs, the patient is referred by the surgeon for postoperative care. The rehabilitation clinician must be aware of the precautions, dangers, and rehabilitation sequences relevant to these patients. Each specific joint replacement has its own precautions and considerations, as discussed next.

Overview

As with most other injuries and surgeries, specific rehabilitation progression occurs in a logical manner. This progression is based on healing times and the fundamental evolution of goals and succession from one sequence to the next. As we have already discussed, relieving the immediate problems of pain, spasm, and swelling occurs first. This process is followed by emphasis on range-of-motion and flexibility gains, then strength and endurance gains. Once these are established, the patient progresses to balance, agility, and coordination before functional and activity-specific exercises. When the patient demonstrates an ability to perform normal functions, the rehabilitation program is complete.

There are some aspects that the various joint replacement surgeries have in common; other aspects of these surgeries are very distinct for each joint. It is important to realize what these similarities and differences are for each joint. The clinician must know the specific type of surgical procedure that has been performed. Precautions must always be respected. If the surgeon has his or her own protocol, it should be followed.

Patients younger than 70 years are now common recipients of total joint surgery.

Hip

Patients begin their rehabilitation the day following THA surgery. If the prosthesis is cemented, the patient is full weight bearing (FWB) or weight bearing as tolerated (WBAT). If the prosthesis is noncemented, the patient may be restricted to either toe-touch weight bearing (TTWB) or touch-down weight bearing (TDWB). Crutches or a walker is usually used for walking for about two weeks, and then the patient advances to a cane for another four weeks before walking without assistive devices (Hartzband, 2006). In-hospital exercises consist of isometric hip abduction, adduction, flexion, extension, and ankle pumps. Other isometric exercises include quad sets and hamstrings sets. These exercises progress to straight-leg raises (SLR), heel slides, and short-arc quadriceps (SAQ) extension exercises. If the patient's incision is on the posterolateral hip, hip flexion is limited to 90° and medial rotation is limited to 0°. If the surgical site is either anterolateral or over the lateral hip, then hip extension, lateral rotation, and adduction beyond 0° are restricted. If the gluteus medius muscle was detached and then reattached, active abduction motion is restricted for about six weeks.

For THA, remember that hip flexion beyond 100°, adduction beyond 0°, and sitting on low seats are restricted for 8 to 12 weeks. Whenever sitting, the patient sits on an elevated surface: A pillow is used for chairs; an elevated seat is used for the toilet, and the patient is asked to avoid soft, cushioned seating such as a sofa during the first three months after surgery. A bolster between the legs is used for sleeping during this time. If the prosthesis is noncemented, FWB is prohibited for the first six weeks after surgery.

Hospital stays for THA patients vary from three to seven days. Some patients may be required to transfer to a rehabilitation unit before being discharged to home. Normally, patients must demonstrate independence in ambulation, be able to transfer in and out of bed, and be able to perform self-care activities before they are discharged from an extended-care facility.

Once the patient is home, the physician will prescribe additional rehabilitation. These treatments are performed either at home or in an outpatient facility. If the right lower extremity is involved, the patient will be unable to drive a car until the right lower extremity is functional, often at least three to four weeks following the surgery.

At the patient's first clinic visit, the clinician will find that the patient has little pain, reduced motion, reduced strength, poor to fair balance, and less-than-optimal gait. Therefore, the goals are to relieve these deficiencies. The patient's hip motion may be limited to less than 50° initially; but by the time the patient is discharged, the hip should have at least 100° of flexion and 0° of extension. The muscles most deficient initially are the hip abductors and hip extensors. If the gluteus medius was cut during the THA procedure, then strengthening the muscle will be delayed until the surgical repair is healed, usually about six weeks; the status of this muscle must be identified by the surgeon before it is rehabilitated.

If the patient's upper extremities are weak, they should be strengthened to provide for greater ease in walking with assistive devices. The upper-extremity muscles active during crutch or walker ambulation include the scapular depressors, rotator cuff, latissimus dorsi, teres major, pectoralis major, triceps, and wrist flexor and extensor muscles. A normal gait pattern is advocated by the rehabilitation clinician. A THA patient typically ambulates with the surgical hip laterally rotated; this technique and any other deviation should be corrected.

Outpatient exercises include range-of-motion exercises for the hip. These are active exercises initially. By week 6, the patient may require passive-motion assistance if goals for motion are not yet achieved. Once the surgical wound is healed, the patient may benefit from aquatic exercises and gait training in the pool. Resistive exercises in the pool and gait activities are beneficial for total joint patients. Early strength exercises advance from standing isotonic hip extension, flexion, abduction, and lateral rotation, first without resistance and then with resistance, to weight-resistive exercises with either machines or free weights in antigravity positions. The weakest muscles tend to be the hip abductors and extensors, so they should be specifically examined and rehabilitated. Quadriceps and hamstrings resistance exercises, as well as ankle resistance exercises, are also incorporated and progressed as tolerated. When the patient is able to bear full weight on the limb, standing balance activities are initiated and progressed as the patient tolerates. Squats, step-ups, lateral step-ups, heel raises, treadmill walking, and other weight-bearing activities are also added once FWB is permitted. Gait-training progression moves from two crutches or a walker to one crutch or a cane and then to no assistive devices on level ground and on stairs.

After the hip flexion precautions are removed, the patient is able to progress to improving strength and motion in the previously avoided portions of motion. A reasonable expectation is to have 110° of flexion and at least 0° hip extension by the time of discharge, although it is even better if the patient is able to achieve 10° of hip extension. Patients may want to resume sport activities such as golf, tennis, or swimming, so additional rehabilitation goals are added for these patients; these patients will also require additional exercises to accomplish these other goals. One study demonstrated that patients who underwent a THA were able to resume golfing less than six months following the surgical procedure (Liem et al., 2006).

Knee

As with THA patients, TKA patients begin their rehabilitation soon after surgery. The patient may be fitted with a continuous passive motion (CPM) machine in the recovery room and be required to use it daily for 6 to 8 h. Motion may begin with motion set at 0° to 40° and increase by 10° each day. Some physicians use CPM as part of their standard postoperative care while others do not. There is evidence to demonstrate that CPM use reduces postoperative pain, swelling, and need for medications; but other studies have shown little long-term difference with or without their use, so the benefits of CPM use are controversial (O'Driscoll and Nicholas, 2000).

As is the case for THA patients, the TKA patient will be walking with crutches or a walker, weight bearing to tolerance, the day following surgery. Inpatient exercises include heel slides, quad sets, gluteal sets, hamstrings isometrics, ankle pumps, and SLR. Once the patient is able to lift the leg independently, ambulates safely with appropriate assistive devices, and is able to care for him- or herself, the patient is discharged from the hospital, usually three to five days following surgery.

Either home care or outpatient rehabilitation begins when the patient is discharged from the hospital. Outpatient goals are to have sufficient quadriceps strength for full active knee extension, knee flexion to at least 110° since most daily activities are possible with this minimum motion, and sufficient strength to ambulate without assistive devices and resume normal activities. Patients may want to resume sport activities such as golf, tennis, or swimming, so additional rehabilitation goals are included for these patients.

Reductions in pain, swelling, and soft-tissue adhesions are immediate goals for rehabilitation. Any of these dysfunctions may limit motion, so alleviating them helps patients to gain motion as well. Total knee arthroplasty patients are frequently able to achieve 120° to 130° of knee motion following joint replacement, so these motions may be reasonable expectations for TKA patients, particularly active patients. Active range of motion is initiated in-hospital and continues in outpatient treatments. The most important motion to regain is full knee extension. Flexion is also important, but if full extension is not regained, premature wearing of the joint will occur during ambulation and other weight-bearing activities. If the patient intends to be sedentary, 110° of flexion allows easy performance of daily activities such as stair climbing and getting in and out of a car; but if the patient wants to resume sport activities, 120° to 130° of knee motion is advisable.

Once the surgical incision is healed, aquatic exercises and gait training are beneficial to reduce swelling, improve gait, and increase strength and cardiovascular conditioning levels. Total knee arthroplasty patients should avoid the breaststroke kick. Examples of good aquatic exercises for TKA patients are taking large steps forward, backward, and sideways; hopping in chest-deep water; walking on toes; squatting; and running in deep water.

The patient may be required to remain WBAT with assistive devices for a minimum of four to six weeks. Assistive devices should not be discontinued until the patient has full active knee extension without an extensor lag and demonstrates a normal gait. The clinician should work to achieve these elements early in rehabilitation.

Hamstring, quadriceps, hip extensor, and hip abductor strength are usually deficient in TKA patients. The long-term pain and gait deviations these patients have lived with prior to their arthroplasty have been directly responsible for the muscle weaknesses they now must overcome. Additionally, the surgery has made the quadriceps even weaker than it was preoperatively. Ankle plantar flexors and dorsiflexors are often weak since the patient has not been using the lower extremity correctly for several months, perhaps years. Strengthening exercises for each of these muscle groups must be incorporated into both the outpatient program and the home exercise program to ensure proper strength gains in these muscle groups. Functional or neuromuscular electrical stimulation will aid the muscles in strength gains, especially the quadriceps, since it will shut down with the presence of edema (Fahrer et al., 1988). The patient should not discontinue the use of assistive devices for gait unless full knee extension and quadriceps control are present. Exercises with more resistance begin around post-op week 4 to 6.

Patellar mobilizations should be performed if patellar mobility is restricted. Patellar restriction reduces the tibiofemoral joint's full flexion motion ability, so lateral, medial, inferior, and superior mobilizations should be performed from day one in outpatient rehabilitation if it does not have normal excursion. After post-op week 6 to 8, tibial mobilization on the femur may be required if the patient does not have desired knee range of motion. Soft-tissue mobilization will also improve knee range of motion if soft-tissue mobility does not coincide with that of the contralateral knee; work on soft-tissue mobility is initiated at the same time as patellar mobilization.

Typical balance exercises such as tandem standing, stork standing, standing on uneven surfaces, and stork standing while performing distracting upper-extremity activities are all good proprioception activities. These begin when the patient is able to ambulate without assistive devices. Strength and balance exercises at this time also include activities such as step-ups, lateral step-ups, lunges, and lunges on a Bosu ball.

Once the patient has motion and flexibility, strength, and control, agility and functional activities precede the sport- and activity-specific exercises in the rehabilitation progression. These specific activities will depend on the individual's goals and ultimate desires. Some of them may be similar to those required for athletes returning to sport while others may be more simple, for example getting up from the floor after doing calisthenics or getting in and out of a car; whatever the patient's goals, the final portion of the rehabilitation program should be geared toward preparing the patient so that these goals are achieved prior to discharge.

Patients usually are able to return to sport activity anywhere from 8 to 10 weeks to four to six months following TKA surgery, depending on the surgeon and individual patient. The sport activities these postoperative patients will likely participate in are low-impact sports such as rowing, swimming, cycling, dancing, and golfing. Patients who wish to participate in impact-loading sports such as running or jumping are advised to discuss this with their physician. The rehabilitation clinician is unable to provide this authorization without consulting with the physician.

Shoulder

Sometimes surgeons use CPM machines for TSA patients. The arm is maintained in a sling for three to six weeks, taken out only for exercises and showering. Early exercises, which are passive, include pendulum exercises and tabletop exercises. The tabletop exercises are performed with the patient's hands in a weight-bearing position on the table. In this position, the patient's body moves from side to side to allow the shoulders to move into horizontal abduction and adduction; trunk flexion moves the shoulders into flexion; and with only the

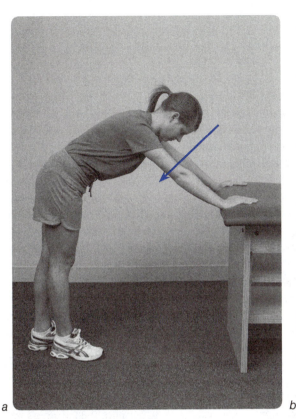
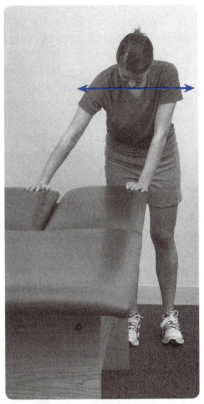
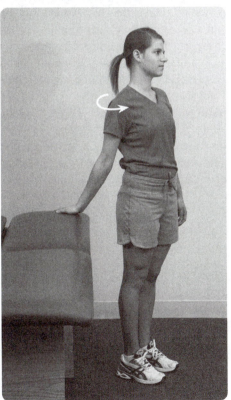
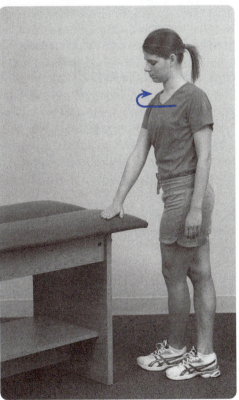

a

b

c

d

▶ **Figure 16.5** Weight-bearing exercises for range of motion for patients with total shoulder arthroplasty. *(a)* Patient anchors hands on table and leans forward to move shoulder into flexion. *(b)* With hands anchored on table, patient moves the body side to side. *(c)* Patient anchors hand and rotates body away from arm to move shoulder into lateral rotation. *(d)* Patient anchors hand and rotates body toward arm to move shoulder into medial rotation.

hand of the involved side on the table, the patient rotates the body toward and away from the hand to provide medial and lateral rotation at the shoulder (figure 16.5). Weight-bearing exercises for the shoulder assist in facilitating proprioception, reduce pain, and stabilize the joint by recruiting cocontraction of agonists and antagonists (McMullen and Uhl, 2000). Passive rather than active motion is used during early rehabilitation to reduce deltoid and subscapularis muscle stress and joint stresses. Passive lateral rotation and active medial rotation are limited in the first several weeks to reduce the pull on the subscapularis tendon. Active exercises for the elbow, wrist, and hand are performed frequently throughout the day.

When the patient is not exercising, the arm is in the sling. At night, the patient should lie supine with a support placed posterior to the arm and elbow (while the arm is in the sling) so that the arm does not move into hyperextension.

The patient may begin outpatient rehabilitation within a couple of weeks following surgery. It is important within the first month to work on motion gains rather than strength gains. By the end of the first month, the patient should have at least 90° of flexion and abduction, around 70° of medial rotation, and at least 45° of lateral rotation (Wilcox, Arslanian, and Millett, 2005). Rotation and abduction motions should be performed in the scapular plane.

Although strengthening exercises for the rotator cuff and other glenohumeral muscles are avoided during the first two months following surgery, scapular muscles can be strengthened during this time. Manual resistance applied directly to the scapula can strengthen scapular muscles in elevation, depression, protraction, and retraction without stressing the glenohumeral joint. Wrist and hand resistance exercises with light to medium weights can be started around the third post-op week.

By the 8th to 10th week, the patient begins light-resistance, high-repetition exercises for the shoulder muscles, including the rotator cuff and deltoid. Light dumbbell weights and rubber tubing exercises are started. The patient is able to remove the sling around this time. Rotation and abduction are performed in the scapular plane. Full shoulder motion should be present by around week 8 to 12. Sudden jerking, lifting, or twisting motions of the shoulder are avoided to reduce the risk of dislocation. Activities such as Swiss ball proprioception motion circles, low-level (under 60° elevation) resistance exercises, and weight-bearing resistance exercises are used to improve both glenohumeral and scapular muscles. After week 12 to 16, the patient should progress in strength levels, making gains similar to those experienced by a rotator cuff repair patient (see chapter 19).

The patient moves to functional and activity-specific exercises by the fourth to sixth month and then on to normal activities. Depending on the specific shoulder joint arthroplasty used, the patient will regain functional but not normal range of motion; final flexion range of motion may vary from 80° to 120° with rTSA (Bourdeau et al. 2007) and to 120° to 150° with TSA.

SUMMARY

More and younger patients are receiving total joint replacements. As surgical techniques and replacement parts improve, individuals receiving joint replacements will have them at earlier ages. Candidates for these procedures have suffered osteoarthritis or rheumatoid arthritis to a the degree that causes pain and dysfunction to interfere with lifestyle. Rehabilitation clinicians will see more total joint patients as the techniques and parts improve in quality and longevity. Even now, hip replacements are seen in individuals in their 20s and knee replacements are estimated to last more than 20 years. Sport activities may be resumed following some total joint surgeries. Although there are many joint replacement models for most of the body's joints, the most commonly replaced ones (the hip, knee, and shoulder) were discussed in this chapter. Each joint replacement has its unique qualities and considerations. The rehabilitation process for most of them begins early, usually the day following surgery, and continues for a couple of months following the procedure. Rehabilitation programs were outlined for the knee, hip, and shoulder.

KEY CONCEPTS AND REVIEW

1. Know the various terms and abbreviations for total joint replacements.

Total joint replacement is also known as arthroplasty. A total joint replacement of a hip is either a total hip replacement (THR) or total hip arthroplasty (THA). Likewise, a total knee replacement is either a TKR or TKA.

2. Identify the progression of osteoarthritis and how it leads to joint replacement.

Osteoarthritis is often the result of trauma to a joint at an earlier age. As the individual gets older, evidence of fraying and thinning of articular cartilage appears, eventually causing a degeneration of the joint surface. Once the articular cartilage is worn, the bone surface has no protection. Since articular cartilage has no pain receptors but bone does, the patient begins to experience gradually progressive and worsening episodes of pain with use or with weight bearing of the osteoarthritic joint.

3. Appreciate the secondary factors that add to debilitation when osteoarthritis occurs.

Pain and reduced function secondary to the pain produce muscle weakness and declining mobility. Muscle weakness and motion loss then become factors in placing more stress on already weakened joints. As the muscles weaken and the joint deteriorates, deformity becomes more evident. Gait patterns deviate, and pain causes a loss of normal function and ability to perform daily activities.

4. Describe the options available to a young person with osteoarthritis of the knee.

In the very early days of joint pain, many people resort to medication for pain relief. Some use anti-inflammatory medication; however, long-term use can be problematic for the liver. Some individuals use an over-the-counter medication, glucosamine chondroitin, to relieve joint pain. As the osteoarthritis progresses, however, relief with medications does not readily occur, and patients find themselves resorting to other methods of pain relief.

Some physicians may inject the joint or refer osteoarthritic patients for rehabilitation (or both) before any discussion of surgery. Various surgical techniques to encourage articular cartilage regeneration or replacement are usually the first surgical procedures used. These measures cause bleeding from subchondral bone to allow entrance of stem cells onto the joint surface. These stem cells then differentiate into articular cartilage cells. Depending on where the lesion is, how large it is, and the postoperative care provided, the repair may provide good protection for a few years. Chondral plugs and autogenous chondrocyte transplantation have also been discussed as a means of substituting for damaged articular cartilage. Patients usually resume full, normal activities after appropriate rehabilitation following these procedures. Arthroscopic debridement is a short-term pain relieving-technique. This procedure usually relieves pain enough to allow the patient more function, but it is not reparative; it will not make the joint better. The last resort, especially in a patient younger than 70 years old, is arthroplasty. If the individual undergoing the arthroplasty is 50 years old or younger, it is likely that a noncement arthroplasty will be performed. Not using cement will allow for an easier arthroplasty replacement when needed, 20 years or so later.

5. Identify the precautions involved in treatment and care following total hip joint replacement surgery.

Hip flexion beyond 100°, adduction beyond 0°, and sitting on low seats are restricted for 8 to 12 weeks. When sitting, the patient is on an elevated surface: A pillow is used for chairs and an elevated seat for the toilet, and the patient is asked to avoid soft, cushioned seating such as a sofa during the first three months after surgery. A bolster between the legs is used for sleeping during this time. If the prosthesis is noncemented, full weight bearing is prevented for the first six weeks after surgery.

CRITICAL THINKING QUESTIONS

1. A 60-year-old patient underwent a right THA six weeks ago. Today is his first time in outpatient rehabilitation. It is his goal to return to golfing, an activity he performs at least twice a week on a league team. You have just completed your examination of him and his abilities. He remains on crutches with WBAT on the right. What will your treatment today include? What exercises will you include? List the precautions you must remember to respect.

2. A 50-year-old tennis player had a left TKA three weeks ago. She is allowed WBAT but remains on crutches because she has an extensor lag of 40°. Flexion range of motion is to 90°. Her hamstrings and gluteus medius and maximus are all at 4–/5 strength, and her quadriceps are 3–/5. What will her exercise program include today? What will you give her for home exercises?

3. Referring to the opening scenario, what do you suspect is limiting Jan's knee extension to only 15°? What do you think would be the best exercises for Floyd to have Jan perform today? What are Jan's problems, and what short-term and long-term goals should Floyd list to relieve those problems?

LAB ACTIVITIES

1. Find two different manufacturers of artificial joints online. Identify the types of joints they manufacture. List how these companies differ in their emphasis of their joints, what the advantages of each are, and the materials from which they are constructed. Make another list indicating how these company's joints are similar. Following your investigation of these two companies, what conclusions can you draw from your research?

2. Identify a surgeon in your community who performs total joint replacement surgeries. Inquire if you are able to observe one of the surgeries. List 5 different observations you made of this surgery that differs from other surgeries you have observed. What was the most intriguing aspect of this experience?

3. If you have a THA patient who is restricted in the amount of hip flexion and hip adduction according to normal post-operative precautions, list the adaptations that would have to be made for the person to be able to sit, get up to standing, and perform daily activities at home and in the clinic where you would treat him. For example, how would you teach him to put his shoes on if he is unable to bend his hip beyond 100°? Think of all the daily activities he must perform at home, getting to your clinic for treatment, and what he would be required to do during your clinic treatment.

4. You have a TKA patient who is coming to you 4 weeks post-op. Her knee motion is 25° to 95°. Her quadriceps is atrophied. She has weakness in the hamstrings, quadriceps, hip abductors, and hip extensors. She continues to walk with two crutches although she is able to get rid of the crutches once she has full knee extension and a good gait. Make a list of the exercises and the progression for each of those exercises that you would use to return this patient to ballroom dancing, her favorite activity. You only need to make a progressive list of exercises to the completion of her rehabilitation program; you do not need to identify a timeline for these exercises.

5. You are working with a THA patient. Make a list of all the exercises and the criteria you would use to advance each of these exercises to the next level of difficulty. Include exercises for the hip, knee, and ankle. You may assume that you have any piece of equipment available to you.

Age Considerations in Therapeutic Exercise

OBJECTIVES

After completing this chapter, you should be able to do the following:

1. Realize why there are more people involved in sport today and therefore more who incur sport injuries.

2. Appreciate why little is known of sport injuries in the very young and the very old.

3. Understand why it is important to know how to manage injuries of preadolescent athletes and athletes who are older.

4. Provide an outline of growth and development based on the Tanner system and understand how boys and girls vary in the process.

5. Identify the problems associated with an anterior cruciate ligament reconstruction for a younger athlete.

6. Explain the precautions that one should take when providing a therapeutic exercise program to an older patient.

> ▶ During his career, Chaz Michaels has worked in a variety of athletic training clinics from high schools to universities to orthopedic settings. His new job at a sport clinic has a variety of clientele, including age groups from 10 years old to patients in their 80s. This is the first time Chaz has worked with any athlete over the age of 35. Although he hasn't been at this clinic long, he is surprised to realize how much he enjoys working with older athletes. One of his favorites is a 70-year-old tennis player, Lorrie. She has played tennis since high school. Chaz is treating her because she suffered a moderate ankle sprain when she ran to the net for a ball and rolled over on her ankle. She is anxious to get back onto the court, but Chaz is hesitant to push her as hard as he does his 20-year-old patients. He realizes that there are physical and physiological considerations he must think about as he progresses Lorrie in her rehabilitation program.

*The great secret that all old people share is that
you really haven't changed in 70 or 80 years.
Your body changes, but you don't change at all.*

DORIS LESSING, 1919- ; British author and Nobel Laureate in Literature

This is the second new chapter for this edition. It deals with age and the various patient populations whom health care workers treat. This is an essential addition to the text since musculoskeletal injuries occur in any age population. Additionally, different age groups require different considerations. Preteen and teen-aged patients are not small adults, just as patients in middle age and those who are older do not possess 25-year-old bodies. The chapter addresses the considerations that are unique to these age groups.

Much has changed in the past half century in the world of sport and leisure activity. First, there is more of both, and secondly, many more individuals participate in both sport and leisure activity than ever before (Kallinen and Markku, 1995; Koester, 2002). It is estimated that around 3 million children and adolescents are injured annually in organized sport activity (Koester, 2002). Clubs and interscholastic competitions for most sports are available for millions of teens and preteen athletes around the country.

Physicians across the United States advocate exercise for both children and older adults to promote individual healthy lifestyles (Fernhall and Unnithan, 2002). With higher expectations of longevity, there are more organized sport activities for older adults than in the past. Senior adults have many opportunities for competitive events. Not only are there municipally organized and club-related events and competitions such as races and tournaments; there are also national and international competitive events such as Senior Olympics for older adults.

STAGES OF LIFE, ACTIVITY LEVELS, AND HEALTH CARE

From birth to death, our bodies are continually changing. Some changes are for the good, some are for maintenance, and some are not so good; but they happen in all of us as we grow, develop, and age. The natural progression is from a stage of growth and development in youth to one of maturation and adaptation in the young adult stage, and then to the final stage of regression in ability and function. In our youth, our bodies learn functions that become automatic for us such as balance, standing, walking, and tossing a ball. Throughout this time, our systems of nerves, muscles, and bones adapt and change along with the stresses we apply to them as we grow and perform. In our young adult stage, our bodies continue to develop and adjust to the things we "teach" them by becoming more refined and adapted to the more sophisticated things we do. These things can be activities that seemed complicated at first but quickly became automatic, such as dancing, driving a car, solving physics equations, or juggling. However, as we approach our older years, we find that some of the activities that were once simple are no longer so. It becomes more difficult to respond as quickly to a stimulus as we once did; falling becomes more frequent because our reactions are slower; it isn't possible to hit a golf ball as far down the fairway as when we were younger; and stretching our hamstrings after we run is more difficult. Some of us move through these maturation stages slowly and others more quickly, and some of us spend more time in one stage than another, but we all move through these stages as we progress from birth to old age.

It is these various stages that the rehabilitation clinician must take into account when presented with a patient. How old is the patient? Where in the maturation process is he or she? How will this influence the rehabilitation program I want to create for this patient? What considerations are necessary because of this patient's age? If I deal with athletes, why do I need to think about my patient's age? These are the questions the chapter answers.

With the explosion of youth leagues for all sports, and with more "baby boomers" who remain active in recreational and leisure activities and are approaching retirement age and beyond, there is perhaps a wider range of ages than ever before in active patients who suffer activity-related injuries. As clinicians in outpatient clinics, we also see several types of work-related injuries in patients over the age of 30. Although we realize that each person is unique, we often do not take into consideration how age influences a body's response to the demands imposed upon it by therapeutic exercise. The body's reaction to those demands can be a direct result of the individual's age. That is why this chapter appears at this point in the book. Once you have acquired the information in this chapter and go on to the chapters in part IV, remember that when you develop a therapeutic exercise program for your patient, your patient's age will be a factor to consider in your rehabilitation program design.

There are organized and competitive activities for all ages in the United States. Athletic trainers may encounter patients from any age group.

Trends in Work and Leisure Time

It wasn't long ago that work was what consumed the waking hours of individuals. Within the last half century, following industrial and computer advances, people now live lives that are more consumed with leisure time than with work time (Ausubel and Grübler, 1995).

This slow but steady evolution from long workdays to more leisure time has led to an increase in the number of types of leisure activity and the number of individuals participating in them. Both sexes and persons of varying economic backgrounds, differing skill levels, and varying degrees of devotion to a seemingly endless number of activities participate in regular activity. These activities include archery, bowling, curling, dancing, fencing, golf, tennis, squash, swimming, ice skating, hockey, racquetball, basketball, soccer, and rowing, as well as various other types of recreational, league, and competitive pursuits.

Impact on Injury and Health Care

Health services are affected by the fact that people are living longer; in addition, health services are among the types of services most frequently used by consumers of all ages (Ausubel and Grübler, 1995). The health professions are called upon to assist not only those who are living longer but also those who have yet to enter the workforce—preadolescents and adolescents (Backx et al., 1989). Among those individuals who participate in athletics, the young and the old are populations that we know little about in terms of injury epidemiology, but we do know that if they participate in sport activities, injuries will occur. We also know that both younger and older athletes differ from early-adult athletes, who are the ones we most commonly refer to when presenting information on treatment and rehabilitation of injuries. These differences are important because they affect the patient's response to injury and to recovery. It is our responsibility as rehabilitation clinicians to know these differences and to understand how they influence the patients we treat in the age groups at either end of the life spectrum.

Physical Activity Throughout Life

The information we refer to in our sport rehabilitation practices is obtained from studies that usually involve subjects in their early-adult years. Since many of the studies are performed on university campuses, the age range of the subjects is from 18 to 25. These subjects are in the physical prime of their lives, having passed through the years of puberty and having yet to enter their declining years. There have been relatively few studies of sport injuries in either older or younger populations. However, there has been a plethora of research on both the progression of physical development and the regression of physical ability associated with aging. The next section deals with the preteen and teen years of puberty when physical change is most evident. It is also during these years that people come to rehabilitation clinicians with first-time sport injuries.

PEDIATRIC CONSIDERATIONS

From the perspective of the medical community, the pediatric population includes anyone between the time of birth and the completion of puberty (Steadman, 1990). A generation ago, before computer technology, children were more engaged in free play activity than in organized sport. The current generation of children engages in a variety of activities from physical education classes to community-based team sports and some free play (Backx et al., 1989), but the majority of their sport participation is through organized sport (Koester, 2002). Koester contends that with the decline of free play, youngsters begin sport activities without first establishing a physical conditioning base that protects them from injury (Koester, 2002). With an increased incidence of pediatric injuries, what considerations must the rehabilitation clinician respect as he or she treats these patients?

General Physiological Considerations

The majority of the physiological considerations relating to a pediatric patient have to do with the patient's developmental stage and the structure injured. The severity of the injury and the way in which the patient responds to the injury and recovery process are elements that we must also take into account.

Kids Are Not Small Adults

Children under 18 years are not adult in either their physiological or their physical maturity. Likewise, they cannot be treated as adults in their rehabilitation programs. Adjustments must be made and consideration given to the individual's physical and physiological maturity level in order to ensure a safe and appropriate progression of injury care and rehabilitation.

Growth and Development

Before we distinguish the unique features of a rehabilitation program and progression for this group, we must identify growth and development factors that influence these features. Although there are several systems for categorizing maturity in youth, one of the more commonly used systems is the Tanner growth chart, presented in table 17.1 (Tanner and Davies, 1985). This is a staging system that was first developed during the mid-1970s (Tanner and Whitehouse, 1976) and later updated to reflect changes in the development rate of children (Tanner and Buckler, 1997). The Tanner system identifies different developmental stages for secondary sexual characteristics, rate of height changes, and muscle development (Tanner and Whitehouse, 1976). A typical pubertal growth pattern begins with a phase of acceleration, which is followed by a phase of deceleration before growth ceases (Abbassi, 1998). Growth stops when the epiphyses close, at approximately 18 years in girls and 20 years in boys (Cronin and Mandich, 2005). Girls begin this growth pattern earlier and end it earlier, usually about two years ahead of their male counterparts in each process. Although the exact age when the

TABLE 17.1   Tanner Stages of Development

Tanner stage	Adolescence level	Male characteristics	Female characteristics
I	Preadolescence	No pubic hair	No pubic hair, flat breasts
II	Early adolescence	Darkening of pubic hair; enlargement of testes	Sparse pubic hair; small, raised breasts
III	Middle adolescence	Coarsening and curling of pubic hair; increased penis size	Coarsening and curling of pubic hair; enlargement and raising of breasts
IV	Middle adolescence	Continued penis growth	Formation of areola and nipple contour separate from breast development
V	End of adolescence	Presence of adult genitalia	Presence of adult genitalia

puberty process begins varies from one individual to another, the average starting age for girls is 9 years and for boys is 11 years (Abbassi, 1998).

Prior to puberty, there are no differences in physical abilities of girls and boys. Once children enter puberty, however, strength and size differences create distinctions in physical abilities between the two sexes. All preadolescents and adolescents, however, have physical qualities that vary greatly from adults. The following discussion focuses on some of the factors that are important considerations for rehabilitation clinicians.

Bone Factors   Children's bones grow until the end of puberty. Longitudinal bone growth occurs at the growth plate, called the physis. A **physis** is a complex cartilaginous matrix that lies near the end of the longitudinal bone and forms new bone, providing growth of the long bone. The epiphysis sits on the distal end of the physis and forms the joint end of the bone (figure 17.1).

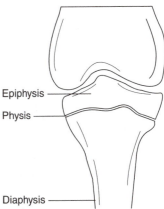

Epiphysis

Physis

Diaphysis

▶ **Figure 17.1**   Long bone growth areas. The physis is the cartilaginous section of long bones that creates greater length of the bone.

Reprinted from R. Behnke, 2005, *Kinetic anatomy*, 2nd ed. (Champaign, IL: Human Kinetics), 5.

TABLE 17.2   Salter-Harris Epiphyseal Fracture Classifications*

Classification	Characteristics	Cause	Notations
I	Separation of the cartilage from the bone without any bone fracture	Avulsion or shearing force	A common epiphyseal injury during the early years. It has the best outcome.
II	A fracture that extends through the physis and into the metaphysis but not the epiphysis	Shearing or avulsion; occurs in children over 10 years old	Most common epiphyseal plate injury. The growing cartilage cells remain intact, so growth still occurs.
III	A fracture through the physis and epiphysis	Intra-articular shearing force	Not a common injury. May require surgery. Prognosis is good as long as circulation to the epiphysis remains intact.
IV	Intra-articular fracture from the epiphysis through the physis and into the metaphysis	Impact or torsional stress	A complete split is present. ORIF (open reduction and internal fixation) is necessary to realign epiphyseal plate and prevent growth stoppage.
V	Compression fracture of the epiphyseal plate	A crushing force during a lateral motion or stress resulting in displacement of the epiphysis; occurs in uniplanar joints	These injuries are commonly dismissed as a sprain. Although weight bearing is restricted for 3 weeks, prognosis is poor.

*From Salter and Harris 1963.

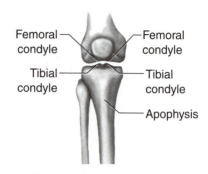

Femoral condyle

Femoral condyle

Tibial condyle

Tibial condyle

Apophysis

▶ **Figure 17.2** Apophysis is an outgrowth of bone to which a tendon or ligament attaches.

Salter and Harris developed an injury classification method for the various degrees of physis injuries (Salter and Harris, 1963). Their classification system is presented in table 17.2. Another segment of the bone that is not present in mature bones is the apophysis. An **apophysis** is an outgrowth of bone where a tendon or ligament attaches (figure 17.2). Until a bone matures, these sites are susceptible to excessive shear or compressive forces. Compressive stress to a physis can result in fractures that damage the bone's growth center, stopping bone growth. Shear stresses to an apophysis create a pulling away of the tendon's bone attachment.

Young bones are more resilient and elastic than adult bones, so young bones are able to tolerate greater stresses before a fracture occurs. Because of this bone elasticity and resilience, fractures in youth are different than fractures in adults. Immature bones may suffer a "greenstick fracture" or partial fracture, in which one side of the bone is broken and the opposite side is only bent. When a fracture involves the epiphysis or physis, bone growth or alignment (or both) may be affected. For this reason, additional care is taken with these fractures.

Articular Cartilage Factors The articular cartilage of children and adolescents is similar to physis in its construction and tolerance to stress, especially shearing forces (Micheli et al., 2006). In other words, it is a structure that is subject to injury. However, there is evidence that articular cartilage in these age groups may heal better than in adults (Riegger-Krugh et al., 2008). What is important is that these injuries be detected immediately and that care following the diagnosis allow for sufficient stress to encourage proper healing but not so much stress as to cause deterioration of healing tissues. In addition, there is evidence to indicate that articular cartilage volume increases in children who are active and involved in vigorous activity compared to those who are sedentary; active children gain twice as much articular cartilage as sedentary children (Jones et al., 2003). This suggests that perhaps children who are active may be less likely to develop osteoarthritis in later years.

Muscle Factors Girls and boys have essentially equivalent muscle proportion and strength prior to puberty. Once children enter puberty, however, muscle size and strength are greater in boys than in girls. The males' greater testosterone levels are primarily responsible for these developing differences. Both groups, however, have the potential for greater muscle strength than bone strength during their growth spurts. It is during this time that apophyseal injuries may occur, especially if the child participates in sport activities. One reason for the occurrence of these injuries is that muscle lengthening is stimulated by bone lengthening, so it occurs after bones begin their growth spurt.

There has been a dispute for several years about whether preadolescent children should engage in strengthening activities. People who argue against such activities are inclined to believe that strength exercises during the preadolescent years place the individual at risk for epiphyseal injuries secondary to unnecessary loading and shear stresses (Faigenbaum et al., 1996). However, a policy statement published by the American Academy of Pediatrics (AAP) indicated that strength-training programs did not have a detrimental effect on young athletes (AAP, 2001). The following is a summary of the AAP strength-training guidelines and recommendations for preadolescents and adolescents:

Guidelines

1. Begin with low-resistance exercises until proper technique is learned.

2. When 8 to 15 repetitions can be performed, add weight in small increments.

3. Exercises should include all muscle groups and should be performed through the full range of motion at each joint.

4. To achieve gains in strength, workouts need to be at least 20 to 30 min long, take place a minimum of two or three times a week, and continue to add weight or repetitions as strength improves.

5. There is no additional benefit to strength training more than four times a week.

Recommendations

1. Strength-training programs can be safe and effective if proper resistance training techniques are used and safety precautions are followed.

2. Competitive weightlifting, powerlifting, bodybuilding, and maximal lifts should be avoided until the individual reaches physical and skeletal maturity.

3. When pediatricians are asked to recommend or evaluate strength-training programs, the following issues should be considered:

    a. Before the beginning of a strength-training program, a medical evaluation should be performed by a pediatrician. If indicated, a referral may be made to a sports medicine physician who is familiar with various strength-training methods as well as risks and benefits.

    b. Aerobic conditioning should be coupled with resistance training if general health benefits are the goal.

    c. Strength-training programs should include a warm-up and a cool-down component.

    d. Specific strength-training exercise should be learned initially with no resistance. Once the exercise skill has been mastered, incremental loads can be added.

    e. Progressive resistance exercise requires successful completion of 8 to 15 repetitions in good form before weight or resistance is increased.

    f. A general strengthening program should address all major muscle groups and should include exercise through the complete range of motion.

    g. Any sign of injury or illness from strength training should be evaluated before the exercise in question is continued.

Tendon Factors   Because muscle lengthening lags behind bone lengthening during growth spurts, the muscle's tendon applies increased tension on the apophyseal attachments. Because of the bone attachment's lesser resilience compared to muscle tissue, the apophyseal plate is usually the site of injury following repetitive-stress occurrences. An additional fact is that with delayed muscle lengthening during growth spurts, inherent tension is applied to the apophyseal plate via tension transmission from the muscle along the tendon to its insertion. Some common apophyseal plates in which we see these types of injuries are the calcaneus with Sever's disease, medial humeral epicondyle with Little League elbow, and tibial tubercle with Osgood Schlatter's disease.

Neurological Factors   The neurological system controls the muscular system with respect to strength and skill execution. Skill execution is assessed as the ability to perform accurately and efficiently. Accuracy and efficiency are achieved through repetition of the specific activity; the skill is corrected and refined as it becomes engrained within the neuromuscular system (Kottke, 1982). Strength gains occur in prepubescent children, but not because of an increase in muscle size as in adults. Essentially, neural changes and neuromuscular recruitment improvement are responsible for strength gains in children prior to puberty (Bar-Or and Rowland, 2004).

Thermoregulatory Factors   Since prepubescent children do not have the sweat mechanisms that adults possess, their ability to release heat is different. Prepubescent children have a higher convection rate than adults (Williams, 2007). This means that their blood is diverted to the surface to reduce heat buildup within the body, as evidenced by increased skin coloration during exercise in this age group.

Children expend more energy per body mass in heat than adults. Greater energy expenditure translates to greater heat output. If a child and an adult are running at the same speed, the child will expend 20% more body heat per kilogram than the adult (Williams, 2007).

Sweating is a primary means of evaporative heat dissipation. Although children older than 2 years have as many sweat glands as adults, this does not mean that they are able to produce sweat as well as adults. Heat dissipation through sweat production is dependent upon how soon the sweat response occurs and the amount of sweat produced. Children produce a little more than half the amount of sweat that adults produce (Williams, 2007). Additionally, boys sweat more than girls, and postpubertal youngsters sweat more than either pre- or midpubertal youngsters (Williams, 2007). Given the importance of sweating in heat dissipation, prepubertal and midpubertal youngsters have a disadvantage when hot environmental conditions are present. Children lose more fluid than electrolytes while sweating in high temperatures, so it is important to take frequent breaks to replace these lost fluids.

Considerations in Therapeutic Exercise

The prepubescent, midpubescent, and postpubescent age groups vary greatly from one another in physical and psychological maturity. As rehabilitation clinicians, we must be cognizant of these variations, as such awareness will help us to provide optimal rehabilitation programs for individuals within these age groups. Given the brief discussion in the preceding sections, it is apparent that many changes occur within the body between the beginning of middle school and the end of high school, the time period when we often see patients' first-time injuries. How we treat these patients and their injuries may have a profound impact on them, both physically and emotionally.

Sport Injuries in School-Aged Patients

More than half of boys and one-fourth of girls in the United States engage in organized sport (Omey and Micheli, 1999). With the profound increase in organized sport for younger athletes, it is likely that rehabilitation clinicians will treat younger patients with athletic injuries since more injuries occur during organized sport than in free play activities (Backx et al., 1989). More schools are employing certified athletic trainers who not only will treat these young patients but also will likely see the injuries occur.

A natural question is, what types of injuries occur in this population? Thirty-six percent of injuries to youngsters occur as a result of sport (Bijur et al., 1995). Contusions and sprains, which are among the most common of these injuries (Backx et al., 1989), occur most frequently in sports such as basketball and field hockey (Backx et al., 1989). A significant number of injuries in this age group also involve overuse syndromes (Andrish, 1984).

Sever's disease, stress fractures, Osgood-Schlatter's disease, jumper's knee, apophysitis, and tendinopathies are common chronic conditions (Andrish, 1984). Often, these injuries occur either during growth spurts while excessive stress is applied to the bones or soft tissues (Draper and Dustman, 1992), or because of poor technique execution (Hutchinson and Wynn, 2004), or both. Most fractures occur in the 13- to 16-year-old age group and are Salter-Harris type II fractures; these occur primarily from a combination of rapid growth and physis weakness (Wasserlauf and Paletta, 2003).

Regardless of the cause, the patient's complaints are similar to those of an adult. Treatment progression, however, is complicated by the fact that the patient may still be growing and the injury site is not mature, such that it is unable to tolerate the same level of stresses as its adult counterpart.

Acute sprains may be severe enough to indicate surgical repair. Anterior cruciate ligament ruptures are occurring with more regularity in teens and preteens (Kocher, 2006). These skeletally immature patients require unique considerations. One of the primary concerns is avoiding the epiphyseal growth plate during the graft implantation. Thus the physician must know the patient's physiological age in order to prevent growth plate damage. As indicated in figure 17.3, Kocher's group varies anterior cruciate ligament (ACL) reconstruction according to the patient's physiological age, classified into one of three groups (Kocher, 2006):

- Prepubescent: Either no surgery is performed and a functional brace is used for protection, or a physeal-sparing and combined intra-articular and extra-articular reconstruction is performed using an autogenous iliotibial band graft.

- Adolescent with significant growth remaining: Surgery features a transphyseal ACL reconstruction using autogenous hamstrings tendons with fixation away from the physes.

- Older adolescent approaching skeletal maturity: Surgery is a conventional adult ACL reconstruction with interference screw fixation using either autogenous central third patellar tendon or autogenous hamstrings.

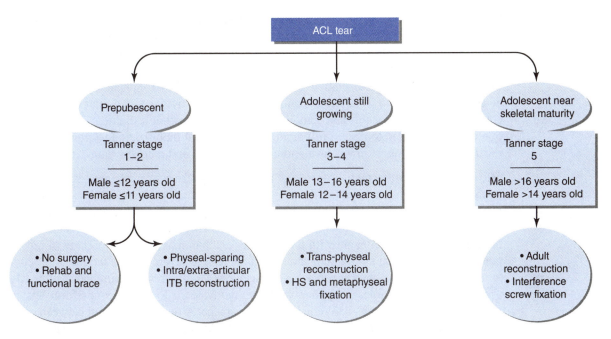

▶ **Figure 17.3** Surgical decision making for anterior cruciate ligament injuries in skeletally immature patients.

Rehabilitation Considerations for Sport Injuries in School-Aged Patients

Just as surgeons must adapt their surgical techniques to accommodate growth and developmental stages, the rehabilitation clinician must make adjustments in the rehabilitation program. Not only do we have the physiological and physical immaturity issues to consider, but it also can be challenging to maintain a young patient's interest in and focus on rehabilitation exercises. Young patients often do not realize the importance of performing exercises correctly; frequently they focus on completing the exercises as soon as possible rather than performing them correctly or conscientiously. With these patients, clinicians need to use their imaginations to make exercises fun while accomplishing the necessary goals of safe and sufficient recovery. Exercises must be carefully monitored for correct execution and proper compliance.

Proper care provided as soon as possible is a key factor in relation to the future and to injury outcome for young athletes. It is during this age that postural deviations are often discovered. Sometimes these deviations result in an athletic injury. The rehabilitation clinician should assess each young patient for possible postural deviations as part of a routine rehabilitation examination. Immediate care involves the use of modalities such as ice and electrical stimulation to relieve inflammation, pain, and edema. Range-of-motion exercises to restore flexibility follow reduction of pain and swelling. Strengthening exercises with primary emphasis on endurance activities are the next part of the progression. The final phase in a youngster's rehabilitation program involves the restoration of proprioception, balance, and agility prior to sport-specific activities.

Preparation and planning for this rehabilitation program must account for the physical variations in younger patients compared to adults. Those factors have already been outlined; next we see how they need to be considered in relation to rehabilitation.

Bone and Articular Cartilage Factors When we are dealing with injuries to bone, epiphysis, physis, or articular cartilage, the primary concern is preventing additional injury to these structures. Bone heals quickly in young patients; but if damage occurs to the growth regions of bone, one must be careful to avoid activities that cause pain, which is a key sign of excessive stress to these structures. Rehabilitation is gradual and progressive. Most epiphyseal injuries have good outcomes (Salter and Harris, 1963). Most are immobilized in either a cast or a splint.

The site of common restriction following immobilization is the elbow joint. Although many fractures in children require little postinjury rehabilitation, elbow joint immobilization often necessitates postimmobilization treatment including joint mobilizations to restore full motion.

Following any immobilization, the clinician's goals are to reduce inflammation and restore motion first. Active range-of-motion exercises are often sufficient for regaining motion. When necessary, assistive motion exercises and other types of activities to facilitate motion gains are used. If the joint is stable and demonstrates a capsular motion restriction, joint mobilization may also be used to restore full motion. Grade II joint mobilization is often used early in rehabilitation to assist in increasing joint fluid mobility and reducing pain.

Muscle and Tendon Factors   Athletes of any age benefit from strengthening exercises. It is important, however, that exercises for prepubescent athletes and young adolescents involve two factors, supervision and endurance. Rather than high weights, these age groups benefit more from high-repetition, low-resistance bouts. It is recommended that any youth below the Tanner stage V level begin with a resistance less than maximal. The number of repetitions should be eight at a minimum and should not lead to severe muscle fatigue. It is better to increase repetitions before increasing resistance when progressing in rehabilitation. My usual routine for preadolescent patients who are motivated is to have them perform sets up to 20 or even 30 repetitions before increasing resistance. A rest of 1 to 2 min between exercises should be incorporated into the program. The clinician must instruct the patient and explain cautions about proper execution of the exercises before having the patient perform any exercise with weights.

Manual resistance and resistance to the opposite extremity are both useful exercises for young injured athletes. There is evidence to demonstrate that exercising one extremity facilitates strength of the contralateral extremity (Hellebrandt and Waterland, 1962). Manual resistance is also an engaging activity for the young patient who may prefer to make a game out of the exercise, attempting to "conquer" the clinician and "win."

Neurological and Thermoregulatory Factors   Recall that prepubescent patients will not increase their muscle bulk but will make strength gains. As these patients continue with repetitions, their accuracy also improves because the repetitions create an engram within the neuromuscular pathways (Kottke, 1982). This factor becomes important as the patient begins the last phase of the rehabilitation program, working on functional and sport-specific activities. Begin the sport-specific activities with exercises that the patient can do successfully in order to enable proper execution. As patients gain accuracy, the exercises become more challenging but they can still be successful.

Because of the thermoregulatory factors previously discussed, children often look red-faced after a workout. This is normal, but on days that are hot or are both hot and humid, extra caution must be taken to ensure more breaks and frequent water breaks. Because a young person's thermal regulation is not as efficient as an adult's, careful observation throughout an exercise program is warranted. Adolescent patients have a more efficient sweating mechanism than prepubescent patients, so the need for this caution is not as great with these youngsters.

GERIATRIC CONSIDERATIONS

Our bodies continue their maturation progression through the adolescent years and reach their peak potential for physical conditioning in our 20s and early 30s. The reversal of this process begins so slowly that it is many years later that we notice a decline in our abilities. This is the normal aging process. Perhaps it is slow to allow us time to mentally adjust to these physical changes. Before we can safely treat older athletes, we must understand the changes their bodies have experienced and realize that our performance expectations cannot be the same as for our younger patients.

General Physiological Considerations

It was Bette Davis who said, "Old age ain't no place for sissies!" She was likely referring to the fact that with age, the body changes in ways that are not always desirable. Older patients deserve our care and attention as much as the younger people we treat in our clinical practices. It may be surprising to realize that although these older patients have typically lived many more years than those of us who treat them, inside they still feel young and even energetic.

Body Changes With Age

Once we move into our 20s and 30s, our bodies begin a decline that proceeds slowly over many years into our old age. Assuming that we hit our peak at age 20 and experience a 1% loss per year, it takes between 50 and 60 years to get to the 40% level at age 75 (Kemp, 2005). Some systems move through this aging process much more slowly than others, but all of our body systems decline as we age. This section briefly reviews the systems pertinent to orthopedic function. The systems we are primarily concerned with are the muscular, skeletal, and neural systems. Generally, connective tissue becomes stiffer. This affects muscles, tendons, joints, and other structures surrounded by connective tissue; flexibility is reduced, and the risk of injuries such as sprains and strains is increased.

Muscular Factors The muscular system declines about 40% from age 20 to 80 (Narici and Maganaris, 2007). **Sarcopenia** is the term used for a decrease in muscle mass secondary to aging. Sarcopenia involves a reduction in both the size and number of muscle fibers, similar to the reductions that occur with muscle disuse (Narici and Maganaris, 2007). After age 25, the number of the body's muscle fibers begins to diminish (Thompson, 2002). Accompanying the reduction in size is a decrease in muscle strength and power. Fewer functioning myosin heads restrict the number of possible bonds between the actin and myosin during muscle activity, resulting in less strength production. Muscle strength is reduced by 15% each decade up to the age of 70 and by 30% each decade after that (Poluri et al., 2005).

Speed of contraction also declines with age, and the point of peak output of the muscle is more delayed as we age (Runnels et al., 2005). The faster type II muscle fibers decline at a faster rate than the type I fibers. In the quadriceps, the fast-twitch fibers diminish about 20% more readily than the slow-twitch fibers during the third and fourth decades (Thompson, 2002). There is also some evidence that the normally reduced output levels of hormones related to aging may have an effect on muscle strength (Ahmed, Matsumura, and Cristian, 2005).

Muscle endurance declines with age as well. This reduced muscle endurance may be the result of reduced contractile function and diminished metabolic activity within the muscle (Thompson, 2002). Capillary density diminishes as we age. Diminished muscle endurance and naturally reduced blood flow may result from this reduced capillary density, and these effects, along with fewer mitochondria in muscle fibers, all diminish glucose availability and result in a less efficient phosphocreatine reconversion mechanism.

On the other hand, older individuals can benefit from exercise and show improved muscle performance with exercise. Evidence consistently demonstrates that muscle strength and endurance can improve with exercise (Frontera, 2006; Reeves, Narici, and Maganaris, 2006). Muscle size, speed, and coordination also increase with exercise (Ahmed et al., 2005).

Skeletal Factors We will include both bones and joints when we consider the skeletal system. The body's synovial joints are made up of fibrocartilagenous ligaments and capsules, while the joint surfaces are covered with articular cartilage that is nourished by the synovium and subchondral bone. The synovial fluid also provides lubrication for the joint. Remember from our discussion in chapter 2 on articular cartilage that proteoglycan aggregates, enmeshed within the type II collagen, bind with the water in articular cartilage to provide protection from compressive forces on joints. As the body ages, the aggregates become shorter, and less proteoglycan is produced (Ahmed et al., 2005). These changes result in less water within the articular cartilage, leading to increased stress on the joint surface. Unfortunately, the thickness of articular cartilage also diminishes with age (Lane and Bullough, 1980). Eventually, cartilage calcification occurs and subsequent osteoarthritic changes become evident (Ahmed et al., 2005).

It is well known that after the onset of menopause, women become more susceptible to osteopenia and osteoporosis. **Osteopenia** is a mild to moderate bone density loss that places the individual at risk for advancing to osteoporosis. **Osteoporosis** is marked bone density loss. Individuals with osteoporosis are at risk for fractures. Both conditions are related to calcium deficiency or bone demineralization.

Loss of bone mass is a naturally occurring event in both men and women. We possess our strongest bones between the ages of 25 and 30. By the time we reach our 40s and 50s, we begin to lose bone density. Bone density diminishes slowly at first but then more rapidly as women enter postmenopausal ages. At this time, bone mass declines since osteoblasts are unable to replace calcium at the same pace that it is reabsorbed.

Exercise, however, positively affects bones and joints. Bone strength improves with weight-bearing activities (Milgrom et al., 2001). Bone health is also improved with exercise (Mazzeo et al., 1998).

Neural Factors Nerves and their excitation change with age. Changes in the neural system affect proprioception, motion sense, and joint position. These, in turn, influence balance. Autonomic reflexes including musculotendinous reflexes become less sensitive, and reaction times become longer from stimulus to response. These changes make it more difficult for older individuals to react to sudden changes in position. Another aspect of neuromuscular decline is the reduced speed of transmission of neural stimuli from sensory receptors to the muscle fibers (Mase et al., 2006; Thompson, 2002). In summary, balance and speed of movement are impaired with aging. These factors are influenced by various changes in the neural input and the rate of input into the neuromuscular system.

When dealing with older patients, we must consider other neurological factors that prevent them from reacting to their environment as they did when they were younger. These factors involve sensory systems besides the proprioceptive system. Loss of hearing is a natural decline in most people. Because of slower synapse neural transmission mechanisms, it takes longer for older individuals to grasp what they hear than it does for younger persons. You may have been told by an older person that he or she has difficulty understanding you because you speak too fast. Moreover, since memory also declines with age, even healthy older individuals may forget instructions given to them only orally.

Additional existing neurological pathologies make it more difficult for an aging individual to respond to a clinician's instructions as would normally be expected of a younger patient. For example, for someone who has reduced sensation secondary to conditions such as diabetic neuropathy or cardiovascular compromise, standing or walking on an unstable surface may be too challenging. If older patients have reduced vision because of cataracts or other optical conditions, they may find it difficult to read home exercise instructions. If patients have difficulty hearing, they may not hear instructions properly.

Rehabilitation Considerations Regarding Injuries in Older Patients

A significant amount of evidence demonstrates that exercise has a positive influence on the aging process (Frontera, 2006; Mazzeo et al., 1998; McDermott and Mernitz, 2006). For this reason, older athletes may show less decline than the average member of their age group. It should not be assumed that an individual who is older is necessarily fragile or is declining at a rapid rate. Exercise improves many physiological and physical parameters in older adults. For example, cardiovascular function, muscle strength, balance and coordination, flexibility, and endurance all increase with regular exercise programs (Hara and Shimada, 2007). Research has also demonstrated that muscle mass increases in older subjects undergoing a strengthening program, albeit at a slower and lower rate than in younger adults (Frontera,

2006). Older persons engaged in a regular exercise program demonstrate less risk of falling than nonexercising older subjects (Shigematsu and Okura, 2006).

The benefits of a regular exercise program and the importance of older Americans' engagement in regular exercise have prompted the American College of Sports Medicine (ACSM) to establish a position stand and recommendations for exercise regimens for older adults (Mazzeo et al., 1998). This text deals with rehabilitation and therapeutic exercise, not conditioning, so the ACSM program is not included here. Guidelines for factors such as heart rate during exercise and strength progression are presented, however, since these and other physical concerns must be considered in a therapeutic exercise program.

Cardiovascular System Because the cardiovascular system of an older athlete is unable to tolerate the same stresses as that of a younger athlete, the clinician should be aware of the patient's heart rate, especially during endurance activities. Until the clinician knows the patient's physiological response to exercises, it may be necessary to monitor heart rate and blood pressure. The American Heart Association's recommendation for older individuals is to establish a heart rate maximum for exercise by subtracting the individual's age from 220, then multiplying that number by 50% to 80%; this product is the maximum target heart rate for that individual. Table 17.3 provides a quick reference for target heart rate for various ages and various intensity levels. If you work with an older athlete who has not exercised for a while, 50% of the maximum heart rate may be a good starting point in the earlier rehabilitation phases. It is likely that older athletes know their normal exercise heart rate and will be able to inform you of this target. As the patient's condition improves, a gradual increase to the normal target heart rate may be indicated.

Neuromuscular System Muscles in older patients can gain strength in response to exercise, though the muscles respond more slowly to exercise than do those of younger patients (Reeves et al., 2006). The tendons of older patients also regain some of their stiffness and strength with exercise (Narici and Maganaris, 2006). These studies seem to indicate that exercise is able to alleviate aging factors to some degree.

Target heart rate for older adults will vary according to age and physical abilities.

TABLE 17.3   Target Heart Rates for Various Ages

Age	Maximum heart rate (MHR)	Target heart rate at 50% MHR	Target heart rate at 55% MHR	Target heart rate at 60% MHR	Target heart rate at 65% MHR	Target heart rate at 70% MHR	Target heart rate at 75% MHR	Target heart rate at 80% MHR	Target heart rate at 85% MHR
40	180	90	99	108	117	126	135	144	153
45	175	88	97	105	114	123	131	140	149
50	170	85	94	102	111	119	128	136	145
55	165	83	91	99	107	116	124	132	141
60	160	80	88	96	104	113	120	128	136
65	155	78	86	93	101	110	116	124	132
70	150	75	83	90	98	105	113	120	128
75	145	73	80	87	94	102	109	116	123
80	140	70	77	84	91	98	105	112	119
85	135	68	74	81	88	95	101	108	115

We know that muscles atrophy and get weaker following injury. This occurs in athletes and other individuals of all ages. The strength and muscle changes we have been discussing in relation to old age are similar to the changes seen following injury or immobilization (Natri et al., 1996). Given that older athletes are able to improve strength and muscle function, and given that the changes seen in muscle during inactivity and aging are similar, it seems intuitive that strengthening exercises used in therapeutic exercise can bring about strength gains in older patients. This is in fact true, so strength training for older patients is advocated (Frontera, 2006).

Although strength gains can be made in older patients, the speed with which these gains are made is slower than in younger patients. In fact, the speed with which gains are made in many muscular parameters is slower in older patients. The rate at which endurance improves is also slower than in younger patients. Speed of muscle contraction is slower as well, so agility exercises are not performed at the speed expected of younger patients.

Through proprioception, the neuromuscular system is a large influence on balance, coordination, and agility. Young individuals should be able to balance in a single-leg stance position for 30 s, but older persons do not usually attain this duration in the single-leg stance. Although age is a variable, otherwise healthy individuals between 65 and 84 demonstrate, on average, an ability to sustain a single-leg stance for around 19 s (Baezner et al., 2008). People toward the higher end of that age range will balance for a shorter time while those toward the younger end of the range will be able to balance longer. We know that injury leads to a reduced ability to perform balance activities, so it is logical to assume that older athletes with injuries will also have deficiencies in balance activities; they will balance for less than 19 s in the single-leg stance exercise.

Considerations in Therapeutic Exercise

Some of the factors we should consider when designing a therapeutic exercise program for an older patient have already been mentioned, and we have alluded to others. This section summarizes these necessary considerations.

Older patients may move more slowly than younger patients, so additional time may be required for an initial examination and evaluation. Since hearing and slower comprehension may both be issues with the patient, speaking slowly and clearly becomes an important element of communication. A lower-pitched voice is usually easier to hear than a high-pitched voice, so make a conscious effort to speak in a low pitch, especially if you are female. Remember that vision can be a problem with older patients. If you provide the patient home exercises, it may be beneficial to use larger-font handouts with diagrams to accompany your verbal instructions. This will also assist in alleviating memory difficulties regarding the specific exercises you provide the patient once she or he is to begin home exercises.

Because older patients may have compromised vascular supply, it may take them longer than younger patients to heal following an injury. As with any patient, it is advantageous to use the patient's response to your program as a guide to progression. If the patient reports increased pain or swelling, the program may be progressing too quickly for his or her body to adjust. Remind the patient that good nutrition and adequate water intake are both important for optimal healing.

Flexibility may be reduced in older patients. Hamstring flexibility is usually less in older groups than in younger patients, with men having less flexibility than women (Youdas et al., 2005). Given that muscle tissue and tendon tissue are weaker in older patients, overstretching should be avoided. Stretching exercises, however, should be used with patients lacking normal flexibility. Ballistic types of flexibility exercises are not recommended for older patients. Slow, controlled stretches for 10 to 15 s repeated four times, as for other age groups, are safe and adequate for this age group.

Strengthening exercises will be a part of an older athlete's therapeutic exercise program. Recommendations for sets and repetitions in strengthening programs for all populations including the elderly have been established by ACSM and other professional groups (Feigenbaum and Pollock, 1999). However, no recommendations have been established for orthopedic- and sport-injured elderly groups. Lacking any research evidence in this area, I have devised a protocol based on my own experiences and existing related evidence. As already mentioned, older individuals normally have diminished muscle strength, muscle endurance, and muscle mass. Because of poorer balance and a thinning of articular cartilage that occurs with age along with these muscle changes, it seems that the best way to improve muscle strength is not to overstress joints and body support with excessive weights but rather to improve muscle function through muscle endurance exercises. Such exercises will improve strength and muscle endurance and will build muscle tissue without overstressing joints. Avoidance of heavy weights will also prevent issues such as the patient's not being able to adjust body balance to the added weight and falling. For example, my preference is to start with two sets of 12 to 15 repetitions and progress to three sets of 12 to 15 repetitions before moving to three sets of 20 to 25 repetitions. When an older patient is able to lift a weight with a given set and repetition goal for a minimum of one to three treatments, then the weight is increased. The number of visits using a particular goal before the weight is increased will depend upon a variety of factors, including the patient's age, fitness level, and long-term goals.

A light weight is advised, with adjustments depending on the patient's response to the weight initially used. If it is apparent that the weight is very light (the patient completes sets and repetitions beyond the goal or even expresses a desire to use more weight), then more rapid adjustments may be made. Lower-extremity closed-chain exercises involving multiple joints and muscles allow greater resistance to be used than when a muscle is isolated in an open chain exercise. For example, a smaller weight such as 5 lb (about 2 kg) may be as much as a patient is able to manage in an open chain knee extension exercise, but the same patient may be able to perform a half-squat with half the body weight on each lower extremity because the ankle and hip muscles are also used.

Reflexes and reaction to changes in body position are not as rapid in older patients. When you use a new exercise that requires balance, it is prudent for you to spot the patient for protection from possible falls. A slower progression may also be beneficial to ensure that the patient is able to manage a new exercise with less risk of falling. For example, if you have been having the patient work on single-leg stance on the floor and want to advance him or her to the trampoline, it may be better to advance to a foam rubber pad before the trampoline. Using small increments between the progressions will help to prevent falls and also give the patient confidence in his or her own abilities. Also, the goal with single-leg stance is not the 30 s expected of younger patients; remember that although some senior-aged patients may be able to achieve 30 s, the average for this age group is 19 s. Progression in balance will be slower than in younger patients. As with strengthening, it is beneficial to have a patient remain at a given level for one to three sessions before advancing to a new, more difficult level.

Warm-up and cool-down are important aspects of an exercise program (Kallinen and Markku, 1995). Keeping in mind the target heart rates in table 17.3 and the patient's individual conditioning level, a warm-up activity such as a 10 min stationary bike or elliptical exercise may be beneficial—more so than a hot pack to warm muscles in preparation for other exercises. Flexibility exercises at the end of a therapeutic exercise program are not only a good way to cool down; they also provide optimal lengthening of warmed muscles (Warren, Lehmann, and Koblanski, 1976).

SUMMARY

Individuals from a wide range of ages participate in sports and life-long exercise. Individuals from youngsters to senior-aged adults, by the mere fact of being active, are at risk for injury. When people within these groups suffer injuries, they turn to clinicians for treatment so they can recover and return to their activities. Clinicians must therefore understand the impact age has on both recovery and rehabilitation progression. Although young athletes may heal faster than older athletes, they are at risk for joint injuries that may affect their growth. Older athletes who suffer injuries similar to younger athletes will not heal nor progress in their rehabilitation programs at the same rate as their younger counterparts. This chapter addressed the important distinctions relevant to injuries and rehabilitation in these groups compared to the group on which most timelines and recoveries are based, the youthful adult population.

KEY CONCEPTS AND REVIEW

1. Account for why there are more people involved in sport today and therefore more who incur sport injuries.

There are more youth leagues and more organized sports than in previous generations. Additionally, people are living longer, and the "baby boomer" generation is more involved in athletic activities throughout their adult years and into their retirement than previous generations.

2. Why is so little known about sport injuries in the very young and the very old?

The information we refer to in our sport rehabilitation practices is obtained from studies that usually involve subjects in their early-adult years. Since many of the studies are performed on university campuses, the subjects' age range is 18 to 25. These subjects are in the physical prime of their lives; they have passed through the years of puberty and have not yet entered their declining years. Relatively few studies have investigated sport injuries in either older or younger populations.

3. So why is it important to know how to manage injuries of preadolescent athletes and athletes who are older?

National statistics on employment of certified athletic trainers in the United States indicate that approximately half of this group works in outpatient clinics. Outpatient clinics are settings in which these two age groups are treated for their orthopedic and sport injuries. These two populations are expanding; related to this population growth will be an increase in the number of injuries seen in outpatient clinics. Rehabilitation clinicians must be aware of how to treat these groups if they are to provide successful rehabilitation programs.

4. Provide an outline of growth and development based on the Tanner system and explain how boys and girls vary in the process.

The Tanner system identifies different developmental stages for secondary sexual characteristics, rate of height changes, and muscle development. A typical pubertal growth pattern begins with a phase of acceleration; this is followed by a phase of deceleration before growth ceases. Growth stops when the epiphyses close, at approximately 18 years in girls and 20 years in boys. Girls begin this growth pattern earlier and end it earlier, usually about two years ahead of their male counterparts in each case. Although the exact age when the puberty process begins varies from one individual to another, the average starting age for girls is 9 years and for boys is 11 years.

5. Identify the problems associated with an ACL reconstruction for a younger athlete.

Because the patient's physis remains open, reconstruction must avoid damaging the still-growing bone. Additionally, instability of the joint because of either ACL injury or injury to the meniscus is likely to result in premature osteoarthritis. Care must be taken both during the surgery and in rehabilitation to ensure optimal healing without damage to articular cartilage or the epiphyseal plate.

6. Explain the precautions that one should take when providing a therapeutic exercise program to an older patient.

Instructions should be given slowly and the voice should be low in pitch if the patient has difficulty hearing. Providing visual instructions with larger-than-normal print and images is advisable for all older patients, especially those with vision problems. Flexibility exercises may be performed as with other age groups. Strength exercises should begin with a low resistance for 12 to 15 repetitions and should progress slowly to three sets of 20 to 25 repetitions. The progression should allow for a few days at one level before the patient advances to the next weight. Balance and coordination exercises should begin at a low level and progress with small increments from one level to the next. Adequate warm-up and cool-down are recommended for each session.

CRITICAL THINKING QUESTIONS

1. An 11-year old competitive cheerleader comes to you with a diagnosis of Sever's disease, with more pain in the left heel than in the right. Her mother indicates that the patient is very competitive at the national level and wants to compete in the upcoming season, which starts in two months. Your examination of her demonstrates extreme tenderness on the left heel and moderate tenderness on the right heel. She is unable to jump because of pain. How will you explain this condition to the patient and her mother? What will you do for her rehabilitation program? What precautions must you consider? What will you tell the patient and her mother regarding the upcoming competitive season?

2. A 15-year-old basketball player underwent an autologous ACL reconstruction three weeks ago. He is still partial weight bearing on the right lower extremity, but the surgeon is having him begin rehabilitation. The surgeon wants the patient to continue partial weight bearing until six weeks post-op. At that time the patient can get rid of his crutches and the brace he is wearing as long as he is able to walk without a limp. What will you do with him between now and the time he is full weight bearing to ensure that he is able to walk normally by six weeks post-op?

3. A 55-year-old competitive golfer tore his rotator cuff while golfing. He hit a large divot and felt a severe pain in his shoulder. He had a rotator cuff repair last week. The surgeon is sending the patient to you to begin his rehabilitation program. She wants the patient to wear the sling he is currently wearing for another three weeks, but she wants you to remove the sling during his exercises. She does not want the patient to move the shoulder to more than 80° of flexion, 45° of abduction, and 0° of lateral rotation for the first six weeks post-op. For the first two weeks with you, the physician has indicated that she wants you to work primarily on relieving the pain, spasm, and swelling and on making sure that the patient does not get a frozen shoulder from wearing the sling. How will you manage this patient for these next two weeks? What will you do to fulfill the physician's requests?

LAB ACTIVITIES

1. Find x-rays of joints of teenagers and older adults. Compare the x-rays and identify how they are different and how they are the same.

2. Create a table with three columns, one for preadolescent, one for adolescent, and one for older adults. Under each of these titles, list the items that must be considered in putting together a therapeutic exercise program for each age group. Include special considerations (such as hearing) and other factors such as rate of progression, precautions, etc.

3. Look up the ACSM recommendations for both the youth and the older adult populations' exercise programs. As in #2, make columns and place a listing of these recommendations for each of the groups in their respective columns. Identify the similarities and differences between the two. How do you explain these differences and similarities?

4. Compare the posture of one of your siblings, one of your parents, and one of your grandparents. How do differences in their ages affect their posture? What exercises should you give each of them to improve their posture?

5. Looking at the opening scenario, Chaz understands the physical and physiological considerations (AAP, 2001; Tanigawa, 1972) as he progresses Lorrie in her rehabilitation program. What are the considerations he must realize if he is to create a safe and successful program for her?

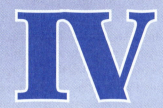
Specific Applications

The quality of a person's life is in direct proportion to their commitment to excellence, regardless of their chosen field of endeavor.

VINCE LOMBARDI, NFL football coach, 1913-1970

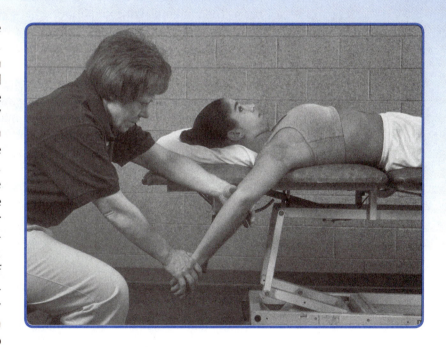

Parts I, II, and III have established the groundwork for this final part of the book. Having acquired the information from the earlier parts, you are now prepared to fully understand and appreciate the information presented in part IV. Part IV is where you will put all the information and knowledge you have gained in the other parts into whole therex programs. Part IV consists of therapeutic exercise programs for each body segment. The programs are not divided by activity, for an ankle sprain is an ankle sprain regardless of whether it occurs in basketball, volleyball, or at work, and regardless of whether it is incurred by a teenager, college student, or other individual. The only point when a treatment program for an injury will deviate from one individual to another is in the final stages of therapeutic exercise, when the patient begins specific functional exercises that will allow return to a specific activity.

Although I will offer timelines of normal progression, part IV is not a cookbook for rehabilitation of injuries. A cookbook is not necessary, nor is it practical. Now that you have the information from parts I, II, and III, you have the tools to design your own rehabilitation programs. Because each patient must have an individualized program, a cookbook approach is irrelevant and useless. The information in part IV provides suggestions for exercises and treatment techniques, but for application, you will depend on the knowledge you have gained throughout this text to put those suggestions together in an appropriate and formidable program for each patient with whom you work.

By now it should be clear that the rehabilitation clinician is a combination of detective, problem solver, innovator, and educator who follows laws of knowledge, skill application, logic, and common sense to achieve the final goal of returning a patient to full participation as efficiently and safely as possible. Detective work involves examination of the injury's status, determination of the underlying causes of the injury to correct these causes and reduce the chance of re-injury, and continual reassessment of the patient's response to the treatment so the results are positive.

As a problem solver, the rehabilitation clinician must be able to adjust treatment programs, exercises, and progression sequences when a patient does not respond according to expectations. The individualized program produces individual results, so the rehabilitation clinician must be alert to problems and must be able to adjust the program as needed for each patient.

As an innovator, the rehabilitation clinician attempts to achieve treatment goals and still make the program interesting and stimulating for the patient to help ensure compliance in the therapeutic exercise program. If equipment is limited, innovation becomes an even more important element, because making the program interesting and challenging using minimal materials presents an even greater test of the rehabilitation clinician's imagination. This situation of limited resources can make a therapeutic exercise program as interesting and challenging for you to design as it is for the patient to perform.

Throughout a therapeutic exercise program, the rehabilitation clinician is an educator. The patient is educated regarding the "dos and don'ts" following an injury—what activities are important to perform and what activities should be avoided to prevent further harm. The patient is educated about what to do to protect the injury and to promote an uneventful healing process. The patient is educated with regard to the injury, the rehabilitation program process, the rationale for specific exercises, and the importance of home exercises; each of these is vital to assuring the patient's compliance and the program's success. The rehabilitation clinician educates the patient throughout the program as the injury changes and the program evolves.

The rehabilitation clinician's knowledge, understanding, observation skills, evaluation skills, application skills, and ability to apply common sense and logic all contribute to the success of the rehabilitation process. Rehabilitation involves applying all these elements to provide a balanced program for the patient—one that provides appropriate stresses with the right degree of protection to advance the patient efficiently and effectively toward the goal of safe return to participation as soon as possible.

Along with all of these caveats on putting a rehabilitation program together, the final one is that the rehabilitation clinician should make the program fun for both the patient and clinician.

The clinician with a good imagination can combine that imagination with all the knowledge and skills that have been learned to create a rehabilitation program to not only achieve the program's goals but stimulate the patient to perform at his or her best in rehabilitation and make the treatment something to look forward to each day.

PROGRAM CONSIDERATIONS

The specific elements and the complexity of a rehabilitation program are determined by a variety of factors. These include the magnitude of the injury, the type of injury, the body segment involved, the patient's activity, the patient's response to the injury (physical, emotional, and psychological), and the patient's goals. All must be considered in the injury examination design and rehabilitation program execution.

Examination

Before providing treatment in a rehabilitation program, the rehabilitation clinician examines the injury to determine where in the healing process the injury is and how irritable it is. If the injury is very irritable, regardless of healing stage, the treatment must begin gently and include primarily modalities to calm the area. If the patient had reconstructive surgery three days ago, the initial treatments are not aggressive with strengthening activities. If, on the other hand, the injury is not very irritable and is well along in the healing process, the rehabilitation clinician can be more aggressive in the first treatment. Whatever the initial treatment includes, careful observation for responses to the treatment is necessary, both during the first treatment session and before the next. The current treatment course is always determined by the injury's response to the previous treatment session.

Modalities

A total rehabilitation program includes the use of modalities to modulate pain and enhance healing. Modalities serve as preliminary adjuncts to the total program and should not be the primary means of returning the patient to full participation. Once pain modulation and healing are under way, therapeutic exercises become the primary emphasis in the rehabilitation process. Since this text includes information specific to therapeutic exercise, you should keep in mind as you read the following chapters that although a complete rehabilitation program may include pain-modulating modalities and efforts to manage and promote the healing process, these are not included in this text.

An injury does not have to become entirely pain free before exercises begin. In fact, most of the time it is not desirable to wait until the patient is completely pain free before starting exercises. Pain and swelling, however, are monitored throughout the rehabilitation process, especially in the first half of the therapeutic exercise program when the newly forming tissue is more susceptible to overstress from exercise than it is later. Both pain and edema act as neural inhibitors, reducing the patient's rehabilitation output and ability to perform therapeutic exercises (Fahrer et al., 1988; Leroux, Bélanger, & Boucher, 1995).

Remember the advice of Hippocrates: "Do no harm." If you are unsure as to whether you should advance a patient's program, do not until you are sure it is appropriate to do so. If you have any doubt about whether an exercise may cause edema or increased pain later, it is advisable to apply ice following the exercise session to reduce the risk for these deleterious effects. As you obtain a more accurate impression of the patient's ability to tolerate the stresses applied during the therapeutic exercise program, and as the injury advances in the remodeling phase, application of ice after a session becomes optional and relates more to the patient's preference or comfort level than to any physiological benefit.

Maintenance of Conditioning Level

Periodically throughout this book, I have emphasized the importance of maintaining cardiovascular health and conditioning levels of non-injured body segments. Although this is a vital aspect of a total therapeutic exercise program, it is not addressed in the chapters in part IV; however, you should always include exercises for these parameters in a rehabilitation program. The exercises discussed in this part of the book include only those relevant to the injured segment.

CHAPTER SEGMENTS

Each chapter in part IV includes specifics on various aspects of topics covered in earlier chapters. The first portion of each chapter in part IV includes general considerations and specific techniques corresponding to concepts, theories, and applications presented in part II: soft-tissue and joint mobilization. The next portion deals with the usual progression of therapeutic techniques for achieving goals of normal range of motion, strength and muscle endurance, and coordination and agility. Once you are familiar with these elements, you will learn to apply them in the next section of the chapter, "Special Rehabilitation Applications." These sections address injuries that require special program considerations, precautions, or unique therapeutic exercise applications, followed by case studies. Specific answers are not given for the questions in these case studies because the studies are meant to stimulate discussion between students and instructor. There is no right answer for each question, because the answer is driven by the particulars of the case and is to some extent flexible, as dictated by the rehabilitation clinician's preferences and the equipment available. Of course, you must take into consideration specific precautions, contraindications, healing timeline, and injury-unique information when creating a program for each case study.

Soft-Tissue Mobilization

You may want to refer to earlier chapters that deal specifically with these techniques to review technique application. Soft-tissue mobilization techniques in the chapters to follow do not include the full range of soft-tissue techniques discussed in chapter 6. The primary techniques discussed are myofascial release and trigger point release. You should realize that these specific techniques or other soft-tissue mobilization techniques may or may not be indicated in individual situations; you must examine the patient's injury to decide whether they may be appropriate. The intent of the discussion of these techniques is to provide examples to help you appreciate the important role that soft-tissue mobilization can play in the total rehabilitation process.

The soft-tissue pain-referral patterns discussed in these chapters are based on the extensive work of Travell and Simons (1983, 1992). Other pain-referral patterns are based on common neurological patterns.

Joint Mobilization

As discussed in chapter 6, joint mobilization is a complex technique entailing either accessory movements or physiological movements. When using joint mobilization, the rehabilitation clinician should remember that the movement is produced not by the rehabilitation clinician's hands but by his or her body; this produces a better perception of the movement by the clinician and a more comfortable sensation for the patient. The hands are the vehicles through which the rehabilitation clinician's body produces the joint motion.

Joint mobilization is not used in all conditions. Positive results in mobilization should usually occur within four to five days (Maitland, 1991). As discussed in chapter 6, joint mobilization is appropriate for treatment of pain using I and II grades of movement or treatment of joint stiffness using grade III or IV. These movements can be oscillatory motions or sustained. Please refer to chapter 6 for review of these techniques if necessary.

Most of the joint mobilization techniques presented in part IV are based on a combination of Kaltenborn's and Maitland's works. Various scholars have developed a number of variations and techniques. At the back of this book is a listing of suggested readings that you can refer to for specific instruction in joint mobilization techniques.

Therapeutic Exercise Phases

The therapeutic exercise phases differ slightly from the rehabilitation phases outlined in chapter 2. The primary difference is that the therapeutic exercise program does not include very early aspects of rehabilitation. Of course, the emphasis in the early stage of rehabilitation is to get the inflammation under control and protect the healing process, as dealt with in earlier chapters. Although the rehabilitation clinician must know what constitutes a total rehabilitation program and know how to administer such a program, only therapeutic exercises and manual techniques are addressed in the following chapters.

If the modalities portion of the rehabilitation program is the first phase, the therapeutic exercise portion of a rehabilitation program can be divided into three additional phases: early (phase II), middle (phase III), and late (phase IV) exercise phases. In administration of a program, the exercise progression is not specifically dictated; but the components of the progression are distinguished here to make the progression easier to comprehend and identify.

Phase I: Inactive Phase

The early part of the rehabilitation program is very important since it influences the injury's secondary problems: pain, muscle spasm, and edema. It is a time of relative inactivity to relieve the problems that occur from injury and insult to tissue. If these factors are controlled and healing is encouraged in an optimal environment, advancement to the remaining phases occurs on schedule.

The goals of this phase are to *relieve* pain, edema, and muscle spasm. Additionally, the goal is to maintain a proper conditioning level of the non-affected body segments and the cardiovascular system. During this phase the injured segment is in the inflammation phase of healing, so caution must be part of the treatment protocol. Aggravating the injury site is contraindicated.

Accomplishing these goals utilizes a number of items such as thermal and electrical modalities, massage, and other manual therapies. Depending on the tissue involved, the specific injury, and its severity, motion may or may not be permitted during this phase. Exercises, if instituted, must not disrupt or threaten fragile healing tissue.

Phase II: Active Phase

Phase II begins once the injured segment is past inflammation and is in the proliferation phase. Tissue strength through the advent of collagen fibers is gradually increasing, and structures are becoming resilient enough to tolerate some stress. Therefore, activity of the injured segment may be permitted. Pain, edema, and muscle spasm are either no longer present or minor issues that are still resolving with various procedures utilized in the inactive phase. During phase II these factors are resolved, if they have not yet been eliminated as problems.

Goals during this phase are to improve range of motion and flexibility, begin strength gains, and improve balance and proprioception. Treatment in this phase includes mobility techniques such as joint and soft-tissue mobilization and range-of-motion exercises. If exercises started during late inflammation, range of motion was likely the only exercise at that time. In the active phase with tissue's increased stability, strength and proprioception exercises begin. The closer to the inflammation phase the injury is, the more cautious the clinician should be in the amount of stress applied to newly developing tissue. In some cases, exercises may not be permitted until three weeks after injury.

Range of motion and flexibility are important factors to restore during phase II. Along with joint and soft tissue mobilization techniques, passive, active, and assistive exercises can also be used to improve motion. Early strengthening exercises vary depending on the severity of the injury and include a range of activities, such as isometrics and concentric, concentric-eccentric, and/or eccentric exercises. Isometric exercises are often performed in either multiple angles, midrange, or in an anatomic position, depending on mobility and medical restrictions for motion. Strength exercises are usually performed in a straight plane, not progressing to diagonal or functional positions until the patient has achieved sufficient strength in straight-plane movement to control the extremity through a functional motion. It is common for strength exercises to begin with high repetitions and low weights. This reduces stress on joints that may not be strong enough to tolerate the shear forces produced by heavy resistance. Proprioception exercises begin at a simple level and do not advance to exercises that are more complex until the patient demonstrates an ability to perform the lower-level activity well.

Phase III: Resistive Phase

By the time the patient progresses to phase III, range of motion is nearly or completely normal. Edema and pain are no longer problems. Strength and muscle endurance have improved but remain deficient. This phase is the resistive phase since our primary goal is to completely restore any deficient parameters in strength, agility, and endurance so the patient can move to the final rehabilitation phase. It is during the resistive phase that tensile strength is significantly greater than in earlier phases, so the clinician and patient is able to focus on restoration of remaining deficiencies.

Phase III begins anywhere from the end of the proliferation phase of healing into the remodeling phase. Determinants on when this phase begins include physician preference for progression and the patient's response to the program. Goals during this phase are to maintain the parameters that have been restored and to restore the patient's strength, muscle endurance, and agility to normal levels.

Exercises include more aggressive strength and muscle endurance exercises than were used previously. Additionally, more aggressive proprioception exercises that evolve to agility activities are included. Even if motion is normal, flexibility exercises should continue in this phase to prevent a loss of motion since continued contraction occurs because of the myofibril activity during the healing process. If flexibility is not yet normal, more assertive stretching exercises occur during this phase. This is the time the patient begins more aggressive exercises, as discussed in chapter 1, including a progression of exercises that continue to make gains in range of motion, strength, muscle endurance, and proprioception. Strength exercises here are in transition. In the beginning of this phase, patients may perform the strength exercises primarily in a straight plane, but as the patient continues towards the end of this phase, many exercises advance to diagonal, functional patterns of movement. This is possible because the muscle strength improves to a level that allows the patient to maintain extremity control while moving the segment.

Proprioception exercises become more complex in this phase. They may include multiple task-activities, and the aim is to help prepare the patient for the stresses of functional activities in the next phase.

Phase IV: Aggressive Phase

Phase III exercises ready the patient for phase IV exercises, when power, strength, and coordination are jointly stressed in agility activities. This time is also called the aggressive phase because exercises during this phase mimic all the stresses that the patient will be facing when he or she returns to normal activities. By the time the patient reaches the final phase, flexibility, strength, and muscle endurance are all at near-normal levels; so the patient is ready for more advanced, aggressive activities that further stress the injured area in preparation for return to normal activities. At this point, the only real deficit lies in the patient's functional activity and performance levels so the goals in this phase are to restore the patient's functional abilities and the activity- and sport-specific activities that will permit the patient to resume all pre-injury participation. Flexibility and strength activities are now at maintenance levels, and the major emphasis is on finely-tuning the patient for a smooth transition and return to normal participation. Although these chapters mention functional activities, they do not fully address activity-specific exercises because these are so numerous and so varied in their demands. You must remember, however, that functional activities are a vital part of the final phase and must always be part of a therapeutic exercise program. Functional activities should evolve to a progression of activity-specific exercises. Functional activities begin with less stress, speed, force, and distance and continue to increase these parameters as the patient's body adjusts to the stresses and the patient acquires better skill and ability to execute his or her performance-specific activities appropriately.

Exercise Continuum

The exercises for each phase lie on a rehabilitation continuum. On the continuum are all the previously presented parameters, as well as exercises corresponding to the phases as seen in the figure in this introduction. The diagram outlines the progression of a therapeutic exercise program according to parameter and divides those parameters according to the exercise phases of a program. The progression is a continuum

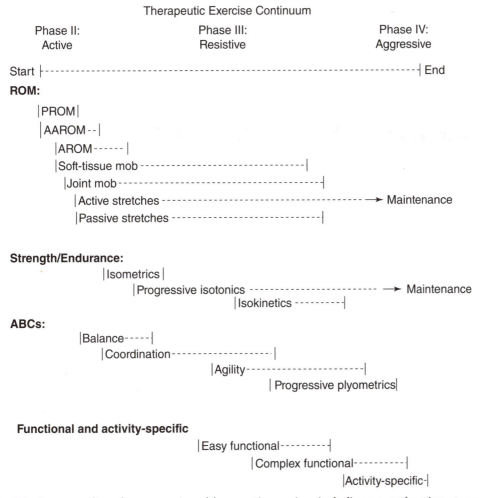

▶ This diagram outlines the progression of therapeutic exercises, including range of motion, strength endurance, proprioception, and functional and activity-specific exercises, in the active, resistive, and aggressive phases of a program.

in that all exercises in a therapeutic exercise program flow from one level to the next. It is sometimes difficult to determine whether an exercise corresponds to the active or resistive exercise phase or to the resistive or aggressive exercise phase, and a particular exercise can correspond to one phase with one injury and another phase with another injury. That is the essence of a continuum.

PUTTING IT ALL TOGETHER

The purpose of the exercise phase continuum is less to delineate a specific program and progression for a patient than to give you a mental image that helps you identify how to advance a patient in a therapeutic exercise program. Knowing to which phase an exercise corresponds is not as important as recognizing the progression and level of difficulty of the exercise and identifying when the patient is able to move from one level to the next.

To make the rehabilitation program progression even less clear cut and more confusing, a patient may be in the active phase with one parameter and in the resistive phase with another parameter. For example, the patient may have good range of motion and grade 4/5 strength, indicating that he or she is in the resistive exercise phase of a therapeutic exercise program, but the balance ability of that patient may still be in the active exercise phase. Each segment must be stressed to its capacity as long as other segments are not overly stressed. As an example, a patient with shoulder impingement and weakness of the scapular rotators should not be advanced to open chain exercises in the higher elevations of motion if such exercises will worsen the injury; if the scapular muscles lack sufficient strength, they will not be able to hold the scapula properly to prevent impingement. In that case, although coordination abilities of the patient may be able to advance, his or her strength remains deficient, so attempting to advance the coordination parameter before strength improves will aggravate the injury.

THERAPEUTIC EXERCISE INDIVIDUALIZATION

As has been mentioned throughout this book, it is important to design the patient's therapeutic exercise program for the individual. Even though two patients have ankle sprains, they will not necessarily progress at the same rate, so expectations of patients following the same timeline are not appropriate. These patients may even have different exercises within their programs. The individual's injury and the body's response to the injury, the patient's abilities and goals, and the way the patient responds to both the program and the clinician all determine the exercises selected, the rate of progression, and the final outcome of the therapeutic exercise program. Using other guidelines for expectations leads to frustration for both the patient and the rehabilitation clinician.

The clinician should continually assess the patient's performance; examine outcomes before, during, and after treatment to see whether the treatment has had the desired effect; and be ready to alter treatments if undesirable effects occur. It is essential to obtain information from the patient regarding post-treatment responses to accurately assess the effects of the treatment program. If increased pain, swelling, and other deleterious effects occur after treatment, the program has been too stressful. Progression without regression should be the rehabilitation clinician's creed. In other words, the program should challenge the patient enough to improve all parameters without overstressing the injury to increase symptoms.

CHAPTER PROGRESSION

Part IV begins with the spine (chapter 18) and then moves to the upper extremities (chapters 19-21); the final chapters (22-24) include therapeutic exercise programs for the lower extremities. The material is presented this way because many upper- and lower-extremity problems can be related to the core, the spine. The spine is also an important consideration in rehabilitation of upper and lower extremities because core strength is vital for both upper- and lower-segment stability and performance.

It would be nearly impossible to list all the exercises in a therapeutic exercise program. Those outlined in these chapters include more commonly used activities, as well as some that are unique for each parameter. As always, the clinician's knowledge of injury healing, appreciation of the patient's abilities, the facilities and equipment available, and his or her own imagination are the only limiting factors of a therapeutic exercise program. A therapeutic exercise program can be fun and challenging for the patient as well as the rehabilitation clinician. The clinician can be imaginative in providing stimulating exercises for the patient so both enjoy the rehabilitation process. So as you read these next few chapters, see whether you can think of exercises in addition to those presented that would challenge and stimulate a patient in a therapeutic exercise program.

Spine and Sacroiliac

OBJECTIVES

After completing this chapter, you should be able to do the following:

1. Explain three flexibility exercises for the cervical spine and lumbar spine.
2. Explain three strengthening exercises for the cervical spine and lumbar spine.
3. Identify three progressive spinal stability exercises.
4. Identify three sacroiliac muscle energy release techniques and the indications for their use.
5. Outline a therapeutic exercise program for a cervical sprain.
6. List precautions for a therapeutic exercise program for disc lesions.
7. Discuss the difference in therapeutic exercise programs for a lumbar strain and a facet injury.
8. Present a sequence of activities to begin a core strengthening program.
9. Outline the exercises in Williams' Flexion program and McKenzie's Back Program.
10. Explain the differences between McKenzie's postural syndromes, dysfunction, and derangement.
11. Explain the various McKenzie derangements.

► About half the patients Rita sees have back injuries. Joey, a high school athlete she is currently rehabilitating, is one of these. While practicing his high-jump maneuver last week, he slipped during his approach and injured his back. Now that the muscle spasms are resolved, Rita is improving Joey's soft-tissue mobility with myofascial release (MFR) across the lumbar area. His sacroiliac came out of alignment when he slipped, so Rita used muscle energy techniques and home exercises to correct the problem. Her initial examination revealed significant weakness of the trunk muscles, so she plans to develop Joey's abdominal and back strength. Rita is confident that this will not only protect Joey's back from further injury but may also improve his high jump.

Courage is the power to let go of the familiar.

RAYMOND LINDQUIST, American pastor, author

This chapter begins the fun part of therapeutic exercise, applying the science that we have been discussing and letting our imaginations create therapeutic exercise programs. We will start the true blending of science and art in rehabilitation. We now have the opportunity to apply our scientific knowledge in an artful manner to provide patients with a complete, stimulating, and challenging therapeutic exercise program that will allow those patients a safe and speedy return to full participation and normal activity.

Oftentimes, the spine is not as familiar to clinicians as the extremities. As a result, clinicians do not enjoy working with patients who suffer injuries of the spine. This chapter will familiarize you with the spine and allow you to realize that spine injuries, like extremity injuries are approachable and treatable.

The spine and sacroilium (SI) are composed of several different segments. Any segment can have separate injuries that do not affect the other spinal regions. They also can have injuries that affect or are affected by other regions. Since the spine and SI are interrelated, we are considering the spine and sacroilium together.

There are both similarities and unique characteristics among regions of the spine. For example, in the thoracic region, each vertebra is joined with a rib; the cervical spine has the atlas and brachial plexus; and the lumbar region has the lumbar plexus, larger vertebral bodies, and is connected to the sacrum. Examples of similarities are that vertebrae in the three regions have spinous and transverse processes and are separated by discs.

This chapter addresses general rehabilitation concepts for the spine. Some of the factors unique to the spine that influence a rehabilitation program are also introduced. Many texts are devoted to spine anatomy and function, so this chapter by no means deals with all there is to know about the spine. The aim is to present key information that will enable you to treat most spine and spine-related injuries that you will encounter as a rehabilitation clinician.

The spine is a complex structure that is often neglected in education programs because of its uniqueness in comparison to the upper and lower extremities. Rather than approach the spine as another body segment that is subject to injury and in need of treatment, many approach the topic with apprehension because of ignorance and fear: ignorance because the spine seems to be a mystifying body segment that is far too complex to understand, and fear because its complexity gets in the way of appreciating its simplicity.

The spine is complex. So is the shoulder. So is the knee. There are many segments of the body that we still have much to learn about and understand, yet we do not hesitate to deal with injuries to these segments. The spine is like any other segment in that, regardless of its complexity, it is often injured and needs to be addressed. This chapter deals with common spinal injuries and outlines typical therapeutic exercise programs for them.

By the end of the chapter, you should view the spine not as a body segment to shy away from, but rather an area that you can approach with an appreciation of both its simplicity and its complexity.

Catastrophic injuries that include spinal cord injury resulting in paralysis are not among injuries seen for therapeutic exercise with the goal of returning the patient to sport participation, so they are not addressed here.

GENERAL REHABILITATION CONSIDERATIONS

It was not long ago that conservative treatment of spine injuries, especially low-back injuries, involved bed rest for extended periods of time. As medical professionals realized how detrimental immobilization and extended rest were and noticed that those individuals who did not rest improved faster than those who did, the standard of care for spine injuries changed. Current treatment applications include minimal rest and progression into activity as quickly as is appropriate for the individual and the specific injury (Kasai, 2006).

Williams' Flexion Exercises

For many years, Williams' flexion exercises were the accepted back-exercise regimen. Paul Williams was an orthopedic surgeon who believed that lordosis was the cause of low back pain. Williams' flexion exercises are a series of six exercises that emphasize flexion and include activities (Williams, 1955). These are the six exercises (figure 18.1):

- Exercise #1: Sit-up in a flexed-knee position to strengthen the abdominals.
- Exercise #2: Pelvic tilt to strengthen the gluteal muscles.

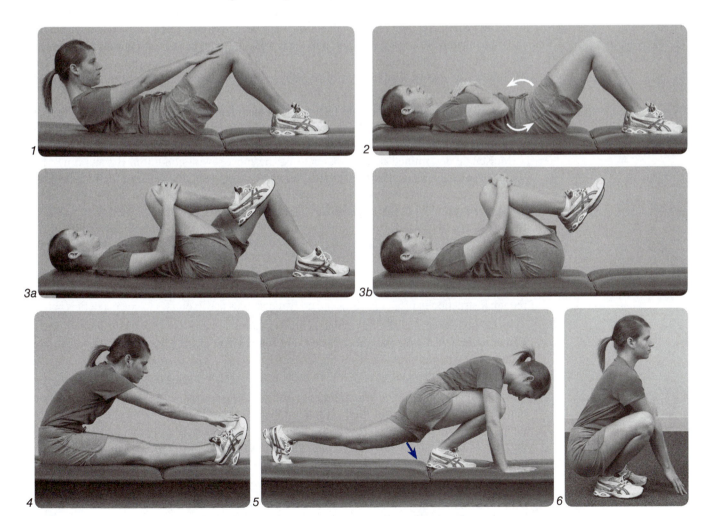

▶ **Figure 18.1** Williams' flexion exercises #1 through 6, see text for descriptions.

- Exercise #3: Single knee-to-chest and double knee-to-chest to stretch the erector spinae muscles.
- Exercise #4: Seated reach to the toes with knees extended to stretch the erector spinae and hamstring muscles.
- Exercise #5: In a quadruped position with one knee forward under the chest and the other hip and knee in extension to stretch the tensor fascia lata and iliofemoral ligament.
- Exercise #6: Starting in standing and moving to a full squat to strengthen the quadriceps muscles.

McKenzie Back Program

Later, extension exercises became the exercises of choice because flexion exercises made many patients with disc injuries worse. Extension exercises, advanced by Robin McKenzie, a New Zealand physiotherapist, emphasize trunk extension aimed at relieving posterior pressure on discs (McKenzie, 1981). His rationale was that the disc is the primary source of back pain. Disc problems occur because people spend a lot of time in sitting positions and other positions of flexion, not moving enough into extension to relieve disc pressures. He, therefore, advocated primarily extension exercises to relieve disc pressures. Additionally, he divided back problems into three progressive syndrome classifications: postural syndromes, dysfunctions, and derangements.

According to McKenzie, postural syndromes are the first step in progressive chronic back pain. This condition is not severe and occurs during one's teen years and early twenties. The patient experiences back, neck, or interscapular pain, especially after prolonged postures in sitting. The pain is intermittent in this stage, and the patient's examination is essentially negative.

Unfortunately, if no steps are taken to correct posture and habit, the condition may progress to the next syndrome, dysfunction. It is during this phase that early changes are noted. There is some loss of accessory joint movement, reduced range of motion, and diminished soft tissue mobility. Neurological examinations during this phase, however are negative. The patient may complain of either intermittent or constant pain and stiffness. It is imperative that posture and deficiencies in soft tissue and joint mobility be corrected to prevent the patient from advancing to the final phase.

McKenzie determined derangements to be the most severe condition. By this time, the source of pain has changed from inflammation of peripheral structures to the disc. Poor posture, over time, changes vertebral positions, leading to advanced stress that produces disc alterations and degeneration. McKenzie further divided derangements into seven different types. The first six deal with posterior disc pathology and the seventh involves anterior disc pathology:

- Derangement #1: There is a mild disc bulge with either central or asymmetrical pain in the back. The pain results from irritation to the posterior annulus and the posterior longitudinal ligament caused by the bulging disc. Usually the pain subsides in a few days, but these patients require instruction in proper posture and body mechanics and exercises to correct deficiencies.
- Derangement #2: The disc bulge is now moderate in size and may cause buttock pain. Examination reveals the patient to have a flat lumbar spine and some pain when changing positions or when in prolonged sitting. In addition to the exercises and posture activities for derangement #1, the patient may find relief when lying in a prone position.
- Derangement #3: The disc bulge is now more prominent, with pain occurring to the buttock or even the posterior thigh. Although there is no deformity visible, the pain is more intense. At this time, the goal is to relieve the pain referral down the extremity and "centralize" the pain, or move it more proximally until the pain is restricted to the central spine. Repetitive exercises of trunk extension in a prone position are added to the previous exercises.
- Derangement #4: The pain is pronounced down one extremity to the knee, and the patient exhibits a shift of the lumbar spine. If the bulge occurs medial to the nerve root (figure 18.2a), the shift is to the same side as the pain, but if the derangement is lateral to the nerve root (figure 18.2b), the shift is towards the contralateral side of pain. This is the body's method of

reducing stress on the nerve root. The first step in treating this derangement is to correct the shift. Following that step, efforts to centralize the pain by providing extension exercises and then follow the treatment program for derangement #1 are included in treatment of this derangement.

■ Derangement #5: Disc degeneration continues now to where the patient experiences unilateral referred pain below the knee. No deformity is noted on examination, but the progressive bulge of the annulus fibrosis causes irritation of the nerve root and the dura. Although the patient's pain is more intense and less positions of comfort may be found, treatment goals are to centralize the pain through repeated extension exercises and continue with other treatment aspects outlined for derangement #1. It is probably necessary to have the patient perform the extension exercises in side-lying or prone, not in extension.

■ Derangement #6: In this derangement, the disc is herniated through the annulus fibrosis. The unilateral extremity pain is below the knee and may go into the foot. The patient reports feelings of paresthesia, weakness, and numbness. Treatment at this time includes reducing any shift that may be present, centralizing the pain, and having the patient avoid flexion for 2 to 3 months to allow the annulus fibrosis to scar over. Treatment also includes those procedures in derangement #1 as the patient tolerates them.

■ Derangement #7: As mentioned, this derangement involves an anterior bulge of the disc and stretching of the anterior longitudinal ligament. This type of derangement occurs infrequently. Buttock and thigh pain may be seen with this condition, and the patient usually has a fixed lumbar lordosis. Treatment involves repeated flexion activities, first in supine and then in standing.

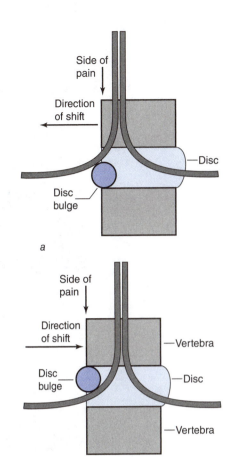

▶ **Figure 18.2** Disc bulge with pressure on nerve roots. *(a)* Bulge with pressure applied medial to nerve root. *(b)* Bulge with pressure applied lateral to nerve root.

McKenzie's approach to treating back pain used a method he identified as *centralizing*, which progressively moves the pain from its more distal region in the extremities to a proximal and central location in the lumbar region. Since low back pain is more tolerable than pain referred into the extremity, *centralizing* the pain is a key factor in his treatment of distal pain referred from the spine. His idea included allowing the patient control over the pain and the use of simple exercises to treat the pain. To that end, McKenzie listed six exercises that are given to the patient in a sequential order (figure 18.3 p. 510):

■ Exercise #1: Prone lying for 5 minutes. If the patient is unable to lie prone, it may be necessary to place a pillow or two under the lumbar and pelvic area. As the patient's pain subsides, the pillows are removed one by one until the patient is able to lie prone without a pillow.

■ Exercise #2: Once the patient is able to lie prone, the patient advances to lying prone on the elbows with the elbows under the shoulders for 5 minutes. The pelvis must be flat on the table. If the patient's ASIS are not on the table, have the patient place the elbows further forward of the shoulders until the pelvis is flat on the table. As flexibility is gained, the elbows are moved until they are directly under the shoulders.

■ Exercise #3: Once the patient has succeeded in lying prone with the elbows in the correct position, the exercise becomes prone press-ups. Once again, the ASIS should be flat on the table as the elbows are extended into a full press-up. The hands start near the shoulders to push the trunk upward, but if the hips cannot remain on the table, adjustments in hand positions will be necessary until flexibility is gained. This exercise is performed for 10 repetitions, for 6 to 8 times a day. Each time the patient moves into the end of the push-up position, the patient remains in that position to relax the spine and gluteal muscles before returning to the start position.

■ Exercise #4: The next exercise is trunk extension in standing. The patient places both hands in the small of the back and extends the trunk backwards from the waist, not the knees. This exercise is performed for 6 to 8 repetitions for 6 to 8 times each day.

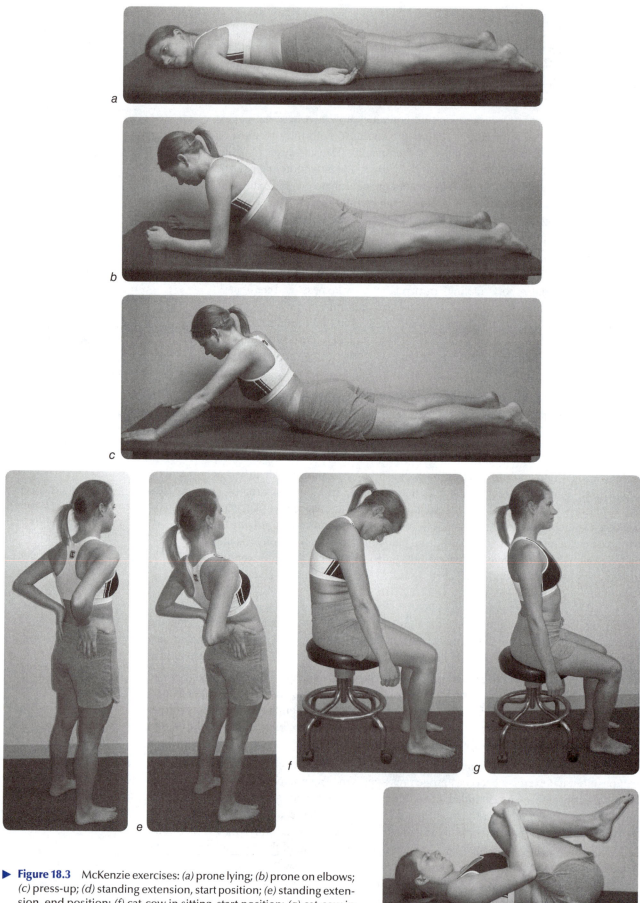

▶ **Figure 18.3** McKenzie exercises: *(a)* prone lying; *(b)* prone on elbows; *(c)* press-up; *(d)* standing extension, start position; *(e)* standing extension, end position; *(f)* cat-cow in sitting, start position; *(g)* cat-cow in sitting, end position; *(h)* both knees to chest.

© Peggy Houglum

■ Exercise #5: This is the seated "cat-cow" exercise. The patient begins in a slumped position with the lumbar spine curved posteriorly. Then, the patient moves into an anterior pelvic tilt. Each position should be in the extreme end of motion. This exercise is repeated 15 to 20 times three times a day.

■ Exercise #6: The final McKenzie exercise is similar to a Williams' exercise. It is bringing both knees to the chest. It is repeated 10 times for 6 to 8 times a day. Each leg is moved to the chest and returned to the start position one at a time with the first leg held to the chest while the other is brought up, then the first leg held in the start position while the second leg is brought down so the back does not arch during the motion.

Many rehabilitation clinicians today do not advocate a purist attitude of either flexion or extension exercises for spine patients. Rather, a program uses a combination of activities and is individualized on the basis of the problems and needs of the patient (Beattie, 1992).

A complete rehabilitation program for the spine typically involves modalities, therapeutic exercise, manual techniques, and patient education. Manual techniques include soft-tissue and joint mobilization. Spinal injuries respond well to Swiss ball, foam roller, and aquatic exercises. As you have learned, it is easy to incorporate these into a therapeutic exercise program.

It is important for spine rehab programs to include cardiovascular exercises (Mannion, Taimela, Müntener, & Dvorak, 2001). The specific injury dictates the requirements for each program. The rehabilitation clinician must identify the patient's deficiencies before deciding on a precise therapeutic exercise program.

In addition to cardiovascular activities, a therapeutic exercise program for the spine should routinely include spinal stability instruction, posture correction, and body mechanics instruction (Rydeard, Leger, & Smith, 2006). It should also include flexibility exercises, strengthening exercises, and muscle endurance activities (Hubley-Kozey, 2005; Liebenson, 2006). Hip tightness and weakness, especially in the rotators, is often correlated with low-back pain; so the program should include flexibility activities for those hip muscles that have been assessed as having restricted motion (McConnell, 2002). The abdominals (transverse, abdominus, and obliques) and spine extensor muscles are key muscle groups that provide support and stability to the spine, so strength exercises for these groups should also be included. Recent evidence has demonstrated that patients with back pain have neuromuscular dysfunction in that the muscles either fire in an incorrect pattern or their firing is delayed (Ebenbichler, Oddsson, Kollmitzer, & Erim, 2001; Radebold, Cholewicki, Panjabi, & Patel, 2000; Zazulak, Hewett, Reeves, Goldberg, & Cholewicki, 2007). Chronic low back pain patients have improved with proprioceptive retraining (Ebenbichler et al., 2001; Kofotolis & Kellis, 2006).

If one segment of the spinal column is hypomobile, it is common for an adjacent segment to be hypermobile (Sahrmann, 2002). One must carefully examine each vertebra's mobility before applying joint mobilization. Random joint mobilization to any segment in the absence of an examination of its mobility may increase, not decrease, the patient's symptoms. If you are ever in doubt whether to use joint mobilization, do not use it.

Although approaches to the various spinal segments have many similarities, and although the symptoms and treatment from one segment to an adjacent segment frequently overlap, this chapter deals with the segments separately to make it easier to identify and discuss treatment for each. You should keep in mind, however, that one segment and its injury are often intimately related to another segment. For example, painful symptoms at T4 are often associated with cervical dysfunctions, and pain in the low back can be related to sacroiliac dysfunctions.

REHABILITATION TECHNIQUES

Soft-tissue mobilization techniques are presented here before joint mobilization techniques; other types of exercises focusing on flexibility, stability, strength, and agility and coordination are presented in subsequent sections. Because there are so many types of soft-tissue mobilization techniques, only a couple are described. Keep in mind, however, that other soft-tissue mobilization techniques may be more appropriate than those presented here, depending on the individual and the specific injury.

Treatment of spine injuries has changed greatly in the last few years. A therapeutic exercise program for the spine typically has many components, including instruction on posture and stability as well as exercises for flexibility, strength, and muscle endurance.

Vertebral Artery Insufficiency

Prior to treating cervical injuries, the clinician should examine the patient for possible vertebral artery insufficiency. Although such a problem is rare in young athletes, injury to the cervical spine or poor posture may create vertebral artery compromise, or insufficiency. Treating patients with such a condition has the potential to create serious complications such as brainstem ischemia.

The ability to detect vertebral artery insufficiency with certainty is disputed (Childs et al., 2005). However, since no definitive tests have yet come to light, clinicians rely on the existing tests as current criteria prior to manual therapy administration on a cervical patient.

To identify possible patients with vertebral artery insufficiency, static and dynamic tests should be performed prior to cervical treatment. These tests are particularly important if the patient reports any symptoms of vertebral artery involvement; these symptoms include dizziness, light headedness, nausea, blurry vision, tinnitus, headaches, or facial sensory deficiencies.

The five static tests are passive and can be performed with the patient sitting, standing, or supine. The clinician maximally rotates the patient's head and neck to the left, to the right, maximally extends the patient's neck with exaggerated lordosis in the mid-cervical region, maximally rotates and extends to the left, and repeats both movements to the right. Each position is held for 10 seconds during which time the clinician observes the patient's eyes for either changes in pupil size or nystagmus, and asks the patient to report any symptoms.

The two active tests are performed with the patient sitting or standing and the clinician behind the patient. In the first test the clinician stabilizes the patient's shoulders and has the patient rotate the head and neck maximally to the left and to the right, holding each position for about 10 seconds. In the second test, the clinician holds the patient's head stable while the patient rotates the body repeatedly to the left and right for about 10 seconds. If the patient reports symptoms in the first test but not the second test, the problem is related to the vestibular system. Symptoms produced with the second test may indicate vertebral artery compromise. A positive test should be reported to the physician, and the patient should avoid positions in cervical rotation until further examination is provided.

Soft-Tissue Mobilization

Although various techniques are available for soft-tissue mobilization as discussed in chapter 6, the techniques emphasized here are trigger point release and myofascial release. If the rehabilitation clinician observes pain-referral patterns identified with these muscles, he or she should use some of these techniques. Trigger points, referred pain, and release techniques presented here are based on the work by Travell and Simons (Travell & Simons, 1983).

Cervical Spine

The upper trapezius, levator scapulae, sternocleidomastoid, scalenes, spleni, and posterior cervical muscles are the primary cervical muscles that often have soft-tissue restriction. The following sections cover treatment of these muscles. Trigger point treatments for the cervical muscles are presented here.

■ Trigger Point Releases for the Cervical Spine

Upper Trapezius

Referral Pattern: Posterior neck, mastoid process, temple, and posterior region of head, occiput, and angle of jaw (figure 18.4a).

Location of Trigger Point: Junction of the angle between the neck and shoulder.

Patient Position for Palpation: Supine.

Muscle Position for Palpation: Slight slack in the muscle with the patient's head tilted slightly toward the shoulder on the side of pain.

Ischemic Treatment: Either grasp the muscle at the juncture between the neck and shoulder portion of the muscle (figure 18.4b) or apply a caudally directed pressure over the trigger point.

Spray-and-Stretch Treatment: Apply a mild stretch by rotating the head to the opposite side and flexing the neck. The direction of the ice strokes is upward from the acromion process toward the base of the skull (figure 18.4c).

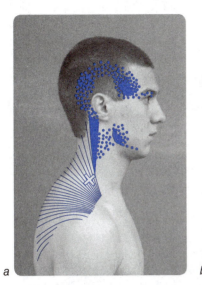
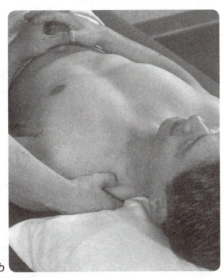
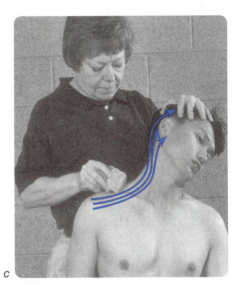

▶ **Figure 18.4** Upper trapezius: *(a)* pain pattern (x indicates trigger point), *(b)* myofascial release, *(c)* ice-and-stretch.

Levator Scapulae

Referral Pattern: The site of most intense referred pain from the levator scapulae occurs at the angle between the neck and the shoulder with occasional referral along the vertebral border of the scapula or to the posterior shoulder (figure 18.5a).

Location of Trigger Point: Either at the distal insertion of the levator scapulae on the vertebral angle of the scapula or at the angle of the neck.

Patient Position for Palpation: Supine or side-lying for ischemic compression. Sitting for spray-and-stretch.

Muscle Position for Palpation: Muscle is slightly relaxed with clinician supporting the patient's head.

Ischemic Treatment: Finger is on the trigger point as in figure 18.5b.

Spray-and-Stretch Treatment: The same-side arm is anchored, and the head is tilted forward and to the opposite side. A steady stretch is applied while the ice is stroked from the base of the skull downward along the path of the muscle (figure 18.5c).

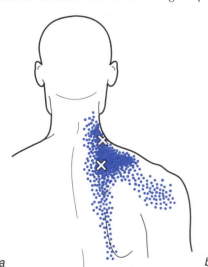
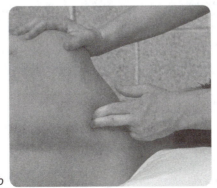
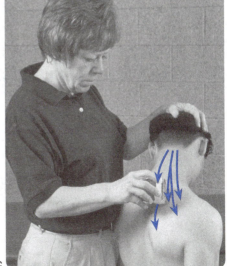

▶ **Figure 18.5** Levator scapulae myofascial release: *(a)* pain pattern (x indicates trigger point), *(b)* trigger point release, *(c)* ice-and-stretch.

Sternocleidomastoid

Referral Pattern: Both the sternal and clavicular heads can refer pain into the face and head. The most common areas are in and behind the ear, around the eye, the forehead, cheek, teeth, tongue, pharynx, and the upper aspect of the sternum.

Location of Trigger Point: There are multiple trigger points for this muscle, as seen in figure 18.6, a and b.

Patient Position for Palpation: Supine.

Muscle Position for Palpation: Head is tilted to the same side.

Ischemic Treatment: A pincer grasp on the muscle at the trigger point or a vertical pressure can be applied to the muscle (figure 18.6c).

Spray-and-Stretch Treatment: Ice-and-stretch is applied with the patient sitting, the same-side arm anchored, and the neck positioned in extension and rotation to the opposite side if the clavicular head is being treated (figure 18.6d). If the sternal head of the muscle is being treated, the neck is rotated to the same side and extended (figure 18.6e). The ice strokes are swept from the clavicle upward toward the head.

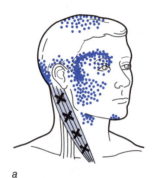

a

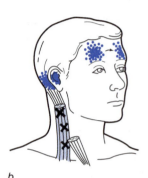

b

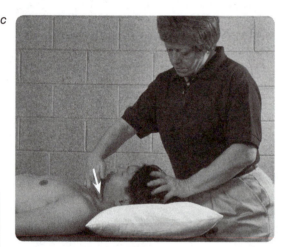

c

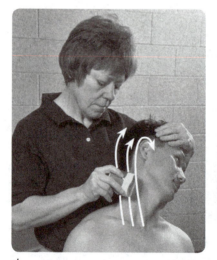

d

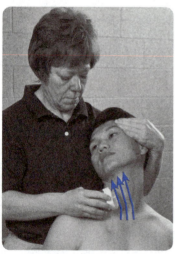

e

▶ **Figure 18.6** Sternocleidomastoid myofascial release: *(a-b)* trigger point pain-referral patterns (x = trigger point), *(c)* release of clavicular head, *(d)* ice-and-stretch of clavicular head, *(e)* ice-and-stretch of sternal head.

Scalenes

Referral Pattern: We will consider the scalene muscles—anterior, medius, and posterior—together. Trigger points of these muscles are seen in people with a forward-head posture. The pain-referral patterns for the scalenes include pain along the anterior chest, lateral shoulder and arm, vertebral border of the scapula, radial forearm and hand, posterior thumb and index finger and metacarpal, and interscapular areas (figure 18.7, a & b).

Location of Trigger Point: Locate the posterior sternocleidomastoid, cephalad to the clavicle. The scalenes lie just lateral to the sternocleidomastoid. Identify the external jugular vein as it crosses over the anterior scalene; the anterior scalene's trigger point is just caudal to the external jugular vein. The scalene medius is deep; it is found just lateral to the anterior scalene and just above the clavicle. The subclavian artery lies between the medius and anterior scalenes and can be palpated as it passes over the first rib behind the clavicle. The cervical transverse processes can be palpated when pressure is applied to the scalene medius.

Patient Position for Palpation: Supine for ischemic compression (figure 18.7c). Sitting for spray-and-stretch.

Muscle Position for Palpation: Have a pillow under the head for comfort and slightly relax the scalenes for ischemic compression. Arm is anchored and neck is in extension for spray-and-stretch.

Ischemic Treatment: Use finger pad to press directly on trigger point. Referral may be reported into the shoulder or arm.

Spray-and-Stretch Treatment: Applied with the patient in sitting and the arm anchored (figure 18.7d). The neck is positioned in extension with the head rotated away from the side being treated. Ice stroking is applied from the cephalad insertion of the muscles downward and along the shoulder and arm.

Notations: Take care to avoid applying pressure over the blood vessels in this area. These muscles are frequent sites of trigger points in people with forward-head postures.

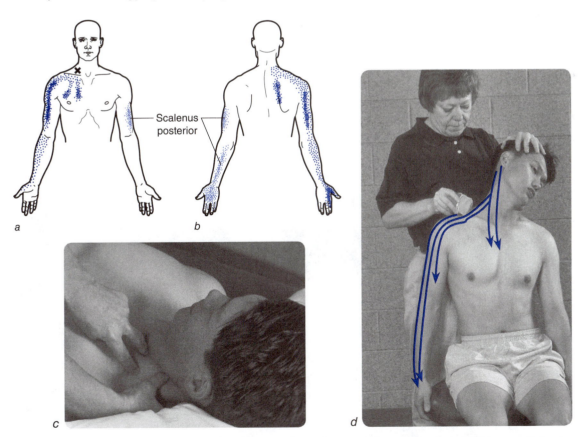

Scalenus posterior

► **Figure 18.7** *(a)* Trigger point pain-referral pattern for scalene anterior and medius. *(b)* Trigger point pain-referral pattern for scalene posterior. *(c)* Scalenes myofascial release: With the two fingers of the left hand on either side of the anterior and medius scalenes, the right thumb is on the groove between these two muscles. *(d)* Ice-and-stretch for scalenes.

Spleni Capitis and Cervicis

Referral Pattern: Pain is referred to the top of the head, behind the eye, to the base of the neck, and along the side of the head (figure 18.8a-d).

Location of Trigger Point: The splenius capitis trigger point is located just distal to its mastoid attachment (figure 18.8d). The cervicis lies posterior to the lower cervical transverse processes; locate it by laterally flexing the neck to the same side to relax the upper trapezius and levator scapulae. The cervicis is palpated over the lower cervical transverse processes. Its trigger point is located between the upper trapezius and sternocleidomastoid.

Patient Position for Palpation: Supine or sitting.

Muscle Position for Palpation: The neck is rotated and laterally flexed to the side opposite the pain.

Ischemic Treatment: Place the flat pad of the finger directly over the trigger point (figure 18.8e).

Spray-and-Stretch Treatment: Spray-and-stretch is performed with the patient in sitting. The ice sweeps are directed from the base of the neck upward and downward (figure 18.8f).

Notations: These muscles are frequent sites of trigger points in people with forward-head postures.

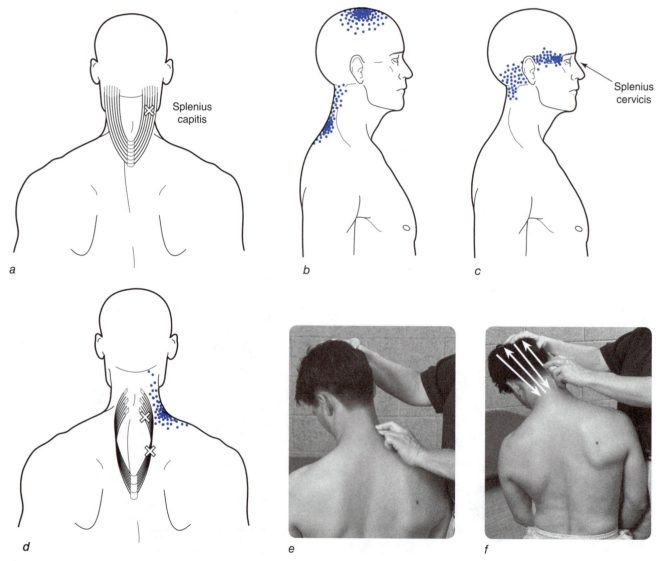

▶ **Figure 18.8** **Splenius** myofascial release: *(a-c)* trigger point pain-referral pattern for splenius capitis, *(d)* upper and lower trigger point pain-referral patterns for splenius cervicis, *(e)* trigger point release, *(f)* ice-and-stretch.

Posterior Cervical Muscles

Referral Pattern: The posterior cervical muscles (figure 18.9a) commonly refer to the base of the neck and upward into the suboccipital area, down the neck to the vertebral border of the scapula, and in a horizontal band to the temple on the same side of the head. The suboccipital muscles refer to the occiput, the eye, and the forehead. They often give the injured patient a sensation of pain inside the skull; sometimes the patient describes either a vague headache or a pain that is all over the head on one side (figure 18.9, b-f).

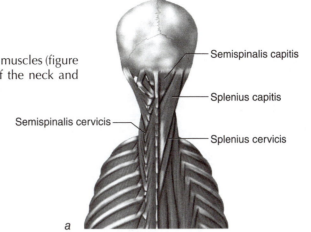

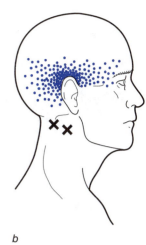

Location of Trigger Point: See figure 18.9, b through f, for images. The trigger points run generally just lateral to the spine from the occiput to the base of the neck.

Patient Position for Palpation: Supine with the clinician at the patient's head for ischemic treatment. Sitting for spray-and-stretch.

Muscle Position for Palpation: In supine, the head is properly aligned in a position of patient comfort. In sitting, the head is in a forward position for treatment of bilateral muscles. For unilateral treatment, the neck is flexed forward and sideward and rotated to the side opposite the pain.

Ischemic Treatment: Direct pressure with the finger pads using the tabletop to provide an upward pressure from the hand on the table (figure 18.9g).

Spray-and-Stretch Treatment: Head and neck position depends on the specific muscle being treated. The parallel semispinalis muscles can be treated bilaterally in a forward-head position. The rotator muscles that are angled from their distal to their proximal insertion are treated with the neck flexed forward and sideward and rotated to place the muscle on stretch (figure 18.9h). The ice is applied from the base of the neck upward toward the head.

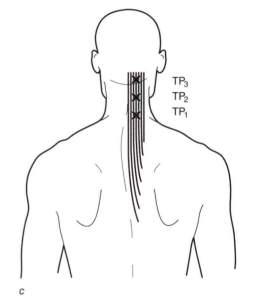

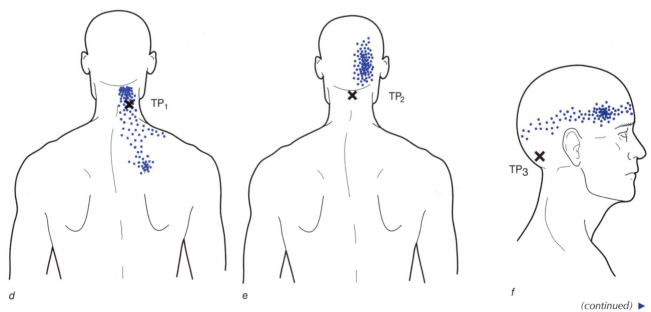

(continued) ▶

▶ **Figure 18.9** Posterior cervical muscles myofascial release: *(a)* muscle positions. Pain-referral patterns for *(b)* suboccipital muscles, *(c)* posterior cervical muscles, *(d)* multifidus, *(e)* semispinalis cervicis, and *(f)* semispinalis capitis.

(a) Reprinted from R. Behnke, 2005, *Kinetic anatomy*, 2nd ed. (Champaign, IL: Human Kinetics), 134.

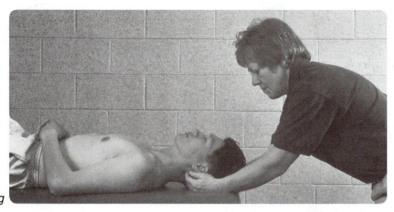

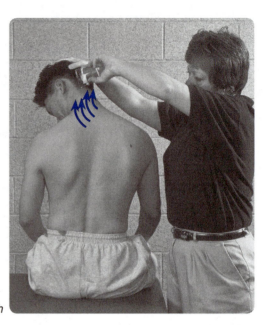

▶ **Figure 18.9** *(continued)* Posterior cervical muscles. *(g)* Trigger point release for posterior cervical muscles. *(h)* Ice-and-stretch to posterior cervical rotator muscles.

Notations: There are two groups of muscles in the posterior cervical region, one superficial and the other deep. The more superficial group is referred to as posterior cervical muscles and includes the semispinalis capitis, semispinalis cervicis, multifidi, and rotatores (figure 18.9a). Beneath the semispinalis muscles are several additional smaller muscles, termed the suboccipital muscles. These include the major and minor rectus capitis muscles and the superior and inferior oblique capitis muscles.

Thoracic and Lumbar Spine

Often the muscles treated with soft-tissue mobilization in the thoracic area are the shoulder and scapular muscles. Those are discussed in chapter 19. Some of the cervical muscles, as you have just seen, can refer into the scapular area, so if a patient describes pain around the scapula without any frank injury to the shoulder or thoracic region, you should examine the neck as a possible source of the pain. Likewise, some lumbar pain is referred from the thigh and gluteal muscles; these areas are discussed in chapters 23 and 24.

Because thoracic muscles commonly refer pain into the lumbar area, and because many lumbar and thoracic muscles are extensions of the same muscles, the thoracic and lumbar muscles are discussed together. It is often very difficult to separate the two regions from each other. Treatment also often overlaps from one area to another, so it is logical to consider the two areas at the same time.

Muscles in the thoracic and lumbar regions that can refer pain into the thoracic, lumbar, and sacral areas include the thoracic and lumbar paraspinals, the quadratus lumborum, and the serratus posterior. The following sections cover their referral patterns, trigger points, and ice-and-stretch treatments.

▪ Trigger Point Releases for the Thoracic and Lumbar Spine

Paraspinals

Referral Pattern: Midthoracic superficial paraspinals can refer pain into the scapula or anterior chest area (figure 18.10, a & b); the lower thoracic superficial paraspinals can refer pain upward into the scapula (figure 18.10c), anteriorly to the lower abdomen (figure 18.10d), or downward to the low back and buttock (figure 18.10, e).

Thoracic multifidi refer pain to the spinous process near the trigger point (figure 18.10, g & h), while the lumbar multifidi can also refer pain into the abdomen (figure 18.10f & i). Multifidi at S1 can refer into the coccyx (figure 18.10h).

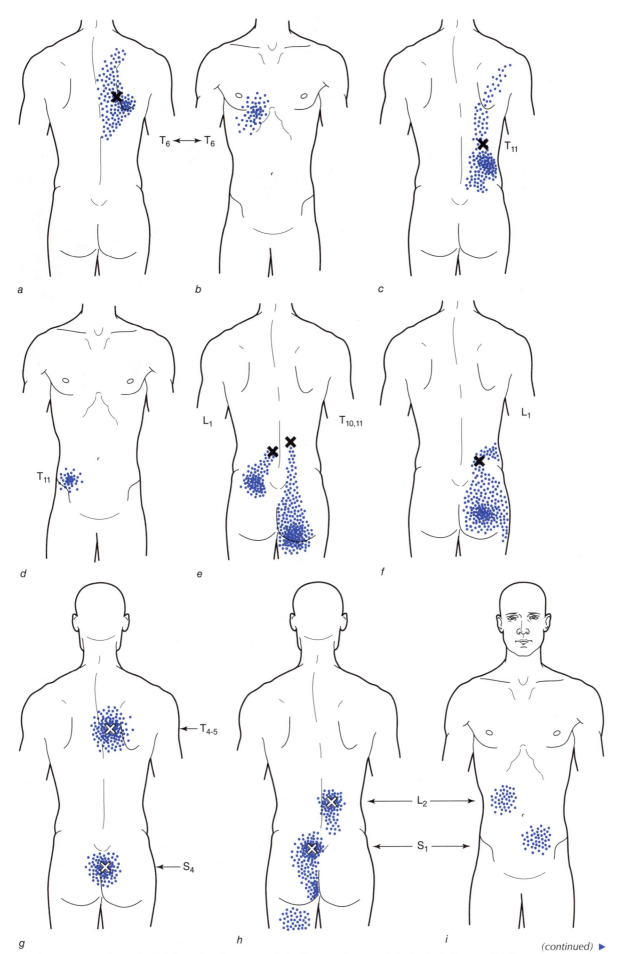

$T_6 \longleftrightarrow T_6$

T_{11}

T_{11}

L_1 $T_{10,11}$

L_1

$\leftarrow T_{4-5}$

$\leftarrow S_4$

$\longleftarrow L_2 \longrightarrow$

$\longleftarrow S_1 \longrightarrow$

a   b   c   d   e   f   g   h   i

(continued) ▶

▶ **Figure 18.10** Paraspinal pain-referral patterns (x indicates trigger point sites): *(a-f)* superficial paraspinals, *(g-i)* deep paraspinals.

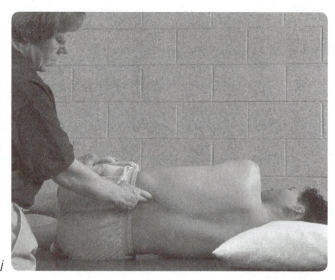

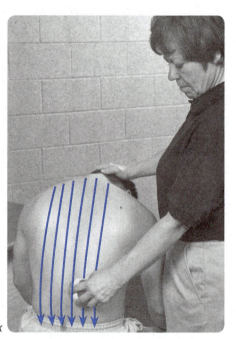

▶ **Figure 18.10** *(continued)* Paraspinal pain-referral patterns: *(j)* myofascial release, *(k)* ice-and-stretch.

Location of Trigger Point: See figure 18.10, a through f, for pain-referral patterns of these muscles. The trigger points are located over the paraspinal muscles and usually proximal to the lumbar spine from the referred pain. Some thoracic trigger points may refer anteriorly as well as either cephalad or caudal to the trigger point site.

Patient Position for Palpation: Prone or side-lying for ischemic compression and sitting for spray-and-stretch.

Muscle Position for Palpation: Position of comfort for ischemic compression. On stretch in forward bending while seated for spray-and-stretch.

Ischemic Treatment: Apply pressure over the site of the trigger point where the patient's referred pain is reproduced.

Spray-and-Stretch Treatment: Ice-and-stretch is applied in a sitting position with the patient in trunk flexion (figure 18.10k). The ice is applied in a cephalad-to-caudal motion from the head to the sacrum. If the deep paraspinals are being treated, the stretch must involve rotation and flexion while the ice stroking is performed at an angle.

Notations: This group of muscles includes deep and superficial paraspinal muscles. The superficial group, the iliocostals and longissimus muscles, is collectively referred to as the erector spinae. The deep muscles include the rotatores, semispinalis, and multifidi; of these, the multifidi group most commonly produces pain.

Quadratus Lumborum

Referral Pattern: Typical quadratus lumborum pain can be either a deep ache or a sharp pain. The superficial fibers can refer pain along the iliac crest or greater trochanter, or the pain can wrap around to the outer groin. The deep fibers refer down to the sacroiliac joint or lower buttock (figure 18.11a).

Location of Trigger Point: The superficial trigger points are located laterally, just cephalad to the iliac crest or distal of the 12th rib. The deep trigger points are located just lateral to the paraspinal muscles.

Patient Position for Palpation: Side-lying on the uninvolved side.

Muscle Position for Palpation: The top arm is placed over the head to elevate the lower ribs, and the top hip and knee are flexed with the knee on the table to lower the ilium (figure 18.11b). If the area is too tight or painful for the patient to lie in this position, the top knee should be placed on the bottom ankle or on a supportive pillow to reduce the stretch of the muscle.

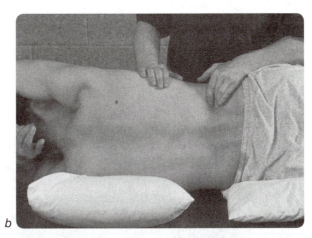

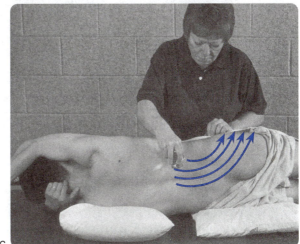

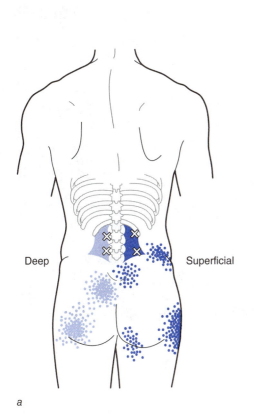

▶ **Figure 18.11** Quadratus lumborum: *(a)* pain-referral pattern, *(b)* trigger point release, *(c)* ice-and-stretch.

Deep / Superficial

a

b

c

Ischemic Treatment: Apply direct pressure over the trigger points that reproduce the patient's referred pain.

Spray-and-Stretch Treatment: Ice-and-stretch treatment is applied with the patient in a position similar to that for trigger point release, but with the top leg forward of the bottom leg and distal thigh and positioned off the table to allow a stretch (figure 18.11c). The ice strokes are swept in a cephalad-to-caudad motion.

Notations: This muscle's pattern often gives the false sign of a disc syndrome and is neglected as a source of low-back pain. The pain, which can be intense, can accompany deep inhalation or can make walking painful.

Serratus Posterior Inferior

Referral Pattern: Pain in this muscle usually remains localized and does not refer to other sites.

Location of Trigger Point: In the lateral region of the muscle close to its rib insertion and lateral to the paraspinal muscles (figure 18.12b).

Patient Position for Palpation: Side-lying for ischemic compression. Sitting for spray-and-stretch.

Muscle Position for Palpation: In a position of comfort for ischemic compression. In forward flexion and rotation of the trunk for spray-and-stretch.

Ischemic Treatment: Apply direct pressure over the trigger point.

Spray-and-Stretch Treatment: The trunk is flexed and rotated, and the ice is applied in upward and outward sweeps from the spine to the lateral trunk (figure 18.12c).

Notations: This muscle causes an annoying ache in the posterior lower rib area in the site of its locale, from the posterior ninth rib medially to the L2 spinous process (figure 18.12a).

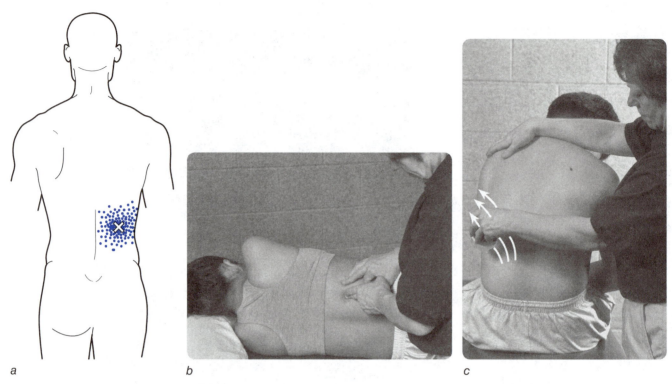

▶ **Figure 18.12** Serratus posterior: *(a)* trigger point (x) with pain referral pattern, *(b)* trigger point release to right serratus posterior inferior, *(c)* ice-and-stretch to left serratus posterior inferior.

Self Soft-Tissue Mobilization

This is a soft-tissue mobilization technique that you can instruct the patient in and that does not require assistance. It uses either one or two old tennis balls that have lost their compression. If two balls are used, they can be either taped together (figure 18.13) or placed together in a sock. The patient lies on the tennis balls, which are placed under a restricted soft-tissue area. The patient lies on the tennis balls until the tenderness is gone and he or she feels only the pressure of the tennis balls. The balls are then moved to another location of restriction and discomfort and the technique is repeated. This technique can be performed in the thoracic and lumbar areas; it can also be used in other soft-tissue restricted areas of the body such as the hip and thigh.

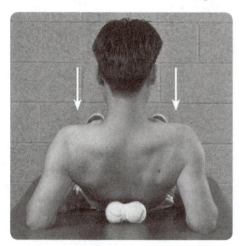

▶ **Figure 18.13** Tennis ball release. The patient relaxes and lies down so body weight pushes balls into trigger point or area of restriction.

Joint Mobilization

Obviously, the degree of movement in spinal joint mobilization accessory motion is very different from that in peripheral joints. Before you acquire the ability to determine normal movement, you will have evaluated many different vertebral movements on many different patients of varying ages and with various conditions. Normal accessory movement in the lumbar spine is different from that in the cervical spine, and joint accessory movement in a 19-year-old patient is different from that in a 40-year-old. You must recognize and consider these normal variations when assessing and treating a patient with joint mobilization.

Joint mobilization is used to reduce pain or improve mobility. Since it is common to find a hypermobile vertebral joint adjacent to a hypomobile joint, each spinal level should be assessed prior to joint mobilization application. The hypermobile joint should not be mobilized, but treatment will be necessary to improve motion of the restricted joint.

It is necessary to outline some basic principles of application before discussing specific application techniques. When the cervical spine and head are in normal alignment, the lower cervical and lower lumbar spines are curved slightly anteriorly. Because the best position for joint mobilization is an open-packed position, these areas of the spine should be placed in slight flexion to place the joints into a mid-position before mobilization is performed. Rotating the head to the non-painful side opens the vertebral foramen of C2 to C7. You can also open these by laterally tilting the patient's head away from the painful side. Mobilization techniques differ for the upper and lower cervical spine.

The clinician should use body weight and weight transfer as the force source, not the force from the fingers, thumbs, or hands. Using the body as the source of force permits a finer sense of touch for joint movement; is more comfortable for the patient; imposes less stress on the fingers, thumbs, and hands; and conserves the rehabilitation clinician's energy.

Initial mobilization techniques should be gentle. There should be no increase in symptoms because of the treatment. Examination before, during, and after the application is necessary in order for you to decide the appropriate depth of treatment. The primary factors restricting the depth of mobilization application are muscle spasm and pain. Frequently, muscle spasm will not permit grades III or IV mobilization. When this occurs, gentle grades I and II mobilization are used. Mobilization that exacerbates distally referred pain should be modified to include reduced amplitude or even discontinued. Refer to chapter 6 for joint mobilization indications, precautions, and contraindications.

Although there are several mobilization techniques for use in the spine, only a few for each area of the spine are discussed here. The primary techniques to be described include central posterior-anterior (PA) and unilateral PA mobilization. The symbols used to record these techniques are ↓ for central PA and ⌐ or ⌐ for right or left unilateral PAs, respectively. The symbols used to record rib mobilization are ⌐ for right-rib and for ⌐ left-rib mobilizations. In this section we will consider additional techniques for some specific sites. I recommend that once you begin practice as a qualified health care provider, you participate in continuing education courses to develop an understanding and appreciation of more complex maneuvers.

Cervical Spine

The most commonly used cervical spine joint mobilization techniques are outlined in the following sections. Description of these techniques will primarily emphasize hand placement. The specific grade to apply is determined by the patient's condition and the treatment goals, but remember that grades I and II are used for pain relief and grades III and IV are used to improve range of motion. Refer to chapter 6 for a review of joint mobilization.

■ Joint Manipulation of the Cervical Spine

Longitudinal Movement

Resting Position: Normal alignment of the head with the body.

Mobilization Technique: Distraction.

Indications: Relaxing technique used to gain patient's confidence.

Patient Position: Supine.

Clinician and Hand Positions: The clinician stands or sits at the top of the table. The patient's head is grasped and supported with one of the rehabilitation clinician's hands behind the head; the thumb and fingers are at the occiput. The other hand is placed under the chin (figure 18.14).

Mobilization Application: While maintaining the position of the upper extremities, the clinician leans back to produce a gentle longitudinal pull of the neck.

Notations: The hand on the chin is for positioning only; no force is directed into the chin. This is often the technique used to initiate a mobilization treatment session.

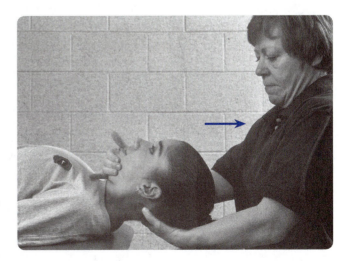

▶ **Figure 18.14** Longitudinal cervical movement joint mobilization.

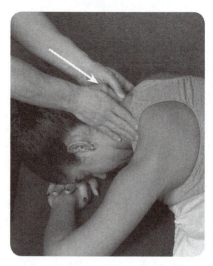

▶ **Figure 18.15** Central PA cervical mobilization.

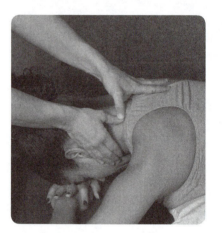

▶ **Figure 18.16** Unilateral cervical mobilization.

Central PA Mobilizations

Resting Position: The cervical spine is in good alignment to allow the clinician to identify the specific level to be treated. Most often this is a position of proper alignment relative to the entire spine or slightly flexed to expose the specific joint.

Mobilization Technique: Anterior glide.

Indications: Midline pain, unilateral pain, or spasm; decreased mobility.

Patient Position: The patient lies prone with his or her hands under the forehead and the chin slightly tucked.

Clinician and Hand Positions: The rehabilitation clinician stands at the head and places the thumbs on the spine with the fingers relaxed, along the sides of the neck (figure 18.15). C1 and C3 are usually too difficult to palpate; but C2, C4, C5, C6, and C7 can usually be readily identified.

Mobilization Application: The clinician applies PA pressure with the thumbs through movement of his or her trunk over the hands.

Notations: The pressure should be gentle initially; adjustments are made using I and II grades according to the patient's response.

Unilateral PA Mobilizations

Resting Position: The cervical spine is in good alignment to allow the clinician to identify the specific level to be treated. Most often this is a position of proper alignment relative to the entire spine or slightly flexed to expose the specific joint.

Mobilization Technique: Anterior glide on one side, usually the painful side.

Indications: For lower cervical spine and for unilateral neck pain; decreased mobility.

Patient Position: The patient lies prone with his or her hands under the forehead and the chin slightly tucked.

Clinician and Hand Positions: The rehabilitation clinician stands on the side that is to be treated. The thumbs are placed on the articular pillar and angled about 30° medially (figure 18.16).

Mobilization Application: The pressure is applied by the thumbs in a PA direction with a constant medially directed pressure to maintain position on the articular pillar.

Notations: The head may nod slightly, but there should be no rotation motion if the pressure is applied correctly.

Thoracic Spine

Look at the bony arrangement on a skeleton to see how the position and relative alignment of the spinous processes change from the cervical to the lumbar spine. The angle of the joint mobilization force must change to produce a force in the plane of the joint. This is a crucial point to keep in mind as you perform mobilization techniques along the spine. Joint mobilizations for the thoracic spine are presented here.

■ Joint Manipulation of the Thoracic Spine

Central PA Mobilizations

Resting Position: The thoracic spine should be relatively parallel to the floor with the patient prone on the treatment table.

Mobilization Technique: Anterior glide.

Indications: Central or unilateral symptoms.

Patient Position: The patient lies prone with his or her hands under the forehead and the chin slightly tucked.

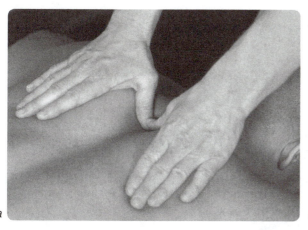

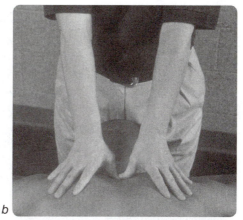

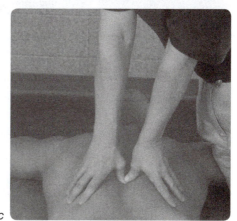

▶ **Figure 18.17** Central PA thoracic mobilization: *(a)* Thumbs are placed over the spinous process. One thumb can be used to reinforce the other thumb. *(b)* Upper thoracic mobilizations are most easily performed while the clinician is standing at the patient's head. *(c)* Lower and middle thoracic mobilizations are performed with the clinician standing at the patient's side.

Clinician and Hand Positions: The specific thoracic segment being treated determines where the rehabilitation clinician stands. His or her position is at the head (figure 18.17b) if the upper segments are treated and at the side (figure 18.17c) if the middle and lower segments are treated. The thumbs are placed directly over the spinous process (figure 18.17a), with the fingertips spread across the back to act as a stabilizer for the thumbs.

Mobilization Application: The pressure is applied at an angle perpendicular to the surface, so the position will change slightly as the hands move along the thoracic spine. The force is transmitted from the trunk through the arms to the thumbs. The fingers should remain relaxed.

Unilateral PAs

Resting Position: The thoracic spine should be relatively parallel to the floor with the patient prone on the treatment table.

Mobilization Technique: Anterior glide.

Indications: Used for unilateral symptoms.

Patient Position: The patient lies prone with the head turned to the side being treated. The arms hang over the side of the table.

Clinician and Hand Positions: The rehabilitation clinician stands on the side being treated and places his or her hands on the patient's back, with the thumb pads on the transverse process and the fingers buttressed over the back (figure 18.18). The clinician's shoulders and arms are directly over his or her hands.

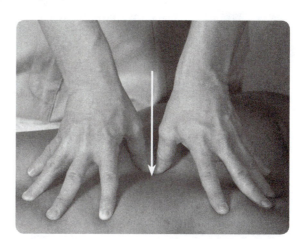

▶ **Figure 18.18** Unilateral PA thoracic mobilization.

Mobilization Application: The force is directed perpendicular to the surface.

Notations: Clinician's hand motion occurs as a result of trunk and leg movement, not thumb movement. The side of treatment is usually the painful side.

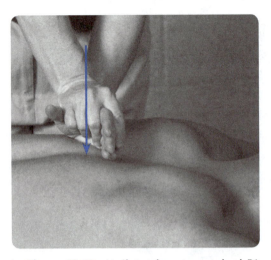

▶ **Figure 18.19** Unilateral costovertebral PA mobilization.

Unilateral Costovertebral PAs

Resting Position: The thoracic spine should be relatively parallel to the floor with the patient prone on the treatment table.

Mobilization Technique: Anterior glide.

Indications: Painful and restricted rib joints.

Patient Position: The patient lies prone with the head turned to the side being treated. The arms hang over the side of the table.

Clinician and Hand Positions: The ulnar border of the rehabilitation clinician's hand is placed along the line of the patient's rib over the costovertebral joint, with the other hand placed on top of the second metacarpal and digit (figure 18.19). Placement of the ulnar border is approximately two finger-widths from the spinous process.

Mobilization Application: The pressure is applied parallel to the joint surface from the trunk through the shoulders and into the hands.

Notations: The two-finger-width positioning for the treatment application is based on the patient's finger width, not the clinician's.

Lumbar Spine and Sacroiliac

Like the cervical and thoracic areas, the lumbar spine can be treated with central and unilateral PA movements. In addition, rotation mobilizations can be performed as a gross technique affecting the lumbar spine as a whole rather than treating individual levels. The following sections describe the various mobilizations for the lumbar spine.

■ Joint Manipulation of the Lumbar and Sacroiliac Spine

Central PA Mobilizations

Resting Position: The lumbar spine should be relatively parallel to the floor with the patient prone on the treatment table. A pillow under the patient's abdomen may be necessary to maintain a level lumbar spine.

Mobilization Technique: Anterior glide.

Indications: For hypomobility and central or unilateral pain and derangements.

Patient Position: The patient lies prone.

Clinician and Hand Positions: The clinician stands to the side of the patient at the lumbar spine level. The ulnar side of one hand, with the other hand reinforcing the treatment hand, may be used to apply the treatment force (figure 18.20). The clinician's shoulders are directly over his or her hands.

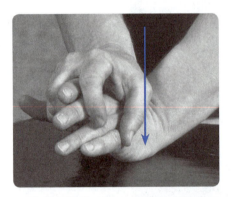

▶ **Figure 18.20** Central PA mobilization using the ulnar border of the left hand with reinforcement from the right hand.

Mobilization Application: Pressure is applied parallel to the joint surface through the shoulders from the trunk.

Notations: Maintain elbow extension while applying the treatment force.

Unilateral PAs

Resting Position: The lumbar spine should be relatively parallel to the floor with the patient prone on the treatment table. A pillow under the patient's abdomen may be necessary to maintain a level lumbar spine.

Mobilization Technique: Anterior glide.

Indications: For unilateral symptoms.

Patient Position: The patient lies prone with the head turned to the side being treated.

Clinician and Hand Positions: The rehabilitation clinician stands on the side to be treated and places the thumbs just lateral to the spinous

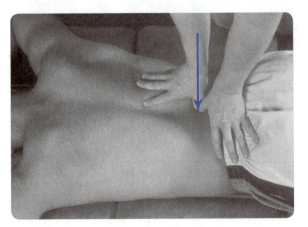

▶ **Figure 18.21** Unilateral lumbar mobilization.

process, at the level being treated, with the fingers spread across the back (figure 18.21).

Mobilization Application: The pressure is applied directly parallel to the joint surface through the shoulders.

Notations: The clinician's shoulders are placed directly over his or her hands with the fingers relaxed.

Rotation

Resting Position: Position for all grades is in side-lying, but specific position depends upon the grade. The lumbar vertebrae are positioned in midrange flexion-extension by the amount of hip flexion.

Mobilization Technique: Gross movement rotational glide.

Indications: Unilateral restriction of movement or unilateral back or leg pain.

Patient Position: The patient lies on the unaffected side with a pillow under the head. The top shoulder is near the side, and the elbow is flexed with the forearm resting on the side. The lower-extremity position depends on the grade of pressure being applied. For grades I and II, the hips and knees are flexed with the top leg slightly more flexed than the bottom leg. In grade III, the top shoulder is rotated slightly more posteriorly so that the chest faces the ceiling and the torso is in a three-quarter position. The bottom leg is more extended than in grades I and II; the top leg is flexed with the medial femoral condyle on the table or just off the edge, and the ankle is hooked around the bottom leg. Grade IV motion is produced with the top leg more extended and off the table (figure 18.22c).

Clinician and Hand Positions: The clinician places his or her hands on the pelvis. For grade III, the rehabilitation clinician places one hand on the patient's shoulder and the other on the pelvis with the fingers pointing forward. If the desired motion is more into extension, then the hand is placed over the iliac crest with the clinician standing near the shoulder (figure 18.22b); but if the desired motion is flexion, the hand is placed over the greater trochanter with the clinician standing near the pelvis. For grade IV, the clinician may need to kneel on the table behind the patient or lower the table so the force can be directed more easily from the clinician's shoulders to the hand on the pelvis. The clinician's knee behind the patient's back can also assist in stabilization.

Mobilization Application: For grades I and II, a gentle rocking motion of the pelvis is produced by the clinician (figure 18.22a). The rocking motion is produced with movement caused by the hand on the patient's pelvis, not the shoulder.

Notations: Motion for each grade should be a rotatory motion of the pelvis, not posterior to anterior or inferior to superior.

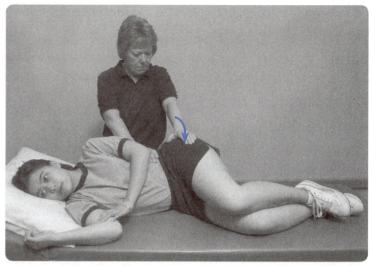

a

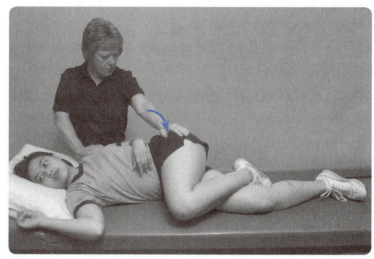

b

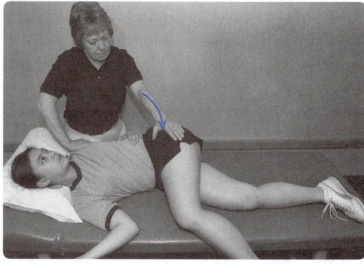

c

▶ **Figure 18.22** Unilateral lumbar mobilization: *(a)* grades I and II rotation, *(b)* grade III rotation, *(c)* grade IV rotation.

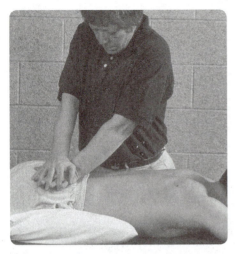

▶ **Figure 18.23** Sacroiliac PA mobilization. The rehabilitation clinician is shown on the opposite side from the side being treated; this is only to allow better visualization of the technique.

Sacroiliac PA Pressures

Resting Position: The sacrum lies in a neutral position with the support of a pillow under the pelvis and lumbar spine.

Mobilization Technique: Anterior glide applied either centrally or unilaterally.

Indications: Pain or restriction of motion.

Patient Position: Prone.

Clinician and Hand Positions: Clinician stands by the side to be treated. One hand is reinforced with the other hand on top of it and is placed over the upper sacrum.

Mobilization Application: Posterior-to-anterior pressure is applied at the S1 level with repetitions moving in a cephalad-to-caudal direction to the distal end of the sacrum (figure 18.23).

Notations: Because of the complexity of the SI joint, the PA pressure can be applied in a cephalic, caudal, medial, or lateral direction or in any combination of these.

Flexibility Exercises

Because the lower cervical spine is related to the upper thoracic spine and the lumbar spine is related to the lower thoracic spine, sacrum, and hips, some of the flexibility exercises for cervical and lumbar regions of the spine overlap into these respective areas. Unless otherwise indicated, the stretch is held for about 15 s and repeated four to five times.

The description of each flexibility exercise in the following sections includes the correct manner of execution and common incorrect substitutions that should be avoided. These substitutions occur as the patient attempts to produce as much motion as possible. You should watch for these patterns carefully and correct them as they occur to prevent the patient from stretching ineffectively.

■ Flexibility Exercises for the Cervical, Thoracic, and Lumbar Spine

Axial Extension

Body Segment: Cervical.

Stage in Rehab: I and II.

Purpose: This exercise helps the patient restore normal cervical alignment and correct posture.

Positioning: The patient lies supine on a firm surface, such as a tabletop or the floor. A pillow is not used.

Execution: The patient places the fingertips of one hand on the cervical spinous processes and the other hand under the chin (figure 18.24). The neck is then pushed into the fingertips as the patient pushes the tucked chin back with the front hand.

Possible Substitutions: Tilting the head rather than moving it straight posteriorly.

Notations: As the patient finds this activity easier to perform, he or she can do it in sitting. The patient places the index finger and thumb of one hand on the chin and the fingertips of the other hand along the upper cervical spine. With the chin tucked, the patient pushes the chin back with the chin hand and feels with the other hand as the cervical spine is pushed into that hand (figure 18.24b).

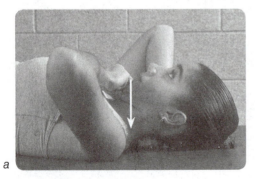

a

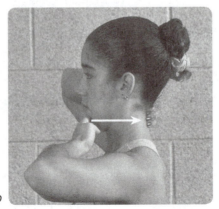

b

▶ **Figure 18.24** Axial extension in *(a)* supine and *(b)* sitting.

Cervical Retraction

Body Segment: Cervical.

Stage in Rehab: I and II and throughout.

Purpose: This exercise is used to stretch the posterior cervical muscles and improve posture.

Positioning: Sitting or supine.

Execution: The chin is tucked, and the head is pulled back while the chin stays at the same level (figure 18.25). The head does not tilt up or down during this activity.

Possible Substitutions: Tilting the head upward and moving the cervical spine into lordosis.

Notations: Also called the turtle exercise because of the motion involved.

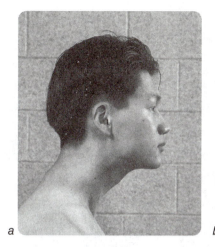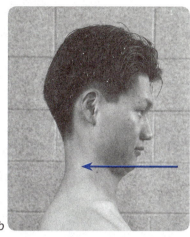

a   b

▶ **Figure 18.25** Cervical retraction: *(a)* forward, starting position; *(b)* retracted, end position.

Cervical Flexion

Body Segment: Cervical.

Stage in Rehab: I and II and throughout.

Purpose: Stretch the posterior muscles.

Positioning: Sitting.

Execution: With the chin tucked, the patient bends the head forward, attempting to touch the chin to the chest.

Possible Substitutions: The common substitution for this exercise is not to curl the neck but to use the lower cervical spine as a fulcrum while the upper cervical spine stays straight. If this occurs, instruct the patient to unwind the neck, beginning with the upper spine and moving downward. Remind the patient not to pull with the arms since this will produce unnecessary force on the posterior neck.

Notations: Slight overpressure can provide additional stretch: The patient places his or her hands on top of the head and relaxes the shoulders. The weight of the arms will provide sufficient stretch, so instruct the patient not to pull the head but to let the arms relax and the elbows hang down (figure 18.26).

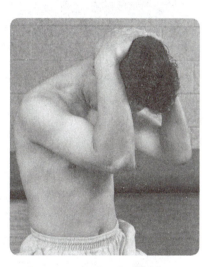

▶ **Figure 18.26** Cervical flexion.

Upper Trapezius Stretch

Body Segment: Cervical.

Stage in Rehab: II and later.

Purpose: Isolate the upper trapezius muscle.

Positioning: Sitting; sometimes it may be necessary to start the patient in a supine position so that rotation and forward flexing are minimized.

Execution: The patient grasps the wrist of the side to be stretched and pulls it across the body. The head is tilted away from the shoulder (figure 18.27a). Leaning the head to the opposite side can increase the stretch.

Possible Substitutions: Common substitutions for this exercise are allowing the shoulder to shrug upward, rotating the neck, or bending the head forward, rather than directly sideways. If these substitutions occur, correct the patient by instructing him or her to stabilize the shoulder by sitting on the hand, and to keep the nose in a forward position.

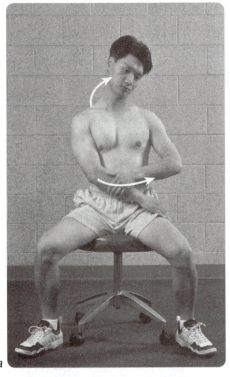
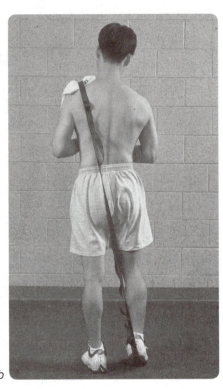

Notations: An alternative stretch uses a stretch strap that is draped over the treated shoulder. The toes of the opposite foot are used to anchor the strap to the floor (figure 18.27b). The patient aligns the strap from the anchoring toes to beneath the elevated heel and takes up the slack using the hands to pull on the strap in the front of the body. A towel or other pad is placed under the strap on the shoulder for comfort. The heel is then moved to the floor so the strap becomes taut, applying pressure on the upper trapezius. While in this position, the neck is laterally stretched away from the strap until the patient feels a stretch from the strap on the side of the neck.

a   b

▶ **Figure 18.27** Upper trapezius stretch: *(a)* active stretch, *(b)* with stretch strap.

Scalene Stretch

Body Segment: Cervical.

Stage in Rehab: II and later.

Purpose: Isolate the scalenes in three different positions.

Positioning: Because the scalenes have three different parts, there are three positions for stretching them. These stretches can be performed in sitting or supine.

Execution: The arm on the side being stretched is anchored under the hip in all positions, and the opposite hand is placed over and across the top of the head and above the ear on the stretch side. For the posterior scalene, the face is turned to the opposite axilla (figure 18.28a). For the medius, the face is kept looking forward while the head is tilted laterally (figure 18.28b). To stretch the anterior scalene, the face is turned to the ipsilateral side and the patient looks to the ceiling (figure 18.28c). The hand over and across the top of the head applies a gentle force that produces a stretch sensation without discomfort or pain.

Possible Substitutions: The common substitutions for this exercise are to move the shoulders or lean sideways during the stretch. If this occurs, have the patient perform the exercises in supine, and make the patient aware of the substitution.

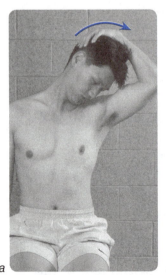
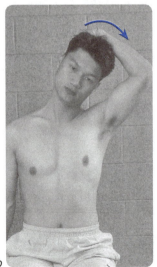
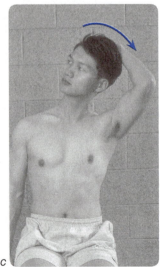

a   b   c

▶ **Figure 18.28** Scalene stretch: *(a)* posterior, *(b)* medius, *(c)* anterior.

Pectoral Stretch

Body Segment: Cervical.

Stage in Rehab: II and later.

Purpose: Stretch the pectoral muscles, a common source of poor cervical posture.

Positioning: The patient stands in a doorway with the forearms on the doorframe and elbows at shoulder level with one foot in front of the other.

Execution: The patient attempts to push through the doorway (figure 18.29). This exercise can also be performed in a corner, although empty corners are often difficult to find.

Possible Substitutions: The common substitution for this exercise is rotating the body toward the tight shoulder, especially if patients are small and the doorframe is too wide. If this occurs, have the patient keep both arms at the same level on the doorframe.

Notations: Using a corner instead of a doorframe may help improve execution of the exercise.

Sternal Raise

Body Segment: Cervical.

Stage in Rehab: I and II and later.

Purpose: For the cervical and upper thoracic spine, to improve posture.

Positioning: Standing or sitting.

Execution: The patient elevates the sternum while moving the scapulae downward toward the back pockets.

Possible Substitutions: Common substitutions in this exercise include taking in a big breath or hyperextending the lumbar spine rather than elevating the sternum. To eliminate substitutions, instruct the patient to simultaneously contract the abdominal muscles to stabilize the lumbar spine.

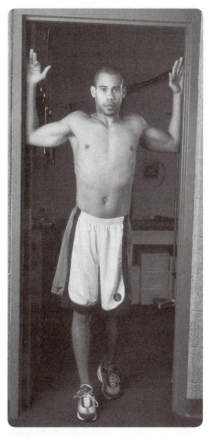

▶ **Figure 18.29** Stretch to middle pectoralis.

Spinal Twist

Body Segment: Thoracolumbar.

Stage in Rehab: II and later.

Purpose: Stretch the middle and low back.

Positioning: Sitting on the ground or in a chair.

Execution: On the ground, the patient crosses one leg over the opposite outstretched leg so that the crossing foot is placed on the outside of the outstretched leg. The elbow on the outstretched-leg side is placed on the outside of the bent knee, and the opposite arm is placed behind the body with the elbow straight. The patient then twists the body around toward the straight arm. If performing this exercise in a chair, the patient uses a straight-backed chair without arms. The feet are firmly planted on the floor, and the trunk is rotated toward the back of the chair. With one hand placed on the chair back, the other hand is placed on the outside of the knee as shown in figure 18.30. The patient uses the hands to pull around and provide the stretch.

Possible Substitutions: A common substitution for this exercise is to allow the hips to rotate with the stretch. Instruct the patient to apply a hand on the outside of the thigh during the chair-twist stretch. To correct the substitution when the stretch is performed on the floor, the patient should use the hand on the thigh to apply a stabilizing force.

Notations: The thighs should not move during the stretch.

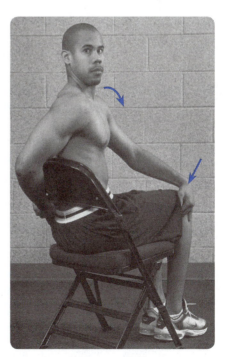

▶ **Figure 18.30** Spinal twist stretch.

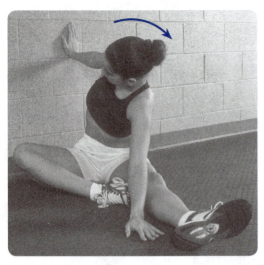

▶ **Figure 18.31** Quadratus lumborum stretch.

Quadratus Lumborum Stretch

Body Segment: Thoracolumbar.

Stage in Rehab: I and II and later.

Purpose: Stretch the quadratus lumborum and latissimus dorsi.

Positioning: The patient sits on the floor. One thigh is parallel to the wall with the knee flexed so that the sole of the foot of that leg is placed on the inner thigh of the opposite leg, which is extended out to the side and close to perpendicular to the wall (figure 18.31).

Execution: The arm farther from the wall is in front of the ipsilateral leg, and the hand nearest the wall is placed on the wall to push the trunk away from the wall. The hips remain on the floor and the pelvis remains in neutral.

Possible Substitutions: A common substitution for this stretch is to move out of pelvic neutral and flex the trunk. Instruct the patient to maintain a pelvic neutral position and lean only as far as possible while in pelvic neutral.

Notations: In an alternative position that offers more stretch, the patient places the wall arm over the head in lateral rotation and full abduction and leans toward the opposite side.

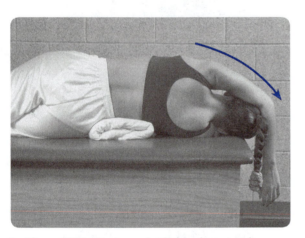

▶ **Figure 18.32** Prolonged side-bending stretch.

Prolonged Side-Bending

Body Segment: Thoracolumbar.

Stage in Rehab: II and later.

Purpose: Stretch the lateral trunk area. This activity can also be used to open a closed facet.

Positioning: The patient is in side-lying with the tight region on the top and a rolled towel or pillow supporting the portion of the trunk that is directly under the tight region.

Execution: The top arm is placed overhead, and the top leg is straight in extension (figure 18.32). Increasing or decreasing the size of the rolled towel or pillow can alter the degree of stretch.

Possible Substitutions: Trunk flexion is a common substitution with this exercise. The patient must remain in a straight-aligned position of the trunk relative to the pelvis to attain optimal results.

Notations: Depending on the position, this exercise can be used to stretch out the middle or lower thoracic area or the lumbar area.

Bent-Over Stretch

Body Segment: Thoracolumbar.

Stage in Rehab: III and later.

Purpose: Stretch the lumbar and thoracic spine.

Positioning: The patient sits in a chair with the feet flat on the floor and shoulder-width apart.

Execution: Starting from the neck, the patient slowly flexes forward and continues to bend the spine as the body flexes forward. The patient can wrap the hands around the ankles from inside the legs to outside the ankles and pull in order to give an extra stretch. When returning to the starting position, the patient places the hands on the knees and pushes with the arms to move upright rather than using the trunk muscles.

Possible Substitutions: Bending from the hips is the most common substitution. Instruct the patient to roll and feel each segment moving as he or she curls to the end position.

Notations: Because the ribs restrict mobility of the thoracic spine, thoracic motion is possible but limited. Abnormally limited motion in the thoracic ribs or spine can reduce shoulder motion and lung inhalation.

Lumbar Rock

Body Segment: Lumbar.

Stage in Rehab: II and later.

Purpose: Stretch the low back and hips.

Positioning: The patient is positioned on hands and knees with elbows straight, hands shoulder-width apart, knees under the hips, and hands under the shoulders.

Execution: The back is arched, and the hips are pushed back toward the ankles as the shoulders go down toward the floor (figure 18.33, a & b). Without moving the hands or knees, the patient then moves forward to the starting position and continues forward until he or she is in a press-up position (figure 18.33c).

Possible Substitutions: A common substitution is to move the hands rather than keeping them stationary. If you observe this, remind the patient to maintain hand positions.

Knees to Chest

Body Segment: Lumbar.

Stage in Rehab: I and II and later.

Purpose: Stretch the low back and hips.

Positioning: Supine with knees and hips flexed and feet on the floor.

Execution: For a single knee-to-chest exercise, the patient first tightens the abdominal muscles to stabilize the pelvis, and then lifts one knee to the chest. The knee is held to the chest passively by the arms. In the more aggressive double knees-to-chest stretch, the patient stabilizes the pelvis by tightening the abdominal muscles, and then raises one knee to the chest. While keeping the knee up, the patient raises the other knee to the chest and pulls both knees to the chest with the arms. To lower the legs, the reverse occurs, with the patient lowering one leg at a time.

Possible Substitutions: The most common substitution is losing pelvic neutral and arching the back. To prevent this, remind the patient to keep the abdominal muscles tight prior to lifting and lowering each leg.

Notations: In the double knees-to-chest stretch, one leg at a time is raised and lowered to prevent the back from arching.

Lateral Trunk Stretch

Body Segment: Lumbar.

Stage in Rehab: II and later.

Purpose: Stretch the lateral lumbar spine.

Positioning: Patient lies supine with the hips and knees flexed, feet flat on the floor and arms away from the sides.

Execution: One knee is crossed over the other, and the top leg pulls the bottom leg toward the top-leg side while both shoulders remain in contact with the floor (figure 18.34).

Possible Substitutions: A common substitution is to allow the ipsilateral shoulder to come off the floor so less stretch is applied. Remind the patient of the importance of shoulder stabilization if you observe this error.

Notations: For a more localized stretch to the lumbar spine, the hip is flexed to approximately 90°.

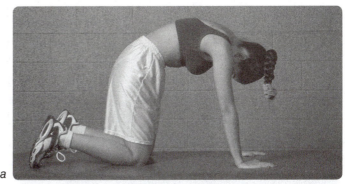
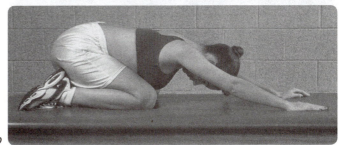
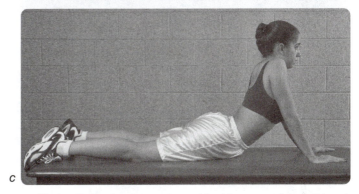

a

b

c

▶ **Figure 18.33** Lumbar rock stretch: *(a)* start position, *(b)* end position for lumbar flexion portion of the lumbar rock, *(c)* end position for lumbar extension of the lumbar rock.

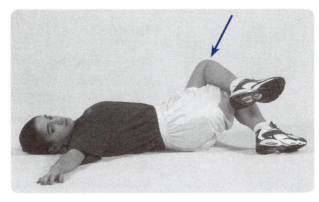

▶ **Figure 18.34** Lateral trunk stretch.

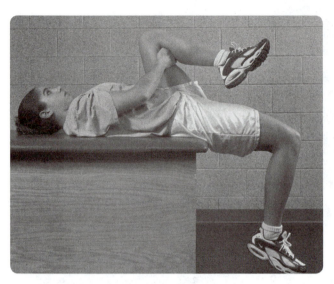

▶ **Figure 18.35** Thomas hip flexor stretch.

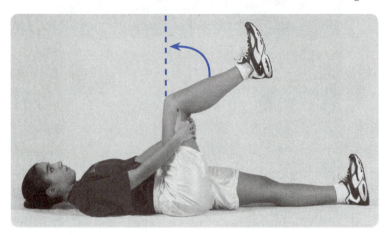

▶ **Figure 18.36** Hamstring stretch.

Thomas Hip Flexor Stretch

Body Segment: Hip.

Stage in Rehab: II and later.

Purpose: Stretch the iliopsoas muscle to reduce lumbar spine stress.

Positioning: The patient sits on a table so that the thigh is halfway off the table. The patient lies supine with both knees to the chest.

Execution: One thigh is grasped behind the knee, and the leg being stretched is lowered. The thigh of the leg being stretched (the lowered leg) should be kept in alignment with the body's midline, without hip rotation or abduction and with knee flexion to 90° (figure 18.35).

Possible Substitutions: Lateral rotation and abduction of the stretch hip are common substitutions. If the patient does not have adequate stability of the flexed hip, the back may still arch off the table. Remind the patient to firmly pull the nonstretched leg to the chest.

Notations: In normal flexibility in the stretch position, the thigh rests comfortably on the table with the back in full contact with the table.

Straight-Leg Raise

Body Segment: Hip.

Stage in Rehab: I and II and later.

Purpose: Stretch the hamstrings.

Positioning: Supine.

Execution: The patient places the hands behind the thigh of one leg while the other leg remains extended. The patient then straightens the knee of the leg that the hands are on until he or she feels a stretch in the posterior thigh or behind the knee (figure 18.36).

Possible Substitutions: The common substitution for this exercise is to flex the opposite hip to relieve the stretch. The patient should keep the other leg in a fully extended position throughout the exercise.

Notations: Hamstring tightness can contribute to low-back inflexibility. Although a variety of methods are available to stretch the hamstrings, this exercise places minimal stress on the spine.

Piriformis Stretch

Body Segment: Hip.

Stage in Rehab: I and II and later.

Purpose: Stretch the lateral rotators, especially the piriformis.

Positioning: The patient lies supine with the knees flexed and feet flat on the floor.

Execution: The knee of the involved leg is crossed on top of the other, and both knees are brought to the chest. The patient grasps the lower knee and pulls both knees toward the chest (figure 18.37a).

Possible Substitutions: A common substitution is to provide less rotation of the stretched hip. The knees should be adequately crossed to aim the knee toward the opposite shoulder when the knees are brought to the chest.

Notations: Piriformis is a common source of low-back pain. In an alternative piriformis stretch, the patient is on hands and knees with the uninvolved leg crossed over the involved leg and behind the involved hip. The patient moves the hips backward, keeping the uninvolved leg extended and flexing the knee of the involved leg (figure 18.37b). A common substitution when

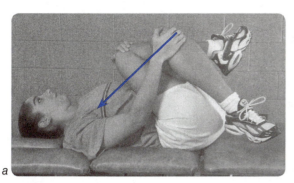

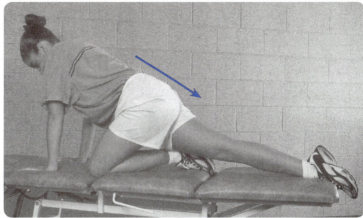

a

b

▶ **Figure 18.37** Piriformis stretch: *(a)* supine, *(b)* quadruped.

this exercise is performed is moving the hips toward the extended leg rather than keeping the weight equally distributed over both hips. Instruct the patient not to rotate but move straight back if you observe this substitution.

Iliotibial Band (ITB) Stretch

Body Segment: Hip and thigh.

Stage in Rehab: I and II and later.

Purpose: Stretch the lateral tight muscles and soft tissue.

Positioning: Supine with the knees extended.

Execution: The extremity to be stretched is crossed over the other so that the foot

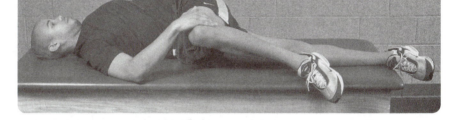

▶ **Figure 18.38** Iliotibial band stretch.

of the top leg lies on the outside of the opposite knee. The hand on the opposite side grasps the crossed-over knee and pulls it toward the floor (figure 18.38).

Possible Substitutions: The common substitution for this exercise is to lift the ipsilateral shoulder off the floor. Instruct the patient in proper stabilization of the trunk for this exercise.

Notations: Tightness in the ITB can affect the low back.

Lateral Shift

Body Segment: Lumbar.

Stage in Rehab: I.

Purpose: Correct a lateral shift and realign the spine.

Positioning: The patient stands next to the wall, with the side that has the lumbar lateral shift farthest from the wall.

Execution: Keeping the shoulders level, the patient shifts the pelvis laterally to the wall (figure 18.39a).

Possible Substitutions: The common substitution for this exercise is a tilting of the shoulders away from the wall or a leaning of the hips into the wall, or both. If this occurs, either have the patient perform the exercise in front of a mirror or place your hands above the shoulders, but not touching them, and instruct the patient to perform the exercise without letting the shoulder touch your hands.

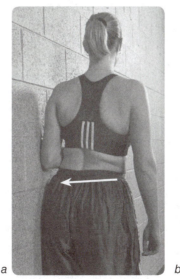

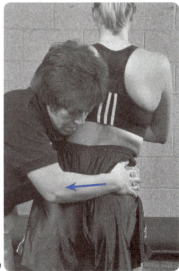

a

b

▶ **Figure 18.39** Lateral shift: *(a)* independent, *(b)* assisted.

Notations: To perform the stretch passively, the clinician stands next to the patient, facing the side that has the shift. The clinician then encircles the patient's waist and clasps his or her hands together on the opposite hip (figure 18.39b). The clinician stabilizes the patient's trunk by leaning his or her shoulder into the patient's waist while pulling the pelvis toward him- or herself.

For links to a wide range of sports medicine resources, see *The Physician and Sportsmedicine* Web site at www.physsportsmed.com.

Standing Extension

Body Segment: Lumbar.

Stage in Rehab: I and II and later.

Purpose: Increase trunk extension and relieve tension in the lumbar spine after prolonged sitting or a prolonged forward-bending position.

Positioning: The patient stands and places both hands in the small of the back.

Execution: The patient then leans backward, leading with the head and keeping the knees and hips extended.

Possible Substitutions: A common substitution is moving the hips posteriorly and flexing the knees to lean backward from the knees. If this occurs, have the patient perform the exercise with his or her back against a kitchen countertop or other firm structure at waist level to stop the hips from moving posteriorly.

Posture, Core, and Pelvic Stabilization Exercises

Any patient with a spinal injury should be examined for posture. Posture plays a vital role in both recovery from and prevention of injuries. If a patient has poor posture and nothing is done to correct it, the poor posture will continue to affect the injury and make recovery difficult. Instruction in techniques to maintain proper posture and use of proper body mechanics should also be a part of the rehabilitation program. Refer to the discussion of posture in chapter 11 as necessary.

Core

We know that the spine by itself is unable to support any significant load; by itself, it collapses with no more than 5 lb (about 2 kg) applied to it (Panjabi et al., 1989). Therefore, it receives a significant amount of support and stability from the surrounding muscles. Trunk stability is often discussed in relation to what is known as the "core." When we speak of the core, we are referring to the trunk muscles and their ability to control and stabilize the trunk for functional movement. On the basis of biomechanical principles discussed in chapter 2, we know that if there is to be power transfer, it has to occur through stable structures. Since the trunk is the means by which power is transferred between the upper and lower extremities, the core is an important factor in performance in both conditioning and rehabilitation programs (Clark, Fater, and Reuterman, 2000).

Interest in the core developed in the latter half of the last century after Kennedy (1967) suggested that the abdominal muscles provide an effectual brace for the spine by increasing intra-abdominal pressure to stabilize the trunk during movement. Since then, we have understood the importance of intra-abdominal pressure in spine support and stability. When intra-abdominal pressure is created, it converts the trunk into a solid cylinder to withstand compressive and shear loads placed on it (Norris, 1995).

For this intra-abdominal pressure to be produced, a coordinated and synchronous effort of the abdominal muscles, pelvic floor, and diaphragm is required (Norris, 1995). Beyond the obvious muscles, the abdominal muscles, the diaphragm, and pelvic floor muscles play an important part in providing intra-abdominal pressure for stability. There is evidence to demonstrate that patients with sacroiliac pain have poor recruitment of these muscles compared to individuals without pain (O'Sullivan et al., 2002).

Stiffness is a factor in prevention and treatment of low-back pain. Stiffness is the result of a combination of active and passive elements. The passive elements are the ligaments, capsules, and fascia that surround the lumbar spine and trunk region. The active elements are the muscles. The superficial and deep muscles play a role in providing stiffness for the spine. A stronger muscle is stiffer than a weak one. If a ligament is injured, then the muscles must compensate for the loss of stiffness from that structure since it will not be restored to its former level. Many back injuries involve inert tissues and secondarily the muscles surrounding the area. Loss of stiffness in any of these tissues will reduce the patient's ability to produce stability through stiffness.

In defining the core muscles, Bergmark (1989) distinguished between the trunk movers and the trunk stabilizers, referring to the trunk stabilizers as local muscles and the trunk movers as global muscles. He identified the local muscles as those muscles close to the center of the body that provide stabilization since their lever-arm lengths are unable to provide little else. On the other hand, he suggested that the global muscles are able to provide for gross trunk motions because they are sufficiently distanced from the center of motion and have longer lever arms that cover many more spinal segments. It was not long after Bergmark's ideas were made known that Panjabi indicated through his development of a biomechanical model that both the local and global muscles are necessary for spinal stability (Panjabi et al., 1989). It may seem irrelevant, then, to distinguish between local and global muscles. However, their functions are different, and we need to understand these differences before we can design a therapeutic exercise program for any patient with low-back pain (LBP).

The global, or superficial, muscles include the rectus abdominis ventrally and the large paraspinal muscles dorsally. These large paraspinal muscles include those muscles spanning several vertebral levels; these muscles are collectively referred to as the erector spinae muscles and include the longissimus and iliocostalis. The local, or core muscles, sometimes known as the stabilizers, are not as clearly identified. Some consider the transverse abdominis and multifidus the only core muscles (Wilke et al., 1995), while others include the obliques as well (Radebold et al., 2000). The internal and external oblique muscles are sometimes discussed as core muscles and sometimes as global muscles. Although they provide trunk motion, they also provide stability—hence the confusion that often arises with attempts to categorize these two groups of muscles. We will come back to this topic shortly when we discuss rehabilitation.

Since the lumbar extensor muscles contain primarily type I muscle fibers, they are designed to provide long-term activity for the spine (Thorstensson and Carlson, 1987). However, it has been shown that people with LBP have less muscle endurance in their local lumbar muscles (Nourbakhsh and Arab, 2002). Additionally, LBP patients demonstrate reduced proprioception and position sense compared to persons without LBP (O'Sullivan et al., 2003). Another important factor related to LBP is a dysfunction in recruitment patterns of low-back and extensor muscles following incidents of back pain (Ebenbichler et al., 2001). The transverse abdominis contracts, and so does its antagonist in normal subjects prior to movement of the trunk or extremities; this is thought to occur to stabilize the spine prior to motion (Radebold et al., 2000). However, when these muscles are not recruited or are delayed in their recruitment as seen in LBP subjects, other muscles are used in their place; this puts additional stresses on the back as well as inert tissue and other muscles that are overstressed in place of the lumbar muscles. In summary, research has demonstrated that patients with LBP either do not use their muscles in a correct sequential pattern or do not recruit them in time for them to be effective in providing stiffness and stability, and that the muscles lack the endurance to offer support to the spine during daily activities.

In addition to the back, lack of lumbar stability places other body segments at risk of injury as well. Core instability has been linked to knee injuries, including anterior cruciate ligament injuries and patellofemoral pain syndrome (Leetun et al., 2004). Other lower-extremity injuries related to instability and imbalances include ankle sprains (Leetun et al., 2004).

When discussing methods of providing trunk stability, we have to consider more than the trunk muscles. Hip muscles are also included since they not only provide hip motion but, because of their attachment to the pelvis, also influence pelvis and trunk motion (Ekstrom, Donatelli, and Carp, 2007). Discussions of trunk stability frequently refer to support from the core muscles, trunk flexor and extensor groups, and pelvis stabilizers. The pelvic stabilizers include the hip muscles, especially the quadratus lumborum, hip extensors, hip abductors, and hip rotators. There is evidence that patients with LBP have deficiencies in hip abductors and rotators (Leetun et al., 2004).

It has been shown that trunk stability is improved with cocontraction of anterior and posterior trunk muscles (Bergmark, 1989). Unfortunately, because of the positions and fiber alignment of the muscles surrounding the trunk, there is no one exercise that facilitates all of these muscles. It has been shown, however, that the transverse abdominis and multifidus are the only muscles that are activated in all trunk motions (Wilke et al., 1995).

Based on what we know of the spine and the importance of stabilization, we realize that several factors must be involved in a rehabilitation program for any patient with LBP. These factors are founded on what we know to be common problems in these patients, including the following:

1. Reduced proprioception. With deficiency in proprioception, we know that balance and activity coordination will be deficient.

2. Reduced muscle endurance. Although strength is a factor, especially in the athletic and blue-collar work population, muscle endurance is perhaps a greater factor; muscle endurance may be more deficient than strength and must be restored for safe functional activity performance.

3. Lack of muscle coactivation. If the trunk muscles do not cocontract during trunk activity, spinal stiffness and stability will be lacking and the risk of injury increased.

4. Delayed recruitment of core muscles. If stabilizers fail to fire when they should, stability is lost and more stress occurs to other supporting structures.

5. Reduced stability. All of these factors create a situation of instability of the trunk. This situation not only increases the individual's injury risk, but also prevents optimal functional performance by limiting force transfer through the trunk.

Given these problems, the goals for treatment of a patient with LBP are designed to resolve them. A therapeutic exercise program for a patient with LBP will include the following:

1. Trunk proprioception and balance activities

2. Core muscle endurance and secondarily strength exercises

3. Core muscle reeducation and retraining for coactivation and recruitment

4. Exercises for trunk movers in all planes of motion

5. Strength exercises for quadratus lumborum and other hip muscles

6. Progression to functional activities that include core stabilization

Basic to any therapeutic exercise program for the spine is the ability to place the spine in a position of low stress. This position is known by many names, as discussed next.

Pelvic Neutral

A stable pelvis serves as a platform from which the extremities are able to perform their activities. It is as basic to running as standing is or as basic to standing as balance is. It must be taught prior to a patient's performing therapeutic exercises. In this section, we will discuss what pelvic neutral is, why it is important, and how to teach it to patients.

Pelvic stability is also referred to as *lumbar stability, trunk stability, core stability, spinal stability,* or *lumbosacral stability*. These various terms will be interchanged throughout this section to bolster their familiarity. Pelvic stability relies on the strength and control of several trunk muscles: abdominal obliques, transverse abdominis, multifidus, the trunk movers, hip rotators, and the gluteal muscle group. The quadratus lumborum and latissimus dorsi also play a role in stability. It is important that the clinician design a program that improves the endurance and strength of these muscles before performance activities are initiated.

Before an individual can have good pelvic stability, he or she must be able to maintain a *pelvic neutral* position. **Pelvic neutral** is a position where the least amount of stress is placed on the lumbar spine. Sometimes the position is called *lumbar neutral,* or *neutral spine.* Pelvic neutral can be difficult to find for someone who is not accustomed to being in this position, especially individuals who have low back pain. I have found the best position for the patient to be in for instruction on how to achieve pelvic neutral is sitting. With the patient sitting, have the patient place his or her fingers on the left and right ASIS. Instruct the patient to rock the pelvis as far as possible posteriorly and note the end position, and then rock the pelvis as far as possible anteriorly, noting the end position. Now the patient rocks between each extreme, moving through a progressively smaller range of motion until he or she is balanced in the mid-position between the ends of motion. This is the patient's pelvic neutral; it is the center of pelvic motion where the spine should be balanced over the pelvis. Pelvic neutral is individualized and dependent upon the person's ability to move the pelvis and the range of motion available.

Once the patient is able to find and hold pelvic neutral, it is important to explain and emphasize to the patient the need to maintain this position during all activities. Maintaining this position will require some contraction of the stabilizing muscles. The exercises presented on the next few pages can be used in the early phase when the patient has difficulty maintaining pelvic neutral with arm and leg motions. The intent of these exercises is to have the patient perform arm and leg motions while maintaining pelvic neutral. Careful attention must be paid to the patient's performance so correction of erroneous performance can be made and encouragement is given for correct performance.

Stabilization Exercise Progression

Two exercises that assist patients in facilitating the inner core muscles are abdominal hollowing and abdominal bracing. There is disagreement as to which is the better exercise since abdominal hollowing recruits the transverse abdominis and multifidus muscles but does not facilitate the rectus abdominis and external oblique (Richardson, Jull, Hodges, & Hides, 1999). The abdominal bracing exercise, however, facilitates the transverse abdominis as well as the internal and external obliques (McGill, 2001). Because, as has been mentioned, use of both local and global muscles is required for optimal core control, it is recommended that both exercises be used in a rehabilitation program.

Transverse Abdominis Recruitment Activities The abdominal hollowing exercise is best initially performed with the patient supine in a hook-lying position with the hips and knees flexed and the feet on the surface. The patient positions himself or herself in a neutral spine. The clinician then instructs the patient to maintain the neutral spine position and hollow the abdomen by pulling in the navel in and up towards the spine (Jull & Richardson, 2000). It is important that the patient not suck in the belly but hollow the abdomen instead. The position is held for 5 seconds to start and repeated. As the patient improves control, the hold duration may be increased up to 30 seconds.

If the patient has difficulty with this exercise, use of a blood pressure cuff may be helpful. With the patient in a supine hook-lying position, the blood pressure cuff is placed comfortably beneath the patient's low back. The cuff is inflated to 40 mmHg. The patient moves into a pelvic neutral position and is instructed to, "Pull your navel up and in toward your spine." The clinician is able to monitor whether the patient has successfully performed the activity by monitoring the blood pressure cuff gauge. If the pressure jumps significantly, then the patient has also lost pelvic neutral and gone into a posterior pelvic tilt; if the pressure decreases significantly, the patient has moved into an anterior pelvic tilt. Allow the patient to see the blood pressure gauge as a visual feedback mechanism. Palpation of the abdominals may also assist the patient in correct muscle recruitment. Once the patient is able to pull the navel to the spine without more than a 3- to 5-degree change in blood pressure gauge reading, correct recruitment of the transverse abdominis has occurred.

Another technique that used to facilitate better transverse abdominis activity and provide the patient tactile feedback is having the patient place fingertips just medial and superior to the anterior superior iliac crest. The patient should feel the abdominal muscles pull in, not out, in the abdominal hollowing exercise. In each of these exercises, strength and control along with development of muscle endurance are goals.

Abdominal bracing is an activation of all the abdominal muscles to create stiffness of the trunk. Because of the intensity of muscle activity, a secondary extensor muscle activation occurs. This anterior, lateral, and posterior muscle tension provides stiffness without restricting motion (Grenier & McGill, 2007). Again, this isometric hold is maintained for 5 seconds initially but may increase to 30 seconds with the patient's improved control.

Use of these two exercises in a therapeutic exercise program is important to facilitate, strengthen and improve the endurance of the core muscles. However, how much activation of these muscles is required for appropriate stability? A maximal contraction is not necessary for most functional activities. It has been found that the amount of force these core muscles are required to exert during functional activities is substantially submaximal as long as the individual maintains a neutral position (Cholewicki, Panjabi, & Khachatryan, 1997). Therefore, a maximal contraction is not necessary, but a sustained submaximal contraction is (McGill, Grenier, Kavcic, & Cholewicki, 2003).

Once a patient is able to create a strong contraction of the transverse abdominis, demonstrating a good hollowing performance, have the patient begin controlling the quantity of the contraction. Contrast between maximal and half-maximal can usually be easily made by the patient, so have the patient contract the transverse abdominis as much as possible, then instruct the patient to relax to 50% of that contraction and hold it. Once the patient is comfortable with that change in contraction level, instruct him or her to go to 50% of the submaximal contraction (50% of the 50%). This is approximately the amount of force necessary to maintain core stability during functional activities (25% of maximal contraction). Of course, with activities that require extreme effort, the core stability requirements also increase, but 25% is an average of what I recommend for daily functional activities. Once the patient is able to adjust and maintain a 25% core contraction, he or she should be encouraged to maintain this tension throughout the day, allowing it to become an automatic and natural condition.

Multifidus Recruitment Activities The multifidus is too deep to palpate, so it may be difficult to determine whether or not the patient is using the muscle correctly. However, we do know that the multifidus is activated when pelvic floor muscles are used. In order to activate the pelvic floor muscles, the verbal cue that is provided to the patient is, "Tighten muscles as if you were stopping urination at mid-flow." Although you will not palpate the multifidus directly, you may be able to feel it tighten indirectly if you place your finger tips adjacent the patient's lumbar spinous processes as you provide the verbal cue. If the muscle is weak, it may feel like a very light pressure into your fingertips.

With the patient in a supine hook-lying position and in pelvic neutral, provide the verbal cue, "Tighten muscles as if you were stopping urination at mid-flow." Once again, the blood pressure cuff inflated to 40 mmHg placed in the lumbar region provides feedback to the clinician and patient as to the patient's quality of performance. As with the transverse abdominis exercise, if the pressure increases or decreases substantially, the patient has lost pelvic neutral. Tension in the muscle should be produced without changing the position of the pelvis. If this is the case, provide the patient tactile feedback by having the patient place finger tips just medial and superior to the anterior superior iliac spine; the patient should feel the abdominal muscles pull in, not out, in the abdominal hollowing exercise. In each of these exercises, strength and control along with development of muscle endurance are goals.

Combining Transverse Oblique and Multifidus Activity Once the transverse abdominis and multifidus are activated individually, the clinician now instructs the patient to activate both, "and now pull your navel to your spine. Tighten your muscles as if stopping urination mid-flow." This combined activity is a type of bracing exercise that recruits abdominals and posterior muscles. The patient is able to perform these activities correctly if there is no change in the blood pressure gauge.

In addition to these two exercises, other basic exercises may be initiated early in the core program. Once the patient finds pelvic neutral and is able to perform the abdominal hollowing and bracing exercises, two other types of exercise progressions may be used, the dead bug exercises and the bird dog exercises. The dead bug exercises involve moving the arms and/or legs in a supine position while maintaining neutral spine, while the bird dog exercises are performed on hands and knees but involve similar activities. The goal of these exercises is to strengthen core muscles and simultaneously have the patient perform simple extremity motions while holding a proper neutral position.

Dead bug exercises should be performed, at least in the early stages, with the blood pressure cuff to provide the patient with feedback on his or her performance. If the patient's pressure gauge indicates a big jump during any of the exercises, it may be necessary to start with a smaller range of movement; the patient should perform an exercise only in the range of motion where pelvic stability is maintained. As greater control is achieved, a greater range of movement will be possible.

The "dead bug exercises," or "bug exercises," are named presumably because of the position in which they are performed and the arm and leg movement that occurs. The same holds true for the "bird dog" exercises. These supine and quadruped exercises, respectively, are outlined here from the easiest to the more difficult. Progression from these moves the patient to standing exercises using rubber band resistance for either upper or lower extremity activities while the patient maintains a pelvic neutral position.

Correct the patient when a neutral spine is not maintained for both the dead bug and bird dog exercises. This correction is completed by telling the patient what is being incorrectly performed and providing instruction on what to do to correct the technique. The hips should not roll; the lumbar spine should not flex or extend; and there should not be an anterior or posterior pelvic tilt. If the patient is unable to maintain stability during any exercise, even with your verbal and tactile cueing, it is necessary to return to exercises at the previous level of difficulty before advancing. The abdominal and buttock muscles should be tensed in each of these exercises to provide hip, pelvis, and spine stabilization necessary for correct performance. You should instruct or remind the patient regarding this proper technique until he or she can perform the exercise without verbal or tactile cueing.

Not all patients with back injuries need to perform these dead bug or bird dog exercises and some may be able to progress rapidly through the earlier-stage exercises. Any difficulty the patient has with any of these exercises indicates that pelvic stabilization is limited and that the patient should do the exercise until he or she is able to perform it correctly.

Once the patient masters one exercise, he or she progresses to the next one. These exercises may appear to be easy, but if you try them, you quickly realize that when they are performed correctly they may not be as simple as they look. These exercises are more difficult with the patient lying on a foam roller during their execution.

Each exercise is prefaced with the verbal cues from the rehabilitation clinician to "Pull the navel to the spine" and "Tighten muscles as if stopping urination mid-flow." Once the patient sets the transverse abdominis and multifidus muscles, the exercises are performed.

Each of these dead bug exercises can be made more difficult by having the patient perform arm and/or leg motions in a diagonal pattern rather than straight-plane motions. This alteration will require recruitment of the oblique muscles.

When the patient is able to perform the supine stabilization exercises, progression can be made to exercises in a quadruped position. As with the dead bug exercises, the quadruped exercises are presented in a progressive manner, from easiest to most difficult. As with the dead bug exercises, these exercises can be further advanced by having the patient perform arm and/or leg motions in a diagonal pattern rather than straight-plane motions to not only make the exercise more difficult but also recruit the oblique muscles.

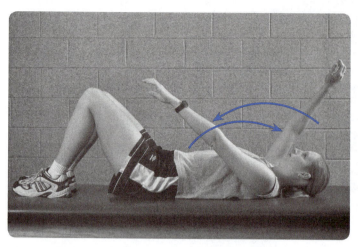

▶ **Figure 18.40**   Dead bug spine stabilization with arms.

■ Dead Bug and Bird Dog Exercises

Supine Stabilization With Arm Movement

Exercise Type: Dead bug.

Stage in Rehab: I and II.

Purpose: Provide arm resistance while the patient is in spinal stabilization.

Positioning: Supine with knees and hips flexed, feet on the table.

Execution: One arm is raised overhead and then the other, in an alternating fashion (figure 18.40). The trunk is stabilized, with no movement occurring in the spine or pelvis while the arms are moving.

Cues and Notations: Cues are given to the patient to take and maintain a neutral spine position. The patient must maintain pelvic neutral and breathe while performing the movement.

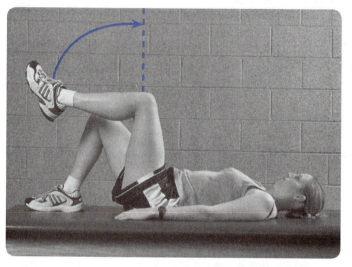

▶ **Figure 18.41**   Dead bug spine stabilization with legs.

Supine Stabilization With Leg Movement

Exercise Type: Dead bug.

Stage in Rehab: I and II.

Purpose: Strengthen lower abdominal muscles and provide increased resistance to spine stabilization.

Positioning: Supine hook-lying position.

Execution: While in a neutral spine position, the patient raises one knee up toward the chest and then extends the leg from the knee without moving the hips as the abdominal muscles are contracted more tightly to maintain pelvic neutral (figure 18.41).

Cues and Notations: The hips should not rise up or rotate, and the back should not arch. The motion should be smooth. The patient returns the leg to the starting position and repeats the movement with the opposite leg.

Supine Stabilization With Arm and Leg Movement

Exercise Type: Dead bug.

Stage in Rehab: I and II.

Purpose: Strengthen the abdominal muscles and stabilize the spine during arm and leg movement.

Positioning: Supine in a hook-lying position.

Execution: One arm and the opposite leg are raised simultaneously and then lowered while pelvic neutral is maintained (figure 18.42). The movement is repeated with the contralateral arm and leg.

Cues and Notations: The movement should be smooth, and no trunk motion should occur. The pelvis is maintained in neutral throughout the exercise. The back should not roll from one side to the other and should not arch off the floor.

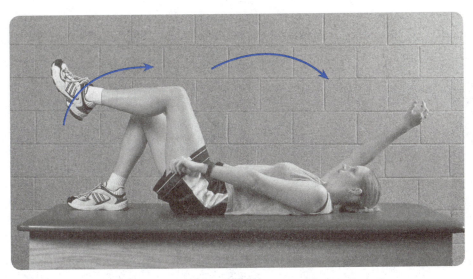

▶ **Figure 18.42** Dead bug spine stabilization with arm and leg movement.

Supine Stabilization With Arms and Unsupported Legs

Exercise Type: Dead bug.

Stage in Rehab: I and II.

Purpose: This is a more severe exercise for strengthening the abdominal muscles and maintaining pelvic neutral during independent arm and leg movement.

Positioning: Supine hook-lying in spinal neutral.

Execution: The neck and shoulders should remain relaxed throughout the exercise. The abdominal muscles remain tightened as the patient lifts the arms and legs off the floor. The patient gradually extends one leg while flexing the arm on the same side, then reverses the position with the extremities on the opposite side (figure 18.43).

Cues and Notations: The back should not lift off the floor, and the hips should not roll.

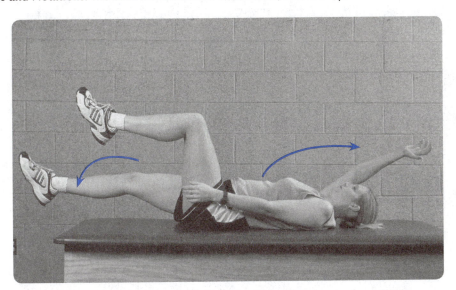

▶ **Figure 18.43** Dead bug spine stabilization with arms and unsupported legs.

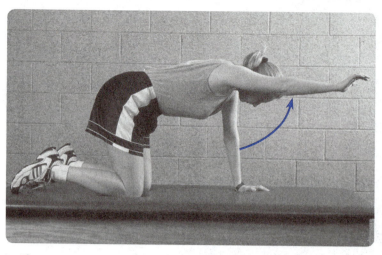

Bird dog exercise in quadruped arm raise.

Quadruped Arm Raise

Exercise Type: Bird dog.

Stage in Rehab: I and II.

Purpose: Spinal stabilization.

Positioning: Quadruped position in spinal neutral.

Execution: One arm is raised and lowered, and the movement is then repeated on the opposite side (figure 18.44).

Cues and Notations: The hips and back should not move throughout the exercise. A good feedback technique to help the patient detect hip motion during these exercises is to place a 0.9- to 1.2-m (3 to 4 ft) stick or dowel across the low back. The dowel should be balanced on the back. If the patient sees the stick drop on one side during the exercise, he or she knows that the hips have rotated and that pelvic neutral has not been maintained.

Quadruped Leg Raise

Exercise Type: Bird dog.

Stage in Rehab: I and II.

Purpose: Enhance pelvic stabilization.

Positioning: The patient is in a quadruped position with the pelvis in neutral.

Execution: The patient extends one leg, rather than an arm, and moves it backward by tightening the buttocks and hamstrings. No movement of the pelvis, trunk, or back occurs throughout the motion.

Cues and Notations: The extremity motion should be smooth and steady. As with the arm exercises, a stick placed across the lumbar spine can provide the patient feedback on unwanted pelvic movement.

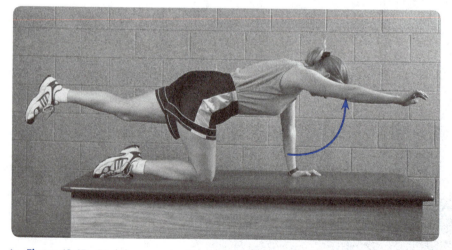

▶ **Figure 18.45** Bird dog exercise in quadruped arm and leg raise.

Quadruped Arm and Leg Raise

Exercise Type: Bird dog.

Stage in Rehab: I and II.

Purpose: Enhance stabilization and strengthen spine extensors.

Positioning: Quadruped position and a neutral spine position.

Execution: The patient lifts one arm and the opposite leg and then repeats the motion with the other arm and leg (figure 18.45). The shoulders, hips, and back should not move throughout the exercise.

Cues and Notations: The hips should not drop or lift, and the back should not roll. Use a stick across the lower back to assist in feedback for the patient during the exercise.

Quadruped Arm and Leg Raise With Manual Resistance

Exercise Type: Bird dog.

Stage in Rehab: I and II.

Purpose: Enhance stabilization and strengthen spine extensors and abdominal muscles.

Positioning: Quadruped position with the lumbar spine in neutral. The patient lifts the arm on the side of the back that is painful and the opposite leg.

Execution: The clinician grasps the hand in a handshake position. The clinician and patient then play "tug of war"; the patient's shoulders move from flexion to extension while the clinician moves his or her body in different positions so that the angle of the force in the tug of war varies; the clinician moves across the patient's right and left sides and in front of the patient's body while providing resistance.

Cues and Notations: The patient should maintain pelvic neutral with proper core tension throughout the activity.

Additional Activities   Once the patient has mastered these movements while maintaining pelvic or spinal neutral, core stabilization exercises progress from these basic exercises to dynamic activities to regain proprioceptive function and neuromuscular control. It is important that the patient maintain good trunk stability during all activities. This protects the spine and allows the patient to perform physical activities more skillfully and with greater force, because with good pelvic stability the lower-extremity forces can be more readily transmitted to the upper extremities.

From the exercises presented above, trunk movements become more aggressive and more multi-planar. For example, the patient begins with simple walking in pelvic neutral. More advanced resistive activities include performing diagonal lower and upper extremity exercises with a resistance band while maintaining a neutral position. Careful observations must occur to assure the neutral position is maintained. Placing a mirror for the patient to see his or her performance may be necessary if your verbal and tactile cues fail to correct the patient's loss of a neutral spine during these activities. The resistance does not need to be severe; a light resistance, especially early in this progression will allow the patient to perform the exercise correctly and maintain proper control but still create a progression.

More advanced exercises for trunk stabilization include strength exercises for the hips, abdominals, and back extensors. These exercises are discussed in the next unit on strengthening exercises and in chapter 24. Careful attention is necessary by the clinician regarding the patient's performance of all these exercises to assure the patient maintains a pelvic neutral position throughout each activity.

Strengthening Exercises

Goals for these exercises are to increase the muscles' strength and endurance. We begin with the mildest and proceed to more challenging exercises, first for the neck and then for the lower back. Keep in mind that other exercises you can use for strengthening include the aquatic exercises discussed in chapter 13 and the Swiss-ball and foam-roller exercises discussed in chapter 14. The patient should maintain a pelvic neutral position throughout each of these exercises.

Strengthening exercises that are in other chapters but should be included for LBP patients involve muscles from both the shoulder and hip that are attached to the back. The latissimus dorsi, rhomboids, trapezius, hamstrings, gluteus maximus, gluteus medius, and hip external rotators should all be strengthened as part of a total lumbar stabilization program.

Cervical Exercises

Distinct advantages of isometric exercises are that they can be initiated early in the therapeutic exercise program and that the patient can perform them independently throughout the day.

Following isometric exercises, more aggressive exercises for strengthening the cervical muscles are instituted. These are labeled "resistive cervical exercises." They are performed with manual resistance or various equipment such as resistance bands, pulleys, or machines. It is important to be careful using the machine exercises, because if applied inappropriately, they can place too much stress on the cervical spine and increase the risk of injury. Proper cervical alignment must be maintained throughout the exercises with movement occurring at each segment—the lower cervical spine should not be used as a fulcrum.

■ Strength Exercises for the Cervical Muscles

Isometrics

Body Segment: Cervical.

Stage in Rehab: II.

Purpose: Early strengthening in all planes.

Positioning: Patient is sitting or supine with neck in a midrange and properly aligned position.

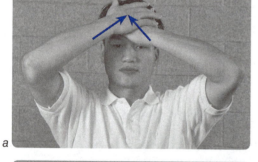

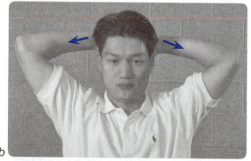

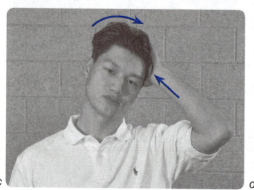

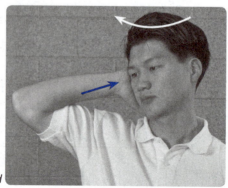

Execution:

1. Forward flexion: Patient places the palms of the hands on the forehead and attempts to touch the chin to the chest while providing resistance to the motion with the hands on the forehead (figure 18.46a).

2. Extension: The patient places both hands behind the back of his or her head while attempting to tilt the head backward, resisting the motion with the hands (figure 18.46b).

3. Lateral flexion: The patient places one hand near the ear, resisting the motion of bringing the ear to the shoulder on the same side (figure 18.46c). Repeat the exercise to the opposite side.

4. Rotation: The patient places one hand on the side of the face and resists the movement of rotating to look over the same-side shoulder (figure 18.46d). Repeat the exercise to the opposite side.

Possible Substitutions: A common substitution for each of these exercises is to perform them out of cervical alignment.

Cues and Notations: Each exercise should be performed with the head and neck in correct postural alignment. If the patient has difficulty identifying correct postural alignment, he or she should perform the exercises in front of a mirror until correct alignment can be maintained during the exercises.

▶ **Figure 18.46** Cervical isometric exercise: *(a)* flexion, *(b)* extension, *(c)* lateral flexion, *(d)* rotation.

Prone Neck Retraction

Body segment: Cervical.

Stage in Rehab: II and III.

Purpose: Strengthen the posterior cervical muscles and encourage correct cervical alignment.

Positioning: Prone with the head off the end of the table.

Execution: Keeping the chin tucked, the patient lifts the posterior head toward the ceiling (figure 18.47). The scapulae can also be squeezed together. At the top of the movement, the position is held for 5 to 10 s.

Possible Substitutions: The neck moves into hyperextension and is tilted upward toward the ceiling.

Cues and Notations: Instructing the patient to keep the chin tucked and describing the activity as "like opening and closing a drawer" may give the patient a visual image that will help.

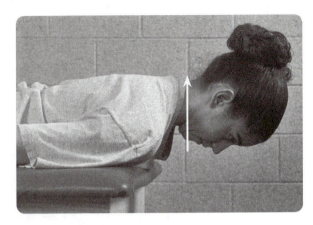

▶ **Figure 18.47** Prone cervical retraction.

Side-Lying Head Lifts

Body segment: Cervical.

Stage in Rehab: II and III.

Purpose: Strengthen lateral neck muscles.

Positioning: Side-lying with the head hanging down to the table or off the end of the table.

Execution: Patient lifts the head toward the top shoulder, going through a full arc of motion.

Possible Substitutions: The neck moves into a forward-head position or does not move in an arc.

Cues and Notations: Give verbal cues for correct alignment and movement.

Upper-Back Exercises

Many upper-back exercises are also shoulder exercises, because many of the shoulder muscles are located in the upper-back region.

■ Strength Exercises for the Upper Back

Prone Fly

Body segment: Upper back.

Stage in Rehab: II.

Purpose: Strengthen the rhomboids, middle trapezius, and cervical and upper thoracic spine extensors.

Positioning: Prone on a bench with the arms hanging down to the floor. Patient can also lie prone at the end of a treatment table with shoulders and head off the end of the table.

Execution: The patient lifts dumbbells toward the ceiling while squeezing the scapulae together (figure 18.48).

Possible Substitutions: People often perform this exercise incorrectly by raising the arms but not squeezing the scapulae together.

Cues and Notations: The patient should be instructed to go through the full scapular retraction motion, squeezing the shoulder blades together.

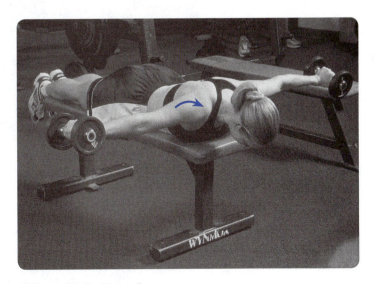

▶ **Figure 18.48** Prone fly.

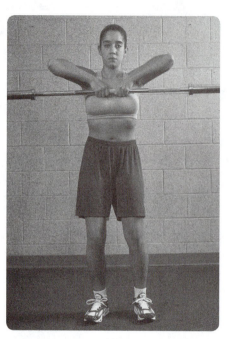

▶ **Figure 18.49** Upright row.

Upright Row

Body segment: Upper back.

Stage in Rehab: II and III.

Purpose: Strengthen upper back, trapezius, and deltoids.

Positioning: The patient uses pulleys, weights, or resistance bands with hands close together while standing erect.

Execution: With the abdominal muscles tightened to maintain a pelvic neutral position, the patient lifts the device upward toward the chin, keeping the elbows higher than the wrists (figure 18.49).

Possible Substitutions: Keeping the elbows down rather than up provides less resistance for the deltoids and rotator cuff.

Cues and Notations: Instruct the patient to keep elbows up and wrists straight.

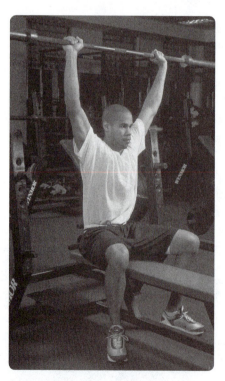

▶ **Figure 18.50** Upright press.

Upright Press (Also Called a Military Press)

Body segment: Upper back and neck.

Stage in Rehab: II and III.

Purpose: Strengthen deltoids, trapezius, and trunk stabilizers.

Positioning: Seated or standing with weights grasped in hands, elbows flexed, and weights positioned at shoulder level.

Execution: The abdominal muscles are tightened to maintain trunk stability and prevent the back from arching as the patient lifts the weight straight up and overhead toward the ceiling (figure 18.50).

Possible Substitutions: Arching the back and shrugging the shoulders are common substitutions.

Cues and Notations: Provide verbal cues to correct for these errors: Instruct the patient to maintain pelvic neutral or abdominal hollowing and "pull the shoulder blades into your back pocket."

Bouhler Exercises

Body segment: Middle and lower back.

Stage in Rehab: II and III.

Purpose: Strengthen the middle back muscles and lower trapezius.

Positioning: Patient stands with the back to the wall, arms overhead with elbows next to the ears, and elbows extended.

Execution:

1. Patient pushes the thumbs to the wall, holds the position for 5 s, relaxes, and then repeats (figure 18.51a).
2. The patient, positioned with the thumbs facing each other, repeats the movement with backs of the hands to the wall (figure 18.51b).
3. The arms are positioned at a 45° angle from the horizontal and then pushed backward to the wall, with the elbows straight and the scapulae retracted together (figure 18.51c).

Possible Substitutions: Common errors include arching the back and standing too far from the wall. Good lumbar stability helps ensure correct execution.

Cues and Notations: In each position the patient must tighten the abdominal muscles to stabilize the trunk and prevent the back from arching. A progression of these exercises is to position the patient in prone to perform the exercises (figure 18.51d) or to add weights while the patient is in prone.

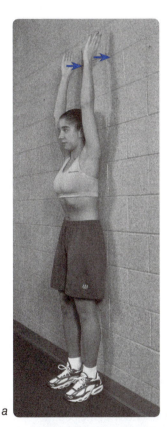
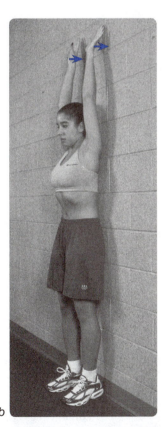
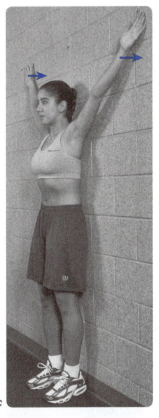
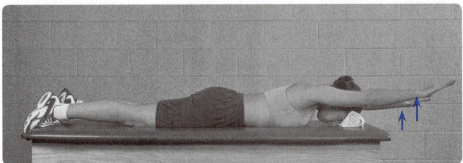

a b c

d

▶ **Figure 18.51** Bouhler exercises: *(a)* thumbs to wall, *(b)* thumbs facing each other, *(c)* 45° angle, *(d)* prone.

Lower-Back, Abdominal, and Pelvic Exercises

You may recall the abdominal and trunk exercises using the Swiss ball and foam roller (chapter 14) and the medicine ball (chapter 9). It is easy to incorporate these exercises into a progressive strengthening exercise program for the abdominal muscles and lower back. You must be able to judge the degree of difficulty of each of these exercises and incorporate them at an appropriate time in the strengthening program. Most of the exercises listed in this section are useful for pelvic or lumbosacral stabilization.

One of the exercises included in this section is the abdominal curl, or sit-up. However, it is listed here with a caveat: It is an exercise that is not recommended for abdominal strengthening because of the high loads the activity places on the spine (Norris, 2001). Therefore, a patient who has LBP caused by disc dysfunction may experience harm with this exercise. Additionally, the exercise does not recruit abdominal muscles as effectively as the crunch exercise does (Norris, 2001).

■ Strength Exercises for the Lower Back, Abdomen, and Pelvis

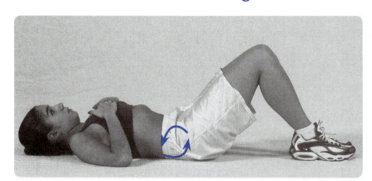

▶ **Figure 18.52** Posterior pelvic tilt.

Posterior Pelvic Tilt

Body Segment: Lumbar.

Stage in Rehab: II.

Purpose: Strengthen gluteals and abdominal muscles and encourage a posterior pelvic tilt position.

Positioning: Supine with hips extended or in a hook-lying position. Arms relaxed at the sides.

Execution: The patient tightens the abdominal muscles, tightens the buttocks, and pushes the back to the floor. The pelvis should roll posteriorly (figure 18.52).

Possible Substitutions: Common errors include using t,he legs rather than the abdominal and back muscles to move the pelvis, arching the back rather than performing a pelvic tilt, and pushing the abdomen outward rather than tensing the abdominal muscles to pull the navel toward the spine.

Cues and Notations: It is not recommended that this exercise be used in standing or lifting since it puts pressure on the posterior discs (Hubley-Kozey, 2005). Exceptions include hyperextension conditions such as spondylosis or facet injuries.

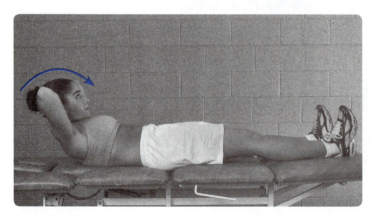

▶ **Figure 18.53** Abdominal curl.

Abdominal Curl

Body Segment: Lumbar.

Stage in Rehab: II and III.

Purpose: Strengthen the rectus abdominis and obliques.

Positioning: Legs are extended with the patient supine.

Execution: The chin is tucked to the chest, and the neck and upper trunk are slowly curled toward a sitting position. The end position is not a full sitting position (figure 18.53). The abdominal muscles should be tensed so that the umbilicus moves toward the spine. A curl should occur throughout the movement. Holding the top of the position for several seconds or holding weights in the hands makes the exercise more difficult. The feet are not anchored in this exercise because that would permit the hip flexors to perform the exercise instead of the abdominal muscles.

Possible Substitutions: The back should not be arched, and movement should occur as a curling up starting from the neck and proceeding to the low back.

Cues and Notations: This exercise is used with caution since the lumbar spine may experience increased pressures.

Abdominal Crunch

Body Segment: Lumbar and lower thoracic.

Stage in Rehab: II and III.

Purpose: Strengthen the rectus abdominis and obliques.

Positioning: The patient lies supine with the knees flexed, feet flat on the floor, and hands on top of the head.

Execution: The abdominal muscles are tightened by pulling the navel to the spine, and the head and shoulders are lifted upward toward the ceiling. There is no curling movement (figure 18.54). The position is held for 10 to 20 s at the top of the motion.

Possible Substitutions: The patient is performing the exercise incorrectly if the trunk moves toward the knees rather than toward the ceiling. Elbows should remain back with the scapulae retracted as the patient lifts the upper trunk upward. If the patient complains of LBP, it is likely that either the muscles are too weak to perform the exercise correctly or the patient is not maintaining enough tension in the abdominal muscles during the motion.

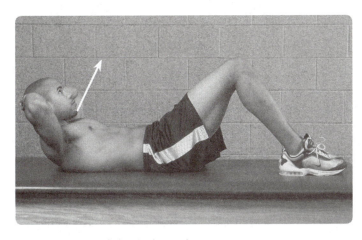

▶ **Figure 18.54** Abdominal crunch.

Cues and Notations: The exercise becomes more difficult if the patient has the legs in an unsupported position with the feet off the floor. This exercise can serve as a progression toward abdominal crunch exercises combined with medicine-ball tosses as introduced in chapter 9.

Oblique Abdominal Curl

Body Segment: Lumbar.

Stage in Rehab: II and III.

Purpose: Strengthen the internal and external obliques.

Positioning: Patient is supine with the hips and knees flexed and feet on the floor.

Execution: The patient rotates the hips to one side so that he or she is lying on the back while on one hip and the other hip is facing the ceiling. With hands on shoulders, or in the more difficult position, on top of the head, the patient curls toward the top hip, attempting to lift the head and shoulders upward and forward as much as possible (figure 18.55). The feet are not anchored.

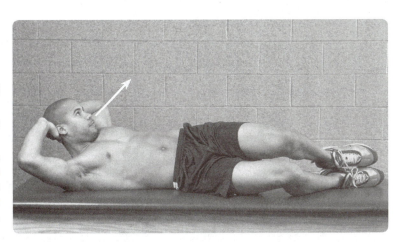

▶ **Figure 18.55** Oblique abdominal curl.

Possible Substitutions: A common error is beginning the rotation at the end of the motion rather than beginning the rotation at the onset and continuing through the range of motion.

Cues and Notations: An alternative method is for the patient to lie supine and rotate one elbow toward the opposite knee while performing a crunch. Difficulties with this method are that hip rotation can be easily substituted for trunk rotation, trunk rotation can begin too early or too late in the motion before the patient lifts the shoulders upward, or the rotation can be performed with too much momentum.

Supine Leg Exercises

Body Segment: Lumbar.

Stage in Rehab: II and III.

Purpose: Strengthen the lower rectus abdominis and facilitate pelvic neutral.

Positioning: Patient lies supine in a hook-lying position. Arms are at the side or across the abdomen.

Execution: The spine is maintained in neutral throughout the exercise.

1. Both legs are passively moved so the hips are at 90°. The patient slowly lowers one flexed leg to the table and returns it to the 90° hip flexion position while holding pelvic neutral. The activity is repeated on the other leg.

2. One hip is flexed with the knee extended, foot pointing toward the ceiling. The leg is slowly lowered to the floor (figure 18.56a).

3. The patient alternately moves one leg out into extension while bringing the other leg toward the starting position so that both legs are moving simultaneously in opposite motions without either foot touching the table (figure 18.56b).

4. In this next progression, the patient starts with both knees in extension and both feet elevated toward the ceiling. The patient slowly lowers the legs to the floor without letting the low back arch (figure 18.56c).

5. A V-sit-up is performed while the back is maintained in neutral (figure 18.56d).

Possible Substitutions: Spinal neutral is lost during the exercise, the pelvis rolls from one side to the other, or the back flexes.

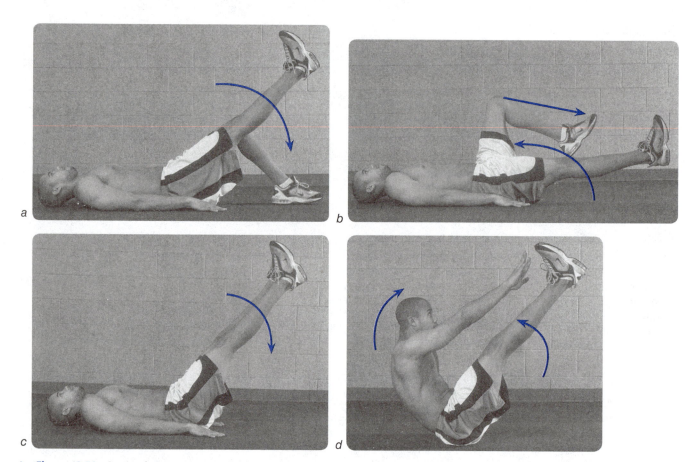

▶ **Figure 18.56** Supine leg exercises: *(a)* leg lowering, single; *(b)* leg thrusts; *(c)* leg lowering, bilateral; *(d)* V-sit-up.

Cues and Notations: Remind the patient to maintain a neutral position and keep the abdominal muscles tense. If the patient is able to advance to the next-level exercise but unable to perform the next exercise correctly, flex the knees to shorten the lever-arm length of the lower-extremity resistance arm so that he or she performs the exercise without losing neutral.

Side Bridge

Body Segment: Lumbar.

Stage in Rehab: II and III.

Purpose: Strengthen obliques and quadratus lumborum.

Positioning: Patient is side-lying in a semireclined position with hips and knees in extension and elbow positioned under the shoulder.

Execution: In a neutral position, the patient lifts the hips so that the body forms one line from the shoulders to the feet. The position is held for 5 s.

Possible Substitutions: Trunk flexion or lateral rotation is often a substitution pattern.

Cues and Notations: Inform the patient that the lower extremities may feel as though they are behind the trunk when they are actually in good alignment. If the exercise is too difficult, reduce the time of the hold or begin with a hip-hike exercise in standing.

Bridging

Body Segment: Lumbar.

Stage in Rehab: II.

Purpose: Strengthen trunk extensors and emphasize stabilization.

Positioning: Patient is in a supine hook-lying position.

Execution:

1. In a neutral position, the patient lifts the hips off the floor until the thighs form a straight line with the trunk (figure 18.57a). The position is held for 15 to 60 s.

2. The next progression of this exercise is to perform the bridge and then lift each leg to march in place while maintaining the bridge in pelvic neutral. The patient must use the abdominal muscles and buttocks while performing this exercise to maintain a straight line from the trunk to the supporting thigh.

3. A more advanced version of this exercise has the patient in the same bridging position, keeping abdominal, buttock, and lower-back muscles in good tension to maintain the position. The patient first brings one knee into full extension without moving the hips, then lowers it, and then performs the motion with the other leg (figure 18.57b).

Possible Substitutions: The hips should not drop or roll to one side.

Cues and Notations: A stick placed across the hips and parallel to the floor will notify the patient if changes in the pelvis position occur. If the stick either falls off or dips on one side, stability is lost.

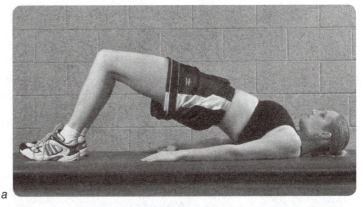

a

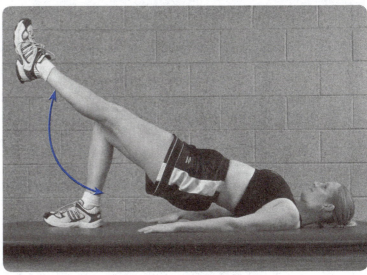

b

▶ **Figure 18.57** Bridging progression: *(a)* bridging, *(b)* leg lift.

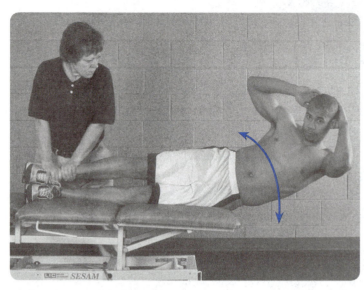

▶ **Figure 18.58**   Side-lying sit-up.

Side-Lying Sit-Up

Body Segment: Lumbar.

Stage in Rehab: III.

Purpose: Strengthen the quadratus lumborum and obliques.

Positioning: Patient is side-lying with the feet anchored and the legs extended and in line with the trunk.

Execution: Hands are placed across the chest or in the more difficult position on top of the head. The patient curls sideways toward the top hip as far as possible, attempting to curl rather than lift from the hips (figure 18.58).

Possible Substitutions: Moving into trunk flexion is the most common substitution.

Cues and Notations: Remind the patient to remain in pelvic neutral throughout the exercise and hold a good alignment between the trunk and legs.

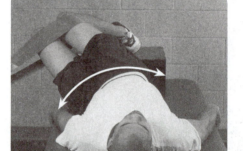

▶ **Figure 18.59**   Lateral trunk rotation: start position—hips and knees flexed with knees together.

Lateral Trunk Rotation

Body Segment: Lumbar.

Stage in Rehab: III.

Purpose: Strengthen the obliques and quadratus lumborum.

Positioning: Patient lies supine in a hook-lying position.

Execution: A resistance band or a pulley system is secured around both knees. The feet are either on a bench or flat on the floor. The patient lets the pulley or band pull the knees downward to the side and then brings the knees upright by tilting the pelvis to flatten the back onto the floor, initiating the movement from the abdominal and back muscles (figure 18.59).

Possible Substitutions: Initiating the movement from the knees rather than the trunk is the most common substitution.

Cues and Notations: Use tactile feedback with your hands on the patient's back and abdomen to facilitate the correct recruitment pattern.

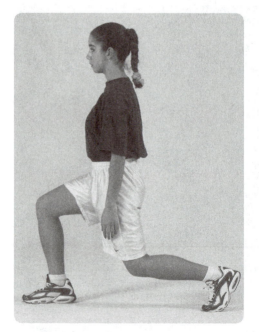

▶ **Figure 18.60**   Lunge.

Lunges

Body Segment: Lumbar.

Stage in Rehab: III.

Purpose: Strengthen the abdominal muscles, thigh, and gluteal muscles. This exercise also facilitates correct trunk stability during lower-extremity activities.

Positioning: Patient is in a standing position with the spine in neural.

Execution: Keeping the abdominal muscles tightened and the back straight, the patient moves to a lunge position, going down smoothly, and then returns to a standing position (figure 18.60).

Possible Substitutions: Flexing the trunk out of neutral, tilting or rotating the trunk, and moving the hips and shoulders out of the same plane.

Cues and Notations: Use verbal cues to remind the patient to keep a neutral position, an erect trunk, and the pelvis in the same plane as the shoulders. If this is difficult to perform, have the patient take smaller lunge steps until control is achieved.

Prone Trunk Extension

Body Segment: Lumbar.

Stage in Rehab: III.

Purpose: Strengthen the lower-back extensors, gluteals, and hamstrings.

Positioning: Patient lies prone over the end of a table, a Swiss ball, or a Roman chair so that the hips are at the edge of the object and are flexed to 30°. Either another person (figure 18.61a) or the equipment (figure 18.61b) anchors the feet. A chair seat below the patient may prevent the patient from flexing too far forward.

Execution: With the hands at the side or in the small of the back, the patient contracts the gluteal muscles to lift the trunk to align with the lower extremities. Moving the hands from behind the back to across the chest and overhead increases resistance and exercise difficulty. Once the patient has mastered the straight-plane extension exercises on the Roman chair, a progression can include trunk rotation during extension exercises. The patient can perform this exercise similarly to a rotational abdominal curl but in reverse motion; or the exercise becomes more difficult if the patient uses a medicine ball, rotating with the ball in the hands while going into extension. Patients cannot perform this exercise until they have good strength in the abdominal muscles and trunk extensors; they must also be able to perform side sit-ups and trunk rotations in standing with a medicine ball without difficulty or pain.

Possible Substitutions: The most common substitutions include arching the back rather than using the hip muscles to lift the trunk, and bending from the back rather than at the hips.

Cues and Notations: Reposition the patient if he or she is unable to flex at the hips. Provide verbal cueing and tactile correction if the back arches.

Prone Leg Lift

Body Segment: Lumbar.

Stage in Rehab: III.

Purpose: Strengthen trunk extensors, abdominal muscles, and gluteal muscles.

Positioning: Patient is in the reverse position of that for the prone trunk lift. This time the trunk is supported on the table or Roman chair, and the legs are off the table or apparatus.

Execution: The patient squeezes the buttocks to lift the legs until they are parallel to the floor. The pelvis must remain in neutral and is supported on the apparatus so flexion occurs at the hips, not the spine (figure 18.62).

Possible Substitutions: Movement is initiated from the back, not the gluteals, and the patient swings the legs upward using momentum so the back hyperextends.

Cues and Notations: Instruct the patient to squeeze the buttocks to lift the legs and control the speed of the lift. If this is difficult, instruct the patient to flex the knees slightly to shorten the lever-arm resistance.

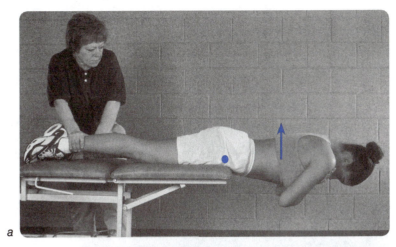

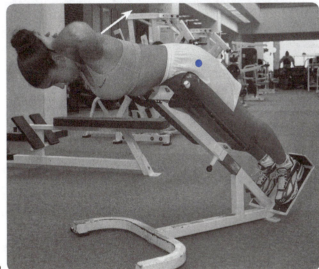

a

b

▶ **Figure 18.61** Prone trunk extension: *(a)* with assist on a table, *(b)* independently on Roman chair. Movement comes from the hip with the contraction of the gluteus maximus. The back should remain straight throughout the exercise, regardless of position of equipment on which it is performed. Dot indicates point from which movement occurs.

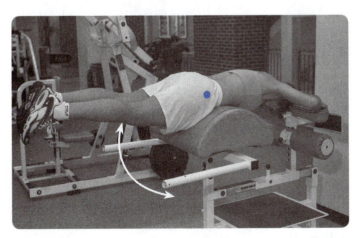

▶ **Figure 18.62** Prone leg lift. Dot indicates point from which movement occurs.

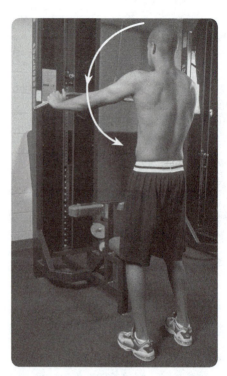

▶ **Figure 18.63** Latissimus pulldown.

Lat Pulldown

Body Segment: Lumbar.

Stage in Rehab: II.

Purpose: Strengthen the latissimus dorsi.

Positioning: The exercise uses an overhead pulley bar, with the patient's hands positioned shoulder-width or slightly farther apart and the elbows extended.

Execution: The abdominal muscles remain taut throughout the exercise and the pelvis remains in neutral. The patient brings the bar downward toward the thighs while keeping the elbows in near-extension (figure 18.63).

Possible Substitutions: Common errors include flexing the elbows too much, shrugging the shoulders, or flexing the lumbar spine.

Cues and Notations: The latissimus dorsi is important in providing stabilization to the thoracolumbar spine because the muscle originates from the lower thoracic spinous processes, lumbar fascia, and iliac crest and has interdigitations with the external oblique muscles.

Agility and Coordination Exercises

Once patients have mastered the strengthening exercises, they should be ready for the trunk rotation and plyometric exercises that involve higher forces, quicker movements, and functional multiplanar motions. Pelvic stability should always be maintained throughout execution of any of these exercises. Two examples of such exercises are explained below.

Resisted Leg Lifts

This exercise is performed with the patient supine on the floor and the rehabilitation clinician standing at the patient's head. The patient's knees are extended, and the hips are flexed to approximately 90°. The patient attempts to lift the legs upward as the clinician attempts to push them back down (figure 18.64). This exercise is performed quickly but with control. It is important that the patient maintain pelvic neutral and that the back not arch throughout the exercise.

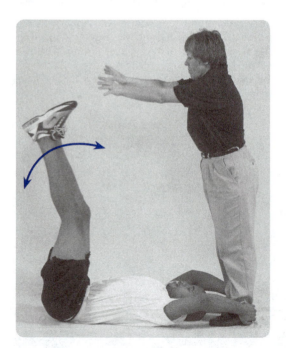

▶ **Figure 18.64** Resisted leg lifts.

Medicine-Ball Exercises

Many of these medicine-ball exercises are listed in chapter 9. As a reminder, figure 18.65 depicts two of them. These exercises include activities such as ball passing low or high, trunk rotations, and abdominal curls with ball catching.

Many other exercises can be used to increase agility and resistance. Additional exercises include ball tossing on the Roman chair to increase trunk extension activity and adding rotation with the medicine ball to the Roman chair exercise.

Rehabilitation techniques for the various segments of the spine include soft-tissue mobilization, joint mobilization, and exercises to improve parameters such as flexibility, postural and pelvic stability, strength, and agility.

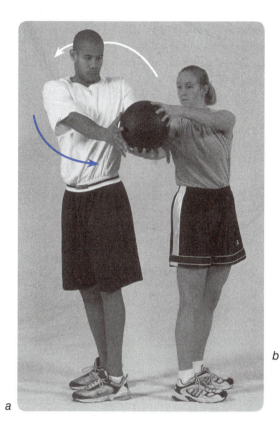

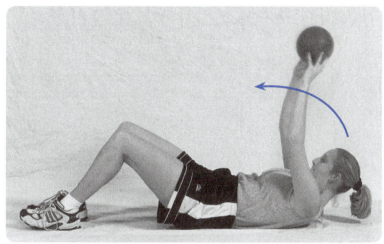

▶ **Figure 18.65** Medicine-ball exercises. *(a)* Trunk rotations. *(b)* Medicine-ball toss can be performed in straight plane to body or rotationally to facilitate oblique activity.

SPECIAL REHABILITATION APPLICATIONS

Before we look at specific injuries and the corresponding programs, let us use our artillery of exercises and progressions to put together a generic outline of a spinal rehabilitation program. We should keep in mind that modalities might be required initially to provide pain modulation and control inflammation. Soft-tissue mobilization and joint mobilization, if appropriate, are also part of the program. Flexibility exercises to improve range of motion of deficient areas are usually incorporated in phases I and II of the program, with instructions to perform the exercises frequently throughout the day. Instruction in neutral positioning, core stabilization exercises, and body mechanics must be part of the early portion of the program. Once the patient is able to maintain pelvic neutral in simple exercises, he or she can progress to other activities such as pool exercises and trunk-strengthening exercises. Phase II trunk-strengthening exercises include abdominal crunches, oblique exercises, bridging, and side-bridging exercises. As has been mentioned, the latissimus pull-down is included as part of the strengthening exercises. As the patient is able to maintain a proper neutral position, he or she performs lower extremity-strengthening exercises for the hip muscles including hamstrings. Swiss-ball exercises such as crunches, bridges, leg lifts, side sit-ups, and progressions of strengthening exercises for the abdomen and trunk can begin in later phase II and early phase III of the program once the patient demonstrates good pelvic stability during arm and leg movements. Recall that endurance and proprioception should be emphasized during these phases.

When the patient is able to demonstrate good control and strength with Swiss-ball and weight exercises in phase III, more aggressive strengthening exercises for the trunk begin. These more aggressive exercises include trunk and leg extension exercises on the Roman chair and abdominal crunches and standing trunk rotations using the medicine ball. Toward the end of phase III, specific exercises required for the individual's normal task demands are added to the program. For example, if the patient is to return to track and field as a hurdler, jumping and bounding exercises for quadriceps power may be added.

Phase IV of the program includes incorporation of drills that mimic sport-specific activities. The patient should be able to maintain good stability and spinal alignment throughout the activities. When the individual is pain free, has good strength and flexibility, and is able to perform functional activities without difficulty, return to full sport participation is the next step. Figure 18.66 presents the goals and treatment schedule for a rehabilitation program for the spine. Specific alterations and considerations required beyond this general program are presented in this section.

Because the spine is subject to a few unique injuries, additional special considerations beyond this general therapeutic exercise program are necessary for each of these injuries. The following sections present these injuries and therapeutic exercise programs to address them.

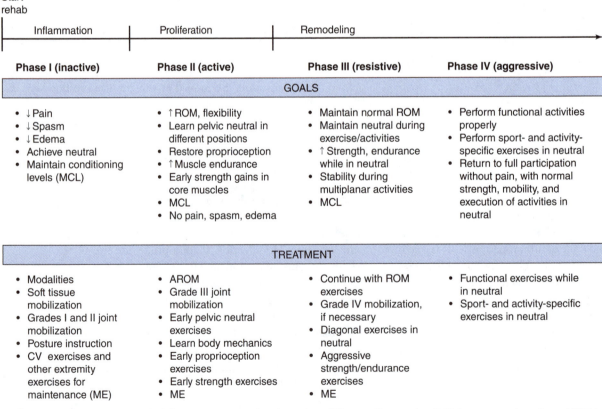

▶ **Figure 18.66** A generic rehabilitation program for the spine. CV = cardiovascular; ROM = range of motion; AROM = active range of motion.

Sprains and Strains

Sprains and strains are among the most common back injuries. If they are not appropriately examined and treated, sprains and strains become frustrating and aggravating injuries because they can linger and cause lasting disability.

The resulting pain and muscle spasm from acute sprains and strains must first be resolved in phase I with modalities and mild stretching exercises. Sometimes these conditions respond to grades I and II mobilization, but early response will depend on the severity of the pain and spasm and on the effectiveness of the modalities in relieving these problems.

Acute conditions require primarily modalities in the initial treatment phase along with limited activity and stretching exercises. As spasm and pain are reduced, soft-tissue mobilization is indicated if restriction is noted with palpation. Joint mobilization may be useful if the restriction is the result of joint hypomobility.

As with all spinal injuries, posture and body mechanics should be assessed and corrected as needed. Spasm will persist if the muscles are required to work more than they should because poor posture or body mechanics is present.

A progression of strengthening exercises should begin once the pain and spasm are under control. The muscles requiring the greatest emphasis are the pelvic stabilizers, abdominals, especially the obliques, lower abdominals, trunk extensors, and gluteals. Figure 18.67 presents a rough timeline of events in a rehabilitation program for a lumbar sprain injury.

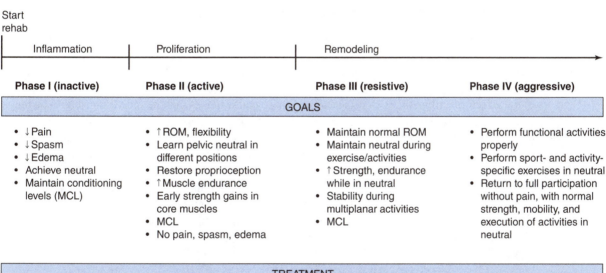

▶ **Figure 18.67** Rehabilitation progression for lumbar sprain or muscle strain. ES = electrical stimulation; PROM = passive range of motion; CV = cardiovascular; AROM = active range of motion; ROM = range of motion; UE = upper extremity; LE = lower extremity.

Case Study

A javelin thrower injured his back last week in practice when he attempted to throw the javelin and felt a sudden pain in the right low-back area. He comes to you stating that he applied ice to the injury when it occurred. The pain is now better than it was last week, but he still has pain when he rotates his trunk to the left and to the right. He has pain when he gets up from a chair and when he gets out of bed in the morning. His pain is worse at the end of the day. He has been taking it easy for a couple of days but is still unable to practice because of the pain. His pain is located on the right side of his low-back area. He has no radiation of symptoms into the lower extremities, but he does get pain in the right buttock. When you examine him, you find that he is unable to bend forward because of pain; sidebending to the left is too painful to perform, but sidebending to the right is better. Trunk rotation is more painful to the left than to the right. His spine has a lateral shift to the right in the lumbar region. Palpation reveals muscle spasm with tenderness in the right paraspinals and quadratus lumborum muscles. Pressure over the right lumbar multifidus reproduces his buttock pain.

Questions for Analysis

1. What stage of the healing process is he in? How severe is the injury?

2. How irritable is his injury? What is the nature of the injury?

3. What is your first treatment?

4. What is your treatment progression and what guidelines will you use to advance this patient from one level to the next?

5. What are some examples of specific exercises, including functional activities you should use before the patient's return to full participation?

Spondylosis, Spondylolysis, and Spondylolisthesis

The following is a brief outline of considerations to keep in mind in a therapeutic exercise program for spondylosis, spondylolysis, and spondylolisthesis.

Although these three conditions differ from one other, they all most often involve the lower lumbar spine and become irritated with extension movement. The two most important factors with patients who have any of these conditions is that the individual should be taught to maintain a posterior pelvic tilt and he or she should avoid hyperextension movements as much as possible. It is vital that these patients establish and maintain pelvic stability in more of a posterior-tilt position and strengthen the abdominals. In spondylolisthesis, the most severe of the three conditions, there is a forward displacement of the vertebrae.

A therapeutic exercise program for these individuals involves the same exercises and progressions. The difference, however, is that their pelvic neutral is in a posterior pelvic tilt position. The least degree of posterior pelvic tilt that the individual achieves without pain is the position he or she should maintain during activities.

Disc Lesions and Sciatica

Disc lesions can be unnerving conditions for both patient and rehabilitation clinician. You should be familiar with the factors identified here and consider them before establishing care.

A protruding or herniated disc can be a serious problem and often causes radiculopathy down one or both extremities, depending on the location of the protrusion. The mere presence of pain or symptoms down the leg does not mean that there is a disc herniation, but you should consider this a possibility until it has been ruled out. Other conditions such as facet injuries, muscle spasm, and myofascial pain can also referred pain.

Patients who have been diagnosed with disc lesions should avoid those positions and motions that aggravate or produce the sciatica symptoms. These motions most commonly are forward flexing or flexing and twisting in the direction that further impinges the disc protrusion.

Patients who have disc lesions must learn to find and maintain pelvic neutral and must strengthen the abdominals, obliques, back extensors, and gluteal muscle groups, as in a general spine program. Likewise, they should learn correct body mechanics and posture and eventually progress to performing all physical activities in a neutral spine position.

■ **Case Study**

A gymnast has seen an orthopedic physician because of persistent complaints of low-back pain that did not resolve after two weeks of modality treatments and reduced activity. The physician's diagnosis is a spondylolysis. The patient needs a rehabilitation program before she can return to competition.

Questions for Analysis

1. What exercises would you have this patient avoid?

2. What progression of exercises and activities should her therapeutic exercise program include to return her to full participation?

Although not all authorities agree on its importance, some advocate the centralization of pain for disc lesions (McKenzie, 1989). What this means is that if the treatment is appropriate, the patient will experience a gradual and progressive retreat of the sciatic pain distally to proximally until the only pain remaining is localized to the back. It is the goal of treatment to also relieve this central pain. Most often, the use of extension exercises, flexibility and strengthening activities, and pelvic-neutral exercises will accomplish this goal. Exercises progress at the patient's own rate. Progression depends on the treatment results and the patient's feedback regarding the pain. If the pain is receding, the progression of exercises can continue; but if the sciatic pain worsens, you must re-evaluate the most recently performed exercises and activities, first for possible incorrect execution and secondly for appropriateness. It may be that the exercise is too soon for the patient to tolerate the severity of the exercise. Use of the wrong exercises or failure to correct body mechanics and posture may aggravate the disc lesion. It is vital that the clinician have a good understanding of the exercises and the stresses that occur with each exercise.

Microdiscectomy

Occasionally, patients are not successful with conservative treatment. In these instances, surgical procedures are necessary. A microdiscectomy is a common procedure where a small incision in the center of the back at the site of the herniated disc is made. Rather than cut through the muscles, they are moved out of the way so post-operative recovery is less involved. The surgeon bypasses the nerve root and cuts through the lamina to remove the part of the disc that is protruding and irritating the nerves.

Those patients who have undergone microdiscectomies follow a course of treatment similar to that for patients who have disc pathology but have not had surgical correction. In a typical timeline, treatment begins about one week postoperatively and follows a logical progression. During the initial phase of rehabilitation care must be taken to keep motion restricted within a pain-free range. Phase I treatment includes pain modulation, flexibility exercises, pelvic stabilization, and instruction in proper posture. Phase II adds more flexibility range of motion and core exercises. The patient may begin short distances to start and gradually increase as muscle tolerance improves. Early strength exercises of increasing difficulty as already outlined may begin if the patient tolerates them without pain. If post-surgical muscle tightness and soft-tissue restriction are present, they are treated with soft-tissue release and modalities. Of all of these factors, it is imperative that disc patients learn to maintain pelvic neutral, use correct posture and body mechanics, and improve muscle endurance and strength of core, latissimus dorsi, and hip muscles to support the spine. Also in phase II, stretching exercises for the hamstrings, piriformis, and quadriceps are added. A cardiovascular program on a stationary bike, treadmill, elliptical, or other equipment is used in a progressive manner, using patient tolerance and heart rate as a guide. As the healing process continues into remodeling, phase III of the rehab program begins. During this time, more intensive strength exercises and agility activities occur and evolve into phase IV where activity-specific routines are used to prepare the patient to return to normal activities.

Spinal Fusion

In more severe cases, a spinal fusion may be indicated. These surgeries are usually reserved for those people with unstable spines, severe disc degeneration, and spondylolisthesis. To fuse two or more vertebral levels, a bone chip from the hip is most commonly placed between the vertebrae. Following surgery, the patient is restricted from range of motion to allow the fusion to heal. For this reason, the clinician must see to it that the patient does not excessively load the spine or rotate the spine to disrupt the fusion site.

During phase I, reducing the inflammation through the use of modalities for pain, swelling, and muscle spasm are used. Pelvic stabilization activities also begin in this phase. In phase II, proper body mechanics instruction using pelvic neutral is used. Daily walking while maintaining pelvic neutral is also started here. Once in phase II, soft tissue mobilization of the scar, proprioceptive exercises, and core stabilization exercises start. Towards the end of phase II, advanced instructions in body mechanics are instituted. These advanced instructions may include techniques on lifting, lateral movements, and pushing and pulling activities. Cardiovascular activities on the treadmill, elliptical, or stationary bike and hip strengthening exercises with the back stabilized also occur later in phase II. By the time the patient approaches phase III, he or she is able to perform strengthening exercises for the body and trunk and begin agility exercises. Phase IV, as with other conditions, begins the progressive activity-specific program to permit the patient's return to normal activities.

As you can see, the programs for the two surgical conditions are similar. The precautions are the primary difference. This difference is present because with the microdiscectomy there is removal but no repair of tissue, but with the fusion there is repair involved. Although both conditions will involve an inflammation phase following the insult to the body of surgery, the fusion requires much more caution because the body must be allowed the necessary time to fuse the bones. The rehabilitation process with the microdiscectomy may last from 6 to 10 weeks, but the fusion recovery may take 3 to 4 months, depending on the patient and the physician.

Case Study

A football lineman injured his back in a game four weeks ago. He was referred to an orthopedic surgeon because of continued low-back and right lower-extremity pain. Magnetic resonance imaging (MRI) revealed that he has a disc bulge of 3 mm at L4-5. The physician indicates that this patient is not a surgical candidate because the problem may be resolved with rehabilitation, corticosteroid injections, or Medrol dose pack. The patient has had two of the three injections and reports significant relief of back and leg pain. He is now coming to you for a rehabilitation program. He moves pretty well when he enters the examination room. He does not appear to hesitate to walk or get up from a chair. When he moves around the room, however, you notice that he has very poor body mechanics, bending from the back to sit down and bending and twisting sideways to retrieve his backpack. His examination reveals a straight-leg raise to 50° on the right and 55° on the left, and his medial hip rotation is 20° bilaterally. In a forward bend, he is able to touch his fingers to his knees; in a side bend he can touch 10 cm above his knee; and in backward bending he has normal motion. Forward bending produces some discomfort. You notice that when he bends, most of the motion occurs in the thoracic spine, with the lumbar spine remaining essentially flat. The neurological examination reveals no deficiencies in sensory, motor, or reflex innervation. The patient's gluteal muscles and abdominals each test at 4/5 strength. He is unable to perform a side sit-up on the right side. The paraspinals, quadratus lumborum, and hip lateral rotators are all tender to palpation, especially on the right, and you are able to palpate restriction of soft-tissue mobility in those tender areas. There is some restriction of joint mobility to PA tests in the lower lumbar spine.

Questions for Analysis

1. What precautions would you observe in treating this patient?

2. What would your initial treatment program include?

3. What techniques would you include in your first three treatment sessions?

4. What progression of exercises would you select for this patient, and what criteria would you use for progression from one level to the next in the program?

Facet Injuries

Facet injuries can be frustrating to treat, especially if you do not consider the factors listed here. Facet injuries can also be difficult to identify. The rehabilitation clinician must use his or her deductive tools to identify the presence of a facet injury.

Before we discuss facet injuries, we must first realize that in the spine, motion in one direction will facilitate motion in a different plane. This is because of the position of the facets. Although the precise motions that go together are of some dispute (Legaspi & Edmond, 2007), they are called *coupled motions*. Coupled motions are motions that occur in a joint together; one motion does not occur without the other. The coupled motions in the spine are lateral bending and rotation. The disagreement centers around the discussion as to whether these coupled motions occur to the opposite or to the same sides (Cook, Hegedus, Showalter, & Sizer, 2006; Legaspi & Edmond, 2007). The problem in finding grounds for agreement is probably multifactorial and includes various methods used in the studies, the original postures of the subjects studied, age factors, and other considerations that could make results variable. In spite of the lack of consensus on normal coupling motions, many agree that during dysfunction, lateral flexion motion in the spine is coupled with rotation to the opposite side.

You can determine your own coupling motions. In a standing position, flex your trunk laterally as far as you can go while keeping your feet flat on the floor. As you reach the end of your motion, notice how your trunk is positioned. Is it rotated to the side you flexed to or to the opposite side? You can also do this in the cervical spine. Standing in a proper cervical alignment, laterally flex your neck as far as possible and notice which direction you rotate to by the end of your lateral flexion. Many people agree that the lumbar spine lateral flexion and rotation coupling occur to the opposite directions, but the same motions in the cervical spine couple in the same direction with each other. If your cervical spine motions were to the same side, now assume a slumped posture position and repeat the exercise. You should notice that the coupling motions are now in opposite directions: lateral flexion is to one side and rotation is to the opposite.

Fryette's Laws of Physiologic Spinal Motion

Coupled motions in the spine originate with concepts brought forth by an osteopathic physician and are named after him. Although they are not actually "laws" of motion as much as they are observations and ideas, they are called "Fryette's Laws of Physiologic Spinal Motion," or more simply, "Fryette's Laws of Motion" (Fryette, 1980). Fryette presented his ideas of coupled motions between facets in both a neutral position and out of a neutral position. He presented three laws that determine coupling motions of the spine.

Fryette's First Law states that when the lumbar or thoracic spine is in neutral, side-bending occurs to the opposite side of vertebral rotation. For example, in a neutral position, if the spine is laterally flexed to the right, it will also rotate to the left. This law does not address the cervical spine since he defined a neutral position as when the facet joint surfaces are not in contact with each other, but the adjacent cervical facet surfaces are always in contact with each other.

Fryette's Second Law deals with pathological positions and coupled motions. Fryette indicated that when the spinal alignment is either in flexion or extension, the side bending and rotation of the vertebrae will be toward the same direction. For example, if the lumbar spine is placed into a lordotic position, and side bending to the left is performed, rotation to the left will also occur at the vertebral level.

Fryette's Third Law states that if motion in one plane occurs in the spine, motion in another direction is diminished. For an example of this, stand erect, rotate the spine to the left, and note the amount of rotation that occurs. Next, forward flex at the trunk and then in that position, repeat the left rotation motion. You will find that the amount of rotation you are able to perform is less than in erect standing.

Facet Impingement and Positional Dysfunction

Fryette's laws help us understand what occurs with facet-restricted motions. Facet restriction can occur from an impingement following a traumatic event where the facet surfaces on one side suffer an injury. A facet can be restricted in either flexion or extension, and this determines whether the motion restriction is to the same side or opposite the site of injury. The position the facet is in is called *positional dysfunction*. A *motion restriction* is what the facet is unable to do. A positional dysfunction position will always be opposite to the direction of its motion restriction. A facet joint in flexion is *open* since the two facet surfaces comprising the facet joint are apart; a facet joint in extension is *closed*. If a facet is restricted in opening (flexing), the facet is stuck in extension and has motion restriction in flexion; extension is the positional dysfunction and flexing is the restricted motion. Since rotation and sidebending are coupled with each other, they will also have motion restrictions in positional dysfunctions. In a positional dysfunction of *(stuck in) extension*, rotation and sidebending are limited on the *opposite side of the problem facet*. In a positional dysfunction of *(stuck in) flexion*, side bending and rotation are limited on the *same side of the problem facet*.

For example, if a left facet has a postural dysfunction of (stuck in) extension, rotation left and sidebending left, the motion restriction will be flexion, right rotation, and right sidebending (figure 18.68). On the other hand, if the positional dysfunction of *(stuck in) flexion* is present, restricted motion in sidebending and rotation will be *ipsilateral*. For example, if a patient had a positional dysfunction of (stuck in) flexion because the right facet will not close, the stuck position will be flexion, rotation right, and sidebending right with motion restricted in extension, left rotation, and left sidebending (figure 18.69). Other signs include radiating pain mimicking dermatomal distribution, tenderness of spinous processes, and reflex muscle spasm.

More trauma causes sprains rather than impingement so tissue injury is greater. A more conservative treatment approach is needed. Additionally, soft tissue around the joint may also have been injured, and swelling and muscle spasm are common. A cervical collar may reduce pain. A forward-head position occurs because extension is painful. If motion loss occurs, a unilateral capsular pattern may develop. The capsular pattern for facets is limitation of rotation to the involved side and sidebending to the opposite side. For example, if a left cervical or lumbar facet has a capsular pattern, left rotation and right sidebending will be restricted but right rotation and left sidebending will be free. Gentle ROM in pain-free movements and

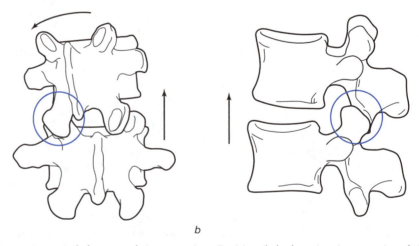

a   *b*

▶ **Figure 18.68** Left facet stuck in extension. Positional dysfunction is extension, left rotation, and left sidebending. Motion restriction is in flexion, right rotation, and right sidebending.

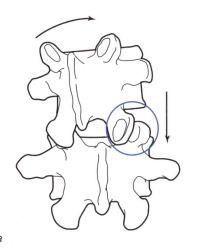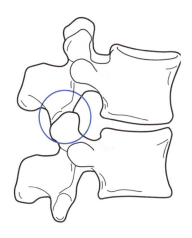

a   b

▶ **Figure 18.69** Right facet is stuck in flexion. Positional dysfunction is flexion, right rotation, and right sidebending. Motion restriction is in extension, left rotation, and left sidebending.

■ **Case Study**

Four days ago, a diver landed poorly in a dive during practice. She has had a stiff neck since that time. This morning she awoke and could not turn her head to the left. She presents to you with her head laterally flexed about 20° to the right and is unable to look straight ahead. Her head is rotated to the right about 15°. It is painful for her to attempt to place her head in an upright and straight position, but she has no difficulty turning her head all the way to the right and looking over her right shoulder. Your palpation reveals tenderness over the C5 and C6 spinous processes, and there is some tightness in the muscles in the same area.

Questions for Analysis

1. What do you believe her problem is; what side of her cervical spine is the location of her problem?

2. Outline your treatment program, sequencing your treatment in a logical progression.

---

joint mobilization following modalities can relieve muscle spasm, pain, and edema. Later, grades III and IV joint mobilization is used for facet mobility.

Sacroiliac Joint

The impact of the SI joint on low back pain is controversial (Cibulka, 1992). There is some evidence to indicate that the SI should be an important consideration in low back pain, and the back can refer pain into the SI joint (Cappaert, 2000). The SI and hip can also refer pain to each other (Rosatelli, Agur, & Chhaya, 2006). An examination of the SI should be part of the examination of any patient who complains of back or hip pain.

As you learned in biomechanics, as the spine flexes forward, the sacroilium rotates posteriorly in extension, and the opposite occurs when the spine extends. During ambulation, the sacrum rotates posteriorly on the same side as heel strike and anteriorly on the same side as toe off. This will assist in also causing a rotation around a diagonal axis. The pubic bones correspond to iliac motion during walking. You may remember from anatomy that the sacrum has an inferior lateral angle (ILA) at its base. The ILA is located most easily by first locating the cornua, the inferior facet of the sacrum that connects to the coccyx. The right and left ILA

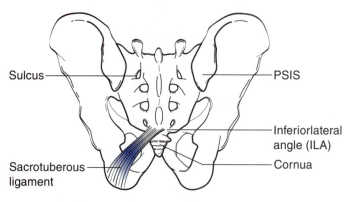

▶ **Figure 18.70** Sacroilium.

are located just lateral to and on either side of the cornua (figure 18.70). The sacrotuberous ligament connects the ischial tuberosity to the inferior sacrum. It is located at about a 45° angle superior to and medial from the ischial tuberosity between the ischium and inferior-lateral sacrum. You will need to identify each of these structures during an SI examination.

Susceptibility to SI pathology increases because of posture or activities that increase SI torque. Patients who have excessive lumbar lordosis with an exaggerated forward pelvic tilt can place excessive stress on the SI joint and cause pain in the area. Patients are susceptible to SI injuries if they have a leg-length discrepancy, fall on the side or buttocks, misstep off a curb while running, run while twisting, or bend and twist the lumbar spine. The patients most susceptible to SI injuries because of the stress of their sports are soccer, basketball, and football players; gymnasts; wrestlers; and track and field athletes. Sacroiliac malalignments can occur with imbalances caused by injury or secondary spasm, weakness, or loss of mobility. Some SI joint injuries result from classic types of injuries.

Because of these stresses, various malalignments of the SI occur. Upslips, inflares or outflares, and pubic subluxations can occur when there is a sudden, sharp jolt to the leg as a person steps off a curb or steps down and does not realize that there is another step. Falling on the buttock can lead to sacral flexion, pubic subluxations, and up-slip injuries. Trunk rotation and bending activities can cause sacroiliac dysfunctions. Knowing the history will help to identify the problem.

Sacroiliac Examination

Before treatment is initiated, an examination to determine the areas of malalignment must be made. A complete sacroiliac examination includes an investigation of posture, alignment, and lumbar range of motion. There are specific factors that are also examined when sacroiliac pathology is suspected. These factors are used to determine either relative alignment or quality and quantity of motion. The three special tests used to determine quality and quantity of motion include the standing forward bend test (StFBT), kinetic test (KT), and seated forward bend test (SitFBT). The relative alignment tests are performed with the patient in supine and prone positions; the supine tests include examination of left and right iliac crest height, leg length (Leg L), distance of the ASIS to umbilicus and the ASIS height (ASIS), and height and springiness of the symphysis pubis (Pube ht, Pube Spring). The prone tests include examination of positions of the sulcus (Sulcus), inferior lateral angle (ILA), and sacrotuberous ligament (St. Lig). See table 18.1.

Standing Forward-Bend Test   The standing forward-bend test is sometimes called the Piedallus test and is performed with the clinician facing the patient's back and placing each thumb on the patient's PSIS and the hands on the iliac crests. The clinician's eyes are at the same level as the patient's pelvis. The patient then bends forward (figure 18.71). If the SI joint is normal, the thumbs will move inferiorly as the patient bends forward; if there is a lesion, the thumb on the side of the lesion will either move upward or not move as the other thumb moves inferiorly. This test only identifies the side of the lesion; it does not identify the kind of lesion.

TABLE 18.1 Sacroiliac Tests

Purpose	Test	Positive results
Quality and quantity of motion	Standing forward bend test (StFBT); also called Piedallus test	Identifies side of lesion.
Quality and quantity of motion	Seated forward bend test (SitFBT)	Identifies side of sacroiliac lesion.
Quality and quantity of motion	Kinetic test (KT)	Identifies side of sacroiliac or iliosacral dysfunction.
Relative alignment in supine	Leg length (leg L)	Sacroiliac dysfunction present only if difference is easily noticed and significant.
Relative alignment in supine	Left and right iliac crest height	Difference in height between the two should be notable if present.
Relative alignment in supine	Distance of ASIS to umbilicus	Dysfunction indicated by obvious difference of 1 to 2 in.
Relative alignment in supine	ASIS height (ASIS)	One will appear more superior if it is positive.
Relative alignment in supine	Height of symphysis pubis (pube ht)	One side is higher than the other.
Relative alignment in supine	Springiness of symphysis pubis (pube spring)	Pain occurs with spring test on one side.
Relative alignment in prone	Positions of left and right sulcus (sulcus)	One side will be deeper than the other.
Relative alignment in prone	Positions of left and right inferior lateral angles (ILA)	One side will be more posterior (relative to sacral alignment) to the other.
Relative alignment in prone	Tension of left and right sacrotuberous ligaments (st lig) (figure 18.80b, p. 570)	One ligament will be looser than the other.

FBT = forward bend test; KT = kinetic test; Pube = pubic bones; ASIS = anterior superior iliac spine; ILA = inferior lateral angle; L = left; R = right; Sit = sitting; ST = standing; Sup = superior; St lig = sacrotuberous ligament; isch tub = ischial tuberosity.

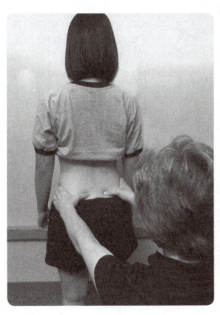 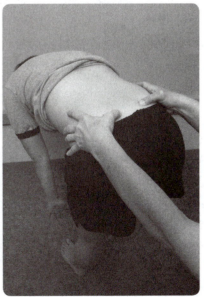

▶ **Figure 18.71** Standing forward bend test.

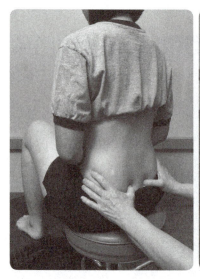

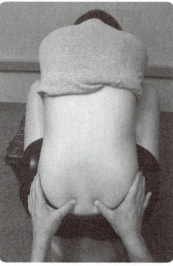

▶ **Figure 18.72** Seated forward bend test.

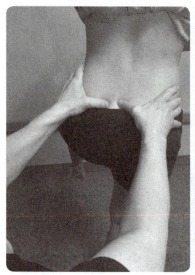

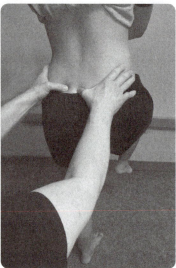

▶ **Figure 18.73** Kinetic test.

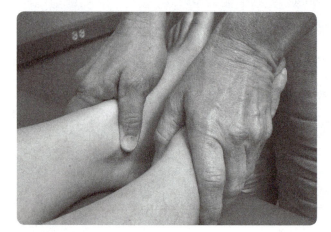

▶ **Figure 18.74** Leg-length difference.

Seated Forward-Bend Test The seated forward-bend test is performed with the clinician's hands as indicated in the standing forward-bend test. The patient is in a seated position with the knees apart and higher than the hips (figure 18.72). The clinician's eyes are at the same level as the patient's pelvis. The patient bends forward; in normal movement, the thumbs should move as they do in the standing forward bend-test. If a thumb either does not move or moves superiorly, the patient has a sacroiliac lesion on that side.

Kinetic Test In the kinetic test (also called the Norwegian test), the patient stands with his or her back to the clinician. To evaluate the left, the clinician places one thumb on the left PSIS and the other thumb at the same level on the mid-superior sacrum (figure 18.73). The clinician's eyes are at the same level as the patient's pelvis. The patient then lifts the left knee toward the chest; if the SI joint is normal, the left thumb moves inferiorly, but it stays at the same level if motion is restricted. This test checks for left iliosacral motion, so if the thumb does not move inferiorly, then the left ilium motion on the left sacrum is restricted. With the thumbs and patient in the same start position, the patient then lifts the right knee toward the chest; if the SI is normal, the right thumb moves inferiorly, but motion is restricted if the thumb stays at the same level; this test checks for left sacroiliac motion. In this instance, if the right thumb does not move inferiorly, the left sacrum motion on the left ilium is restricted. The clinician then places the thumbs in a reverse position with the right thumb on the right PSIS and the left thumb on the mid-superior sacrum and repeats the two tests. Lifting the right leg and watching right thumb movement assesses right iliosacral motion (iliac motion on the sacrum), and lifting the left leg while watching left thumb movement assesses right sacroilial motion (sacral motion on the ilium).

Leg length test Pain with pressure on a palpation point during supine or prone tests is a positive sign. Before performing the supine tests, the patient performs a bridge then moves both hips and knees into extension. Leg length is assessed by comparing levels of medial malleoli; if leg length discrepancy is present secondary to SI dysfunction, the difference will be readily apparent (figure 18.74).

Iliac crest and ASIS tests The clinician stands on the same side of the patient as the clinician's dominant eye. For example, if the clinician's dominant eye is right, then he or she stands on the patient's right side. The clinician then determines iliac crest (figure 18.75) and ASIS height (figure 18.76a). Placing the hands at the top of each iliac crest, the clinician looks directly down at the crests; obvious differences must exist to classify it as dysfunctional. When palpating the ASIS, the clinician places a thumb on each ASIS and visualizes them from eye level. Each ASIS should be equal in height from the table top and to each other when compared to each other. If one ASIS is more posterior than the other, it will appear more superior. The distance between each ASIS and navel should be determined by placing a thumb on each ASIS and rotating the hands to place the index finger at the navel (figure 18.76b); obvious differences between the distances will be approximately 1 to 2 inches, if present.

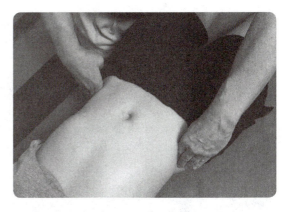

▶ **Figure 18.75** Iliac crest height test.

Pubic symphysis tests

Springiness of the pubic bones is tested by first locating the pubic symphysis by placing the palm of the hand on the patient's abdomen and moving the hand caudally until the heel of the hand contacts the superior portion of the symphysis pubis. Once the pubic bones are located, the clinician's hands are repositioned so the index fingers are place about 2 cm (<1 in.) laterally from the superior symphysis pubis joint to light on the pubic tubercles. The clinician then presses down on the left then the right pubic tubercle (figure 18.77); pain or restricted mobility is a positive sign. Differences in height between the right and left pubic bones is assessed by placing a finger or thumb on each bone, observing the bones at eye level, and noting differences.

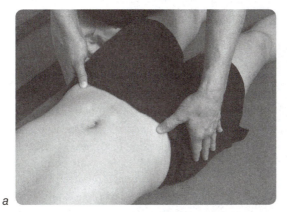
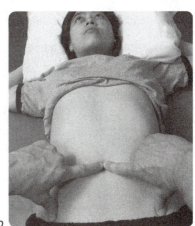

a

▶ **Figure 18.76** ASIS *(a)* height and *(b)* to-navel tests. *b*

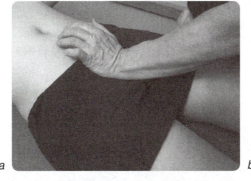

a   *b*

▶ **Figure 18.77** Pubic symphysis test. *(a)* Locating symphysis pubis and *(b)* testing for springiness and height of left and right.

Prone examination is made of the position of the right and left PSIS (figure 18.78a); they should be of equal height from the table to each other. If dysfunction is present, one will appear more superior or inferior than the other. Prone examination is also made of the position of the left and right sulcus (figure 18.78b). The left and right sulcus are located immediately medially and about 30° caudally from the left and right PSIS, respectively (figure 18.79); the position of each should be equal, but if one is more posterior or anterior, it should be noted since this is abnormal (figure 18.78b). The height of right and left ILA are then examined (figure 18.80). To locate the ILA, the cornua, or the very end of the sacrum as it meets the coccyx, are palpated; the ILA are about 1.5 to 2 cm lateral to their respective cornua. The ILA should be level with each other, but if one is more anterior or more posterior than the other is, this should be noted. There should be no pain with palpation or pressure of any of these landmarks; pain is an abnormal response.

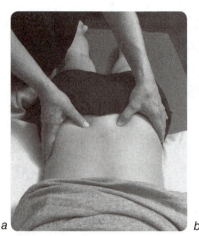 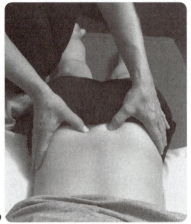

▶ **Figure 18.78**   *(a)* PSIS examination and *(b)* location of right and left sulcus.

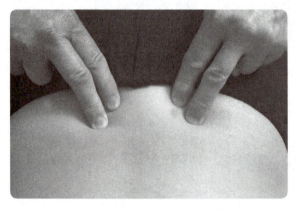

▶ **Figure 18.79**   Sulcus and PSIS. The middle fingers indicate the location of the left and right PSIS and the index fingers show the location of the left and right sulcus, 30° medial and inferior to their respective PSIS.

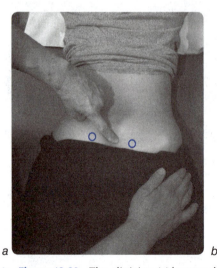 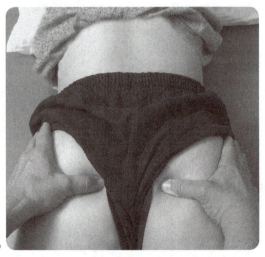

▶ **Figure 18.80**   The clinician *(a)* locates the cornua and moves thumbs laterally to palpate the ILA (open circles), and *(b)* palpates sacrotuberous ligaments (medial and superior to ischial tuberosities).

Additional Tests   Additional examinations include trunk range-of-motion tests for quality and quantity of motion and pain during any motion. If lateral flexion is limited and accompanied with signs of SI dysfunction, the problem is probably of sacroiliac origin. If flexion-extension motion is limited, the problem may be iliosacral in origin.

Sacroiliac and Iliosacral Lesions   The pathological patterns that can develop occur because either the sacrum is malaligned on the ilium or the ilium is malaligned on the sacrum. When the sacrum is malaligned on the ilium, it is a sacroiliac (SI) dysfunction; the sacrum is malaligned between the two iliac bones to result in either bilateral or unilateral restriction of motion. On the other hand, when either ilium is out of alignment from the sacrum, it is a iliosacral (IS) dysfunction.

All of the dysfunctions with their common causes and symptoms are listed in table 18.2. The iliosacral and sacroiliac pathologies are in table 18.3. Once you have examined a patient for possible SI lesions, compare your results with table 18.3. If your patient has a SI lesion, your findings should correlate with the findings of one of the pathologies in these tables. The iliosacral and sacroiliac pathologies are listed along with the examination results for each condition. Treatment is directed toward relieving and correcting the SI joint alignment, stabilizing the joints, and correcting posture or faulty techniques. The techniques used to correct alignment are muscle energy techniques. The specifics of theory and application for these are presented in chapter 6. The muscle energy techniques discussed here are treatments for specific SI and IS dysfunctions.

Muscle Energy Treatment Techniques

Muscle energy techniques are a form of manual therapy that lend themselves well to the sacroiliac region. As was mentioned in chapter 6, muscle energy techniques treat either the spine or the extremities. Isometric contractions are used with muscle energy spinal techniques while isotonic contractions are used for the extremities. Muscle energy techniques for the SI and IS will be presented here.

When muscle imbalances occur, malalignments result and cause restriction of movement. These issues have been previously discussed. These restrictions, in muscle energy terminology, are *barriers* to movement. A barrier is not an end of movement but rather a resistance to movement. The objective of muscle energy is to relieve these barriers and restore balance. Muscle energy allows the patient

TABLE 18.2 Dysfunctions and Symptoms

Type of dysfunction	Dysfunction	Common causes	Signs and symptoms
Iliosacral	Pubic subluxation	Soccer; after pregnancy and delivery	Groin pain, buttock pain; patient may have only low-back pain.
	Iliac inflare	Direct blow; soccer	Groin pain; patient may or may not have leg pain.
	Iliac outflare	Falls; direct blow; soccer	Groin pain; patient may or may not have hip pain or leg pain.
	Anterior iliac subluxation (R upslip)	Past history of falling on buttock; sudden step off curb; hockey; basketball; motor vehicle accident (MVA)	Always on right (right upslip); pain often on opposite side; leg pain; low-back pain; coccygeal pain; nerve-root pain.
	Posterior iliac subluxation (L upslip)	Same as for anterior iliac subluxation	Always on left (left upslip); often occurs with other spinal problems that haven't responded to treatment; often occurs with spinal flexion.
	Anterior iliac rotation	Usually occurs with other lesions	Long leg on side of lesion; should be the last to be treated.
Sacroilial	Sacral flexion	Occurs with bending and twisting activities or push–pull activities; MVA	Pain often on side opposite lesion; patient may report feeling as if back popped at the time of injury.
	Forward torsion: same letters (1st letter = sacral motion; 2nd letter = axis)	Bending with twisting motion; getting out of car quickly	Most common sacroiliac injury. Back or leg pain; buttock pain. Pain may be on side opposite lesion. Indicated as a right-on-right (RonR) or left-on-left (LonL) forward torsion.
	Backward torsion: opposite letters (1st letter = sacral motion; 2nd letter = axis)	Bending with twisting motion	Not as common as the forward torsions. Patient is flexed in trunk flexion 2° to pain and waddles like a duck; painful during movement into extension; may appear to have a disc lesion or may have pain in the buttock and lumbosacral region; indicated as a right-on-left (RonL) or a left-on-right (LonR) backward torsion

to control the muscle contraction, but the clinician must first place the patient's segment in the correct alignment and correctly instruct the patient to produce a specific muscle contraction in a specific direction to promote optimal results.

Caution must be taken by the clinician to avoid common errors that will reduce optimal outcomes of the treatment. These errors include the following:

1. Not controlling the joint position or direction of movement
2. Not applying a counterforce to the patient's force in the correct direction
3. Not allowing enough time between the contractions to achieve complete muscle relaxation prior to moving the segment to a new barrier
4. Not providing the patient with sufficient instructions for him or her to perform the activity correctly.

On the other hand, patients also make errors in their muscle energy performance. Some of the patient errors include:

1. Using too much force
2. Not contracting in the correct joint or segment position
3. Not holding the contraction long enough
4. Not completely relaxing after the contraction.

TABLE 18.3 Iliosacral and Sacroiliac Pathologies

Pathology	Sit FBT	ST FBT	KT	Leg length	Pube ht	Pube spring	ASIS	PSIS	Sulcus	ILA	St lig
ILIOSACRAL											
R sup pubic subluxation	Neg	Pos R	Pos R	Short R	R sup	Pain R					
R iliac inflare	Neg	Pos R	Pos R		R ant	Pain R	↓ Dist R ASIS to umbilicus	R is lat			
R iliac outflare	Neg	Pos R	Pos R		R post	Pain R	↑ Dist R ASIS to umbilicus	R is med			
R upslip: ant iliac subluxation (always on R)	Neg	Pos R	Pos R	Short R	R sup	Pain R	R sup	R is sup	Varies	Shorter R	R is slack with high R isch tub. tension in L st lig.
L upslip: post iliac subluxation (always on L)	Neg	Pos L	Pos L	Short L	L sup	Pain L	L sup	L is sup	Varies	Shorter L	Tension in R st lig L is slack.
R ant iliac rotation	Neg	Pos R	Pos R	Long R	R inf	Pain R	R inf				
SACROILIAC											
L sacral flexion	Pos L	Pos L	Pos L	L long	Varies	Varies	Varies	Varies	L deep	L post	
Forward torsion L on L (same)	Pos L	Pos L	Pos L				L inf	L is sup	R deep	L post	
Backward torsion L on R (opp)	Pos R	Pos R	Pos R				L inf	R is sup	R deep	L post	

FBT = forward-bend test; KT = kinetic test; Pube = pubic bones; ASIS = anterior superior iliac spine; PSIS = posterior superior iliac spine; ILA = inferior lateral angle; L = left; R = right; Sit = sitting; ST = standing; Sup = superior; St lig = sacrotuberous ligament; Isch tub = ischial tuberosity; Inf = inferior; Ant = anterior; Post = posterior; Opp = opposite; Neg = negative; Pos = positive.

Application of muscle energy techniques involves some very precise applications. The clinician must remember and perform these correctly for optimal results. An isometric contraction is held for 3 to 10 s, and the amount of the contraction is only 2 ounces of force. Typically, the patient attempts to produce a maximal contraction, but the clinician must establish the importance of a light resistance force application by the patient. Once the contraction is relaxed, the clinician should pause to allow full relaxation of the muscle before applying the stretch. As the segment is moved, the clinician pays attention to where the new barrier is felt, for motion goes only to that point and not beyond. Once the new barrier is reached, the process is repeated for 3 to 5 times.

Listed here are a few, but not all, muscle energy techniques. These techniques are used to treat some of the more common SI and IS lesions.

Anterior Iliac Subluxation: Upslip This treatment is for an iliosacral lesion—an upslip of the ilium whereby the ilium on the right is higher than the one on the left. This injury can occur when someone falls on the buttock or steps down off a curb. It also occurs in sports such as basketball and hockey. Although it always occurs on the right, the pain is sometimes on the left. Pain can also be located in the low back or coccyx or can mimic nerve root pain. The right leg appears shorter than the left leg, and the right iliac crest is higher. When palpated, the right sacrotuberous ligament feels slack compared to that on the left side.

The muscle energy treatment is to have the patient lie prone with the right leg in 30° of abduction and extension. The rehabilitation clinician grasps the tibia and fibula above the ankle to maintain the leg position and takes up the slack of the leg. The patient takes in a deep breath and blows it out as the rehabilitation clinician takes up the slack of the leg again (figure 18.81). This is repeated three or four times. On the last repetition, the clinician has the patient cough twice and simultaneously provides a quick pull on the leg along the long axis of the leg.

Posterior Iliac Subluxation: Upslip This treatment is for an iliosacral lesion. This upslip always occurs on the left. It commonly occurs with other spinal problems and should be investigated if the pain does resolve with treatment. The left leg is the short leg this time, and the left sacrotuberous ligament is slack when palpated. The left iliac crest appears higher than the right.

In this treatment the patient is supine and the left leg held by the rehabilitation clinician, proximal to the ankle in 30° of abduction and flexion (figure 18.82). The slack is taken out of the leg, and the patient is instructed to take a deep breath in and then let it out as the clinician takes out additional slack. After the final repetition, the patient is asked to cough, and simultaneously with the cough the clinician provides a quick longitudinal pull on the leg.

Sacral Flexion This treatment is for a sacroiliac lesion that can occur with a bending-and-twisting activity. Push-pull activities can also cause a sacral flexion injury. This injury occurs more commonly on the left than on the right, but it can occur on either side. The pain may sometimes be on the side opposite the injury. If the injury is on the left side, the left sulcus will appear deeper (more anterior) than the right, and the left inferior lateral angle of the sacrum (ILA) is palpated more posteriorly.

Treatment is to have the patient lie prone with the leg in 30° abduction and medially rotated. The patient's thigh is stabilized on the clinician's thigh, and the clinician's hand applies pressure to the left ILA (if the injury is on the left) (figure 18.83). The patient takes a deep breath in and holds it, then breathes out while the clinician continues to exert constant pressure over the left ILA. The pressure is maintained as the patient breathes in again. This technique is performed three times. Sometimes a click can be palpated or heard on the maneuver.

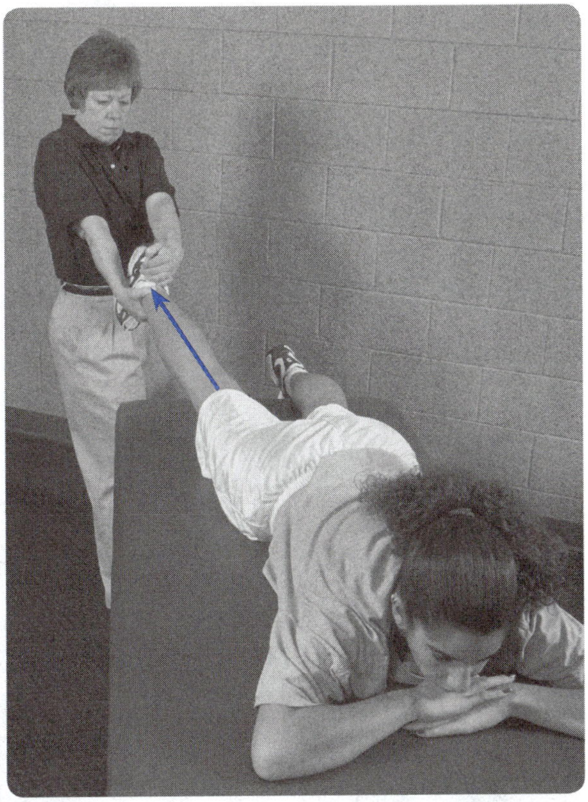

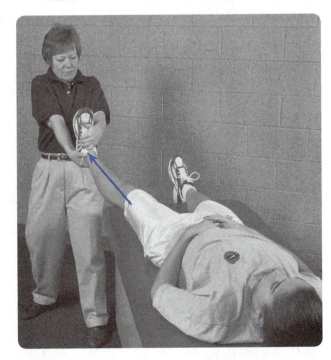

▶ **Figure 18.81** Anterior iliac subluxation: upslip treatment.

▶ **Figure 18.82** Posterior iliac subluxation: upslip muscle energy treatment.

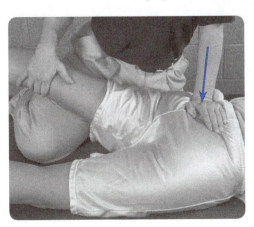

▶ **Figure 18.83** Sacral flexion muscle energy treatment.

In a home exercise that can accompany this treatment, the patient lies with both knees to the chest. This facilitates sacral extension because the sacrum moves in the opposite direction of the lumbar spine: As the lumbar spine moves into flexion, the sacrum extends; and vice versa.

Forward Torsion   The sacroiliac lesion of a forward torsion occurs primarily on the left and is more common than a backward torsion. Simultaneous bending and twisting is the most common mechanism for this injury. The pain may be present in the back, buttock, or leg, and it may occur on the opposite side. Because this is a torsion injury, one side of the sacrum is twisted on the other. For example, if the torsion is on the left, the left ILA is more posterior than the right ILA; but the right sulcus lies deeper than the left sulcus. The left piriformis is tight.

Treatment is delivered with the patient lying on the side of the injury, usually the left, with the knees and hips flexed to 90°. The patient then pushes up with his or her top hand to lift the trunk off the table and places the bottom arm behind the back. The patient then lies back down with the top arm hanging over the table toward the floor. The rehabilitation clinician places a hand in the L5-S1 joint space to monitor and maintain the spine in neutral (figure 18.84). The patient's thighs are supported on the table to the knee, and the lower legs are off the table. The clinician provides light resistance at the distal legs as the patient produces an isometric lift of the feet toward the ceiling. The muscles relax, and the clinician lowers the patient's legs to the floor until a new barrier is felt.

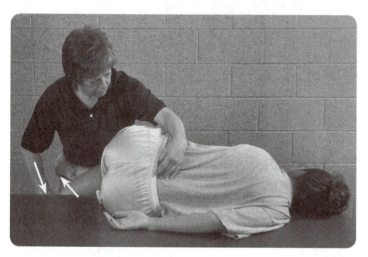

▶ **Figure 18.84**   Forward torsion muscle energy treatment, using right rotation on a right axis (R on R).

The exercise that helps correct a forward torsion is similar to the treatment. The patient assumes a sidelying position; the bottom arm is behind the trunk and the top arm hangs to the floor while the knees and hips are flexed to 90° with the lower legs over the edge of the bed or table. This position is held for 5 to 10 min. This exercise is performed until the area is stable.

Backward Torsion   This treatment is for a sacroiliac impairment that has very unique and classic signs. The patient is unable to stand upright because extension is too painful. He or she may waddle like a duck in a forward-flexed position and is unable to walk normally. Pain may be in the low back or buttock or may mimic nerve root pain.

Treatment for this injury has the patient standing facing a table and leaning onto it with the anterior superior iliac spine (ASIS) on the edge of the table. The trunk

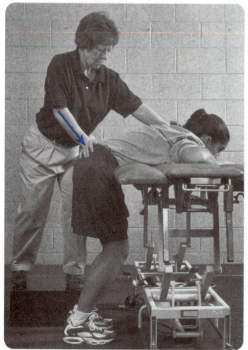

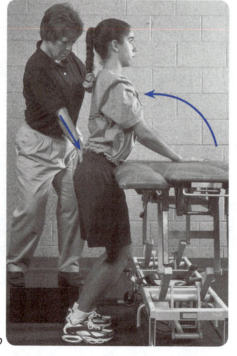

▶ **Figure 18.85**   Backward torsion muscle energy treatment: *(a)* start position, *(b)* end position.

is supported on top of the table. The rehabilitation clinician applies firm pressure on the sacrum, with the heel of the hand at the base and the fingers pointing toward the sacral apex (figure 18.85a). The pressure should be downward and firm throughout the motion. The patient then walks with the hands on the table to a standing position (figure 18.85b). The movement may be uncomfortable, but the patient should be encouraged to continue to the end of the motion.

The exercises that the patient should do to promote correction of the backward torsion are press-ups or standing trunk extensions. If standing extensions are too painful, start with press-ups. If press-ups are too uncomfortable, the patient can begin by lying prone on a pillow (figure 18.86a), progressing to lying prone without a pillow (figure 18.86b), and then progressing to lying prone on elbows (figure 18.86c) before advancing to a press-up (figure 18.86d) and then to standing trunk extensions.

Anterior Iliac Rotation The dysfunction known as anterior iliac rotation usually occurs with other lesions. It is an iliosacral lesion and is also called an anterior innominate lesion. It usually occurs on the right, and the patient complains of cervical or lumbar symptoms. The iliac crest may be low on the same side as the injury, whereas the (PSIS) is high and the ASIS is low.

For treatment of this injury, the patient lies prone along the edge of the table with the leg of the involved side positioned over the side of the table and the foot on the floor. The rehabilitation clinician places his or her thumb in the sacral sulcus to monitor the SI joint. For control of the leg, the foot is placed on the clinician's thigh and the knee is grasped (figure 18.87). The patient's 3 to 10 s isometric contraction toward extension is resisted. The patient is instructed to relax, and the leg is moved into flexion until its barrier is felt. This exercise is repeated three to five times.

There are two home exercises for this iliosacral lesion. These exercises include a pelvic tilt and both knees to chest.

Posterior Iliac Rotation This iliosacral lesion is a posterior iliac rotation, or a posterior innominate lesion. It usually occurs on the left side and is seen following a fall or sudden hamstring contraction. The patient may use an antalgic gait and walk with reduced hip extension movement on the involved side. Patients with this injury usually complain of a lot of pain in the buttock or knee. The ilium is posteriorly rotated, and the ASIS, PSIS, and iliac crest can appear high. There may also be a short-leg appearance on the same side as the lesion.

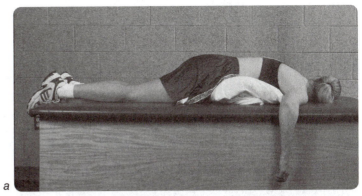
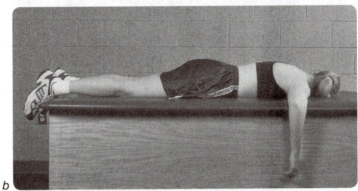
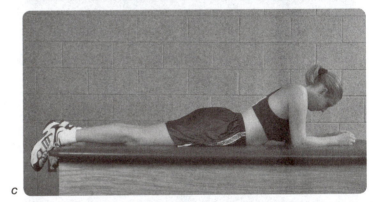
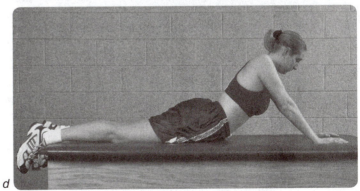

▶ **Figure 18.86** Extension progression: *(a)* prone with pillows, *(b)* prone without pillows, *(c)* prone on elbows, *(d)* press-ups.

For treatment, the patient lies in a prone position. The rehabilitation clinician places one hand on the ilium to monitor joint movement and the other on the anterior thigh proximal to the knee. The hip is extended while the pelvis maintains neutral until the barrier is felt (figure 18.88). The barrier occurs when the monitor hand feels ilium movement as the hip is extended. The patient is instructed to attempt to push the thigh to the table isometrically for 3 to 10 s. The patient then relaxes, and the thigh is passively moved into extension to the next barrier. The procedure is repeated three to five times.

There are two home exercises for this iliosacral dysfunction. These exercises include press-ups and hip-flexor stretches.

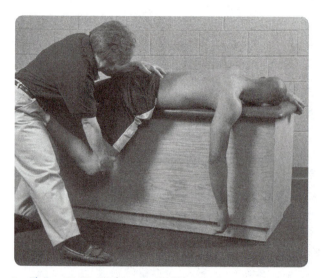

▶ **Figure 18.87** Right anterior iliac rotation muscle energy treatment.

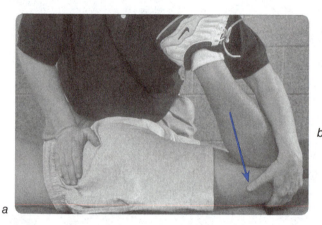

a

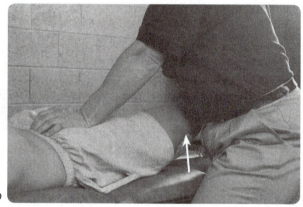

b

▶ **Figure 18.88** Left posterior iliac rotation muscle energy treatment: *(a)* Start position—patient is prone; rehabilitation clinician's monitor hand is on the ilium and the movement hand is under the patient's knee. *(b)* Once relaxed after isometric hip flexion, the thigh is passively moved into extension to the new barrier.

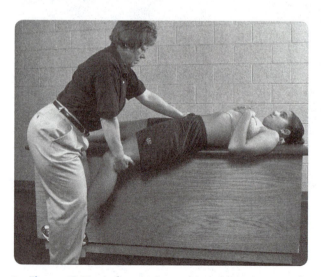

▶ **Figure 18.89** Left superior pubic subluxation muscle energy treatment.

Pubic Subluxation This is an iliosacral lesion that occurs in soccer players. It occurs also during pregnancy or delivery of a child. This lesion commonly occurs in combination with other SI lesions, especially upslips, or low back injuries. The patient may complain of only low-back pain or may have groin or buttock pain. Pushing down on the left or right pubic bones (spring test) produces pain. If it is a superior lesion, the leg will appear shorter, but if it is an inferior lesion, the leg will appear longer.

Treatment depends on whether the pubis is superior or inferior and involves a contract-relax-stretch technique. For a superior subluxation, the patient lies supine with the leg on the involved side over the edge of the table. The rehabilitation clinician supports the hanging leg under the patient's thigh and stabilizes the ASIS on the opposite side (figure 18.89). The patient performs isometric hip flexion for 5 to 10 s against the clinician. The leg is relaxed and the hip is then passively moved into extension to its new barrier.

For an inferior subluxation, the patient lies supine with the hip in flexion while the clinician places a hand under the ischial tuberosity to monitor its stability. The patient performs isometric hip extension against the clinician's hand on the proximal lower leg (figure 18.90). A passive movement into hip flexion to the new barrier is performed after the patient has relaxed the muscles.

Occasionally, a treatment technique specific to superior subluxations or one specific to inferior pubic subluxations can be successful for either problem. The patient is supine with the hips and knees flexed and the feet on the table. The patient performs a series of isometric abduction exercises of both legs simultaneously as the rehabilitation clinician resists the movement (figure 18.91a). This is followed by a series of isometric adduction exercises with the clinician's forearm placed between the patient's knees during the isometric exercise (figure 18.91b). Sometimes a pop of the pubic bones may be heard.

Exercises the patient should perform for superior pubic subluxation include a Thomas stretch. The inferior pubic subluxation exercise is a single-knee-to-chest stretch.

Inflares and Outflares Inflares and outflares are also referred to as innominate medial and lateral rotations, respectively. These iliosacral conditions often produce groin pain. Leg and hip pain may or may not be present as well. They occur in soccer players and can result from a direct blow on the ilium. In an inflare, the distance from the ASIS to the umbilicus is shorter on the affected side. In an outflare, the distance is greater on the affected side than on the opposite side.

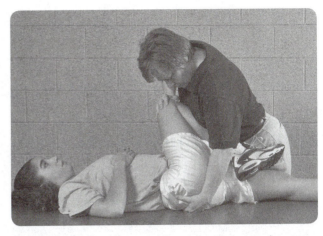

▶ **Figure 18.90** Inferior pubic subluxation muscle energy treatment.

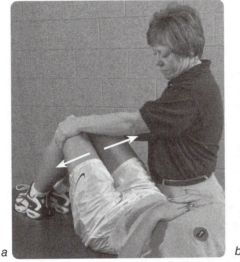 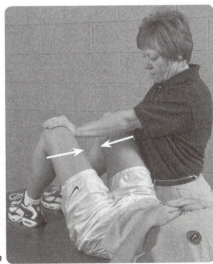

a   b

▶ **Figure 18.91** Inferior or superior pubic subluxation muscle energy treatment: *(a)* isometric abduction, *(b)* isometric adduction.

Treatment for an inflare is to have the patient lie supine with the leg of the involved side flexed and across the opposite knee. The rehabilitation clinician's hand is either on the medial malleolus, with the forearm against the lower leg or on the medial aspect of the knee. The patient's lateral thigh rests against the rehabilitation clinician's hip (figure 18.92). The clinician's other hand is used to stabilize the opposite ASIS. The patient performs an isometric hip adduction exercise for 5 to 10 s. When the muscle relaxes, the patient's leg moves passively into hip abduction until the new barrier is felt. When the exercise series is complete, the patient's leg is passively moved into extension by the clinician.

The home exercise position for an inflare is supine with the leg flexed at the hip and knee and the leg across the contralateral thigh. In this position, knee is dropped out to the side to move the hip into abduction and external rotation.

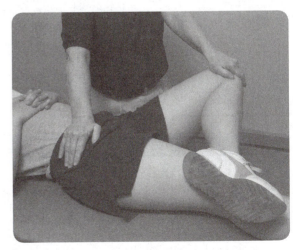

▶ **Figure 18.92** Inflare muscle energy treatment.

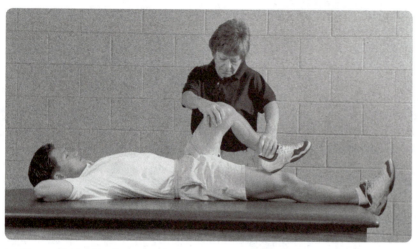

▶ **Figure 18.93** Outflare muscle energy treatment.

An outflare is treated with the patient in supine and the knee of the affected side brought toward the opposite shoulder. The rehabilitation clinician places his or her hand on the sulcus of the involved side. The hip is medially rotated passively. While maintained in this position, the patient performs a series of isometric exercises in hip flexion, adduction, and medial rotation (figure 18.93). Following the isometric contraction, the clinician moves the extremity into greater hip flexion, adduction, and medial rotation until the barrier is felt. Once the repetitions are completed, the extremity is returned passively to full extension.

To perform the home exercise for this dysfunction, the patient moves the knee to the opposite shoulder and produces a series of hold-relax techniques, using the arms to position the lower extremity in the stretch.

Program Considerations

When the sacroiliac joint is treated, the low back and hip areas should also be addressed to eliminate other sites of injury or referral. Muscle energy techniques are used in combination with flexibility and strengthening exercises. The cause, if it was not a traumatic injury, is also corrected to prevent a recurrence.

If the SI joint is the source of pain, muscle energy techniques are usually very effective in relieving or reducing the pain. If the problem has not been long-standing, the patient usually experiences significant resolution within a few treatments. Following muscle energy techniques, core exercises, specific strengthening exercises designed for the patient's needs, functional training for maintenance of pelvic neutral, and agility activities are part of the therapeutic exercise program before activity-specific exercises.

Thoracic Outlet Syndrome

Thoracic outlet syndrome (TOS) can be classified as a cervical injury or a shoulder injury. The classification depends on your orientation. Because the syndrome can be caused by structures in the neck region, some feel it is related to the cervical spine. Many of the structures contributing to it, however, are shoulder based, and certainly many of the exercises used to correct the problem are shoulder exercises. Therefore, it is logical to include TOS in a discussion of either cervical or shoulder injuries. The syndrome is discussed here, but you should keep in mind that examination of shoulder injuries and development of shoulder rehabilitation programs

■ Case Study

In last week's game, a basketball player was going in for a layup when she collided with an opponent whose knee hit her on the front of the left hip. She had an initial bruise over the anterior ilium but since then has noticed persistent left groin pain. She also has pain that goes into the left leg. Examination shows that she has normal lumbar range of motion. There is no spasm or pain in the low back area. In supine, the distance from the umbilicus to the ASIS is 0.5 cm (1/5 in.) longer on the left than on the right.

Questions for Analysis

1. What do you suspect this patient has, and what is your treatment program?

2. What exercises would you include in her home program?

should also include consideration of possible TOS manifestations, particularly if the patient does not respond as expected to the shoulder rehabilitation program.

Although the diagnosis of TOS can be difficult and the signs and symptoms complex, the treatment program is simple. Symptom control is the first goal; this should include the use of modalities as needed and instruction in positions

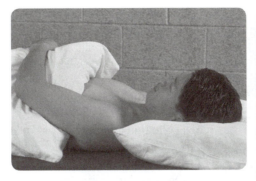

▶ **Figure 18.94**   Resting position for TOS.

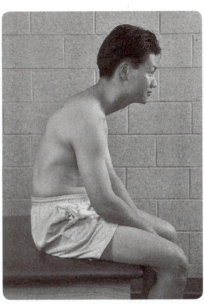

▶ **Figure 18.95**   Poor posture associated with TOS.

that relieve the tension or compression on the brachial plexus. The position that best relieves TOS in a supine sleeping position is with the scapula in protraction and elevation and the shoulder in medial rotation and adduction. Pillows should be used to support and position the shoulder and scapula as seen in figure 18.94. In severe cases, it may be necessary for the patient to wear a sling during the day. In less severe cases, the patient can obtain relief during the day by placing his or her hand in a front pant pocket or in the waistband when standing and by supporting the arm when sitting.

Correction for posture and body mechanics is vital to correcting and preventing recurrence of TOS. A typical posture held by persons with TOS is a forward-head, round-shoulder posture as seen in figure 18.95. The patient should be made aware of his or her current posture and receive instruction in how to correct it. Instructions in proper posture may begin early, but keep in mind that because of soft tissue and joint restrictions along with muscle weakness, the patient may not be able to hold a proper posture for prolonged periods. Additionally, a change in posture is dependent upon the patient remembering to correct posture, so provide the patient with a cue to remember to reposition into a proper posture position throughout the day. Any number of items may be used, such as a small colorful dot on a notebook or watch face, a small piece of tape on the patient's hand, or an alarm on the watch that goes off periodically throughout the day. As the patient's motion and strength improve, the ability to maintain a better posture for longer times should also improve. Nevertheless, it is important to use verbal cues for posture correction throughout the treatment sessions.

■ Case Study

A 20-year-old wrestler reports that for the past week he has had trouble sleeping at night. He awakens with severe numbness and tingling in the right hand and a feeling of pressure in the forearm. The problem has been getting progressively worse since it started. He has pain if he carries many books between classes, but feels all right when he is sitting in class. He does not recall any specific injury. He has been wrestling for eight years and lifts weights during the preseason. His shoulder weight program includes bench press, military press, push-ups, flys, and biceps curls. Your examination confirms the doctor's diagnosis of TOS; although the Military brace and Allen tests are negative, you can reproduce his hand's tingling symptom when you perform an Adson test. His posture is one of forward-head and round-shoulder alignment. He has limited shoulder range of motion in elevation and lateral rotation, and he is unable to move his elbow behind his

shoulder in horizontal extension without discomfort in the chest. He has well-pronounced pectoralis and anterior deltoid muscles, but his rhomboids appear diminished and his rotator cuff muscles are weak.

Questions for Analysis

1. What instructions on posture will you give this patient?

2. What flexibility exercises will you give him, and what guidelines will you use in determining when to begin them?

3. What are his strength deficiencies and muscle imbalances, and what exercises will you use to restore muscle balance?

4. What core exercises would you provide as part of his therapeutic exercise program?

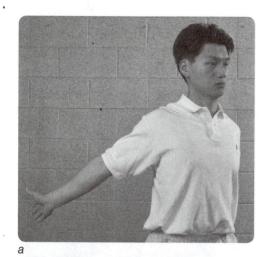

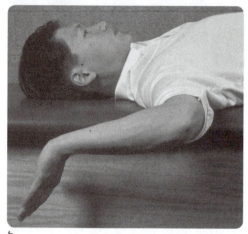

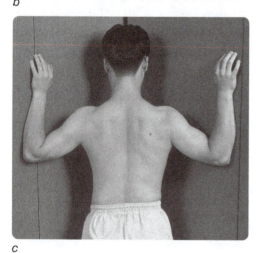

▶ **Figure 18.96** Brachial plexus stretches for TOS: *(a)* ULTT with elbow extended, *(b)* ULTT with elbow flexed, *(c)* ULTT with elbow flexed into a corner.

Soft-tissue mobilization of the cervical spine and scapular muscles—especially the upper trapezius, scalenes, pectoralis minor, and occasionally the cervical paraspinal muscles—is often effective in relieving pain and tenderness if the muscle tension in these muscles is contributing to the symptoms.

Improving joint mobility of the first rib may also help to relieve symptoms if the rib is restricted and impinging on the brachial plexus. If the rehabilitation clinician is comfortable with spine mobilization techniques, he or she should perform cervical spine and thoracic spine mobilization if areas of restriction are present.

Once the inflammation has subsided, flexibility and strengthening exercises should begin. The brachial plexus is stretched using the upper-limb tension tests (ULTT) described in chapter 6. These are reviewed in figure 18.96. These stretches are performed to the point of pain, not beyond, because pushing into the pain may re-inflame the nerve.

Flexibility exercises for the cervical and thoracic spine should also be included. Axial extension and cervical retraction exercises (figures 18.24 and 18.25) are simple beginning exercises. Additional flexibility exercises include cervical extension, lateral flexion, and forward flexion exercises. Cervical extension is performed with the neck maintained in a slightly retracted position as the patient extends the neck beginning from the upper spine and moving through the lower spine. If tolerated, overpressure with the hand on the chin can be added (figure 18.97). Lateral flexion is essentially an upper trapezius stretch as seen in figure 18.27. The patient may find it more comfortable to perform the lateral flexion exercise in supine, but it is also effective when performed either in sitting or supine.

Because thoracic mobility can influence cervical range of motion, flexion and extension flexibility exercises of the thoracic spine should also be part of a program for TOS. These are performed sitting with the hands clasped behind the neck. A rolled towel can be placed around the neck at the restricted level and pulled downward from the front with the hands as the neck is extended. For extension, the elbows are raised toward the ceiling and the patient looks upward (figure 18.98). For flexion, the patient lowers the elbows toward the chest with hands clasped together at

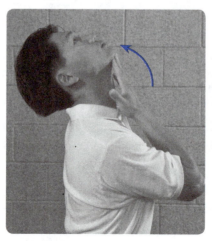

▶ **Figure 18.97** Cervical extension with overpressure.

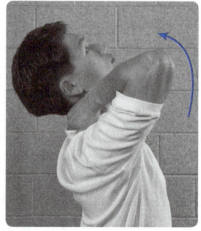

▶ **Figure 18.98** Thoracic extension with overpressure.

the base of the neck. The movement should come from the thoracic spine without pressure on the neck from the hands.

Because shoulder positioning with associated scapulothoracic and glenohumeral soft-tissue tightness can restrict brachial plexus mobility, shoulder flexibility exercises should also be included in a TOS program if there are deficiencies in the shoulder motions of lateral rotation, medial rotation, or flexion or scapulothoracic motions of retraction, rotation, and elevation. Stretches for these muscles are presented in chapter 21.

Strength exercises are designed to restore correct muscle balance of the neck and upper back so that normal movement of the brachial plexus and related soft tissue can occur and stress is reduced. The clinician should assess balance of respiratory muscles by determining how the patient breathes. It is common for patients with TOS to breathe using primarily upper respiratory muscles, the sternocleidomastoid and scalenes. These patients should be taught how to do diaphragmatic breathing, or belly, breathing in addition to using a combination of upper and lower respiratory muscles.

Additional strengthening and muscle balance activities include exercises for the rotator cuff, especially lateral rotators; rhomboids, and middle trapezius for scapular retraction; and cervical and thoracic extensors. These are commonly the weakest muscle groups in patients with TOS and should be strengthened to create a balance with their opposing muscles.

Specific types of back injuries call for particular kinds of exercises. Back problems that the rehabilitation clinician often encounters include sprains and strains; spondylosis, spondylolysis, and spondylolisthesis; disc lesions; facet injuries; sacroiliac joint injuries; and thoracic outlet syndrome.

SUMMARY

This chapter presented some of the more frequently seen trigger points of the cervical and lumbar muscles, common joint mobilization techniques for the spine and ribs, and progressions of exercises for the spine. Before any manual techniques are applied to the cervical spine, tests for vertebral artery compromise should be performed. McKenzie's and Williams' exercises were also included in the exercise programs presented. Since the spine is important in extremity function, core stabilization techniques and exercises were included in this chapter. Sacroiliac examination and muscle energy techniques were included as part of this chapter since the SI joint and pelvis are so intimately related with the lumbar spine.

KEY CONCEPTS AND REVIEW

1. Explain three flexibility exercises for the cervical spine and lumbar spine.
   - Cervical flexion: Bring the chin down to the chest, attempting to move one cervical level at a time.
   - Rotational stretch: While sitting in a chair, reach behind to grasp the back of the chair with the near hand, and use the opposite hand to keep the legs stable.
   - Both knees to chest: In a supine position, bring one leg to the chest, then the other leg; return to the starting position by reversing the procedure.

2. Explain three strengthening exercises for the cervical spine and lumbar spine.
   - Isometrics: In a proper posture, place the right hand along the right side of the head; push the head against the hand while not allowing any movement.
   - Prone leg lift: Lying prone in a neutral spine position, squeeze the buttocks and lift the legs upward.
   - Abdominal crunch: In a hook-lying supine position with hands behind the head, lift the chest and head toward the ceiling.

3. Identify three progressive spinal stability exercises.

Dead bug, quadruped, and abdominal exercises.

4. Identify three sacroiliac muscle energy release techniques and the indications for their use.

- Upslip: Upslip is always on the right and often accompanies other spinal problems. A leg pull is performed with the patient in prone and the leg positioned in 30° abduction and extension.

- Forward torsion: This occurs primarily on the left and occurs with twisting and bending motions. With the patient lying on the involved side, the legs are off the table, where resistance is provided to leg movement toward the ceiling.

- Posterior iliac rotation: This occurs primarily on the left side because of a fall or sudden hamstring contraction. With the patient prone, the hip is passively extended; the isometric force occurs in hip flexion.

5. Outline a therapeutic exercise program for a cervical sprain.

The program should begin with modalities for pain and spasm, soft-tissue mobilization, and joint mobilization if there is soft-tissue or joint restriction. Range-of-motion exercises begin with active motion within a pain-free range of motion. Overpressure can occur as the tissue continues to heal. Isometric exercises can be initiated after pain and spasm are relieved. Other exercises can include strengthening exercises such as machine resistance and manual resistance through a full range of motion. Strengthening exercises should address the abdominals, trunk extensors, and gluteals for a foundation for the cervical spine. Agility and coordination exercises with medicine balls for the upper extremity and abdominals are included once strength and endurance are good. Functional exercises are the final phase of the program and depend on the patient's specific activity requirements.

6. List precautions for a therapeutic exercise program for disc lesions.

Avoid positions that aggravate the sciatica; rule out other causes of sciatica; strengthen abdominals, gluteals, and back extensors; have the patient maintain a pelvic neutral position during activities; exercises should progress at the patient's own pace; and the rehabilitation clinician should have a good understanding of the exercises and the stresses that are imposed by each exercise.

7. Discuss the difference in therapeutic exercise programs for a lumbar strain and a facet injury.

Facet injury treatment includes gentle rotation and sidebending in a pain-free range of motion, as well as avoiding extension activities (pain will occur in rotation to one side and sidebending to the opposite side). Extension exercises do not have to be avoided in lumbar strains; rotation and sidebending are painful in the same direction and should occur in pain-free motions.

8. Present a sequence of activities you would use to begin a core strengthening program.

Identify the patient's neutral position. Use hollowing exercises to facilitate the transverse abdominis. Add abdominal bracing to incorporate other abdominal muscles. Facilitate multifidus activity by incorporating pelvic floor muscles. Improve muscle endurance and muscle strength and flexibility as individually determined, based on deficiencies and need.

9. Outline the exercises in Williams' Flexion program and McKenzie's Back Program.

Williams' Flexion Program includes 6 exercises:

- Exercise #1: Sit-up in a flexed-knee position to strengthen the abdominals.

- Exercise #2: Pelvic tilt to strengthen the gluteal muscles.

- Exercise #3: Single knee-to-chest and double knee-to-chest to stretch the erector spinae muscles.

- Exercise #4: Seated reach to the toes with knees extended to stretch the erector spinae and hamstring muscles.

- Exercise #5: In a quadruped position with one knee forward under the lata and ilio-femoral ligament.

- Exercise #6: Starting in standing and moving to a full squat to strengthen the quadriceps muscles

McKenzie's Back Program has 5 progressive exercises:

- Exercise #1: Prone lying for 5 minutes

- Exercise #2: Lying prone on the elbows with the elbows under the shoulders for 5 minutes.

- Exercise #3: Prone press-ups.

- Exercise #4: Trunk extension in standing.

- Exercise #5: The seated "cat-cow" exercise.

10. Explain the differences between McKenzie's postural syndromes, dysfunction, and derangement.

Postural syndromes are the first step in progressive chronic back pain. This condition is not severe and occurs during the teen years and early twenties. The patient experiences back, neck or interscapular pain, especially after prolonged postures in sitting. The pain is intermittent in this stage, and the patient's examination is essentially negative. Unfortunately, if no steps are taken to correct posture and habit, the condition may progress to the next syndrome, dysfunction. It is during this phase that early changes are noted. There is some loss of accessory joint movement, reduced range of motion, and diminished soft tissue mobility. Neurological examinations during this phase, however are negative. The patient may complain of either intermittent or constant pain and stiffness. It is imperative that posture and deficiencies in soft tissue and joint mobility be corrected to prevent the patient from advancing to the final phase. Derangements are the most severe condition. By this time, source of the patient's pain has changed from inflammation of structures to the disc. Over time with poor posture, vertebral positions and advanced stress have changed to produce disc alterations and degeneration. Derangements are divided into seven different types. The first six deal with posterior disc pathology and the seventh involves anterior disc pathology.

11. Explain the various McKenzie derangements.

- Derangement #1: There is a mild disc bulge with either central or asymmetrical pain in the back. The pain results from irritation to the posterior annulus and the posterior longitudinal ligament caused by the bulging disc. Usually the pain subsides in a few days.

- Derangement #2: The disc bulge is now moderate in size and may cause buttock pain. Examination reveals the patient to have a flat lumbar spine and some pain when changing positions or when in prolonged sitting

- Derangement #3: The disc bulge is now more prominent with pain occurring to the buttock or even the posterior thigh. Although there is no deformity visible, the pain is more intense.

- Derangement #4: The pain is pronounced down one extremity to the knee, and the patient exhibits a shift of the lumbar spine. If the bulge occurs medial to the nerve root, the shift is to the same side as the pain, but if the derangement is lateral to the nerve root, the shift is towards the contralateral side of pain. This is the body's method of reducing stress on the nerve root.

- Derangement #5: Disc degeneration continues now to where the patient experiences unilateral referred pain below the knee. No deformity is noted on examination, but the progressive bulge of the annulus fibrosis causes irritation of the nerve root and the dura.

- Derangement #6: In this derangement, the disc is herniated through the annulus fibrosis. The unilateral extremity pain is below the knee and may go into the foot. The patient reports feelings of paresthesia, weakness, and numbness.

- Derangement #7: This derangement involves an anterior bulge of the disc and stretching of the anterior longitudinal ligament. This type of derangement occurs infrequently. Buttock and thigh pain may be seen with this condition, and the patient usually has a fixed lumbar lordosis.

CRITICAL THINKING QUESTIONS

1. Regarding the scenario presented at the beginning of this chapter, identify a myofascial release technique Rita probably used on Joey. Why did you select this technique?

2. What exercises would you give Joey to strengthen his core and trunk muscles? What progression would you include for each exercise, and what are your criteria for progression?

3. With reference to the example of the gymnast with spondylolysis mentioned in the chapter, extension exercises should be avoided. How can you strengthen her back muscles without aggravating her injury? Will your attempts to strengthen her abdominals irritate the spondylolysis? Why or why not?

4. A football lineman who has been diagnosed with a disc herniation is attempting conservative rehabilitation to avoid surgery. What will your program of therapeutic exercises include? What will you avoid in the exercises? Body mechanics affect his injury, but how? What will you do to assure that he uses proper body mechanics both in his everyday activities and when he returns to football?

LAB ACTIVITIES

1. Have your lab partner lie prone; be sure to have him or her positioned comfortably and in a neutral position from the cervical to the sacral area. Start at the cervical spine and palpate each the spinous process to the L5. Locate L4; first examine your partner's joint excursion at L4-5, and then apply grades 1, 2, 3, and 4 PA joint mobilizations to the joint. Determine mobility of each joint throughout the spine. Where is there laxity and where is there restriction? Now examine another lab partner and repeat the process. How do they differ, or are they similar? Have each person on whom you performed a joint mobilization examination stand and bend forward while you observe the spine from a posterior view. Do the areas of restriction you found during joint mob examination correlate with the range of motion restrictions you see during active physiological motion? What does this indicate for you in terms of patient motion related to joint mobility?

2. Locate the trigger points for the following muscles on your lab partner:
   a. Upper trapezius
   b. Levator scapulae
   c. Sternocleidomastoid
   d. Scalenes
   e. Spleni
   f. Quadratus lumborum
   g. Lumbar multifidus

   Where were your partner's most sensitive trigger points? Perform a spray-and-stretch technique on the most sensitive areas after you have determined for active range of motion of the muscle. After the treatment, have your partner repeat the active range of motion so you can determine the effectiveness of your treatment. How did the AROM change from before to after the treatment? Why?

3. Demonstrate two flexibility and strength exercises for each of the muscles or muscle groups listed below:
   a. Scalenes
   b. Upper trapezius
   c. Sternocleidomastoid
   d. Quadratus lumborum
   e. Erector spinae
   f. External obliques

4. Find your pelvic neutral position while sitting. Now find pelvic neutral while supine, and then while standing. In which of these positions was it most difficult to identify your neutral position? Why do think that is?

5. Perform a progression of supine lumbar stabilization exercises outlined in the chapter. Now attempt the lumbar stabilization exercises in a quadruped position. Perform a sit-to-stand motion while in pelvic neutral. While your lab partner observes you, maintain pelvic neutral while you walk and then while you perform a jump. If you are unable to maintain pelvic neutral during these activities, have your partner provide you with cues and instructions that will improve your performance.

6. Have your partner perform abdominal hollowing and abdominal bracing exercises in supine. Now have your partner perform them in a quadruped and then in a sitting position. During each exercise, correct your partner when the neutral position is lost. During which of the three positions did your partner have the most difficult time maintaining neutral while performing the exercises? Was it more difficult to maintain neutral in the hollowing or in the bracing exercise?

7. Instruct your partner in one sport activity and incorporate pelvic neutral into the activity. Be sure you provide feedback and correction cues if your partner loses neutral during the activity. When you both performed this exercise, which errors did you both make most often? Do you know why?

8. Examine your partner's sacroiliac joint for proper alignment using all the examination techniques outlined earlier in the chapter. Be sure to locate each landmark appropriately.

9. Perform the following muscle energy techniques:
   a. Anterior iliac subluxation
   b. Sacral flexion
   c. Forward torsion
   d. Anterior iliac rotation
   e. Pubic subluxation
   f. Inflare
   g. Outflare

   What will the malalignments be for each of these conditions? What home exercise will you provide a patient who presents with these problems? How will you know if your treatment has been effective?

10. Case Study: A 21-year-old male discus thrower began having left low back pain after a long workout last week. He presents to you today with complaints of left low-back pain that goes into his left buttock. He does not remember a frank injury. Your examination reveals a deep sulcus and a posterior left ILA. He is tender to palpation of the left sulcus. What do you suspect is his problem? What will your treatment with him today include? What home exercise will you give him? What therapeutic exercises would you provide as part of his treatments? What other things would you include in his rehabilitation program?

ADDITIONAL SOURCES

Corrigan, B., and G.D. Maitland. 1989. *Practical orthopaedic medicine.* Boston: Butterworth-Heinemann.

Erhard, R.E., Delitto, A., and M.T. Cibulka. 1994. Relative effectiveness of an extension program and a combined program of manipulation and flexion and extension exercises in patients with acute low back syndrome. *Physical Therapy* 74:1093-1100.

Foster, D.N., and M.N. Fulton. 1991. Back pain and the exercise prescription. *Clinics in Sports Medicine* 10:197-209.

Hodges, P.W., and C.A. Richardson. 1997. Contraction of the abdominal muscles associated with movement of the lower limb. *Physical Therapy* 77:132-144.

Hopkins, T.J., and A.A. White. 1993. Rehabilitation of athletes following spine injury. *Clinics in Sports Medicine* 12:603-618.

Johannsen, F., Remvig, L., Kryger, P., Beck, P., Warming, S., Lybeck, K., Dreyer, V., and L.H. Larsen. 1995. Exercises for chronic low back pain: A clinical trial. *Journal of Orthopaedic and Sports Physical Therapy* 22:52-59.

Kaltenborn, F.M. 2003. *Manual mobilization of the joints.* Vol II. *The spine.* 4th ed. Minneapolis: OPTP.

Kuzmich, D. 1994. The levator scapulae: Making the con-NECK-tion. *Journal of Manual and Manipulative Therapy* 2:43-54.

Lee, H.W.M. 1994. Progressive muscle synergy and synchronization in movement patterns: An approach to the treatment of dynamic lumbar instability. *Journal of Manual and Manipulative Therapy* 2:133-142.

Maitland, G.D. 1990. *Vertebral manipulation.* Boston: Butterworth-Heinemann.

Oliver, J. 1994. *Back care. An illustrated guide.* Boston: Butterworth-Heinemann.

Saudek, C.E., and K.A. Palmer. 1987. Back pain revisited. *Journal of Orthopaedic and Sports Physical Therapy* 8:556-566.

Smith, K.F. 1979. The thoracic outlet syndrome: A protocol of treatment. *Journal of Orthopaedic and Sports Physical Therapy* 1:89-99.

Tan, J.C., and M. Nordin. 1992. Role of physical therapy in the treatment of cervical disc disease. *Orthopedic Clinics of North America* 23:435-449.

Walker, J.M. 1992. The sacroiliac joint: A critical review. *Physical Therapy* 72:903-916.

Watkins, R.G. 1996. *The spine in sports.* St. Louis: Mosby.

CHAPTER 19

Shoulder and Arm

OBJECTIVES

After completing this chapter, you should be able to do the following:

1. Explain how knowledge of the mechanics of sport performance impacts the establishment of a therapeutic exercise program.
2. Discuss the importance of stability in shoulder rehabilitation.
3. Explain the role of scapular stabilization in shoulder function.
4. Describe two soft-tissue mobilization techniques for the shoulder.
5. List three joint mobilizations for the shoulder.
6. Identify three strengthening exercises for the scapula and three for the gleno-humeral muscles.
7. Discuss the general progression of strengthening exercises for the shoulder.
8. List precautions for a therapeutic exercise program following a rotator cuff repair.
9. Outline key factors for a program for a biceps rupture.

▶ Bob George, certified athletic trainer for the local baseball farm team, sees several shoulder injuries each season. He is very familiar with the shoulder rehabilitation process, having successfully treated many players over the years.

His latest patient, P.G. Pamaloo, is one of the more promising pitchers Bob has seen in recent years. P.G. began having shoulder pain as a result of scapular muscle weakness and fatigue. Although he didn't have any shoulder capsular tightness that would have necessitated joint mobilization techniques, he did have the lateral rotator tightness that pitchers often acquire. Bob has provided P.G. with a good rehabilitation program that has resolved the shoulder's motion and strength deficits, and P.G. is about to begin a plyometric exercise program before beginning throwing activities.

Bob likes to make the rehabilitation program interesting for the baseball players. On different days, he provides different exercises that can produce the same result. He uses rubber bands, manual resistance, and medicine balls instead of machine weights or dumbbells, because he feels that his patients find these more interesting and fun than weights.

Life is a test: The test of life is open-book, take-home, and multiple choice. Your test is personalized. Not all problems make sense. Some problems are very difficult, but solutions are always simple. Mistakes can be fixed until the test is over. You must help others solve their problems. If you need help, you can call the instructor at any time. Don't quit – only the instructor knows how many problems there are and how long the test will last.

TED GIBBONS *(This Life is a Test)*

The shoulder is a complex multiplex. Its complexity makes it a difficult region to comprehend from both a functional and a rehabilitation perspective. This chapter will assist you in understanding its complexity and appreciating rather than fearing it.

The purpose of the shoulder is to position the hand for function. The shoulder provides the impetus for propelling objects from the hand; it also places the hand in a position that enables you to catch or propel an object or to make contact with an object or surface. For these activities to occur, the entire shoulder complex, including its related joints and muscles, must operate with precise timing, intensity, positioning and speed of movement.

The shoulder has more mobility than any other joint in the body. Differentiated into one-degree increments, there are approximately 16,000 different possible shoulder positions (Perry, 1978). The shoulder is designed for large ranges of motion, making thousands of hand placements possible. People who participate in overhead sports, such as baseball; softball; golf; football; swimming; volleyball; racket sports; and field events including javelin, discus, and shot put, utilize the shoulder's expansive mobility repetitively throughout each day of practice and participation. Overhead sports entail the use of tremendous forces to produce great upper-extremity velocity. During the acceleration phase of pitching, for example, arm movement at a velocity of around 7500°/s has been recorded (Pappas, Zawacki, & Sullivan, 1985). Rotational velocity in a tennis serve is 1500°/s, and hand speed at ball impact has been clocked at 75.6 kph (47 mph) (Kibler, 1995). These velocities are generated from the shoulder starting essentially at rest in the cocking phase of a movement, accelerating to these top speeds and then suddenly decelerating in the follow-through, all in the space of less than 180° of rotation and milliseconds of time. For the shoulder to withstand these repeated stresses, the joints and muscles must all work as a highly synchronous, well-balanced unit. If a joint fails to move correctly or the muscles are imbalanced, an injury is sure to occur.

The risk of injury makes it vital for the rehabilitation clinician to understand the mechanics of normal shoulder motion and to have the knowledge, wisdom, and good judgment for appropriate rehabilitation progression. Before presenting specific therapeutic exercises for the shoulder, this chapter introduces the mechanics of overhead activities and basic considerations that are unique to the shoulder. As a clinician, you must be aware of these elements to design appropriate functional and sport-specific elements of a shoulder rehabilitation program.

MECHANICS OF OVERHEAD SPORT ACTIVITIES

All overhead activities impart stress to the shoulder and other upper extremity segments. An appreciation of these stresses and of the biomechanics in overhead sports can help you develop suitable rehabilitation programs.

The muscles to be discussed in relation to each motion include only those that have been investigated by researchers. Even though the research on shoulder biomechanics and muscle activity is extensive, we still have much to learn before we will have a complete picture of the shoulder in overhead activities. Meanwhile, you need to realize the importance of your own observations, understanding of shoulder function, and knowledge of the muscles that produce those functions. Even though research may not have yielded all the answers you need, your clinical skills, knowledge, and observations will help you identify and correct a patient's deficiencies to permit a safe return to full participation.

Common athletic activities in this section involve the shoulder joints and muscles. These athletic activities include baseball pitching, tennis strokes, freestyle swimming stroke, and golf. Analysis of these activities are inserted here so that when you design a therapeutic exercise program for an athlete involved in one of these sports, you may understand the joint and muscle requirements for your patient to return to the activity. Functional and sport-specific therapeutic exercises included in the program are based on these specific requirements and demands.

Baseball Pitching

Pitching has been investigated more thoroughly than any other overhead activity, with the shoulder most often the primary focus. It is recognized that the baseball pitcher uses the entire body in the pitching motion, beginning with the lower extremities and advancing to the trunk, shoulder, elbow, wrist, and hand. An alteration in any segment of this chain can affect the outcome. Consistent accuracy through repetition of coordinated high-velocity activity is the key to successful pitching. It is also the source of injury.

Pitching is a smooth, continuous motion that occurs during a relatively brief period. Depending on the investigator, baseball pitching is divided into three (Pappas et al., 1985), four (Jobe, Moynes, Tibone, & Perry, 1984), five (Braatz & Gogia, 1987), or six (Park, Loebenberg, Rokito, & Zuckerman, 2002/2003a) phases. Of these studies, the most commonly used phases include windup, early cocking, late cocking, acceleration, and follow-through (figure 19.1).

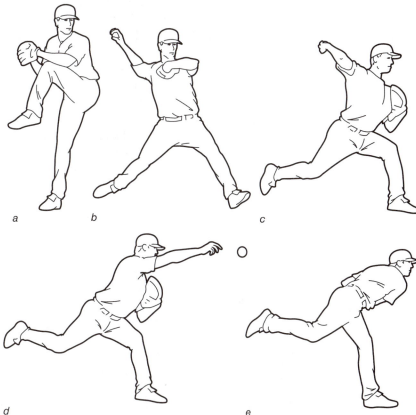

▶ **Figure 19.1** Throwing motion: *(a)* windup, *(b)* early cocking, *(c)* late cocking, *(d)* acceleration, *(e)* follow-through.

Windup

Windup, the setting phase of the pitching motion, occurs when the individual positions the body such that the glove (non-throwing) side is facing the target. The purpose of the windup is to set a rhythm that establishes a synchronized timing of the body parts (Braatz & Gogia, 1987). At the start, the two hands are together and near the body anywhere from the belt to the head as he takes a step back with the leg contralateral to the throwing arm. This contralateral leg is the stride leg while the ipsilateral leg is the support leg (Dillman, Fleisig, & Andrews, 1993). With the weight transfer, the body rotates 90° as the stride leg flexes at the hip and knee so the pelvis rotates towards the throwing shoulder and the lumbar spine flexes slightly. The body winds up so that all segments of the body from the legs to the arms are able to contribute to the ball's propulsion (Pappas et al., 1985). This phase is a minimally demanding portion of the pitching motion. Speed, energy expenditure, and forces generated are all at low levels.

Cocking

Cocking begins when the hands separate and ends when abduction and maximum lateral rotation of the shoulder is achieved (Pappas et al., 1985). Cocking is divided into early cocking and late cocking according to the contact of the forward foot on the ground. In early cocking, the scapula is retracted and the humerus is abducted, laterally rotated, and horizontally extended. The elbow flexes. The stride leg begins to extend the knee; abduct, medially rotate and extend the hip; and evert and plantar flex the ankle (Braatz & Gogia, 1987). The non-throwing shoulder is abducted and its elbow is extending. The body's center of gravity is lowered because the support knee and hip are flexing and the hips and pelvis begin to rotate forward.

Late cocking begins when the stride foot hits the ground (Jobe et al., 1984). At the time of foot contact, both arms are elevated about 90° and in line with each other along the plane of the shoulders. Anterior stress on the glenohumeral joint is predominant at this time, with the body in front of the arm. The deltoid is strongly active during early cocking. When maximum shoulder lateral rotation and abduction to at least 90° occur, the static stabilizers of the shoulder, the glenohumeral capsule and ligaments, serve to limit further motion. Active stabilizers, including the forward flexors, lateral rotators, the subscapularis, pectoralis major, and latissimus dorsi, act as additional restraints to control motion. Scapular stabilizers such as the pectoralis minor and serratus anterior are also active in late cocking. Reciprocal inhibition of the other rotator cuff muscles, the teres minor, supraspinatus, and infraspinatus, is also taking place as these muscles attempt to resist the superior subluxating forces that occur when the trunk is in a forward lean and the shoulder is maximally laterally rotated (Jobe et al., 1984). At the end of late cocking, the lumbar spine hyperextends to add to the shoulder's lateral rotation (Braatz & Gogia, 1987). The supraspinatus and infraspinatus are particularly active in late cocking. By the end of this phase, the shoulder medial rotators are on maximum stretch, the body is "wound" optimally for the elastic energy transfer, and the pelvis leads the shoulders to face the target legs and trunk begin their acceleration for energy transfer to the arm. Right before the end of this phase, the body laterally tilts to the non-throwing arm side. Shoulder rotation to the target and lateral trunk motion are facilitated by the non-throwing arm's motion from a position of abduction at the start of late cocking to adduction and extension at the end (Braatz & Gogia, 1987).

Acceleration

Acceleration starts with maximum shoulder lateral rotation and abduction and ends when the ball leaves the fingers (Jobe et al., 1984). The movements in this phase include scapular protraction, humeral horizontal flexion and medial rotation, and elbow extension. Just prior to ball release, the shoulder is still at about 90° of abduction. The glenohumeral joint's capsule is wound tight to provide an elastic force release and the accelerator muscles are also maximally stretched (Perry, 1983). During this phase the speed of the arm has increased significantly in a relatively brief period, beginning from almost 0°/s at the end of cocking to 7500°/s by the end of acceleration, a time of 50 msec (Pappas et al., 1985). The serratus anterior and pectoralis major are strongly active during this phase as the arm moves forward and the scapula protracts (Jobe et al., 1984). The subscapularis and latissimus dorsi are contracting concentrically as the arm moves into medial rotation during acceleration (Jobe et al., 1984).

Follow-Through

Follow-through occurs from the point of ball release to the completion of the motion when the support leg moves forward and contacts the ground to stop forward body motion (Jobe, Tibone, Perry, & Moynes, 1983). It is divided into early and late follow-through according to the point of maximal shoulder medial rotation. Early follow-through is completed rapidly, in less than 0.1 s (Moynes, Perry, Antonelli, & Jobe, 1986). Trunk rotation and scapular motions occur and are diminished to a varying extent from one style to another, depending on the individual thrower. The deltoid is strongly active during early follow-through (Jobe et al., 1984). The rotator cuff, especially the lateral rotators, must decelerate the arm after ball release and work against the momentum distraction forces occurring at the shoulder. The biceps is also working at high levels eccentrically to reduce distraction forces at the elbow (Jobe et al., 1984). Some of the forces produced during acceleration are absorbed by the stride leg; it is planted during acceleration and flexed knee position absorbs some of the forces (Braatz & Gogia, 1987). After the ball is released, the throwing arm continues to move across the body toward the opposite hip with the scapula continuing to protract; this cross-body motion helps to minimize irritation to the rotator cuff since the concomitant scapular motion keeps the coracoacromial arch structures from impinging on the rotator cuff (Braatz & Gogia, 1987).

It is during the follow-through that injuries to the posterior shoulder occur. The body must now dissipate the energy that has been developed to accelerate the ball. This is one reason it is important for the body to continue to move after the ball is released. An abrupt stop in arm motion will prevent this energy dissipation and cause these tremendous forces to be absorbed primarily by the shoulder. Flexing the trunk, flexng the support knee, and allowing the arm to continue along its path of movement across the body and to the opposite leg all assist in dissipating this energy and reducing distraction forces on the shoulder (Braatz & Gogia, 1987).

Tennis

The repetitive motions and forces applied to the shoulder in tennis are a frequent cause of tennis injuries. Overhead serves and hits require more muscle activity of the shoulder than other motions and are the leading cause of shoulder injuries in this sport. The three main strokes in tennis are the serve, the forehand groundstroke, and the backhand groundstroke. Each deserves a brief discussion because the rehabilitation clinician must understand the motions involved and the demands placed on the shoulder to effectively and safely advance the patient in a functional therapeutic exercise program.

Serve

The serve is divided into four phases-windup, cocking, acceleration, and follow-through (Ryu, McCormick, Jobe, Moynes, & Antonelli, 1988) (figure 19.2).

Windup Windup, the setting phase of the serve, takes place when the athlete prepares for the motion. The serve stance is taken in preparation for the ball toss. The body is

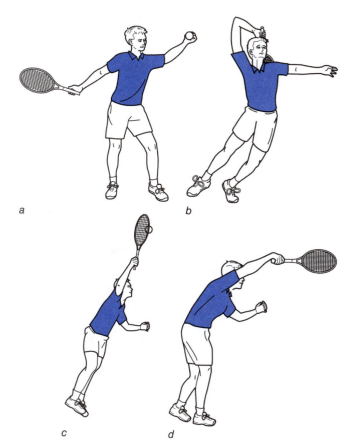

▶ **Figure 19.2** Tennis serve: *(a)* windup, *(b)* cocking, *(c)* acceleration, *(d)* follow-through.

perpendicular to the service line, with the weight on the back leg and the front leg facing the target. The shoulder muscles are relatively quiet. The shoulder is in slight abduction, extension, and lateral rotation. The trunk is slightly laterally flexed and rotated, and the legs are rotated.

Cocking   Cocking begins with ball release from the opposite arm and continues to the point at which the racket shoulder is at maximum lateral rotation (Ryu et al., 1988). The scapula is upwardly rotated and adducted, the shoulder is abducted and laterally rotated, and the elbow is flexed. The supraspinatus, infraspinatus, and subscapularis muscles are very active, stabilizing the humerus in the glenoid and positioning the shoulder. The subscapularis also works to decelerate lateral rotation in preparation for acceleration. The serratus anterior is active to stabilize the scapula on the thoracic wall and simultaneously rotate the scapula into the correct position to serve as a platform from which the glenohumeral joint moves (Ryu et al., 1988). The posterior deltoid and trunk lean produce shoulder abduction. Biceps activity is moderately high during this phase so that the racket is held in the correct position with the elbow flexed overhead.

Acceleration   Acceleration begins with medial rotation movement of the shoulder and ends with ball contact (Ryu et al., 1988). Glenohumeral medial rotation is rapid and forceful, occurring with shoulder adduction, elbow extension, and trunk flexion. It is the quickest and briefest phase of the serve. The subscapularis is very active to produce medial rotation. The pectoralis major and latissimus dorsi adduct the arm. Scapular stabilizers, performing a critical function, are active as they continue to maintain good scapular positioning and stabilization on the thoracic wall. The biceps is eccentrically controlling elbow extension and pronation.

Follow-Through   The last phase of the serve, follow-through, occurs from ball impact to the end of the motion (Ryu et al., 1988). As with pitching, the rapid change from accelera-tion to deceleration places tremendous stress on the shoulder and causes the scapular and glenohumeral muscles to work at moderate to high levels primarily to decelerate and protect the shoulder. Most of these muscles work intensely in the early part of follow-through, their activity declining as the motion continues. The latissimus dorsi and pectoralis major decelerate forward shoulder motion; the rotator cuff muscles work eccentrically to provide deceleration of the forward momentum and distraction pull on the humerus in the glenoid; the serratus anterior (the most thoroughly investigated scapular rotator) is active eccentrically; and the biceps continues its eccentric control of the elbow (Ryu et al., 1988).

Forehand Ground Stroke

The forehand ground stroke is divided into three phases—racket preparation, acceleration, and follow-through (figure 19.3).

Racket Preparation   The racket prepa-ration phase begins with the shoulder turn and ends with the initiation of weight transfer onto the front foot (Ryu et al., 1988). The trunk and hips are rotated away from the front foot. The arm is positioned into abduction and lateral rotation, and the weight is on the back foot. The shoulder positioning is primarily the result of hip and trunk rotation; little muscle activity occurs in the shoulder.

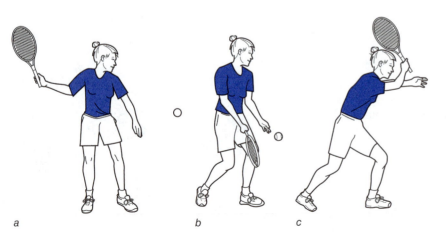

a   *b*   *c*

▶ **Figure 19.3**   Forehand ground stroke: *(a)* racket preparation, *(b)* acceleration, *(c)* follow-through.

Acceleration   This phase begins with weight transfer onto the front foot and ends at ball impact (Ryu et al., 1988). During this phase the body and racket are moved forward, and the hips and trunk begin to rotate. A rapid medial rotation of the shoulder and adduction occur. Medial rotation results from strong concentric contraction of the subscapularis; adduction occurs because of the pectoralis major (Ryu et al., 1988). The serratus anterior also works actively to continue protraction and scapular stabilization. The biceps works to keep the elbow slightly flexed.

Follow-Through   Follow-through occurs from ball contact to the end of the motion (Ryu et al., 1988). The serratus anterior, biceps, infraspinatus, and supraspinatus are highly active as during other follow-through motions (Ryu et al., 1988).

Backhand Ground Stroke

The backhand ground stroke is similar to the forehand ground stroke in having three phases: racket preparation, acceleration, and deceleration (figure 19.4).

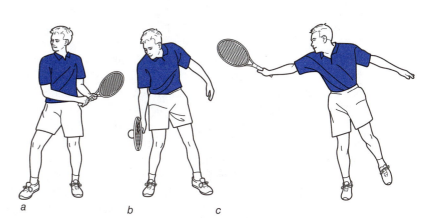

▶ **Figure 19.4**   Backhand ground stroke: *(a)* racket preparation, *(b)* acceleration, *(c)* follow-through.

Racket Preparation   This phase begins with shoulder turned to place the racket shoulder to the net and ends with weight-transfer initiation to the front foot (Ryu et al., 1988). The trunk and hips are rotated with the weight primarily on the back foot, the shoulder is in medial rotation and adduction, and the elbow is flexed. As with other preparatory phases, shoulder muscle activity is relatively quiet.

Acceleration   Acceleration begins with weight transfer to the front foot and ends with ball contact (Ryu et al., 1988). The hips and trunk begin rotation, and as the weight is transferred, the scapula retracts, the shoulder abducts and laterally rotates, and the elbow extends. This movement occurs with strong, forceful shoulder lateral rotation caused by the rotator cuff (supraspinatus, infraspinatus, and teres minor). The middle deltoid is also active as the shoulder is abducted. The serratus anterior, acting as a scapular stabilizer, and the biceps, working as an elbow decelerator, are also active during this phase (Ryu et al., 1988).

Follow-Through   Follow-through takes place from ball contact to the end of the stroke (Ryu et al., 1988). The most active muscles during this phase are the middle deltoid, biceps, supraspinatus, and infraspinatus (Ryu et al., 1988).

Swimming

Shoulder pain is common in swimmers. The shoulder provides the propulsive force to permit use of the hand as a paddle for moving the body through the water (Perry, 1983). The legs provide less propulsion than the arms in swimming, and they are important for smoothing out the stroke and making it more efficient. The legs also provide a base for body roll during the stroke, so therapeutic exercise programs for injured swimmers should include lower-extremity exercises.

Each of four primary swimming strokes—the freestyle, the backstroke, the breaststroke, and the butterfly—has unique characteristics, but they all have two phases of motion, pull-through and recovery. With the exceptions of the backstroke and the recovery phase in the breaststroke, which are performed out of the water, all are performed in a prone position. Because most shoulder injuries in swimming are seen with the freestyle stroke, we will consider this stroke here.

Pull-Through

The pull-through phase is the propulsive phase of the freestyle stroke and is similar to the acceleration phase in throwing. In contrast to the acceleration phase in throwing, though, pull-through is the longest phase in swimming. This requires sustained activity of the muscles producing the movement. Pull-through occurs during 65% to 70% of the freestyle stroke (Nuber, Jobe, Perry, Moynes, & Antonelli, 1986). The shoulder begins in lateral rotation and abduction at hand entry into the water and ends medially rotated and adducted just before leaving the water. The elbow moves from flexion to extension. The body rolls to a maximum of 40° to 60° from horizontal, and the shoulder is at 90° abduction and neutral rotation during the middle of the pull phase (Richardson, Jobe, & Collins, 1980). In the early portion of pull-through, the arm reaches forward underwater with the hand lateral to the head but medial to the shoulder and is ready for the pulling aspect of the phase. The fingers enter the water first. Pulling begins after the arm is positioned in the water and continues until the hand is near the thigh, before the hand exits the water. During the most propulsive portion of the pull-through phase, the arm moves in an S-shaped curve: The hand moves across the chest as the shoulder adducts, then moves laterally as it passes by the pelvis. Before lifting the hand out of the water, the shoulder medially rotates to turn the palm to reduce drag. During hand entry and early pull-through when the hand crosses the body, the shoulder is in adduction, flexion, and medial rotation; this position can produce mechanical impingement on the biceps tendon and the supraspinatus tendon.

Muscles active during the early pull-through phase include the upper trapezius to upwardly rotate the scapula, the rhomboids to retract the scapula, and the supraspinatus and anterior and middle deltoids to work as a force couple to stabilize the humerus. During later pull-through, the pectoralis major and latissimus dorsi act as the propulsive muscles; the deltoids lift and place the arm in preparation for hand exit from the water; the serratus anterior stabilizes the scapula and the teres minor and the subscapularis both stabilize the humerus in the glenoid and provide humeral motion; the teres minor assists with shoulder extension, and the subscapularis medially rotates the humerus (Pink, Perry, Browne, Scovazzo, & Kerrigan, 1991). The rhomboids downwardly rotate the scapula as the shoulder moves into extension (Pink et al., 1991).

Recovery

The recovery phase begins when the arm leaves the water and continues until hand entry. This phase, used as a preparation for the pull phase, is equivalent to the cocking phase in pitching. During recovery, the shoulder abducts and is in medial rotation but moving into lateral rotation as the elbow is lifted and the body rolls to the opposite side, as during early pull-through (Richardson et al., 1980). It is during this time that impingement can occur. This is especially true if weakness or fatigue prevents the swimmer from lifting the elbow out of the water first or if weak or fatigued rotator cuff and biceps muscles prevent adequate humeral head depression. By mid-recovery, the shoulder is abducted to 90° and in lateral rotation. The body roll reaches its maximum of 40° to 60° as the athlete breathes. By the time the hand enters the water, the shoulder is maximally laterally rotated and abducted, and the body roll is back to a neutral position.

Early recovery is initiated by the muscles abducting and rotating the humerus (middle deltoid and supraspinatus, respectively) and rotating the scapula (trapezius and serratus anterior) (Richardson et al., 1980). As recovery progresses, the rhomboids retract the scapula, and the subscapularis medially rotates the shoulder from a maximally laterally rotated position at middle recovery and assists the infraspinatus in depression of the humerus in the glenoid before hand entry.

The subscapularis and the serratus anterior are essentially active throughout the entire swimming stroke (Pink et al., 1991). The range of activity varies according to the arm position and the activity occurring, but the sustained activity of these muscles is significant and should be taken into account in the design of a therapeutic exercise program. Therapeutic exercise programs for these two muscles must include both high-endurance and strength exercises to provide proper shoulder positioning during swimming and to prevent fatigue.

Golf Swing

There are four phases of the golf swing: take-away, forward swing, acceleration, and follow-through (figure 19.5). Research on the golf swing has expanded in recent years. Jobe, et al (Jobe, Moynes, & Antonelli, 1985) were early investigators of the golf swing. Their research looked only at the supraspinatus, subscapularis, infraspinatus, latissimus dorsi, pectoralis major, anterior deltoid, middle deltoid, and posterior deltoid. Other investigators since have looked at other muscles, forces, and equipment. We will deal primarily with limb segment motions and muscle activity and only in a full swing.

The shoulders do not elevate in golf as they do in other overhead sports. For this reason, the deltoids do not play as important a role in golf as they do in throwing, tennis, and swimming. The major muscles in golf, according to the investigation by Jobe et al. (Jobe et al., 1985), include the rotator cuff (especially the subscapularis), latissimus dorsi, and pectoralis major.

Phases involved in the golf swing include the set-up or address of the ball, take-away or wind-up, forward swing, and follow-through (Hume, Keogh, & Reid, 2005). Each one will be briefly presented.

Set-Up

The purpose of the set-up is to set a proper grip on the club and align the golfer with the target in a good biomechanical alignment (Hume et al., 2005). Approximately 50% to 60% of the golfer's weight is on the back foot and the knees are flexed slightly, about 30°. Since the dominant hand is lower on the club grip, the shoulders will be laterally tilted to the dominant side.

Take-Away

This phase begins when the golfer begins to move the club back and away from the ball, and it ends at the top of the backswing (Hume et al., 2005). An important purpose of the take-away is to wind the body up to put muscles and joint structures on stretch so kinetic energy is available to produce power for the forward swing (Hume et al., 2005). As the club is pulled backward and upward, the shoulders rotate and the pelvis follows the rotation of the shoulders.

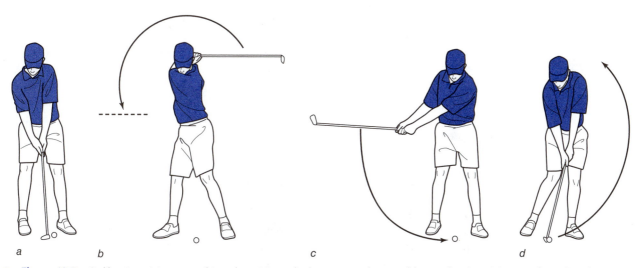

a   b   c   d

▶ **Figure 19.5** Golf swing: *(a)* set-up, *(b)* end position of take-away and start of forward swing, *(c)* start of acceleration, *(d)* start of follow-through.

Overhead motions, such as those that athletes perform in baseball, tennis, swimming, and golf, place stresses on the shoulder.

As the hands reach the hip level, the target shoulder is adducted and medially rotated while the back shoulder is abducted and laterally rotated with a flexed elbow (Hume et al., 2005). During take-away, the front shoulder has low-level activity except in the subscapularis. The primary activity of the back shoulder is in the supraspinatus (Jobe et al., 1985). At the top of the backswing, the back arm is abducted around 90° and laterally rotated about 90° (Hume et al., 2005). The target shoulder is medially rotated and horizontally adducted along with its scapula which is also abducted but laterally rotated (Hume et al., 2005). This end take-away position places the rotator cuff in an impingement position (Hume et al., 2005).

Forward Swing

This phase begins at the end of backswing and continues until the club hits the ball (Hume et al., 2005). Jobe et al. (Jobe et al., 1985) preferred to define the forward swing from the end of the backswing to when the club is parallel to the ground; they defined the next phase, acceleration, as the point between when the club is parallel to the ground and ball contact. The purpose of the forward swing is to provide a biomechanically accurate and solid impact between the ball and the club head, utilizing the cumulative forces to move the ball as fast as possible. The target arm has moderate activity of the subscapularis and latissimus dorsi, whereas the back arm has more activity of the other rotator cuff muscles—the infraspinatus and subscapularis—and less of the supraspinatus (Jobe et al., 1985). The pectoralis major and latissimus dorsi of the back arm also increase their activity.

Acceleration

Acceleration occurs from the time the club becomes horizontal to the time of ball contact (Jobe et al., 1985). The target and back arm muscles that are highly active at this time are the same; these include the pectoralis major, latissimus dorsi, and subscapularis (Jobe et al., 1985).

Force during the forward swing that is applied when the club head makes contact with the ball is the result of the summation of forces from the legs, hips, pelvis, and upper extremities. As the body unwinds, starting at the upper extremities and progressing distally, the optimal forces are delivered when the unwinding occurs in this sequential order from proximal to distal body segments (Hume et al., 2005).

Follow-Through

Follow-through begins with ball contact and continues to the end of the stroke (Hume et al., 2005). The purpose of the follow-through is to decelerate the body. This deceleration process occurs through eccentric muscle activity. The target shoulder's subscapularis continues at high activity levels, but the activity of the pectoralis major and latissimus dorsi subsides. The infraspinatus produces increased activity during this phase (Jobe et al., 1985). In the back arm, the subscapularis, pectoralis major, and latissimus dorsi continue high activity output (Jobe et al., 1985). As the target arm abducts and laterally rotates, the back arm adducts and medially rotates. Once the elbows are at shoulder level, both elbows flex to decelerate shoulder and trunk motion (Hume et al., 2005). The target lower extremity medially rotates and supinates so the body faces the target with the spine in hyperextension and some lateral flexion towards the target arm (Hume et al., 2005).

GENERAL REHABILITATION CONSIDERATIONS

The shoulder is a unique area that is composed of several joints: the sternoclavicular, acromioclavicular, scapulothoracic, and glenohumeral joints. Not only must these joints possess appropriate mobility and provide stability, but also the muscles that surround and control these joints must all work synchronously to provide normal shoulder function and timing of movement.

Stability

Fundamental to normal joint function is stability. When an injury occurs, normal joint stability is compromised, and full recovery is threatened unless the stability is restored (Myers, Wassinger, & Lephart, 2006). Joint stability is provided by static and dynamic factors. Static stability is provided by the inert structures. In the shoulder, these inert structures include the joint capsule, ligaments, and glenoid labrum. Dynamic stability is the responsibility of the nerves and muscles, providing appropriate input from the afferent receptors to the central nervous system to impart timely support through balanced muscle activity as discussed in chapter 8. When the joint's ligaments are injured, the afferent receptors located in those ligaments are unable to provide adequate sensory input (Myers et al., 2006). This creates insufficient neural input and, in turn, inappropriate muscle responses. The result is a deficiency in static stability because of the injury itself, and a secondary dynamic instability caused by the damage to the afferent receptors (Myers et al., 2006). These conditions set up a continuous injury cycle in which continued dynamic and static instability causes functional instability. The cycle continues and leads to progressive injury (figure 19.6).

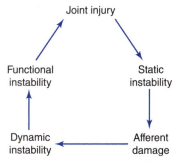

▶ **Figure 19.6** Joint instability cycle.

Dynamic instability results if muscles surrounding the shoulder are imbalanced. If the agonist and antagonist groups are not balanced, there is loss of proprioceptive and kinesthetic control, leading to dynamic instability (Borsa, Lephart, Kocker, & Lephart, 1994). Muscle imbalance, if not corrected, can be the primary cause of shoulder injury.

The rehabilitation clinician is able to break this cycle by designing a rehabilitation program to restore dynamic stability. Rehabilitation programs include reeducation of the neuromuscular system and exercises to reestablish balance between agonists and antagonists. Sometimes, this is enough to restore the patient to full sport participation. When the static instability is too great, surgical intervention is necessary. Rehabilitation of dynamic stabilizers is just as important after surgical correction of static instability as it is in cases without surgical intercession.

Scapular Muscles

Fundamental to all shoulder rehabilitation is rehabilitation of the scapular stabilizers. These muscles control scapular motion. Their strength and control are crucial to the shoulder because the scapula serves as a platform from which the shoulder moves (Burkhart, Morgan, & Kibler, 2003a). Weak scapular muscles will produce insufficient scapular stabilization for shoulder movement. The difference between a stable and an unstable scapula for the shoulder is similar to the difference between running on firm ground and running on a suspended wood-and-rope footbridge. The ground provides the runner with a stable base from which to move the body forward smoothly and efficiently. Running on an unstable footbridge places high energy demands on the individual's leg muscles, causes incoordination and inefficiency of movement, and increases risk of injury. So, too, a shoulder with an unstable scapula moves inefficiently and is at risk for injury. With an unstable scapula, the glenohumeral joint tends to migrate superiorly. This leads to impingement and biceps or rotator cuff tendinopathy. It is imperative, then, that all therapeutic exercise programs for the shoulder include exercises for the scapular stabilizing muscles.

Fatigue of scapular muscles can also affect shoulder motion and performance. The scapular muscles' role as a stabilizer is disrupted when the muscles are fatigued. This disruption occurs because of changes in normal scapulohumeral rhythm with fatigue of the scapular muscles, as shown by McQuade et al. (McQuade, Dawson, & Smidt, 1998). The results of their study point to the importance of scapular muscle endurance activities in a therapeutic exercise program. It is advisable to use high repetition, low resistance exercises for scapular muscles, especially for patients who will be returning to activities that require high levels of endurance from the lower trapezius and serratus anterior muscles. Activities that require extended outputs from these muscles include repetitive throwing such as for baseball and softball pitchers and catchers; swimmers, especially distance swimmers; gymnasts, especially on upper body apparatus; volleyball hitters; oarsmen; tennis players; and racquet sports athletes.

Because scapular muscle strength is so important to the function and stability of the shoulder, exercises for these muscles begin early in the rehabilitation program, even after surgical repair. Strengthening exercises for these muscles may start early since exercising them is possible without stressing the glenohumeral joint with the use of manual resistance to all scapular motions. In many cases, the upper trapezius and levator scapulae muscles are not weak, but the other scapular muscles are and, therefore, need reeducation and rehabilitation. Scapular depression, protraction, retraction, and upward and downward rotation are all motions that can and should be manually resisted early in the rehabilitation process.

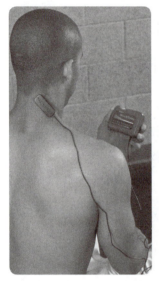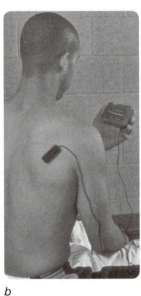

a   *b*

▶ **Figure 19.7** Biofeedback: electrode placement *(a)* for upper trapezius inhibition to decrease activity, and *(b)* for infraspinatus facilitation to increase activity.

If the upper trapezius and levator scapulae are weak, of course, strengthening of these muscles is in order. Often, however, these muscles overpower weak shoulder muscles during scapular rotation so muscle imbalances become more pronounced if they are strengthened along with the deficient scapular muscles. If the rotator cuff is weak, the upper trapezius commonly substitutes for the rotator cuff and works with the deltoid to elevate the shoulder, further encouraging muscle imbalances and incorrect mechanics, and continue to perpetuate the shoulder injury. Two techniques that can control and retrain the upper trapezius are biofeedback and taping. Biofeedback can be used to either facilitate rotator cuff activity or reduce upper trapezius activity during shoulder elevation exercises (figure 19.7). The specific application depends on the electrode placement, machine settings, and motions desired. Refer to Denegar et al. (Denegar, Saliba, & Saliba, 2010) for specific applications.

Scapular taping can be useful in cases of secondary impingement in which faulty positioning of the scapula during overhead movements causes impingement of the rotator cuff tendons. The taping must be accompanied by retraining exercises to reeducate the scapular muscles so that they position the scapula correctly during shoulder motions. The taping technique was introduced by Jenny, an Australian manipulative physiotherapist. Limited research by McConnell has demonstrated that tape application inhibits upper trapezius and facilitates lower trapezius activation (Selkowitz, Chaney, Stuckey, & Vlad, 2007). This can improve scapular stability by facilitating muscle balance during motion to permit arm movement without impingement pain; it can also enhance muscle reeducation for normal scapular alignment and positioning (Host, 1995). One of two methods of taping may be selected to encourage lower trapezius facilitation and inhibit upper trapezius activity. Both methods use the same two types of tape. The tape applied adjacent to the skin is a protective stretch tape called Cover-Roll stretch, and the "treatment" tape is a support tape, Leukotape P (both distributed by Beiersdorf, Inc., Norwalk, CT). In both methods of application, the patient is positioned in a proper thoracic and cervical posture and two to three strips of the protective stretch tape are laid down on the skin over the shoulder from anterior to the upper trapezius insertion on the clavicle and over the posterior aspect of the upper trapezius, ending at the lower thoracic spinous processes at the distal insertions of the lower trapezius. In the first tape option, the treatment tape is applied in two to three strips from the mid-anterior clavicle in a direction downward and medially toward the lower thoracic spinous processes (figure 19.8). As the tape is

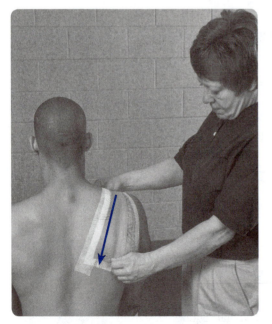

▶ **Figure 19.8** Scapular taping support to improve lower trapezius facilitation.

brought downward, the rehabilitation clinician supports and lifts the patient's shoulder from under the axilla so that the upper trapezius stays relaxed during the tape application (Selkowitz et al., 2007). The tape is snug but still permits scapular motion during shoulder elevation.

In the second tape option, not only is the patient aligned in proper cervical and thoracic posture, but the patient is also instructed to retract and depress the scapula while the tape is applied (Lewis, Wright, & Green, 2005). The tape application uses only the protective tape on the skin as the treatment tape. Mirroring strips are placed on the right and left sides of the back, two on each side of the back. The first treatment strip is similar to the treatment strip placement in the first option, but the upper trapezius is not passively relaxed by the clinician. The second strip runs between the thoracic spinous processes and the vertebral border of the scapula starting superiorly at the superior angle of the scapula and ending lateral to the T12 spinous process. Tape is applied on the contralateral side of the back (figure 19.9). Tension is taken out of the treatment tape as it is applied, so it is not uncomfortable for the patient.

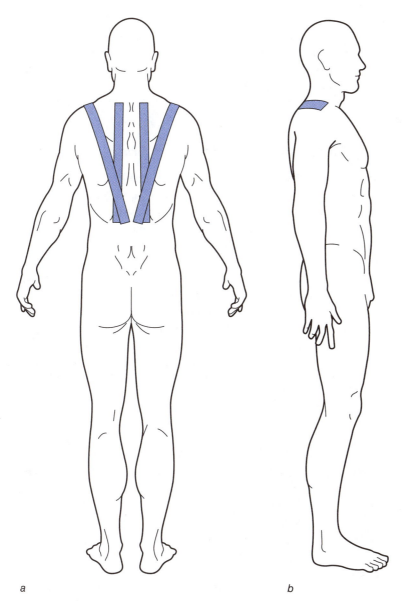

a   *b*

▶ **Figure 19.9** Alternate taping for shoulder to reduce upper trapezius activity and facilitate lower trapezius activity.

Force Couples

Force couples are two equal forces acting in opposite but parallel directions to produce rotatory motion. The shoulder has several force couples that function during arm movement. It is important that the muscles within each of these force couples are balanced to provide optimal function. The shoulder complex has four force couples, two for the glenohumeral joint and two for the scapulothoracic joint. In the glenohumeral joint, the infraspinatus and teres minor form a force couple with the subscapularis to produce downward translation of the humerus in the glenoid. This movement prevents compression of the humeral head against the coracoacromial arch and allows for greater motion during overhead activities. The second glenohumeral force couple is between the entire rotator cuff and the deltoid. The anterior and posterior rotator cuff muscles (subscapularis, infraspinatus, and teres minor) depress the humeral head. The supraspinatus assists in this depression and compression force of the humeral head into the glenoid as the glenoid elevates the humerus (Goldstein, 2004). The scapular force couples include the upper and lower trapezius and serratus anterior. These muscles work together to upwardly rotate the scapula. The other scapular force couple includes pectoralis minor, levator scapulae, and rhomboids; these muscles work together to downwardly rotate the scapula against resistance. The muscles within each force couple must work cooperatively in timing and level of intensity to produce the desired activity or injury results. For example, if the deltoid overpowers the rotator cuff, the glenohumeral joint is elevated without humeral depression, and impingement of superior glenohumeral soft tissues occurs. If the upper trapezius is stronger than the lower trapezius and serratus anterior, the scapula is not positioned correctly during arm elevation, and impingement of the rotator cuff occurs.

Relationship Between Trunk/Hip and Shoulder

Just as scapulothoracic stability, strength, and endurance are important for glenohumeral function, trunk and lower-extremity stability and strength are important for scapular function. The trunk must have the strength to maintain a stable base for the functioning of the scapula. The legs and trunk provide 51% to 55% of the total kinetic energy and total force for overhead activities (Kibler, 1995). The shoulder contributes 13% to the total energy production and 21% of the total force (Kibler, 1995). For this reason, exercises for hip rotators, extensors, and abductors, as well as transverse abdominis, obliques, and multifidus, should all be included in a shoulder rehabilitation program.

The forces generated from the legs, hips, trunk, shoulder, and arm are delivered through summation via the body's kinetic chain and are ultimately delivered to the hand and transferred to the object within the hand (Braatz & Gogia, 1987). These forces must be timed, directed, and applied in a specific sequence if the body is to work efficiently and effectively (Cools, Witvrouw, Declercq, Danneels, & Cambier, 2003). This requires a balance of muscle strength throughout all the delivery systems involved.

Posture

Any patient with a shoulder injury should have a posture examination. Correct posture is crucial to shoulder balance and function. If a patient has a forward-head posture with a thoracic kyphosis, the shoulders are drawn forward and medially rotated (figure 19.10). This causes a protraction, elevation, and posterior tilt of the scapula and medial rotation of the humerus (Lukasiewicz, McClure, Michener, Praff, & Senneff, 1999). With prolonged kyphotic posture, secondary weakness of the scapular retractors and shoulder lateral rotators and tightness of the scapular protractors and shoulder medial rotators occurs. These deficiencies prevent full elevation of the shoulder and lead to subacromial impingement to cause rotator cuff tendinopathy. In short, muscle imbalance with shortening of the anterior muscles and lengthening and weakness of the posterior muscles develops. Posture must be corrected if the rehabilitation program is to be successful.

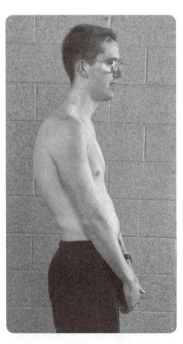

▶ **Figure 19.10** Forward-head, kyphotic posture.

Cervical Influence

There is an intimate relationship between the cervical spine and shoulder beyond the posture factor. Patients who complain of shoulder pain without a frank shoulder injury should be examined for cervical involvement. Cervical disc pathology can refer pain along the medial border of the scapula, into the shoulder joint, or down the arm. If shoulder symptoms increase with movement, palpation, or joint mobilization of the spine, the cervical spine is likely the source of shoulder pain. It is sometimes difficult to determine whether the cervical spine or the shoulder is the primary source of pain. A quick quadrant test can rule out the possibility of cervical involvement. If the test is negative, the neck may not be the source of pain; however, if the patient does not respond to shoulder treatment, reassessment of the cervical spine is in order. Reproducing the patient's pain is a key component of the rehabilitation assessment for determining the origin of the patient's complaints.

Thoracic Influence

Shoulders lacking full range of motion may have joint mobility restriction in the ribs and or thoracic spine. If a patient lacks full elevation of the glenohumeral joint and the shoulder complex presents with normal mobility, the thoracic spine and costothoracic joints should be examined for hypomobility. Restricted costothoracic and thoracic spine mobility can restrict the shoulder's movement by limiting the expansion of the trunk that is necessary for full shoulder motion. This is particularly true if the patient has habitually poor thoracic and or cervical posture. Application of posterior-anterior mobilization of the thoracic spine or rib mobilization techniques, or both, should restore normal shoulder mobility when thoracic hypomobility is a factor in a patient's difficulty achieving the last few degrees of glenohumeral motion. If poor posture is contributing to the thoracic motion reduction, it must be corrected with stretching of the tight soft tissue structures and strengthening of the weak structures.

Scapular Plane

It is important to exercise the rotator cuff in the scapular plane. This is a position about 30° forward of the coronal plane. In this position, the arm is in line with the scapula as it lies on the ribs. It is a functional position for the rotator cuff and shoulder. Often, exercises for the rotator cuff performed in the coronal plane are too uncomfortable for the rotator cuff and encourage impingement of its tendons. Placing the arm in a scapular plane reduces this possibility and is generally more comfortable for the patient.

When medial and lateral rotation exercises are performed, a towel roll should be placed between the arm and the ribs (figure 19.11). This positions the shoulder in a scapular plane. This position also reduces the tension on the supraspinatus tendon, lessening irritation to the tendon (Kelly, Kadrmas, & Speer, 1996). In addition, this position may improve the subscapularis alignment to more effectively depress the humeral head.

Exercise Plane and Height Progression

Strength exercises may begin as isometrics and progress to concentric and eccentric exercises. When agonists are weak and are imbalanced with their antagonists, the exercises should be initially performed in straight-plane motions. As strength and control of motion improve, the exercises progress to diagonal, multiplane, functional motions. Patients should not perform diagonal motions until they have adequate muscular strength of weakened muscles in straight planes. Without proper muscle balance, it is too easy for stronger muscles to overpower weaker muscles and perform the movement in lieu of activity with a properly executed and balanced motion, and thereby further encouraging a continuation of the imbalances the clinician is attempting to correct.

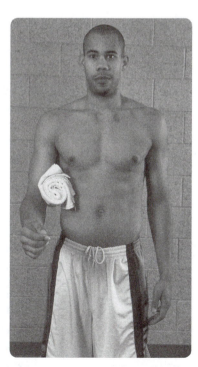

▶ **Figure 19.11** Using a rolled towel under the arm helps to position the shoulder in the scapular plane during medial and lateral rotation exercises.

Exercises should be kept to less than 60° elevation in the initial strengthening stages; since little scapular motion occurs in the first 60° of glenohumeral motion, scapular muscles exercised below 60° work primarily as stabilizers, not scapular movers (Sagano, Magee, & Katayose, 2006). Elevation higher than 90° is an unstable position for the glenohumeral joint, and scapular muscle strength in the early stages is not adequate to keep the shoulder stabilized. The scapular muscles are also not strong enough in their shortened range to provide the scapular stabilization necessary for glenohumeral motion above 60° elevation. Once scapulothoracic and glenohumeral muscles have adequate strength to control shoulder motion and provide the stabilization necessary for activity at 80° to 110°, progression of exercises to the fully elevated ranges is the next step. It is at ranges of terminal elevation where the scapular rotators are not only at their shortest length but also are at their highest output demands (Ryu et al., 1988), so strengthening of these muscles is reserved until lower elevation strengths are achieved.

REHABILITATION TECHNIQUES

As in chapter 18, manual therapy techniques including soft tissue mobilizations and joint mobilizations are presented in this section, followed by the various exercises that may be included in rehabilitation of the shoulder complex. The manual therapy techniques are placed ahead of the exercises since those usually precede exercises in a treatment session. The exercises also follow a typical sequence, starting with flexibility and ending with activity-specific exercises.

Soft-Tissue Mobilization

Because of the intimate relationship between the cervical spine and the shoulder, some of the muscles discussed in the preceding chapter are also relevant here. Refer to chapter 6 for details on soft-tissue mobilization theory, physiology, and application. Trigger point release and spray-and-stretch techniques are the primary treatment approaches discussed here. These techniques and the pain referral patterns described here are based on the work of Travell and Simons (Travell & Simons, 1983).

Rotator Cuff Muscles

Each rotator cuff muscle has distinct pain-referral patterns. The rehabilitation clinician should be aware of these differences to make an accurate differential diagnosis and correctly treat the patient's injury. The following sections describe the trigger points and their treatments for the supraspinatus, infraspinatus, teres minor, and subscapularis muscles.

■ Trigger Point Releases for the Rotator Cuff

Supraspinatus

Referral Pattern: Can refer pain into the arm. The referred pain pattern is a deep ache that occurs around the lateral shoulder in the middle deltoid area down to the deltoid insertion (figure 19.12, a & b).

Location of Trigger Point: There are two sites that are most common for this muscle. One is at the juncture of the middle third and lateral third of the muscle and the other is at the junction of the middle third and medial third of the muscle. Of these, the more tender site is the trigger point site just above the clavicular spine, 2 to 3 cm (0.8-1.2 in.) lateral to the vertebral border.

Patient Position for Palpation: Seated or side-lying.

Muscle Position for Palpation: Relaxed with the arm at the side.

Ischemic Treatment: Sustained pressure is applied over the trigger point site just above the scapular spine, 2 to 3 cm (0.8-1.2 in.) lateral to the vertebral border (figure 19.12c).

Spray-and-Stretch Treatment: Ice strokes are swept from the proximal supraspinatus insertion, across the muscle and acromion, over the deltoid, and down the arm to the elbow (figure 19.12d).

Notations: The clinician applies the stretch by raising the patient's hand behind the back upward toward the opposite scapula.

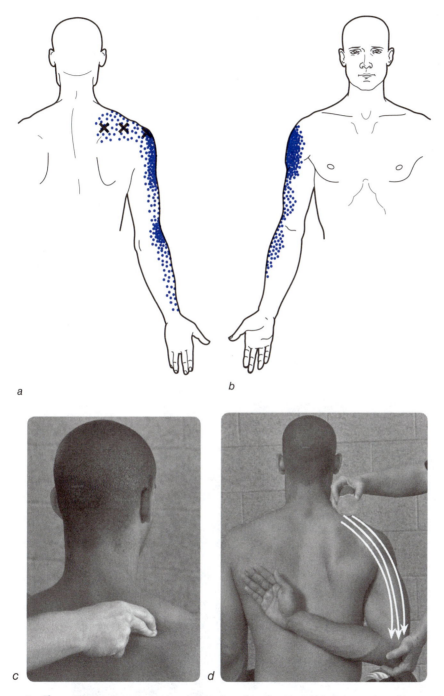

▶ **Figure 19.12** Supraspinatus: *(a-b)* pain-referral pattern, *(c)* trigger point release, *(d)* ice-and-stretch.

Subscapularis

Referral Pattern: The subscapularis refers pain to the posterior wrist and in the inferior aspect of the posterior shoulder region where the arm meets the trunk. It can also occasionally refer pain into the scapula, down the posterior arm to the elbow, and circumferentially around the wrist (figure 19.13, a & b).

Location of Trigger Point: Lateral anterior region of the scapula.

Patient Position for Palpation: Supine.

Muscle Position for Palpation: The arm is abducted comfortably away from the body to about 60° to 90°. The clinician supports the patient's arm while applying traction to keep the scapula away from the ribs.

Ischemic Treatment: The finger pads of the clinician's treatment hand are moved past the teres major and latissimus dorsi to palpate the anterior surface of the scapula. A sustained pressure in a cephalic direction toward the spine is applied once the trigger point has been located (figure 19.13c).

Spray-and-Stretch Treatment: Spray-and-stretch is applied with the patient supine and the arm in partial abduction and lateral rotation. Sweeps start at the side and move over the axilla and along the posterior arm. As the sweeps are repeated, the arm is moved into more abduction and lateral rotation until it is positioned overhead in full abduction and lateral rotation (figure 19.13, d & e).

Notations: This is a very tender trigger point on most people, but it is especially tender on pathological shoulders.

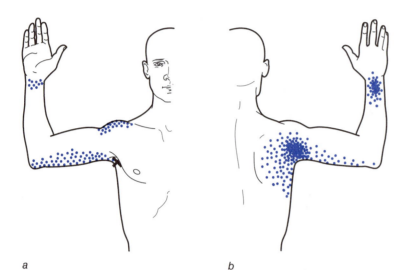

a   b

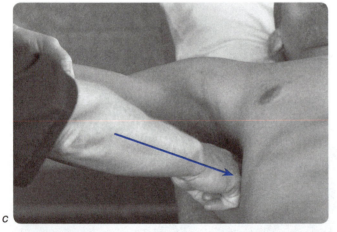

c

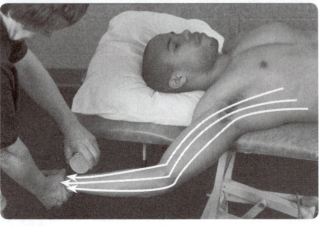

d

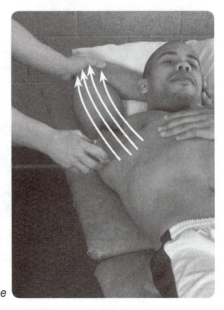

e

▶ **Figure 19.13** Subscapularis: *(a-b)* pain-referral pattern, *(c)* trigger point release, *(d)* ice-and-stretch in moderate stretch position, *(e)* ice-and-stretch in full stretch position.

Teres Minor

Referral Pattern: Refers pain to the upper posterior arm, just proximal to the posterior deltoid attachment, where the area of referred pain less than 5 cm (2.0 in.) in diameter (figure 19.14a). The pain is frequently described as deep and sharp. The spillover area of pain referral remains in the proximal aspect of the posterior upper arm and the lateral arm from the acromion downward.

Location of Trigger Point: In the teres minor muscle belly along the lateral scapular border between the teres major inferiorly and the infraspinatus superiorly.

Patient Position for Palpation: Side-lying on opposite side.

Muscle Position for Palpation: Arm is in a comfortable position at the side.

Ischemic Treatment: A finger or thumb pad locates the trigger point and applies direct pressure over the point (figure 19.14b).

Spray-and-Stretch Treatment: The ice sweeps begin low on the side and move along the lateral border of the scapula over the teres minor and along the posterior arm. As the ice is applied, the arm is moved overhead and medially rotated (figure 19.14c).

Notations: Be sure to move the muscle through its full motion as it responds to the spray-and-stretch.

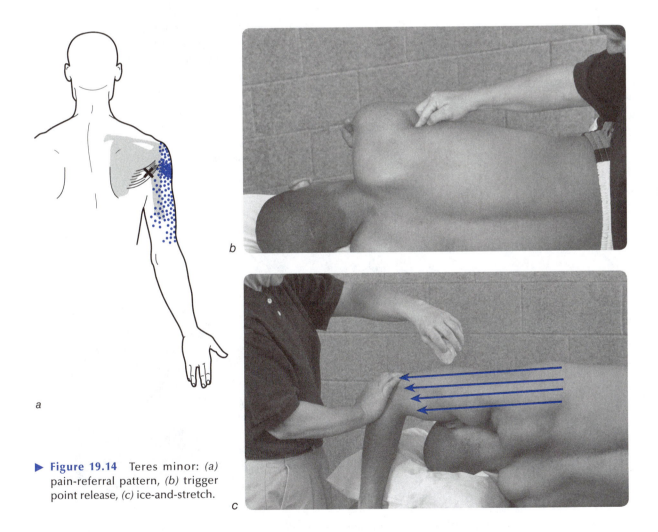

a

b

c

▶ **Figure 19.14** Teres minor: *(a)* pain-referral pattern, *(b)* trigger point release, *(c)* ice-and-stretch.

Infraspinatus

Referral Pattern: Most often refers to the anterior shoulder, to the anterior arm, to the wrist, and to the radial fingers (figure 19.15, a & b). On occasion, vertebral border scapular pain or pain at the base of the skull can also occur. Pain can be felt deep in the anterior shoulder as well.

Location of Trigger Point: The superior aspect of the muscle inferior to the scapular spine and along the vertebral border.

Patient Position for Palpation: Side-lying on opposite side.

Muscle Position for Palpation: Arm is relaxed at the patient's side.

Ischemic Treatment: Sustained pressure by the finger pads is applied over the central knot located along the tender bands within the muscle (figure 19.15c).

Spray-and-Stretch Treatment: Sweeps are applied from the vertebral border upward to the shoulder and then either up to the head or down the arm (figure 19.15d).

Notations: Progressively stretch the muscle by moving the arm either behind the back with the shoulder in medial rotation or horizontally in front and across the body with medial rotation.

Scapular Muscles

Although the scapular muscles refer pain primarily to the upper back, they can also refer pain to the chest and upper extremity. As with the rotator cuff muscles, the scapular muscles have pain-referral patterns that are unique for each muscle. The following sections describe the trigger points and their treatments for the serratus anterior, rhomboids, and pectoralis minor. Trigger points and treatment of the upper trapezius and levator scapulae muscles are described in chapter 18. Refer to figures 18.4 and 18.5 for details.

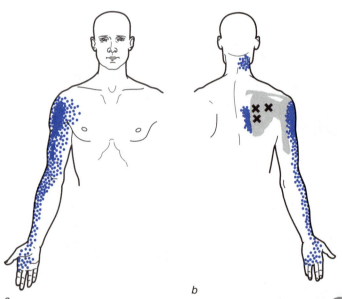

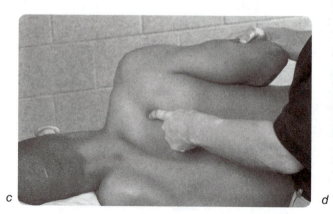

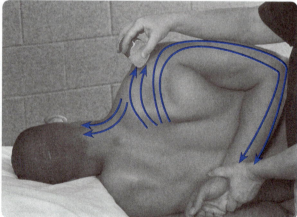

▶ **Figure 19.15** Infraspinatus: pain-referral patterns, *(a)* anterior and *(b)* posterior; *(c)* trigger point release; *(d)* ice-and-stretch.

■ Trigger Point Releases for the Scapular Muscles

Serratus Anterior

Referral Pattern: Laterally to the midchest area or to the inferior angle of the scapula (figure 19.16, a & b). Spillover referral pain can also be experienced as abnormal breast sensitivity, pain down the anteromedial forearm to the palm and ulnar digits, or pectoralis major pain.

Location of Trigger Point: Level of the fifth or sixth rib just anterior to the midaxillary line at the nipple level (figure 19.16c).

Patient Position for Palpation: Supine for ischemic compression and side-lying on opposite side for spray-and-stretch.

Muscle Position for Palpation: Shoulder and scapula are relaxed with the arm resting in some extension and abduction away from the side.

Ischemic Treatment: Sustained pressure is applied over the trigger point (19.16c).

Spray-and-Stretch Treatment: With the patient side-lying, sweeps are applied from the trigger point outward anteriorly and posteriorly over the muscle while a progressive stretch is applied with backward and downward pressure on the arm (figure 19.16d).

Notations: An additional stretch can be applied to the muscle if the patient takes a deep breath and holds it during the stretch.

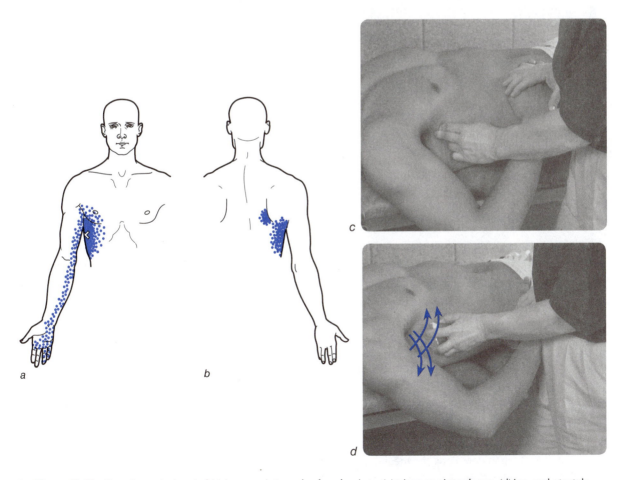

▶ **Figure 19.16** Serratus anterior: *(a-b)* trigger points and referral points, *(c)* trigger point release, *(d)* ice-and-stretch.

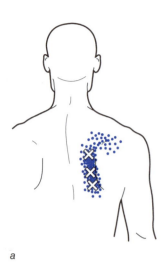

a

Rhomboids

Referral Pattern: Similar to those of the levator scapulae except that there is no neck component. The pain-referral pattern is along the vertebral border of the scapula, with some pain possible into the medial supraspinatus area (figure 19.17a).

Location of Trigger Point: Tender bands are located along the vertebral border of the scapula. Locate the nodule within each tender band identified.

Patient Position for Palpation: Prone or sitting.

Muscle Position for Palpation: Arm is in a comfortable position at the side.

Ischemic Treatment: Identify the nodule and apply sustained pressure until it relaxes. Repeat until all nodules are resolved (figure 19.17b).

Spray-and-Stretch Treatment: The patient is in a relaxed sitting position with the thoracic spine flexed and the arms hanging forward or across the chest to protract the scapula. Ice sweeps are made in parallel strokes across the back in the direction of the muscle's fibers from the vertebral border and upward to the shoulder (figure 19.17c).

Notations: Spray-and-stretch is applied with the muscle on stretch at the start of the treatment.

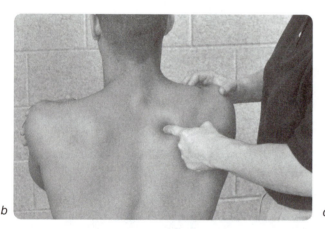

b

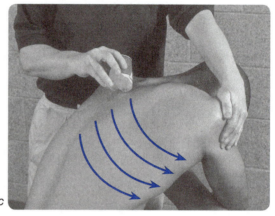

c

▶ **Figure 19.17** Rhomboids: *(a)* pain-referral patterns, *(b)* trigger point release, *(c)* ice-and-stretch.

Pectoralis Minor

Referral Pattern: Pain over the anterior deltoid with some spillover into the subclavicular area; entire pectoral area; and ulnar aspect of the arm, forearm, palmar hand, and fingers (figure 19.18a).

Location of Trigger Point: Directly below the concavity of the clavicle at the third and fourth ribs.

Patient Position for Palpation: Supine.

Muscle Position for Palpation: Forearm is supported by the clinician overhead or on the patient's abdomen.

Ischemic Treatment: Palpate the taut band in the muscle in the region of the third and fourth ribs directly down from the concave portion of the clavicle. Apply direct pressure until a release is palpated (figure 19.18b).

Spray-and-Stretch Treatment: Spray-and-stretch is performed with the patient seated or supine with shoulder over table edge. The arm is abducted, and the shoulder is pulled posteriorly in horizontal extension and lateral rotation to elevate and retract the scapula to put the pectoralis minor on stretch. Ice sweeps are made from the anterior chest region upward to the anterior shoulder, along the medial upper arm and forearm to the ulnar fingers (figure 19.18c).

Notations: If the patient has a well-developed pectoralis muscle, palpation of the trigger point is easier with the arm relaxed overhead.

Large Glenohumeral Muscles

Some of the large glenohumeral muscle pain-referral patterns can closely resemble those of other shoulder muscles, including the rotator cuff and scapular rotators. Careful observation and testing are necessary in order to focus in on the proper muscle to treat. The following sections describe the trigger points and their treatments for the latissimus dorsi, teres major, pectoralis major, and deltoid.

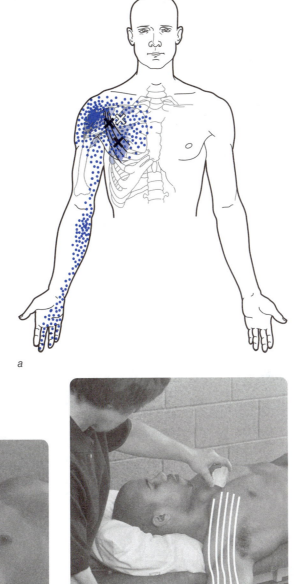

a

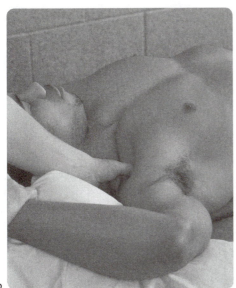

b

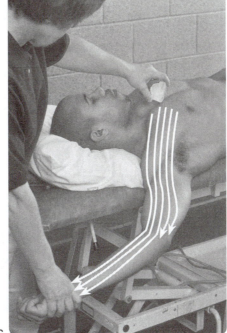

c

▶ **Figure 19.18** Pectoralis minor: *(a)* pain-referral patterns and trigger points, *(b)* trigger point release, *(c)* ice-and-stretch.

■ Trigger Point Releases for Large Glenohumeral Muscles

Latissimus Dorsi

Referral Pattern: A constant aching in the inferior angle of the scapula and midthoracic area is typical of a pain referral with this muscle. Spillover pain referral can also occur in the posterior shoulder, down the posterior or medial arm and forearm, and to the ulnar hand and fingers (figure 19.19a-c).

Location of Trigger Point for Palpation: Muscle a couple of centimeters below the top of the arch of the posterior axillary fold at the midscapular level (figure 19.19d).

Patient Position for Palpation: Supine.

Muscle Position for Palpation: Arm is abducted to about 60° to 90°.

Ischemic Treatment: A pincer grasp is used to locate and treat the trigger point within the myofascial bands.

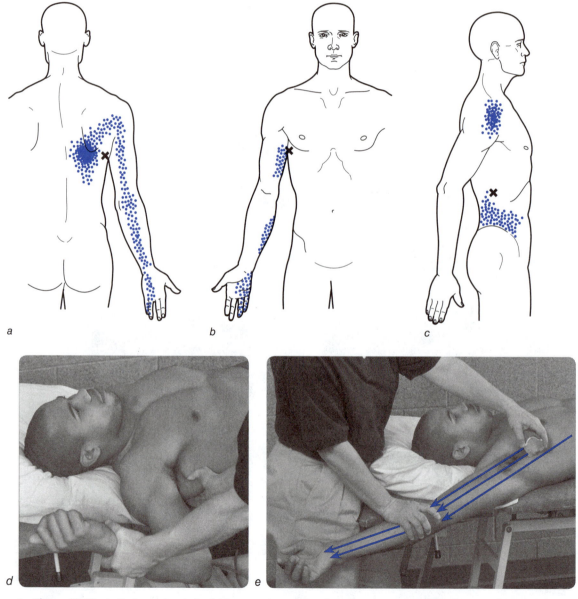

▶ **Figure 19.19** Latissimus dorsi: *(a-c)* trigger points and pain-referral patterns, *(d)* trigger point release, *(e)* ice-and-stretch.

Spray-and-Stretch Treatment: Ice sweeps are performed in parallel strokes, from the distal insertion of the muscle upward over the axilla and along the arm and ulnar aspect of the forearm to the hand (figure 19.19e).

Notations: The muscle is stretched upward so the arm is eventually placed behind the ear by the end of the motion.

Teres Major

Referral Pattern: Pain over the posterior deltoid, over the triceps long head, and occasionally into the posterior forearm (figure 19.20, a & b).

Location of Trigger Point: At the inferior angle of the scapula if the patient is side-lying. If sitting, the trigger point is located with an index-finger-and-thumb grasp anteriorly in the groove between the lateral lower edge of the scapula and the axillary fold (in this position, the hand's web space surrounds the latissimus dorsi).

Patient Position for Palpation: Side-lying or sitting.

Muscle Position for Palpation: The arm is supported at the side in side-lying and in some abduction in sitting.

Ischemic Treatment: In side-lying, a finger or thumb pad applies pressure over the trigger point (figure 19.20c). In sitting, a finger-and-thumb grasp from an anterior position maintains pressure on the trigger point until a release is palpated or the patient reports no pain.

Spray-and-Stretch Treatment: Spray-and-stretch is performed with the patient supine or side-lying and with the arm overhead in shoulder abduction and lateral rotation and elbow flexion. Ice strokes are swept from the lateral inferior border of the scapula along the triceps as the arm is moved into medial rotation (figure 19.20d).

Notations: If the latissimus dorsi is large, it may be difficult for a clinician with small hands to grasp the teres major trigger point with a pincer grasp.

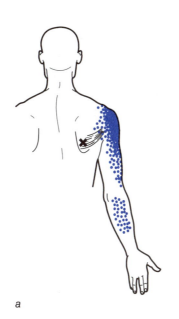

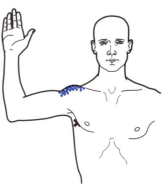

b

a

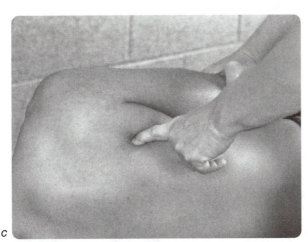

c

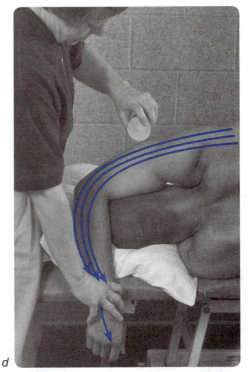

d

▶ **Figure 19.20** Teres major: *(a-b)* pain-referral patterns and trigger points, *(c)* trigger point release, *(d)* ice-and-stretch.

Pectoralis Major

Referral Pattern: This muscle refers pain to the anterior chest, anterior deltoid, medial epicondyle, sternum, and breast. Overspill referral pain can also occur in the medial arm and ulnar digits (figure 19.21, a-c).

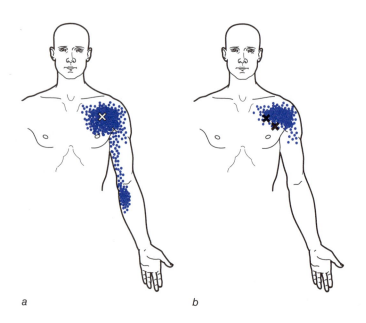

a   *b*

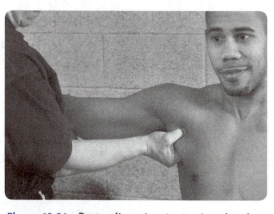

c

Location of Trigger Point: Between the fifth and sixth ribs (figure 19.21d). Locate the site by first finding the tip of the xiphoid process and drawing a horizontal line laterally that intersects with an imaginary vertical line between the lateral sternum and nipple; the point of intersection of these two lines is the site of a common trigger point. Other areas of localized tenderness can be treated in the trigger point regions of the muscle identified by "x" in figure 19.21, a through c.

Patient Position for Palpation: Supine or sitting.

Muscle Position for Palpation: Arm is supported at 90° of abduction.

Ischemic Treatment: Consistent upward pressure with a finger pad is applied to the muscle between the fifth and sixth ribs.

Spray-and-Stretch Treatment: Spray-and-stretch is applied with the patient either supine or sitting. The various heads of the pectoralis major are stretched in different positions. The clavicular portion is stretched with the patient in sitting, with the shoulder in 90° of abduction and horizontally extended (figure 19.21e). The sternocostal portion is stretched in sitting or supine, with the shoulder in abduction and lateral rotation moving into full flexion. Ice strokes are swept from the sternum to the shoulder, along the medial arm, to the ulnar aspect of the hand as the stretch is applied.

Notations: Traction should be applied to the arm throughout the treatment. If the application is performed with the patient supine, care must be taken to keep the scapula unimpeded during the treatment.

Deltoid

Referral Pattern: The anterior and posterior deltoid portions can refer pain over the anterior, posterior, and middle deltoid locations with some spillover into adjacent areas of the arm (figure 19.22, a & b).

Location of Trigger Point: The anterior trigger point is located in about the center of the anterior deltoid just inferior to the lateral end of the clavicle. The posterior trigger point is posterolateral and superior to the deltoid tuberosity of the humerus.

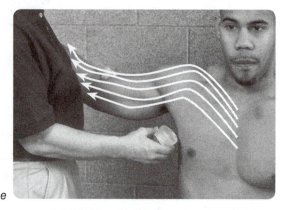

d   *e*

▶ **Figure 19.21** Pectoralis major: *(a-c)* pain-referral patterns and trigger points; *(d)* trigger point release; *(e)* ice-and-stretch, clavicular portion.

Patient Position for Palpation: Sitting.

Muscle Position for Palpation: Arm is comfortably positioned in 30° to 90° of abduction.

Ischemic Treatment: Once the trigger point within the taut band is located, direct pressure with a finger or thumb pad is applied until release of the trigger point occurs (figure 19.22c).

Spray-and-Stretch Treatment: The arm is positioned in horizontal flexion and medial rotation to stretch the posterior deltoid, and in horizontal extension at 90° abduction and lateral rotation to stretch the anterior deltoid (figure 19.22d). As the muscle is being stretched, the ice strokes are swept from the origin of the specific muscle portion, and over the shoulder and arm along the pain-referral pattern. For the posterior deltoid ice strokes, move from posterior to anterior; reverse the direction for the anterior deltoid.

Notations: Since the deltoid trigger point pain pattern can be similar to rotator cuff muscle pain-referral patterns, care should be taken to eliminate those muscles as potential sources of referred pain before treating the deltoid.

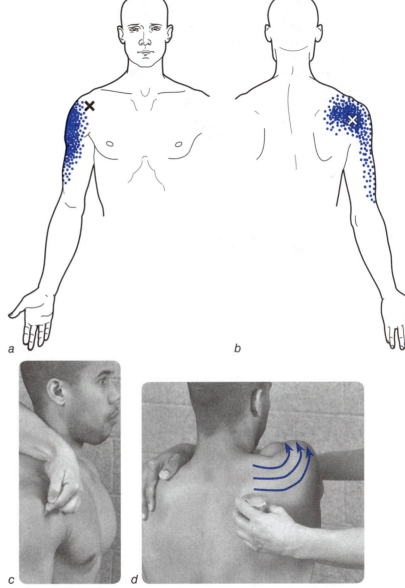

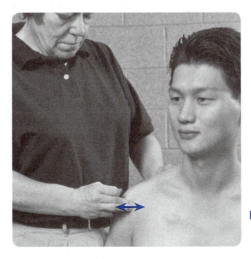

▶ **Figure 19.22** Deltoid: *(a-b)* trigger points and pain-referral patterns for the anterior and posterior deltoid, *(c)* trigger point release, *(d)* ice-and-stretch of posterior deltoid.

Supraspinatus Friction Massage This massage technique is used to treat supraspinatus tendinopathy. The patient is sitting with his or her hand behind the back to expose the supraspinatus tendon. The rehabilitation clinician's index finger is reinforced by the middle finger and placed on top of the tendon about two finger-widths inferior to the acromion. Cross-friction pressure is applied to the tendon for 1 to 2 min or until the tenderness subsides (figure 19.23).

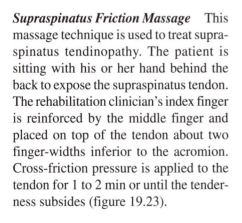

▶ **Figure 19.23** Cross-friction massage to supraspinatus tendon.

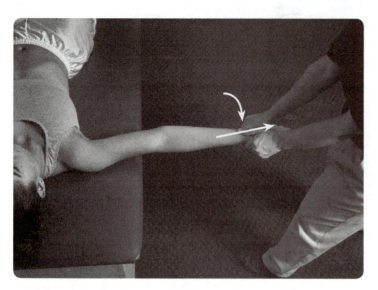

▶ **Figure 19.24** Arm pull in abduction and lateral rotation.

Myofascial Stretch: Arm Pull This technique is a general myofascial stretching technique for stretching or mobilizing soft tissue. With the patient in supine, the clinician grasps the patient's hand to apply a longitudinal traction. While traction is applied, the arm is passively placed in lateral rotation, and a gradual, passive movement of the arm into abduction occurs (figure 19.24). When the clinician feels a barrier to motion, the position is held until a release is felt.

This procedure is repeated with the arm in horizontal adduction. For the horizontal adduction pull, the scapula is protracted, and the patient rolls to the side.

A final arm-pull technique is performed with the patient supine. As traction is applied to the arm, the arm is medially rotated and adducted. For each pull, the clinician moves the arm until the barrier is felt and holds that position until the barrier releases before moving into a greater range of motion.

Joint Mobilization

Joint mobilization can be performed on all joints of the shoulder complex. Findings from the initial examination will determine the specific joints requiring mobilization treatment. Shoulder joint mobility is also influenced by the mobility of the ribs and thoracic spine. As mentioned earlier in this chapter, if a shoulder lacks full range of motion and appears to have good mobility in its joints, examination of rib and thoracic spine mobility may demonstrate restriction of these joints. If this proves to be the case, thoracic and rib mobilization techniques discussed in chapter 18 for these areas may be helpful in restoring full shoulder motion.

Capsular restriction of the glenohumeral joint follows a capsular pattern: more restricted motion in lateral rotation than in abduction, more restricted motion in abduction than in medial rotation. For example, if a patient's shoulder has 70° medial rotation, 90° abduction, and full lateral rotation, the joint capsule is not the primary structure limiting full motion. However, if the joint measures 70° medial rotation, 90° abduction, and 50° lateral rotation, the joint capsule is probably restricting full motion. If a patient's shoulder presents with this loss-of-motion profile, the capsule is restricted, and joint mobilization is needed to restore glenohumeral motion. If a shoulder does not demonstrate this capsular pattern, capsule tightness is not the primary cause for the patient's loss of motion.

Glenohumeral mobilizations are initially applied with the joint in resting position—55° flexion and 20° to 30° horizontal abduction. As additional motion is achieved but full mobility is still lacking, the joint may need to be mobilized out of its resting position and in other loose-pack positions. The extreme close-packed position for the glenohumeral joint is full abduction with full lateral rotation.

While applying joint mobilization, the rehabilitation clinician always uses proper body mechanics. The hand applying the force is positioned as close to the joint as possible. The mobilization force is directed from the legs, not the arms.

The rehabilitation clinician needs to remember the principles of glide, roll, and spin so that the force application is proper for the desired movement. The humerus is a convex surface moving on the glenoid fossa's concave surface, so the convex-concave rule applies. The joint mobilization techniques presented here are the most commonly used techniques. As with any joint mobilization procedure, it is important for the clinician to visualize the joint surfaces and apply the mobilization force parallel or perpendicular to the plane of the surface. As the arm is moved into different positions, the plane of the glenoid changes; you must consider this as you determine the angle of force application.

Precautions and contraindications are respected. The timeline for tissue healing and the status and strength of new tissue must be considered when one is deciding whether to apply joint mobilization and how much force to use. Joint mobilizations applied to hypermobile joints can increase instability and cause further damage, and are contraindicated. Improper technique, incorrect force application, excessive force, and inappropriate timing of application can all result in unnecessary injury or damage to the joint's structures.

Glenohumeral Joint

During some mobilization techniques for the glenohumeral joint, a sustained joint distraction force is applied in addition to the mobilization force. The techniques are usually named according to the direction of the mobilization force. The following sections provide instructions for joint mobilization of the glenohumeral joint.

■ Joint Mobilization of the Glenohumeral Joint

Oscillation

Resting Position: 55° flexion and 20° to 30° horizontal abduction.

Mobilization Technique: Oscillation of the shoulder.

Indications: For general relaxation of the shoulder muscles prior to and after other joint mobilization techniques.

Patient Position: Supine and relaxed with shoulder near edge of table.

Clinician and Hand Positions: Clinician stands on the side of the patient, facing the patient's shoulder, and grasps the patient's distal forearm and wrist with two hands.

Mobilization Application: Mild distraction force perpendicular to the glenohumeral joint plane as oscillations are performed (figure 19.25).

Notations: Distraction force is applied by the clinician's body weight on the back foot while the clinician gently pulls on the shoulder with the hand grasp on the forearm and wrist.

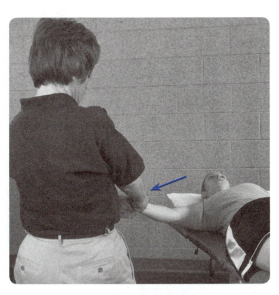

▶ **Figure 19.25** Joint mobilization: distraction with oscillation.

Distraction

Resting Position: 55° flexion and 20° to 30° horizontal abduction.

Mobilization Technique: Longitudinal distraction.

Indications: To improve inferior capsular mobility.

Patient Position: Supine with the involved shoulder as close to the edge of the table as possible.

Clinician and Hand Positions: For a right shoulder, the rehabilitation clinician places his or her right hand in the axilla to stabilize the glenoid. The left hand grasps just above the elbow joint.

Mobilization Application: A distraction force is applied to the humerus (figure 19.26).

Notations: Good initial technique. A prolonged force is more effective, but oscillation combined with distraction can also be used.

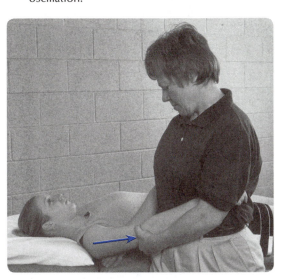

▶ **Figure 19.26** Joint mobilization: longitudinal distraction.

Inferior Capsular Stretch

Resting Position: 55° flexion and 20° to 30° horizontal abduction.

Mobilization Technique: Inferior capsule glide or caudal glide.

Indications: To improve inferior capsular mobility and glenohumeral abduction.

Patient Position: Supine with involved shoulder as close to the end of the table as possible.

Clinician and Hand Positions: The stabilizing hand is on the proximal humerus and the mobilizing hand is on superior aspect of the humerus as close as possible to the acromion. The mobilizing hand web space should be over the superior humeral head.

Mobilization Application: The stabilizing hand maintains the shoulder in a resting position with some distraction as the mobilizing hand applies a glide force in a caudal direction parallel to the joint's surface (figure 19.27a).

Notations: A stabilization belt around the patient's chest may be used to stabilize the scapula. The arm can be abducted to a maximum of 60°, but initial glides should be performed in the resting position. Once approximately 120° of flexion has been attained, an inferior glide can be performed with the arm in an elevated position. As the shoulder's position changes, the glenoid joint surface changes. Likewise, the mobilization force direction changes as the joint plane changes: The force is directed inferiorly (figure 19.27b).

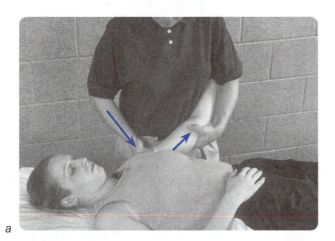
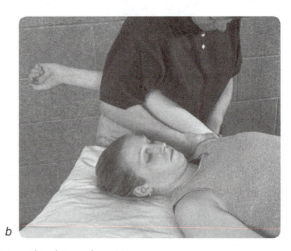

a

b

▶ **Figure 19.27** Joint mobilization—inferior glide: *(a)* initial position, *(b)* advanced position.

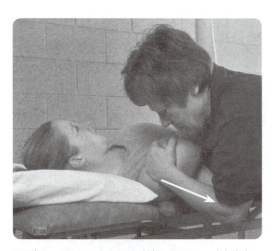

▶ **Figure 19.28** Joint mobilization: caudal glide.

Alternative Inferior Capsular Stretch

Resting Position: Shoulder flexion to 90°. The upper arm rests on the clinician's shoulder.

Mobilization Technique: Inferior capsule glide or caudal glide.

Indications: To improve inferior capsular mobility and glenohumeral abduction.

Patient Position: Supine with involved shoulder as close to the end of the table as possible.

Clinician and Hand Positions: The rehabilitation clinician's hands grasp the humerus as close as possible to the shoulder joint with the patient's upper arm resting on the rehabilitation clinician's shoulder.

Mobilization Application: An inferior force is applied to the proximal humerus (figure 19.28).

Notations: A prolonged mobilization or oscillation technique can be used.

Lateral Glide

Resting Position: 90° flexion with some horizontal abduction.

Mobilization Technique: Lateral glide.

Indications: To increase all motions of the glenohumeral joint.

Patient Position: Patient is supine with involved shoulder as close to the edge of the table as possible.

Clinician and Hand Positions: The clinician faces the patient at shoulder level and grasps the patient's humerus as proximally as possible with the patient's shoulder flexed to 90° and the patient's upper arm resting on the rehabilitation clinician's shoulder.

Mobilization Application: Lateral force is applied to the proximal humerus (figure 19.29).

Notations: The clinician should remember to use proper body mechanics, keeping the back straight and using the legs.

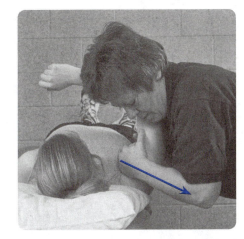

▶ **Figure 19.29** Joint mobilization: lateral glide.

Posterior Glide

Resting Position: 55° flexion and 20° to 30° horizontal abduction.

Mobilization Technique: Posterior glide or dorsal glide.

Indications: To improve shoulder flexion and medial rotation by improving posterior capsular mobility.

Patient Position: Supine with shoulder as close to the edge of the table as possible. A towel roll or wedge is placed under the scapula for stabilization.

Clinician and Hand Positions: The clinician abducts the patient's arm in order to stand between the patient's arm and trunk; the clinician places the stabilizing hand at the elbow and the mobilizing hand just distal to the acromion, as close to the humeral head as possible.

Mobilization Application: The mobilizing hand applies a downward and slightly lateral force, and the stabilizing hand applies slight traction of the patient's glenohumeral joint at the patient's elbow (figure 19.30a).

Notations: An alternative technique is performed with the patient's shoulder in medial rotation to gain additional motion in that direction (figure 19.30b). An advanced flexion technique can be performed with the patient's shoulder flexed to 90° and adducted with the elbow flexed. In this position the rehabilitation clinician stabilizes the arm with a hand on the proximal humerus. A downward mobilization force is applied with the mobilizing hand on the patient's elbow and the clinician's forearm in line with the patient's arm (figure 19.30c).

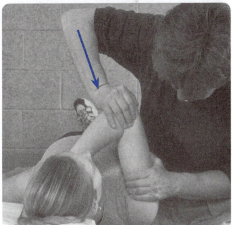

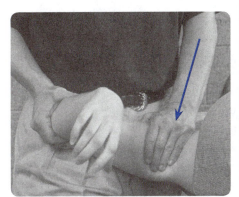

a

b

c

▶ **Figure 19.30** Joint mobilization: *(a)* posterior glide, *(b)* posterior glide with medial rotation, *(c)* advanced posterior glide with flexion.

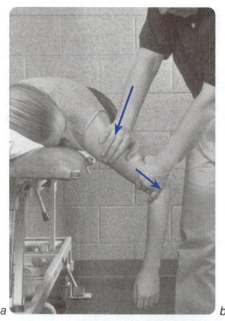
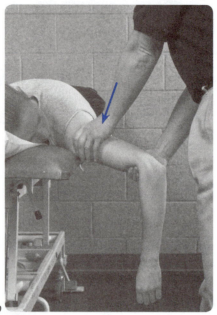
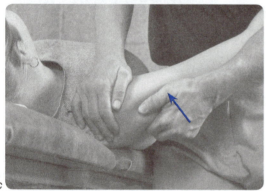

a

b

c

▶ **Figure 19.31** Joint mobilization—anterior glide: *(a)* initial position, *(b)* alternative position, *(c)* supine position.

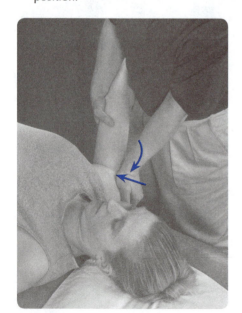

▶ **Figure 19.32** Joint mobilization: lateral rotation.

Anterior Glide

Resting Position: 55° flexion and 20° to 30° horizontal abduction.

Mobilization Technique: Anterior glide or ventral glide.

Indications: To increase anterior capsule mobility so that glenohumeral extension and lateral rotation improve.

Patient Position: Prone with a towel or wedge support under the anterior clavicle and coracoid process to stabilize the shoulder. The glenohumeral joint is off the edge of the table, and the arm is placed in the resting position.

Clinician and Hand Positions: The rehabilitation clinician stands between the patient's arm and side, facing the shoulder, and places the stabilizing hand on the distal humerus and the mobilization hand on the posterior aspect of the humeral head just distal to the acromion.

Mobilization Application: As the stabilizing hand applies a distraction force, the proximal mobilizing hand applies an anterior and slightly medial mobilization force (figure 19.31a).

Notations: As additional motion is achieved but restriction in the anterior-inferior capsule remains, an alternative position for mobilization is with the arm in elevation (figure 19.31b). An alternative technique can be used to increase lateral rotation by positioning the arm in additional lateral rotation during the mobilization. With another technique, one that is less comfortable for the clinician, the patient is supine and a force from the posterior aspect of the shoulder is applied (figure 19.31c).

Lateral Rotation

Resting Position: 55° flexion and 20° to 30° horizontal abduction.

Mobilization Technique: Lateral rotation.

Indications: To improve lateral rotation of the glenohumeral joint.

Patient Position: Supine with the arm in the scapular plane.

Clinician and Hand Positions: Clinician places the distal hand over the distal humerus and the heel of the proximal hand over the humeral head.

Mobilization Application: As the distal hand stabilizes the arm in lateral rotation, the proximal hand applies a simultaneous lateral rotation and inferior glide force (figure 19.32).

Notations: As more motion is gained, the technique can be applied in other open positions closer to the end of motion.

Scapulothoracic Joint

The mobilization techniques described in the following sections are possible only if the patient remains relaxed. If a patient is not relaxed, the rehabilitation clinician will be unable to position his or her hands between the scapula and ribs to apply the techniques.

■ Joint Mobilization of the Scapulothoracic Joint

Scapular Distraction

Resting Position: The scapula is resting against the thoracic cage.

Mobilization Technique: Distraction of the scapula from the thorax.

Indications: To increase movement between the scapula and thoracic ribs.

Patient Position: Side-lying with the involved arm on top.

Clinician and Hand Positions: Clinician's lower hand is placed between the patient's arm and rib cage, and the inferior angle of the scapula is grasped with the clinician's web space and index finger. The upper hand grasps the scapula's upper vertebral border.

Mobilization Application: For personal comfort and professional consideration, a pillow should be placed between the patient and the clinician. As the shoulder is stabilized by the clinician's abdomen against the anterior shoulder, both hands apply a force to tilt the vertebral border of the scapula posteriorly away from the ribs (figure 19.33a).

Notations: An alternative position is with the patient prone. The patient's arm is extended alongside the body, supported on the table. The clinician stands beside the patient, facing the patient's head, cups one hand around the anterior humeral head, and places the other hand under the inferior angle of the scapula as shown in 19.33b. The hands are moved simultaneously toward each other, the hand under the humerus lifting upward and medially and the hand under the scapula moving laterally under the scapula.

Inferior Glide

Resting Position: The scapula is resting against the thoracic cage.

Mobilization Technique: Inferior glide of the scapula.

Indications: To improve downward rotation of the scapula.

Patient Position: Side-lying with the involved arm on top.

Clinician and Hand Positions: The clinician's cephalad hand is placed over the superior scapula, and the caudal hand is positioned with the web space cradling the inferior angle of the scapula.

Mobilization Application: As the superior hand pushes the scapula in a caudal direction, the inferior hand moves under the inferior angle of the scapula (figure 19.34).

Notations: The patient must be relaxed for this technique to be successful.

Clavicular Joints

Because clavicular motion contributes 60° to glenohumeral motion, it is important for clavicular joint mobility to be intact. After shoulder immobilization, these joints may become restricted if hypomobility is present.

Four mobilization techniques are used at the sternoclavicular and acromioclavicular (AC) joints: inferior, superior, anterior, and posterior glides. The force is applied with the thumb pad of one hand, reinforced with the other thumb. Mobilization techniques for these joints are described in the following sections.

The resting position for the AC and sternoclavicular (SC) joints is called the physiological position; it is the position the joints are in when the arm is resting at the side. The close-packed position for the sternoclavicular joint is with the arm in full elevation overhead. The close-packed position for the AC joint is with the arm abducted to 90°.

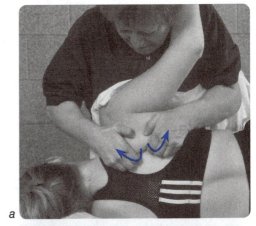

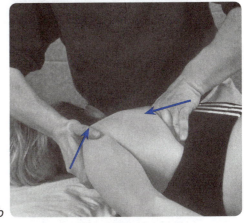

▶ **Figure 19.33** Joint mobilization—scapular distraction: *(a)* in side-lying, *(b)* alternative technique in prone.

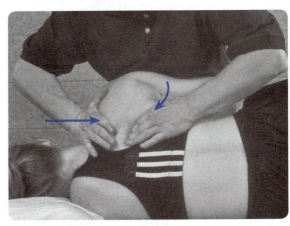

▶ **Figure 19.34** Joint mobilization: scapular inferior glide.

■ Joint Mobilization of the Clavicular Joint

Acromioclavicular Inferior Glide

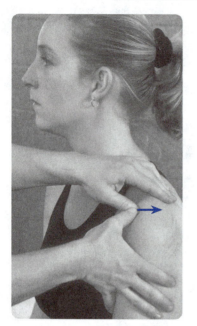

▶ **Figure 19.35** Joint mobilization—AC glide: *(a)* posterior glide.

Resting Position: Joint is in its physiological position with the arm at the side.

Mobilization Technique: Inferior glide or caudal glide.

Indications: Hypomobility of the AC joint.

Patient Position: Supine with the arm relaxed at the side.

Clinician and Hand Positions: Clinician stands at the patient's head. The clinician's thumb is positioned on the superior aspect of the acromion.

Mobilization Application: A superior-to-inferior mobilization force is applied to the distal acromion. Force is applied parallel to the joint plane.

Notations: This technique may also be performed with the patient sitting.

Acromioclavicular Posterior Glide

Resting Position: Joint is in its physiological relaxed position with the arm at the side.

Mobilization Technique: Posterior glide or dorsal glide or anterior-to-posterior glide.

Indications: Hypomobility of the AC joint.

Patient Position: Supine with the arm relaxed at the side.

Clinician and Hand Positions: When the patient is supine, the clinician stands at the waist for superior glides, at the head for inferior glides, and at the side for posterior glides. One thumb is reinforced by the clinician's other thumb over the distal acromion while the fingers are used as buttresses to support thumb motion on the AC joint.

Mobilization Application: An anterior-to-posterior mobilization force is applied to the distal anterior acromion. Force is applied parallel to the joint plane (figure 19.35a).

Notations: This technique may also be performed with the patient sitting and the clinician facing the patient to perform posterior and inferior glides or behind the patient to perform anterior glides.

Acromioclavicular Anterior Glide

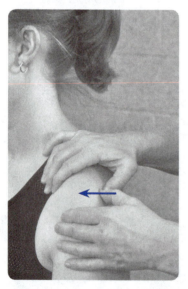

▶ **Figure 19.35** Joint mobilization—AC glide: *(b)* anterior glide.

Resting Position: Joint is in its physiological position with the arm at the side.

Mobilization Technique: Anterior glide or ventral glide or posterior-to-anterior glide.

Indications: Hypomobility of the AC joint.

Patient Position: Seated with the arm relaxed at the side.

Clinician and Hand Positions: Clinician stands behind the patient. The clinician's thumb is positioned on the posterior aspect of the acromion.

Mobilization Application: A posterior-to-anterior mobilization force is applied to the distal posterior acromion. Force is applied parallel to the joint plane (figure 19.35b).

Notations: This technique may also be performed with the patient supine.

Sternoclavicular Inferior Glide

Resting Position: Arm is relaxed at the side of the body.

Mobilization Technique: Inferior glide or caudal glide.

Indications: Hypomobility of the SC joint or reduced clavicular rotation.

Patient Position: Supine.

Clinician and Hand Positions: Clinician's thumb is placed on the proximal clavicle just lateral to the manubrium at its superior aspect.

Mobilization Application: Force is applied inferiorly toward the patient's waist (figure 19.36a).

Notations: Force is applied parallel to the joint surface.

Sternoclavicular Posterior Glide

Resting Position: Arm is relaxed at the side of the body.

Mobilization Technique: Posterior glide or dorsal glide or anterior-to-posterior glide.

Indications: Hypomobility of the SC joint or reduced clavicular rotation.

Patient Position: Supine.

Clinician and Hand Positions: Clinician's thumb is placed on the proximal clavicle just lateral to the manubrium on its anterior aspect.

Mobilization Application: Force is applied posteriorly down toward the table (figure 19.36b).

Notations: Force is applied parallel to the joint surface. Clinician may also stand at the patient's side.

Sternoclavicular Superior Glide

Resting Position: Arm is relaxed at the side of the body.

Mobilization Technique: Superior glide or cranial glide.

Indications: Hypomobility of the SC joint or reduced clavicular rotation.

Patient Position: Supine.

Clinician and Hand Positions: Clinician stands at the patient's side near the waist, facing the patient. Clinician's thumb is placed on the proximal clavicle just lateral to the manubrium at its inferior aspect.

Mobilization Application: Force is applied superiorly.

Notations: Force is applied parallel to the joint surface.

FLEXIBILITY EXERCISES

The stretch force for all flexibility exercises should be sufficient to produce a stretch sensation without pain. Pain indicates that the stretch force is too aggressive and should be reduced. Stretches can be either short term or prolonged. Recent injuries with newly formed scar tissue can be effectively treated with short-term stretches. Injuries that occurred several months before treatment and contain scar tissue that is more mature will benefit from prolonged stretches. The following sections present exercises that are by no means exhaustive lists of flexibility exercises for the shoulder complex, but they provide a start of exercises that you will learn to expand upon as you gain more experience in shoulder rehabilitation.

Active Stretches

Selection of these stretches is based on areas of the capsule that are tight. These exercises are often used in conjunction with joint mobilization.

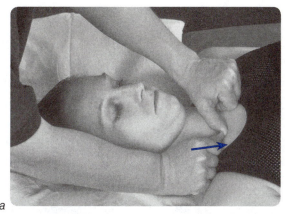

▶ **Figure 19.36** Joint mobilization—SC glide: (a) inferior glide.

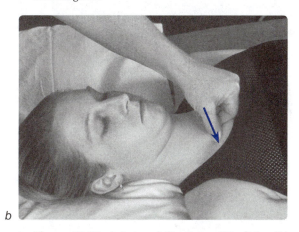

▶ **Figure 19.36** Joint mobilization—SC glide: (b) posterior glide.

Two rehabilitation techniques for the shoulder are soft-tissue mobilization and joint mobilization. Trigger point release and myofascial release are soft-tissue mobilization techniques used to improve parameters in the rotator cuff muscles, the scapular muscles, and the large glenohumeral muscles. The rehabilitation clinician uses joint mobilization techniques to improve mobility in the glenohumeral joint, the scapulothoracic joint, and the clavicular joints.

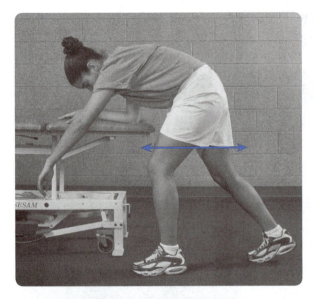

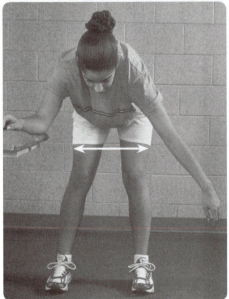

▶ **Figure 19.37** Codman's exercises: *(a)* flexion-extension, *(b)* horizontal flexion-extension.

■ Active Shoulder Flexibility Exercises

Pendulum Exercises or Codman's Exercises

Passive motion of the shoulder occurs because of weight transfer back and forth between the left leg and the right leg while the arm remains relaxed.

Body Segment: Glenohumeral joint.

Stage in Rehab: I and II.

Purpose: Gain early motion, relax muscles, distraction of the glenohumeral joint, pain modulation.

Positioning: The patient is flexed forward at the waist with the involved arm hanging in a resting position away from the body; the body weight is supported by the uninvolved arm on a table.

Execution: Involved arm motion is initiated from the hips, not the shoulder. The arm should remain relaxed throughout the motions. Passive flexion-extension motion of the shoulder occurs with the patient's legs in a forward-backward straddle position; body weight is transferred from the front to the back leg to provide momentum for arm movement (figure 19.37a). Horizontal flexion-extension movement occurs with the patient standing in a side-to-side straddle position; body weight is transferred from the left leg to the right leg to produce sideward arm motion (figure 19.37b). Circular motion of the shoulder is produced by the hips as the patient moves the body in a circular direction while the arm hangs passively, swinging with momentum produced from the hips. Circular motion can occur in a clockwise or counterclockwise direction.

Possible Substitutions: Using shoulder muscles to move the joint rather than hip and leg muscles.

Notations: Patient must not use shoulder muscles to move the shoulder; motion comes from the lower extremities. If a weight is used for additional joint distraction, it should be a cuff weight, not a dumbbell weight, so that the muscles remain relaxed. This is a passive exercise.

Inferior Capsule Stretch

Body Segment: Glenohumeral joint.

Stage in Rehab: II through IV.

Purpose: Increase mobility of the inferior capsule to improve shoulder elevation.

Positioning: The patient positions the arm overhead with the elbow flexed and the forearm behind the head.

Execution: The uninvolved hand, placed on the elbow, pulls the elbow behind the head (figure 19.38).

Possible Substitutions: A common substitution with this exercise is lateral trunk lean away from the shoulder being stretched. If this occurs, the patient should perform the exercise in front of a mirror to monitor and correct trunk position. The patient should not shrug the shoulder as it is stretched.

Notations: This is an active stretch.

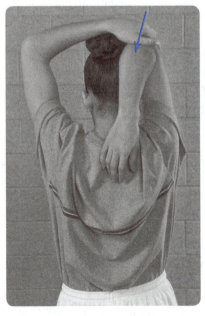

▶ **Figure 19.38** Flexibility exercise: inferior capsule stretch.

Posterior Capsule Stretch

Body Segment: Glenohumeral joint.

Stage in Rehab: II through IV.

Purpose: Gain medial rotation and horizontal flexion of the glenohumeral joint and stretch out the posterior rotator cuff.

Positioning: The patient positions the involved arm at shoulder level and grasps the elbow with the opposite hand.

Execution: The patient pulls the arm across the body, attempting to place the hand of the involved shoulder behind the opposite shoulder and the elbow close to the chin (figure 19.39).

Possible Substitutions: A common error is to rotate the trunk rather than pull the arm across the body. The patient may also tend to lower the elbow below shoulder level. The clinician uses verbal cueing to correct for proper execution. If necessary, the patient can also stand in front of a mirror to receive visual feedback.

Notations: If the exercise is not performed correctly, stretch results will not be optimal.

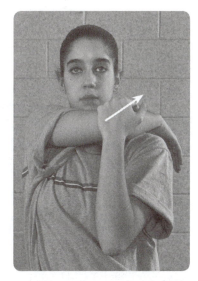

▶ **Figure 19.39** Flexibility exercise: posterior capsule stretch.

Anterior Capsule Stretch

Body Segment: Glenohumeral joint.

Stage in Rehab: II through IV.

Purpose: Gain horizontal extension and lateral rotation. This exercise stretches the anterior capsule and pectoralis major.

Positioning: The patient stands in a doorway with the elbows and forearms on the door jamb.

Execution: To stretch upper pectoralis fibers, the elbows are positioned below the shoulders (figure 19.40a). To stretch middle fibers, the elbows are positioned at shoulder level. To stretch lower fibers, the elbows are positioned above the shoulders (figure 19.40b). With one foot placed in front of the other, the patient pushes from the back foot to lean through the doorway and feel a stretch in the anterior chest area.

Possible Substitutions: Common substitutions include arching the back, moving the elbows off the door jamb, and keeping the involved shoulder behind the uninvolved shoulder so that the trunk is at an angle to the doorway. Verbal cueing for proper technique should be used to correct these substitutions.

Notations: This stretch can also be performed in a corner, but it is often difficult to find an available corner that is not occupied with furniture or other difficult-to-move objects.

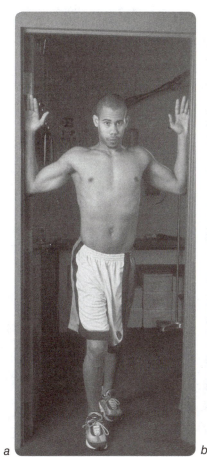
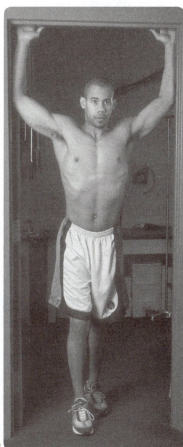

a   *b*

▶ **Figure 19.40** Flexibility exercise—anterior capsule stretch: *(a)* upper, *(b)* lower.

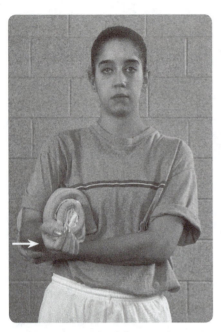

▶ **Figure 19.41** Flexibility exercise: superior capsule stretch.

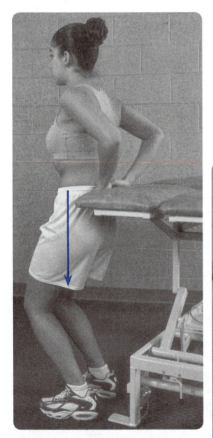

▶ **Figure 19.42** Flexibility exercise: medial rotation stretch.

Superior Capsule Stretch

Body Segment: Glenohumeral joint.

Stage in Rehab: II through IV.

Purpose: Increase superior capsule mobility and shoulder extension.

Positioning: In standing, the patient places a rolled towel under the arm and positions the elbow next to his or her side.

Execution: With the uninvolved hand, the patient pulls the elbow toward the side (figure 19.41).

Possible Substitutions: A common error is to use a roll that is not large enough to provide adequate stretch.

Notations: Applying the stretch force too high on the arm delivers less stretch force.

Medial Rotation Stretch

Body Segment: Glenohumeral joint.

Stage in Rehab: II through IV.

Purpose: Increase medial rotation and stretch the glenohumeral joint capsule.

Positioning: Patient stands with his or her hands behind the back and grasps the countertop. The feet are shoulder-width apart.

Execution: Patient squats down while maintaining a grasp on the countertop (figure 19.42).

Possible Substitutions: The most common substitutions are bending over at the waist, looking down at the floor, and flexing the wrist. The wrist should remain straight, and the patient should maintain an erect position. Giving the patient a verbal cue to keep the head up or to look at the ceiling will help correct the posture.

Notations: The hands may start in a shoulder-width grip, but the patient should move the hands closer together as flexibility is gained until one hand is on top of the other.

Rhomboid Stretch

Body Segment: Scapula.

Stage in Rehab: II through IV.

Purpose: Improve rhomboid flexibility and posterior capsule mobility.

Positioning: Patient stands facing the edge of an open door, with the feet placed on either side of the door and the hands on the doorknobs.

Execution: With the legs straight, the patient pushes the hips backward. The arms should remain straight and relaxed as the body weight moves backward (figure 19.43).

Possible Substitutions: A common error is not allowing the body weight to stretch the shoulders. If this error occurs, instruct the patient to relax the arms and let the hips move backward and downward, attempting to sit on the floor while the legs are kept straight.

Notations: Keeping the shoulders relaxed allows for a better stretch.

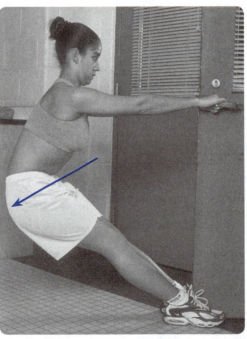

▶ **Figure 19.43** Flexibility exercise: rhomboid stretch.

Supraspinatus Active Stretch

Body Segment: Glenohumeral joint.

Stage in Rehab: II through IV.

Purpose: Increase supraspinatus flexibility and superior capsular mobility.

Positioning: The patient positions the involved arm behind the body with the elbow flexed and grasps a chair back with the hand.

Execution: The patient leans away from the hand.

Possible Substitutions: Twisting the body and bending the trunk rather than leaning.

Notations: An alternative technique is to grasp the hand behind the back with the opposite hand and pull the involved arm toward the uninvolved side (figure 19.44).

Assistive Stretches

Most of these stretches require the assistance of the clinician. These stretches may be combined with contract-relax-stretch techniques to give the stretch a proprioceptive neuromuscular facilitation (PNF) element. Improper technique and substitutions should be corrected so that the intended structures are appropriately stretched. The PNF techniques are described in later sections.

If PNF is not used with these exercises, the shoulder is brought to the end range and held in that position for 10 to 15 s; this is repeated at least four times. It is preferable if these exercises are repeated two to four times throughout the day in the early rehabilitation phases. Once the desired range of motion is achieved, the exercise is continued once or twice daily in order to maintain the motion.

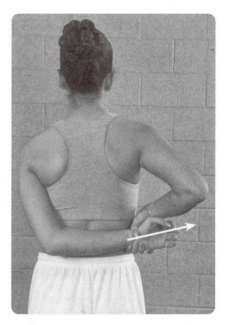

▶ **Figure 19.44** Flexibility exercise: supraspinatus stretch.

▪ Assistive Stretches for the Shoulder

Supraspinatus Stretch

Body Segment: Supraspinatus.

Stage in Rehab: II through IV.

Purpose: Increase supraspinatus motion and improve superior capsular mobility.

Positioning: Patient is standing with the involved arm behind the back. The uninvolved hand grasps the wrist of the involved arm.

Execution: The arm is pulled across the back to bring the involved hand to the opposite side. The patient maintains medial rotation of the shoulder.

Possible Substitutions: Lateral flexion of the trunk and trunk rotation.

Notations: This can also be performed with the clinician providing the stretch.

Infraspinatus Stretch

Body Segment: Infraspinatus.

Stage in Rehab: II through IV.

Purpose: Increase infraspinatus flexibility and improve posterior capsular mobility.

Positioning: Patient is sitting. The involved arm is placed in front of the body in medial rotation with the elbow flexed.

Execution: The clinician grasps the elbow or wrist and pulls the arm across the body while maintaining medial rotation (figure 19.45).

Possible Substitutions: Trunk lean and trunk rotation. Place a hand on the patient's shoulder to stabilize the trunk.

Notations: If the patient performs the stretch, the uninvolved hand is placed on the elbow to pull the arm across the body.

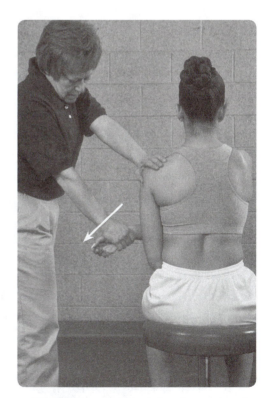

▶ **Figure 19.45** Assistive infraspinatus stretch.

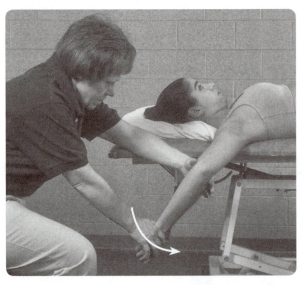

▶ **Figure 19.46** Assistive subscapularis stretch.

Subscapularis Stretch

Body Segment: Subscapularis.

Stage in Rehab: II through IV.

Purpose: Increase subscapularis flexibility and improve inferior capsular mobility.

Positioning: Patient is supine. Arm is in abduction and at the end of lateral rotation.

Execution: Clinician applies a stretch force into lateral rotation (figure 19.46).

Possible Substitutions: Arching the low back is a common substitution. Verbal cueing to the patient and flexing the hips and knees will prevent the back from arching.

Notations: Care must be taken to avoid excessive elbow stress during the stretch.

Teres Minor Stretch

Body Segment: Teres minor.

Stage in Rehab: II through IV.

Purpose: Increase teres minor flexibility and stretch the inferior capsule.

Positioning: Patient is sitting with the arm in abduction and medial rotation.

Execution: Clinician stabilizes the scapula to isolate teres minor and then applies a medial rotation stretch (figure 19.47).

Possible Substitutions: Scapular rotation may occur if the scapula is not stabilized.

Notations: An alternative position can be used with the arm overhead in end-range abduction with medial rotation; the scapula must be stabilized by the clinician in this stretch.

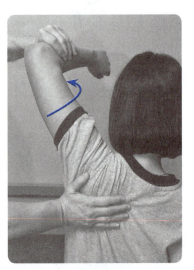

▶ **Figure 19.47** Assistive teres minor stretch.

Teres Major Stretch

Body Segment: Teres major.

Stage in Rehab: II through IV.

Purpose: Increase teres major flexibility.

Positioning: Patient is supine with the arm overhead in flexion and lateral rotation.

Execution: Clinician applies the stretch force moving into additional flexion and lateral rotation (figure 19.48).

Possible Substitutions: The spine should not rise up from the table. Instruct the patient to lie with the hips and knees flexed, with the back flat on the table, to prevent lumbar hyperextension.

Notations: Clinician may stand either at the head or at the side of the patient.

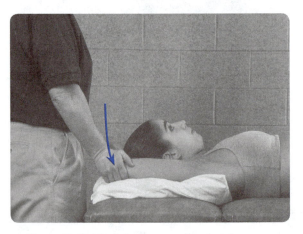

▶ **Figure 19.48** Assistive teres major stretch.

Latissimus Dorsi Stretch

Body Segment: Latissimus dorsi.

Stage in Rehab: II through IV.

Purpose: Increase latissimus dorsi flexibility.

Positioning: Patient lies prone with the arm overhead.

Execution: Clinician grasps the forearm and then distracts the shoulder and laterally rotates the shoulder as the arm is lifted toward the ceiling (figure 19.49).

Possible Substitutions: Trunk rotation and elbow flexion are substitutions.

Notations: If the patient has a history of elbow or wrist injury, the force is applied just proximal to the elbow joint.

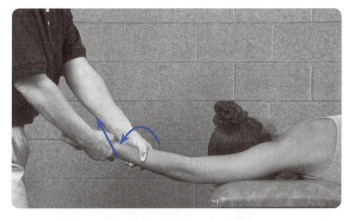

▶ **Figure 19.49** Assistive latissimus dorsi stretch.

Wand Exercises

The following exercises, performed with a wand, use the uninvolved contralateral arm to provide the stretch force. Commercial wands and T-bars can be used, but a dowel (2.5 cm [1 in.] in diameter), broom handle, cane, and other similar items are readily available, inexpensive, and easy to use.

The patient uses the uninvolved arm to guide the wand in the desired direction to provide the stretch force needed to increase motion. He or she holds the end position 5 to 10 s and repeats each motion several times. The advantage of these exercises is that the patient can perform them independently several times throughout the day. These exercises are detailed in the following sections.

▧ Wand Exercises for the Shoulder

Wand Flexion Stretch

Body Segment: Shoulder flexion.

Stage in Rehab: II.

Purpose: Increase glenohumeral flexion motion.

Positioning: Patient may be sitting, standing, or supine.

Execution: Patient grasps the wand in each hand, with the hands shoulder-width apart. He or she moves the arms overhead, keeping the elbows straight throughout the exercise (figure 19.50).

Possible Substitutions: Arching the back, bending the elbows, and hyperextending the wrists.

Notations: It is advisable that the exercise start in a supine position to eliminate need for strength in later ranges of motion.

▶ **Figure 19.50** Wand flexion.

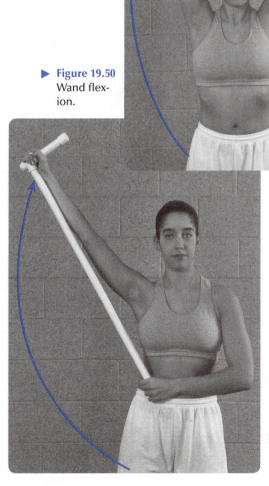

Wand Abduction Stretch

Body Segment: Shoulder abduction.

Stage in Rehab: II.

Purpose: Increase glenohumeral abduction motion.

Positioning: Supine or standing. Patient grasps the end of the wand with the involved hand and places the uninvolved hand toward the other end of the wand.

Execution: The uninvolved arm pushes the involved arm upward into abduction (figure 19.51).

▶ **Figure 19.51** Wand abduction.

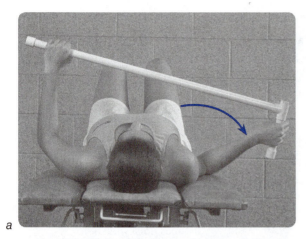

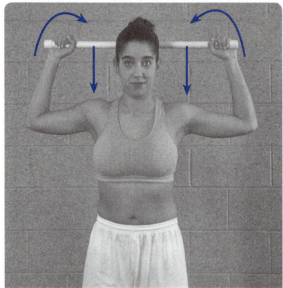

▶ **Figure 19.52** Wand lateral rotation: *(a)* supine, *(b)* advanced.

Possible Substitutions: Leaning sideways, moving the shoulder into the flexion plane, and flexing the elbow.

Notations: Placing the involved hand in an underhand grasp may reduce shoulder soft-tissue impingement in higher elevations.

Wand Lateral Rotation Stretch

Body Segment: Shoulder lateral rotation.

Stage in Rehab: II.

Purpose: Increase glenohumeral lateral rotation motion.

Positioning: The patient lies supine with the involved hand on one end of the wand and the uninvolved hand toward the other end. The involved elbow is kept next to the side at 90° flexion throughout the exercise.

Execution: With the wand, the patient pushes the involved hand away from the body to laterally rotate the shoulder (figure 19.52a).

Possible Substitutions: Extending the elbow as the wand is pushed laterally and abducting the involved shoulder.

Notations: A more advanced lateral rotation exercise can be performed with the hands shoulder-width apart on the wand. The patient raises the wand overhead and then bends the elbows to attempt to place the wand behind the neck (figure 19.52b). Neck flexion, trunk flexion or rotation, elbow extension, and wrist hyperextension are common substitutions with this exercise.

Wand Medial Rotation Stretch

Body Segment: Shoulder medial rotation.

Stage in Rehab: II.

Purpose: Increase glenohumeral medial rotation.

Positioning: The patient stands with the wand behind the waist; hands are placed shoulder-width apart.

Execution: The wand is raised along the back as high as possible (figure 19.53a).

▶ **Figure 19.53** Wand medial rotation: *(a)* initial position, *(b)* alternative position.

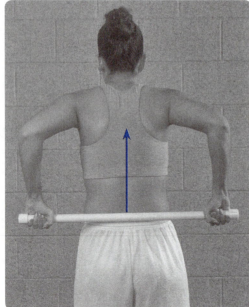

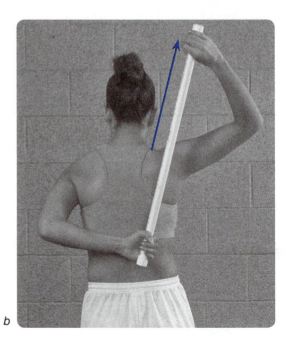

Possible Substitutions: Excessive wrist flexion and trunk lean.

Notations: An alternative stretch is with the wand placed vertically behind the back. The involved hand is at the waist, and the uninvolved hand is at the top of the wand. The wand is pulled upward with the top hand (figure 19.53b). Trunk flexion is a common substitution with this alternative stretch.

Wand Glenohumeral Horizontal Flexion-Extension Stretch

Body Segment: Shoulder horizontal flexion and extension.

Stage in Rehab: II.

Purpose: Increase horizontal motions.

Positioning: The patient lies supine with the hands overhead, shoulder-width apart on the wand, and the elbows straight.

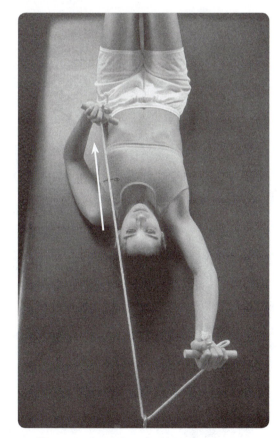

▶ **Figure 19.54** Wand horizontal flexion-extension.

Execution: The uninvolved arm pushes the involved arm away from the body as far as possible, and then pulls the arm across the body as far as possible (figure 19.54).

Possible Substitutions: Elbow flexion, trunk rotation, moving the shoulders into extension, and shoulder rotation.

Notations: Throughout the exercise the hands remain at shoulder level and the elbows remain straight.

Pulley Exercises

These exercises can be performed with a pulley, rope, or stretch strap. They are easy to incorporate into a home exercise program that the patient can perform independently. The patient must be careful to avoid driving the humeral head into the glenoid socket, especially when using the pulleys for frozen-shoulder exercises. The patient is instructed to maintain the scapula in a depressed position throughout the motion.

Shoulder Flexion

For this exercise, an overhead rope and pulley or a stretch strap and hook are attached in a doorway or on a wall. The patient sits with his or her back to the door or wall. The hands are positioned with the thumbs facing upward. The uninvolved arm pulls the rope or strap down to elevate the involved arm into flexion as high as possible. The involved arm is lowered and the motion is repeated several times.

One alternative stretch uses a stretch strap placed over the top of a door. The patient reaches up as high as possible on the strap, and then bends the knees to lower the body and apply the stretch force to the shoulder. Another alternative position is with the patient supine and the pulley attached to the wall or doorjamb (figure 19.55).

Shoulder Abduction

This exercise is similar to the shoulder flexion exercise except that the arm is raised in abduction from the side of the body.

▶ **Figure 19.55** Pulley: shoulder flexion.

Flexibility exercises for the shoulder include pendulum exercises, active and assistive stretches, wand exercises using the uninvolved extremity, and pulley exercises.

STRENGTHENING EXERCISES

These exercises incorporate a broad spectrum of degrees of difficulty and of stresses applied to the shoulder. They are presented here from easiest to more advanced exercises, beginning with early-phase isometric exercises and progressing to later-phase plyometric exercises. As the exercises become more difficult, they advance from straight-plane to diagonal exercises. We will consider the diagonal exercises, which combine movement planes to stress muscles for all the shoulder joints, in terms of their function and goals within a therapeutic exercise program. The rehabilitation clinician should note and correct substitution patterns to achieve optimal strengthening of intended muscles and facilitate appropriate muscle firing patterns.

Isometrics

Isometrics begin early in a rehabilitation program when the patient is limited in shoulder mobility and strength. They help to minimize atrophy during times when use or motion of the shoulder is limited. They are performed in a pain-free position and may be performed at multiple angles of a motion, if motion is permitted. If motion is limited, the exercises are performed in non-aggravating, acceptable positions. Each isometric contraction is gradually increased to a maximum contraction, held at the maximum, and then decreased gradually until the muscle is relaxed. The patient must be instructed to avoid sudden maximal contractions to avoid injury or undue strain of the muscle. The patient should maximally contract only if no pain occurs. If pain occurs, effort should be limited to a submaximal contraction until the greater force is non-irritating. Each isometric is held for 5 to 10 s and repeated 10 times. These exercises are performed frequently throughout the day. The following sections describe these exercises.

■ Isometric Exercises

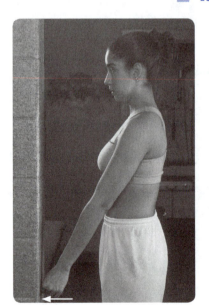

▶ **Figure 19.56**   Isometric flexion.

Isometric Shoulder Flexion

Body Segment: Glenohumeral joint.

Stage in Rehab: II.

Purpose: Strengthen shoulder flexors.

Positioning: Patient stands facing a doorway or wall; the involved arm is slightly forward with the radial hand on the doorframe or wall.

Execution: Patient attempts to move the arm forward while pushing the hand against the doorframe or wall (figure 19.56).

Possible Substitutions: Elbow flexion.

Notations: The patient should keep the elbow straight. If the hand is uncomfortable from the pressure, he or she should apply a towel between the hand and the wall.

Isometric Shoulder Abduction

Body Segment: Glenohumeral joint.

Stage in Rehab: II.

Purpose: Strengthen shoulder abductors.

Positioning: Patient stands with the involved side facing a wall or doorway. The arm is positioned in slight abduction with the dorsum of the hand against the wall.

Execution: The patient keeps the elbow extended and pushes the arm against the wall, attempting to move the arm into abduction.

Possible Substitutions: Elbow flexion and shoulder flexion.

Cues and Notations: Patients should keep the arm in line with the body rather than forward of it. If the hand is uncomfortable from the pressure, they should apply a towel between the hand and the wall.

Isometric Shoulder Extension

Body Segment: Glenohumeral joint.

Stage in Rehab: II.

Purpose: Strengthen shoulder extensors.

Positioning: Patient stands with the back to the wall and positions the arm slightly behind the body, with the ulnar hand against the wall.

Execution: The patient pushes the hand backward to the wall, keeping the elbow extended (figure 19.57).

Possible Substitutions: Elbow flexion and trunk lean.

Cues and Notations: Patients should keep the body and arm straight. If the hand is uncomfortable from the pressure, they should apply a towel between the hand and the wall.

Isometric Shoulder Medial Rotation

Body Segment: Glenohumeral joint.

Stage in Rehab: II.

Purpose: Strengthen medial rotators.

Positioning: The patient stands facing a doorway with the elbow flexed to 90° and the anterior distal forearm placed against the surface of the doorframe.

Execution: Patient attempts to roll the forearm inward toward the abdomen.

Possible Substitutions: Elbow extension and shoulder abduction.

Cues and Notations: Patients should keep the elbow at their side.

Isometric Shoulder Lateral Rotation

Body Segment: Glenohumeral joint.

Stage in Rehab: II.

Purpose: Strengthen lateral rotators.

Positioning: Patient stands facing a doorway with the elbow flexed to 90° and the posterior distal surface of the forearm against the doorframe.

Execution: Patient attempts to roll the forearm outward (figure 19.58).

Possible Substitutions: Elbow extension and shoulder flexion.

Cues and Notations: Patients should keep the elbow at their side.

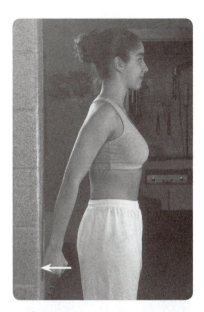

▶ **Figure 19.57** Isometric extension.

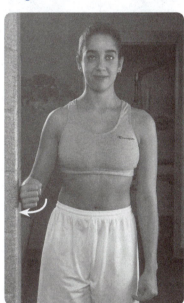

▶ **Figure 19.58** Isometric shoulder external rotation.

Isolated-Plane Isotonic Exercises

As mentioned previously, initial strengthening exercises should include primarily straight-plane activities. Once strength is sufficient to control the joint during motion, multiplane and diagonal exercises can begin. Here we look first at straight-plane exercises and then move to multiplane exercises. Keep in mind that although this section includes many of the commonly used exercises, the listing here is far from exhaustive.

Although shoulder motion includes function of scapulothoracic and glenohumeral muscles, patients can and should perform isolated exercises of the muscles for each joint until the muscles have sufficient strength to control the joints during functional motions. To make it easier to identify specific exercise functions, the straight-plane exercises for the scapulothoracic and glenohumeral muscle groups are presented separately and identified as such in the following sections. Most are considered relative to the specific motion and muscles they address and are presented from easiest to more difficult.

Scapulothoracic Exercises

If the patient has pain with the shoulder in elevated positions, it is best to provide manual resistance with the shoulder in the lower planes of motion. An advantage of offering manual resistance to the scapulothoracic muscles is that these exercises can be performed without affecting the glenohumeral joint, so they may begin early in the rehabilitation program.

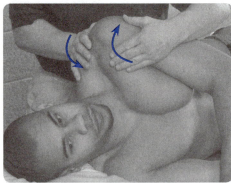

a

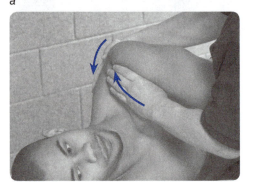

b

▶ **Figure 19.59** Manual resistance to scapula: *(a)* with hand on table, *(b)* with arm supported in non-weight-bearing position.

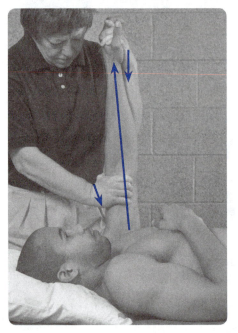

▶ **Figure 19.60** Serratus anterior.

■ Isotonic Isolated-Plane Strength Exercises

Manual Resistance to Scapular Retractors and Protractors

Body Segment: Scapulothoracic.

Stage in Rehab: II.

Purpose: Strengthen scapular retractors and protractors.

Positioning: Patient is side-lying on the uninvolved side. The involved arm is along the side of the body.

Execution: The clinician faces the patient and places his or her hands on the medial scapular border posteriorly to resist the combined movements of retraction and depression of the scapula; he or she places the other hand on the anterior shoulder to resist protraction and elevation of the scapula in the opposite direction (figure 19.59, a & b).

Possible Substitutions: Trunk rotation.

Cues and Notations: For greater patient comfort, a rolled towel may be placed between the arm and side. If there is a recent anterior surgical scar on the shoulder, a towel between the shoulder and clinician's hand may increase patient comfort.

Manual Resistance to Serratus Anterior

Body Segment: Scapulothoracic.

Stage in Rehab: III.

Purpose: Strengthen serratus anterior for glenohumeral elevation stability.

Positioning: Patient lies supine with the arm flexed to about 110° to 120° and the elbow extended.

Execution: The hand is pushed toward the ceiling, with the movement coming from the scapula as it moves forward and anteriorly around the ribs. This motion can be resisted manually (figure 19.60), with a dumbbell in the hand, or on a bench-press machine with the bar lifted into position by the clinician.

Possible Substitutions: Incomplete range of motion, shoulder extension, use of upper trapezius to hold arm above 90°.

Cues and Notations: Patients should keep the shoulder blade pulled down toward their back pocket. This exercise should not be performed in this position until the shoulder joint has greater than 120° flexion.

Push-Up Plus

Body Segment: Scapulothoracic.

Stage in Rehab: II and III.

Purpose: Facilitate serratus anterior strength.

Positioning: This exercise starts in push-up position with the hands shoulder-width apart, the elbows extended, and the hands above shoulder level on the wall. The feet are far enough from the wall that the patient leans forward with trunk and hips extended to reach the wall.

Execution: Patient pushes the body away from the hands while maintaining hand contact on the surface and body alignment as in the start position. The scapulae slide forward on the rib cage (figure 19.61). From a wall push-up, the patient progresses to a modified push-up on the floor, then a regular push-up, and finally to a decline push-up position with the feet higher than the hands. With the feet higher than the hands, the serratus anterior and the upper trapezius are particularly facilitated (Lear and Gross, 1998).

Possible Substitutions: Trunk lean into the wall; elbow flexion, hands close together.

Cues and Notations: Patients with anterior instability or those who have had recent shoulder surgery should avoid lowering the body to the point where the shoulders move in front of the plane of the elbows during push-ups in order to prevent undue stress on the anterior shoulder.

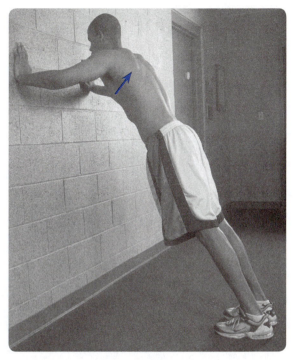

▶ **Figure 19.61** Push-up plus.

Scapular Protraction With Pulleys or Resistance Bands

Body Segment: Scapulothoracic.

Stage in Rehab: II and III.

Purpose: Strengthen serratus anterior.

Positioning: The bands or pulleys are anchored just below shoulder level, and the patient stands or sits with his or her back to the anchor. The elbow begins the exercise in flexion with the upper extremity next to the body (figure 19.62a).

Execution: The patient pushes the band forward and slightly upward, reaching as far as possible, extending the elbow and punching the scapula forward (figure 19.62b).

Possible Substitutions: Using the trunk to rotate the arm forward rather than using the serratus anterior to punch the scapula forward.

Cues and Notations: An alternative exercise using rubber tubing or a resistance band can be performed

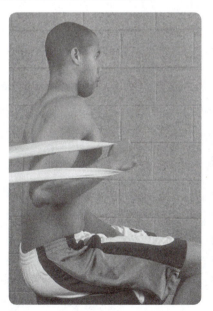
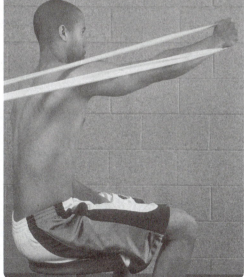

a   *b*

▶ **Figure 19.62** Serratus anterior with a resistance band: *(a)* start position, *(b)* end position.

with the patient supine and the tubing or band under the shoulders and back area. The patient grasps the ends of the tubing or band and starts with the elbows extended and the shoulders flexed to 90° so that the hands are toward the ceiling and the tubing or band is taut. The patient punches the hands toward the ceiling, protracting the scapulae.

Scapular Squeeze

Body Segment: Scapulothoracic.

Stage in Rehab: I and II.

Purpose: Strengthen rhomboids and middle trapezius.

Positioning: Patient sits with elbows at the sides.

Execution: Patient squeezes the scapulae together, keeping the elbows at the sides, and holds for 5 to 10 s at the end of the range of motion.

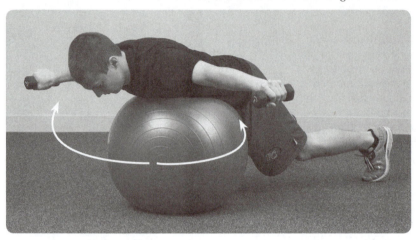

▶ **Figure 19.63** Reverse fly.

Possible Substitutions: Shrugging the shoulders and extending the shoulders without retracting the scapulae.

Cues and Notations: This is the first level of exercise for retractors. The next two exercises are progressions of this one.

Prone Flys

Body Segment: Scapulothoracic.

Stage in Rehab: II and III.

Purpose: Strengthen rhomboids and middle trapezius.

Positioning: Patient is prone with the arms hanging over the table.

Execution: The patient lifts a weight in horizontal extension as the scapulae are squeezed together. The elbows remain extended but not locked throughout the movement (figure 19.63). Although the patient need perform the exercise with only the involved extremity, a greater facilitation of the muscles occurs if both arms perform the exercise simultaneously.

Possible Substitutions: Shoulder horizontal extension without scapular retraction.

Cues and Notations: An alternative position is shown in figure 19.63, with the patient flexed at the hips and trunk supported on an exercise ball so that the back is straight.

Rows With Pulleys or Resistance Bands

Body Segment: Scapulothoracic.

Stage in Rehab: II and III.

Purpose: Strengthen rhomboids and middle trapezius.

Positioning: In sitting, the patient faces resistance bands or pulleys that are anchored to a door at or below shoulder level. The patient leans forward from the hip, keeping the back straight, with the scapulae in a protracted position, and then moves to an erect position (figure 19.64a).

Execution: Maintaining proper trunk position, the patient pulls to retract the scapulae, squeezing them together and keeping the elbows at the sides (figure 19.64b).

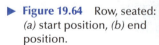

▶ **Figure 19.64** Row, seated: *(a)* start position, *(b)* end position.

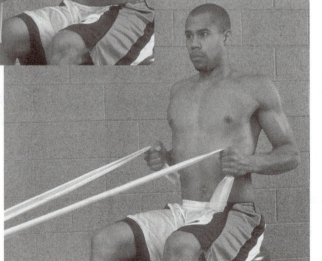

a

b

Possible Substitutions: Extending the trunk and hips; using shoulder extensors without retracting the scapulae.

Cues and Notations: Patient may sit on a Swiss ball to make the exercise more challenging.

Seated Push-Up (Sometimes Called a Press-Up or a Press-Down)

Body Segment: Scapulothoracic.

Stage in Rehab: Late III.

Purpose: Strengthen lower trapezius and pectoralis minor. Latissimus dorsi is also strengthened.

Positioning: Patient is seated with hands alongside the hips on the chair seat. If patient has sufficient strength and the chair has arms, the hands may be placed on the chair arms.

Execution: The patient pushes down to lift the hips off the chair (figure 19.65a). The elbows must extend, and then the patient pushes down additionally to depress the scapulae.

Possible Substitutions: Using legs to lift body up, leaning forward to tilt trunk forward.

Cues and Notations: If the patient complains of shoulder joint pain, the rotator cuffs are not strong enough to stabilize the glenohumeral joint during this exercise. In this case, begin with the exercise listed next.

Press-Downs Using Pulleys or Resistance Bands

Body Segment: Scapulothoracic.

Stage in Rehab: III.

Purpose: Strengthen scapular depressors.

Positioning: The pulley or band is positioned high overhead, and the patient grasps the handle or band with an extended elbow and the shoulder in flexion (figure 19.65b).

Execution: Keeping the shoulder and elbow joints in their start positions throughout the exercise, the patient depresses the scapula downward toward the buttocks.

An alternative exercise can be performed with use of a latissimus bar: Using both hands, the involved arm positioned at the end of the bar and the uninvolved arm positioned closer to the middle of the bar, the patient begins with the elbows extended overhead and the scapulae elevated. The motion comes only from the scapulae as it goes into full depression; the elbow positions do not change.

Possible Substitutions: Lateral trunk lean; going through a partial range of motion; extending the shoulder and flexing the elbow.

Cues and Notations: An alternative for this exercise can be performed with the resistance device anchored to the shoulder; in this position the shoulder is not placed in an elevated position (figure 19.65c). This exercise isolates the depressors and does not put stress on the glenohumeral joint.

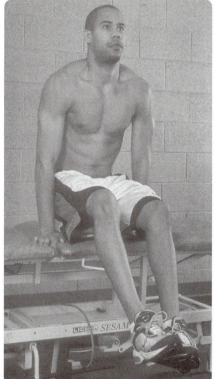

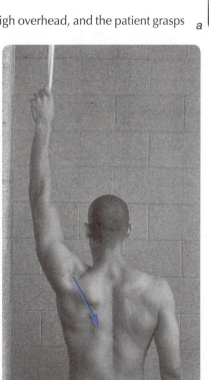

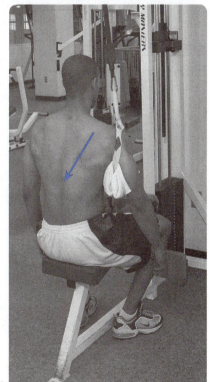

▶ **Figure 19.65** Scapular depressors: *(a)* seated press-up, *(b)* overhead depression, *(c)* alternative scapular depressor exercise position.

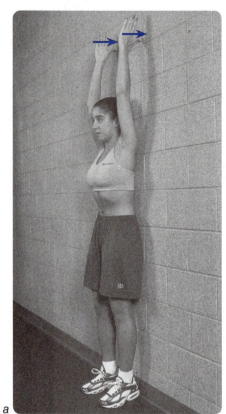

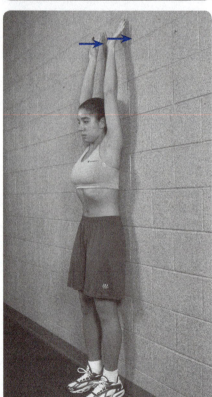

Bouhler Exercises

Body Segment: Scapulothoracic.

Stage in Rehab: III.

Purpose: Strengthen lower trapezius as an upward rotator.

Positioning: Patient stands with the back and buttocks to the wall and the heels about 1 in. (2.5 cm) from the wall.

Execution: With the abdominal muscles tightened to prevent the back from arching, the patient raises the arms overhead with the elbows straight and close to the ears. In the first exercise, the thumbs face the wall and are pushed to the wall (figure 19.66a). In the second exercise, the arms are in the same position as in the first exercise, but the thumbs face each other as the arms are moved to the wall (figure 19.66b). In the last exercise, the arms are positioned at a 45° angle from the body and are moved to the wall as the shoulder blades are squeezed together (figure 19.66c). In each exercise the patient holds the position for 5 to 10 s and repeats several times.

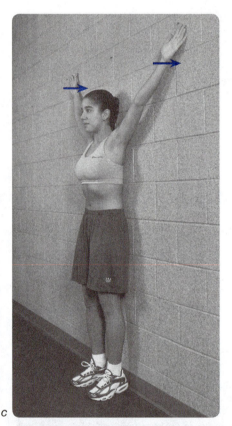

Possible Substitutions: Arching the back, moving the elbows away from the head, and flexing the elbows.

Cues and Notations: It may be necessary to add one of these exercises at a time on separate days since the lower trapezius may fatigue quickly. To perform these exercises at a more advanced level, the patient is prone, either on a table or on a Swiss ball. Weights can be added to the hands for additional resistance (figure 19.66d).

Scapular Elevation

Body Segment: Scapulothoracic.

Stage in Rehab: II and III.

Purpose: Strengthen upper trapezius and levator scapulae muscles.

Positioning: Patient stands with arms at sides.

Execution: Patient pulls shoulders up to the ears.

Possible Substitutions: Cervical extension.

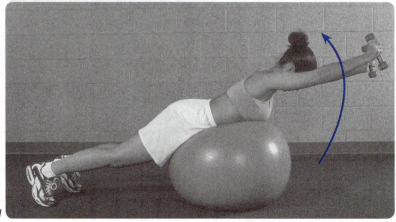

▶ **Figure 19.66** Bouhler exercises: *(a)* thumbs to the wall, *(b)* thumbs facing each other, *(c)* arms at 45° angle, *(d)* progression in an antigravity position with weights.

Cues and Notations: These muscles are normally not weak and often overpower their synergists and their antagonists, resulting in a muscle imbalance. They are often used incorrectly during shoulder elevation as substitution for weak rotator cuff muscles, contributing to faulty mechanics, further muscle imbalances, and prolonged injury recovery. In patients who have weakness of these muscles, initial strengthening can include shoulder shrugs and manual resistance to shrugs. A more advanced exercise uses dumbbell weights during shrugs.

Upright Press (Also Known as the Overhead Press or Military Press)

Body Segment: Scapulothoracic.

Stage in Rehab: III.

Purpose: Strengthen upper trapezius and levator scapulae.

Positioning: Patient stands, elbows flexed, with weights in hands. Hands are at shoulder level.

Execution: Patient pushes weights straight up to end with hands above the head and elbows fully extended but not locked.

Possible Substitutions: Arching the back; using momentum to lift the weight by swinging the weights upward.

Cues and Notations: This is a later exercise that is not always included in rehabilitation because of the stress it may place on the glenohumeral joint. It also strengthens the upper trapezius, a muscle that is not often deficient. Scapular rotator muscles and rotator cuff muscles should have good strength before this exercise is used.

Scapular Upward Rotation

Body Segment: Scapulothoracic.

Stage in Rehab: III.

Purpose: Strengthen scapular upward rotators.

Positioning: Patient is standing. With weight in hand, the thumb faces forward.

Execution: The elbow is maintained in extension and the upper extremity is lifted in a scapular plane, moving through a full range of motion and then returning to the start position (figure 19.67). The patient must maintain scapular control and correct glenohumeral positioning.

Possible Substitutions: Hyperextending the back; shrugging the shoulder to initiate movement.

Cues and Notations: Full range-of-motion exercise for scapular rotation also includes glenohumeral motion, so it is important for the rehabilitation clinician to be sure that glenohumeral joint stability is adequate before including these full-motion scapular activities in the rehabilitation program.

Scapular Downward Rotation

Body Segment: Scapulothoracic.

Stage in Rehab: Later II and III.

Purpose: Strengthen downward rotators of the scapula.

Positioning: Patient is prone with the shoulder over the edge of the table. Weight is in the hand, and the hand is in a neutral position.

Execution: Keeping the scapula depressed, the patient moves the upper extremity into full hyperextension at the shoulder (figure 19.68).

Possible Substitutions: Elbow flexion and shoulder shrugging.

Cues and Notations: Latissimus pulldowns are an advanced exercise for downward rotation. The hands are shoulder-width apart on the lat bar, and the elbows are kept straight throughout the exercise. Keeping the scapulae set, the patient brings the arms down to the front of the thighs.

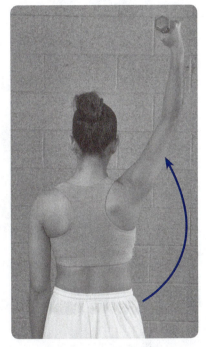

▶ **Figure 19.67** Scapular upward rotation.

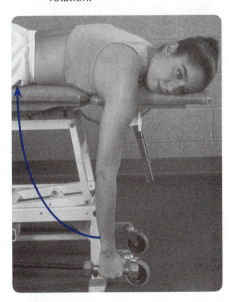

▶ **Figure 19.68** Scapular downward rotation.

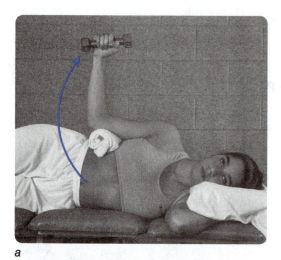

a

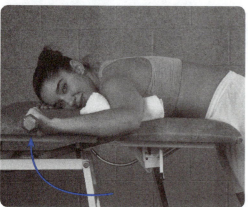

b

Glenohumeral Lateral Rotation

Body Segment: Glenohumeral joint.

Stage in Rehab: II and III.

Purpose: Strengthen teres minor, infraspinatus, and posterior deltoid.

Positioning:

1. In side-lying on the uninvolved side with a towel roll placed under the arm, the patient positions the elbow at 90° (figure 19.69a).

2. The patient is in prone with the shoulder at 90° abduction (figure 19.69b).

3. The patient is in standing with an elastic band or rubber tubing, with the elbow at the side (figure 19.69c).

In all positions, a rolled towel is placed between the elbow and the side.

Execution:

1. For 1 above, patient lifts the weight upward until the forearm is parallel to the floor. As motion improves, the weight may be lifted toward the ceiling.

2. For 2 above, patient lifts the weight toward the ceiling.

3. For 3 above, patient pulls the band away from the abdomen, keeping the upper arm parallel to the floor.

Possible Substitutions: Elbow extension in positions 1 and 3, elbow flexion in position 2. Shoulder extension in position 1 and 3, shoulder horizontal extension in position 2. Rolling the trunk in all three positions.

Cues and Notations: Exercise should be performed in the scapular plane. Once scapular stability is achieved, this exercise can be performed with the arm abducted to 90°. Initially, it may be necessary to support the elbow (figure 19.69d); but as strength improves, elbow support becomes unnecessary (figure 19.69e). In the elevated position, the elbow remains elevated and the shoulder is maintained at 90° abduction without horizontal adduction or abduction.

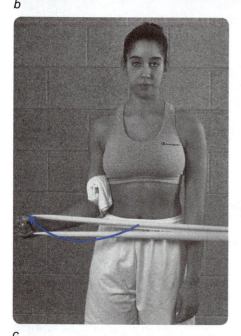

c

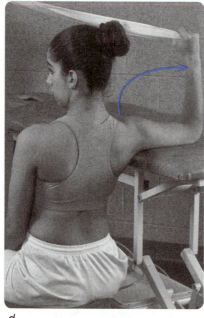

d

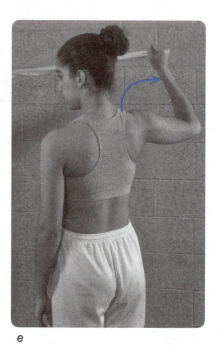

e

▶ **Figure 19.69** Lateral rotation: *(a)* side-lying, *(b)* prone, *(c)* standing, *(d)* in 90° of abduction with support, *(e)* without support.

Medial Rotation of the Glenohumeral Joint

Body Segment: Glenohumeral joint.

Stage in Rehab: II and III.

Purpose: Strengthen subscapularis. This exercise also strengthens the teres major, latissimus dorsi, anterior deltoid, and pectoralis major.

Positioning: The patient can be sidelying on the involved side or supine. In either position, the elbow is flexed to 90°. If the patient is supine, the arm is abducted slightly. If the patient is sidelying, the elbow is next to the side and a towel roll is used to hold the arm in the scapular plane.

Execution: The hand moves toward the abdomen (figure 19.70).

Possible Substitutions: Elbow flexion to 90° is not maintained throughout the motion. Other substitutions include rotating the trunk and flexion of the shoulder.

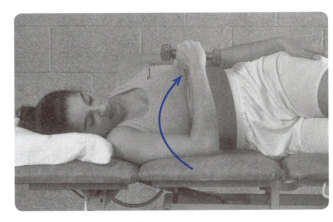

▶ **Figure 19.70** Medial rotation.

Cues and Notations: Once scapular stability is achieved, as with the previous exercise, this exercise can be performed with the arm abducted to 90°. Initially, it may be necessary to support the elbow as is done in figure 19.69d for medial rotation; but as strength improves, elbow support becomes unnecessary. In the elevated position, the elbow remains elevated and the shoulder is maintained at 90° abduction without horizontal adduction or abduction.

Glenohumeral Abduction in the Scapular Plane

Body Segment: Glenohumeral joint.

Stage in Rehab: II and III.

Purpose: Increase supraspinatus strength.

Positioning: Patient stands or sits with a weight in the hand (figure 19.71a).

Execution: The arm is raised in the scapular plane to 90°.

Possible Substitutions: Shoulder flexion, trunk lateral flexion, shoulder shrugging, and elbow flexion.

Cues and Notations: If the patient is unable to control the glenohumeral joint to 90°, the exercise may be performed in side-lying with the involved arm on top. Instructions are to pull the scapula down toward the back pocket while elevating the shoulder. As scapular control improves, the shoulder moves to full elevation (figure 19.71b).

Horizontal Abduction or Horizontal Extension

Body Segment: Glenohumeral joint.

Stage in Rehab: II and III.

Purpose: Strengthen teres minor and infraspinatus muscles. This exercise also strengthens posterior deltoid and scapular stabilizers.

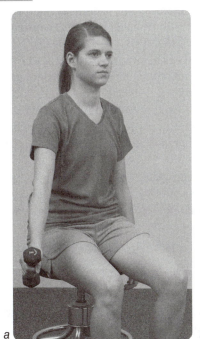
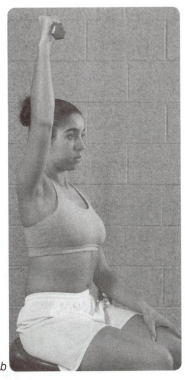

a b

▶ **Figure 19.71** Shoulder abduction in scapular plane (scaption): *(a)* start position with thumbs up and lateral rotation, *(b)* end position with thumbs up and lateral rotation.

Positioning: Patient lies prone with the arm over the edge of the table. Weight is in the hand.

Execution: The arm is lifted toward the ceiling into horizontal extension (abduction) with the shoulder in lateral rotation.

Possible Substitutions: Rolling the trunk rather than lifting the arm, moving out of the plane of motion, placing the hand closer to the hip, flexing the elbow.

Cues and Notations: This is similar to the prone fly but concentrates more on the rotator cuff lateral rotators.

Glenohumeral Exercises

Glenohumeral exercises performed in the lower levels of shoulder elevation emphasize the glenohumeral muscles. Once the shoulder is elevated, scapular muscles are also stressed with the exercise to maintain the shoulder position. Early strengthening of the shoulder start in the lower levels of elevation (first 60°) until sufficient scapular muscle strength is present for stabilizing the shoulder in its correct position. I divide shoulder exercises into three levels: below 60°, 60° to 100°, and above 100°. As shoulder elevation increases, scapular muscles must work harder to provide both scapular stabilization and scapular motion simultaneously (Bagg & Forrest, 1988). Because scapular stabilization is a prerequisite to good glenohumeral motion, scapular muscle strength is achieved in the low ranges of motion first and then in the middle ranges of shoulder motion before advancing to end ranges of motion.

Glenohumeral abduction motion occurs through force-couple activity of the deltoid with the supraspinatus. The other rotator cuff muscles also play an important role during shoulder abduction and flexion as they co-contract during abduction to depress the humeral head into the glenoid. Thus, the rotator cuff and deltoid collectively stabilize the glenohumeral joint during elevation activities. It is important that the scapular stabilizers also work to position the scapula during abduction. In the early strengthening stages it may be necessary to remind the patient to fix or "set" the scapula before moving the humerus so that proper sequencing of shoulder motion occurs.

Abduction can be performed in the coronal plane, but the recommendation is to perform this movement in the scapular plane, approximately 30° forward of the frontal plane. This position maximally facilitates the rotator cuff muscles. This position of the humerus in the plane of the scapula is called **scaption,** a term originally created and defined by Jacqueline Perry, M.D. (Perry, 1993a, 1993b).

Studies have demonstrated that the best position to strengthen the supraspinatus is with the hand in a full-can position rather than an empty-can position (Blackburn, McLeod, White, & Wofford, 1990; Reinold et al., 2007). The full-can exercise is commonly performed in one of two positions, prone or standing. However, the deltoid muscle works more when the patient lies prone than when the patient stands, so the best position in which to strengthen the supraspinatus is in a standing position using the open-can hand position (Reinold et al., 2007). The elbow is maintained in an extended position as the arm is elevated in the scapular plane.

The empty-can exercise is also performed in the scapular plane, but the shoulder is medially rotated. Although this position facilitates the supraspinatus and deltoid (Reinold et al., 2007), it may also aggravate the supraspinatus tendon by impinging it if the rotator cuff is not strong enough to counterbalance the deltoid (Reinold et al., 2007).

Key Shoulder Exercises

For several years, many clinical researchers have looked at various exercises to identify which exercises are most important for shoulder and scapular muscle strength gains. Because there are so many muscles and even more exercises, most investigators focus on one or a few muscles. Hence, many investigations are required before all answers as to what exercises should be used are provided. Occasionally, there is a conflict between research findings because protocols and methods of exercise execution, number of subjects studied, or any other number of variables are different between studies. The information in table 19.1 provides a summary of the results from several investigations (Bradley & Tibone, 1991; Decker, Hintermeister, Faber, & Hawkins, 1999; Ekstrom, Bifulco, Lopau, Andersen, & Gough, 2004; Hardwick, Beebe, McDonnell, & Lang, 2006; Hintermeister, Lange, Schultheis, Bey, & Hawkins, 1998; Kuechle et al., 2000; McCabe, Orishimo, McHugh, & Nicholas, 2007; Moseley, Jobe, Pink, Perry, & Tibone, 1992; Reinold et al., 2007; Reinold et al., 2004; Townsend, Jobe, Pink, & Perry, 1991; Uhl, Carver, Mattacola, Mair, & Nitz, 2003).

Exercises for strengthening the shoulder begin with isometric activities and straight-plane isotonic exercises, then progress to multiplane and diagonal exercises.

TABLE 19.1 Summary of Optimal Shoulder Rehabilitation Exercises

Shoulder complex segment	Muscle	Exercises
Scapula	Serratus anterior	Push-up plus, scaption elevation, dynamic hug, shoulder abduction, seated rowing
Scapula	Lower trapezius	Press-up, bilateral scapular retraction, scaption elevation, seated rowing, shoulder abduction
Scapula	Middle trapezius and rhomboids	Horizontal abduction, seated rowing
Scapula	Upper trapezius	Scaption elevation, seated rowing
Scapula	Pectoralis minor	Push-up plus, scaption elevation, press-up
Humerus: rotator cuff	Supraspinatus	Scaption elevation, horizontal abduction at 100° in prone, military press
Humerus: rotator cuff	Infraspinatus and teres minor	Lateral rotation in side-lying, horizontal abduction, scaption elevation, abduction (both); weight-bearing exercises (infraspinatus)
Humerus: rotator cuff	Subscapularis	Medial rotation, scaption elevation
Humerus: large movers	Anterior deltoid	Scaption elevation, military press, shoulder abduction
Humerus: large movers	Middle deltoid	Scaption elevation, seated rowing, shoulder abduction, military press
Humerus: large movers	Posterior deltoid	Seated rowing, horizontal abduction, shoulder extension
Humerus: large movers	Pectoralis major	Press-up, push-up
Humerus: large movers	Latissimus dorsi	Press-up

Based on data from Bradley and Tibone 1991; Decker, Hintermeister, Faber, and Hawkins 1999; Ekstrom, Bifulco, Lopau, Andersen, and Gough 2004; Hardwick, Beebe, McDonnell, and Lang 2006; Hintermeister, Lange, Schultheis, Bey, and Hawkins 1998; Kuechle et al. 2000; McCann, Wooten, Kadaba, and Bigliani 1993; Moseley, Jobe, Pink, Perry, and Tibone 1992; Reinold et al. 2007; Reinold et al. 2004; Townsend, Jobe, Pink, and Perry 1991; Uhl, Carver, Mattacola, Mair, and Nitz 2003. Exercises are listed only if they were used in more than one research study.

STABILIZATION EXERCISES

The importance of stability during shoulder motion cannot be overstated. As previously discussed, trunk or core stabilization must provide a firm base from which the scapula can operate. Scapular stabilization must provide a firm foundation for shoulder movement. Rotator cuff stabilization allows the humerus smooth, synchronous glenohumeral motion for functional upper-extremity activity.

Trunk stabilization exercises are discussed in chapter 18. A few will be mentioned later in this chapter, but only as they relate to shoulder exercises. Refer to chapter 18 for specific trunk stabilization exercises.

Shoulder stabilization exercises are important in that they aid strength development. They also facilitate neuromuscular reeducation of the shoulder. They stimulate the afferent receptors to provide appropriate feedback into the central nervous system, to reeducate and reactivate the proprioceptive pathways that will eventually lead to proper functional performance.

Although some of these exercises are open kinetic chain activities, many are closed kinetic chain activities. One can argue that because most people involved in physical activity do not perform closed kinetic chain activities, use of closed kinetic chain exercises for the upper extremities is not germane in a rehabilitation program. However, closed kinetic chain exercises are useful for the upper extremity for a couple of reasons. In a closed-chain position, the shoulder has more stability through increased joint congruity; less stress is applied to the ligaments, and joint proprioceptors are stimulated (Myers et al., 2006). Closed kinetic chain exercise also facilitates cocontraction of muscles around the joint (Zhang, 2007). This cocontraction during closed kinetic chain exercises permits stabilization activities to be initiated with less shear force applied to the static structures and also facilitates dynamic stabilization of the joints (Lephart & Henry, 1996).

It is not necessary that every exercise mimic functional motions. In fact, in the early and middle stages of rehabilitation, it is important to improve muscle strength before functional movements are safely executed. Neither straight-plane exercises nor pure closed kinetic chain exercises are necessarily functional; they do not mimic most of the shoulder's functional movements. They are crucial in a therapeutic exercise program, though, in that they facilitate, develop, and improve specific muscle activity that permits progression to functional shoulder movement.

Scapular Stabilization

Because scapular stability is vital to functional shoulder motions, scapular stabilization exercises should begin early in the rehabilitation program, in late phase II or early phase III. Scapular stabilization exercises should be included in any shoulder rehabilitation program. A variety of scapular stabilization exercises are provided in the following sections.

The progression begins with isometric stabilization exercises and advances to stabilization during arm movement, first in simple planes and then in diagonal planes. The progression also begins with movements in the lower shoulder positions (30°-60° elevation) where the scapula has relatively little motion and its muscles work to primarily stabilize, or set, the scapular for glenohumeral motion and advances to middle-range positions of shoulder elevation (60°-100°) where the scapular muscles must work to stabilize and move the scapula simultaneously (McCabe et al., 2007). Exercises in shoulder positions over 100° are initiated only after strength and control in the lower ranges are achieved; it is in the higher ranges of motion that the scapular muscles are most stressed as they must continue to provide glenohumeral stability and also work to move the scapula in its final degrees of motion when the muscles are at their shortest and weakest positions (McCabe et al., 2007). In the final phases of stabilization, movements include a combination of high (over 100° elevation) and low joint positions, use increased resistance, and are performed with greater speeds. These activities then become more functionally based.

■ Scapular Stabilization Exercises

Swiss Ball Stabilization

Body Segment: Scapula.

Stage in Rehab: II.

Purpose: Basic exercise to improve scapular stabilization early in rehab.

Positioning: Ball is placed on a table or on the floor.

Execution: Patient bears weight through the shoulder as the ball is moved from side to side, forward and backward, and in circles.

If the patient does not have 90° of shoulder motion so the Swiss ball activity is not possible, the patient can begin in lower degrees by placing the ball on a table, on the floor, or on a wall. The patient bears weight on the upper extremity and rolls the ball in varying patterns.

Possible Substitutions: Using the trunk to move the ball rather than the shoulder.

Cues and Notations: The patient should move his or her body forward and back and from side to side on the ball while maintaining weight bearing through the upper extremities (figure 19.72a).

A more advanced weight-bearing exercise with the Swiss ball has the patient's lower body on a table and the hands placed on the ball while the upper body is over the edge of the table. The patient moves the ball out and away from the body as far as possible, then moves the ball closer (figure 19.72b).

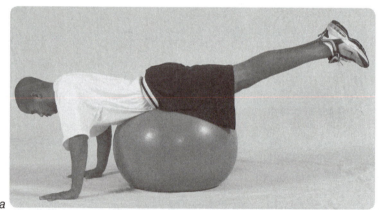

a

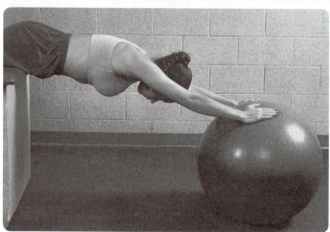

b

▶ **Figure 19.72**   Swiss ball weight-bearing exercises: *(a)* prone on a ball, *(b)* prone on a table.

Rhythmic Stabilization 1

Body Segment: Scapula.

Stage in Rehab: II.

Purpose: Reeducate the proprioceptors and improve kinesthetic awareness.

Positioning: Patient is supine with the arm in a scapular plane and elevated to 100°.

Execution: The patient holds a weight in the hand with the shoulder in a specific position, maintaining the angle with the eyes closed (figure 19.73a). As an alternative, the clinician can offer manual resistance in different directions while the patient provides an isometric resistance to the movements.

Possible Substitutions: Flexing the elbow, lowering the shoulder to below 100°.

Cues and Notations: The exercise can be repeated in different positions, each time requiring the patient to maintain the desired position of the shoulder with the eyes closed.

Rhythmic Stabilization 2

Body Segment: Scapula.

Stage in Rehab: II.

Purpose: Reeducate the proprioceptors and improve kinesthetic awareness.

Positioning: Patient stands and bears weight on the arms on a tabletop.

Execution: The clinician provides resistance to the patient as the patient shifts weight from one arm to the other, attempting to move the patient off balance (figure 19.73b).

Possible Substitutions: Using the legs more than the arms to provide stability.

Cues and Notations: Progression can advance to using only the involved upper extremity on the table.

Rhythmic Stabilization in Quadruped 3

Body Segment: Scapula.

Stage in Rehab: II and III.

Purpose: Reeducate the proprioceptors and improve kinesthetic awareness.

Positioning: Shoulders are directly over the hands, and the hips are forward of the knees so the weight is primarily on the upper extremities.

Execution: The simplest exercise is to have the patient shift weight from the left to the right arm. The clinician offers manual resistance as the patient attempts to stabilize in the quadruped position, attempting to move the patient off balance (figure 19.73c). Once the patient can stabilize without difficulty, he or she balances in a tripod position with the uninvolved arm off the table (figure 19.73d). From this exercise the patient can advance to a biped position, with the involved arm and the opposite leg bearing the weight (figure 19.73e).

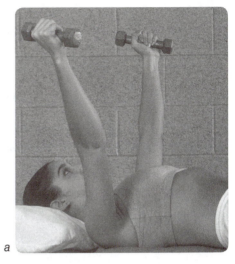

a

▶ **Figure 19.73** Rhythmic stabilization: *(a)* open kinetic chain.

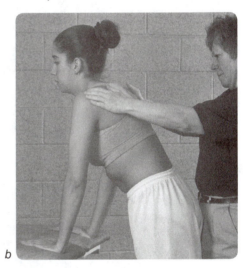

b

▶ **Figure 19.73** Rhythmic stabilization: *(b)* weight bearing in standing.

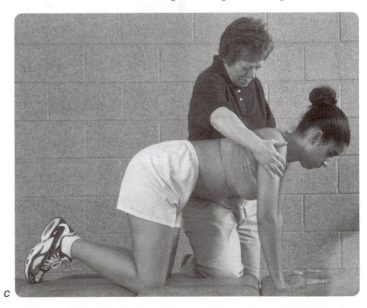

c

▶ **Figure 19.73** Rhythmic stabilization: *(c)* quadruped weight bearing.

Possible Substitutions: Using the legs more than the arms to stabilize the trunk.

Cues and Notations: If the patient is unable to hold this position, the hips may be positioned directly over the knees to equalize weight distribution between the upper and lower extremities.

For additional challenge, you can provide resistance to the uninvolved arm using a pulley or resistance band while the involved arm maintains balance (figure 19.73f), or you can apply PNF manual resistance to the uninvolved arm (figure 19.73g).

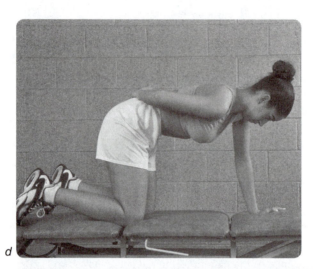

d

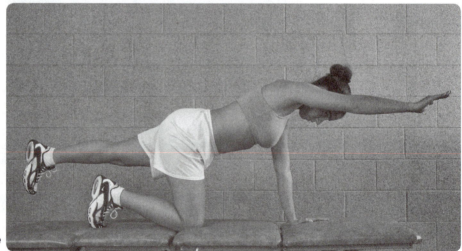

e

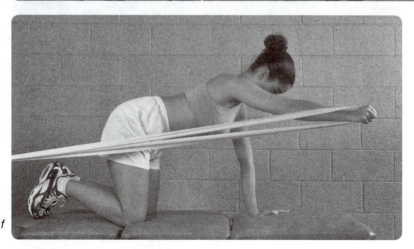

f

▶ **Figure 19.73** Rhythmic stabilization: *(d)* tripod weight bearing, *(e)* bipod weight bearing, *(f)* with a resistance band providing resistance to uninvolved extremity.

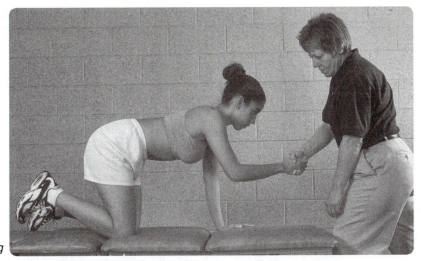

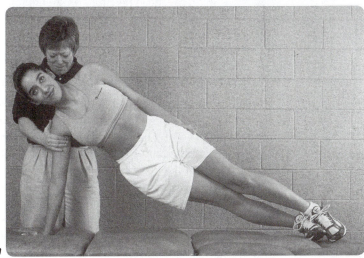

▶ **Figure 19.73** Rhythmic stabilization: *(g)* with proprioceptive neuro-muscular facilitation manual resistance to uninvolved extremity, *(h)* unilateral weight bearing.

Rhythmic Stabilization 4

Body Segment: Scapula.

Stage in Rehab: III.

Purpose: Reeducate the proprioceptors and improve kinesthetic awareness.

Positioning: Patient is in a sidelying position. The involved upper extremity and its ipsilateral lower extremity are on the floor with the patient's lower extremities in full extension and one leg on top of the other. The patient then lifts the body upward into a side-bridge position so the body's weight is on the involved upper extremity's hand and the ipsilateral foot (figure 19.73h).

Execution: The clinician provides manual resistance as the patient attempts to maintain balance.

Possible Substitutions: Flexing at the trunk, placing the knees on the floor.

Cues and Notations: This is a difficult exercise that may not be indicated for all patients.

Distal Movement Stabilization

These activities involve movement of the distal extremity, requiring movement control and strength as well as stabilization of the shoulder. You must be careful to have the patient maintain correct scapular position throughout each of these exercises. Verbal cueing may be necessary as a reminder to maintain proper scapular positioning. In one activity the patient

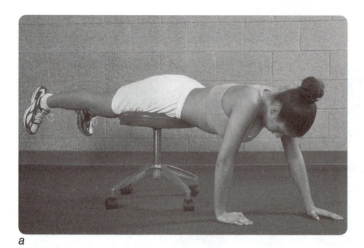

a

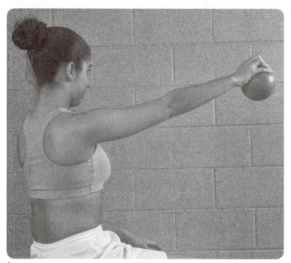

b

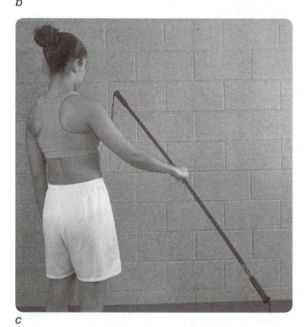

c

lies prone with a roller stool under the hips or pelvis; feet are off the floor and hands are on the floor. The patient then moves across the floor, using only the arms to move the roller stool (figure 19.74a). Another distal movement activity is performed with a weighted ball in the hand. The patient stands or sits with the arm outstretched at from 60° to 110° elevation in the scapular plane. In this position, the patient spells out the alphabet with the ball (figure 19.74b). Heavier balls provide additional resistance.

The Body Blade (Hymanson, Inc., Los Angeles, CA), B.O.I.N.G. (exclusively distributed by OPTP, Minneapolis, MN), and other commercially available rhythmic-wand equipment are useful in rhythmic stabilization exercises. They can be used in different positions, beginning in the scapular plane at 30° elevation (figure 19.74c) and advancing to overhead positions as strength improves.

Upper-body ergometers are another means of offering distal movement and proximal stabilization. These machines also provide cardiovascular exercise.

Proprioceptive Neuromuscular Facilitation

Proprioceptive neuromuscular facilitation (PNF) is useful in shoulder rehabilitation. There are a number of advantages to using PNF. There is no cost because this form of exercise uses the clinician's manual resistance; PNF is appropriate throughout most of the program. In the early rehabilitation stages, PNF can enhance neuromuscular control, and at later stages it can improve strength and coordination of muscle firing. Techniques include isometrics, concentrics, eccentrics, and rhythmic stabilization. Proprioceptive neuromuscular facilitation incorporates functional positions because it uses multiplane motions.

In the early rehabilitation stages, PNF is commonly used for rhythmic stabilization (figure 19.75). This assists in reeducating synchronous muscle firing and providing joint stability. Moving

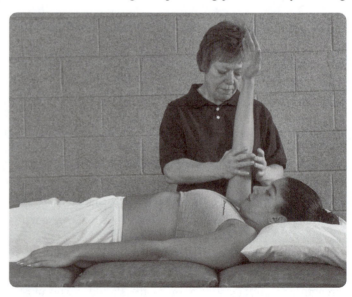

▶ **Figure 19.74** Distal movement stabilization exercises: *(a)* walk while prone on roller stool, *(b)* alphabet with distal weight, *(c)* rhythmic wand.

▶ **Figure 19.75** Proprioceptive neuromuscular facilitation: rhythmic stabilization.

through functional patterns can stimulate neuromuscular control for stability and synchronous patterns of movement. The rehabilitation clinician provides isometric resistance at points in the range of motion that are weak.

In later rehabilitation stages, PNF can increase coordination through use of eccentric resistance in functional planes and through use of combinations of eccentric with concentric and isometric resistance as the arm moves through its motion patterns. In this activity, the patient attempts to move the arm through either a D1 or D2 flexion-extension pattern at a constant rate of speed as the rehabilitation clinician provides various types of resistance—eccentric, concentric, and isometric.

Advanced Open Chain Exercises

These exercises can incorporate various types of equipment. They are performed unsupported, first in straight-plane and then in diagonal positions. The unsupported position is the primary distinction between these and earlier exercises.

Isokinetic Exercises

Many rehabilitation facilities have isokinetic machines. These machines can be useful for monitoring and advancing shoulder strength. Unless the unit is used for range of motion or isometrics, isokinetic machines are generally not introduced into a rehabilitation program until the later stages after healing is to a level where injured structures will tolerate the stresses that these machines produce. Early exercises are performed in straight-plane motions, isolating specific muscles to perform the desired activity. As the patient's strength improves, diagonal patterns are used and the patient performs a more normal movement pattern using a summation of trunk and hip forces to produce normal shoulder motion (figure 19.76).

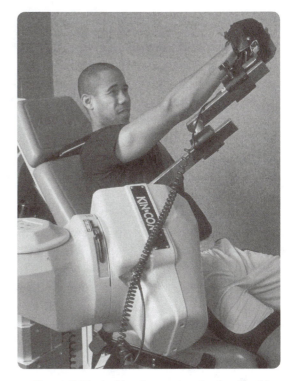

▶ **Figure 19.76** Isokinetic exercises for the shoulder.

Open Chain Elastic-Band Exercises

Elastic-band or rubber-tubing activities in an open kinetic chain provide another type of resistive exercises to challenge the patient. The challenge is to maintain stability during resisted arm movement. This is the next step after closed kinetic chain stabilization exercises. The patient is now required to execute resistive exercises without the feedback of the clinician in PNF and without the feedback of joint compression that closed kinetic chain activities provide. These exercises include a combination of concentric and eccentric resistance. The need for dynamic stabilization during these exercises more closely resembles functional activity demands, and these exercises prepare the shoulder for the next level of resistive exercises, plyometrics.

Straight-Plane Exercises

By now the patient should be able to maintain joint stability with the arm in at least 45°-60° of elevation. Straight-plane exercises include medial and lateral rotation with the elbow at shoulder level and in the scapular plane. As control is achieved, the arm is elevated to 90° (figure 19.77). You must correct errors in execution. Common errors include dropping the elbow, horizontally extending the arm during lateral rotation and horizontally flexing it during medial rotation, and flexing the elbow during lateral rotation and extending it during medial rotation.

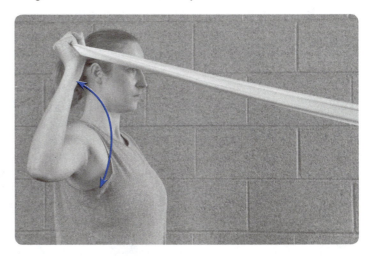

▶ **Figure 19.77** Straight-plane external elastic-band exercises.

Diagonal-Plane Exercises

These exercises are performed once the patient demonstrates proper stabilization and control in straight-plane exercises. Proprioceptive neuromuscular facilitation movements in D1 and D2 flexion and extension patterns are used (figure 19.78). It is important for the patient to execute the motion correctly and to maintain appropriate joint stability throughout the motion. Joint stability is not maintained if the patient shrugs the shoulder during activity or initiates the activity with a shoulder shrug.

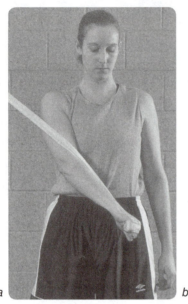
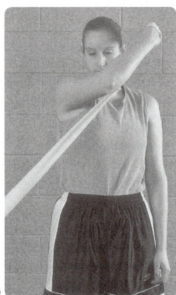
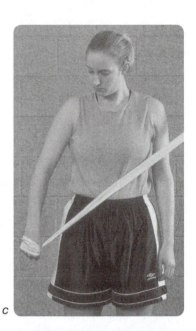

a b c

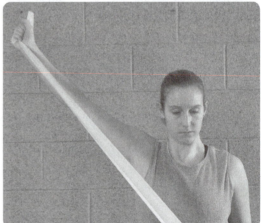

d

▶ **Figure 19.78** Diagonal-plane exercises: *(a)* D2 extension, *(b)* D1 flexion, *(c)* D1 extension, *(d)* D2 flexion.

PLYOMETRIC EXERCISES

For shoulder-related fact sheets and patient information brochures and booklets, see the American Academy of Orthopaedic Surgeons Web site at: http://orthoinfo.aaos.org/menus/arm.cfm

Once the patient has achieved strength and static and simple dynamic stabilization control, he or she progresses to plyometric exercises before performing functional activities. Plyometrics are the most demanding in the series outlined because they require maximum strength, optimal joint stabilization during high-level dynamic activities, and agility and coordination throughout the activity. The following sections provide some examples of plyometric exercises for the shoulder girdle.

The medicine-ball exercises begin with a lightweight ball—approximately 0.9 kg (2 lb)—and can progress as the patient is able to maintain control and still execute the exercise correctly.

■ Plyometric Exercises for the Shoulder Girdle

Dynamic Stabilization on Unstable Surfaces

Body Segment: Upper extremity.

Stage in Rehab: III.

Purpose: Challenge muscles to provide stability to the shoulder during motion.

Positioning: A slide board, Fitter, Swiss ball, or other apparatus may be used to challenge balance.

Execution: Patient places the hands on the surface of the slide board, Fitter, Swiss ball or other apparatus and attempts to maintain balance while moving the arms (figure 19.79a-c). Depending on the apparatus used, arm motions may include lateral, up-and-down, or circular motions.

Possible Substitutions: Using the trunk to move the arms or the hips to control the motion.

Cues and Notations: One progression includes having the patient move from weight bearing on the knees to weight bearing on the feet, and a more difficult progression consists of making both the hand surface and the lower-extremity surface unstable.

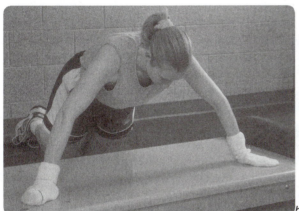

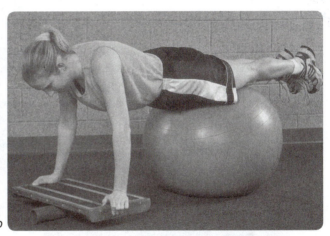

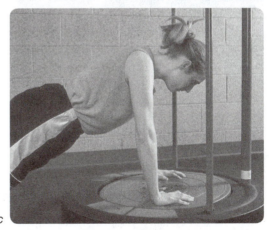

▶ **Figure 19.79** Unstable surface exercises: *(a)* slide board while on knees, *(b)* balance board, *(c)* commercially available balance system.

Plyometric Push-Ups

Body Segment: Upper extremity.

Stage in Rehab: III.

Purpose: Prepare muscles for functional activity with sudden eccentric-concentric exercises while maintaining control of the shoulder.

Positioning: The progression of plyometric push-ups begins with a wall push-up. The patient stands farther than an arm's length from the wall and places the hands at shoulder level on the wall.

Execution: The patient pushes him- or herself away from the wall with enough force to remove the hands from the wall. When the patient's hands come off the wall, the rehabilitation clinician pushes the patient back toward the wall, and the patient stops the movement toward the wall by "catching" him- or herself with both hands on the wall. The impact force is absorbed by bending of the elbows as the body returns to the starting position.

This exercise progresses to an incline push-up. The patient pushes off the incline support, such as a tabletop or counter, to lose hand contact and is pushed back to the start position by the clinician as done with the wall push-ups.

An additional progression involves having the patient perform a regular or modified push-up, first with the uninvolved hand on a medicine ball and the involved hand on the floor, then with both hands on the ball (figure 19.80, a & b).

Possible Substitutions: Flexing at the trunk, not flexing the elbows to absorb the force. Not standing far enough from the wall to perform a good plyometric exercise.

Cues and Notations: Plyometric push-ups can also be performed on a trampoline. With the patient in a regular push-up position and the hands on the trampoline, the individual "jumps" the hands off the trampoline and lands them out to the side, then "jumps" them back to the center on the next push-up movement. The most difficult plyometric push-up is performed with boxes (figure 19.80c). Two boxes of the same height are placed on either side of the patient. The recommended starting height is 10 to 15 cm (3-6 in.). The patient begins with the hands on the floor in either a modified or regular push-up position and pushes up and away from the floor to position each hand on the adjacent box. Progressions include having the patient move his or her lower-extremity support from the knees to the feet and making both the hand surface and the lower-extremity surface unstable.

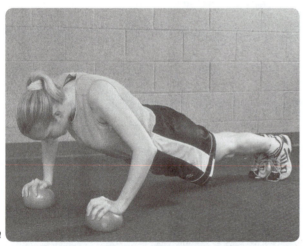

a

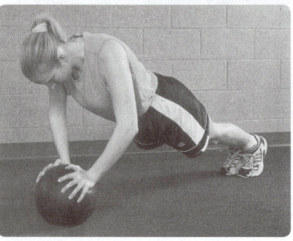

b

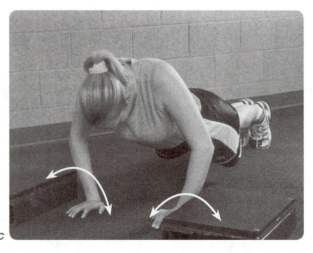

c

▶ **Figure 19.80** Plyometric push-up variations: *(a)* push-up with hands on small medicine balls, *(b)* push-up with both hands on one large medicine ball, *(c)* box jump.

Resisted Movements in Weight Bearing

Body Segment: Upper extremity.

Stage in Rehab: III.

Purpose: Facilitate muscle control, endurance, and coordination.

Positioning: The patient begins with hands on the machine and knees on the floor.

Execution: The patient "walks" the hands as the treadmill belt or stair machine steps move (figure 19.81, a & b).

Possible Substitutions: Shoulder shrugging.

Cues and Notations: A stair machine, treadmill, or step machine may be used. The speed of the machine depends on the patient's abilities. The recommendation is to use a manual setting initially, but a random setting may be appropriate as the patient progresses. Bouts of 30 s to 1 min provide the patient ample challenge initially. As the patient improves, speed, time, and resistance may be increased. Wearing gloves during the exercise will protect the patient's hands.

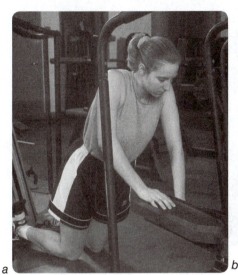 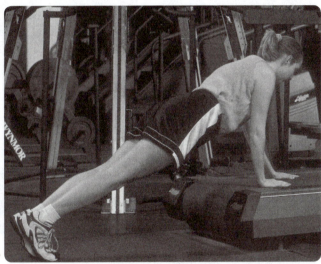

a   b

▶ **Figure 19.81** Resisted movement in weight bearing: *(a)* on stair machine on knees, *(b)* on treadmill on toes.

Medicine-Ball Rotation Progression

Body Segment: Upper extremity.

Stage in Rehab: III.

Purpose: Progress eccentric levels of lateral rotators from a supported to an unsupported position.

Positioning:

1. The patient is in supine and the shoulder at 90° abduction and laterally rotated with the entire arm supported on the table. The forearm should be supported on the table to prevent excessive lateral rotation during the initial phases of this progression.

2. The patient is in the same position as just described.

3. The patient stands, kneels, or sits on a Swiss ball. The patient must maintain an elevated elbow at 90° of shoulder abduction and elbow flexion.

Execution:

1. The medicine ball is dropped from the level of the rehabilitation clinician's shoulder to the patient's hand. Initially, the patient only catches the ball but should quickly advance to catching and tossing the ball back to the clinician (figure 19.82a).

2. The clinician stands away from the patient toward the patient's feet and tosses the ball to the patient. The patient catches the ball and returns the toss, keeping the shoulder at 90° abduction and allowing the shoulder to laterally rotate as the ball is caught. The arm moves into medial rotation when the ball is thrown back to the rehabilitation clinician (figure 19.82b).

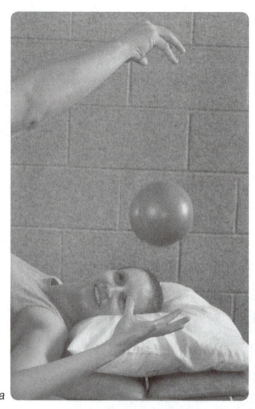

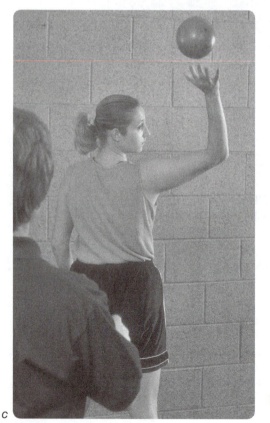

▶ **Figure 19.82** Medicine-ball progression: *(a)* drop-and-catch, *(b)* standing forward toss.

3. Tosses continue without support to the elbow or arm. Motion is smooth from eccentric external rotation to concentric external rotation.

Possible Substitutions: Flexing the elbow, dropping the elbow, moving the shoulder in front of the body.

Cues and Notations:

1. When the individual can perform this exercise without pain and through good motion for the desired repetitions, the next level of exercise begins.

2. Progression to the next level occurs when the patient performs the exercise for the desired repetitions with good control and good lateral rotation during the catch and shows a smooth transition to medial rotation.

3. This exercise increases the eccentric and concentric requirements of the shoulder.

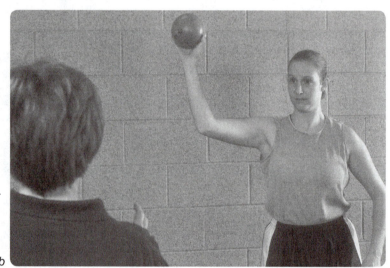

Medicine-Ball Rotation

Body Segment: Upper extremity.

Stage in Rehab: III.

Purpose: Eccentric-concentric activity for the shoulder lateral rotators.

Positioning: The patient stands, kneels, or sits on a Swiss ball with his or her back to the clinician. The patient must maintain an elevated elbow at 90° of shoulder abduction and elbow flexion.

Execution: The clinician tosses the medicine ball to the patient; the patient catches the ball with the shoulder in lateral rotation, then allows the weight of the ball to pull the shoulder into medial rotation before throwing the ball back to the clinician (figure 19.82c).

Possible Substitutions: Dropping the shoulder, twisting the body too much, using too much elbow flexion.

Cues and Notations: Increasing the distance and repetitions increases the difficulty of the exercise. The patient must maintain an elevated elbow with the shoulder at 90° of abduction.

▶ **Figure 19.82** Medicine-ball progression: *(c)* backward toss.

Rotational Tosses

Body Segment: Upper extremity and trunk.

Stage in Rehab: III.

Purpose: Enhance coordination of the trunk and shoulder.

Positioning: Patient stands with the back to the wall. The arms are maintained at a low level initially (figure 19.83a), then raised as shoulder strength and control improve.

Execution: Standing far enough from the wall, the patient tosses the ball to the wall as trunk rotation occurs. He or she catches the ball and winds the trunk away from the wall, then repeats the toss.

Possible Substitutions: Stopping between trunk rotation and ball toss.

Cues and Notations: As strength improves, the arms are elevated higher (figure 19.83b). Overhead toss exercises can be performed in standing or kneeling.

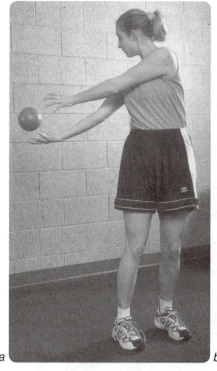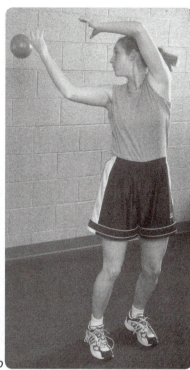

a   b

▶ **Figure 19.83** Rotational medicine-ball tosses: *(a)* backward with arms at low level; *(b)* backward overhead toss, standing.

Overhead Tosses

Body Segment: Upper extremity and trunk.

Stage in Rehab: III.

Purpose: Enhance trunk and shoulder coordination and strength.

Positioning: Patient is supine on the floor with the knees and hips flexed. The hands are overhead.

Execution: The patient tosses the ball to the clinician and moves into a sit-up position as the ball is released. The patient stays in the sit-up position until the clinician tosses the ball back, aiming overhead so that the patient must reach overhead to catch the ball. The patient simultaneously catches the ball and returns to the start position (figure 19.83c).

Possible Substitutions: Using the legs to curl up rather than the abdominal muscles; moving the trunk and shoulders as two separate entities rather than together.

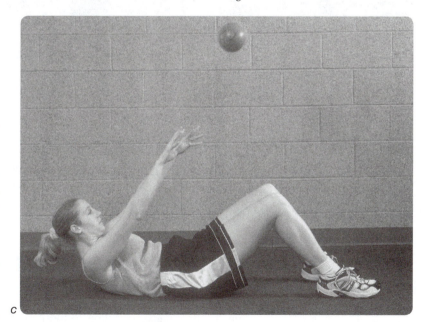

c

▶ **Figure 19.83** Rotational medicine-ball toss: *(c)* overhead toss, supine.

Cues and Notations: Trunk rotation can also be incorporated by having two people, one on either side of the patient (about 30° to 45° to the side), catch the ball. The patient tosses to one and receives the ball, then tosses to the other.

Patients who have achieved strength and stability of the shoulder can go on to perform plyometric exercises on unstable surfaces, plyometric push-ups, weight-bearing activities, and medicine-ball exercises.

FUNCTIONAL AND ACTIVITY-SPECIFIC EXERCISES

By the time functional activities become the emphasis of a therapeutic exercise program, the specifics of the program are dictated by the patient's normal activity demands. If a patient participates in a throwing sport, during the plyometric exercise phase he or she can begin throw-

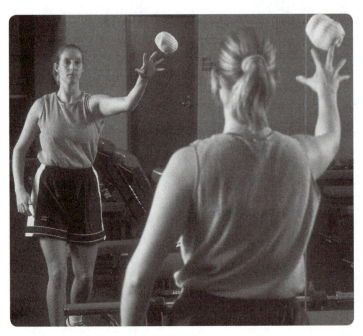

▶ **Figure 19.84**   Mirror feedback.

ing a foam rubber ball or knotted sock toward a mirror, watching for form and motion pattern (figure 19.84). A tennis player can begin forehand and backhand strokes in the same manner in front of a mirror. This helps to promote proprioception and correct technique through the additional afferent feedback that comes from the visual system.

Chapter 10 covers progressive functional programs, outlining specific sequences of exercises as a guide for setting a patient on a course of functional return to full activity participation. The most important point to remember is that the program must present a gradual progression of time, resistance, and/or distance. One element of an activity is increased at a time to allow the body time to adjust to new stresses. For example, if a pitcher increases throwing speed from 50% to 75% of his or her normal speed, throwing distance or repetitions remain unchanged for the session. An increase in the program is usually added only every third day of activity, so after the third day of increased speed, the pitcher's throwing distance can increase. This allows the body the time it needs for adjustment to new levels of stress before application of additional levels. For example, if a golfer is now able to perform a full swing with the long irons, it will be three days before he or she advances to using the woods.

In overhead events, the patient progresses through a program of low- and medium-height movements and attempts high movements last. For example, a tennis player begins functional activities with forehand and backhand groundstrokes. It is not until the individual accomplishes full-distance and full-force hits with these strokes that he or she progresses to overhead strokes. Because serves are the most strenuous activity, they are the last stroke the patient resumes. Partial force is used in the initial stages of serve activities, with progression to normal serves.

Functional exercises for patients with shoulder injuries progress gradually in time, resistance, or distance. For overhead activities, the progression is from lower to higher movements.

SPECIAL REHABILITATION APPLICATIONS

The combination and progression of exercises used in each rehabilitation program are determined individually according to the patient and the injury. Some injuries dictate special concerns for the rehabilitation clinician. Some of these injuries and the concerns unique to them are addressed here.

Shoulder Instability

The shoulder has two systems of stability, the **static restraints** and the **dynamic restraints.** The static restraints include the ligaments, capsule, and glenoid labrum. The dynamic restraints are the neuromuscular components. If the static restraint is damaged by joint sprains, sub-luxations, or dislocations, the neural input from the proprioceptors located within the injured static structures is compromised (Myers et al., 2006). Damage to static restraints also causes a deficiency in muscle function. Instability is the result. A secondary problem that can result from instability is rotator cuff tendinopathy that can lead to rotator cuff tears with repetitive impingement and breakdown. If instability is not corrected either by surgery to reinforce static structures, or by rehabilitation to restore dynamic structures, or both, reinjury is perpetuated with continued activity until the joint becomes so unstable that it may sublux or dislocate or the impinged soft tissues break down and tear with relatively little stress.

Before you design a therapeutic exercise program for a patient with shoulder instability, you must consider several factors. The most common instability is anterior instability, which occurs when anterior structures become damaged. Inferior instability is the result of injury and laxity of the inferior capsule and support structures. Posterior instability, which is less common, occurs with damage to the posterior joint structures.

Two acronyms, AMBRI and TUBS, indicate the difference between non-traumatic and traumatic shoulder instability and present guidelines for treatment. The acronym **AMBRI** stands for "**A**traumatic, **M**ultidirectional, **B**ilateral, **R**ehabilitation effective, **I**nferior capsular shift required." Patients with this condition usually have bilateral shoulder laxity, as well as hypermobility in most joints. The instability is multi-directional but usually responds well to the conservative treatment of rehabilitation. If surgery is necessary, an inferior capsular shift is usually the procedure of choice. More recently, some surgeons have used an electrothermally assisted capsular shift to relieve multi-directional instability (Miniaci & Codsi, 2006).

Anterior Instability

Shoulders with **TUBS** (**T**raumatic, **U**nilateral, **B**ankart lesion, **S**urgery required) are shoulders that have incurred a traumatic injury. A **Bankart lesion,** or tear of the anterior capsulolabral complex, is present and surgery is required to relieve the problem.

Patients in overhead-throwing sports commonly develop anterior instability because the throwing motion places repetitive stresses on the anterior joint structures. Often accompanying and encouraging this problem is a concomitant posterior capsule and rotator cuff tightness of the medial rotators. In these patients, the rehabilitation program for instability should include stretching of these structures.

The rehabilitation processes for surgically corrected anterior instability and non-repaired instability are similar. The greatest differences may be their timelines, but the exercise sequence is essentially the same. A non-repaired shoulder may require longer immobilization time and, thus, a delay in the total rehabilitation process.

Surgical patients undergoing an anterior capsulolabral reconstruction (ACLR) repair have two options, open procedure and an arthroscopic surgical procedure. In the open procedure, an axillary incision over an inch long is made and the muscles are separated rather than cut to view and repair the glenohumeral joint structures, so there is more post-operative pain with the open repair than the arthroscopic repair. In the arthroscopic procedure, the redundancy in the capsule is taken up and the capsule is usually tightened with a pants-over-vest overlap of the redundant capsular portions and secured with either sutures or staples that are attached through an arthroscope. With recent advances in arthroscopic repair of anterior shoulder instability, results are similar for open and arthroscopic repairs (Dietz & Dreese, 2007).

The shoulder is immobilized in a sling for approximately three weeks for the surgically repaired shoulder, but the time in a sling can be longer for the non-repaired shoulder. Older patients are the exception. Patients over 30 are usually started on early postoperative exercise intervention because a frozen shoulder is a common complication if motion is not initiated soon after any surgical shoulder procedure. The time required for a complete rehabilitation program varies from younger to older patients and from one sport to another. Patients in overhead sports such as baseball or volleyball may require a longer rehabilitation process than those whose shoulder demands are minimal, such as soccer players. An average program may take anywhere from 15 to 26 weeks.

After the first week following surgery or injury, the shoulder is taken out of the sling to permit active–assistive range of motion in straight-plane motion. Gentle, passive motion to no more than 0° lateral rotation with the elbow at the side can also begin. Abduction to 30° is also permitted. Isometrics in non-stressful positions begin after the first week. Care must be taken to avoid lateral rotation greater than 20° to 30° and abduction greater than 30° to 40°. The anterior shoulder joint should be minimally stressed during the first three weeks. Manual resistance to scapular stabilizers, avoiding stress to the glenohumeral (GH) joint, should begin early in the program. The most stressful position for the anterior joint is lateral rotation with abduction; this position is avoided for the first several weeks.

During the first two weeks, grade I and II joint mobilization techniques to the GH joint in its resting position may provide pain relief. Simple, mild distraction with oscillation may be beneficial.

During the time the patient is wearing a sling, he or she may develop trigger points in the upper trapezius and levator scapulae as well as other neck and shoulder muscles. These trigger points are identified and treated during this time.

By the end of the second week, elevation in the scapular plane is approximately 135° and by the sixth week, passive shoulder flexion range of motion should be normal. By the sixth week, passive lateral rotation should be approximately 50° to 60° with the elbow at the side. By the 8th to 10th week, full passive range of motion should be present in all motions except lateral rotation, which should be at approximately 75°. Between weeks 10 and 12, full passive motion should be possible in all movements.

After the third week, gentle, active-resistive isotonic exercises for medial rotation, lateral rotation to about 20° to 30° with the elbow near the side, and abduction to 20° can begin in a scapular plane. Scapular exercises should advance as tolerated without the imposition of additional stress on the glenohumeral joint. By the fourth week, horizontal abduction exercises begin.

Joint mobilizations in the grade III range can begin in the third week. These should begin in the resting position. If a capsular pattern is present, the clinician should identify those portions of the capsule that are restricted and perform joint mobilizations to improve mobility in the appropriate ranges. Joint mobilization stress to the anterior capsule should be mild and start at III–.

By the end of the third or fourth week, the shoulder sling is removed. This can be a time of apprehension for the patient. The lack of shoulder support can also be initially fatiguing for the shoulder muscles. The patient should be encouraged to support the extremity throughout the day by placing the forearm on top of a table or desk while sitting, and by putting the hand in a pocket when standing. These actions will provide some muscle rest. With increased muscle demands, trigger point treatment during this time may be effective if trigger points are a source of the patient's discomfort.

By the sixth to tenth week, rotator cuff strength exercises can go through increased ranges of motion as long as the anterior joint is not excessively stressed. The program should continue with low weights and high repetitions. The elbow is kept near the side, but lateral rotation can progress to approximately 45°. Mild isokinetic exercises with the shoulder stabilized can begin during this time.

Joint mobilization by the sixth week can be any grade. By this time, repaired structures are of sufficient strength to withstand joint mobilization forces. It is important that the clinician emphasize attaining full range of motion in all planes by this time. If necessary, the clinician may apply joint mobilization in other loose-pack positions besides the resting position. Home exercises for range of motion gains can also be more aggressive at this time.

When the patient has full lateral rotation, eccentric exercises can begin. These start with the arm in the low position, less than 60°, and progress to the higher positions as tolerated. Once strength and control of the joints during motion are achieved, overhead activities, plyometrics, and finally functional activities can be added to the therapeutic exercise program.

Active-assistive exercises that do not stress the anterior capsule begin within the first two weeks following surgery, according to the patient's tolerance and physician's instructions. Scapular exercises that do not stress the glenohumeral joint are also incorporated early in the program. Rubber tubing or band resistance exercises for the glenohumeral rotators start around the third week and progress to weights as tolerated. Progressive scapular strengthening also continues. Isotonic exercises are well engrained in the program by the third month when the patient should have about two-thirds normal strength in the shoulder. Once the involved shoulder is around 75% strength compared to the contralateral extremity, functional and then sport-specific activities are added to the program.

Throughout the program, the clinician must receive feedback from the patient about the shoulder's response to activity. Pain should not be present with any activities. Scapular stability must be present before the patient advances to activities that place the arm above shoulder level. If this precept is not respected, rotator cuff tendinopathy may occur and delay the patient's return to sport participation.

Sport-specific progressions will depend upon the specific sport and the individual. Throwing, pitching, golf, swimming, tennis, volleyball and any other overhead sport will require the clinician to develop a progressive program. Speed or force, distance, repetitions, and types of throws or hits are all variables that are altered as the patient progresses in the sport-specific progression. Every session should include a warm-up and cool-down of easy performance activities. Speed or force is usually the last factor to increase after the other factors have improved without pain.

Posterior Instability

Traumatic posterior instability most often occurs from a fall on an outstretched, adducted and medially rotated shoulder. Impact forces are directed through the extremity, forcing the humeral head posteriorly. Football linemen, swimmers, pitchers, and tennis players are more susceptible to posterior instability problems because of chronic anterior-to-posterior forces applied to the shoulder during their specific activities.

Following a posterior instability injury, positions that put stress on the posterior capsule are initially avoided: flexion with adduction and medial rotation. The rehabilitation process follows a similar routine presented above for anterior instability, but different motions are restricted. Excessive medial rotation and horizontal adduction are performed carefully after the first three to four weeks, but active assisted lateral rotation and abduction can begin on post-op day 3 to 7, depending on surgeon's preference. Isometric exercises for shoulder flexion, extension, abduction, adduction, and lateral rotation can begin after post-op day 7. Weight-bearing activities in a quadruped position are avoided initially. This position puts undue additional stress on the posterior capsule. Other exercises that are modified or avoided because of the posterior capsule stress they impose include chest flys, bench press, and push-ups. These activities are added to the program carefully and not until the later stages of the therapeutic exercise program.

In phase II, exercises are performed with the shoulder in some lateral rotation and abduction. Glenohumeral lateral rotation exercises begin with the patient supine and progress to performing the exercise in sitting. In the sitting position, joint stability is more difficult to maintain than it is in supine. Seated weight-bearing exercises, such as a press-up, do not stress the posterior capsule, so they can occur earlier in the program than quadruped weight-bearing exercises. Medial rotation exercises are performed from full lateral rotation to neutral in the early phases. Horizontal adduction exercises are avoided early in the program. When added later, they begin with horizontal adduction limitations to approximately 45° forward of the frontal plane. Gradually, full horizontal adduction is instituted in the later stages.

Quadruped weight-bearing exercises for the shoulder begin in the later part of phase III after the patient has achieved stabilization, adequate strength, and appropriate tissue-healing time has passed. When the bench press is initiated in the later phases, it is performed with a wide grip so that the shoulders are in abduction and horizontal extension.

■ Case Study

A 16-year-old basketball player was seen by the physician after experiencing a right shoulder subluxation. The injury occurred as he was going under the basket for a layup and his arm was caught by an opponent and pulled into horizontal extension with lateral rotation. He has no history of prior injury. The physician has placed the arm in a sling and instructed you to begin a rehabilitation program for this patient. It has been one week since the injury. The patient reports some difficulty sleeping at night; he cannot get comfortable as a result of the pain. He reports that he wears the sling all the time except for showers, as the physician has instructed. On examination, you find some discoloration in the upper arm, but the swelling of last week is gone. There is some muscle spasm and tenderness to palpation of the infraspinatus, supraspinatus, teres minor, rhomboids, upper trapezius, and levator scapula. You notice that atrophy of the supraspinatus is already evident after one week. Range of motion of the shoulder is 20° medial rotation, 20° abduction, and unable to achieve lateral rotation by 10° from neutral (remains in medial rotation).

Questions for Analysis

  1. What will be your initial treatment?

  2. Outline the exercises you will use for this patient during the first week of treatment.

  3. What precautions must you take with his treatments?

  4. Give a general outline of progression for his rehabilitation program, specifying what guidelines you will use to move from one stage to the next.

The timeline used for posterior shoulder instability repair is similar to that outlined for anterior instability repair. As with any injury, pain is avoided with the exercises. Full motion is expected at around 2 months. Once 75% strength compared to the contralateral limb is present in the involved shoulder, functional exercises begin and progress to sport-specific activities.

Inferior Instability

Shoulder inferior instability is cared for similarly to anterior and posterior instability. The only caveat is that it is common to have multi-planar instability when inferior instability is present. In these cases, the clinician must be cognizant of all the positions and movements that may put the shoulder joint at risk and take care to avoid these positions, especially in the early phases of rehabilitation.

Initial positions to avoid with inferior instability injuries include placing the arm overhead and allowing it to hang at the side unsupported. The upright press and shrugs are exercises that the patient should avoid until later in phase III because of the stress they place on the inferior capsule.

Shoulder Impingement

Shoulder impingement is associated with unique factors that you must consider in developing and executing a therapeutic exercise program. These are discussed as program considerations before the case study is presented.

The subacromial space is not a large area—a little wider than a pencil. Because the space is small, even a slight alteration in its normal structures can have significant consequences, especially to a patient who places great stress on the joint.

There are two types of impingement, primary and secondary. Primary impingement is the result of structures present within the subacromial space that narrow the normal size of the space to compromise the soft-tissue structures within it—the rotator cuff tendons (supraspinatus and infraspinatus), biceps tendon, and subacromial bursa. Among these structural factors are a congenital anomaly of the acromion structure, an osteophyte on the distal acromion, a narrower-than-normal subacromial space, and a larger-than-normal tendon. All these structural variations narrow an already small space and cause the soft-tissue structures to become impinged. Most often, the cause of primary impingement is either a congenital anomaly in the distal acromion configuration or a bone spur.

Acquired or secondary impingement reduces the subacromial space because of alterations in the shoulder's function that lead to instability. These factors can include capsular laxity or tightness, postural deviations, rotator cuff weakness, and scapular rotator muscle imbalances. Cervical radiculopathy can also result in impingement if muscle weakness occurs, resulting in muscle imbalances during shoulder motion. If the capsule is loose, the humerus moves forward during follow-through of throwing motions. If the posterior capsule is tight, it tends to push the humerus upward and anterior into the anterior joint during shoulder motions, narrowing the subacromial space. Normal function of the rotator cuff is to depress the humeral head during shoulder elevation motions to provide for adequate subacromial space; but if the rotator cuff is weak, the humeral head will ride higher than it should in the glenoid, causing impingement. When the scapular rotator muscles are imbalanced, the upper trapezius and levator scapulae usually overpower the weaker lower trapezius. This causes poor scapulohumeral rhythm and narrows the subacromial space under the coracoacromial arch during shoulder motion because scapular elevation and upward rotation will not occur with shoulder elevation (Kamkar, Irrgang, & Whitney, 1993). Poor posture causes the shoulders to round forward so that the greater tubercle is more directly under the acromial arch to cause impingement earlier in the range of motion (Lewis et al., 2005). Related to posture is the position of the scapula on the thorax. If shoulder rotation is lacking medially, the scapula is positioned such that impingement occurs at the end of medial rotation (Borich et al., 2006). Finally, if the scapular stabilizers become fatigued, biomechanics of the glenohumeral joint are altered, leading to impingement of the glenohumeral soft tissue structures under the coracoacromial arch (Ebaugh, Karduna, & McClure, 2006). Each of these secondary problems can result in subacromial impingement. Uncorrected secondary impingement leads to a gradual, progressive shredding of the rotator cuff tendon and ultimately results in rotator cuff tears. Although the problem may begin at a young age, manifestations of secondary impingement and rotator cuff tears are more common in athletes over the age of 30 than in those who are younger.

Secondary and primary impingement both result in inflammation of the soft-tissue structures in the subacromial space. This inflammation most commonly includes the supraspinatus tendon. The infraspinatus tendon and subscapularis tendon can sometimes be affected as well. The subacromial bursa and biceps tendon can also be involved. Impingement, then, causes tendinopathy or bursitis. Inflammation of the rotator cuff tendons weakens the tendon and can lead to tendon rupture if the condition is poorly managed or untreated.

Secondary impingement can be resolved through conservative efforts if the cause of the impingement is corrected. The cause must be determined before treatment can be successful. Secondary factors of muscle imbalance and asynchronous shoulder motion are commonly seen in primary impingement, leading to pain and rotator cuff tendinopathy. Primary impingement is surgically corrected, but both primary and secondary problems should be treated with rehabilitation whether surgery is performed or not. The most common surgical correction is either removal of the osteophyte (if present) or an anterior acromioplasty.

Early rehabilitation emphasizes control of the inflammation, correction of the secondary cause, and restoration of normal shoulder function. Initially, the focus is on pain and inflammation control and achievement of full range of motion. Placing the shoulder in a resting position with the arm slightly abducted and flexed helps to provide optimal circulation to the tendons. Gentle grade I and II mobilizations are helpful in relieving pain. If inferior capsule tightness is present, inferior glenohumeral glide mobilizations will increase general capsule mobility, permitting the rotator cuff to position the humerus caudally during arm elevation. The rehabilitation clinician can massage the supraspinatus tendon by placing the patient's hand behind the hip to expose the anterior humerus and providing deep cross-friction to the tender area until the pain subsides (figure 19.24). Strengthening exercises for scapular stabilizers can begin early and do not stress the rotator cuff tendons. Early on, the program should

---

■ Case Study

A 40-year-old, competitive tennis player reports to you that she has had shoulder pain since the first half of the tennis season. She is now unable to serve without pain. She has pain in the beginning of her warm-ups but before a match begins, the pain goes away. About 2 h after a match, her pain is significant. She has pain in the deltoid insertion area. The doctor has ruled out primary impingement but feels that a course of rehabilitation is necessary before the patient returns to tennis. On examination this patient has full range of motion except that she is lacking about 10° in elevation. Pain occurs in the end ranges of movement and above 90° of elevation. She has a forward-head, round-shouldered posture. Her glenohumeral rotators and abductors are weak and painful. She has weakness in the lower trapezius and rhomboids.

Questions for Analysis

1. What is the cause of her secondary impingement?
2. What will you do to relieve the causes?
3. What will your first treatment include?
4. How will you help the patient progress in her rehabilitation program?
5. What guidelines will you use for her progression?
6. What functional program will you use to prepare her for her return to tennis?

---

incorporate simple neuromuscular reeducation techniques for proprioception and improved kinesthetic awareness of the scapular rotators for correct scapular positioning during shoulder movement. Rotator cuff exercises in a pain-free range of motion are important at this time as well. Most rotator cuff exercises should be performed in the lower positions (below 60°), and the scapula should be in a "set" position. The "set" position is achieved with simple instructions to the patient: "pull your shoulder blade down towards your back pocket." Resistive exercises should begin with high repetitions and lower weights.

Progression of exercises is based on the patient's pain and strength. Exercises that produce pain are avoided. In the early stages, these exercises include activities that place the arm above 60° to 90° or behind the back, as well as diagonal-plane motions. As the tendon's inflammation subsides and the patient achieves scapular stabilization strength, he or she performs glenohumeral exercises at higher shoulder positions, and more challenging exercises are added to the rehabilitation program. Finally, the plyometric and functional exercises are incorporated into the program before the patient returns to full activity.

Traumatic Rotator Cuff Conditions

Traumatic rotator cuff injuries are different from degenerative tears that occur in older patients. You must take into account several unique factors associated with traumatic rotator cuff injuries before developing a therapeutic exercise program for a patient with this type of injury.

Traumatic rotator cuff conditions include an acute rotator cuff strain, a partial tear, a complete tear, and post-surgical conditions. Although rotator cuff tears are more commonly seen in older individuals, patients now begin sport participation at an earlier age and at a greater intensity level than earlier generations did, so rotator cuff tears are increasingly seen in younger patients as well. A sudden traumatic event such as a shoulder dislocation or a fall on the outstretched, laterally rotated arm can cause rotator cuff tears at almost any age, and may occur in a healthy rotator cuff or in one with minor asymptomatic changes. Tears can also occur in rotator cuff muscles that have undergone repetitive stresses over time. These conditions are associated especially with overhead physical activities in which the musculotendinous unit has encountered chronic stress and tissue fiber damage. An open repair is necessary for most rotator cuff tears in patients who wish to remain active. Following surgical repair, the starting point, duration, and progression of the rehabilitation process depends on the size of the tear, the extent of the surgical repair, the state of integrity of the deltoid (whether it was cut or preserved in surgery), and the age of the patient. A sling or abduction brace may be used immediately postoperatively and continued for about six weeks. After 7 to 10 days of immobilization, mild passive and active assistive range-of-motion exercises may be possible, but this depends on the surgeon's preference. Early exercises include passive and active assistive elevation and lateral rotation, extension, and medial rotation. Pendulum exercises are also appropriate early in rehabilitation. Joint mobilization for pain relief (grades I and II) can be used. Active lateral and medial rotation can be performed with the elbow at the side and extended. Sidelying on the uninvolved shoulder, manual resistance to scapular rotators with the involved arm at the side can be useful. Trigger point treatments may be necessary, if indicated. Distal joint movements such as elbow and wrist flexion and extension and ball squeezes are performed to minimize atrophy of the muscles in the distal segments. At the end of the first three weeks, a resistance band or manual-resistance glenohumeral medial and lateral rotation with the elbow at the side, and rhythmic stabilization with the arm at 100° to 120° flexion, can begin.

The time to start active exercises depends on the size of the tear and the type of repair, but an average time is approximately four to eight weeks after the surgery. At this time, joint mobilization for increased mobility (grades III and IV) can begin. Active range of motion is performed in the scapular plane and is accompanied by isometric exercises in different arm positions as long as the motion is pain free. Resistive exercises such as those done with a resistance band should continue for the rotator cuff with the arm kept at the side. If scapular stabilization is adequate, gentle guided medial and lateral rotation with the arm at 90° abduction also begins. Biceps and triceps exercises are performed against resistance. Antigravity shoulder extension, supine fly, and prone fly to no more than a horizontal neutral position, as well as weight-bearing scapular stabilization exercises, are suitable at this time. Exercises are performed in a straight plane.

At 10 to 12 weeks, the patient should have nearly full range of motion. More vigorous stretching exercises, such as overhead hangs, are permissible if full motion is not present. Exercises should remain in a pain-free range. Sidelying exercises for the lateral and medial rotators can begin; these should initially use low resistance and high repetitions. Isokinetic exercises in the scapular plane are appropriate once the patient has sufficient single-plane strength in the rotator cuff and scapular stabilizers. Proprioceptive neuromuscular facilitation patterns of resistance can be used.

After 12 weeks, the scapular stabilizers should have adequate strength to control the scapula in planes higher than 60° to 90° of elevation. The shoulder should be able to tolerate an aggressive strengthening program. Resisted diagonal movements begin in the lower levels, progress to shoulder level, and then progress to above shoulder levels. Plyometrics such as medicine-ball exercises are started at this time.

At 15 to 18 weeks, resisted rotation exercises with the arm at 90° abduction can be performed, as can aggressive resistive exercises for all shoulder muscle groups. Toward the end of this time when the patient has full pain-free motion, normal strength of all shoulder muscles, and normal scapulohumeral synchronized motion a progression of functional exercises is started. By 21 to 26 weeks, the patient should be able to return to full participation.

The difference in rehabilitation for a conservatively managed and postoperative rotator cuff injury lies primarily in the initial treatment and the progression rate. In conservative treatment, the inflammation following injury must be initially treated with modalities and activity modification. Isometric exercises begin earlier for conservatively treated injuries, and active motion can be initiated early as long as the shoulder remains pain free and scapular strength is sufficient to maintain proper scapular stabilization during shoulder motion. Early shoulder medial and lateral rotation motions are performed with the elbow near the side in a scapular plane. Shoulder elevation can occur to 90° as long as the shoulder is pain free and scapular stabilization is maintained. Resistance exercises begin with high repetitions and low resistance and progress to higher resistance with increased scapular and glenohumeral control.

■ **Case Study**

An 18-year-old baseball pitcher with shoulder instability underwent a glenohumeral capsular shift reconstruction one week ago. The surgeon wants you to begin the rehabilitation process today. The patient's shoulder is supported on a bolster with the arm in partial abduction and medial rotation. Examination reveals a nicely healing surgical scar over the anterior-inferior aspect of the shoulder. Passive range of motion measures 70° medial rotation, 80° abduction, and lateral rotation stops at 10° from neutral (unable to achieve lateral rotation). There is tenderness over the supraspinatus muscle belly, and the upper trapezius and levator scapula muscles are tense and tender to palpation.

Questions for Analysis

1. What will your treatment session today include? What precautions must you consider?
2. Give this patient an outline of your rehabilitation program with an estimate of how long it will be before he begins a pitching program.
3. Outline his pitching progression program.

Arthroscopic Decompression

The advancement of arthroscopic procedures to improve subacromial arch space has permitted a relatively rapid recovery following surgery to relieve subacromial impingement (Sauers, 2005). Simple debridement without the need for additional repairs provide for an uncomplicated and relatively rapid post-surgical process.

Debridement of rotator cuff tendons and decompression of the subacromial space via an **arthroscopy** permits early rehabilitation because there has been no disruption of the deltoid and the surgical insult is less than with open surgical repairs and techniques. A decompression relieves primary impingement, and debridement relieves chronic tendinitis or synovitis.

Rehabilitation following arthroscopic decompression can begin immediately after surgery. The first week or two involves primarily pain and swelling modulation and range-of-motion exercises. Grade I and II joint mobilization can be used to achieve pain relief. Early motion exercises can include Codman's exercises and active assistive range-of-motion exercises with a wand, pulley, or the rehabilitation clinician. Medial and lateral rotation motion exercises start with the elbow near the side with a towel roll between the side and elbow and progress to positioning the shoulder at 45° and then 90° of abduction during rotation exercises. Motion activities also include capsular stretches and joint mobilization. Submaximal isometric exercises begin in the first two weeks postoperatively. Scapular stabilization exercises and biceps and triceps exercises are important in the early program as well. Early neuromuscular control exercises such as proprioception drills for glenohumeral positioning with eyes closed are started early.

Once pain is under control and near-full motion is possible, straight-plane resistive exercises are added, first below 60° in the scapular plane. As scapular stabilization improves, lateral and medial rotation are performed at 90° of abduction, first with the arm supported, and then with the arm unsupported during exercise. Isokinetics in the scapular plane can begin. Full range of motion and good capsular mobility should be present before the patient moves to the next step of the progression. Once scapular stabilization and straight-plane strength are performed well at the desired strength levels, diagonal-plane exercises using pulleys or resistance bands can begin. These are followed by first low-level, then higher-level (about 90°), and finally overhead medicine-ball activities. Plyometrics are followed by functional exercises before the patient finally performs sport-specific activities prior to return to normal activities. The entire rehabilitation process may average three to five months.

Case Study

A 19-year-old volleyball player underwent an arthroscopic decompression of her right-dominant shoulder after an eight-week course of rehabilitation did not alleviate her shoulder pain. The surgery was two days ago. The surgeon wants her to begin a rehabilitation program today. On examination she reports normal postoperative shoulder pain, but no more rotator cuff pain. There is minimal ecchymosis around the shoulder. The surgical portal sites are covered with adhesive suture strips. There is some spasm in the rotator cuff muscles and upper trapezius. Range of motion of the shoulder is 150° flexion, 100° abduction, 80° lateral rotation, and 90° medial rotation. Her strength has diminished from preoperative levels and is now 3/5 in the rotator cuff muscles, 3–/5 in shoulder abduction, 3/5 in shoulder flexion, and 4–/5 in the scapular rotators. The patient tends to shrug her shoulder when she elevates the arm.

Questions for Analysis

1. What will you include in your treatment today?
2. What instructions will you give the patient today?
3. What will the next three treatment sessions include?
4. Explain what you will use as guidelines to determine when she is ready to progress from straight-plane to diagonal-plane exercises, from diagonal plane to plyometrics, and from plyometrics to functional exercises.
5. List four exercises for each exercise level and indicate your justification for their inclusion.
6. Describe the functional program you will use before the patient's return to volleyball.

Glenoid Labral Tears

Glenoid labral tears are difficult to identify. Nevertheless, when they are diagnosed, and whether an anterior or posterior tear is present, special considerations are warranted in the execution of a therapeutic exercise program. We look at these considerations first and then at a case study.

Glenoid labrum tears are primarily the bane of throwing athletes. The large compression and shear forces generated during deceleration in throwing are mainly responsible for causing degenerative tears, abrupt tears, or detachments of the glenoid labrum. The labrum frequently tears superiorly either on the posterior or anterior glenoid in throwers. This type of lesion is referred to as a **SLAP** lesion—**S**uperior **L**abrum tear **A**nterior and **P**osterior in location. The anterior-superior lesion occurs because of the tremendous throwing deceleration forces applied in this area where the long head of the biceps tendon attaches to the labrum. The posterior-superior lesions are thought to occur because of glenohumeral joint instability. If a glenoid labrum tear is present, instability is frequently an accompanying problem and should be examined and treated as part of the total rehabilitation process.

Labral tears often involve the long head of the biceps, especially during deceleration and follow-through throwing phases. When the biceps-labral complex is involved, the labrum can be torn from the superior aspect of the glenoid, and the biceps tendon can be either avulsed with the labrum or suffer a partial tear at its proximal insertion. One surgeon's group noted that 83% of labral tears also involved the biceps-labral complex (Andrews, Carson, & McLeod 1985). Based on this information, it may be presumed that the majority of glenoid labrum tears do not merely involve the labrum.

Whether or not instability is present, the usual treatment choice is to try a conservative approach with rehabilitation first. If this is unsuccessful, excision of the torn segment may be

---

■ Case Study

A 17-year-old lacrosse player injured his right-dominant shoulder when another player ran into him while his arm was abducted. He suffered a torn glenoid and was in rehabilitation for three weeks following the injury. The following winter, he slipped on the ice and landed on an outstretched arm, causing his shoulder to sublux. He underwent an open debridement and anterior capsular reconstruction last week and is now ready for rehabilitation. The arm is in an abduction bolster harness, but the surgeon wants it removed during therapeutic exercises. Shoulder motion is 60° medial rotation, 60° abduction, and lateral rotation stops at 10° from neutral (unable to achieve lateral rotation). Rotator cuff strength in the middle of available range is 3+/5. The surgical scar is well healed, but there is ecchymosis surrounding the anterior shoulder area and into the upper arm. The upper trapezius and pectoralis major muscles are tender to palpation and in spasm.

Questions for Analysis

1. What will be your first treatment?
2. What will be included in your first two weeks of treatment?
3. When will you begin passive range of motion?
4. When will you begin resistive exercises, and what will they first include?
5. What precautions must you be aware of in this case?

---

necessary. If instability is present, open reduction to remove the avulsed segment and stabilize the joint may be necessary. A variety of surgical repairs are used for this problem, including a Bankart repair and capsulolabral reconstruction.

If the patient undergoes an arthroscopic excision, the rehabilitation process follows the program used for arthroscopic debridement presented earlier with full recovery in approximately 3 to 5 months. If an open repair is necessary, the rehabilitation process will be delayed because of the required additional time of immobilization; the rehabilitation program proceeds more slowly and cautiously because of the greater shoulder area involved and the risk of damaging the surgical repair if the rehabilitation is too aggressive. An open repair will damage more proprioceptors than an arthroscopic procedure, so rehabilitation for these procedures should emphasize proprioceptive activities once active motion is possible. The open surgical cases will more closely follow the timeline outlined for the rotator cuff repair program discussed previously; refer to that program for guidelines on procedures and timelines.

Adhesive Capsulitis

Adhesive capsulitis is more commonly seen in patients over the age of 30 than in younger patients but does occur in younger age groups, especially those with metabolic disorders. Understanding the condition is essential to designing a therapeutic exercise program. Elements unique to this injury are discussed and a case study is then presented.

Adhesive capsulitis is commonly referred to as a frozen shoulder. The generic term for adhesions in the capsule is arthrofibrosis. An idiopathic frozen shoulder occurs spontaneously with no known trauma or aggravating incident. Idiopathic frozen shoulder occurs predominantly in middle-aged patients—usually over 30, usually female—and typically in the non-dominant shoulder. Although adhesive capsulitis is a malady of older patients, the shoulder can become restricted in its motion in younger patients because of a variety of predisposing factors. These factors can include surgery that changes the biomechanics of the shoulder; prolonged immobilization of the shoulder; scar-tissue adhesions in the capsule or ligaments surrounding the shoulder; and prolonged inflammation of the tendons, bursa, and other soft tissue around the shoulder. This condition is termed traumatic or secondary adhesive capsulitis since there is a sudden onset of injury or immobilization causing loss of motion (Sheridan & Hannafin, 2006).

Immobilization causes adhesions in connective tissue that can reduce muscular tissue mobility. Reduced muscle tissue mobility decreases the number of sarcomeres present in the muscle (Akeson, Woo, Amiel, Coutts, & Daniel, 1973). The additional changes that occur with immobilization in muscle, joints, and supportive tissue were discussed in chapter 2. When the joint capsule is affected, loss of motion is most notable in lateral rotation, abduction, and flexion of the shoulder. A capsular pattern of motion loss in the glenohumeral joint is evident with lateral rotation more limited than abduction, abduction more limited than flexion, and flexion more limited than medial rotation (Cyriax, 1982).

When adhesive capsulitis is in stage I, hallmark signs include shoulder pain, pain at end ranges of movement, difficulty sleeping on the shoulder, and progressive loss of motion. It is during this stage that the capsular scar tissue is forming and maturing. Lateral rotation will demonstrate loss of available motion, but other movements may or may not show evidence of lost motion. The most effective treatment at this time is active range-of-motion exercises. Joint mobilization should not be painful and should be oriented more toward pain relief (grades I and II) than mobility gains. Stronger mobilization grades only aggravate the capsule and may promote an inflammatory response or cause a reactive muscle spasm that will increase pain. Active range-of-motion exercises maintain muscle length. Attempts at stretching the capsule at this time cause pain but little change in mobility.

By stage II, adhesive capsulitis has become mature, the glenohumeral joint has lost its normal mobility, and the shoulder is very stiff. Pain is present at the end of available motion. The patient may complain of pain in the elbow and is unable to lie on the shoulder. At this time, more aggressive joint mobilization is used as long as an inflammatory response does not result. Continued active stretches are also used. Strengthening exercises in the available ranges are a part of the program. Ultrasound before joint mobilization may permit more optimal results from the mobilization.

In the third stage, the patient's pain is evident before the end of capsular restriction. The primary area of pain is distal on the arm, not in the shoulder. Pain is present at rest as well as during activity. Passive range-of-motion assessment demonstrates a hard, leathery end-feel with more profound motion loss in a capsular pattern. Scapulohumeral rhythm is lost because glenohumeral capsular restrictions prevent normal motion between the scapulothoracic and

■ Case Study

A 45-year-old golfer had noticed a gradual loss of motion in his left non-dominant shoulder over the past several months. He went to the physician when he was unable to retrieve his wallet out of his back pocket and was diagnosed with a frozen shoulder. He is unable to lie on the left side and has pain with sudden movements and when just sitting. He is concerned about getting his shoulder ready for golf season, which begins in three months. On examination, you find that he has 120° of flexion, 80° of abduction, 35° of lateral rotation, and 60° of medial rotation and that he is able to reach across in horizontal adduction to get his elbow even with his left ear. He has pain about 10° to 15° before the end range of all motions, and you observe a stiff end-feel at the end of each movement. Joint mobilization assessment indicates tightness throughout the capsule, especially the inferior and posterior capsule. Palpation reveals tenderness in all the rotator cuff muscles and some tension in the pectoralis major, upper trapezius, and levator scapulae. The patient's posture is good, but when he moves the arm there is no scapulohumeral rhythm, and he shrugs the shoulder toward his ear to initiate shoulder flexion motions.

Questions for Analysis

1. What stage of adhesive capsulitis is he in?

2. What will be your first treatment for him?

3. What home exercises will you give him on the first day?

4. Outline a progressive program for him including modalities, exercises, mobilization techniques, and functional progression for returning to golf.

glenohumeral joints. Because glenohumeral rhythm is lost, shoulder elevation is replaced with shoulder shrugging, and the scapula moves at the same time and rate as the humerus. Grades III and IV joint mobilizations are used at this time. Continued range-of-motion exercises and active stretches are performed throughout the day to promote mobility gains. Self-mobilization techniques are taught to the patient. Strength exercises for the scapular rotators, rotator cuff, and large glenohumeral muscles (deltoid, pectoralis major, teres major, and latissimus) are included in a progressive program. If the patient is not seen until the third stage, a 3 to 6 month treatment program may be necessary to resolve the condition. Figure 19.85 outlines a timeline for rehabilitation of adhesive capsulitis.

Without treatment, the adhesive capsulitis takes longer to resolve, perhaps at least 18 and 24 months. During this time, the shoulder presents in the fourth stage, the "thawing" stage (Sheridan & Hannafin, 2006). A gradual decrease in pain is observed during this time. Additionally, a slow but progressive increase in motion is also obtained. It is neither practical nor reasonable, however, to expect a patient to wait for this length of time to obtain relief from an adhesive capsulitis without treatment intervention.

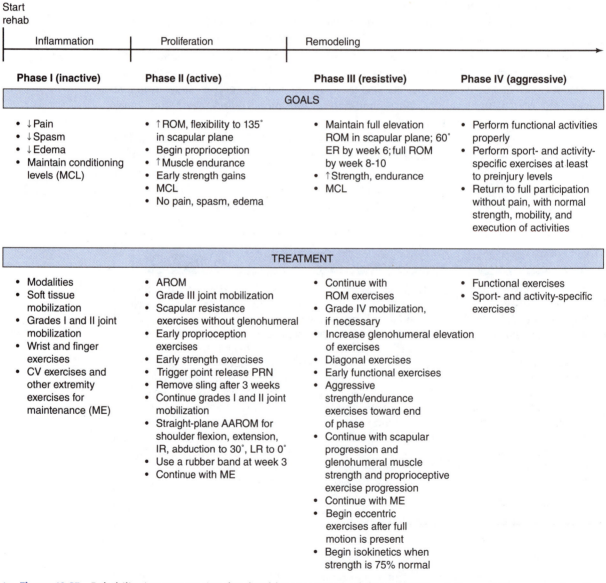

▶ **Figure 19.85** Rehabilitation progression for shoulder anterior instability. AAROM = Active assistive range of motion; CV = cardiovascular; AROM = active range of motion; LR = lateral rotation; ROM = range of motion; PRN = as needed.

Electrothermally Assisted Capsular Shift

Electrothermally assisted capsular shift is a procedure for which long-term results have not been defined because of its newness to medicine. There remain many unanswered questions regarding the proper rehabilitation course. There is little research on postoperative treatment procedures. One study indicated that early range of motion and a slow but progressive strengthening program produce successful results over a 12-week therapeutic exercise treatment course (Ellenbecker & Mattalino, 1999). This section presents the information currently available about the procedure and the postoperative course.

The electrothermally assisted capsular shift procedure is a relatively new arthroscopic technique used to address glenohumeral instability. The long-term effects of the procedure are still being investigated and are at this point unknown because the technique has been used only since the late 1990s (Gerber & Warner, 2002; Miniaci & Codsi, 2006). The arthroscopic technique incorporates the use of a thermally assisted coagulator probe that is set at 65-80 °C (Hayashi & Markel, 2001; Miniaci & Codsi, 2006) and is swept along the capsule between the glenoid and the humeral head to denature the capsule (Hayashi et al., 1997; Miniaci & Codsi, 2006). The capsule immediately shrinks like a plastic shrink-wrap, reducing the joint's laxity.

It is thought that the heat causes the collagen to denature and fuse when fibroblasts invade the area (Hayashi & Markel, 2001; Hayashi et al., 1997). The fibroblasts are thought to use the denatured collagen as a scaffold in the new collagen matrix formation during the inflammatory healing phase (Hayashi & Markel, 2001; Hayashi et al., 1997). It is during this time that immobilization of the shoulder must occur so that the collagen matrix formation will result in appropriate capsular tightening.

The shoulder is immobilized for 7 to 14 days, although wrist and elbow motions are permitted. Active abduction begins about 10 to 14 days postoperatively. Lateral rotation to 45° with the elbow at the side and to 90° abduction occurs after about two weeks. Forward flexion is kept to 90°, and extension is limited to 20° hyperextension. Some physicians allow active motion three days after the procedure with lateral rotation to 0° and scapular plane flexion to 90° for the first four weeks (Gerber & Warner, 2002).

Since joint proprioceptors may have been damaged during the surgery, it is important to include exercises to restore proprioception. These can begin with early-stage activities within the allowed ranges of motion early in the program and advance as mobility and proprioception increase.

Submaximal isometric strengthening exercises start after the first week or two as long as the patient stays within the range-of-motion restrictions and lateral rotation is kept at 0°. Scapular stabilization exercises are performed without placing undue stress on the glenohumeral joint. Resisted elbow and wrist motions are also a part of the program. Joint mobilization to the AC, SC, and scapulothoracic joints are allowed. Scapular strengthening and proprioceptive exercises are emphasized in this phase. Proprioceptive exercises within the patient's motion and tolerance are also included.

At four to eight weeks, all motions should be within normal limits except lateral rotation, which is limited to 15° less than that on the contralateral side. Posterior capsular stretching begins at this time. Light resistive exercises with high repetitions and low resistance occur at this time as long as the patient remains pain free. Strenuous overhead activities are avoided, but controlled diagonal movements can be initiated towards the end of this phase. After week 8, the patient should have full range of motion except in lateral rotation in 90° of abduction. This motion may be less than normal but continuing to progress to normal by week 8 to 10. More aggressive strength exercises and exercises that emphasize scapular control of glenohumeral positions in higher elevations occur in this phase as long as the patient remains pain free. Wall push-ups begin as the patient nears the 12-week mark.

After week 12, the patient should be able to tolerate plyometric exercises. The progression is the usual one previously discussed, starting with low-level movements and progressing to overhead movements once control is achieved at the lower elevation levels. The final step consists of functional activities and drills before return to full participation and normal

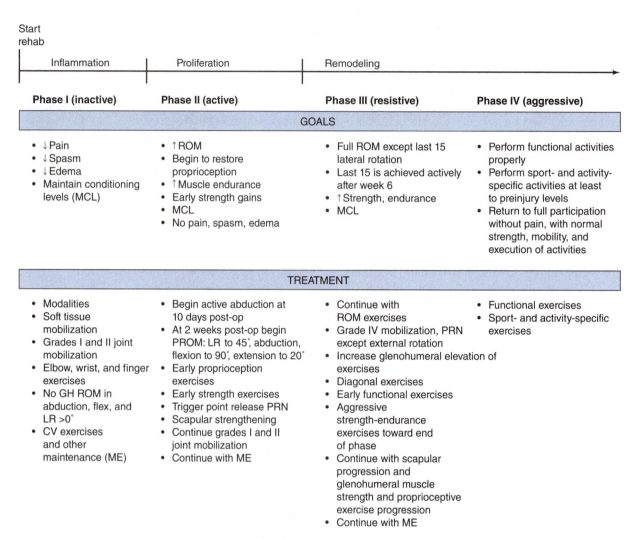

▶ **Figure 19.86** Rehabilitation progression for shoulder electrothermally assisted capsular shift procedure. PROM = passive range of motion; CV = cardiovascular; ROM = range of motion; LR = lateral rotation.

activities. Figure 19.86 outlines a timeline for rehabilitation after a shoulder electrothermally assisted capsular shift procedure.

Acromioclavicular Sprain

Although first-degree sprains are not usually difficult to manage, the treatment approach for more severe acromioclavicular (AC) sprains is more complex. Considerations for the various degrees of AC sprains are presented, followed by a case study.

Most AC sprains, regardless of severity, are not surgically repaired and are treated conservatively. Surgery is resorted to in those rare cases where the individual's injury remains painful and demonstrates persistent joint instability (Bishop & Kaeding, 2006). The speed with which conservative care is advanced depends on the severity of the injury. In mild sprains, the shoulder may be immobilized in a sling for a few days to relieve the traction discomfort caused by the weight of the arm pulling on the AC joint. Modality use relieves pain, swelling, and muscle spasm. Active and active–assistive range of motion exercises are initiated on day 1 or 2 following the injury. Isometrics to tolerance also begin immediately. Once full motion is restored, a progression of strengthening exercises is used until the patient has full function without pain and is able to return to full sport participation.

■ **Case Study**

A 21-year-old swimmer underwent an electrothermal capsular shift 10 days ago for anterior instability. The physician reports that the patient had no other joint damage and that no other surgical procedure was necessary. She is now to begin rehabilitation. She has some mild postoperative pain, but nothing unusual. She is to wear a sling for another four weeks but is permitted to remove the sling for rehabilitation. Her shoulder range of motion is 40° flexion, 30° abduction, and –5° lateral rotation (unable to achieve neutral rotation from medial rotation by 5°). The rotator cuff and scapular rotators are grossly 4–/5 in strength, but there is more weakness in the scapular rotators than in the rotator cuff.

Questions for Analysis

1. What will be your first day's treatment?
2. What precautions will you provide this patient?
3. Outline your treatment progression for her.
4. What will you include in your functional program before her return to full sport participation?

In type II and III sprains, the AC ligament is torn. In type II sprains the coracoclavicular ligament is intact, but in type III sprains it is not. Some deformity is present in both type II and type III sprains. Attempts at immobilization are made, but they are often unsuccessful because of the discomfort and restriction of the immobilizing device and the difficulty in stabilizing the AC joint. The benefits of surgical repair for type III sprains are disputable. Most often the treatment option selected is non-surgical: A sling is used to relieve the distraction force of the weight of the arm on the AC joint. Some deformity usually persists, but this is a cosmetic issue and does not interfere with activity and shoulder function. The more severe injuries (types IV, V, and VI) are often surgically repaired, especially in overhead throwing athletes, because significant damage to both static and dynamic structures around the joint has occurred (Mazzocca, Arciero, & Bicos, 2007).

In the type II and III injuries, the shoulder may be immobilized for one to three weeks. Active–assistive range of motion of the glenohumeral joint may begin early. If proprioception is deficient, basic exercises to restore it can begin early in the program and advance as pain subsides and motion and strength improve. Strengthening exercises (below 60°) follow a normal progression from stabilization, straight-plane, and low-level exercises to higher-level exercises and diagonal movements. Plyometric exercises are followed by functional exercises. Normal progression to heavy lifting occurs at about 8 to 12 weeks post-injury, and the patient returns to full participation after having performed functional exercises correctly.

SLAP Lesion

A **s**uperior **l**abrum tear **a**nterior and **p**osterior in location (SLAP) lesion is an injury to the glenoid labrum. These SLAP lesions may occur either as a frank injury or repetitive stress (Wilk, Reinold, Dugas, Arrigo, & Andrews, 2005). Acute lesions may occur from falling on an abducted arm, causing compression of the joint (Synder, Karzel, Del Pizzo, Ferkel, & Friedman, 1990). In throwers, it often occurs secondary to excessive stress applied by the long head of the biceps tendon, the structure that attaches to the superior glenoid labrum rim. Various theories regarding etiology identify the biceps tendon's attachment to the glenoid labrum as a primary contributing factor to SLAP lesions. One theory indicates that during overhead throwing motion, the biceps' attachment on the glenoid is twisted at the end of the wind-up with the shoulder in abduction and maximal lateral rotation; this position places

■ **Case Study**

A 17-year-old wrestler incurred a type II sprain of his right AC joint in last week's match. He is to begin rehabilitation today. The shoulder has been in a sling for the past week. The patient is able to take the arm out of the sling for brief periods of time, but he reports that keeping the sling off for longer than 4 h causes an ache in the top of the shoulder. The muscles also feel tired. Examination reveals 150° of shoulder flexion, 120° of shoulder abduction, 60° of lateral rotation, and 75° of medial rotation. Strength tests reveal grades of 4–/5 in the pectoralis major and rotator cuff; 3+/5 in the rhomboids, lower trapezius, and serratus anterior; and 4/5 in the deltoid and latissimus dorsi. You can palpate trigger points in the upper trapezius, pectoralis major, and supraspinatus muscles.

Questions for Analysis

1. What will your first treatment session include?
2. What are your goals for the first treatment session?
3. What instructions will you give the patient before he leaves today?
4. Outline the rehabilitation course, including a timeline you anticipate for program changes and four examples of each type of exercise.
5. What will your functional exercise program include before return to sport participation?

torsional stress on the tendon's attachment to the labrum (Burkhart, Morgan, & Kibler, 2003; Kuhn, Lindholm, Huston, Soslowsky, & Blasier, 2003). Another theory supports the idea that deceleration stresses of the biceps during release and follow-through applies tension forces on the bicep tendon's insertion and, over time, causes the labrum to tear away from the glenoid fossa (Andrews, Carson, & McLeod, 1985). There are others who caution the presence of SLAP lesions secondary to glenohumeral instability (Chan & Lam, 2006; Park, Lin, Yokota, & McFarland, 2004).

SLAP lesions are placed in four categories, depending upon the amount of injury to the biceps tendon and the glenoid labrum to which it attaches (Chan & Lam, 2006). According to Snyder et al. the first group to use the term, SLAP lesion (Synder et al., 1990), a type I lesion has fraying of the superior labrum where the biceps attaches but the labrum and biceps tendon remain intact. A type II lesion has both the superior labral fraying and some detachment of the glenoid labrum and biceps tendon off the glenoid neck. Type II lesions are further subdivided into three categories, anterior, posterior, and a combination of anterior and posterior (anteroposterior) involvement. In type III lesions, the biceps tendon and labrum remain attached at their peripheral margins on the fossa but there is a bucket-handle tear of the central section of the labrum. In type IV lesions, there is both a bucket-handle tear of the labrum as well as a tear of the biceps tendon at its attachment site so portions of the labrum and tendon appear as a flap that may shift within the joint. Arthroscopic fixation is usually performed on type III and type IV lesions while arthroscopic debridement is the usual treatment for type I and II SLAP lesions (Chan & Lam, 2006). If there is a substantial biceps tendon tear of more than 30% of its substance in a Type IV lesion, the surgeon will use sutures in an arthroscopic repair of the tendon along with fixation of the tendon and labrum to the glenoid (Mileski & Synder, 1998).

The rehabilitation of SLAP lesions is unique since the biceps is important to function of both the shoulder and the elbow. In addition, various degrees of lesions can occur, so the severity of injury and the physician's choice to approach the problem surgically or non-surgically further complicate therapeutic exercise choices. A final complicating factor for clinicians performing rehabilitation on patients with SLAP lesions is that SLAP lesions are often associated with other shoulder lesions such as rotator cuff tears, Bankart lesions, Hill-Sachs lesions, chondral lesions, and instability (Park, Loebenberg, Rokito, & Zuckerman, 2002/2003b).

Specific rehabilitation techniques and their rate of progression are dependent upon the extent of the injury and the type of surgical treatment performed. Rehabilitation following a debridement is much more aggressive and faster than one to treat a repair.

Rehabilitation for a SLAP lesion debridement begins within the week following surgery. The patient likely wears a sling for the first 3 days or so, primarily for comfort. Since the first three days following surgery involve the most discomfort, the patient finds that the sling is not as necessary after this time. Although it may be uncomfortable, passive and active range of motion exercises may begin within a day of the surgery since only debridement without repair was performed. Sometimes patients find that moving the shoulder actually reduces the normal post-operative discomfort. Motion activities are more comfortable when performed in the scapular plane. Full range of motion in all planes should be normal within two weeks.

Strengthening exercises can also begin early when only debridement has been the surgical procedure. During the first week, easy isometrics for the glenohumeral muscles and scapular muscle strengthening using manual resistance to scapular rotators are also incorporated into the exercises. Proprioception exercises for the glenohumeral joint begin with early joint position sense activities. After the first week, isotonic exercises with resistance begin for the glenohumeral muscles. More active proprioception exercises including weight-bearing activities begin after the first week as well. As with other shoulder rehabilitation programs, elevation of the shoulder against resistance occurs in a progressive manner as the patient is able to maintain good glenohumeral position and stability through scapular muscle control during glenohumeral activities.

Between weeks four and six, plyometric exercises using medicine balls begin. By this time, the patient has good control of the glenohumeral joint and is able to recruit the scapular muscles so impingement or hyperactivity of the upper trapezius are not evident. The last phase of rehabilitation occurs in the third to fourth month. Sport-specific and activity-specific portions of the program in this phase prepare the patient to return to former activities without difficulty in transition from rehabilitation to normal activities.

When a repair of the SLAP lesion occurs, the rehabilitation progression is more conservative. A big consideration is the status of healing tissue. The effects of the program should be to move the patient in an efficient and progressive manner to normal activities, not disrupt the healing tissues. Postoperatively, the patient's arm is placed in a sling for three to four weeks. During this time, the clinician controls inflammation, swelling, and pain with modalities and manual techniques effective for those purposes. The patient is given a rubber ball or sponge ball to perform squeezes throughout the day. After one week, the arm is removed from the sling for exercises. These exercises are initially passive range of motion and are limited to 90° elevation in the scapular plane, 0° lateral rotation, and medial rotation to the waist. The patient can also start pendulum exercises a few times a day and perform elbow and forearm range of motion activities. After the first two weeks, passive lateral rotation to 15° is permitted.

Strength activities as isometrics begin in the first week but should not be painful. Scapular stabilization using manual resistance to scapular protractors, retractors, and depressors with the shoulder in a comfortable resting position are also started the first week. Rhythmic stabilization for proprioception and co-contraction is started during the first two weeks.

During weeks 3 to 6, the patient continues to work on scapular muscles as long as the exercises do not stress the glenoid or biceps, isometric and rhythmic stabilization exercises, and proprioception training. Resistance-band exercises for medial and lateral rotation with the elbow at the side, shoulder extension, shoulder flexion to 90°, and shoulder abduction to 45° in the scapular plane can begin as long as the exercises are pain free.

By the sixth week, the shoulder should have motion in all positions except lateral rotation, which should be about 45°. Full lateral rotation should be present and pain free by week 8. Early biceps strengthening exercises can start at week 6.

Posterior capsular stretches begin at weeks 7 to 8. Strengthening exercises using weights for the rotator cuff, deltoid, pectoralis major, and scapular muscles begin at this time as well. This is when weight-bearing exercises are introduced for the first time. The caveat is that these exercises must be pain free. Strengthening of the muscles surrounding the shoulder continue to progress as tolerated during this 8 to 12 week time. As long as the scapular muscles are able to control the glenohumeral position, the arm can also be raised overhead for full motion resistance exercises at this time. By 12 weeks the biceps is sufficiently stable to be able to tolerate more aggressive resistance and exercises, so the bench press, military press, and latissimus pulldowns are added at this three-month mark. During this 3 to 4 month time, stretches continue to maintain full motion and exercises become more specific to the patient's needs. For example, if the patient requires power and strength, then a program is designed with high resistance and fewer repetitions, but if the patient will return to an endurance activity, then low resistance with higher repetitions is used in his or her program.

By the 4 to 5 month timeframe, the patient progresses to functional activities, once all other goals for flexibility, strength, endurance, and agility are acquired. The transition from the functional phase of the program to the sport-specific or activity-specific program is dependent upon the patient's response to the exercises and the physician's objectives. Throwers usually begin easy throwing during the fourth post-operative month. A progressive program of activity-specific routines must be monitored for gradual progression without pain or other deleterious effects of the activities. It may take a patient six to eight months to fully recover and resume normal activities following a SLAP lesion repair.

Biceps Tendon Injuries

Although it might seem appropriate to deal with the biceps tendon in the chapter on the elbow, the biceps-long tendon plays an important role in shoulder stabilization. For this reason, injuries to the biceps tendon that occur at the shoulder are discussed here.

The most common injury seen in the biceps tendon is tendinopathy. Tears, subluxations, and dislocations can also occur. Bicipital tendinopathy occurs primarily in the long head and is usually secondary to shoulder instability, impingement, rotator cuff pathology, or other inflammations of the shoulder. The patient reports tenderness in the bicipital groove. Cervical pathology can refer into the biceps area and must be ruled out if no frank injury has occurred to cause the pain.

Biceps-long tendon ruptures are often associated with rotator cuff pathology, and most occur in middle-aged individuals. A sudden muscle contraction while the muscle is on stretch is a common mechanism of injury. Complete ruptures may display a "Popeye" muscle, but partial ruptures are not as obvious. Pain, spasm, and swelling are immediate signs. If the long head of the biceps is ruptured in a young patient, surgery may be indicated. The same

---

■ Case Study

Three days ago, a 21-year-old gymnast experienced a ruptured biceps injury while practicing on the rings. He is now ready to begin a rehabilitation program. There is ecchymosis in the distal arm and into the forearm. The area has swelling, and the biceps muscle feels tight from spasm. Elbow motion is lacking 15° of extension and has 120° of flexion. The patient has full passive supination but actively supinates to 45°. Elbow flexion is 3+/5 and painful. The patient admits to having had shoulder pain last season that kept him out of competition for one month. This season the pain has been present but tolerable. He indicates that he has never injured his neck but that sometimes it feels stiff.

Questions for Analysis

1. What will your first treatment include, and what are your goals for the first treatment?
2. What other areas should you investigate before deciding on your course of treatment?
3. When do you expect to achieve full range of motion in the elbow?
4. When will you begin strengthening exercises, and what will your first week of exercises include?

injury in an older patient may or may not require surgery. Because the long head of the biceps provides glenohumeral stability, its surgical repair can be important in the younger and more active population.

Rehabilitation treatment must include an examination of the rotator cuff, because its pathology is often related to biceps pathology. Control of pain, swelling, and inflammation is an initial goal of treatment. Use of modalities, anti-inflammatories, and rest initially may be beneficial. Rest is usually accompanied by active–assistive range-of-motion exercises. Therapeutic exercises progress as tolerated to include an exercise sequence similar to that listed for conditions discussed earlier. It should also obviously include supination and elbow flexion exercises.

Among the types of shoulder injuries that raise special concerns and call for particular exercise approaches are instability, impingement, traumatic rotator cuff conditions, glenoid labral tears, adhesive capsulitis, acromioclavicular sprains, and biceps-long tendon injuries.

SUMMARY

The shoulder undergoes tremendous stresses during its use, especially in upper extremity sport activities such as throwing. This chapter detailed the mechanics of overhead sport activities for activities including pitching, tennis strokes, swimming, and golf. Shoulder area trigger point treatment and joint mobilization techniques were presented. Exercises from flexibility through to functional activities were presented in a progressive manner throughout the chapter. Some of the more common injuries seen in rehabilitation of the shoulder complex were presented with suggested rehabilitation progressions. Of special concern in the shoulder area is stability of the joint during functional activities. The two primary muscle groups providing this stability are the scapular muscles, which anchor the glenohumeral joint to the trunk to provide a stable platform from which the joint functions, and the rotator cuff, which provides glenohumeral stability so the larger "mover" muscles such as the deltoid, pectoralis, and latissimus can perform their activities at the shoulder.

KEY CONCEPTS AND REVIEW

1. Explain how knowledge of the mechanics of an activity impacts the establishment of a therapeutic exercise program.

The shoulder is a complex structure composed of several joints and many muscles that must work synchronously to produce injury-free motion. When activity is not synchronous or when trauma occurs, the result is an injury that can affect the entire shoulder function. During specific motions such as pitching, swinging a golf club, swimming, or performing hits and serves in tennis, the shoulder and its joints and muscles must work in a specifically timed and synchronous manner to produce the desired effect with minimal risk of injury. The rehabilitation clinician must have an awareness and appreciation of these activities to properly rehabilitate the patient for return to full participation.

2. Discuss the importance of stability in shoulder rehabilitation.

Stability of the glenohumeral and scapulothoracic joints is crucial to performance and to reduced injury risk for the shoulder. Central to stabilization of the glenohumeral joint are strong scapular muscles to move and hold the scapula in position advantageous for glenohumeral function. Studies have demonstrated the significance of good stabilization of these joints and the importance of good therapeutic exercise programs to permit restoration of stability to these areas.

3. Explain the role of scapular stabilization in shoulder function.

Basic to shoulder function is scapular stabilization during shoulder activities. Scapular muscles serve as the foundation from which the shoulder moves, so, when scapular muscles do not function properly, because of weakness, loss of motion, or reduced endurance, the shoulder is at great risk of injury.

4. Describe two soft-tissue mobilization techniques for the shoulder.

Cross-friction massage to the biceps tendon and anterior rotator cuff muscles is commonly performed with tendinopathy injuries. Trigger point releases to rotator cuff muscles, such as the supraspinatus in the supraspinatus fossa or the teres minor at the lateral border of the scapula, are commonly performed to relieve pain and improve motion.

5. List three joint mobilizations for the shoulder.

Shoulder joint mobilization techniques should include techniques for the specifically restricted joints. If the AC joint is restricted, PA, AP, and inferior glides can be used. If the scapula is restricted, scapular distraction is appropriate. If the glenohumeral joint is restricted, an arm pull is a gross technique, and an inferior glide is a more specific technique for improving joint mobility. Joint mobilization must be performed in grades III and IV to gain motion.

6. Identify three strengthening exercises for the scapulae and three for the glenohumeral muscles.

Scapular muscle-strengthening exercises can include maneuvers such as push-up plus, prone fly, and Bouhler exercises. Glenohumeral muscle strengthening exercises can include medial and lateral rotation exercises starting with isometric exercises and moving to resistance-band and free-weight exercises, as well as abduction in the scapular plane.

7. Discuss the general progression of strengthening exercises for the shoulder.

The specific progression depends on the specific injury and its severity. A general progression of strengthening exercises begins with scapular stabilization exercises and isometric rotator cuff exercises. Manual resistance to the scapular muscles can begin early in the program. From there the exercises include active resistive exercises in the lower third of shoulder motion until the scapular muscles are strong enough to provide scapular control in the middle ranges of motion and finally in motion over 100°, so overhead exercises can be performed without loss of control of scapular and glenohumeral positioning. Eccentric exercises for the rotator cuff using resistance bands, medicine balls, and even manual resistance begin in straight planes and progress to diagonal planes. Exercises in both weight bearing and non-weight bearing are used for stabilization and strengthening. Plyometric activities begin slowly and progress as the patient gains proficiency. Functional exercises using sport equipment such as a tennis racket or golf club then begin, at first in low ranges of motion with reduced force until control and proficiency have been demonstrated. Exercises next progress to greater ranges of motion and begin to mimic the actual activity. Functional overhead activities are the last item to be added to the program. In addition to the shoulder, the biceps, triceps, and abdominal muscles must also be included in the program.

8. List precautions for a therapeutic exercise program following a rotator cuff repair.

Care must be taken to allow tissue healing before exercises begin. Range of motion usually begins at 7 to 10 days. If immobilization continues for an extended period of time, there can be complications such as adhesive capsulitis, especially in patients over age 30. Range-of-motion exercises begin with activities such as Codman's and must progress on the basis of the status of the healing tissues. Strength exercises begin slowly with high endurance and low resistance, progressing as the patient gains control and strength. Scapular exercises can be initiated early, but rotator cuff exercises begin with submaximal isometrics. Range-of-motion gains in lateral rotation occur slowly and cautiously.

9. Outline key factors for a program for a biceps rupture.

Active range of motion for shoulder, elbow, and forearm is followed by strengthening exercises for motions including elbow flexion, supination, and shoulder flexion and extension. Progression of exercises follows a pattern similar to that for other shoulder programs, according to considerations regarding pain, control, and tissue healing.

CRITICAL THINKING QUESTIONS

1. If you were Bob in the opening scenario for this chapter, what techniques would you have used to relieve PG's posterior shoulder tightness and the scapular muscle weakness? What plyometric progression would you have used to advance him to functional activities? What criteria would you have used to begin his functional activities, and what would your throwing progression have been?

2. If an injured wrestler who experienced a shoulder dislocation two weeks ago comes to you to begin rehabilitation, what must be your greatest precaution with him? How much elevation can you safely place the shoulder in? What is your reasoning for this amount of motion? What exercises should you be able to do with him at two weeks post-injury?

3. If the rehabilitation process and the results for electrothermally assisted capsular shift procedures have not yet been fully documented, what guidelines can you use when a patient comes to you after this procedure has been performed on his or her shoulder? Based on your knowledge of healing and the shoulder, what precautions should be taken, and what exercises can you perform in the first three to six weeks postoperatively?

4. Recall the case of the 40-year-old tennis player presented in the section on impingement in this chapter. Have you figured out the cause of her problem? If posture is a primary contributing factor, what instructions will you give her to relieve the cause? What exercises will reinforce your efforts to change her posture? If her posture has been incorrect for some time, what soft-tissue changes would you expect will need to be treated?

5. If you have a patient whose diagnosis has been narrowed down to a rotator cuff tendinopathy, shoulder instability, shoulder impingement, capsulitis, and cervical radiculopathy, how will you determine which diagnosis is correct? What tests will you use to differentiate between these diagnoses? Would the rehabilitation program change with different diagnoses? Why or why not?

6. A sophomore softball pitcher is diagnosed with a Type II SLAP lesion. She is scheduled to have surgery tomorrow. She wants you to outline for her what she will be doing and how long her rehabilitation will take. She knows that the surgeon has already spoken with you and wants you to start her on rehabilitation two days after surgery, but she is concerned that she will be too sore and painful to do anything. She has never had an injury before that has required surgery, so she is obviously apprehensive about the surgery and concerned that she will not be able to pitch again. What will you say to her and how much will you outline of what lies ahead for her? What will you say to reduce her fears about the surgery and her pitching career?

LAB ACTIVITIES

1. With your lab partner as a patient, perform grades I, II, III, and IV joint mobilization on all shoulder complex joints. For the glenohumeral joint, apply an inferior glide to determine joint mobility. Identify how large the movement is for each of the grades as you go through the joint's total mobility range. Now repeat the examination on another person. How does the range of mobility of each joint compare between the individuals?

2. Apply the following joint mobilization techniques on your partner. While applying each technique, notice where the resistance to movement occurs and where movement stops. Why are these items important to assess for each motion and joint?
   a. Glenohumeral anterior glide
   b. Glenohumeral posterior glide

    c. Glenohumeral lateral glide

    d. Scapulothoracic glides

    e. Acromioclavicular inferior glide

    f. Acromioclavicular anterior-posterior glides

    g. Sternoclavicular AP glide

    h. Sternoclavicular PA glide

3. Locate the trigger points for the following muscles on your lab partner:

    a. Subscapularis

    b. Supraspinatus

    c. Infraspinatus

    d. Teres minor

What muscles contained your lab partner's most sensitive trigger points? Perform an ice-and-stretch technique on the most sensitive areas after you have examined for active range of motion of the muscle. After the treatment, have your partner repeat the active ROM so you can determine the effectiveness of your treatment. How did the AROM change from before to after the treatment? Why?

4. If your partner has a tight anterior and inferior capsule, list the flexibility exercises you would give him. Have your partner go through them and tell you where he feels the stretch.

5. If your partner has a tight posterior capsule, list the flexibility exercises you would give her. Have your partner go through them and tell you where she feels the stretch.

6. Go through wand exercises to increase shoulder flexion, abduction, horizontal abduction, and lateral rotation with your partner. List all possible substitution patterns he performs and the verbal cues you use to correct these patterns.

7. Perform isolated scapular exercises using manual resistance on your partner in all possible planes in sidelying and supine. How many repetitions for each exercise was she able to perform before fatigue occurred? How were you able to identify when she fatigued?

8. Have your partner perform a progression of push-up exercises beginning with wall push-ups and ending with box jumps on the floor (use footstools). List the progression you used and the number of repetitions your partner was able to do. What are you looking for in terms of his performance? How are you determining when he has performed enough repetitions to acquire adequate fatigue levels?

9. Have your partner perform one exercise each for the lower trapezius, middle trapezius, serratus anterior, and rhomboids. List the exercise and how many repetitions your partner was able to perform. What would be a progression for each exercise and when would you advance your partner to the next level?

10. Have your partner perform one exercise for the shoulder abductors, MR, and LR. Describe the exercise you have selected, why you have selected it, how many repetitions your partner was able to perform, possible substitution patterns to watch for, and your next progression for each exercise.

11. Have your partner perform any two of the scapular stabilization exercises in this chapter. What muscle did you partner feel the exercise working, and what possible substitution patterns could have been used?

12. Have your partner perform any two of the plyometric or functional exercises in this chapter. What purpose do they serve (goals for the exercise), and what substitution patterns could be used for each? How will you determine when she should advance to the next level of exercise (what are your criteria)? Can you think of another plyometric or functional exercise that is not in this chapter?

Elbow and Forearm

OBJECTIVES

After completing this chapter, you should be able to do the following:

1. Discuss why you should avoid overstretching the elbow, especially during the inflammation phase of healing.
2. Describe the convex-concave rules for the various elbow joints.
3. Identify the resting positions for the elbow joints.
4. Identify three soft-tissue mobilization techniques for the elbow.
5. List three joint mobilizations for the elbow.
6. Explain three strengthening exercises for the elbow and their purpose.
7. Discuss the general progression of strengthening exercises for the elbow.
8. Outline a therapeutic exercise program for epicondylitis.
9. Indicate precautions to consider in a Little League elbow therapeutic exercise program.
10. List precautions, following an ulnar nerve transposition, for a therapeutic exercise program.
11. Explain the differences in rehabilitation programs for an arthroscopic debridement and a medial collateral reconstruction.

▶ Joan Rennay has worked as the certified athletic trainer in the local high school for the past 10 years. Occasionally a parent brings a preteen athlete to her, knowing that she has worked successfully with the child's older sibling. She normally provides an evaluation of the youngster's injury and makes recommendations to the parents for first-aid treatment or referral to the family physician.

Today, she is visited by a parent who is familiar to Joan because he has had two teenagers pass through Joan's athletic training facility during their high school careers. Mr. Turner reports that his youngest son, 10-year-old Steve, developed medial elbow pain while pitching in a Little League baseball game last week. Although it had been bothering him for a couple of weeks before last week's game, Steve hadn't complained about it until the pain became too intense.

From her past experience, Joan suspected Little League elbow. But she knew she should not assume anything and should perform an examination with an open mind before she came to any conclusions.

A man would do nothing if he waited
until he could do it so well that no one could find fault.

CARDINAL NEWMAN, 1801-1890, English theologian and writer

Like the spine and the shoulder, the elbow has special and distinct characteristics that must be considered in developing rehabilitation programs for elbow injuries. As the joint between two long lever arms, the elbow can experience large force applications from its proximal and distal arms. Open chain activities apply large velocities with sudden acceleration and deceleration forces from the proximal arm of the joint, while closed chain activities apply compressive stresses and torsional forces from the distal arm. The elbow muscles must work synchronously with adjacent structures, and the joint and muscles must have the flexibility necessary to withstand these forces.

Because the elbow lies between the shoulder and wrist, some muscles that traverse the elbow also affect the shoulder or wrist. It is difficult to separate these and thus was difficult to decide which chapter some of the techniques and exercises should be delegated to. It may seem that some of the techniques and exercises presented in this chapter would be better suited to the shoulder chapter or the wrist chapter. That may be the case, but how best to classify the exercise depends on the injury. For example, if a patient has a tennis-elbow injury, exercises and techniques for wrist extensor muscles are appropriately discussed in the context of the elbow. However, if a patient has a wrist sprain, those same techniques and exercises for wrist extensor muscles are best addressed in a discussion of wrist injuries. For this reason, some of the techniques and exercises you read about in this chapter are also referred to in the next chapter on the wrist and hand.

This chapter outlines basic considerations for elbow rehabilitation and then presents soft-tissue and joint mobilization techniques, flexibility and strength exercises, and plyometric and functional considerations. Distinctive considerations for some of the more commonly seen elbow injuries are discussed, and case studies for these injuries are presented so that you can problem solve and devise your own rehabilitation program.

Although there are some aspects to elbow injuries that can make them difficult to manage, as Cardinal Newman suggests, the key to approaching them is not to feel you must be perfect in your management. Using the knowledge and skills you acquire through education and clinical practice allows you to be confident in your rehabilitation of elbow injuries.

GENERAL REHABILITATION CONSIDERATIONS

The elbow is unique in several ways, and the rehabilitation clinician needs to understand its distinctive characteristics to properly design and execute a therapeutic exercise program. The following sections focus on these characteristics.

Joint Stresses

As mentioned in chapter 19, overhead motions are actually a total body movement that includes a summation of forces and properly timed execution of movement that start in the lower extremities and trunk and transfer forces to the shoulder, elbow, and hand. As the summation of forces accelerates the extremity in throwing sports, the elbow and forearm velocity must occur at high rates to successfully propel the hand or object it holds at the desired speed. Researchers have reported different angular velocities for different sports. Baseball pitching produces the highest velocity at 2300°/s (Feltner & Dapena, 1986). Javelin athletes experience an angular velocity of 1900°/s (Mero, Komi, Korjus, Navarro, & Gregor, 1994); the tennis serve has been recorded at 982°/s (Kibler, 1995); and in fast-pitch softball, 680°/s velocities have been recorded (Ellenbecker & Mattalino, 1997).

Most of these overhead motions place additional valgus or varus stress on the elbow joint. The greatest force applications occur during acceleration and deceleration phases of movement. High demands are placed on the biceps, brachioradialis, and brachialis during deceleration to slow forearm motion and prevent overextension and injury to the elbow. During acceleration, the elbow experiences compressive forces laterally and distraction forces medially. The medial stresses can result in injuries such as neuritis, tendinopathy, and medial joint sprains and muscle sprains. The lateral compressive stresses can cause osteochondritis dissecans in young athletes, and bony osteophytes, articular damage, and degeneration in older athletes. It is common for athletes with an extended throwing career to develop flexion contractures because of articular and muscular changes. Proper mechanics, timing, and balanced joint and muscle function are crucial in the prevention of elbow injuries. If biomechanics are altered because of these deficiencies, the stresses become magnified. In pitching, the forces applied are a valgus distraction stress medially with a lateral compressive force (Loftice, Fleisig, Zheng, & Andrews, 2004). Tennis produces stress over the lateral epicondyle during the backhand stroke and medial epicondyle stresses during overhead serves and late-hit forehand strokes (Hume, Reid, & Edwards, 2006). Gymnastics, an upper-extremity weight-bearing sport, places excessive lateral stress on the joint because of the elbow's normal valgus position. Golfers with incorrect mechanics can place excessive medial force on the trailing elbow or excessive lateral force on the leading elbow (Light, 2008). Pitchers with inflexibility of hips, trunk, or shoulder open up too soon and increase the elbow's medial joint stress. If tightness, weakness, or fatigue causes the elbow to drop, increased medial joint stresses are placed on the elbow during the cocking phase in pitching (Kibler & Sciascia, 2004). In tennis, increased lateral stress is placed on the elbow when the player leads with the elbow on the backhand, and increased medial stress is applied on the forehand stroke when the ball is hit late.

It is important for the rehabilitation clinician to understand these concepts because the rehabilitation program should include an assessment of the patient's skill execution. Incorrect techniques may be the underlying cause of the problem, and the program must include correction of those techniques to prevent recurrence of the injury.

Unique Structure

The elbow has unique anatomical characteristics that can be advantageous or disadvantageous. The joint has a high degree of congruency within the humeroulnar joint. That makes it stable. One of the more distinctive characteristics is that a muscle, not its tendon, traverses the joint.

The brachialis muscle traverses the joint and inserts onto the ulna. The biceps tendon not only attaches to the radial head but also extends fibers that insert into the bicipital aponeurosis, blending with the fascia covering the medial proximal forearm muscles. This anatomical attachment must be considered when elbow immobilization is required following injury. Scarring and limitation of motion can easily occur in this area. Immobilization must be used cautiously, and extended periods of immobilization should be avoided. More than two weeks of immobilization can cause severe restrictions of the elbow's joint mobility. Complicating the reality that adhesions occur relatively easily in the elbow is the fact that the joint's anterior capsule is relatively thin and can easily incur damage with aggressive stretching, resulting in additional scarring. For this reason, it is important that aggressive, high-intensity stretching at the elbow be avoided. This is particularly crucial during the inflammation phase when the area is weaker and more easily aggravated than will be the case later. Soft-tissue tearing, scarring, and loss of joint motion can occur with passive overstretching. Early stretching techniques should include primarily active stretches. Passive range-of-motion exercises are permissible, but they should be pain free and performed in controlled and monitored situations.

Joint Mobility

The elbow has three joints that should be examined for joint mobility: the humeroulnar, humeroradial, and radioulnar joints. Each elbow joint has a different **resting** and **close-packed position** that are important to know when performing mobilization techniques. The humeroulnar joint's resting position is at 70° elbow flexion with 10° supination, and its close-packed position is in full extension. The humeroradial joint's resting position is at full extension and full supination, and its close-packed position is at midflexion with midpronation. The radioulnar joint's resting position is at 70° elbow flexion with 35° supination, and its close-packed position is at full pronation or full supination. Joint mobilization is initially performed in the resting position, where there is the greatest mobility and the least stress is applied to the joint. In later rehabilitation phases, it may be necessary to move the joint into other loose-packed positions to perform mobilizations. The close-packed position can also be used as an exercise position for unstable joints to provide increased stability during resistance activities.

Because the humeroulnar and humeroradial joints have the concave ulna and concave radius moving on the convex humerus, the **concave-convex rule** applies for mobilization techniques to these joints. Therefore, the mobilization force application should be in the same direction as the restricted movement. Joint distraction applied in a resting position will stretch the anterior and posterior capsule. If the elbow is placed in flexion, and distraction is applied, the posterior capsule is stretched to increase elbow flexion; but if distraction is applied with the joint in extension, the anterior capsule is stretched to increase elbow extension.

The radius and ulna are connected by two joints, the proximal radioulnar joint distal to the elbow and the distal radioulnar joint proximal to the wrist. Both joints must have normal movement to produce full forearm supination and pronation. The proximal joint is formed by the convex radial head in the concave ulnar notch. This joint abides by the convex-concave mobilization rule. Therefore, the mobilization force application is in the opposite direction of restricted movement. For example, to improve supination, the force is applied anterior to posterior; to improve pronation, the force is applied posterior to anterior.

Force Applications

Depending on the specific injury, the clinician may need to take special precautions with some strength exercises. Stresses applied to the elbow during strengthening can be excessive, depending on the arm position and the weight lifted. Lifting weights with the elbow extended places more stress on the anterior elbow, while lifting weights with the elbow flexed places more stress on the posterior elbow. Because of lever-arm lengths, a resultant force of up to three times body weight occurs when the elbow is flexed 30° (Ellenbecker & Mattalino, 1997). Lighter weights or cuffs attached to the mid-forearm reduce these stresses and should be used, especially with earlier strengthening exercises.

A weight-bearing exercise such as a push-up delivers stress to the elbow, but the arm position determines the degree of stress. In a normal push-up position, the greatest compression force at the elbow is 45% of body weight, but the compression force is decreased if the hands are moved farther apart (Donkers, An, Chao, & Morrey, 1993). In a superior position, the compression force is decreased in the elbow, but the valgus torque is increased by 54% (Ellenbecker & Mattalino, 1997).

Low-resistance, high-repetition strength exercises are used in the early phases of elbow rehabilitation to reduce excessive stresses such as these on the joint. Once healing of tissue has occurred and neuromuscular control and strength gains are such that good joint control is possible, increased weights can be used.

> The design and execution of a therapeutic exercise program for the elbow must take into account the types of joint stresses incurred by the elbow, its unique structure, the mobility of its joints, and the amount of force application that is appropriate.

REHABILITATION TECHNIQUES

The soft tissue techniques of the elbow covered in this section are complementary alternative medicine applications. These techniques include trigger point release and cross-friction massage. Descriptions of joint mobilization techniques follow the sections on soft tissue mobilization. From these manual therapy techniques, a variety of exercises, beginning with flexibility exercises and continuing through to activity-specific exercises, are discussed.

Soft-Tissue Mobilization

The techniques addressed here are primarily trigger point release, ice-and-stretch, and cross-friction massage techniques. The trigger point referral patterns, trigger point releases, and ice-and-stretch procedures described here are based on the work of Travell and Simons (Travell & Simons, 1983). The muscles mentioned here are also muscles that are addressed in chapter 21 on the wrist and hand, because most of the muscles originating at the elbow function at the wrist and hand.

It is important to note the locations of the patient's pain. Pain assessment necessitates investigation and elimination or confirmation of trigger points, neurological pathology, or localized injury as the source of the pain. If pain is not neurologically based, trigger points may often be the source, especially when the site of injury is different from the location of pain and the complaints do not align with typical neurological symptoms.

Elbow Movers

Along with pure elbow muscles, elbow movers also include muscles that cross the shoulder, the biceps, and triceps, but whose primary function is at the elbow. The trigger point locations and treatments for these muscles are found in the following sections.

■ Trigger Point Releases for the Elbow

Biceps Brachii

Referral Pattern: To the anterior deltoid and antecubital space, as well as into the suprascapular and distal biceps regions (figure 20.1, a & b).

Location of Trigger Point: Anterior arm over the distal third of the muscle.

Patient Position for Palpation: Supine or seated.

Muscle Position for Palpation: Elbow slightly flexed and forearm supinated.

Ischemic Treatment: Strumming of the taut band or a deep pressure over the trigger point.

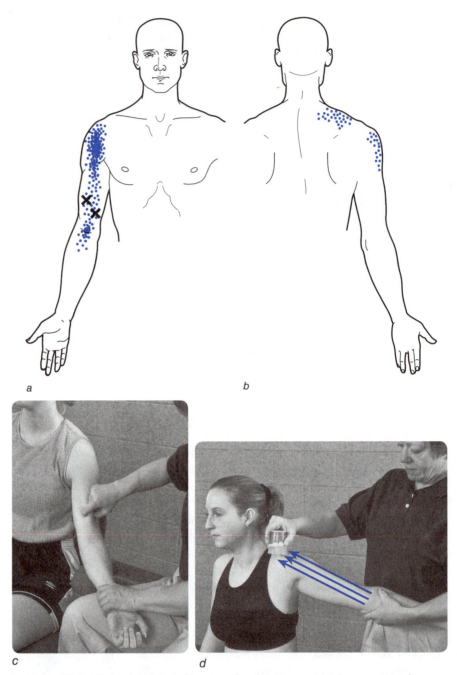

▶ **Figure 20.1** Biceps brachii: *(a-b)* pain-referral patterns, *(c)* trigger point release, *(d)* spray-and-stretch.

Spray-and-Stretch Treatment: Performed with the patient sitting. The shoulder is abducted to 90°, laterally rotated, and horizontally abducted. The elbow is extended and the forearm pronated to put the biceps on stretch as ice sweeps are made from distal to the elbow proximally along the upper arm and to the shoulder (figure 20.1d).

Notations: A pincer grasp may also be used to apply the ischemic treatment (figure 20.1c).

Brachialis

Referral Pattern: To the anterior carpometacarpal thumb joint and thumb's dorsal web space (figure 20.2a). Can also refer to the anterior arm and antecubital space (figure 20.2b). The distal trigger points most commonly refer to the thumb or antecubital space, and the more proximal points refer to the arm.

Location of Trigger Point: Lateral to the biceps muscle on the lateral distal third of the brachialis and over the antecubital space.

Patient Position for Palpation: Supine or sitting.

Muscle Position for Palpation: Elbow flexed about 45°.

Ischemic Treatment: The biceps muscle is pushed medially to gain access to the brachialis (figure 20.2c), and direct pressure is applied to the trigger point.

Spray-and-Stretch Treatment: With the muscle on stretch and the patient in sitting or supine, the elbow is extended with support behind it as ice is stroked in the direction of pain referral from the elbow, either proximally along the arm or distally along the forearm to the thumb (figure 20.2d).

Notations: Use a support to prevent the elbow from hyperextending.

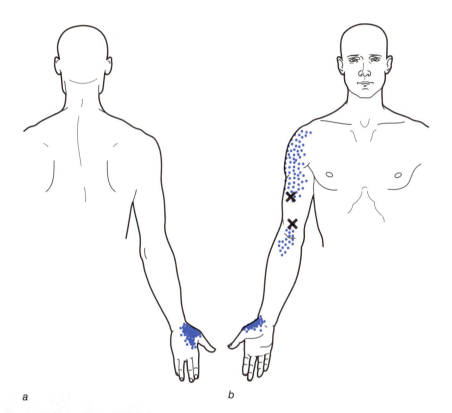

a   b

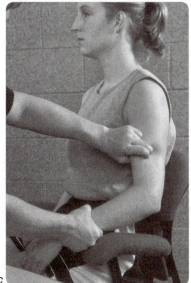

c

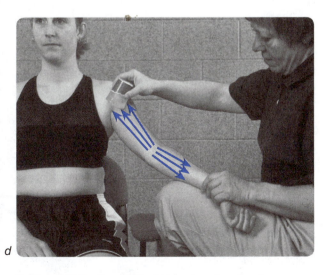

d

▶ **Figure 20.2** Brachialis: *(a-b)* pain-referral patterns, *(c)* trigger point release, *(d)* spray-and-stretch.

Triceps Brachii and Anconeus

Referral Pattern: The three heads of triceps refer pain along the posterior arm to the shoulder and sometimes into the upper trapezius. They can refer pain into the lateral epicondyle, medial epicondyle, and olecranon process; along the lateral, posterior, or posterior forearm; along the posterior arm to the posterior shoulder; and to the fourth and fifth digits (figure 20.3, a-c). The anconeus muscle refers pain locally to the lateral epicondyle (figure 20.3d).

Location of Trigger Point: Clusters of trigger points are often located in the medial and long triceps heads.

Patient Position for Palpation: Supine.

Muscle Position for Palpation: Triceps is relaxed with the elbow in slight flexion.

Ischemic Treatment: Pincer grasp or deep pressure over the trigger point (figure 20.3e).

Spray-and-Stretch Treatment: With the patient supine or sitting, the triceps is placed on stretch with the shoulder and elbow flexed as the ice is applied from the scapula along the posterior arm and forearm (figure 20.3f).

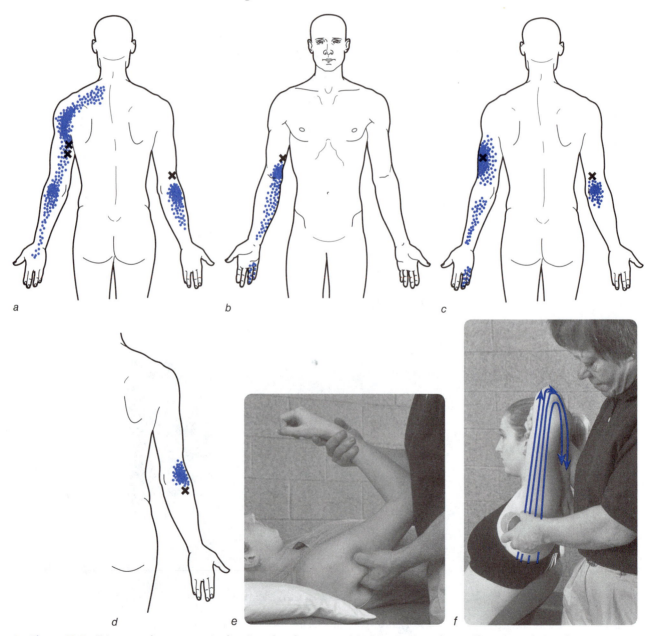

▶ **Figure 20.3** Triceps and anconeus: *(a-d)* pain-referral patterns, *(e)* trigger point release, *(f)* spray-and-stretch.

Notations: If the patient has good passive motion in a relaxed position but is unable to place the elbow next to the ear while the shoulder is in an end-flexion position and the elbow is fully extended, it is likely that the patient has a triceps trigger point. Another position the patient will not achieve if a triceps trigger point is present is with the hand touching the scapula, with both the shoulder and elbow fully flexed to achieve that position.

Supinator

Referral Pattern: Around the lateral epicondyle and lateral elbow region (figure 20.4a). The supinator can also refer to the dorsal thumb web space (figure 20.4b).

Location of Trigger Point: With the forearm in supination, the trigger points lie over the radius between the biceps tendon and brachialis muscle.

Patient Position for Palpation: Supine or sitting.

Muscle Position for Palpation: Elbow is slightly flexed and fully supinated.

Ischemic Treatment: The brachioradialis muscle is pushed laterally, and deep pressure is applied to the supinator between the biceps tendon and brachioradialis muscle (figure 20.4c).

Spray-and-Stretch Treatment: With the elbow in extension and the forearm in pronation, ice or spray strokes are swept from the elbow in the direction of referred pain, either superiorly along the lateral arm or inferiorly along the radial aspect of the forearm to the thumb (figure 20.4d).

Notations: The most common site of pain referral for this muscle is locally around the lateral epicondyle. A patient with lateral epicondylitis who does not respond to treatments should be evaluated for supinator trigger points.

Wrist and Finger Movers

It may seem odd to discuss wrist and finger muscles in the elbow chapter, but the long wrist and finger muscles also act on the elbow because they insert proximal to the elbow joint. Although their main function is in the distal upper extremity, the location of their proximal insertion necessitates attention to these muscles in the context of the elbow. The following sections provide information about trigger points and their treatments.

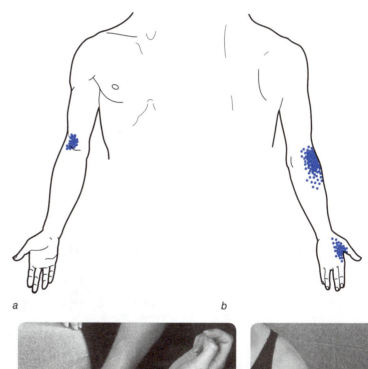

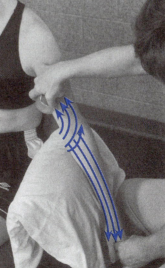

▶ **Figure 20.4** Supinator: *(a-b)* pain-referral patterns, *(c)* myofascial release, *(d)* spray-and-stretch.

■ Trigger Point Releases for the Wrist and Finger Muscles

Brachioradialis and Wrist Extensors

Referral Pattern: Radial extensors refer pain to the lateral epicondyle, to the hand's dorsum, and in the anatomical snuffbox area (figure 20.5, b & c). The ulnar extensors refer pain to the posterior ulnar wrist (figure 20.5a). The brachioradialis refers pain to the lateral. epicondyle, to the thumb's web space, and less often along its muscle belly (figure 20.5d).

Location of Trigger Point: Trigger points for the brachioradialis and extensor carpi radialis longus (ECRL) lie about two inches distal to the bend in the elbow while the extensor carpi ulnaris (ECU) lies a little more distal to the ECRL. The brachioradialis is found with a pincer grasp of the muscle while the ECRL is a little more ulnar to the brachioradialis muscle.

Patient Position for Palpation: Supine or seated.

Muscle Position for Palpation: Forearm is supported in partial flexion and full pronation. The wrist rests in some flexion.

Ischemic Treatment: The trigger points can be treated with either direct pressure (figure 20.5, e-g) or a pincer grasp (figure 20.5h).

Spray-and-Stretch Treatment: The forearm is supported. For the wrist extensors, the elbow is placed on stretch in an extended position, forearm pronated and wrist flexed as the ice strokes are swept from just above the elbow downward along the posterior forearm and past the wrist (figure 20.5i). For the brachioradialis, the stretch and ice sweeps are similar except that the wrist is placed in flexion with ulnar deviation and forearm pronation (figure 20.5j).

Notations: Although the extensor carpi radialis rarely has active trigger points, the other muscles here are often activated with lateral epicondylitis.

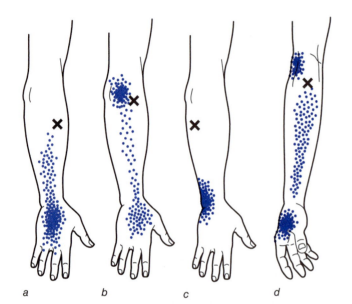

a   b   c   d

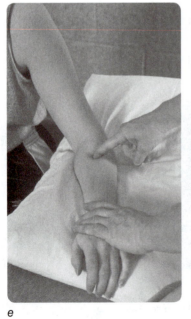

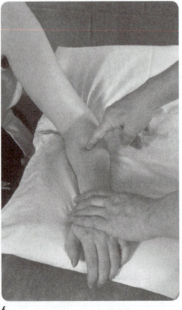

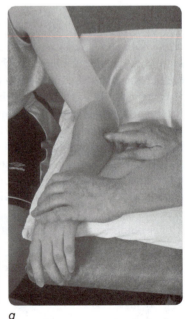

e   f   g

▶ **Figure 20.5** Brachioradialis and wrist extensor myofascial release: *(a)* pain-referral patterns for extensor carpi radialis brevis, *(b)* extensor carpi radialis longus, *(c)* extensor carpi ulnaris, *(d)* brachioradialis. Trigger point release of *(e)* extensor carpi radialis longus, *(f)* extensor carpi radialis brevis, *(g)* extensor carpi ulnaris.

▶ **Figure 20.5** Brachioradialis and wrist extensor myofascial release: *(h)* brachioradialis using pincer grasp. *(i)* Ice-and-stretch of wrist extensor, *(j)* brachioradialis.

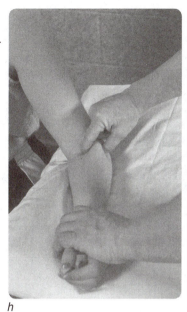
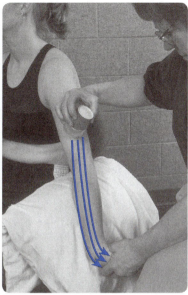
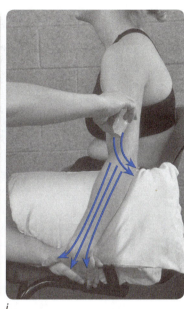

h   *i*   *j*

Finger Extensors

Referral Pattern: The finger extensors refer pain down the forearm along the back of the hand and to the fingers they move (figure 20.6, a-c).

Location of Trigger Point: The middle-finger extensor trigger point is located about 3 to 4 cm (1.2-1.6 in.) distally from the radial head. The ring- and little-finger extensor trigger points are located deep and lateral to the extensor carpi ulnaris. The extensor indicis trigger point is distal on the forearm between the radius and ulna.

Patient Position for Palpation: Supine or seated.

Muscle Position for Palpation: Forearm is pronated with the elbow in flexion and wrist flexed.

Ischemic Treatment: Can be treated with direct pressure or a pincer grasp (figure 20.6d).

Spray-and-Stretch Treatment: With the forearm supported, the elbow extended, and the wrist and fingers flexed as ice is swept distally from the muscle's proximal insertion on the lateral epicondyle toward the fingers (figure 20.6e).

Notations: These muscles can refer pain during injuries such as lateral epicondylitis. The lateral epicondyle is a common pain-referral site. Pain and stiffness of the fingers and hand can also be present even though the source of pain is more proximal.

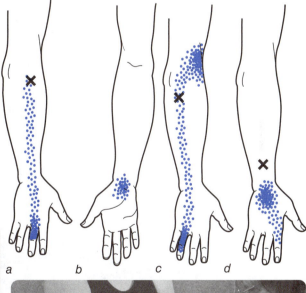

a   *b*   *c*   *d*

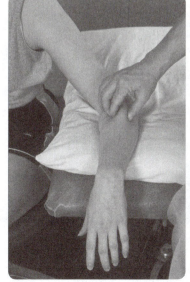

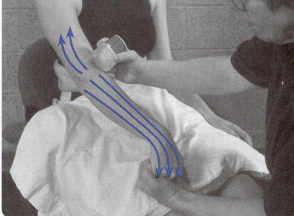

▶ **Figure 20.6** Finger extensor myofascial release: *(a)* middle-finger extensor, *(b)* ring-finger extensor, *(c)* extensor indicis, *(d)* trigger point release, *(e)* ice-and-stretch.

d   *e*

Finger and Wrist Flexors, Pronator Teres

Referral Pattern: Finger flexors refer into and beyond the end of the digits they move. The wrist flexors refer to the side of the wrist they flex, and the pronator teres refers to the radial wrist with overflow along the radial aspect of the anterior forearm and into the base of the thumb (figure 20.7, a-e).

Location of Trigger Point: Most trigger points are located in the distal portion of the upper one-fourth to one-third of the anterior forearm in the midbellies of the muscles. Flexor pollicis longus is located in distal-lateral forearm where the middle and distal thirds of the forearm meet.

Patient Position for Palpation: Supine or seated.

Muscle Position for Palpation: Forearm is supported and in supination. Wrist is in relaxed extension.

Ischemic Treatment: Deep pressure is applied to the trigger points (figure 20.7f).

Spray-and-Stretch Treatment: Strokes are swept from proximal to the medial epicondyle to distally along the anterior forearm to the wrist and into the digit being treated. An extension stretch is applied to the wrist and fingers while ice-and-stretch is performed (figure 20.7g).

Notations: Patients commonly complain of an exploding, lightning-like pain that shoots out the end of the finger.

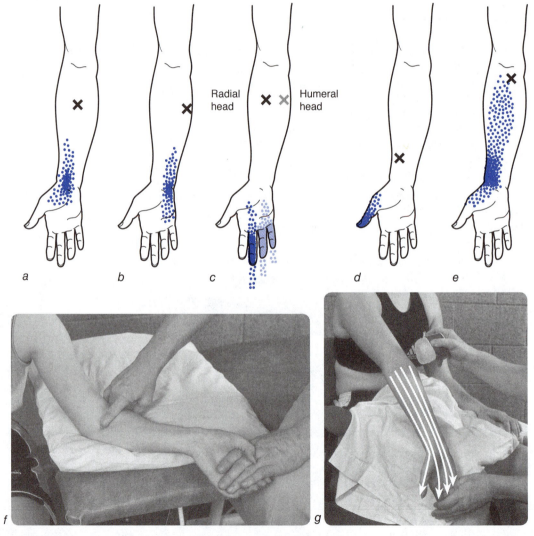

▶ **Figure 20.7** Pain-referral patterns for *(a)* flexor carpi radialis, *(b)* flexor carpi ulnaris, *(c)* flexor digitorum superficialis (dark = radial head, light = humeral head), *(d)* flexor pollicis longus, *(e)* pronator teres. *(f)* Pronator teres and wrist and finger flexor trigger point release about 3 cm (1.2 in.) distal and slightly lateral to the medial epicondyle, *(g)* spray-and-stretch.

Cross-Friction Massage

This technique is most often performed over the lateral or medial epicondyle as part of the treatment for tendinopathy. It may be beneficial in relieving pain and enhancing mobilization of connective tissue restrictions (Denegar, Saliba, & Saliba, 2010). The area of tenderness is isolated with a finger or thumb pad. Pressure over the area is maintained while deep friction is applied to the area. The finger or thumb moves the overlying soft tissue against the underlying bone in a direction perpendicular to the fiber direction: Figure 20.8 shows application over the lateral epicondyle. Sometimes it may be necessary to pull the skin taut with the other hand while applying the cross-friction massage to maintain pressure over an isolated area. Mobile skin and subcutaneous tissue can easily cause the finger or thumb to move off the site.

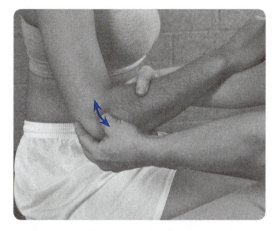

▶ **Figure 20.8** Transverse friction massage.

JOINT MOBILIZATION

This is the capsular pattern demonstrating capsular tightness in the elbow: flexion is more limited than extension, and supination and pronation are equally limited. A patient who presents with this type of motion loss is effectively treated with joint mobilization. Since three joints are enclosed in one capsule, capsular restriction can affect all the joints.

If the elbow is very irritated, initial joint mobilization techniques are mild (grades I and II) for pain relief. Application of more aggressive grades (IIIs and IVs) are postponed until the elbow pain is under control. Aggressive techniques applied too soon may cause additional damage to the weak capsule.

Joint mobilization is performed in the resting position when grades I and II are being applied, and in later stages during the initial applications of the more aggressive grades. This maximizes the effects of the mobilization techniques without aggravating the joint. If joint mobilization techniques to gain motion are required later in the rehabilitation program, other open-packed positions may be used.

While applying joint mobilization, the clinician should always use good body mechanics. The hand applying the force should be positioned as close to the joint as possible. Keep in mind the principles of glide, roll, and spin so you apply forces properly to achieve the desired movement. Both the radial head and ulna are concave surfaces and move on a convex capitulum and convex trochlea, respectively, so mobilization force applications are in the same direction as the restricted movement. In the proximal radioulnar joint, however, the force applied is in the direction opposite the restricted movement because the convex-concave rule applies at this joint.

The joint mobilization techniques presented here are the most commonly used techniques for the elbow. As with any joint mobilization procedure, it is important to visualize the joint surfaces and apply the mobilization force parallel to the surface. You must respect precautions and contraindications, and you must consider the healing-tissue timeline and new tissue strength when deciding whether to apply joint mobilization and how much force to use. As always, application of joint mobilization to hypermobile joints is contraindicated. Improper technique, incorrect force application, excessive force, and inappropriate timing of application can all result in unnecessary injury or damage to the joint's structures. You must be aware of the appropriateness or inappropriateness of accessory and physiological joint mobilization application before you decide to use the techniques. If you are unsure, it is better to refrain from using joint mobilization. Details for elbow and forearm joint mobilization techniques are described in the following sections.

A therapeutic exercise program for the elbow includes trigger point release, ice-and-stretch, and cross-friction massage for the elbow movers and the wrist and finger movers, as well as cross-friction massage for elbow tendinopathy.

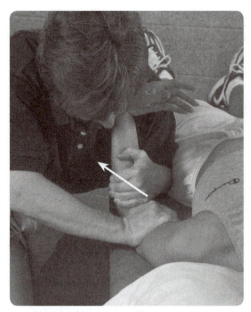

▶ **Figure 20.9** Humeroulnar joint distraction mobilization.

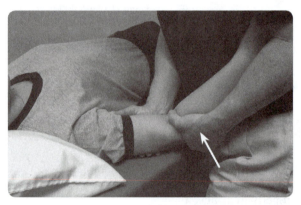

▶ **Figure 20.10** Medial humeroulnar glide mobilization.

Humeroulnar Joint

This joint is also referred to less commonly as the ulnohumeral joint. Although the elbow has three joints, the humeroulnar joint is often considered the primary elbow joint. Even though all three joints lie within the same capsule, joint mobilization for each joint can produce significant range-of-motion gains. The resting position for the humeroulnar joint is 70° flexion with 10° supination.

■ Joint Mobilization of the Elbow and Forearm Joints

Distraction

Joint: Humeroulnar joint.

Resting Position: 70° flexion with 10° supination.

Indications: To relieve pain, generally increase motion.

Patient Position: Supine with elbow in resting position.

Clinician and Hand Positions: The patient's wrist rests against the clinician's shoulder. The humerus is fixated with a stabilization strap, with the help of an assistant, or the rehabilitation clinician's hand. The rehabilitation clinician's hands are placed on top of each other around the proximal forearm near the elbow joint, or one hand is used if the other hand is stabilizing the patient's arm.

Mobilization Application: The clinician applies a distraction force around the humeral axis by leaning backward (figure 20.9).

Notations: The clinician's weight transfer from front to back foot provides the distraction force; clinician's arms should be relaxed.

Medial Glide

Joint: Humeroulnar joint.

Resting Position: 70° flexion with 10° supination.

Indications: To relieve pain, improve elbow flexion or extension.

Patient Position: Patient is supine or sitting.

Clinician and Hand Positions: The rehabilitation clinician faces and stands alongside the patient. The patient's forearm is positioned in the humeroulnar joint's resting position and placed along the rehabilitation clinician's rib cage. The rehabilitation clinician's stabilizing hand's thenar eminence is placed against the patient's medial epicondyle, and the mobilizing hand is on the proximal forearm near the elbow joint.

Mobilization Application: The mobilizing hand applies a sustained 10 s pressure against the radius to create a medial glide of the ulna with the humerus stabilized (figure 20.10).

Notations: An oscillation may also be used with this technique. The pressure against the medial elbow may cause discomfort or injury to the ulnar nerve and must be applied with caution or with the use of a towel for padding.

Lateral Glide

Joint: Humeroulnar joint.

Resting Position: 70° flexion with 10° supination.

Indications: To reduce pain, improve elbow flexion and extension.

Patient Position: Patient is supine or sitting, similar to the medial glide position.

Clinician and Hand Positions: The clinician's hand placement is reversed from the positions for the medial glide, so the stabilizing hand is on the patient's lateral epicondyle and the mobilizing hand is on the medial forearm immediately distal to the joint.

Mobilization Application: The mobilizing hand applies a lateral pressure against the proximal ulna on the medial forearm.

Notations: This mobilization may be applied either as a sustained or as an oscillation technique.

Humeroradial Joint

The humeroradial joint is also referred to less commonly as the radiohumeral joint. The humeroradial joint lies lateral to the humeroulnar joint and should not be ignored when elbow capsular restriction is present. Mobilization of this specific joint can make significant differences in overall elbow mobility. The resting position for the humeroradial joint is full extension with full supination.

Distraction

Joint: Humeroradial joint.

Resting Position: Full extension with full supination.

Indications: To reduce pain, improve elbow extension and radial motion.

Patient Position: Supine or sitting in a chair with the arm slightly abducted and supported on the table.

Clinician and Hand Positions: Rehabilitation clinician stabilizes the arm with a hand on the distal humerus and the index finger palpating the humeroradial joint space. The mobilizing hand is placed around the distal radius but not on the distal ulna.

Mobilization Application: The mobilization force is applied when the clinician moves weight to the back foot; the clinician's body is used to distract the elbow while applying a medially arched distraction at the distal radius (figure 20.11).

Notations: A traction force can be simultaneously applied to the joint.

Anterior Glide

Joint: Humeroradial joint.

Resting Position: Full extension with full supination.

Indications: To increase flexion.

Patient Position: Supine with arm supported on a towel roll on the table.

Clinician and Hand Positions: The rehabilitation clinician places the stabilizing hand on the medial distal humerus and the mobilizing hand on the proximal radius, with the fingers on the posterior aspect and the thenar eminence on the anterior aspect.

Mobilization Application: Finger pads move the radial head upward in a posterior-to-anterior direction (figure 20.12).

Notations: Also called ventral glide or posterior-anterior glide.

Posterior Glide

Joint: Humeroradial joint.

Resting Position: Full extension with full supination (see figure 20.12 in the previous section).

Indications: To increase extension.

Patient Position: Supine with arm supported on a towel roll on the table.

Clinician and Hand Positions: The rehabilitation clinician places the stabilizing hand on the medial distal humerus and the mobilizing hand on the proximal radius, with the fingers on the posterior aspect and the thenar eminence on the anterior aspect.

Mobilization Application: The thenar eminence on the anterior radius moves the radial head posteriorly.

Notations: Also called a dorsal glide or an anterior-posterior glide.

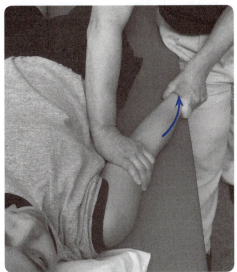

▶ **Figure 20.11** Humeroradial distraction mobilization.

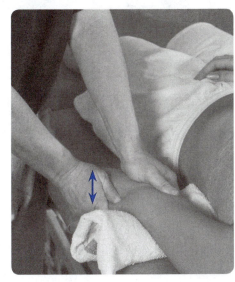

▶ **Figure 20.12** Humeroradial anterior-posterior and posterior-anterior mobilization.

Proximal Radioulnar Joint

Although this joint is not actually part of the elbow's flexion-extension joint, the fact that it lies within the same capsule as the other two elbow joints means that it is part of the elbow. In fact, restriction of this joint can affect overall elbow movement and should not be ignored.

Dorsal Glide

Joint: Proximal radioulnar joint.

Resting Position: 70° flexion with 35° supination.

Indications: To improve pronation.

Patient Position: Sitting or supine with arm supported on the table.

Clinician and Hand Positions: The rehabilitation clinician faces the patient. The proximal ulna is stabilized by the medial hand, and the mobilizing hand is wrapped around the radial head with the thenar eminence on the anterior aspect.

Mobilization Application: A downward pressure is exerted from the rehabilitation clinician's shoulder to move the radial head posteriorly (figure 20.13).

Notations: Also called an anterior-posterior glide or a posterior glide.

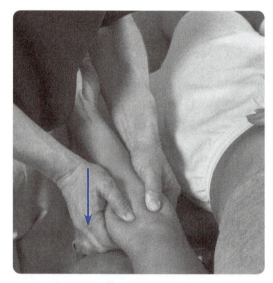

▶ **Figure 20.13** Radioulnar dorsal glide mobilization.

Ventral Glide

Joint: Proximal radioulnar joint.

Resting Position: 70° flexion with 35° supination.

Indications: To improve supination.

Patient Position: Sitting or supine with arm supported on the table.

Clinician and Hand Positions: The stabilizing hand is placed around the proximal ulna, and the mobilizing hand is placed around the head of the radius with the palm on the dorsal surface and the fingers anteriorly positioned.

Mobilization Application: Radial head is moved with a posterior-to-anterior force, using primarily the heel of the hand (figure 20.14).

Notations: Also called an anterior glide or a posterior-to-anterior glide. The elbow can be placed either in the resting position in early treatments or closer to the closed-pack position for a more aggressive application in later treatments.

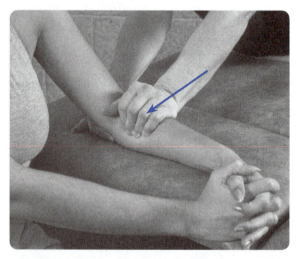

▶ **Figure 20.14** Radioulnar ventral glide mobilization.

Joint mobilization for the elbow addresses the humeroulnar joint, the humeroradial joint, and the proximal radioulnar joint.

FLEXIBILITY EXERCISES

The best way to achieve normal elbow flexibility is to prevent loss of motion. Methods of doing this include the use of continuous passive motion (CPM) machines, early mobilization following injury, and abbreviated periods of immobilization when appropriate. When loss of motion occurs, a variety of methods can be used to regain normal motion. The elbow heals as other areas of the body do, producing collagen that becomes scar tissue. As the collagen matures, stretching techniques and forces must change to influence the collagen arrangement and ultimately its strength. Short, active stretches can be used early to improve motion, but prolonged stretches are necessary later when the collagen matures. These principles and guidelines are discussed in chapters 2 and 5.

Prolonged Stretches

Prolonged stretches to the elbow must be applied with caution. Light forces are applied so as not to disrupt the anterior capsule and still achieve greater joint motion. Prolonged stretches are used only after active stretches have not been successful in restoring elbow motion.

Night Splints

For patients whose motion gains are either difficult to achieve or are progressing slower than normal, a night splint can provide prolonged, low-level forces to effectively increase connective tissue lengthening. The patient wears the brace while sleeping but usually not during the day because the brace prevents the individual from using the arm. The force and angle of the brace can be adjusted to meet the individual patient's needs. It may take a couple of nights for the patient to adjust to the brace; however, continued wear, if tolerated, can significantly improve range of motion.

Equipment Stretches

Although they are not as long as the night-splint stretches, the stretches described in this section are prolonged stretches. The mere fact that they use equipment makes it more likely that application may be too aggressive. You must be careful to use less force than you think is needed, because a longer stretch duration has a significantly greater impact on tissues than a brief stretch using the same force (Kottke, Pauley, & Ptak, 1966). Rather than applying too much force and creating capsular damage, you should begin with a force lighter than you think necessary and increase it if the results and patient response indicate that this is appropriate.

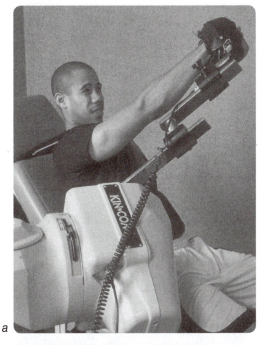

Flexion-Extension Stretches

Often a variety of machines are readily available in the clinic to provide a prolonged stretch. These can be applied for at least 10 to 15 min and longer, if the patient is able to tolerate them. A few pounds of force are applied while the shoulder is stabilized. As discussed earlier, the elbow is unique in that a muscle belly crosses the joint and can complicate attempts to regain lost motion in the joint. You must be careful not to apply too much force and overstretch the soft tissue to cause more scar-tissue formation. The recommendation is to apply no more than 1.8 kg (4 lb) of force to a stretch to increase flexion range of motion. An isokinetic machine can be used to position the elbow on stretch in either flexion or extension with the speed set at zero to maintain the desired angle (figure 20.15a). An Iso-quad exercise unit can also be used to apply a prolonged stretch. If neither of these machines is available, the patient can use free weights in the supine position: a 4.5 kg (10 lb) weight at the shoulder to prevent the shoulder from elevating off the table, and up to a 1.8 kg (4 lb) weight attached to the wrist. The distal arm should have a towel roll under it to protect the elbow from excessive posterior pressure on the table (figure 20.15b).

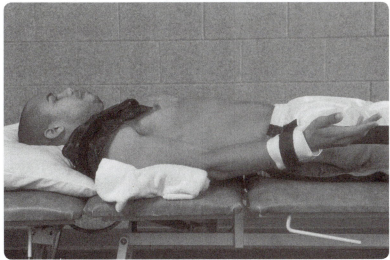

▶ **Figure 20.15** Flexion-extension equipment stretches: *(a)* using an isometric machine set at zero speed to produce a prolonged stretch, *(b)* using a free-weight equipment stretch with 4.5 kg (10 lb) at the shoulder to stabilize it, and no more than 1.8 kg (4 lb) at the wrist to produce the stretch.

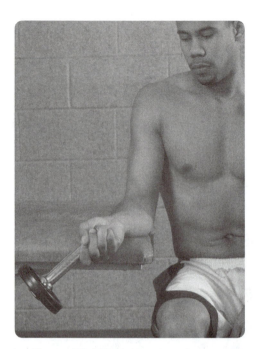

▶ **Figure 20.16** Supination equipment stretches.

Pronation-Supination Stretches

A weighted bar can be used to increase either supination or pronation. The patient sits with the elbow supported on a table; the elbow is positioned directly under the shoulder. A bar, wand, or broom handle is held in the patient's hand with the forearm positioned at end range in either supination or pronation (figure 20.16). A more effective stretch is produced if the bar is secured in place with a strap wrapped around the hand and bar; this permits muscle relaxation to improve the stretch results. The position is maintained for at least 5 min.

Active Stretches

Active stretches are performed by the patient throughout the day. They do not require a great deal of equipment so are convenient and easy to apply. Active stretches can affect both muscle and joint structures. These stretches are explained in the following sections.

■ Flexibility Exercises for the Elbow and Forearm

Active Elbow Flexor Stretch

Body Segment: Elbow.

Stage in Rehab: II and III.

Purpose: Increase elbow extension motion.

Positioning: Patient is supine or sitting with the uninvolved forearm across the abdomen and the hand's dorsum placed just proximal to the involved elbow's posterior joint.

Execution: With the forearm supinated and maintained in this position, the patient extends the elbow actively as much as possible and holds that position for 10 s.

Possible Substitutions: Scapular protraction, forward trunk lean, and shoulder extension.

Notations: This exercise is performed frequently throughout the day with 5 to 10 repetitions at each session.

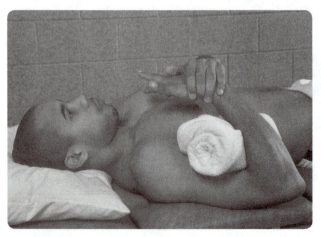

▶ **Figure 20.17** The elbow extensor stretch can be performed in supine or sitting.

Active Elbow Extensor Stretch

Body Segment: Elbow.

Stage in Rehab: II and III.

Purpose: Increase elbow flexion motion.

Positioning: Patient sits or stands. The involved forearm is held by the contralateral hand. The elbow is stabilized next to the side or on a tabletop.

Execution: Patient pulls the involved forearm toward the shoulder with the contralateral hand (figure 20.17).

Possible Substitutions: Shoulder extension and scapular retraction.

Notations: The exercise is performed for 5 to 10 repetitions throughout the day. This stretch can be made more effective and more comfortable if a rolled-up towel or pad is placed in the antecubital fossa; the pad provides a distraction on the joint during the stretch.

Active Pronator Stretch

Body Segment: Forearm.

Stage in Rehab: II and III.

Purpose: Improve supination and stretch the pronators.

Positioning: The patient sits with the elbow flexed to 90° and stabilized at the side. The forearm is positioned in as much supination as possible. The uninvolved hand is placed in an underhand grasp on the distal forearm so that the finger pads are on the volar aspect of the radius and the base of the hand is on the dorsal aspect of the ulna.

Execution: The finger pads pull the radius downward as the base of the hand pushes the ulna upward (figure 20.18).

Possible Substitutions: Movement inward by the elbow, and trunk lean toward the arm. The arm should be placed securely against the ribs to prevent movement during the stretch.

Notations: The patient should perform this stretch several times throughout the day.

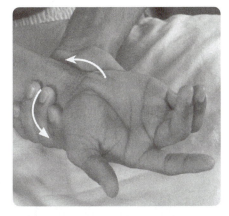

▶ **Figure 20.18** Pronator stretch.

Active Supinator Stretch

Body Segment: Forearm.

Stage in Rehab: II and III.

Purpose: Increase pronation by stretching the supinators.

Positioning: The patient sits with the elbow stabilized at the side and flexed to 90°. The forearm is actively positioned in as much pronation as possible. The patient grasps the distal forearm with the uninvolved hand in an overhand grasp by placing the finger pads around the ventral aspect of the ulna and the base of the hand on the dorsal aspect of the radius.

Execution: The finger pads are pulled upward as the base of the hand is pushed downward (figure 20.19).

Possible Substitutions: Elbow moves away from the side as the shoulder abducts, and trunk leans away from the arm. The elbow must remain in contact with the lateral trunk.

Notations: The stretch is performed frequently throughout the day. Instruct the patient to relax the shoulder and perform only to the point that he or she feels a stretch without pain.

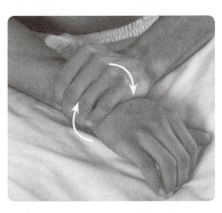

▶ **Figure 20.19** Supinator stretch.

Assisted Stretches

The clinician should apply any stretch to the anterior joint cautiously. Overstretching this area can result in more adhesions or myositis ossificans. Contract-relax-stretch techniques with active contraction of the antagonists can be used in assistive stretches. These stretches are presented in the following sections.

Assistive Stretch to the Elbow Extensors

Body Segment: Elbow.

Stage in Rehab: II and III.

Purpose: Increase elbow flexion motion.

Positioning: Patient is sitting or supine. Clinician stabilizes and supports elbow and places other hand on patient's wrist.

Execution: The clinician moves the patient's hands toward the patient's shoulder (figure 20.20a).

Possible Substitutions: If not properly stabilized, the shoulder can elevate to give a false impression of improved range of movement.

Notations: Placing the clinician's other hand or a rolled-up towel in the antecubital fossa provides joint distraction to make the stretch more comfortable and more effective. To stretch the long head of the triceps, the elbow is flexed by the clinician's hand on the distal forearm. The shoulder is then flexed overhead by the other hand on the patient's elbow.

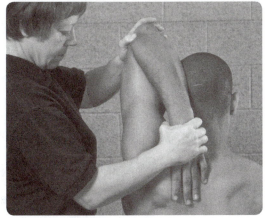

▶ **Figure 20.20** Assisted elbow flexion-extension stretch: *(a)* stretch for long head of the triceps.

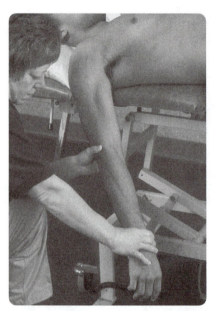

▶ **Figure 20.20** Assisted elbow flexion-extension stretch: *(b)* stretch for the biceps.

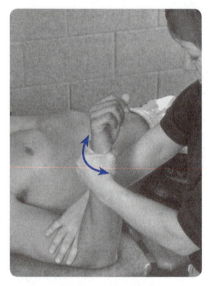

▶ **Figure 20.21** Assisted supination-pronation stretch.

Assistive Stretch to the Elbow Flexors

Body Segment: Elbow.

Stage in Rehab: II and III.

Purpose: Increase elbow extension motion.

Positioning: Patient is sitting or supine. Clinician supports the elbow.

Execution: Clinician applies the stretch as the elbow is extended and the shoulder is moved into hyperextension (figure 20.20b). This stretches the biceps and other anterior elbow structures.

Possible Substitutions: Scapular protraction, scapular tilting.

Notations: The biceps is stretched when the forearm is in pronation, but the stretch should also be applied in supination.

Assistive Forearm Stretches

Body Segment: Forearm.

Stage in Rehab: II and III.

Purpose: Increase forearm supination and forearm pronation.

Positioning: Patient is sitting or supine, and the elbow is flexed to 90°. Clinician grasps the distal arm to stabilize it and places the stretch hand on the patient's wrist.

Execution: The radioulnar joints are moved to end range with overpressure in supination and then in pronation. The stretch is held by the clinician for several seconds and repeated (figure 20.21).

Possible Substitutions: Shoulder abduction with pronation and shoulder adduction with supination. The force is applied to provide the stretch at the radioulnar joints, not twisting the hand.

Notations: It is more comfortable if this stretch is performed under warm water. Results are improved if all supination stretches are performed and then all pronation stretches are performed, as opposed to alternating.

Normal flexibility of the elbow is restored through use of prolonged stretches, as well as active and assisted stretching.

STRENGTHENING EXERCISES

As with other joints, the most basic elbow strengthening exercises include isometrics. Isotonic exercises in straight-plane motions advance to diagonal-plane motions before plyometric exercises become a part of the strength progression. The final part of the therapeutic exercise program includes the functional exercises before the patient's return to full participation.

Isometric Resistance Exercises

The patient can perform the following resistance exercises independently and frequently throughout the day. Each exercise is held for 6 s and repeated around 10 times each session. The patient should demonstrate correct execution of the exercises before performing them independently.

Elbow Flexion

The involved elbow is flexed, and the patient's contralateral hand is placed on the distal forearm. The patient attempts to move the elbow into flexion while using the opposing hand to resist the movement (figure 20.22). This exercise should be performed in supination, pronation, and neutral, as well as at several different angles of elbow flexion.

Elbow Extension

For this exercise, the resistance is applied to the distal forearm as the patient attempts to extend the elbow. This exercise should be performed at several different positions in the range of motion.

Manual-Resistance Exercises

Straight-plane manual resistance is provided by the rehabilitation clinician. It is important that the elbow move through the full range of motion in these exercises. The movement should be smooth, so the clinician needs to alter the resistance force he or she provides according to changes in the patient's strength as the elbow moves through its range of motion. If a point of weakness within the range of motion is present, the rehabilitation clinician can offer an isometric resistance at that point in the motion before proceeding through the remaining motion; if an isometric is used in this case, the patient should be informed prior to performing the exercise. You can begin manual resistance early and use it throughout the rehabilitation program because you can easily alter the resistance to meet the patient's abilities and still respect tissue-healing precautions.

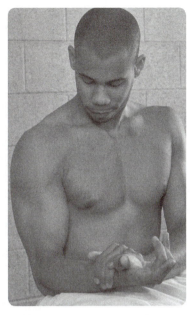

▶ **Figure 20.22** Isometric flexion.

Elbow Flexion-Extension

The best position for strengthening exercises is with the forearm in an antigravity position. This position utilizes the weight of the forearm as additional resistance. For elbow flexion, the patient is sitting or supine. Supine position is preferred because the elbow is more easily stabilized and able to go through a full range of motion. The rehabilitation clinician stabilizes the shoulder with one hand and resists elbow flexion with the other hand over the distal forearm (figure 20.23a). To resist primarily the biceps, the forearm is supinated. To eliminate the biceps and resist primarily the brachialis, the forearm is pronated. To add more resistance to the brachioradialis, the forearm is in neutral. Common substitutions in this exercise include shoulder flexion, shoulder shrugging, and scapular retraction.

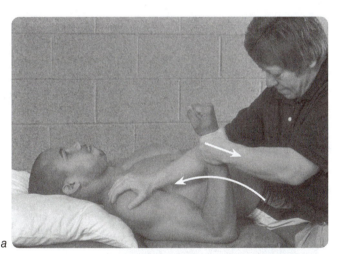

▶ **Figure 20.23**
Manual resistance: *(a)* resisted elbow flexion in supination, *(b)* resisted elbow extension.

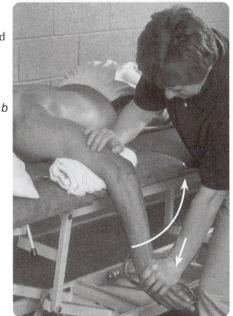

Elbow extension is performed with the patient in a prone position to maximize gravity's effect at end-range extension. The arm is abducted and supported on the table, with the forearm hanging over the side. A towel support is placed under the distal arm to increase patient comfort and elevate that arm to a level position on the table. The rehabilitation clinician stabilizes the arm with one hand and provides resistance to elbow extension at the distal forearm with the other (figure 20.23b). This exercise can also be performed with the patient in sitting with the shoulder fully elevated and the elbow overhead. This position provides maximal gravity resistance in the middle of the range of motion, and because the long head of the triceps is on stretch in this position, it will allow greater force production of the triceps. A common substitution in triceps resistance exercises is scapular protraction.

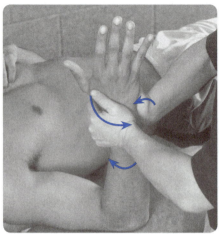

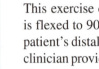

▶ **Figure 20.24** Manual resistance to supination and pronation.

Supination-Pronation

This exercise can be performed with the patient sitting or supine. The elbow is flexed to 90°, and the rehabilitation clinician places both hands around the patient's distal forearm. As the patient supinates the forearm, the rehabilitation clinician provides resistance to the movement. Resistance occurs in the opposite direction for pronation (figure 20.24). The elbow is secured at the patient's side to prevent shoulder abduction with pronation and adduction with supination.

Straight-Plane Resisted Exercises

It is important for the patient to perform these exercises through a full range of motion in a slow and controlled manner. Straight-plane resistance exercises are described in the following sections.

■ Strength Exercises for the Elbow and Forearm

Elbow Flexion

Body Segment: Elbow.

Stage in Rehab: II and III.

Purpose: Strengthen various elbow flexors.

Positioning: Patient stands with the uninvolved hand behind the involved distal arm just above the elbow. The weight is held in the hand in a supinated, pronated, or neutral position as the patient slowly flexes the elbow (figure 20.25a).

Execution: Elbow flexion occurs in a smooth, controlled motion.

Possible Substitutions: The contralateral hand is positioned behind the involved elbow to stabilize the arm and prevent use of the shoulder to lift the weight, the most common substitution in this exercise. Another substitution is to heft the weight up with a sudden shrug movement of the shoulder or the use of momentum. If this occurs, lower the resistance.

Notations: Depending on the forearm position, the biceps, brachialis, or brachioradialis (or more than one of these) is strengthened. Supination emphasizes the biceps, pronation emphasizes the brachialis, and neutral works the brachioradialis. An alternative position is with the shoulder flexed to 90° and the arm supported to maintain this position while the elbow is flexed against resistance (figure 20.25b). This position provides maximum resistance in the beginning of the exercise. This exercise can also be performed with resistance bands or pulleys. The pulley or

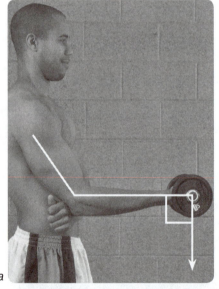

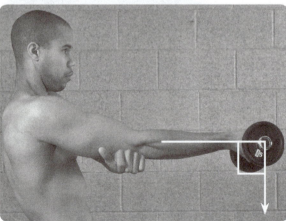

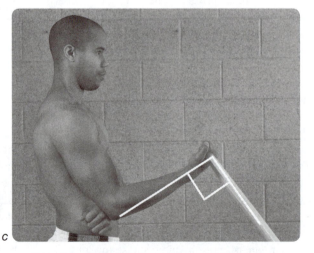

▶ **Figure 20.25** Elbow flexion: *(a)* Maximum resistance occurs at 120° elbow flexion; *(b)* maximum resistance occurs at the start of elbow flexion; *(c)* maximum resistance can change in the range of motion, depending on where the rubber band or pulley is positioned relative to elbow motion.

band is anchored low, near the ground, if maximum resistance is to occur at midrange. Changing the anchor position changes the point in the motion where maximum resistance occurs. Refer to chapter 7 for additional information on joint positions and maximum resistance. It is important to stabilize the arm by placing the opposite hand behind the upper arm as seen in figure 20.25c.

Elbow Extension

Body Segment: Elbow.

Stage in Rehab: II and III.

Purpose: Strengthen triceps and anconeus.

Positioning: Shoulder is elevated with elbow directly over the shoulder.

Execution: Elbow is extended while elbow maintains its position overhead. The contralateral hand maintains the elbow position with support on the posterior arm (figure 20.26a).

Possible Substitutions: Shoulder flexion, shoulder abduction.

Notations: If the long head of the triceps is to be emphasized less, the exercise can be performed with the patient supine (figure 20.26b). To emphasize resistance at end range, the patient leans over at the waist in standing or lies prone on a table with the arm parallel to the floor and the elbow flexed. The elbow is extended alongside the body in either the trunk flexion or prone position (figure 20.26c). Equipment such as the latissimus pulldown bar can also be used to strengthen elbow extensors (figure 20.26d). The patient positions the bar so that the elbows are at the sides and flexed. Maintaining this arm position, the patient lowers the bar by extending the elbows (figure 20.26d).

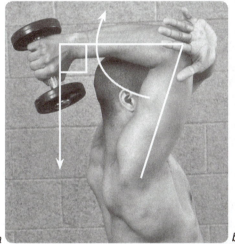
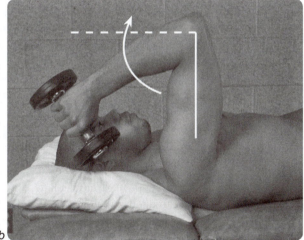
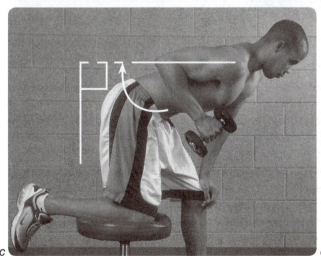
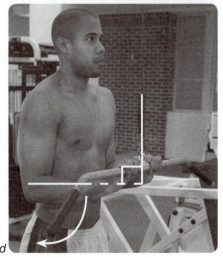

▶ **Figure 20.26** Elbow extension: *(a-b)* Maximum resistance occurs at 70°; *(c)* maximum resistance occurs at end range; *(d)* using the latissimus pulldown bar to strengthen triceps.

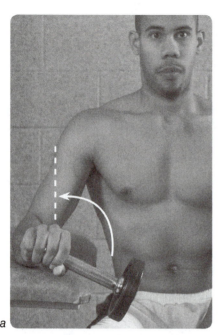

a

▶ **Figure 20.27** *(a)* Supination.

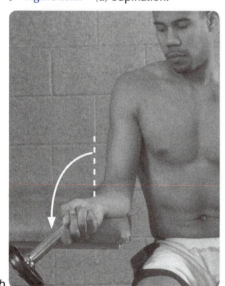

b

▶ **Figure 20.27** *(b)* Pronation.

Supination

Body Segment: Forearm.

Stage in Rehab: II and III.

Purpose: Strengthen forearm supinators.

Positioning: This exercise is performed with the patient sitting and the forearm supported over the end of a table. A weighted bar is held at one end with the forearm in pronation.

Execution: The patient rotates the bar upward until the bar is pointing toward the ceiling for a concentric exercise (figure 20.27a).

Possible Substitutions: Letting the weight fall rather than controlling its movement and speed, shoulder adduction, and elbow extension.

Notations: To perform an eccentric exercise, the patient slowly lets the bar's weight return it to the start position with the palm turned down.

Pronation

Body Segment: Forearm.

Stage in Rehab: II and III.

Purpose: Strengthen forearm pronators.

Positioning: Patient is seated as in the supination exercise just described.

Execution: Patient rotates the bar into forearm pronation to the midposition for a concentric exercise and then returns to full supination for an eccentric exercise (figure 20.27b).

Possible Substitutions: Shoulder abduction, elbow flexion.

Notations: The weight should be controlled throughout the range of motion. It is incorrect to use a dumbbell to perform this exercise and the supination exercise, because one end of the dumbbell will act as a counterbalance force for the other end, making the exercise ineffective.

Plyometric Exercises

The patient progresses to diagonal-plane (multiplane) activities after good strength in straight-plane exercises is achieved. These exercises are more strenuous since they demand simultaneous muscle performance in multiple planes, continued control of the extremity, and accuracy of performance. These exercises serve as a transition phase and prepare the elbow and its surrounding structures for the next phase, functional activities.

Carryover Shoulder Exercises

Many of the closed kinetic chain exercises discussed in chapter 19 are appropriate for the elbow. Instead of repeating details here, I suggest that you refer to chapter 19 for a listing and for information about progression of these exercises. The push-up, seated push-up, Swiss-ball weight-bearing exercises, rhythmic stabilization activities, and distal movement stabilization exercises are all appropriate for the elbow.

Resistance-band diagonal patterns in D1 and D2 flexion and extension can incorporate elbow movements of flexion or extension, or can maintain a stationary elbow position throughout the patterns. Which pattern to use depends on the patient's sport. For example, a pitcher or tennis player should use D2 flexion and extension patterns, because those patterns most closely mimic the motions in those sports. A breaststroke swimmer, on the other hand, should use D1 flexion and extension patterns.

Unstable-surface activities as discussed in chapter 19 are recommended for phase II and III elbow rehabilitation. Resisted movements using the treadmill or stair machine, and medicine-ball exercises and their progressions, are also applicable for elbow therapeutic exercise progressions.

Isokinetics

Isokinetic equipment is used initially in straight-plane exercises with stabilization and isolation of desired motions during phase III rehabilitation. Elbow flexion-extension and forearm pronation-supination motions can all be performed on the equipment. As the patient progresses, diagonal patterns serve as a progression into more functional exercises.

FUNCTIONAL AND ACTIVITY-SPECIFIC ACTIVITIES

Once the patient is able to meet the challenge of plyometric exercises, functional activities and then activity-specific challenges are the next logical steps before one allows a full return to normal activities. Many of the functional programs discussed in chapters 10 and 19 can be used very appropriately for the elbow. Of course, specific applications, once the patient qualifies to move onto sport-specific or activity-specific challenges, depend on the patient's sport or activity.

Functional exercises and sport/activity-specific challenges should include warm-up and cool-down activities. Overhead activity progressions for both groups of exercises should begin with easy activities at diminished distances, forces, and speeds and should gradually increase only one component at a time until the patient performs all activities at normal performance levels. Increases should occur no more often than every third exercise session to permit adequate adaptation to increased stress levels. If a patient experiences pain with any increase, he or she should return to the previous level of exercises for an additional three days before attempting to try the next level again.

Examples of functional activities might include medicine ball tossing for a javelin thrower, plyometric push-ups for a football guard, or resistance-band pull activities for a swimmer. Rather than repeat other programs that have already been described, I suggest that you refer to chapters 10 and 19 for details on programs, their progressions, and the precautions that guide those progressions.

SPECIAL REHABILITATION APPLICATIONS

We will now look at rehabilitation programs for some of the more common elbow injuries. For each injury, specific aspects unique to that injury and the rehabilitation program for that injury are presented. These discussions are followed by a case study for you to solve that will enable you to apply your new knowledge of elbow rehabilitation.

Epicondylitis

Epicondylitis is commonly seen in the elbow. As discussed in chapter 15, among the most important aspects of treatment of these conditions are discovering and correcting the cause of the problem. If you do not correct the cause of the injury, the risk of its recurring is very high. Because elbow motion applies torsion stress to the medial elbow, it is susceptible to tendon pathology, especially when the forces applied are exaggerated because of poor technique.

Lateral epicondylitis is often referred to as tennis elbow, and medial epicondylitis is commonly known as golfer's elbow. These both come under the general heading of tendinopathy and usually result from cumulative trauma (Ciccotti, Schwartz, & Ciccotti, 2004). Lateral

Strengthening exercises for the elbow use isometric resistance, manual resistance, straight-plane resistance, plyometrics, carryover shoulder exercises, and isokinetics in a careful progression.

Functional activities for the elbow, progressing in distances, forces, and speeds, prepare the patient for return to normal activities.

epicondylitis commonly involves the extensor carpi radialis brevis. It is likely the result of various improper techniques on the tennis backhand, including hitting the ball too late or flipping the wrist into extension. Medial epicondylitis is seen in golfers who throw the club down with the back arm to hack at the ball rather than moving the club through from the trunk and lower extremities. Tennis players who hit a forearm stroke with the elbow ahead of the racket and gymnasts who bear weight on hyperextended elbows are also subject to epicondylitis.

In either tennis elbow or golfer's elbow, the patient experiences a gradual onset of epicondylar pain. It may begin with pain only after activity. Then it may progress to some pain at the start of activity that resolves as the activity continues but returns after activity. Eventually, pain occurs with daily activities and then at rest. Grasping objects and shaking hands are painful. Extending the wrist against resistance in lateral epicondylitis and flexing the wrist against resistance in medial epicondylitis are painful. The pain is localized to the epicondyle, but if left untreated, can extend more distally on the forearm. Pronation or supination activities can become painful. Grip strength weakens, as does wrist flexion and extension. Pain can restrict full range of wrist motion, especially when it is combined with elbow extension.

As with other tendinopathy treatments, the cause of the injury must first be determined and corrected to diminish the risk of re-injury. Although there is no consensus on modalities most effective for epicondylitis, some evidence shows effectiveness of shock wave therapy and manual therapy (Kohia et al., 2008). Cross-friction massage to the tender epicondylar areas is used to reduce tissue adhesions and increase local circulation. Weakness and loss of flexibility are often secondary occurrences with epicondylitis. Elbow, wrist, and finger flexion and extension and forearm supination and pronation should be returned to normal ranges of motion through a variety of flexibility exercises. If joint motion presents with a capsular pattern, mobilization techniques are indicated. End-range stretches and mobilizations should not be aggressive, especially in the early rehabilitation phases when pain is significant. Patients who have been long-term participants in tennis or throwing sports may have developed flexion contractures and valgus deformities. These occur from repetitive microtears, scarring, and possible ossification of the flexor muscles and anterior capsule or hypertrophic bone changes (Ellenbecker & Mattalino, 1997). In the presence of these ossification changes, attempts to stretch the elbow are frustrating and are not advised. During rehabilitation phase I and early phase II, stretching exercises should be active and within the patient's comfort range.

If normal range of motion is still lacking in phase II after 3 to 4 weeks following injury onset, mobilization should be initiated. If a bony end-feel is palpated at less than normal extension, the patient may have structural changes that prohibit full extension. If the end-feel is capsular, however, joint mobilization techniques are indicated. In addition to elbow mobilization, joint mobility of the wrist and forearm is a consideration for epicondylitis treatment because muscles originating on the epicondyle affect movement of these segments. If the muscles are not moved through their full range of motion, restricted mobility occurs. Specific wrist mobilizations and flexibility exercises are discussed in chapter 21. In addition to mobilization techniques, active assistive and passive stretching exercises can be used to improve wrist, forearm, and elbow motion in phases II and III.

Strengthening exercises include isometrics, eccentrics, concentrics, and plyometrics, each provided in a logical progression. Chapter 15 contains information on the rationale for and progression of exercises in the treatment of tendinopathy. Isometrics are used in the early rehabilitation phase if motion in other strength exercises are too painful. Effective strengthening exercises for tendinopathy include an eccentric exercise program (Croisier, Foidart-Dessalle, Tinant, Crielaard, & Forthomme, 2007; Rees, Wilson, & Wolman, 2006). Such a program starts with submaximal eccentric exercises using weights or resistance bands and progresses to more aggressive use of heavier weights with increased speeds as tolerated by the injury. In phase I of the rehabilitation program, shoulder and trunk exercises should be included to maintain conditioning levels in these areas.

Rehabilitation phase III includes the use of increased resistance, diagonal motions, and more functional patterns of movement to prepare the injury for plyometric exercises. Many exercises in this phase are those listed in the shoulder rehabilitation program in chapter 19. Motions begin in a slow and controlled manner and progress to faster movements while the patient maintains control of the entire upper extremity throughout the motion. Closed kinetic chain exercises and neuromuscular facilitation exercises are used in phases II and III. Isokinetic exercises, first in straight planes and then in diagonal planes, are suitable in phase III. Isokinetic exercises should be at higher speeds and should emphasize muscle endurance. In later stages of phase III, the patient can use the isokinetic equipment to perform full-body initiated and diagonal activities that mimic normal motions. All exercises should remain pain free with no associated post-exercise discomfort.

Plyometrics in the final aspect of phase III emphasize functional movements that prepare the patient for functional and sport/activity-specific exercises before returning to full participation. These exercises are discussed in chapter 19. The progression is the same as that presented for the shoulder, beginning with easier plyometrics and advancing to higher-speed and/or more resistance as the injured segment adapts and the patient is able to tolerate increased stresses. It is during this phase that the isokinetic exercises are performed in functional patterns, using total-body performance positions. They should mimic normal activity patterns of movement as closely as possible.

Sport-specific activities are individually determined and are based on the patient's sport and activity requirements. Guidelines for these activity-specific progressions are universal and are based on the patient's response to the exercises. As a rule, increases occur no more frequently than every third day. Only one parameter is increased at one time. In other words, if a pitcher increases throwing distance on a particular day, speed of the throw is not changed on the same day. In fact, it may sometimes be prudent to reduce the speed when increasing distance and to gradually build up the throwing speed to the levels that were being attained before the distance increase. If the patient experiences pain with any program increase, he or she returns to the immediately preceding program level for another three sessions before advancing.

Bracing may assist the patient in pain-free performance. A counter-force brace is approximately 5 cm (2 in.) wide or slightly larger and is made of nonelastic strapping, usually secured with Velcro (figure 20.28). Its purpose is to reduce wrist extensor activity and disperse the stresses applied to the extensor tendons (Groppel & Nirschl, 1986). The brace is worn during the treatment phase and also when the patient returns to normal participation.

Before the racket-sport patient begins sport-specific activities prior to returning to competition, his or her equipment should be examined for appropriateness. Racket weight, stiffness, and size should be evaluated. A heavy racket requires greater strength, energy expenditure, and muscle endurance. A stiff racket allows the patient to exert greater power on the ball, but it also absorbs less impact stress and transfers the unabsorbed force to the patient's arm. A tightly strung racket also increases impact-stress transfer to the arm, so a patient returning to participation may be advised to reduce the string tension of the racket slightly. A combination of a less stiff racket and less string tension permits more force absorption in the racket because the ball is in contact with the racket longer (Newton's second law of motion). As the impact force is spread out over a longer period of time, it is reduced.

Grip size is another factor that requires assessment before the patient uses a racket. A grip that is too small may increase the strength requirements, add stress to the epicondyles, and increase fatigue of the forearm muscles. To measure grip size, place the hand flat on a table top with the palm facing up and fingers extended. Extend a tape measure from the proximal lateral crease in the palm to the end of the fourth finger (figure 20.29). This distance to the

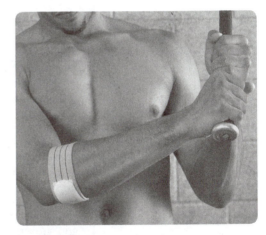

▶ **Figure 20.28** Counterforce brace.

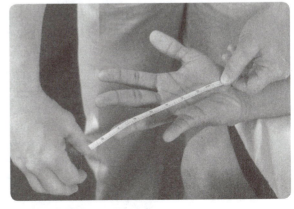

▶ **Figure 20.29** Racket-grip measurement.

nearest eighth of an inch between the proximal palm crease and the end of the fourth finger tip is the person's grip size (Nirschl, 1977).

Occasionally, surgery is necessary to completely resolve more persistent cases of epicondylitis. In lateral epicondylitis surgery, the extensor carpi radialis brevis tendon is detached from the lateral epicondyle, and debridement of the area is the common procedure. Medial surgical release commonly involves the pronator teres and flexor carpi ulnaris tendons.

Postoperative rehabilitation includes the use of an elbow immobilizer immediately after surgery, continuing for about one week. The brace may be continued for occasional support when the elbow gets fatigued, for up to three weeks postoperatively. Active range-of-motion exercises for the wrist and fingers can start after surgery, although the patient will probably not want to begin these until at least the second postoperative day. Gentle active and active assistive range of motion of the elbow can begin around day 5. By the third week, the patient should have full range of motion.

At two weeks, active exercise against gravity without resistance can begin, as can squeezing a soft ball. Pronation and supination motion exercises for the forearm, as well as flexion and extension motion exercises for the wrist and elbow, should continue.

The patient is at the end of phase II and into early phase III by three weeks post-op, so the patient progresses from isometrics to low-resistance, low-repetition exercises in straight-plane exercises. Full motion should be present by this time. The patient progresses as tolerated into higher-repetition exercises before moving into heavier weights.

Diagonal-plane exercises begin at four to eight weeks, depending on the patient's pain tolerance and strength. Once the patient displays good strength and control without pain in diagonal motions, it is appropriate to begin plyometrics in phase III.

■ Case Study

A 24-year-old, right-hand-dominant female tennis player has been playing with tennis elbow for the past six months. It started when she bought a new Kevlar tennis racket and began putting more topspin on her serve. The condition has advanced to a level such that she now has pain throughout her game; she is not playing well any more, has a difficult time opening doors and turning the key to start her car, and is unable to carry her gym bag in the right hand. The forearm feels stiff most of the time. Examination reveals tenderness over the lateral epicondyle extending into the proximal forearm along the radial wrist extensors. Resisted wrist extension is weak and painful. Grip strength measured with a grip dynamometer on the right is 15.8 kg (35 lb) and painful compared to the pain-free left grip strength of 34 kg (75 lb). Her wrist flexion range of motion is limited to 45° because of pain. There is no restriction of joint accessory movements. Passive elbow extension increases the wrist flexion pain.

Questions for Analysis

1. What will your first treatment session include?
2. What are your initial treatment goals?
3. What will be your instructions to the patient in the first treatment?
4. How do you plan to increase her range of motion?
5. Outline your program for strengthening the wrist and identify the guidelines you will use to determine her rate of progression.
6. What suggestions regarding equipment will you make to the patient?
7. Describe functional and sport-specific activity progressions for the patient and identify the criteria you will use to determine when she is ready to return to full participation in tennis.

By three to four months, the patient can begin functional activities if there is no pain with plyometrics and if normal strength, muscle endurance, and flexibility are present. Patients undergoing medial epicondylar releases may not be able to return to full participation for five to six months, but those undergoing lateral epicondylar releases may return to function four to five months postoperatively.

Little League Elbow

Little League elbow is another chronic condition of the elbow, but it is unique because it occurs only in youngsters. Its name comes from the population it most frequently affects, pitchers of Little League baseball. It has been a common enough problem that youth league governing bodies now regulate pitching in this population, but the problem remains. Special issues surrounding this injury are presented before a case study is provided for you to solve.

Little league elbow is unique to the preadolescent population. It involves a number of conditions that have the common thread of elbow pathology secondary to pitching. The most common site of pathology is the medial elbow because of the excessive traction forces applied to the medial epicondyle epiphyseal plate during the late cocking phase (Sabick, Kim, Torry, Keirns, & Hawkins, 2005). The rotation of the humerus during this phase places excessive torque forces on the elbow by producing either humeral retrotorsion or proximal humeral epiphysiolysis after repetitive excesses (Sabick et al., 2005). Curves and breaking pitches increase the demands on wrist flexion and pronation, increasing the medial epicondyle stresses. Injury to the inherently weak epiphyseal plate may begin as an inflammation and progress to an avulsion of the plate if repetitive trauma persists. In severe cases, osteochondritis dissecans of the radioulnar joint can also occur.

Less frequently, the lateral, anterior, or posterior elbow is affected by excessive stresses applied during throwing. The pronator teres suffers increased stresses laterally during extreme pronation, and increased hyperextension forces on deceleration after ball release can increase anterior and posterior joint stresses (Loftice et al., 2004).

In the more common medial Little League elbow, the athlete experiences progressive medial elbow pain with activity, pain with end-motion finger and wrist extension, tenderness to medial epicondyle palpation, and pain and weakness with resisted wrist and finger flexion. Swelling and, in more severe cases, ecchymosis, can be present over the medial epicondyle.

Common causes for Little League elbow are improper warm-up or lack of warm-up, improper or insufficient conditioning, poor pitching mechanics, inadequate rest between games, pitching too many innings, and pitching curves and breaking-ball pitches. It is recommended that adequate conditioning programs and proper warm-up and cool-down procedures be included in a team's program, and that adherence to Little League baseball pitching rules be enforced for practices as well as games. Those rules include permitting an adolescent to pitch no more than six innings and mandating rest of three days between pitching rotations. Patients should avoid those activities that produce little league elbow. If an injury occurs, it becomes even more important for the patient to adhere to recommendations that minimize elbow stresses.

If growth plate damage is evident with the injury, the individual should be advised to stop pitching for the rest of the baseball season. Early phase I treatment for little league elbow includes rest, ice, and in advanced cases, immobilization. Active range-of-motion exercises to tolerance are encouraged. Passive stretches should be avoided. Because of the age of the patient, using heavy weights is not advisable because these could aggravate sensitive growth plates. Exercises are neither as aggressive nor as intensive as they are for adult patients, but the program should follow the same progression. This progression emphasizes range of motion and pain relief in the initial rehabilitation phase, with advancement to a progressive strengthening program before functional and sport-specific activities are initiated. Valgus stress is avoided until it does not cause pain. A gradual throwing progression is included when the elbow is pain free and has full range of motion and normal muscle strength and muscle endurance.

> ### ■ Case Study
>
> A nine-year-old baseball pitcher is in the middle of his season. For the past month he has experienced progressive medial elbow pain on his left throwing elbow. He is the team's top pitcher and usually pitches three days a week. An invitational tournament his team is competing in is planned for next weekend, and he wants to pitch. His parents are reluctant to allow him to do so, but they want your opinion. He has full range of motion of the elbow, but wrist extension is painful in the last 10°. Resisted pronation and wrist flexion are weak and painful. The medial epicondyle is tender to palpation and edematous.
>
> *Questions for Analysis*
>
> 1. What will be your recommendation to the patient regarding the weekend invitational tournament?
> 2. What will be your recommendations on future pitching?
> 3. What treatment procedure will you recommend he follow to reduce the pain and inflammation? Given his age, what precautions must you consider?
> 4. What will be your instructions about exercises he should perform?
> 5. How much information will you give the patient's parents about the injury and potential harm?

Sprains

Sprains in the elbow commonly occur as hyperextension injuries. Capsular injury of the elbow can be frustrating if not treated correctly at the outset. Special considerations relating to this type of injury are presented followed by a case study.

Program Considerations

Sprains in the elbow usually occur as either a hyperextension injury or a medial collateral ligament sprain. A hyperextension sprain can occur when a football opponent runs into and past an outstretched blocking arm or when a gymnast does a handstand with a locked elbow. Any sudden valgus force such as a sidearm throw by a shortstop, or a wrench of the elbow by a wrestling opponent, can also cause a sprain. In a hyperextension injury, the anterior capsule is injured; but in a medial collateral stress injury, the medial (ulnar) collateral ligament (UCL), the primary stabilizing unit for the elbow, is injured.

Hyperextension injuries cause pain in the anterior joint and can also cause a bone contusion and pain of the olecranon or olecranon fossa. Ulnar collateral ligament sprains cause medial joint pain. A support brace may be used during the first couple of weeks following injury to support and protect the area. Initial phase I rehabilitation includes treatment to relieve pain and swelling. Cross-friction massage to adherent scar tissue in the area can also relieve pain but should not be performed within the first 7 to 10 days following injury. Active and active-assistive ranges of motion are used in late phase I and early phase II, along with mild straight-plane strengthening exercises. Pain during activity is avoided. Strengthening exercises should include the biceps and triceps, as well as wrist and finger flexors and extensors and forearm pronators and supinators. Following hyperextension injuries to the inert anterior structures, the biceps, brachialis, brachioradialis, and supinator play an important role in providing dynamic stability anteriorly, and the triceps and biceps co-contract to provide weight-bearing stability. Following a UCL sprain, the supinators assist in providing stability lost by the ligamentous injury. Resistance to the flexor carpi ulnaris may aggravate the UCL in early rehabilitation and should be deferred until the second rehabilitation phase. By the last half of phase II, full range of motion of the elbow should be present. Strengthening exercises for the flexor carpi ulnaris in wrist flexion and ulnar deviation should be instituted at this time if they haven't yet been initiated. Straight-plane exercises continue, and their resistance and repetition levels can increase. Eccentric and concentric exercises are used. By the end of phase III, diagonal-plane movements begin with proprioceptive neuromuscular facilitation stabilization activities and closed kinetic chain exercises; resistance-band exercises are added as long as the stresses do not cause pain either during or after the exercise. Isokinetics are appropriate, beginning with straight-plane movement and progressing to diagonal planes of movement.

In late phase III, plyometric exercises begin. These are the same exercises as those described for epicondylitis. Functional planes of movement are used during these exercises. The patient should be able to maintain good joint stability during all activities. The goal in the final aspect of this phase is to prepare the injury site for phase IV sport-specific activities.

Ulnar Collateral Ligament Repair/Reconstruction

Instability of the elbow occurs primarily following severe injury to the elbow joint's primary stabilizer, the UCL, especially the anterior portion of the ligament (Alcid, Ahmad, & Lee, 2004). In these cases, surgical repair may be required if conservative care does not resolve the instability. Postoperative rehabilitation depends on the surgical technique used. Surgical reconstruction is performed using an autogenous graft with detachment of the flexor/pronator tendon group if the ligament lacks any viable tissue for repair. This situation requires a longer postoperative rehabilitation process than when the ligament contains viable tissue and can be salvaged without detaching the flexor/pronator mass. Since Jobe (Jobe, Stark, & Lombardo, 1986) first developed a surgical reconstruction to allow athletes to return to sport participation after surgery, modifications in reconstruction methods have made surgical reconstruction success commonplace (Nassab, Mark, & Schickendantz, 2006).

Following surgery, the elbow is locked at 90° in an adjustable elbow flexion splint for the first week. During this time, the patient performs active wrist and finger motion exercises. Submaximal isometric exercises for the biceps and the shoulder occur as long as the patient avoids shoulder lateral rotation, a motion which increases valgus elbow stress. The patient can also squeeze a ball.

By the end of the second week, the brace's motion stops are positioned 30° from extension and at 100° of flexion. Submaximal wrist and elbow isometrics can start after the second week. The patient now starts to actively move the elbow in the range of motion allowed by the brace. The brace is adjusted each week to increase motion in both flexion and extension until it is set to full motion by the sixth week. With each change in brace positions, the patient's active motion is also improved through active exercises.

After three weeks, a gradual progression of strength exercises is added to the program. These exercises include mild resistance to wrist and elbow flexion and extension and forearm pronation and supination. Early proprioception exercises for joint-position sense with eyes closed is appropriate, but valgus stress to the elbow is avoided. Proprioceptive exercises that avoid valgus stresses advance as tolerated. Shoulder exercises, with the exception of lateral-rotation motions, are performed as well. Lateral rotation exercises start after the sixth week. Concentric, eccentric, and mild isokinetics are used in straight-plane movements. Co-contraction exercises for the biceps and triceps are also started as long as valgus stress is avoided. Closed kinetic chain exercises and other stabilization exercises are permissible once the patient has strength and control of the elbow.

Full range of motion should be present by week 6 to 8. The muscles providing dynamic stability—the biceps, pronators, and wrist flexors—are important for assisting the UCL and should be well strengthened. After the sixth week, diagonal movements can begin if adequate strength and control without pain are present in the elbow. Work on proprioceptive neuromuscular facilitation patterns, resistance-band exercises, more aggressive stabilization exercises, and diagonal isokinetics at high speeds can all be started at this time.

Plyometric activities begin in the final phase after week 9. As with other plyometric exercises, these begin with lower-stress activities at reduced speeds and resistance, and then increase to higher speeds and place additional stress on the elbow. Medicine ball tosses, push-up progressions, and functional isokinetic motions are included.

Functional exercises can begin in week 10 to 14. The timing depends on the patient's response to these functional exercises and the patient's progression into sport- and activity-specific reconditioning events in the rehabilitation program. For example, a pitcher may need to wait longer before beginning throwing activities because of the higher elbow stresses in pitching compared with those in a less-intense sport, such as golf, or less-intense work activities, such as computer programming. The progression of functional activities and the precautions to observe are the same as for other injuries. Following UCL reconstruction surgery, it is common for a patient to return to full participation by week 22 to 26. These timelines are based on averages, and you must always remember that actual time for recovery will vary from one patient to another. Figure 20.30 describes this rehabilitation progression.

Ulnar Nerve Injury

Injury to the ulnar nerve can occur in any setting but seems most prevalent in repetitive throwing sports such as baseball (pitching). The most frequent cause in this population is incorrect mechanics. This injury is treated with both operative and nonoperative techniques. Considerations in therapeutic exercise for both treatments are presented here.

Repetitive overhand throwing activities, especially in patients whose shoulder lateral rotation in the cocking phase is reduced, places excessive stress on medial elbow structures. The ulnar nerve can become stretched, mechanically irritated, or even subluxed out of its sulcus.

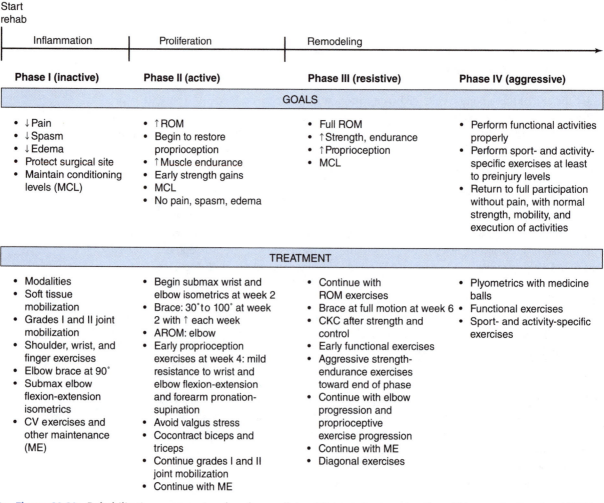

▶ **Figure 20.30** Rehabilitation progression for ulnar collateral ligament reconstruction. CV = cardiovascular; AROM = **active range** of motion; ROM = range of motion; CKC = closed kinetic chain.

■ Case Study

A 30-year-old right-handed golfer injured his right elbow when he hit a divot and tore his ulnar collateral ligament. He attempted to continue playing through the season, but pain persisted. The elbow became unstable, and he underwent a medial collateral reconstruction. The surgery was 10 days ago, and he has been instructed by the surgeon to begin rehabilitation. The elbow is in a functional brace's motion blocks that are at 30° from extension and 100° flexion. Supination is possible to neutral. Your examination reveals mild discoloration still present in the forearm and distal upper arm medially. There is spasm in the upper trapezius and biceps. Active range of motion out of the brace is 60° from extension to 100° into flexion. Wrist extensors have 4/5 strength, the shoulder grossly has 4–/5 strength, the biceps and triceps are also 4–/5, and the wrist flexors are 3–/5. There are active trigger points in the forearm on the flexor and extensor surfaces.

Questions for Analysis

1. What will your first treatment session include?
2. What precautions will you give the patient?
3. When will you start pronation and supination motion activities? What considerations must be made before these exercises are added?
4. What strengthening exercises will you include in the first week, and how will you advance them (what will your criteria be)?
5. At what motion limits will you set the brace in week 5?
6. When will you start shoulder external-rotation exercises?
7. What functional-exercise program will you will establish for the patient, and when will you start it?

Adjacent soft-tissue structures can also compress the nerve. The patient commonly complains of fourth- and fifth-digit numbness or tingling and posteromedial elbow pain. Nonoperative care includes initial treatments to reduce the inflammation and pain. Exercises to improve range of motion and strength are similar to those for other elbow injuries. Mobilization is performed if the joint is hypomobile. Strength exercises are initially low-resistance, high-repetition loads in straight-plane motions. Muscles for all shoulder, elbow, wrist, and forearm motions are strengthened. If shoulder inflexibility, shoulder weakness, or poor athletic technique is contributing to the elbow injury, these deficiencies must be corrected. Initial exercises should not place valgus stress on the elbow. As strength improves, valgus stress is gradually introduced. The final phases of the program include a progression from diagonal motions to plyometrics to functional and then sport- or activity-specific functions before resuming normal and unrestricted participation.

When operative repair is necessary for a subluxating or dislocating ulnar nerve, the surgical technique most commonly used is the creation of fascial slings to support the ulnar nerve and/or a nerve transposition (Keefe & Lintner, 2004). Postoperatively, the elbow is placed in a hinged elbow brace that is positioned at 90° flexion for two weeks. After the first week, the brace motion stops are positioned at 30° to 15° from extension and at 100° to 120° flexion. The brace is discontinued by the third week. By about the sixth week, the patient should have full range of motion in all planes. Gentle gripping exercises using a foam ball start during the first postoperative week along with isometric exercises for the shoulder. Active range-of-motion exercises for pronation, supination, and wrist and finger flexion and extension are also included.

By week 2, isometrics for the elbow and wrist can begin. The splint is removed to permit active and passive range-of-motion exercises. Early proprioceptive exercises for position sense start in week 2. Mild manual-resistance exercises and light weights for the wrist are also added. By the third week, resistance exercises for the wrist, forearm, and elbow include low-

---

■ Case Study

A 19-year-old right-handed volleyball frontline player suffered a subluxed ulnar nerve at the end of the season. She underwent ulnar nerve transplantation two days ago. The surgeon wants her to begin her rehabilitation program today. She has a posterior splint set at 90°. She has some pain over the surgical site, but nothing significant. There is some tension in the upper trapezius muscle, and it is tender to palpation. Wrist extension and supination movements cause some medial elbow pain at the end range. Wrist flexion motion is lacking about 10°, and the patient reports that the wrist feels weak and sore from the surgery. Pronation is also weak. Shoulder flexion is lacking about 10°, lateral rotation is lacking about 20°, and there is some weakness in the rotator cuff.

Questions for Analysis

1. What will your first treatment session include? What will be the goals of this treatment session?
2. What home exercises will you give the patient in the first week?
3. What exercises will the program include for the next three weeks?
4. Outline a functional-exercise program that the patient will use when she is ready for functional activities.

---

resistance, high-repetition exercises in all planes. Exercises begin in straight-plane motions and progress to diagonal planes as strength and motion control improve.

By the eighth week, plyometrics begin with a normal progression from low-load, controlled movement to increased loads with higher speeds of movement. Functional activities progressing to sport- and activity-specific maneuvers begin at week 10 to 12 with full return to normal activities after week 12 to 16.

Dislocation

When an elbow dislocation occurs, the deformity makes it an obvious injury. If there has been no vascular compromise and surgery is not required, a therapeutic exercise program can follow the course described next. As occurs with many therapeutic exercise programs involving serious injury, modalities to relieve pain and swelling and promote healing are applied in phases I and II of the therapeutic exercise program.

Elbow dislocations occur primarily posteriorly and follow sudden hyperextension and abduction force applications. Suggestions for a therapeutic exercise progression following initial and immediate care is presented here.

The elbow is placed in a posterior immobilizing splint at 90° for about a week. Active wrist and shoulder motion in the splint is desirable. Isometric exercises to the elbow and mild resistive exercises to the wrist are used initially. The patient squeezes a ball throughout the day. After about five days, the splint is removed for gentle active range of motion to tolerance in all elbow and forearm planes. Passive motion is avoided.

After the first week, the splint is removed during the day but used as needed when fatigue occurs. After two weeks, the splint is discarded and active range-of-motion exercises are continued. Mild resistive exercises for the elbow with emphasis on high repetitions and low resistance begin at this time. Straight-plane exercises are used initially and advance to diagonal-plane exercises when the patient demonstrates good control, strength, and coordination. By week 6, the patient should have full range of motion in all planes. Joint mobilization is added by week 4 to 6 if additional capsular-motion gains are required.

Strength exercises progress in the same way as for other elbow injuries, from isometric to isotonic to isokinetic. Emphasis is on strengthening the elbow flexors to provide dynamic stabilization against hyperextension. Resistive exercises begin in straight planes and progress

---

> ### ■ Case Study
>
> A 20-year-old right-handed gymnast fell off the balance beam and landed on her left hyperextended elbow, dislocating the elbow, five days ago. Surgery was not necessary, but the orthopedist has placed the elbow in a 90° splint and wants you to begin rehabilitation on it today. Elbow range of motion lacks 50° of extension and can flex to 100°. Supination is 10°, and pronation is 20°. Edema and ecchymosis surround the elbow and extend into the mid-forearm and mid-upper arm. Spasm is present in the biceps, triceps, and upper trapezius. Strength is difficult to test in the elbow because the patient complains of pain and offers minimal resistance to resisted elbow flexion and extension. Wrist movements demonstrate 4/5 strength, and grip strength is 75% compared to that on the right. Shoulder strength overall is 4+/5.
>
> *Questions for Analysis*
>
> 1. What will your first treatment session include? What will your goals be for today's treatment?
> 2. What instructions for home exercises will you give the patient during the first week?
> 3. What exercises will you include as part of the first week's treatment program?
> 4. What are your goals for the first week?
> 5. What will be your progression of flexibility and strength exercises?
> 6. What functional-exercise program will you include for rehabilitation?

to diagonal planes, to plyometrics, and finally to functional and then sport-specific activities by week 8 to 10. A hyperextension brace may be necessary to offer the patient additional protection against hyperextension forces. It may take the patient 16 to 26 weeks to return to full participation.

Arthroscopy

Although arthroscopic surgery is less complicated than an open procedure and leads to less tissue damage, respect for tissue healing is still warranted. As the therapeutic exercise program begins, the rehabilitation clinician must not lose sight of the fact that the patient has had surgery and that tissue healing is a necessary ongoing process.

The most common arthroscopic procedure performed on the elbow is debridement of synovitis and removal of loose bodies. Postoperative rehabilitation following this procedure is more accelerated than with open procedures, because less tissue damage and insult have occurred. The arm is often placed in a sling for one or two days (or three days if pain warrants it) following the surgery. In addition to pain and edema control, initial treatment includes active and mild passive range of motion activities and joint mobilization for pain modulation. Shoulder and wrist range-of-motion exercises are also performed. Gripping exercises are also used in the first two or three postoperative days.

Full range of motion should be present by the third postoperative day. The sling is discarded, and mild resistive exercises to the elbow begin. If debridement has occurred in the posterior elbow, it may be uncomfortable for the patient to perform end-range flexion-extension exercises. These exercises are performed in a straight plane within a pain-free range of motion, especially during the first three to four weeks. Shoulder strengthening and wrist and forearm strengthening are also performed within pain-free limits. Proprioception exercises begin within the first week.

By week 3 to 4, the patient begins phase III rehabilitation; isokinetic exercises can begin in straight planes, advancing as indicated to diagonal planes. Rubber band resistance and other eccentric exercises are added. Diagonal planes with resistive exercises are used once good strength and control are seen in straight-plane exercises.

■ Case Study

A 35-year-old, right-handed, recreational baseball pitcher underwent arthroscopic removal of loose bodies from the posterior elbow yesterday. The surgeon wants him to begin rehabilitation today. The patient reports mild postoperative pain, but nothing unusual. He is wearing an arm sling, but he has been told he can remove it throughout the day. There is swelling around the surgical site. The dressing does not indicate any unusual postoperative drainage. The elbow range of motion is lacking 30° in extension and flexes to 100°. Pronation is 70° and supination is 50°. Wrist flexion and extension are each 60°. There is some spasm in the triceps. Manual muscle testing reveals 4–/5 strength in the biceps and triceps with some tenderness to triceps resistance, 4–/5 wrist flexion and extension without pain, and 4/5 strength throughout the shoulder.

Questions for Analysis

1. What will your first treatment be? Justify you would provide this treatment.
2. What instructions will you give the patient before he leaves today?
3. Outline your expected progression of exercises for the next two weeks. What guidelines will you use to determine when the patient should begin a progressive throwing program?
4. What will you tell him when he asks you how soon he can get back to playing baseball?

Common elbow injuries that warrant special considerations in therapeutic exercise program design are epicondylitis, Little League elbow, sprains, ulnar nerve injury, dislocation, and postarthroscopy conditions.

Plyometric exercises start once the patient shows good control and strength in diagonal-plane activities. These activities may be as early as the third week but may not be possible until the fifth or sixth week, depending on the extensiveness of the surgery and the patient's response to the surgery and exercises. Functional activities begin once plyometric exercises are completed and are followed by sport-specific and activity-specific tasks. By around week 8, the patient may be ready to return to resume normal participation.

SUMMARY

The elbow is a structure that is unique in several ways. It has three joints encased in one capsule, so if capsular restriction occurs with one of these joints, it is likely that it will also affect the other two joints. Trigger points, joint mobilization techniques, and progressive exercises for the elbow region were presented in this chapter. The more common injuries seen in rehabilitation were also presented along with an outline of rehabilitation programs for each of them. The elbow encounters compressive stresses applied to the lateral joint and distraction stress on the medial joint, so injuries seen at this joint often reflect these stresses, especially in repetitive stress injuries. Bony and joint compressive injuries occur laterally, but inflammations and soft tissue irritations from repetitive stretches occur more medially.

KEY CONCEPTS AND REVIEW

1. Discuss why overstretching the elbow should be avoided, especially during the inflammation phase of healing.

The biceps insert onto the forearm's fascia, adhesions occur relatively easily in the elbow, and the anterior capsule is relatively thin. Therefore, soft tissues can be easily damaged with aggressive stretching, resulting in additional scarring.

2. Describe the convex-concave rules for the various elbow joints.

The radial head and ulna both are concave surfaces and move on a convex capitulum and convex trochlea, respectively, so force applications are in the same direction as the restricted movement. In the proximal radioulnar joint, the force is applied in the direction opposite the restricted movement because this joint is a convex surface moving on a concave surface.

3. Identify the resting positions for the elbow joints.

As outlined in table 6.3, the resting position for the humeroulnar joint is 70° elbow flexion and 10° supination. The resting position for the humeroradial joint is full elbow extension with full supination. The radioulnar joint's resting position is 70° elbow flexion with 35° supination.

4. Identify three soft-tissue mobilization techniques for the elbow.

Cross-friction is used for the biceps tendon; trigger point release is used for the brachialis; and trigger point release is used for the triceps.

5. List three joint mobilizations for the elbow.

Distraction of the humeroulnar joint is used for general relaxation and pain relief; posterior glide of the humeroradial joint is used to increase extension; and ventral glide of the radioulnar joint is used for increasing supination.

6. Explain three strengthening exercises for the elbow and their purpose.

Elbow flexion in a supinated position for primarily increasing strength of the biceps, elbow flexion in pronation for primarily strengthening brachialis, and elbow flexion in neutral for primarily strengthening brachioradialis.

7. Discuss the general progression of strengthening exercises for the elbow.

Range of motion begins with cautious active motion and incorporates low-intensity long-term stretches only if active exercises cannot restore range of motion. Isometric strengthening exercises are followed by light-resistance exercises and then more-intense strengthening exercises as strength increases. Eccentric exercises are preceded by concentric exercises, using careful stabilization to isolate the correct muscles. Shoulder, forearm, and wrist exercises are included in the program. Exercises are performed initially in straight plane and advanced to diagonal plane as strength and control improve. Plyometric exercises are added after strength and motion are adequate, and functional activities that prepare the patient for return to sport are the last exercises included.

8. Outline a therapeutic exercise program for epicondylitis.

Basic to any tendinopathy program is discovering the underlying cause and correcting it. Pain and edema relief with modalities is initiated before therapeutic exercises. Soft-tissue mobilizations such as friction massage and myofascial release are used for soft-tissue-related restrictions and pain, and joint mobilization is used with capsular pattern losses of motion. Active range-of-motion exercises can be performed during the soft-tissue and joint mobilization applications. Isometric and manual resistance in straight-plane exercises are followed by greater-resistance and diagonal-plane activities as strength progresses. Plyometric exercises with medicine balls and rubber resistance are followed by functional activities that begin at low resistance and low intensity and progress as the patient's control and execution improve.

9. Indicate precautions that should be considered in a Little League elbow therapeutic exercise program.

If growth-plate damage is evident when an injury occurs, the patient should be advised to stop pitching for the rest of the baseball season. Active range-of-motion exercises (only to tolerance) are encouraged. Passive stretches should be avoided. Use of heavy weights is not advisable, because this could aggravate sensitive growth plates. Exercises should be neither as aggressive nor as intensive as they are for older patients. Valgus stress should be avoided until it does not cause pain.

10. List precautions for a therapeutic exercise program following an ulnar nerve transposition.

Tissue healing must be respected. Exercises begin more slowly than they do with nonoperative treatment for nerve injuries. Straight-plane exercises precede diagonal-plane exercises. While the elbow is in a postoperative sling, handgrip exercises can be used to start early strengthening. Active exercises should be used for stretching. Gentle cross-friction massage should be used only after three weeks if a loss of range of motion persists.

11. Explain the differences in rehabilitation programs for an arthroscopic debridement and a medial collateral reconstruction.

Because the medial collateral reconstruction is an open procedure, rehabilitation is a much slower process than with some alternative procedures. The period of immobilization is longer, and exercises are less aggressive in the early stages of the program. Loss of motion is a more significant factor, so motion and mobility activities are more prominent in the early phases.

CRITICAL THINKING QUESTIONS

1. Joan is faced with a probable Little League elbow tendinopathy in the opening scenario. What other possible diagnoses could Steve have? What tests should Joan perform to determine what the problem is? What recommendations should she make to Mr. Turner for care? What precautions should Joan take in making recommendations to him?

2. How does the rehabilitation program for an elbow differ for a dislocation as compared to a sprain? How are the precautions different and why? Is the progression of exercises different, and if so, how and why?

3. Can you identify the differences between a medial and a lateral epicondylitis? What structures are affected? How are the mechanisms of injury different? Would the rehabilitation programs be different? If so, how?

LAB ACTIVITIES

1 Locate the trigger points for the following muscles on your lab partner:
   a. Biceps
   b. Brachialis
   c. Triceps
   d. Brachioradialis

   Where were your partner's most sensitive trigger points? Perform a spray-and-stretch technique on each of them and provide your partner with a home exercise for each tender trigger point.

2. Locate the lateral epicondyle where the long finger extensors insert on the humerus. Can you palpate each extensor tendon as they come off the epicondyle? Can you locate the tendon that is most often the source of lateral epicondylitis? Explain why an individual with lateral epicondylitis has pain when grasping.

3. Examine your lab partner's various elbow joints using joint mobilization techniques for all three joints. How does the mobility of each one compare to the others? Which of the three joints has the greatest mobility; which one has the least amount of movement? Visualize in each joint's motion where the resistance to movement begins. Is it before or after half of the total joint mobility?

4. Perform the following joint mobilizations on your lab partner and identify what restriction would be best treated with each mobilization:

    a. Humeroulnar joint
- Distraction
- Medial glide
- Lateral glide

    b. Humeroradial joint
- Distraction
- Dorsal glide
- Ventral glide

    c. Proximal radioulnar joint
- Dorsal glide of radial head
- Ventral glide of radial head

5. Have your partner perform two stretches each for elbow flexion, elbow extension, pronation, and supination. Identify possible substitutions you must watch for with each exercise.

6. Apply manual resistance to your partner for each of the motions listed with your partner in supine. Have him or her go through 10 repetitions for each exercise. Be sure to apply a maximum resistance but produce a smooth concentric movement throughout the full range of motion. After the repetitions are completed, apply eccentric resistance to the same motions for 10 repetitions each. Which was more fatiguing for your partner? Which was more difficult for you to perform? Why?

    a. Elbow flexion
    b. Elbow extension
    c. Pronation
    d. Supination

7. Using a dumbbell or cuff weight, have your partner perform a triceps extension exercise in three different antigravity positions, 10 repetitions in each position. Repeat the activity for the elbow flexors. Which position was the most difficult to perform and why?

8. Have your partner use a free weight to perform a supination-pronation exercise while sitting. As your partner goes through the range of motion slowly, have him identify what muscles are being used at various portions of the range of motion. If you wanted to work only supinators in both concentric and eccentric motions, explain how you would have the patient perform the exercises.

9. If your partner has tennis elbow, what specific activities would you have her perform? You should concentrate on eccentric activities. What would they be, and how many repetitions and sets would you have her do today? Provide a rationale for your answers. Have your partner perform them as you state them. Have you changed your mind on the goals you set before the exercises were performed? What made you either keep them or change them from your original goals?

10. Develop a series of three plyometric exercises you would use for an elbow patient's rehabilitation program. Have your partner perform them and identify the easiest and most difficult exercise. What substitution patterns could he develop as fatigue occurred? What would you set as your criteria for progression from one exercise to the next? Justify why you have set these criteria.

11. List three sport-specific exercises you would have an elbow patient who is a softball left fielder perform before you allowed her to return to full play. Justify why you have selected these criteria.

Wrist and Hand

OBJECTIVES

After completing this chapter, you should be able to do the following:

1. Explain the pulley system of the fingers.
2. Explain why reducing edema in the hand is important.
3. Discuss the trimuscular system of the hand and explain its importance to hand function.
4. Identify the precision pinches and power grips of the hand.
5. Explain the difference between static and dynamic splints.
6. Identify what motion increases with carpal radial glide joint mobilization.
7. Explain the force application sequence to improve long finger flexor and extensor motion.
8. Explain how the intrinsic stretches differ from the extrinsic stretches.
9. Discuss the difference in gliding exercises for the flexor profundus and superficialis tendons.
10. Present the differences between long flexor and long extensor tendons.
11. Explain what procedures should be used to eliminate an extensor lag of a distal phalanx.
12. Identify the early signs of CRPS.

▶ Three weeks ago Danny Macky was playing soccer with his friends when he was tripped and fell, landing on his outstretched hands. His right hand was severely cut by a piece of broken glass hidden in the grass. The surgeon repaired his lacerated long finger flexor tendons and placed the hand in an extension-restricted splint, but now wants Deanna Murray, rehabilitation clinician, to begin the rehabilitation process on the hand.

Deanna has had experience with repaired tendons and appreciates the precautions she must consider, especially because the repair is only three weeks old. She is concerned about the adhesions that have begun to form between the long flexor superficialis and profundus tendons and other soft tissue in the anterior finger region, and is concerned about the impact those adhesions might have on the finger's hood mechanism. If the hood mechanism is harmed, the intrinsic muscles can be affected, which will impair the hand's function; so Deanna understands she has to proceed cautiously with Danny's rehabilitation program.

Problems are only opportunities in work clothes.

HENRY J. KAISER, 1882-1967, American industrialist ship builder for the U.S. Navy and creator of America's first HMO, Kaiser Permanente.

We use our hands daily for hundreds of activities, not thinking of it as anything beyond the ordinary. However, if we reflect on the hand at all, we realize that it is an extremely complex structure and vital to our daily tasks. Many health care professionals have little regard for finger and hand injuries, but these can be among the most devastating injuries if not properly cared for, if only because the hand plays such an important role in everyday activities. On the other hand (no pun intended), when an athlete suffers a complex hand injury, the athletic trainer is quick to realize just how much of a problem not being able to use the hand can be. It is my hope that by the end of this chapter you will gain an appreciation for hand and finger injuries to realize that a finger sprain is not *just* a sprain.

The hand is much more complex than many think, and a seemingly minimal imbalance in the hand can cause profound problems in hand function. These problems provide the rehabilitation clinician with challenges that must be addressed before the patient is able to resume normal activities. However, before we can discuss rehabilitation techniques for the wrist and hand, we must review their unique function and structure. It is important to gain an understanding of the wrist's and hand's structure and function, because they play a vital role in the techniques and applications of therapeutic exercises in a rehabilitation program.

Many texts have been written on the anatomy, biomechanics, and function of the wrist and hand. We will be only skimming the surface of this body of knowledge. A complete investigation of the hand's structure and function is beyond the scope of this chapter, but information vital to establishing a safe and appropriate rehabilitation program for the wrist and hand is presented. I refer you to the suggested readings at the end of this chapter for additional information.

This chapter includes structural and functional information that you will need in order to create an appropriate rehabilitation program for wrist and hand injuries. A presentation of soft-tissue and joint mobilization techniques includes information organized similarly to that in previous chapters. The exercises presented are limited to flexibility, strengthening, and coordination exercises for the wrist and hand. You should realize, however, that the wrist is intimately connected to the elbow and closely associated with the shoulder, so a therapeutic exercise program should also include activities for these areas. Specific injuries commonly seen in the wrist and hand are discussed, along with rehabilitation programs used to treat these injuries.

Although the wrist and hand are complex and injuries to them present unique problems to the patient and clinician, these challenges are overcome with informed application of biomechanics and rehabilitation. These challenges should be looked at as Mr. Kaiser suggests, not as problems but as opportunities to use that knowledge and your acquired skills to create and provide successful wrist and hand rehabilitation programs for your patients.

GENERAL REHABILITATION CONSIDERATIONS

The wrist and hand are a complex unit composed of 29 bones, more than 30 tendinous insertions, and an involved neurological system that is vital to the unit's function. Twenty-five percent of the entire body's Pacinian corpuscles' sensory endings are located in the hands. The hand's many compactly arranged muscles, including nine for the thumb and seven for the index finger alone, hint at the complexity of its function. The thumb and index finger primarily provide for fine activities requiring dexterity, whereas the middle, ring, and little fingers act primarily as a stabilizing vise for grasping activities. It is important that all of the structures within the hand work in a balanced, coordinated manner for the hand to function optimally.

Skeletal Structure

Three flexion arches, the proximal and distal transverse arches and a longitudinal arch, are formed by the wrist and hand bones. The carpals and metacarpals form the proximal and distal transverse arches, respectively. The longitudinal arch runs from the carpals out to the ends of the fingers (figure 21.1). These arches form an equiangular spiral that provides for tremendous adaptation in grasping activities. If these equiangular structures are impaired because of joint restriction or muscle weakness, the hand loses its adaptability.

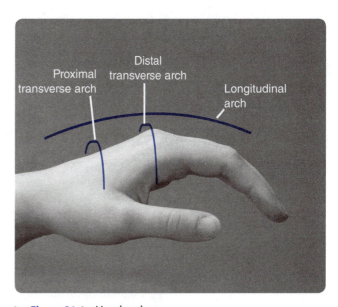

▶ **Figure 21.1** Hand arches.

The concave radius joins with the convex proximal carpal row to form the wrist joint. This joint has motions of flexion, extension, abduction, and adduction. Adduction is commonly referred to as ulnar deviation or *ulnar flexion,* and abduction is referred to as radial deviation or *radial flexion.* These four motions combine to produce circumduction of the wrist. The distal ulna and radius are supported by the distal radioulnar ligament and the interosseus membrane, and allow forearm supination and pronation movement along with the proximal radioulnar joint. Restricted mobility at either joint prevents full supination-pronation motion.

The carpal bones also form several joints with each other, and the distal row forms the carpometacarpal joints with the metacarpals. The intercarpal joints are irregular in structure and are strongly held in place by ligaments, making it difficult to dislocate any carpal. The carpometacarpal joints are, for the most part, saddle joints that permit various degrees of flexion, extension, abduction, and adduction of the metacarpals. The thumb and fourth and fifth metacarpals also rotate to provide opposition of the thumb and little finger and thereby allow the hand to create a conforming grasp on objects.

The metacarpophalangeal (MCP) joints are formed by the distal convex metacarpal surfaces and the corresponding concave proximal phalange surfaces. The interphalangeal (IP) joints are named as either proximal (PIP) or distal (DIP) interphalangeal joints. Collateral ligaments provide stability to these joints. In a relaxed position, the fingers are in partial flexion at the IP and MCP joints. The relaxed finger arrangement is such that it forms a cascade of progressive flexion from the second through the fifth digits; there is pathology present if this cascade is not seen.

Fascia and Ligaments

In addition to the ligaments connecting and supporting the joints throughout the wrist and hand, several other static structures add support to the area. The thick palmar fascia has two layers, superficial and deep. The superficial layer, an extension of the flexor retinaculum (transverse carpal ligament) and the palmaris longus tendon, when it is present, expands over the volar hand and runs into each of the fingers. The deep layer covers the floor of the palm and runs between the thenar and hypothenar eminences. The fascia on the hand's dorsum is in two layers as well but is not as thick as the palmar fascia. The palmar fascia serves to cushion and protect the hand's structures and to assist in maintaining the hand's concavity.

The retinacula is positioned throughout the wrist and hand and serves to hold the flexor and extensor tendons in place. At the wrist, the transverse carpal ligament prevents the flexor tendons from bowstringing away from the wrist. This ligament forms the roof of the carpal tunnel and maintains all of the finger flexor tendons in the carpal tunnel except the palmaris longus and flexor carpi ulnaris, the nerves, and the arteries. The extensor retinaculum on the dorsal wrist keeps the extensor tendons from bowstringing away from the wrist.

An extracapsular ligament, the transverse metacarpal ligament, connects the volar plate of one metatarsal head to the volar plate of its adjacent metatarsal heads (figure 21.2a). This ligament is important in maintaining the distal transverse arch, and its normal flexibility is vital to hand functions such as prehensile grip and grasping activities. There are several fascial restraints in the digits that maintain alignment of the tendons in the fingers that also provide the pulley system for the tendons.

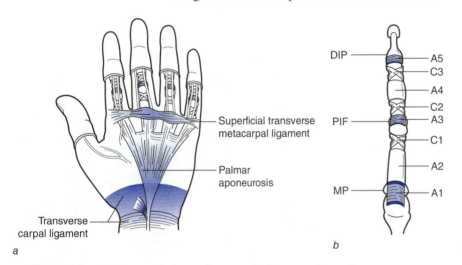

▶ **Figure 21.2** *(a)* Palmar soft-tissue elements *(b)* flexor tendon pulley system.

Tendon Sheaths and Pulleys

The flexor tendons are surrounded by a complex system of sheaths that serve to protect and nourish the tendons. The sheath system of the extensor tendons is not as elaborate; the extensor tendons are enclosed in sheaths at the wrist when they travel under the extensor retinaculum, but otherwise they are extrasynovial. The flexor sheaths begin proximal to the wrist and extend to the distal digits.

There is an elaborate pulley system on the flexor aspect of the fingers. This system is a series of fibrous tunnels that extends from the metacarpal head of each digit to the insertion of the distal finger flexor tendons. These pulleys are similar to the hoops along a fishing rod, positioned to keep the fishing line in place as it travels along the pole. There are five annular pulleys and three cruciate pulleys along the fingers (figure 21.2b). Disruption of the key pulleys can cause bowstringing of the flexor tendons. The pulleys that are key to preventing bowstringing are A2 and A4 (Doyle & Blythe, 1975). When the pulley system of any finger is disrupted, the mechanical advantage of the tendon is impaired and normal function is lost.

Muscles

Hand muscles are divided into two major categories, extrinsic and intrinsic. Extrinsic muscles originate outside the hand whereas intrinsic muscles originate and terminate within the hand. Extrinsic muscles are further divided into flexor muscles and extensor muscles. There are

20 extrinsic muscles and 19 intrinsic muscles. The extrinsic muscles are attached to the long tendons that enter the wrist and hand from muscles originating from the elbow or forearm. The thenar eminence contains the four intrinsic muscles of the thumb, and the hypothenar eminence contains the three intrinsic muscles of the fifth finger. If the hand is to operate well and avoid deformity following an injury, a balanced system must exist between the intrinsic muscles and extrinsic flexor and extensor muscles (von Schroeder & Botte, 2001).

The long finger extensors run to the second through fifth fingers. At the distal metacarpal area they are connected by the juncturae tendinum, a fibrous band that limits independent motion of the extensor tendons. The extensor tendons are connected to the proximal phalanx by sagittal bands that attach on the volar plate to keep the extensor tendons from bowstringing and transmit the extensor tendons' extension force to the metacarpophalangeal joints. Distal to the MCP joints, the extensor tendons split into three segments: the central slip, which attaches to the base of the middle phalanx, and two lateral bands that insert when they rejoin at the distal phalanx (figure 21.3).

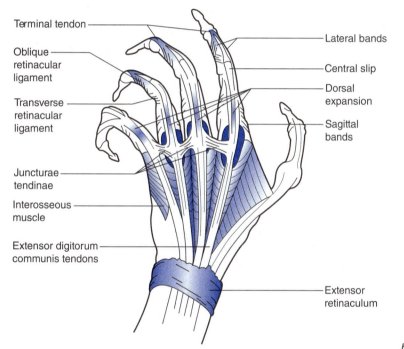

Terminal tendon

Oblique retinacular ligament

Transverse retinacular ligament

Juncturae tendinae

Interosseous muscle

Extensor digitorum communis tendons

Lateral bands

Central slip

Dorsal expansion

Sagittal bands

Extensor retinaculum

a

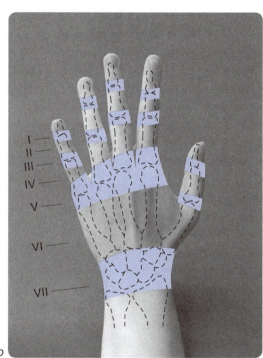

b

▶ **Figure 21.3** *(a)* Dorsal soft-tissue elements and *(b)* zones.

The long finger flexors include the flexor digitorum superficialis (FDS) and the flexor digitorum profundus (FDP). Both tendons pass deep in the hand. The FDS flexes the PIP joint. Each FDS tendon has its own separate muscle belly, so each can operate independently of the other. Each superficialis tendon splits before it attaches to the base of the middle phalanx and permits the deeper FDP tendon to emerge and attach to the distal phalanx (figure 21.4). The tendons of the FDP, unlike those of the FDS, do not possess separate muscle bellies, so distal phalanx flexion of the fingers cannot be isolated in their movements.

Whereas the long finger muscles are used for gross-motor activity, the intrinsic muscles are used for fine-motor activities. They control the more intricate movements of the fingers. The lumbricals and interossei have unique attachments and arrangements with the long flexor and extensor tendons and the ligaments of the fingers. The lumbricals originate from the deep flexor tendons in the palm and insert on the extensor tendon expansion. This unique arrangement allows the lumbricals to function as MCP flexors and IP extensors because their line of force is anterior to the MCP joint, causing flexion at this joint, and their line of force is posterior

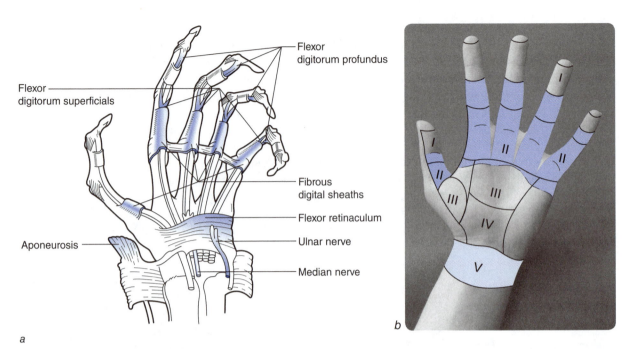

Flexor digitorum superficials

Flexor digitorum profundus

Fibrous digital sheaths

Flexor retinaculum

Ulnar nerve

Median nerve

Aponeurosis

a

b

▶ **Figure 21.4** Palmar surface of the hand and zones.

to the IP joint, resulting in IP extension. The dorsal and palmar interossei are responsible for finger abduction and adduction, respectively. Because they are more superficial than the lumbricals, they can be palpated.

Edema

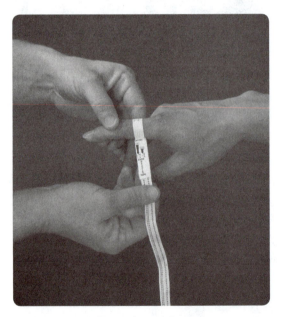

▶ **Figure 21.5** Circumferential gauge.

Skin covering the volar hand is thick, inelastic, and hairless and attaches to the palmar fascia to allow for grasping objects without their slipping out of the hand. The dorsal skin is elastic, mobile, and easily separated from the underlying fascia to permit skin mobility during grasping activities. Because the dorsal skin is loose and pliable compared to the volar skin, edema frequently accumulates in the dorsum of the hand. Pooled edema rich in proteins easily leads to contractures. Excessive swelling on the back of the hand can cause the hand arches to collapse anteriorly and adduct the thumb. Excessive swelling also requires a greater excursion of the skin to flex the fingers. If the skin is already stretched because of the edema, the ability to move the fingers through their full motion is impaired because the skin extensibility is already used by the edema. Fibrous tissue formation secondary to prolonged edema can cause reduced mobility and function of the hand.

Efforts by the rehabilitation clinician to reduce early edema are crucial. A circumferential gauge clinically quantifies edema of the hand and fingers (figure 21.5). A string wrapped around the finger or hand and then measured for its length can also be used to measure finger edema. Compressive dressings, elevation, ice, compressive machines, and other modalities to reduce edema formation and reduce disability secondary to edema effects are important in phase I.

Tendon Zones

The flexor and extensor surfaces of the hand are divided into zones as a means of surgical reference. Each zone has characteristics that are unique and impact both the physician's surgical approach and the clinician's rehabilitation approach. For this reason we consider them briefly here. There are five flexor and seven extensor zones of the wrist, hand, and four medial digits. The thumb has three flexor and five extensor zones. The zones are numbered with the lowest numbers most distal. Keep in mind that when connective tissue in the form of either sheaths or retinaculae surrounds these tendons in either the flexor or extensor zones, the risk of adhesions occurring with immobilization increases significantly. You will notice in the sidebar that the repercussions of injury in extensor zone VII is similar to an injury in flexor zone II for this very reason. Tendon adhesions can result in loss of normal motion, strength, and function. Tendon gliding exercises that assist in preventing these adhesions are presented later in this chapter. The following sidebar lists the tendon zones, and figures 21.3 and 21.4 present them pictorially.

Surgical Zones of the Hand

Flexor Zone V
- **Location:** Forearm at musculotendinous junction of extrinsic muscles to the wrist.
- **Characteristics:** Tendons are surrounded by loose tendon sheaths.
- **Problems:** Tendons can become adherent to the sheath and surrounding soft-tissue structures.
- **Treatment Concerns:** Prevent adhesions and restore normal tendon gliding.

Flexor Zone IV
- **Location:** At the wrist.
- **Characteristics:** Carpal tunnel is located here. Several tendons, nerves, and blood vessels are present in this area.
- **Problems:** Adhesions between tendons are a common problem following surgery or injury.
- **Treatment Concerns:** Prevent adhesions.

Flexor Zone III
- **Location:** In the palm after the flexor tendons leave the carpal tunnel.
- **Characteristics:** Lumbricals attach to the FDP in this region.
- **Problems:** Because the extrinsic tendons have more room, they often heal without difficulty or complications. The intrinsic muscles, however, can have adhesions and contractures from prolonged flexor positioning of the palm.
- **Treatment Concerns:** Gentle passive range-of-motion (ROM) exercises for the intrinsics can help prevent these complications.

Flexor Zone II
- **Location:** From the distal palmar crease to the middle phalanx where the split slips of the FDS insert on the phalanx and near where the FDP traverses anteriorly below the superficialis.
- **Characteristics:** Flexor tendon sheaths are in this region.
- **Problems:** Adhesions can seriously inhibit normal tendon gliding and prevent full restoration of function. This area has been called "no man's land" because of the inhibition of normal function after injury or surgery to this area, but more recent advances in surgical techniques permit improved function following surgery.
- **Treatment Concerns:** Flexor tendon gliding exercises reduce the risk of adhesions.

Flexor Zone I
- **Location:** Area of the DIP joint.
- **Characteristics:** The only tendon involved here is the FDP as it inserts on the distal phalanx.
- **Problems:** Tendons are commonly ruptured from this location.
- **Treatment Concerns:** These injuries require careful rehabilitation because complications such as poor tendon gliding, contractures, and repair failures can occur.

Flexor Zone Thumb I, II, and III
- **Location:** Anterior thumb region.
- **Characteristics:** These zones are comparable to zones I, II, and III, respectively, of the fingers.

(continued) ▶

(continued)

- **Problems:** Tendon injuries in these zones do not carry with them as great a risk of adhesions, because the only tendon enclosed in a sheath is the flexor pollicis longus.
- **Treatment Concerns:** Care must be taken to preserve function since the thumb accounts for the majority of hand function.

Extensor Zone VII

- **Location:** At the wrist joints.
- **Characteristics:** This area contains both wrist extensors and extrinsic finger extensors.
- **Problems:** The tendons in this area have synovial sheaths, are close together, and are covered by the dorsal retinaculum. This can be an area of adhesion formation after injury or immobilization.
- **Treatment Concerns:** If an injury in this area involves only the wrist extensors, the wrist is the only joint in need of immobilization and should be positioned in approximately 45° of extension. However, if the long finger extensors are also involved, the wrist and MCP joints should both be positioned in extension. The rehabilitation clinician must be cognizant of the risks of losing tendon gliding capabilities and should take steps to prevent and treat this complication.

Extensor Zone V and VI

- **Location:** From the hand distal to the extensor sheaths in the carpometacarpal (CMC) joint region to the MCP joints at the start of the extensor hood.
- **Characteristics:** Include extensor tendons and sheaths and other soft-tissue structures.
- **Problems:** Extensor tendons and sheaths can adhere to other surrounding soft-tissue structures, especially because they are close to the skin. Edema formation in the hand is usually seen in this area more predominantly than in the palmar aspect.
- **Treatment Concerns:** Control of edema will help reduce the risk of adhesion formation. Wrist immobilization for this area is approximately 45° extension at the wrist with the MCP and IP joints at 0° extension.

Extensor Zone III and IV

- **Location:** Proximal and middle fingers.
- **Characteristics:** Include extensor tendons that have split into central and lateral slips and PIP joints.
- **Problems:** When injuries occur to the extrinsic extensor tendon's central slip, what results is a boutonniere deformity. The PIP is positioned in flexion and the DIP in extension with the unbalanced pull of the intact lateral bands (see figure 21.63, page 764).
- **Treatment Concerns:** Although stiffness of the PIP joint with loss of joint motion is a complication, immobilization of the digit is necessary, as discussed later in this chapter.

Extensor Zone I and II

- **Location:** Middle and distal finger segments.
- **Characteristics:** Middle phalanx and DIP joints.
- **Problems:** Mallet deformity is the most common injury in this region. If untreated, a mallet deformity may lead to a swan-neck deformity, in which the PIP joint is hyperextended and the DIP joint is flexed. This occurs in the presence of a lax volar plate as the extensor mechanism slides proximally without its anchor at the distal phalanx.
- **Treatment Concerns:** Splinting, and in some cases surgery, is necessary to correct this injury. Care must be taken during this time to guard against an extensor lag and local ischemia. Treatment of this injury is discussed in detail later.

Extensor Zone Thumb I Through V

- **Location:** Extensor surface of the thumb.
- **Characteristics:** The thumb zones coincide with the zones of the finger, and injuries to those zones can be treated similarly to the corresponding finger zones. T I and T II coincide with zones I and II of the fingers. Zones T III and T IV coincide with zones V and VI of the fingers.
- **Problems:** Zone T V, like zone VII of the fingers, can suffer adhesions following injury. Web space contracture, extensor pollicis longus adhesions, and reduced excursion of the thumb are common problems.
- **Treatment Concerns:** The clinician must be aware of secondary problems that may occur with thumb injuries and take a proactive stance to prevent them. The thumb is the most important digit of the hand and must be cared for appropriately.

Excursions

For the hand to close into a fist, a large excursion of the extensor tendons and dorsal surface of the hand and wrist must be possible. Adhesions betweens structures within the hand or wrist can restrict this necessary mobility and reduce hand function. For this reason, early controlled passive motion of tendon injuries is vital to restoring full hand function. Care must be taken to maintain good tendon glide without risking injury.

As a tendon glides within its sheath, adhesions are stretched. The normal excursion of a tendon is variable from one finger to another and is a matter of some dispute. The most commonly repeated values are based on the work of Bunnell reported by Boyes (Boyes, 1970). The significance of these numbers for rehabilitation is twofold: They indicate how much excursion must be restored following injury or immobilization, and how much each healing tendon can move during immobilization without incurring damage. Many investigators have looked at a number of factors regarding tendons, motion, and their excursions. For example, it is now known how far a tendon can be stretched while it is immobilized without endangering its integrity (Duran & Houser, 1975), and how many degrees of motion these distances translate to (Evans & Burkhalter, 1986) so that splints are appropriately designed for the hand after tendon repair. Clinicians specializing in hand splinting must know these values. The rehabilitation clinician should appreciate that there are differences between each of the digit's extensor tendon's excursions, and these differences do not necessarily change in a successive order from the first to the fifth digit, nor do they each change proportionately for each tendon; for example, the thumb's extensor longus tendon has the greatest overall excursion, but it does not have the greatest excursion of all the other extensor tendons at the wrist or the MCP joint (Boyes, 1970).

Use of the Hand

The hand is a trimuscular system that uses the three muscle groups, the extrinsic flexors, the extrinsic extensors, and the intrinsic muscles, to provide balanced, controlled function. If any of these muscle groups does not function normally because of either weakness or loss of mobility, balance is lost and the hand is unable to function normally.

Because of the hand's complex system of joints and muscles, uses of the hand as a tool are numerous. The hand transmits forces or provides movement to produce a desired effect. About 20% (Bowers & Tribuzi, 1992) to 30%-45% (McFee, 1987) of its responsibility involves force transmission. Power grips provide force transmission. Power grips, also known as palmar grips, include the clenched fist, the cylinder grasp, the spherical grasp, and the hook (figure 21.6). In these grasps, the thumb is positioned in opposition to the other fingers to permit a firm grasp of an object. The majority of daily hand activities involve these palmar grips. Because palmar grasping is so vital to hand function, the

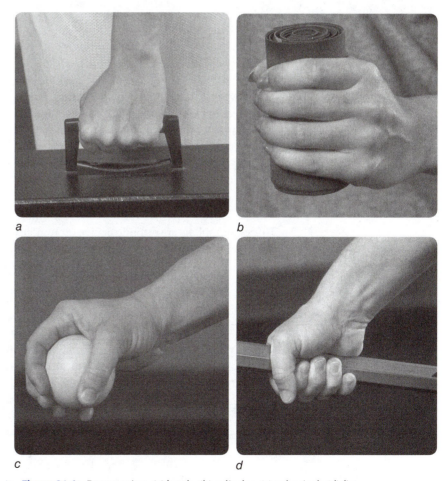

▶ **Figure 21.6** Power grips: *(a)* hook, *(b)* cylinder, *(c)* spherical, *(d)* fist.

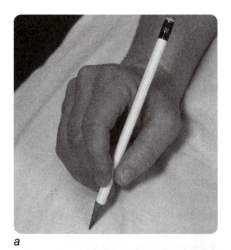

a

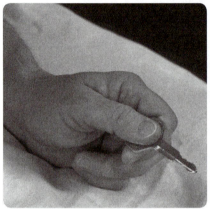

b

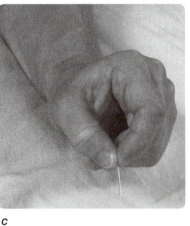

c

▶ Figure 21.7 Prehension pinches: *(a)* digital, *(b)* lateral, *(c)* tip-to-tip.

hand is most commonly splinted in a palmar position with the thumb in slight opposition, facing the other fingers.

The majority of the time, the hand provides movement to accomplish intricate tasks. These tasks include many activities, such as typing, sewing, or writing. These intricate grips, or pinches, include prehensile positions in which the thumb and finger muscles co-contract to produce a desired activity. The three pinches are the digital prehension pinch (also known as 3-jaw chuck), the lateral prehension pinch (also known as key pinch), and the tip-to-tip prehension pinch (figure 21.7). The digital prehension pinch is a grip used to handle and maneuver small tools in intricate activities. The lateral prehension pinch places the thumb tip against the side of the index finger to grasp objects such as a key or book. The tip-to-tip prehension pinch uses thumb opposition to position the tip of the thumb facing the tip of another finger. It is used most often to pick up small objects.

In the precision pinches, the fingers are flexed and abducted at the MCP joints with some opposition present. Unless the object being manipulated is heavy or large, primarily the radial digits are involved in precision activities. The movements involved in power activities vary in excursion and number of digits involved, but usually include the motions of flexion and rotation with some ulnar deviation. The power grips use the ulnar aspect of the hand to grasp the object and deliver the power and stability while the radial aspect of the hand provides the precision for the activity. Golf presents an example of this utilization of the power grip. In a power grip, the fingers flex and rotate and move into ulnar deviation so that the fingertips point toward the thenar eminence to hold the object in the hand and stabilize the thumb in abduction.

All motions and grips must be restored to the injured hand. The clinician accomplishes this through awareness of the component motions these activities require, restoration of joint mobility, attainment of normal tendon glide, and balance of strength and flexibility.

Splinting

Braces and splints are orthotic devices commonly used in the treatment of hand injuries. They are either static or dynamic. Static splints are used to restrict motion and to support and protect the hand. Dynamic splints are used to increase motion or allow motion of the hand. The aim in using these devices is either to prevent damage and maintain balance or to improve balance. Splint design is based on a three-point pressure system whereby two points of application are on one side of the hand, wrist, or forearm, and the fulcrum, or other point of application, is on the opposite side (figure 21.8). This system should be familiar because it was presented as a force system in chapter 3.

Splints are applied for varying amounts of time, depending on the structure injured, the splint's intent, the repair, the adjacent structures and their influence on the injured tissue, and healing of the injured tissue. They may be applied for periods of 1 to 8 weeks. It is common for patients to continue to use a night splint after they have reduced or discontinued splint use during the day. Use of night splints may continue for 10

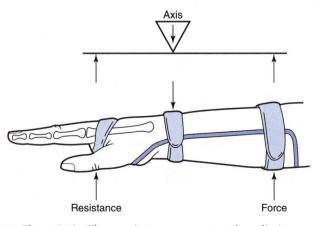

▶ Figure 21.8 Three-point pressure system for splinting.

to 12 weeks postinjury. Complex injuries commonly advance from an initial splint to a less restrictive splint during the day before removal of any day support occurs.

Static Splints

Static splints do not have any moving parts (figure 21.9). They immobilize a joint to protect it from deleterious movement. Periods of immobilization are frequently indicated following injury; the static splint can prevent movement to allow scar-tissue formation to restore joint stability. If a joint has lost its mobility, a different type of static splint places the joint on stretch by applying a low-level prolonged stretch, thus improving joint mobility. Static splints are also designed to maintain ROM gains resulting from other rehabilitation techniques; these are called static progressive splints.

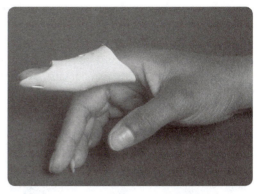

▶ **Figure 21.9** Static tendon splint to restrict ROM.

Although there are some exceptions, most often the hand is placed in a functional position with the wrist in slight extension, the fingers slightly flexed at the MCP and IP joints, and the thumb in slight opposition to the other fingers before splinting (figure 21.10). Only as many joints as necessary are immobilized so that mobility of the unaffected joints is optimized.

Dynamic Splints

Dynamic splints incorporate a system of movement with springs, rubber bands, or other elastic elements. These devices produce passive or passive assistive motion in one line of pull and active resistive motion in the opposite direction.

Dynamic splints can also promote mobility by providing a continual, low-level stretch force to a joint. They are used when the patient lacks normal motion and is unable to achieve the desired mobility independently. The patient perceives the stretch force applied with the splint but

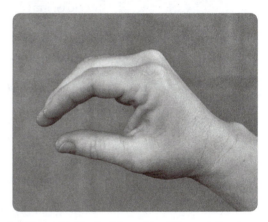

▶ **Figure 21.10** Position of hand immobilization.

should not find it painful. Because the device is worn for a prolonged period to influence scar-tissue remodeling, the force applied is low. These devices are usually worn at night so they do not interfere with hand function throughout the day. How long it is worn depends on the patient's tolerance, but the longer it is in place, the more successful the results. As the joint's ROM increases, adjustments in the splint are necessary.

A special type of dynamic splint is frequently used following tendon surgery to permit protected, guided movement of the tendon so tendon glide is maintained without risking tendon rupture. The device permits the appropriate degree of tendon motion based on the numbers discussed earlier. The tendon is held in its shortened position by rubber bands, and the splint keeps the opposing tendon from moving the digit beyond the designated degree of movement. The opposing tendon must work against the force of the rubber band to move the finger in the direction permitted, and the rubber band passively returns the finger to the resting position.

Fit, design, and purpose must be considerations when splints are designed for the hand. The purpose will determine what type of orthotic is used. The fit is individually determined, based on the hand size and dimensions. The design is based on a combination of fit, purpose, and precautions.

Precautions in the design and construction are primarily two: friction and pressure. Whether the device is static or dynamic, friction can occur between the splint and the skin and must be avoided. When a splint does not fit correctly, it will move from its intended position and cause friction. The device should be held firmly, yet comfortably, in position by its straps and other structures; it may require periodic adjustments for maintenance of proper alignment and reduction of friction, especially as edema and muscle size change.

Pressure is particularly a problem when the splint is over bony prominences. The hand's most susceptible areas are the ulnar and radial styloid processes, pisiform, base of the fifth metacarpal, and metacarpal heads. Padding over these susceptible areas can be applied during

The hand's many special characteristics include its skeletal structure, its tendon sheaths and pulleys, its fascia and ligaments, and two categories of muscles. Edema is an important consideration in the hand, as are the tendon zones, tendon excursion, the various ways the hand is used, and splinting principles.

splint construction and removed when the splint is worn to prevent pressure. If padding or relief is added after the splint is made, it may change the alignment and intended force application of the device.

The patient's skin should be routinely checked for redness; this is a sign of pressure or friction. Adjustments may be necessary as the patient's condition changes. Wrist and hand splint construction can be complicated, depending on the injury. In complex cases, an occupational therapist, orthopedic technician, or other hand specialist typically constructs the orthotic. In these cases, the rehabilitation clinician plays an important role in reporting on the patient's tolerance of the device and can reinforce wear compliance.

SOFT-TISSUE MOBILIZATION

Although soft-tissue treatment of many of the intrinsic muscles of the wrist and hand occurs in chapter 20, other treatments for some of the other extrinsic wrist and hand muscles have yet to be introduced. The soft-tissue mobilization techniques in this chapter are limited to trigger point release and spray-and-stretch techniques based on the work of Travell and Simons (Travell & Simons, 1983). The pain-referral patterns and information presented here are also based on their work. These items are introduced below and presented in the following sections.

Extrinsic Muscles

Although there are several extrinsic muscles of the wrist and hand, they are grossly divided into two groups: flexors and extensors. The flexors are described first in the following sections and are followed by the extensors.

■ Trigger Point Releases for the Wrist and Hand Muscles

Palmaris Longus

Referral Pattern: Pain into the palm but not the digits, and to a lesser extent along the distal anterior forearm.

Location of Trigger Point: The trigger point is a palpable band that is located in the medial aspect of the proximal anterior forearm as seen in figure 21.11a.

Patient Position for Palpation: Sitting or supine.

Muscle Position for Palpation: Forearm is relaxed and supinated.

Ischemic Treatment: Direct pressure over the trigger point location or rolling across the band (figure 21.11b).

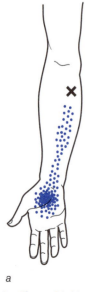

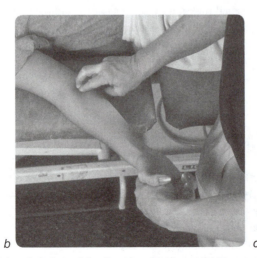

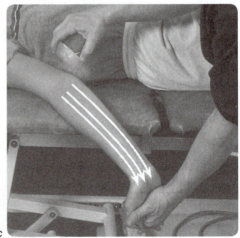

a   b   c

▶ **Figure 21.11** Palmaris longus: *(a)* pain-referral pattern, *(b)* trigger point release, *(c)* ice-and-stretch.

Spray-and-Stretch Treatment: Spray-and-stretch is applied with the muscle on stretch. The elbow is supported on a padded surface while the fingers and wrist are extended. The spray is applied in parallel sweeps from the medial elbow along the medial forearm and into the palm as the elbow and fingers are passively moved into extension (figure 21.11c).

Notations: Because the palmaris longus inserts superficially, the pain is usually a prickly superficial sensation rather than the deep sensation of most muscle pain-referral patterns.

Pronator Teres, Wrist Flexors, and Long Finger Flexors

Referral Pattern: The wrist flexors and pronator teres refer pain into the wrist: the flexor carpi ulnaris to the ulnar aspect, the flexor carpi radialis to the radial aspect, and the pronator teres to the radial wrist. The long finger and thumb flexors refer pain into the digits they activate and extend the sensation of pain shooting out beyond the end of the digits (figure 21.12a). Pain patterns between the finger flexor superficialis and profundus have not been differentiated.

Location of Trigger Point: Within the forearm near the midbelly portion of each muscle. The exception is the flexor pollicis longus, whose trigger point is located on the distal forearm.

Patient Position for Palpation: Sitting or supine.

Muscle Position for Palpation: Forearm is relaxed and supinated.

Ischemic Treatment: Each muscle is treated with direct pressure over the tender trigger point until the discomfort subsides. Each trigger point elicits a local twitch response and produces a pain-referral pattern.

Spray-and-Stretch Treatment: Spray-and-stretch is applied with the muscle on stretch and a support under the elbow (figure 21.12, b & c). The ice sweeps are made from the medial elbow downward to the specific digit being treated.

Notations: Locate each trigger point by identifying the band and then seeking the nodule within the band for each muscle.

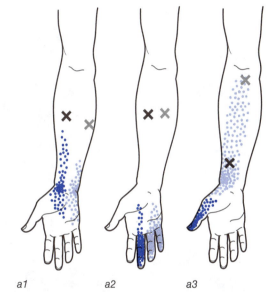

a1   a2   a3

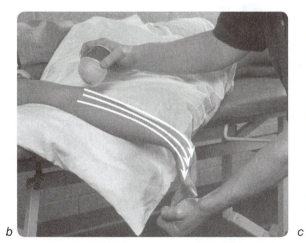

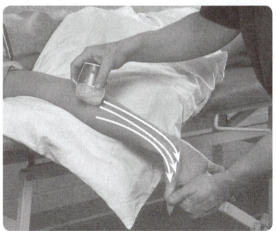

b   c

▶ **Figure 21.12** Pronator teres, wrist and finger flexors: *(a)* pain-referral patterns; *(a1)* dark = flexor carpi radialis, light = flexor carpi ulnaris; *(a2)* dark = long finger flexors radial head, light = long finger flexors humeral head; *(a3)* dark = flexor pollicis longus, light = pronator teres; *(b)* ice-and-stretch to wrist and finger flexors; *(c)* ice-and-stretch to flexor pollicis longus and pronator teres.

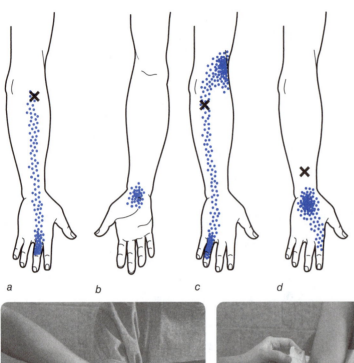

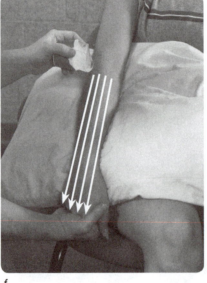

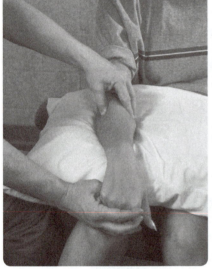

a   *b*   *c*   *d*

e   *f*

▶ **Figure 21.13** Long finger extensors: pain-referral patterns for *(a-b)* middle-finger extensor, *(c)* ring-finger extensor, *(d)* extensor indicis, *(e)* trigger point release, *(f)* ice-and-stretch.

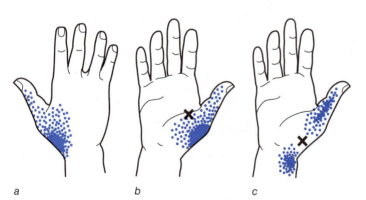

a   *b*   *c*

▶ **Figure 21.14** Thumb intrinsics: pain-referral patterns for *(a-b)* adductor pollicis, *(c)* opponens pollicis.

Long Finger Extensors

Referral Pattern: The pain is referred along the posterior forearm, with the primary pain occurring into the digit. The middle-finger extensor can also refer to the lateral epicondyle. The extensor indicis refers to the ulnar wrist and into the dorsum of the hand but not the digit (figure 21.13, a-d).

Location of Trigger Point: The trigger points are located in the belly of each muscle.

Patient Position for Palpation: Supine or seated.

Muscle Position for Palpation: Relaxed with the forearm in supination.

Ischemic Treatment: Extensor tendon trigger points are easily located as they produce a twitch response, especially the tendon to the long finger. The trigger point is located about 3 to 4 cm (about 7.5-10 in.) distal and dorsal to the radial head. Because the little- and ring-finger fibers are the deeper fibers of the muscle, they are more difficult to palpate but produce a twitch response when located. Deep pressure applied over these trigger points while the muscle is relaxed diminishes the discomfort (figure 21.13e).

Spray-and-Stretch Treatment: Spray-and-stretch is performed with the forearm supported and the elbow extended. Ice sweeps, made from the elbow, move distally to the fingers with the wrist and fingers placed on stretch (figure 21.13f). If pain is referred to the lateral epicondyle, ice sweeps upward toward the epicondyle are also performed.

Notations: In contrast with the long finger flexors, the long extensors refer pain into their digits short of the last phalanx.

Intrinsic Muscles

The intrinsic muscles are divided into three groups based on where they function: (1) at the thumb, (2) at the little finger, and (3) at the other finger muscles—the interossei and lumbricals. The thumb muscles lie within the thenar eminence, and the little-finger muscles lie within the hypothenar eminence. Between these two prominences lie the interossei and lumbricals. Trigger point releases for the most commonly affected muscles are presented next.

Thumb Muscles

Referral Pattern: The adductor pollicis refers pain to the base of the thumb, and the opponens pollicis refers pain to the radial volar wrist and along the palmar aspect of the thumb (figure 21.14, a-c).

Location of Trigger Point: Each trigger point is near the middle aspect of the muscle belly.

Patient Position for Palpation: Supine or sitting.

Muscle Position for Palpation: Relaxed with the forearm in supination.

Ischemic Treatment: Trigger point release of each muscle is applied with the muscle relaxed and pressure over the trigger point until a release is palpated or the discomfort diminishes (figure 21.14d).

Spray-and-Stretch Treatment: Spray-and-stretch is applied with the muscle on stretch. The sweeps are applied across the thenar eminence and over the thumb (figure 21.14e).

Notations: Either of these muscles may have activated trigger points with injuries or immobilization.

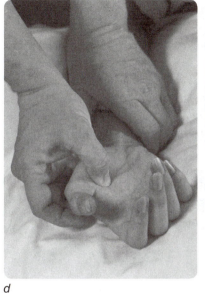
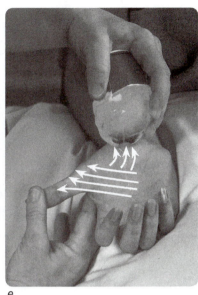

d

e

▶ **Figure 21.14** Thumb intrinsics: pain-referral patterns for *(d)* trigger point release to adductor pollicis, *(e)* ice-and-stretch.

Interossei and Abductor Digiti Minimi

Referral Pattern: The dorsal interossei produce a strong pain referral along the radial side of the index finger, especially at the DIP joint. The other interossei refer pain along the side of the digit to which they attach (figure 21.15, a-d).

Location of Trigger Point: Each trigger point is near the middle aspect of the muscle belly.

Patient Position for Palpation: Supine or sitting.

Muscle Position for Palpation: Relaxed with the forearm in supination.

Ischemic Treatment: While applying pressure on the dorsal surface, the rehabilitation clinician applies counterpressure on the palmar surface.

Spray-and-Stretch Treatment: Spray-and-stretch is applied with the patient relaxed and the forearm supported. Only the first dorsal interossei can be reached with ice-and-stretch. With the thumb in abduction, the index finger is adducted toward the middle finger as an ice sweep is performed from proximal to the wrist and along the index finger (figure 21.15e).

Notations: These intrinsic muscles are a little more difficult to identify than those of the thumb.

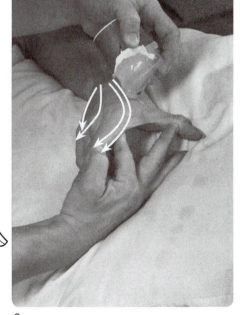

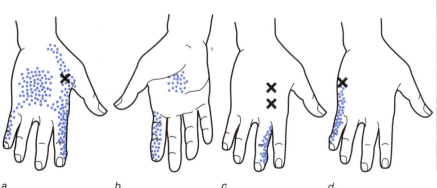

a　　　　　　b　　　　　　c　　　　　　d　　　　　　e

▶ **Figure 21.15** Interossei and abductor digiti minimi: pain-referral patterns for *(a-b)* first dorsal interosseus, *(c)* second dorsal interosseus, *(d)* abductor digiti minimi, *(e)* ice-and-stretch.

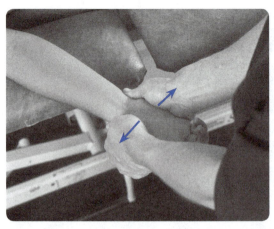

▶ **Figure 21.16** Palmar myofascial release.

Myofascial Release to Palmar Fascia

Lastly, the palmar fascia myofascial release technique is used to mobilize palmar fascia and the wrist retinaculum. The patient sits facing the rehabilitation clinician or lies supine with the forearm resting comfortably on the table. With the patient's hand in a supinated position, the rehabilitation clinician grasps the patient's hand with the thumbs adjacent to each other over the base of the wrist and the fingers wrapped around the hand with the finger pads on the dorsum of the wrist (figure 21.16). The rehabilitation clinician applies a lateral traction of the palmar soft tissue with his or her thumbs and their thenar eminences, as an upward force is applied by the finger pads on the wrist's dorsum. This technique provides the patient with a pleasant myofascial release while simultaneously improving palmar mobility.

JOINT MOBILIZATION

Soft-tissue mobilization techniques used for the extrinsic and the intrinsic muscles of the hand include trigger point release and ice-and-stretch techniques.

Most of the joint mobilization techniques discussed here are for joint accessory movements. They are based primarily on Maitland's (1991) work. There are certainly more movements available, but the movements presented in the following sections are the techniques commonly used to improve joint mobility of the distal forearm, wrist, hand, and fingers.

Distal Radioulnar Joint

As with any elbow injury, both the proximal and distal radioulnar joints should be examined for restricted mobility. If any restriction is present, the joints should be mobilized according to restrictive findings.

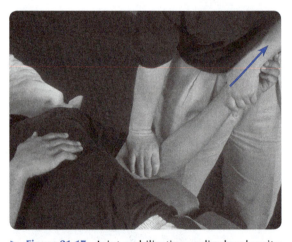

▶ **Figure 21.17** Joint mobilization: radioulnar longitudinal distraction.

■ Joint Mobilization of the Elbow and Forearm Joints

Longitudinal Distraction

Motion: General mobilization of distal radioulnar joint.

Resting Position: 10° supination.

Indications: Used prior to other mobilization techniques. Can be used at end range to improve motion.

Patient Position: Sitting or supine.

Clinician and Hand Positions: With the clinician facing the patient, the clinician's stabilizing hand is just proximal to the patient's elbow with the web space wrapped around the patient's distal arm. Mobilizing hand wraps around anterior wrist (figure 21.17). Forearm of mobilizing arm is in line with the patient's forearm.

Mobilization Application: Soft-tissue slack is taken up, and either an oscillating longitudinal pull or a sustained traction is applied with the mobilizing hand.

Notations: This technique may be performed with the forearm in any position of comfort.

Distal Radioulnar Anteroposterior (AP) and Posteroanterior (PA) Glides

Motion: Radioulnar motion.

Resting Position: 10° supination.

Indications: To increase pronation and supination.

Patient Position: Sitting or supine.

Clinician and Hand Positions: One hand is used to grasp the ulnar head and the other to grasp the radial head.

Mobilization Application: The pad on one thenar eminence is used to apply the AP force on one bone; the fingers of the opposite hand, on the patient's posterior forearm, are used to apply the PA force on the other bone (figure 21.18).

Notations: The vertical forces applied by the two hands should be equal in timing and degree. An AP force on the radius with a PA force on the ulna increases supination, and an AP force on the ulna with a PA force on the radius increases pronation.

Wrist Joint

Wrist mobilizations are performed with the patient in a comfortable position, either sitting or supine. The rehabilitation clinician is sitting or standing. A towel roll is placed under the patient's distal forearm with the wrist over the table edge.

Traction

Motion: Radiocarpal and ulnocarpal joints.

Resting Position: Neutral with slight ulnar deviation.

Indications: General mobilization.

Patient Position: Supine on table or supine with forearm resting on table and towel under distal forearm.

Clinician and Hand Positions: Clinician stabilizes the distal forearm with one hand around the radial and ulnar styloids and places the mobilizing hand over the distal carpal row.

Mobilization Application: A traction force in a longitudinal direction is applied with the mobilizing hand (figure 21.19).

Notations: The force can be either a sustained application or a traction oscillation.

Dorsal Glide

Motion: Wrist.

Resting Position: Neutral in flexion-extension and supination-pronation.

Indications: To increase wrist flexion.

Patient Position: As for the previous motion.

Clinician and Hand Positions: Clinician places the stabilizing hand over the radial and ulnar styloids and the mobilizing hand over the distal carpal row.

Mobilization Application: An AP mobilizing force is applied by the distal, mobilizing hand (figure 21.20).

Notations: The force should be applied at an angle parallel to the wrist joint.

Volar Glide

Motion: Wrist

Resting Position: Neutral in flexion-extension and supination-pronation (see figure 21.20 in the previous section).

Indications: To increase wrist extension.

Patient Position: Patient's forearm in pronation and the wrist in neutral.

Clinician and Hand Positions: The rehabilitation clinician places the stabilizing hand over the radial and ulnar styloids and the mobilizing hand over the distal carpal row.

Mobilization Application: A PA force is applied by the distal, mobilizing hand.

Notations: The force should be applied at an angle parallel to the wrist joint.

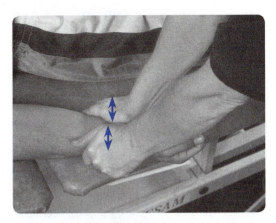

▶ **Figure 21.18** Joint mobilization: distal radioulnar AP and PA glides of either the radial or ulnar heads.

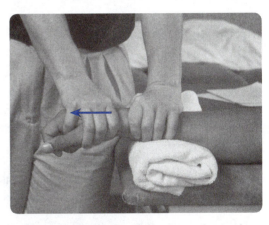

▶ **Figure 21.19** Joint mobilization: wrist traction.

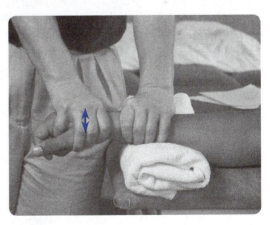

▶ **Figure 21.20** Joint mobilization: dorsal and volar glides of the wrist.

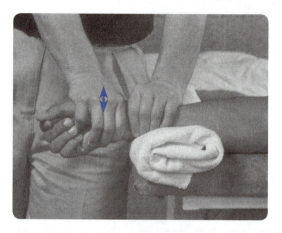

▶ **Figure 21.21** Joint mobilization: radial and ulnar glides of the wrist.

Radial Glide

Motion: Wrist.

Resting Position: Neutral in flexion-extension and supination-pronation.

Indications: To increase ulnar deviation.

Patient Position: Patient's forearm is positioned with the ulnar side upward and the wrist in neutral.

Clinician and Hand Positions: The rehabilitation clinician places the stabilizing hand over the radial and ulnar styloids and the mobilizing hand over the distal carpal row (figure 21.21).

Mobilization Application: A vertically downward mobilizing force is applied.

Notations: Keep the hands relaxed with the mobilizing force coming from the shoulders.

Ulnar Glide

Motion: Wrist.

Resting Position: Neutral in flexion-extension and supination-pronation (see figure 21.21 in the previous section).

Indications: To increase radial deviation.

Patient Position: Patient's forearm is positioned with the radial side upward and the wrist in neutral.

Clinician and Hand Positions: The clinician places the stabilizing hand over the radial and ulnar styloids and the mobilizing hand over the distal carpal row.

Mobilization Application: A vertically downward mobilizing force is applied.

Notations: Keep the hands relaxed with the mobilizing force coming from the shoulders.

Specific Carpal Glides

Each of the carpals in the proximal and distal rows can be mobilized with each other and with the radius and ulna to improve flexion or extension motion in the wrist. Sometimes when individual carpal joints are restricted, individual joint mobilization techniques are necessary. The concave-convex rule applies to these joints, so it is important to know the joint's configuration before deciding whether a PA or an AP mobilization force is appropriate (figure 21.22).

The radius and ulna are concave surfaces, and the proximal carpal row provides the convex surfaces for the radiocarpal and ulnocarpal joints. To increase extension in the radiocarpal joints, the carpals are glided in a volar (anterior) direction. To increase flexion in the radiocarpal joints, the radius is glided in a volar direction. The ulnocarpal joint is mobilized by gliding the ulna in an anterior direction to unlock the articular disk that can obstruct wrist motion.

In the radial intercarpal joints, the convex scaphoid joins with the concave trapezium and trapezoid; this means that flexion is increased with a volar glide of the trapezium and trapezoid on a fixed scaphoid, and extension is increased with a volar glide of the scaphoid on the distal carpal row. Because the capitate is the convex surface and the lunate is the concave surface of the capitate-lunate joint, flexion is increased by a volar glide of the lunate on the fixed capitate, and extension is increased by stabilizing the proximal lunate and performing a volar glide of the distal capitate.

The mobilization techniques for each of these joints are similar. The forearm is unsupported so that the weight of the arm can provide a slight traction force on the joints. In each case mobilization is performed with

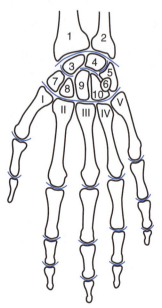

Key

1 = Radius
2 = Ulna
3 = Scaphoid
4 = Lunate
5 = Triquetrum
6 = Pisiform
7 = Trapezium
8 = Trapezoid
9 = Capitate
10 = Hamate

▶ **Figure 21.22** Convex-concave arrangement of carpal bones.

the forearm in pronation, using a pinch grasp with both the stabilizing and mobilizing hands with the thumbs on the dorsal surface. The stabilizing finger and thumb grasp the bone that is to remain stationary, and the mobilizing finger and thumb grasp the bone to be mobilized (figure 21.23). Because the joints are small, the clinician's thumbs may be in contact with each other. The thumbs apply a vertically downward force in a volar direction.

Carpometacarpal Joints

Hand placements for stabilization and mobilization are similar for both the fingers and the thumb carpometacarpal (CMC) joints. The stabilizing hand uses a thumb-and-index-finger pinch grasp over the carpal bone, and the mobilizing hand is placed in a similar grasp around the base of the metacarpal. Some distraction is applied to the joint while the mobilizing force is simultaneously applied. It is important to avoid squeezing the carpal yet grasp it firmly enough to provide adequate mobilization force. Because the CMC joints have a convex carpal and a concave metacarpal, flexion is increased with a volar (PA) glide of the distal segment, and extension is increased with a dorsal (AP) glide of the distal segment of the joint.

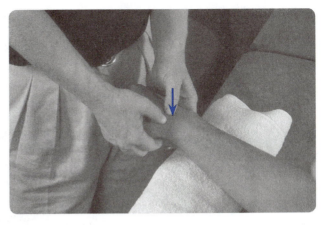

▶ **Figure 21.23** Joint mobilization: specific carpal glides.

Finger Carpometacarpal Joints

Loss of mobility in these joints can restrict the individual's ability to make a fist and can reduce grip capabilities. Joint mobilization is often required to restore motion in these joints. Some of the most common techniques are presented in the following sections.

Traction

Motion: Finger CMC joints.

Resting Position: 20° flexion.

Indications: To relieve pain and provide a general increase in joint mobility.

Patient Position: Supine on table or supine with forearm resting on table and towel under distal forearm.

Clinician and Hand Positions: Clinician is seated or standing. The carpal is stabilized with a finger-pinch grasp. The mobilizing hand uses a lateral finger-pinch grasp at the proximal metacarpal.

Mobilization Application: Metacarpal is pulled in the direction of its long axis (figure 21.24).

Notations: The lateral surface of the index finger makes sufficient contact to provide adequate tension to the joint's capsule.

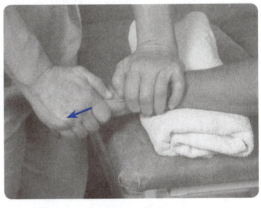

▶ **Figure 21.24** Joint mobilization: CMC distraction.

Anteroposterior Glide

Motion: Carpometacarpal joint.

Resting Position: 20° of flexion.

Indications: To increase CMC joint extension.

Patient Position: Supine on table or supine with forearm resting on table and towel under distal forearm.

Clinician and Hand Positions: Clinician is seated or standing. Clinician stabilizes the patient's carpal with the thumb and index finger of one hand, and then places the thumb and index finger of the other hand over the metacarpal to be treated, with the thumb on the volar surface (figure 21.25).

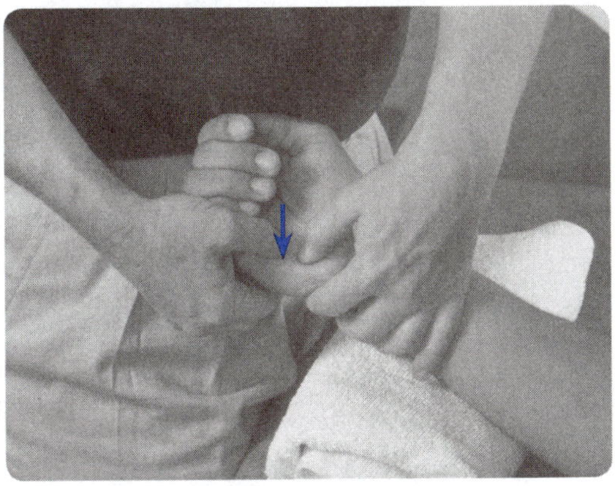

Mobilization Application: An AP force is applied by the thumb on the metacarpal.

Notations: Carpometacarpal joints 4 and 5 normally have more mobility than joints 2 and 3.

▶ **Figure 21.25** Joint mobilization: CMC AP glide joint mobilization.

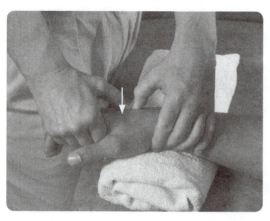

▶ **Figure 21.26** Joint mobilization: CMC PA (dorsal) glide.

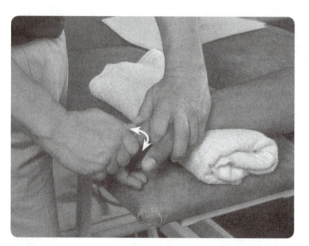

▶ **Figure 21.27** Joint mobilization: MCP rotation.

Posteroanterior Glide

Motion: Carpometacarpal joint.

Resting Position: 20° of flexion.

Indications: To increase CMC joint flexion.

Patient Position: Supine on table or supine with forearm resting on table and towel under distal forearm.

Clinician and Hand Positions: Clinician is seated or standing. The clinician's grasps are similar to those described for AP glides except that the thumbs are placed on the dorsal surface and the fingers are placed on the volar surface (figure 21.26).

Mobilization Application: PA force is applied to the metacarpal.

Notations: If mobilizing the radial side, the clinician's fingers grasp around the first web space of the patient's hand. If mobilizing the ulnar hand, the rehabilitation clinician grasps the ulnar border of the hand.

Rotation

Motion: Finger MCP joints.

Resting Position: 20° of flexion.

Indications: To improve accessory motion of rotation of the joints.

Patient Position: MCP is in 90° of flexion.

Clinician and Hand Positions: With stabilizing hand on the metacarpal head and mobilizing grasp at base of first phalange.

Mobilization Application: Distraction force is applied, followed by a medial and lateral rotation of the distal segment of the joint (figure 21.27).

Notations: This is not a motion that can be performed actively, but it must be present if normal motion is to be possible. If the finger is lacking the last few degrees of motion or the hand cannot make a complete fist, it may be that rotation of the MCP is limited.

Thumb Carpometacarpal Joint

As with CMC techniques for fingers 2 through 5, mobilization of the thumb is applied with the stabilizing hand using a thumb-and-index-finger pinch grasp over the carpal bone and with the mobilizing hand placed around the metacarpal bone, close to the joint margin.

Traction

Motion: Thumb CMC joint.

Resting Position: Midposition between flexion-extension and abduction-adduction.

Indications: General mobilization of the joint.

Patient Position: Supine on table or supine with forearm resting on table and towel under distal forearm.

Clinician and Hand Positions: Stabilizing hand uses a thumb-and-index-finger pinch grasp over the carpal bone, and the mobilizing hand is placed around the metacarpal's proximal region adjacent to the joint margin.

Mobilization Application: Distraction of the joint.

Notations: Distraction can be either sustained or oscillating.

Posteroanterior Glide

Motion: Thumb CMC joint.

Resting Position: Midposition between flexion-extension and abduction-adduction.

Indications: To increase thumb adduction.

Patient Position: Supine on table or supine with forearm resting on table and towel under distal forearm. Palm faces down.

Clinician and Hand Positions: Clinician stabilizes the trapezium and trapezoid at the proximal aspect of the joint, using the thumb and index finger of one hand; the clinician holds the patient's first metacarpal with the opposite thumb along the posterior aspect and the index finger around the anterior aspect.

Mobilization Application: Slight traction to the joint is applied, followed by a PA glide to the metacarpal (figure 21.28).

Notations: Both the trapezium and trapezoid are stabilized in the proximal joint segment.

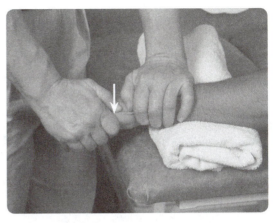

▶ **Figure 21.28** Joint mobilization: thumb CMC PA glide.

Anteroposterior Glide

Motion: Thumb CMC joint.

Resting Position: Midposition between flexion-extension and abduction-adduction.

Indications: To increase thumb CMC abduction.

Patient Position: Supine on table or supine with forearm resting on table and towel under distal forearm. Palm faces down.

Clinician and Hand Positions: Clinician stabilizes the trapezium and trapezoid at the proximal aspect of the joint, using the thumb and index finger of one hand; the clinician holds the patient's first metacarpal with the opposite thumb along the posterior aspect and the index finger around the anterior aspect.

Mobilization Application: This time, instead of the thumb's providing the mobilizing force, the index finger on the metacarpal's volar surface provides an AP glide.

Notations: Clinician stabilizes the trapezium and trapezoid at the proximal aspect of the joint, using the thumb and index finger of one hand; the clinician holds the patient's first metacarpal with the opposite thumb along the posterior aspect and the index finger around the anterior aspect.

Ulnar Glide

Motion: Thumb CMC joint.

Resting Position: Midposition between flexion-extension and abduction-adduction.

Indications: To increase flexion.

Patient Position: The forearm, wrist, and thumb are positioned in neutral. Ulna rests on table.

Clinician and Hand Positions: With the proximal aspect of the joint stabilized with the thumb and index finger of one hand, the rehabilitation clinician grasps the metacarpal with the other hand (figure 21.29).

Mobilization Application: Radial-to-ulnar glide is applied parallel to the joint surface.

Notations: The thumb's CMC joint is convex at its proximal joint surface.

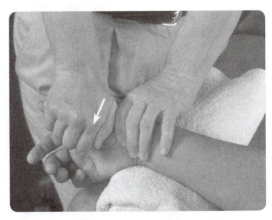

▶ **Figure 21.29** Joint mobilization: thumb CMC ulnar glide.

Metacarpophalangeal and Interphalangeal Joints

The configuration of each of these joints is similar, so the mobilization techniques are similar. Each mobilization described can be used on any of these joints. As outlined in previous sections, traction is applied during each mobilization technique to make the technique more comfortable and produce better results. The grasps should be firm enough to administer the mobilization force effectively but not tight enough to cause discomfort.

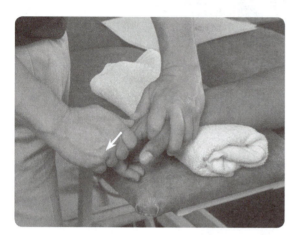

▶ **Figure 21.30** Joint mobilization: MCP distraction.

Traction

Motion: MCP and IP joints.

Resting Position: 20° of flexion.

Indications: General mobilization and relaxation.

Patient Position: Supine on table or supine with forearm resting on table and towel under distal forearm.

Clinician and Hand Positions: The proximal aspect of the joint is grasped with the stabilizing hand while the distal aspect of the joint is grasped by the index finger and thumb of the mobilizing hand (figure 21.30).

Mobilization Application: Traction force in line with the longitudinal axis is applied perpendicular to the joint's surface.

Notations: Since the configurations of these joints are similar, this technique may be applied to any of the IP or MCP joints.

Rotation

Motion: MCP and IP joints.

Resting Position: 20° of flexion.

Indications: To improve accessory rotation motion of the joints.

Patient Position: Supine on table or supine with forearm resting on table and towel under distal forearm.

Clinician and Hand Positions: The proximal aspect of the joint is grasped with a lateral pinch of the thumb and index finger.

Mobilization Application: Traction is maintained while a medial rotation is applied, then a lateral rotation.

Notations: Rotation is an accessory motion that must be restored in order for the patient to have full function of the joint.

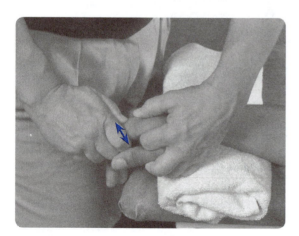

▶ **Figure 21.31** Joint mobilization: MCP AP and PA glides.

Posteroanterior and Anteroposterior Glides

Motion: MCP and IP joints.

Resting Position: 20° of flexion.

Indications: PA glide increases flexion motion; AP glide increases extension motion.

Patient Position: Supine on table or supine with forearm resting on table and towel under distal forearm.

Clinician and Hand Positions: The proximal aspect of the joint is stabilized while the distal aspect receives traction (figure 21.31).

Mobilization Application: While traction is maintained, either a PA force or an AP force is applied.

Notations: Because the joints are a concave surface moving on a convex surface, the mobilization force is in the same direction as the joint's roll or movement.

Lateral Glides

Motion: MCP and IP joints.

Resting Position: 20° of flexion.

Indications: To improve abduction and adduction of the MCP and IP joints.

Patient Position: Supine on table or supine with forearm resting on table and towel under distal forearm.

Clinician and Hand Positions: The proximal aspect of the joint is stabilized while the distal aspect receives traction.

Mobilization Application: A radial or ulnar glide force is applied to the distal aspect of the joint, depending on the finger and movement desired (figure 21.32). Radial glide improves abduction of MCPs 1 and 2, adduction of MCPs 4 and 5, and radial abduction of MCP 3. Ulnar glide improves adduction of MCPs 1 and 2, abduction of MCPs 4 and 5, and ulnar abduction of MCP 3.

Notations: Abduction and adduction occur as physiological motions at the MCP joints and accessory motions at the IP joints.

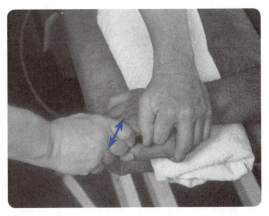

▶ **Figure 21.32** Joint mobilization: MCP lateral glides.

FLEXIBILITY EXERCISES

Range-of-motion exercises are divided into those for the intrinsic muscles and those for the extrinsic muscles. The two groups require different considerations for correct stretch application. Because extrinsic muscles cross multiple joints, the rehabilitation clinician must know these muscle insertion locations to apply appropriate stretches. Each joint the muscle crosses must be placed on stretch to produce optimal ROM changes, but the force should be applied precisely and in sequence from the most distal to the most proximal joint. When one joint is stretched, the other joints need to be stabilized. This is particularly important when considering stretching the fingers since multiple joints are involved. For example, if the proximal finger joints are not stabilized when the distal interphalangeal joint is stretched, the stretch force and surrounding tissue tension can cause any of the proximal joints to buckle, making for an ineffective stretch application. The force applied should be a slow, gentle, and sustained stretch to avoid either incorrect stretch application or excessive force that can damage the small structures of the hand and fingers.

Various joint mobilization techniques are used to improve movement in the distal radioulnar joint, the wrist joint, and the carpometacarpal joints.

One finger is stretched at a time. Joint mobilization is used before stretching so that the stretch of soft-tissue structures is more effective. If joint motion is restricted by extrinsic tightness, each joint is placed on stretch in the sequence just described, distal to proximal, to affect extrinsic structures but not intrinsic muscles. If joint motion is restricted by intrinsic muscle tightness, then the focus is on stretching only the intrinsic muscle. To perform an isolated stretch to the intrinsic muscle, the distal joint is stretched and the proximal joint is placed in the opposite direction to avoid stretching the extrinsic muscles and focus the stretch on the intrinsic muscles. For example, when the PIP joint is placed in flexion and the MCP joint is placed in extension, the intrinsic muscles extending the PIP are stretched, but the extrinsic extensor muscles are not; however, when the PIP and MCP joints are placed in flexion, the extrinsic extensor muscles are stretched but the intrinsic muscles are not. If both structures have limited flexibility, stretch exercises in both positions are necessary.

Joints and Ligaments

As already mentioned, mobilization techniques—both accessory and physiological techniques—should be applied before joints are stretched. The accessory techniques are those already discussed, including motions that are not actively possible but that must take place for full motion to occur. These should be applied before the physiological motions. The physiological motions are those that can be actively produced, such as joint flexion and extension. Techniques used to produce the physiological motions are stretch exercises.

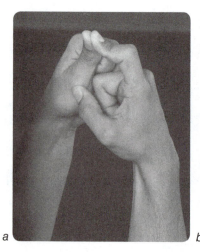
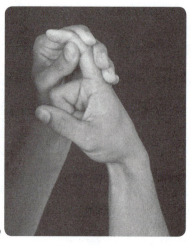

▶ **Figure 21.33** Stretch force application. *(a)* Incorrect: Force is applied on the digit's distal segment. *(b)* Correct: Force is applied at the distal joint first, then moves one joint at a time to the most proximal joint.

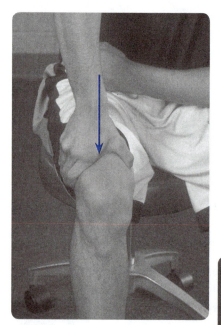

▶ **Figure 21.34** Thumb abduction stretch.

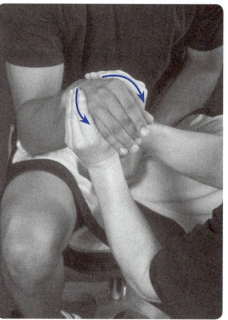

▶ **Figure 21.35** Range of motion of CMC and intermetacarpal joints.

Only one joint is stretched at a time. The other joints are positioned in neutral and kept relaxed to reduce soft-tissue tension on the joint being treated. When you apply a stretch force, the distal portion of the joint's distal segment is the location of the stretch. You need to be careful, however, to apply the force on the joint's distal portion of the bone's shaft and not on the next distal joint. For example, when stretching a PIP joint, your force is on the distal portion of the middle phalanx, not on the DIP joint or on the distal phalanx. Proper stabilization of the proximal phalanx must also occur for the stretch application to be correct (figure 21.33).

Abduction movements are crucial to maintaining vital web space flexibility of the thumb and MCP extension movement of the fingers. Abduction of the fingers can assist in stretching the MCP collateral ligaments. Soft tissue of the web space is stretched using thumb abduction overpressure. These movements are performed either actively and passively. Passive movements are performed by the clinician or the patient. The patient can stretch the finger MCPs by intertwining the fingers of the two hands together as in a praying position. The thumb's web space can be stretched by actively abducting the thumb or applying an abduction force at the CMC joint. As mentioned, care must be taken to apply the force on the distal segment of the CMC joint, not over the MCP joint. The patient can also stretch the thumb's web space by placing the hand over the top of the knee, with the fingers separated from the thumb, and applying a downward force from the shoulder to push the hand on the knee (figure 21.34).

As mentioned earlier, the CMC and intermetacarpal joints form the palmar arches that are vital to hand formation and function. The second and third metacarpals have little mobility and form the peak of the palmar arches. The fourth, and especially the fifth, metacarpals move into flexion as the hand is formed into a fist; this motion is crucial to normal hand function and permits a firm grasp. The rehabilitation clinician can stretch these joints by placing his or her thumbs in the palm of the patient's hand and his or her fingers on the dorsum over the metacarpals. The thumbs are stabilizers as the fingers roll the metacarpals around the thumbs (figure 21.35). The palmar fascia can be stretched using the technique demonstrated in figure 21.16.

Wrist joint stretches are done with the fingers relaxed and the force applied proximal to the MCP joints. The patient can apply the stretches passively in all wrist motions (figure 21.36).

The distal radioulnar joint stretches are the same as those for the proximal radioulnar joint. These are discussed in chapter 20 and are shown in figures 20.19 and 20.20. The stretch is applied at the distal radioulnar joint. The hand is not included in the stretch.

The oblique retinacular ligament acts on the IP joints similarly to the way the intrinsics act on the MCP and PIP joints. When the PIP joint is flexed, it extends the DIP joint. If passive DIP flexion is greater with the PIP joint flexed than with the PIP extended, the oblique retinacular ligament is restricted. Tightness limits DIP flexion particularly during PIP extension. To stretch this ligament, the PIP joint is passively maintained in extension while the DIP joint is stretched into flexion.

Extrinsic Muscles

As mentioned previously, the stretch applied to extrinsic muscles begins with the distal joint and proceeds in sequence, moving distally to proximally. The force is applied slowly and deliberately without excessive stress to the structures. Contract-relax-stretch techniques can improve results of the stretch because reflex inhibition plays a role in these techniques. Application of a slight traction force on the joints makes the stretch more comfortable by reducing compressive forces on the joints.

Because of the easy accessibility of the hand and wrist joints and the relatively small force required to stretch them, the patient can learn proper stretching techniques and apply them frequently throughout the day.

Stretching either extrinsic extensor or extrinsic flexor muscles starts distally and moves proximally. For example, improving flexion motion involves applying a stretch at the DIP joint while stabilizing the PIP joint as the DIP is brought into flexion. Once the DIP joint is moved to its end position, the PIP joint is then moved into flexion. The MCP joint is then moved into flexion while the IP joints are held in their flexed positions. Finally, the wrist is brought into flexion to its end range with the finger maintained in its fully flexed position. Stretch to increase flexion is seen in figure 21.37. Stretches to increase motion of these extrinsic muscles are each applied in both elbow flexion and extension. The patient should feel a stretch on the posterior forearm.

Since the long finger muscles can also influence wrist mobility, wrist stretches are applied with the fingers on stretch. To increase wrist extension motion, the patient extends the fingers first and then moves the wrist into extension (figure 21.38a). As with stretches to the fingers, the wrist is stretched with the elbow in flexion and in extension. The stretch should be felt on the anterior forearm.

A slow sustained stretch is applied to the finger and wrist extensors to increase wrist flexion. The stretch begins at the fingers and is applied last to the wrist (figure 21.38b). The stretch is applied with the elbow flexed and extended until a stretch on the posterior forearm occurs.

Flexibility exercises for the hand are used to stretch the joints and ligaments, the extrinsic muscles, and the intrinsic muscles.

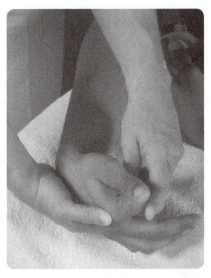

▶ **Figure 21.36** Wrist stretches.

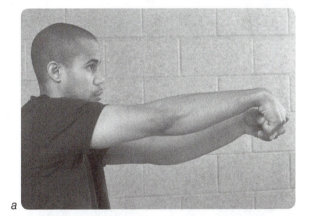

▶ **Figure 21.37** Extrinsic finger extensor stretch. In sequence: DIP, PIP, MCP, wrist elbow.

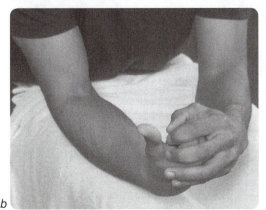

a

b

▶ **Figure 21.38** Independent stretches to increase flexion (a) with elbow extension and (b) with elbow flexion.

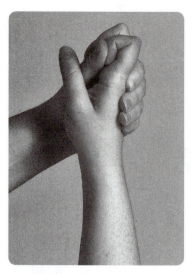

▶ **Figure 21.39** Intrinsic stretch: IPs are flexed, MCP is extended, wrist is in neutral.

Intrinsic Muscles

Because the lumbricals and interossei flex the MCP joint and extend the IP joints, the stretch is applied in the opposite direction of their movement. The IP joints are maintained in a flexed position while a stretch to increase MCP extension is applied (figure 21.39). The wrist is stabilized in neutral during this activity to prevent extrinsic muscle influences on the stretch.

STRENGTHENING EXERCISES

During periods of immobilization, isometric exercises can be used for all wrist and hand muscles. Active exercises are good for maintaining motion and early strengthening. As the patient progresses, various equipment including weights, putty, and rubber bands can be used to further increase strength gains. In the early stages, the muscles may fatigue quickly, so the patient must be cautioned against overdoing it, causing undue stress. Since little functional hand activity is eccentric, concentric exercises, rather than eccentric exercises, for the fingers are the primary emphasis.

Tendon Gliding Exercises

When restriction of normal tendon gliding occurs because of adhesions of tendons or their sheaths, you must restore the normal tendon glide to achieve full motion. Adhesions can occur anywhere along the tendon and can restrict tendon motion proximally and distally to the point of adhesion. Friction massage assists in reducing adhesions of superficial tendons, and exercises improve mobility of both superficial and deep tendons. Muscle activity aids in restoring proximal glide of the tendon. Active and passive exercises and splinting can restore distal glide of the tendon. Because active exercises can restore both proximal and distal tendon gliding, it is advisable to use these whenever possible. The effectiveness of these exercises, however, is limited by the muscle's strength and endurance. Passive stretching and massage may be useful to improve tendon gliding when these parameters are restricted.

Flexor Tendons

Gliding exercises for the long flexor tendons necessitate differentiating between the profundus and superficialis. You must isolate each tendon to facilitate gliding, because adhesions between these tendons restrict movement of both. To show whether or not the tendons are gliding properly, the patient maintains the MCP joint in extension while flexing the PIP joints. With the fingers in this position, the clinician passively extends the DIP joint and should meet no resistance. If there is no resistance, it is normal and only the superficialis is being used, as it should be. If the patient maintains this position but both flexor muscles are tense (clinician cannot passively move the DIP joint), normal tendon gliding between the profundus and superficialis tendons is restricted. The gliding exercise for these tendons occurs with the MCP and PIP joints stabilized in flexion while the patient attempts to flex and extend the DIP (figure 21.40a). To isolate the superficialis from the profundus tendon, the proximal phalanx is stabilized and the PIP joint is flexed and extended: Either one digit is stabilized at a time as shown in figure 21.40b, or all digits except the one being treated are stabilized. In this exercise, the other IP joints are maintained in extension while the digit of interest is

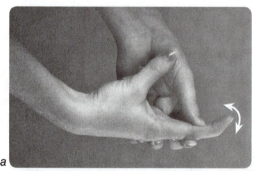

a

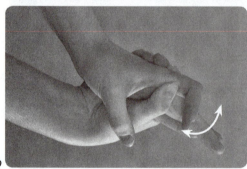

b

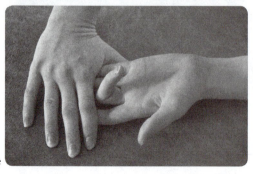

c

▶ **Figure 21.40** Isolation of tendons for gliding exercises: *(a)* flexor digitorum profundus, *(b)* flexor digitorum superficialis, *(c)* elimination of flexor digitorum profundus activity.

flexed. Because the profundus tendons all originate from the same muscle belly, it is easy to eliminate profundus activity by restricting movement of the other digits (figure 21.40c).

There are three functional flexor tendon gliding exercises that belong in a therapeutic exercise program to either prevent gliding restrictions or improve flexor tendon gliding when it is restricted. They are presented in figure 21.41. The first one enhances gliding between the two long finger flexor tendons; this is the hook position exercise and involves keeping the MCP extended while flexing the IPs (figure 21.41a). The second exer-

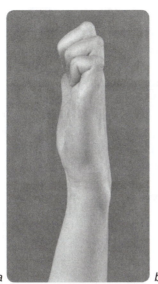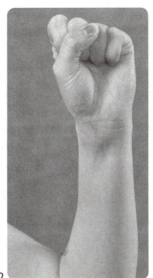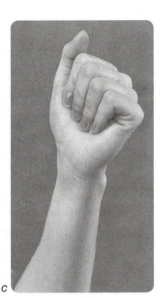

▶ **Figure 21.41** Flexor tendon gliding exercises: *(a)* Hook enhances gliding between FDS and FDP. *(b)* Fist enhances gliding of FDP. *(c)* Modified fist enhances gliding of FDS.

cise produces gliding of the profundus tendons within their sheath. This is the fist formation and is performed with the IP and MCP joints in full flexion and then moving all the joints into extension (figure 21.41b). The third exercise is a modified fist exercise. It occurs with the MCP and PIP joints flexed and the DIP joints extended and provides optimal gliding of the superficialis tendons in their sheath (figure 21.41c). The start position for each of these flexor tendon gliding exercises is with all the fingers in full extension. As the patient performs each specific exercise, controlled digit movements are used throughout the entire motion.

Flexor pollicis longus gliding exercises are performed in a similar manner by moving the IP and MCP joints through a full range of flexion and extension. These exercises are initially performed with the wrist in neutral, but as the patient progresses, the wrist should be moved into flexion with finger flexion and into extension with finger extension.

Extensor Tendons

Because the extensor tendons are flatter and wider than their flexor counterparts and because they have an intimate relationship with the intrinsic muscle system, they are more susceptible to adhesions. Adhesions or weakness can cause an extensor lag of the finger. If full extension occurs passively but not actively, weakness may be the cause. If the digit's passive flexion is also limited, it is because adhesions restrict full tendon excursion during a stretch.

On the other hand, care must be taken in stretching the extensor tendons following tendon repairs or fractures. The rehabilitation clinician must keep a close eye on increases in the extensor lag throughout the stretching process. If the extensor lag increases, it may be that the tendon is actually elongating (dehiscing) or tearing from its attachment. Emphasizing the use of active exercises to reduce extensor lag rather than passive forces to increase flexion motion helps to minimize this risk.

If an extensor lag is present at the MCP joint because of adhesions, the adhesion is of the extensor digitorum communis (EDC) tendon. This tendon is the only extensor of the MCP joint. A gliding exercise for the EDC is performed by moving the hand from a hook to a fist formation as seen in figure 21.42. In this gliding exercise, the MCP joint is moved from flexion to extension while the IP joints are kept in flexion to eliminate the intrinsic muscles. If the patient has difficulty maintaining flexion of the IP joints during this exercise, he or she can facilitate the activity by grasping a drinking straw or pencil in the fingers while moving the MCP joints. Wrist flexion and extension should also be added to the exercise when it is easy to perform with the wrist in neutral.

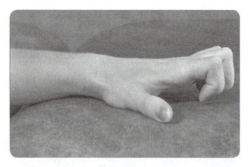

▶ **Figure 21.42** Extrinsic extensor gliding exercises: Keeping the IPs in flexion, the MCPs are moved into flexion and extension.

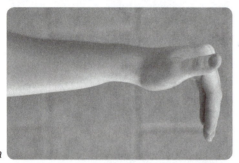

a

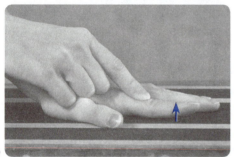

b

▶ **Figure 21.43** Extensor gliding exercises. *(a)* Intrinsic: MCP flexion with IPs in extension. *(b)* Terminal extension: IP extension with MCP in extension.

If the extensor lag at either IP joint is the result of adhesions within the extensor mechanism, then it can include both intrinsic and extrinsic structures—the interossei, lumbricals, and EDC. To isolate the intrinsic muscles and restore their function of IP extension, the MCP is stabilized in flexion while the IP joints move through active extension (figure 21.43a). As this exercise becomes easier, the MCP joint should be moved into extension. In its final progression, the most difficult position for this exercise is with the hand flat on a table and the proximal phalanx stabilized; in this position the patient lifts the middle and distal phalanxes off the table while stabilizing the metacarpal on the table (figure 21.43b).

Resistive Exercises

There are many possible resistive exercises for the wrist and hand. Specific exercises are limited only by the rehabilitation clinician's imagination. A few of the more commonly used resistive exercises are outlined in the following sections. Common substitution patterns for the exercise are also listed. You should correct any errors in the patient's technique.

■ Strength Exercises for the Wrist

Extension

Body Segment: Wrist.

Stage in Rehab: II and III.

Purpose: Strengthen wrist extensors.

Positioning: The forearm rests on a tabletop in pronation with the hand over the end of the table.

Execution: Patient lifts a dumbbell, moving through a full ROM from wrist flexion to wrist extension (figure 21.44).

Possible Substitutions: Flexing the elbow or moving the weight through a partial ROM.

Notations: The forearm must stay in contact with the tabletop throughout the exercise; it may be necessary to stabilize the forearm with a hand across the proximal forearm.

Flexion

Body Segment: Wrist.

Stage in Rehab: II and III.

Purpose: Strengthen wrist flexors.

Positioning: The patient sits next to a table with the forearm resting on the table in supination and the hand over the end of the table.

Execution: Patient moves a dumbbell weight through a full ROM from wrist extension to flexion (figure 21.45).

Possible Substitutions: Partial ROM of wrist movement and elbow flexion.

Notations: Forearm should remain on the table. A rolled towel under the wrist may make the position more comfortable.

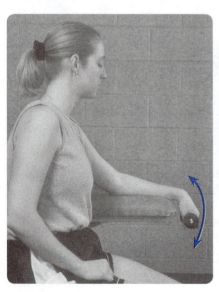

▶ **Figure 21.44** Wrist extension resistance exercise.

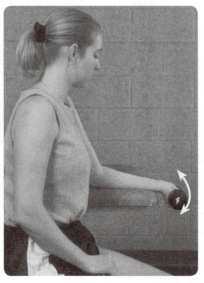

▶ **Figure 21.45** Wrist flexion resistance exercise.

Ulnar Deviation

Body Segment: Wrist.

Stage in Rehab: II and III.

Purpose: Strengthen ulnar wrist flexors.

Positioning: A bar with a weighted end is placed in the hand; the weight is on the ulnar side. The patient stands with the elbow extended.

Execution: The patient moves the wrist into ulnar deviation, lifting the weight as high as possible (figure 21.46a).

Possible Substitutions: Finger motion and shoulder extension are common substitutions.

Notations: Patient should maintain a firm grasp on the bar so that the wrist rather than the fingers is used to produce the motion.

Radial Deviation

Body Segment: Wrist.

Stage in Rehab: II and III.

Purpose: Strengthen radial wrist flexors.

Positioning: Patient's position is the same as for ulnar deviation, but the weighted bar is positioned with the weight on the radial side of the hand.

Execution: The weight is lifted upward as high as possible toward the thumb (figure 21.46b).

Possible Substitutions: Elbow flexion and motion from the fingers rather than the wrist are the most common substitutions.

Notations: Maintaining a firm grasp on the bar will reduce substitutions.

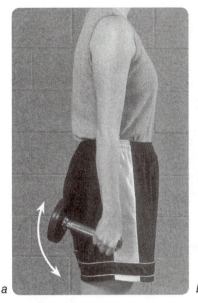
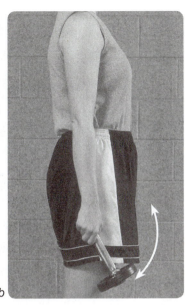

a b

▶ **Figure 21.46** *(a)* Ulnar deviation resistance exercise.

▶ **Figure 21.46** *(b)* Radial deviation resistance exercise.

Forearm Supinators

Body Segment: Forearm.

Stage in Rehab: II and III.

Purpose: Provide eccentric resistance to forearm supinators.

Positioning: A resistance band is attached to a handle or weighted bar and anchored to the side of the table. Patient grasps the weight handle with the forearm stabilized on the table.

Execution: The patient then controls the bar as the resistance band pulls the forearm into pronation (figure 21.47a).

Possible Substitutions: Shoulder adduction.

Notations: Concentric exercises for these muscles are shown in chapter 20, figure 20.25. They can also be used to provide additional eccentric activity with resistance bands.

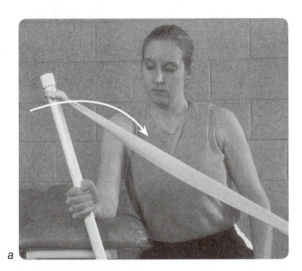

a

▶ **Figure 21.47** Eccentric resistance exercise: *(a)* supination.

Flexion exercises can be performed against manual resistance, rubber bands, putty, or other objects. You can adjust these exercises according to the availability of your equipment.

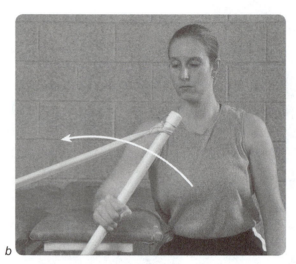

▶ **Figure 21.47** Eccentric resistance exercise: *(b)* pronation.

Forearm Pronators

Body Segment: Forearm.

Stage in Rehab: II and III.

Purpose: Provide eccentric resistance to forearm pronators.

Positioning: A resistance band is anchored to the table on the same side as the injured wrist. Patient grasps the weight handle with the forearm stabilized on the table.

Execution: The bar is passively positioned with the forearm in pronation, and as the resistance band pulls the bar, the patient controls the supination motion of the forearm (figure 21.47b).

Possible Substitutions: Shoulder abduction.

Notations: Exercises for these muscles are shown in chapter 20, figure 20.25. They can also be used to provide additional eccentric activity with resistance bands.

A number of finger exercises can be designed using putty of different strengths to provide a progressive resistive program. These are discussed next.

■ Putty Exercises for the Wrist and Hand

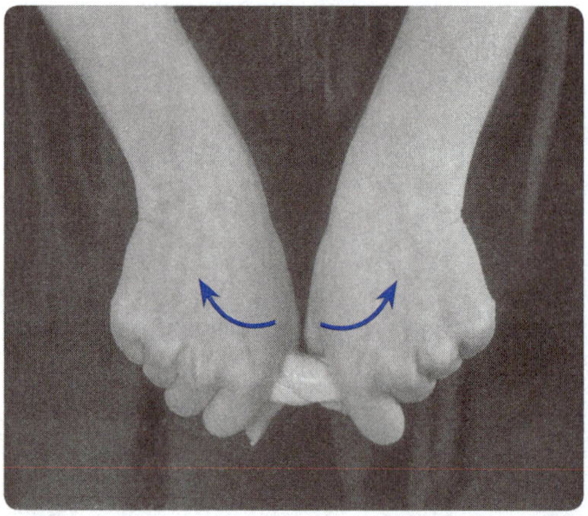

Ulnar Deviation

Body Segment: Wrist.

Stage in Rehab: II.

Purpose: Strengthen ulnar deviation of wrist muscles.

Positioning: Patient grasps the putty in both hands and places the two hands with the lateral sides of the index fingers and thumbs adjacent to each other.

Execution: Using only wrist motion, the patient moves the hands laterally against each other as the wrists move into ulnar deviation (figure 21.48a).

Possible Substitutions: Wrist flexion.

Notations: To emphasize the involved wrist, stabilize the uninvolved wrist while the involved wrist performs the exercise.

▶ **Figure 21.48** Theraputty wrist exercise: *(a)* ulnar deviation.

Radial Deviation

Body Segment: Wrist.

Stage in Rehab: II.

Purpose: Strengthen radial deviation of wrist muscles.

Positioning: The putty is formed into a tube shape and is grasped by both hands. The patient positions the little finger of the involved hand on top of the thumb of the other hand.

Execution: Stabilizing the uninvolved hand and the involved forearm and elbow, the patient moves the involved wrist into radial deviation.

Possible Substitutions: Wrist extension.

Notations: Putty exercises may be used as a home program.

Pronation and Supination

Body Segment: Forearm.

Stage in Rehab: II.

Purpose: Strength exercises for forearm pronators and supinators.

Positioning: The uninvolved arm provides the stabilizing hand to anchor the putty.

Execution: The patient uses the stabilizing hand to hold the putty. Grasping the end with the hand of the involved forearm, she moves the forearm into supination and pronation while stabilizing the elbow next to her side (figure 21.48b).

Possible Substitutions: Wrist motion.

Notations: This is an early strengthening exercise for supinators and pronators.

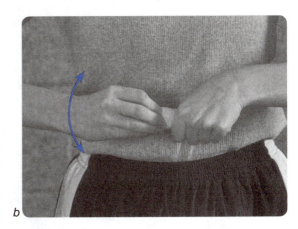

▶ **Figure 21.48** Theraputty wrist exercise: *(b)* supination-pronation.

Power-Grip Exercises

Body Segment: Hand.

Stage in Rehab: II and III.

Purpose: Strengthen finger flexors used in power grips.

Positioning: The hand is placed in various positions, depending upon the grip-strength exercise. All three may be indicated, depending upon the patient's condition.

Execution: Patient squeezes the putty using the different power grips for emphasis on different digits (figure 21.49, a-c).

Possible Substitutions: Wrist flexion rather than stabilization of the wrist in slight extension.

Notations: Strength progression occurs by advancing to more difficult types of putty.

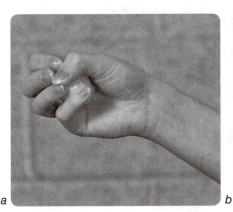
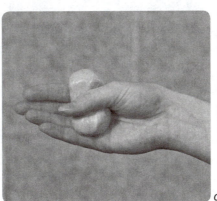
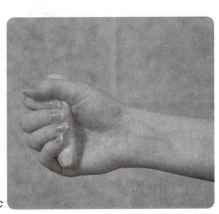

▶ **Figure 21.49** Theraputty power-grip exercises: *(a)* spherical, *(b)* hook, *(c)* cylinder.

Precision Grip Exercises

Body Segment: Fingers.

Stage in Rehab: II.

Purpose: Strengthen intrinsic muscles.

Positioning: The phalanx is in slight flexion. The IP joints are not locked in extension.

Execution: Patient performs the different precision grips against the putty (figure 21.50, a-d).

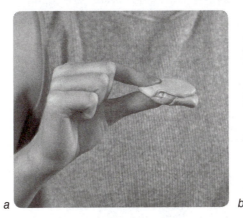
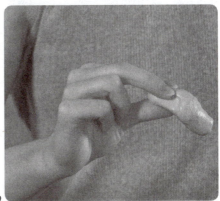

▶ **Figure 21.50** Theraputty precision-grip exercises: *(a)* tip to tip, *(b)* digital prehension.

Possible Substitutions: Locking the IP joints so that the intrinsic muscles are not performing the task.

Notations: The putty is squeezed, then reshaped, and the exercise is repeated. Precision-grip exercises can also be performed with clothespins. Wrapping rubber bands around the end of the clothespin provides additional resistance. As with the putty exercises, the patient should grasp the clothespins with the IP joints in slight flexion. Don't allow extension of any IP joint.

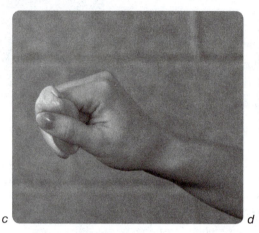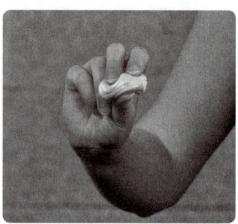

c   d

▶ **Figure 21.50**   Theraputty precision-grip exercises: *(c)* lateral prehension, *(d)* three-prong chuck.

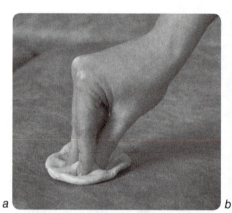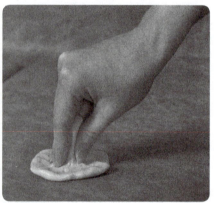

a   b

▶ **Figure 21.51**   Gross opposition exercise for the intrinsic muscles: The patient places all the finger pads on the putty and pulls the finger pads together *(a)*. A cone should be formed in the middle *(b)*.

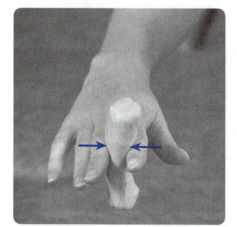

▶ **Figure 21.52**   Finger adduction exercise.

Opposition Exercise

Body Segment: Fingers.

Stage in Rehab: II.

Purpose: Strengthen intrinsic muscles of the hand.

Positioning: The putty begins in a pan-cake shape on a tabletop. The patient places all the finger pads on the putty.

Execution: The patient's finger pads pull the putty up into a cone shape (figure 21.51a-b).

Possible Substitutions: Using the wrist or long finger flexors rather than the intrinsic muscles.

Notations: The intrinsic muscles are worked if the IP joints are kept in extension during the exercise. The extrinsics are worked if the IP joints are flexed during the exercise.

Finger Adduction

Body Segment: Fingers.

Stage in Rehab: II.

Purpose: Strengthen intrinsic adductors.

Positioning: The putty is placed between any two fingers or between the index finger and thumb.

Execution: The patient pulls the fingers toward each other, against the putty (figure 21.52).

Possible Substitutions: IP and MCP flexion.

Notations: The IP and MCP joints should remain extended.

Finger Extension, Thumb and Finger Abduction

Body Segment: Fingers.

Stage in Rehab: II.

Purpose: Strengthen intrinsic muscles.

Positioning: Putty or a rubber band is placed around the fingers and thumb (figure 21.53a).

Execution: The patient spreads the fingers apart as far as possible.

Possible Substitutions: Careful observation is required to detect performance by muscles other than the desired ones.

Notations: These exercises can be used either on the entire group or on individual fingers (figure 21.53, b-f).

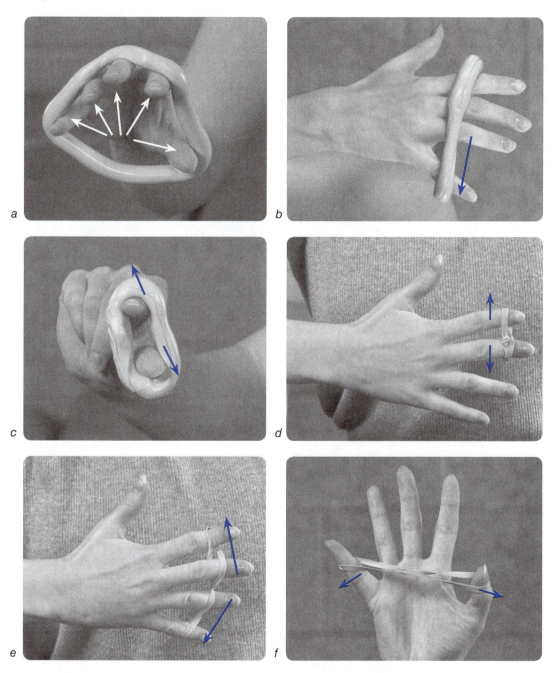

▶ **Figure 21.53** *(a)* Multiple-finger and thumb extension with putty, *(b)* finger abduction with putty, *(c)* index finger and thumb extension with putty, *(d)* two-finger abduction with rubber band, *(e)* multiple-finger abduction with rubber band, *(f)* thumb and fifth-finger abduction with rubber band.

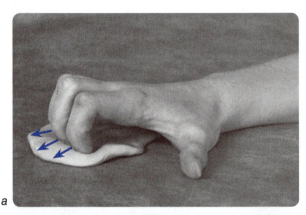

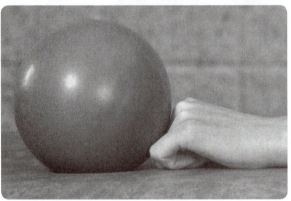

▶ **Figure 21.54** Extensor lag exercise: *(a)* with putty, *(b)* with medicine ball.

🔑 Strengthening exercises are used to restore normal glide of the hand's flexor and extensor tendons; a large variety of resistive exercises promote strength of the wrist extensors, ulnar and radial extensors, and supinators and pronators.

🔑 In addition to plyometric exercises that are also used for the shoulder and elbow, plyometrics for the hand include activities using a medicine ball and isokinetic activities.

Extensor Lag Exercises

Body Segment: Fingers.

Stage in Rehab: II and III.

Purpose: Strengthen finger intrinsics to eliminate extensor lag.

Positioning: The patient places the putty on a tabletop, with the palm facing down and the MCP and IP joints flexed.

Execution: The fingers push outward against the putty as the fingers move into extension (figure 21.54a).

Possible Substitutions: Finger abduction.

Notations: A medicine ball, pushed while the MCP joints remain in flexion and the IP joints move from flexion into extension, provides an alternative resistance exercise to the intrinsic muscles (figure 21.54b). Using heavier medicine balls or increasing surface friction increases the challenge.

Isokinetic Exercises

Wrist-strengthening exercises progress from straight plane to more functional diagonal planes, just as with other isokinetic protocols. Fast and slow speeds are used to enhance strength and muscle endurance. All exercises should remain pain free.

PLYOMETRIC EXERCISES

Many of the plyometric exercises for the shoulder and elbow are also used for the wrist and hand. A couple of additional exercises can be used for the hand. For specific information on the plyometric exercises for the shoulder and elbow, refer to chapters 19 and 20.

Ball Drop and Catch

This exercise uses a medicine ball small enough to be grasped in one hand. The patient stands with shoulder at 90° flexion, the arm outstretched in front of the body, and the hand positioned palm down. The patient grasps the medicine ball in the hand and allows it to drop, then immediately retrieves the ball before it reaches the floor by catching with the hand in the palm-down position. As the exercise becomes easier, a heavier ball is selected. The patient should grasp the ball with all the fingers tightly around the ball.

Other Plyometric Activities

Numerous other activities can be used as plyometric exercises for the hand. Some of these are bouncing a medicine ball against the wall or incline trampoline, boxing against a medicine bag, plyometric push-ups, and volleyball passes with a medicine ball.

FUNCTIONAL AND ACTIVITY-SPECIFIC EXERCISES

Because the hand has such a wide variation of function, it is nearly impossible to define functional activities for the hand. Specific demands for functional activities are determined by the requirements of the patient's sport or activity. A football quarterback's needs for hand function differ from those for the football lineman. A golfer's hand functions vary greatly from those of a basketball player's. The range of demands can include variations in grips, grip positions, rapid or slow hand movements, sustained or changing grips, and forceful or light grasping. The rehabilitation clinician must understand the demands of each patient's activities and outline a functional exercise progression based on those requirements. Once a selection of exercises is made, a progression is designed using a planned program of increasing difficulty until the exercises mimic the stress levels the patient will encounter in full participation.

SPECIAL REHABILITATION APPLICATIONS

Because the hand is so complex and has many structures in close contact with each other, an injury to one area or tissue can impact adjacent tissues and other segments within the wrist and hand. The rehabilitation clinician must not only be cognizant of this and keenly aware of the possibility of secondary involvement of other segments, but also must do everything possible to attempt to prevent these complications.

Some of the more common injuries requiring rehabilitation are addressed here. Tendon rupture and repairs are not often seen in musculoskeletal injuries, but the rehabilitation programs for them are outlined here since the clinician must take additional precautions when they do occur and necessitate a rehabilitation program.

Fractures

There are many bones in the wrist and hand. Which bone is fractured has a great impact on the rehabilitation process. This section presents some general concepts, applicable to all fractures, before addressing specific fractures. Although there are exceptions, a fracture is generally immobilized in a position so that the ligaments of the joints are placed on some stretch. This positioning helps reduce the risk of contractures. Immobilization is typically maintained for two to three weeks unless the fracture is unstable, displaced, or comminuted. Fractures that are unstable are often corrected with open reduction and internal fixation (ORIF), followed by immobilization. Open reduction and internal fixation is advantageous when the fracture is unstable, because it provides needed stability. However, because of the disruption of blood flow and increased soft-tissue damage that occurs with ORIF procedures, healing time can be delayed.

Splints used to immobilize fractures should affect only as many joints as necessary to maintain good fracture alignment. Joints proximal and distal to the fracture site and not included in the splint immobilization should be moved through their ranges of motion regularly.

Distal Forearm and Wrist Fractures

The most common distal forearm fracture is the Colles fracture. The distal radius proximal to the wrist is fractured and is displaced dorsally. A Smith's fracture also involves the radius, but the distal radius fragment displaces volarly. Surgical repair is common with Smith's fractures but does not take place as often with a Colles fracture. A Barton's fracture occurs at the radial articular region and results in wrist subluxation as well as the fracture. While the Colles and Smith's fractures are most often the result of falling on an outstretched hand, the Barton's fracture occurs with a sudden violent wrist extension and pronation. The likelihood of its being unstable makes the need for ORIF highly probable.

As with all fractures, whether treated with open or closed reduction, management of pain and edema is the goal of early rehabilitation in phase I. Coban wrap or other compressive wrap is useful for controlling edema in the fingers and hand. Isotoner gloves may also be used to reduce edema once the wrist cast is removed. Modalities are useful in controlling pain as well as edema. Early rehabilitation exercises in phase II include the use of active range-of-motion (AROM) exercises of the uninvolved joints. These exercises will encourage good tendon gliding, reduce edema, and relieve joint stiffness.

Immobilization casts or splints used for these fractures should permit full MCP flexion motion and full thumb opposition. Active range-of-motion exercises for the extrinsic and

The great range of uses for the hand in sports means that the rehabilitation clinician working with a hand injury must understand the particular demands of each patient's sport and position.

intrinsic finger muscles should be permitted while the patient's hand is in the splint or cast during phase I. The patient should be able to perform three exercises: MCP joint full flexion with IP extension, MCP joint extension with full IP flexion, MCP joint full flexion combined with IP joint full flexion.

It should be possible for AROM to approach passive range-of-motion (PROM) excursion. If full PROM is significantly greater than full AROM, the muscle may be atrophied and may lack sufficient strength, or the tendon is being restricted by adhesions, or both influences may be present. Active exercises, electrical stimulation for facilitation, friction massage in regions where it is appropriate, proprioceptive neuromuscular facilitation, or biofeedback can be used to restore active motion while the wrist is immobilized. Active exercises, such as place-and-hold exercises where the digit is passively placed at an end range of motion and then the patient actively holds that position for five seconds, are used to improve strength during this phase. Massage is used where swelling is present to relieve it; in areas where swelling is resolved but has left residual adhesions, friction massage is used to restore tissue mobility. Although the wrist and hand may be immobilized, upper extremity PNF exercises may facilitate strength of the immobilized structures.

It is common for distal radial fractures to be immobilized for three to six weeks. Once immobilization is discontinued, the clinician attempts to regain full wrist motion and long tendon mobility. Joint mobilization with active stretching is used in late phase II. Grades I and II joint mobilization relieve pain and are used early in phases I and II. Grades III and IV joint mobilizations are not incorporated into the program until the fracture is healed enough to withstand the stress in phase III. Range of motion in all planes is emphasized. Many clinicians neglect to address radial and ulnar deviation, but these must be restored if the patient is to have full wrist function.

In phase III after cast or splint removal, the patient begins low-resistance, low-repetition isotonic activities, progressing to higher repetitions and resistance as tolerated. If pain or swelling increases with exercises, these exercises are too aggressive and should be reduced in intensity or number of repetitions. Exercises for both the intrinsic and extrinsic muscles are introduced in this phase to strengthen all groups.

Once strength gains are near-normal, the patient begins functional activities in phase IV. Functional activities are designed to stress those muscles that will be tested when the patient returns his or her normal activities. Following function activities, the activity-specific program is designed to mimic the patient's normal activities; each patient's exercises during this part of phase IV will be different. For example, tennis has different requirements for the wrist than golf does, and golf and ballet likewise differ in their demands. Similarly, in the work environment, a computer analyst's requirements are different from those of an auto mechanic. The rehabilitation clinician should be aware of the demands required of the patient in his or her normal setting and design a progressive activity-specific program that will lead the patient to an appropriate return to his or her sport or activity.

Carpal and Metacarpal Fractures

The carpal most frequently fractured is the scaphoid. Because of the bones' variability in blood supply, healing time is extremely varied, from 4 to 20 weeks, and depends primarily on the location and type of fracture. The area remains immobilized until radiography demonstrates signs of healing.

Edema control should be aggressive, and the patient should perform ROM of the uninvolved segments of the shoulder, elbow, and hand immediately and continually throughout the immobilization period. Pain should be avoided with these exercises.

Once the cast or splint is removed, ROM for the thumb begins. These exercises should be active. If joint mobility is restricted in a capsular pattern, joint mobilization is added to the program. The patient performs active exercises with the proximal joint stabilized passively to ensure correct movement of the digit.

The hook of the hamate and the pisiform can incur fractures from impact with sport implements such as a baseball bat, golf club, or racket or from a fall on an outstretched arm. Because they are not often unstable, these fractures heal well most of the time with cast immobilization. As with other fractures in this area, ROM exercises for the shoulder, elbow, and other hand joints are routine while the splint is on, and restoration of full ROM for all joints should be the goal following cast removal. If pain occurs with hand and wrist activity following cast removal, a protective splint may be used at night and throughout the day to relieve the stress of motion and use. Progression of flexibility exercises continues until full motion is achieved.

Joint mobilization of restricted metacarpal and carpal joints is used to provide full physiological and accessory movements that are necessary for full hand and wrist function. Strengthening exercises are initiated in phase III after motion is restored. Grip exercises are used early and even in phase II, because they help to mobilize the metacarpals and to restore the normal palmar arches. Wrist strengthening is also incorporated. The patient is weaned from the splint as pain and edema subside and motion and strength are restored.

Because the neck of the metacarpal is the weakest aspect of the metacarpal bone, it is the most frequent site of metacarpal fractures. These fractures most commonly occur in the fourth and fifth metacarpals. Fractures here result primarily from compressive forces like those that occur when a fist is used to administer a direct blow. For this reason they are referred to as boxer's fractures. The alignment of the fingers determines whether the fracture can be treated with immobilization or whether it requires an ORIF. Normal oblique flexion of the digits with the MCP and PIP joints flexed causes an alignment of the digits such that they point toward the scaphoid tubercle (figure 21.55). If digit angulation is off by more than 20° to 30°, an ORIF may be necessary.

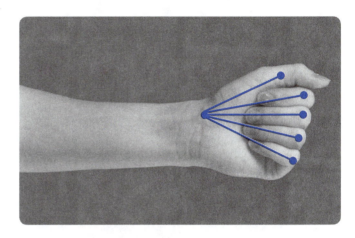

▶ **Figure 21.55** Finger alignment with MCP and PIP flexion.

Two to four weeks of immobilization may be necessary for carpal and metacarpal fractures. Range-of-motion exercises while the cast is on are recommended for the uninvolved areas. Once the cast is removed, the patient enters phase II and ROM exercises for the entire hand and wrist begin immediately. Active range-of-motion exercises are used for the metacarpal joints, and passive and active-motion exercises are used for the digits. This helps to reduce tendon adhesions. Intrinsic and extrinsic ROM exercises should be incorporated. Support for the metacarpals during finger ROM exercises should be provided either manually or with a splint. The patient progresses to PROM exercises to all areas once the fracture is well healed. The patient progresses to resistive exercises from PROM exercises in phase III. During this phase, the patient also performs dexterity exercises, grip exercises for both power and precision, and progressively increases all parameters of flexibility, strength, and agility. From there, phase IV occurs where the patient performs more functional activities in preparation for the final aspect of phase IV, the activity-specific program. Joint mobilization is used to increase joint mobility in restricted segments when capsular mobility is restricted in the later portion of phase II and early phase III. Resistive exercises in phase III begin with light weights and progress to heavier weights and more repetitions, using pain and edema as guidelines for advancing the patient.

A Bennett's fracture involves the first metacarpal. Because the thumb is responsible for at least 50% of hand function, appropriate management and treatment of thumb injuries are crucial. Proper angulation must be ensured with either closed or open reduction to ultimately permit good function of the thumb. The immobilization period is usually four weeks. During this time, treatment efforts to control edema and pain are important. The rehabilitation clinician realizes that adhesions may occur in the first web space and takes steps to maintain appropriate web spacing during immobilization. If the web space is compromised, full thumb motion is limited. Cast removal allows initiation of AROM exercises. Once union of the fracture site is observed on X-ray, usually about 6 to 8 weeks post-injury, PROM exercises are used to regain motion as the patient starts phase II of rehabilitation. If PROM is significantly more than AROM, it is likely that tendon adhesions are present. Friction massage, electrical stimulation, and active and passive ROM exercises assist in reducing adhesions and restoring tendon glide. Dynamic splinting may be necessary when full ROM is not restored by 8 to 10 weeks post-injury. As with other fractures, resistive exercises begin in phase III after healing is apparent and motion gains have occurred. Strengthening exercises should include both precision and power grasping activities and also incorporate other segments that have lost strength secondary to reduced use of the hand. As with other injuries, after strength, mobility, and agility are regained, the patient progresses to phase IV where the emphasis is on functional activities, and then, into the activity-specific program.

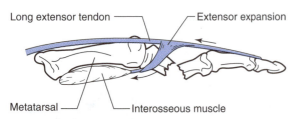

▶ **Figure 21.56** Forces affecting proximal phalanx fracture.

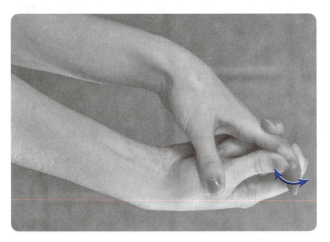

▶ **Figure 21.57** Restraining exercise: The MCP and PIP joints are restrained while the DIP is moved.

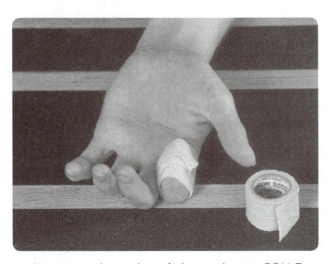

▶ **Figure 21.58** Aggressive techniques to increase ROM: Tape is applied in a prolonged stretch to increase IP joint flexion range of motion.

Phalangeal Fractures

Because of the long finger tendon forces affecting normal finger balance, fractures of the proximal and middle phalanges often result in imbalance and associated displacement and instability. Proximal phalanx fractures occur because of falls or direct blows to the phalanx, most often in the thumb and index finger. Middle phalanx fractures are not as common; these fractures result from a crush injury such as occurs when a hand is stepped on. Distal phalanx fractures are common and account for half of hand fractures. Proximal phalanx fractures typically result in flexion of the proximal bone segment from the pull of the interossei muscles, and extension of the distal segment occurs because of the long extensor tendon's pull on it (figure 21.56). A proximal phalangeal fracture is reduced and immobilized with either open or closed reduction; the use of external wires in an open repair is common. If the fracture is stable, buddy taping the fingers immobilizes the fracture and still permits tendon movement to minimize tendon gliding problems.

If the fracture is stable, motion exercises begin as early as the first to second week after the injury. If the fracture is displaced, motion is usually started three to four weeks post-injury. Finger fractures are seldom immobilized for more than four weeks because of the deleterious effects of prolonged immobilization on surrounding soft-tissue structures.

One of the greatest complications of phalangeal immobilization is tendon adhesions, resulting in restriction of normal tendon gliding. As previously discussed adhesions of the extensor tendon can cause an extensor lag with limited IP flexion. Adhesions of the long flexor tendons will also prevent full extension of the digit. Scar massage minimizes and treats these adhesions. Exercises can isolate tendon function and reduce tendon adhesions. For example, if the FDP tendon is restricted, the exercise to treat this tendon passively places the MCP and PIP joints in flexion and blocks them from moving while the DIP is moved into flexion and extension (figure 21.57).

Once the fracture is healed sufficiently to be stable, more aggressive PROM exercises and joint mobilization are used to improve ROM, especially in the latter half of phase II or early phase III. Dynamic splints provide a continual low-level stress to tight structures for more restricted cases. One can also apply tape to position digits into a stretch position (figure 21.58). These prolonged tape techniques are applied during later phase III if motion is not yet restored and are used for 15- to 20-min

---

Case Study

A 21-year-old hockey forward suffered a fracture of the neck of his dominant hand's fourth MCP when he engaged in a fight during a game and hit an opponent. The hand was placed in a cast for two weeks and then in a splint that could be removed for his rehabilitation activities. The fracture is now stable, so the physician wants to wean him from the splint over the next two weeks. The clinician's initial examination reveals mild swelling in the hand and fingers. Wrist flexion is 50° and wrist extension is 65°. Ulnar deviation and radial deviation are 10°. Supination is 70° and pronation is 90°. MCP flexion is 45°, PIP flexion is 80°, and DIP flexion is 60°. The patient is unable to make a complete fist. The MCP and IP joints can extend passively to 0°. He is unable to simultaneously flex the MCP and extend the IP joints.

Questions for Analysis

1. What do you suspect this patient's primary problems are?
2. What will be included in your first three treatment sessions with him, assuming no regression with your treatments?
3. What will your initial goals during the first week be for him?
4. What precautions must you be aware of when you treat him?
5. Describe three home exercises you will give this patient at the time of your first treatment.
6. List four strengthening exercises you will use with him in the first month.
7. What functional exercises will you incorporate into his rehabilitation program before he returns to hockey?

---

periods throughout the day, as tolerated, to improve scar-tissue mobility and gain ROM. Caution is necessary in force application for prolonged stretching, especially with the extensor tendons, since it is relatively easy to overstretch the flat, broad extensor tendon. A low-level tension force is all that is required for prolonged stretching using taping techniques. The result from overstretching the extensor tendon is an extensor lag. If an extensor lag develops, an extension splint worn continuously for 3 to 6 weeks is required to correct it.

Stretching exercises should involve both intrinsic and extrinsic muscles. Intrinsic muscle stretching exercises are performed with the IP joints in flexion and the MCP joints moving from flexion to extension, as seen in figure 21.39. Extrinsic muscles are stretched with the IP and MCP joints in various combinations of flexion and extension. Refer to figures 21.37 and 21.41 for these exercises.

Once the patient achieves full ROM, resistive exercises, including those using therapeutic putty and rubber bands and other exercises listed earlier, are used to restore full strength of the long finger flexors, long finger extensors, and the intrinsics. Wrist, elbow, and shoulder strength are included in the program. Finger exercises begin with light resistance, increasing in intensity or repetitions as the patient progresses. Exercises should emphasize full tendon and joint functions that incorporate normal movement.

Triangular Fibrocartilage Complex Lesion (TFCC)

The TFCC contains the ligaments and cartilage structures between the distal radioulnar joint and between the distal ulna and carpal bones. The fibrocartilage disc in this complex is sometimes referred to as the "meniscus of the wrist." It serves as a shock absorber for the wrist and provides a gliding surface for wrist motion. The TFCC is injured with either repetitive rotational loading of the wrist or by a direct fall onto an outstretched wrist. The patient typically reports persistent pain in the ulnar wrist during gripping and forearm supination-pronation activities. A click may be heard or palpated occasionally over the sight, and palpation pressure applied directly over the disc produces pain.

These injuries are usually treated conservatively first with rehabilitation. The upper extremity is placed in a cast or splint with the elbow at 90° of flexion, the wrist in ulnar deviation and extension for up to six weeks. This extreme step is taken with these injuries because the TFCC is a vital structure to the distal radioulnar joint and absorbs almost 20% of compressive forces applied to the wrist (Buterbaugh, Brown, & Horn, 1998). Following removal of the cast, the first two to three weeks emphasize regaining wrist flexion & extension and radial & ulnar deviation, and forearm pronation & supination. Strength exercises begin after this time and include straight-plane strengthening without torsion forces to the wrist during the first four to six weeks. The TFCC is not attached to ligaments and is able to rotate freely with the distal ulna, so rotation of the forearm performed too soon may re-aggravate the injury (Buterbaugh et al., 1998).

If the TFCC is not satisfactorily stable following the conservative approach, surgical debridement and/or repair may be necessary. If an arthroscopic debridement is performed, rehabilitation begins one to two weeks following surgery. If an open reduction with repair is required, longer immobilization up to four weeks may be necessary. In rare but severe cases, 10 weeks of immobilization may be required.

During the one to two weeks of immobilization following arthroscopic debridement, the patient participates in exercises for the non-involved segments. Early phase II rehabilitation begins within the week following surgery and includes range of motion exercises and modalities or manual therapies to relieve pain and swelling and to encourage frequent sessions of pain-free active wrist motion. Tendon-gliding exercises may be used if it is apparent that the long finger tendons are losing motion. The splint is worn when not performing ROM exercises. After two weeks, active ROM exercises continue, but active-assistive motion exercises are added to gain additional motion. Once the scar is sufficiently healed, soft tissue mobilization to prevent adhesions is added to the program. The end of phase II is approached at about 3 to 4 weeks; at this time passive stretches are used to gain full motion of the wrist. Forearm pronation and supination motion is also improved actively and passively. Finger grip exercises can begin towards the end of phase II. Phase III begins at week 6 when strengthening exercises begin with putty exercises and progress to weights. Toward the end of phase III, about week 8, the patient should have full motion in all planes and near-normal strength. In phase IV, functional and then activity-specific exercises are instituted to return the patient to normal activities.

Dislocations and Sprains

Because dislocations are a severe form of sprain, sprains and dislocation injuries are addressed together. A dislocation, the most severe type of sprain, is immobilized for longer periods of time than a sprain. Dislocations and sprains occur primarily in the IP joints, and more commonly in the PIP than the DIP joints. A term commonly used for a finger sprain is "jammed finger." Sprains usually occur in ball-handling sports when the ball hits the end of the finger.

When a phalangeal dislocation occurs, the joint's supporting structures—the radial and ulnar collateral ligaments and the volar plate—have been damaged either individually or in any combination. Fractures can frequently accompany dislocations. If the dislocation is unstable, surgical repair using either a Kirschner wire or a pin is often the standard course of treatment. This surgical repair is accompanied by a postoperative cast or splint for three to five weeks. The wire or pin may be removed after three weeks, although use of the splint may continue. Removal of the splint to perform gentle active and passive PIP extension is initiated with the surgeon's approval. Exercises include activities that permit tendon gliding while protecting the injured joint. A gradually progressive program of strengthening exercises starts at six to eight weeks once the patient has achieved full motion.

If the dislocation is stable, the finger is immobilized similarly to the way it is for an unstable dislocation, with the PIP joint in 20° to 40° of flexion to permit maximal collateral ligament length and to control edema. Efforts are made to control edema and pain in phase I, even before motion exercises begin. In 7 to 10 days, AROM is initiated in early phase II

■ Case Study

A 16-year-old, right-handed volleyball setter suffered a dislocated dominant-hand middle finger three weeks ago. The finger has been in a partial flexion splint for the past three weeks. The physician has instructed the patient to tape the finger to her ring finger throughout the day except when in rehabilitation. She has been moving the wrist and MCP joint, but the finger has been immobilized since the injury. The edema is gone, but the finger is stiff in the IP joints. Passive DIP extension lacks 15° and flexion is to 30°, and PIP extension lacks 30° and flexion is to 50°. Active DIP extension lacks 20° and flexion is to 25°, and PIP extension lacks 40° and flexion is to 50°. The patient is unable to make a complete fist because the middle finger does not flex into the palm. Her grip strength measurement is 13.6 kg (30 lb) on the right and 31.7 kg (70 lb) on the left. There is tenderness over the PIP collateral ligaments, especially on the radial side.

Questions for Analysis

1. What will your first treatment goals be for this patient today?
2. What will you attempt to accomplish in the next three treatments? How will you accomplish those goals?
3. What precautions should you consider in the treatments?
4. What are two exercises you will send home with the patient today?
5. What strengthening exercises will you use?
6. What functional activities will you eventually include in her therapeutic exercise program?

---

to prevent tendon-gliding restrictions. These exercises are restricted by blocking individual joints. The exercises promote distal and proximal tendon gliding and emphasize both intrinsic and extrinsic muscles. Splinting is often discontinued after three weeks, with buddy taping applied to continue to protect the joint. Full active extension should be achieved within six to eight weeks. Resistive exercises begin at around eight weeks in the latter half of phase III.

If a finger is sprained, the immobilization and rehabilitation process follows that outlined above for the stable dislocation, but the process may be accelerated. If the sprain is minor, the process will take less time, but when the sprain is more severe, longer time will be required for a full recovery.

Overuse Injuries

The two most common overuse injuries of the wrist and hand are carpal tunnel syndrome and De Quervain's disease. *Overuse* is the term commonly used to describe these injuries, because trauma accumulates over a period of time and produces stress at a greater rate than the structures can accommodate. Microscopic damage occurs and the structure is unable to rebuild before additional stress is applied. If insult to the tissues continues, scar tissue develops and chronic pain occurs, making it a difficult injury to manage. These injuries can be frustrating and challenging for the rehabilitation clinician, especially when the patient does not seek treatment until the injury has become advanced. The key to succinct and successful treatment is early intervention and correction of the causes.

Carpal Tunnel Syndrome

This condition is also known as median nerve compression syndrome. The median nerve is compressed as it passes through the carpal tunnel, under the transverse carpal ligament. Compression of the median nerve results in loss of sensation over its distribution in the hand, as well as weakness and pain. Pain occurs primarily at night, when the wrist is placed in flexion while the patient sleeps. Prolonged flexion positioning of the wrist causes compression on the nerve, venous congestion, and pain. This problem often results from prolonged or repeated wrist extension positioning during daily activities. A gymnast with weak wrists who performs on the bars with the wrists in hyperextension can develop carpal tunnel syndrome. Conditioning athletes whose tendons enlarge as part of the conditioning results may also develop carpal tunnel syndrome since larger tendons will essentially make the carpal tunnel space smaller (figure 21.59).

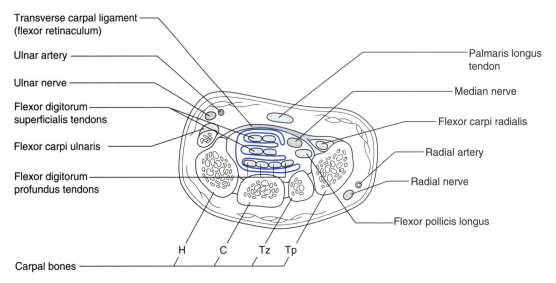

▶ **Figure 21.59** Cross-section of a wrist showing carpal tunnel.

If carpal tunnel syndrome complaints occur bilaterally, the cervical region may be the source of the problem rather than the carpal tunnel. Cervical radiculopathy is a differential diagnosis that should be ruled out for any upper-extremity injury not specifically related to an incident. Obtaining an accurate history is important to correctly determining the cause of the patient's symptoms. If passively placing the neck in a quadrant position (extension with lateral flexion and rotation to the involved side) reproduces the patient's symptoms, cervical radiculopathy cannot be ruled out; further evaluation of the neck is necessary.

When treatment begins early, it can often succeed in relieving symptoms. Use of a splint to position the wrist in neutral, especially at night, is helpful in reducing median nerve compression and night pain. Modalities can be used to relieve the inflammation. Ice, contrast baths, phonophoresis, iontophoresis, or electrical stimulation can be helpful. Flexibility exercises for the wrist and long finger flexors, restriction of aggravating activities, and remedy of incorrect techniques all assist in relieving the pain. Strengthening exercises for all wrist, thumb, and finger movements—beginning with isometrics and advancing to isotonics, eccentric exercises, and concentric exercises—should progress when the inflammation is under control. Endurance, speed, and coordination all should be included in the progression of exercises.

If conservative treatment does not resolve the patient's carpal tunnel syndrome, surgical intervention for release of the transverse carpal ligament may be necessary. Gentle AROM may begin within three to seven days postoperatively with the wrist motion limited to either a neutral or functional position. Once the sutures are removed, scar-tissue management and desensitization through massage and soft-tissue mobilization can begin. The patient starts doing progressive resistive exercises in phase III, usually around three weeks postoperative. By this time, the scar across the carpal tunnel arch has sufficiently healed so stress to the tissue will not allow bowstringing of the tendons under the scar tissue to occur. Prior to this time, the patient performs AROM and isometric exercises so the scar tissue has time to properly heal. The progression of exercises follows a course similar to that discussed earlier for other wrist injuries. A more complete program following surgical release of a carpal tunnel is outlined in figure 21.60.

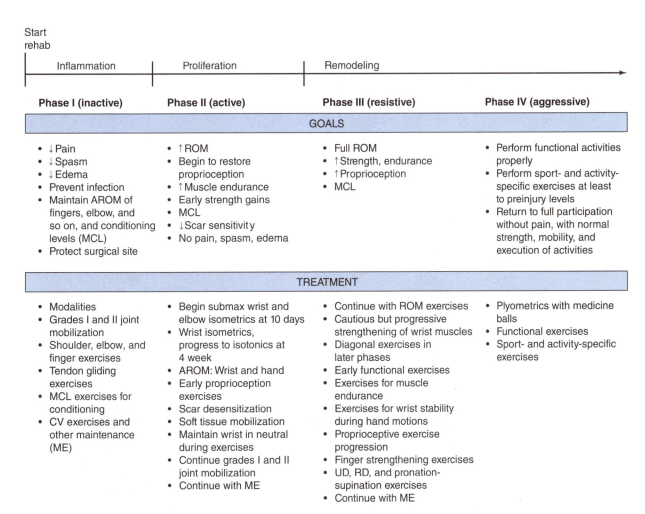

Start
rehab

Inflammation	Proliferation	Remodeling	
Phase I (inactive)	**Phase II (active)**	**Phase III (resistive)**	**Phase IV (aggressive)**

GOALS			
• ↓ Pain • ↓ Spasm • ↓ Edema • Prevent infection • Maintain AROM of fingers, elbow, and so on, and conditioning levels (MCL) • Protect surgical site	• ↑ ROM • Begin to restore proprioception • ↑ Muscle endurance • Early strength gains • MCL • ↓ Scar sensitivity • No pain, spasm, edema	• Full ROM • ↑ Strength, endurance • ↑ Proprioception • MCL	• Perform functional activities properly • Perform sport- and activity-specific exercises at least to preinjury levels • Return to full participation without pain, with normal strength, mobility, and execution of activities

TREATMENT			
• Modalities • Grades I and II joint mobilization • Shoulder, elbow, and finger exercises • Tendon gliding exercises • MCL exercises for conditioning • CV exercises and other maintenance (ME)	• Begin submax wrist and elbow isometrics at 10 days • Wrist isometrics, progress to isotonics at 4 week • AROM: Wrist and hand • Early proprioception exercises • Scar desensitization • Soft tissue mobilization • Maintain wrist in neutral during exercises • Continue grades I and II joint mobilization • Continue with ME	• Continue with ROM exercises • Cautious but progressive strengthening of wrist muscles • Diagonal exercises in later phases • Early functional exercises • Exercises for muscle endurance • Exercises for wrist stability during hand motions • Proprioceptive exercise progression • Finger strengthening exercises • UD, RD, and pronation-supination exercises • Continue with ME	• Plyometrics with medicine balls • Functional exercises • Sport- and activity-specific exercises

▶ **Figure 21.60** Rehabilitation progression for surgical release of carpal tunnel syndrome. CV = cardiovascular; AROM = active range of motion; ROM = range of motion; UD = ulnar deviation; RD = radial deviation.

De Quervain's Tenosynovitis

Long extensor tendons of the hand travel in the wrist region in compartments. There are six dorsal compartments that are identified by consecutive numbers beginning on the lateral hand (figure 21.61). De Quervain's tenosynovitis affects the first dorsal compartment and involves the abductor pollicis longus and the extensor pollicis brevis. These tendons travel together in the same synovial sheath in the first dorsal compartment and pass around the bony radial styloid process, a site of friction for the tendons. The term tenosynovitis in this case refers to both inflammatory and non-inflammatory conditions (Moore, 1997). Repetitive stress and inflammation from friction of these tendons occur with activities such as weight training and rowing or other repetitive activities where the tendons's sheath becomes irritated or damaged. The result is a thickening of the sheath, adding further irritation to the tendon within the sheath. The tendon reacts by becoming narrowed or developing nodules (Moore, 1997).

As with carpal tunnel syndrome, modalities can be useful conservative treatment for relief of the inflammation. A thumb spica splint is used to place the wrist in 15° of extension. The thumb is positioned in abduction, with the MCP joint in 10° flexion to put the affected tendons on slack. Although the splint is worn continually, it should be removed at times throughout the day for AROM exercises for the wrist and thumb. The patient performs active range of motion of the fingers throughout the day.

Once pain and edema diminish, mild strengthening and endurance activities begin. The patient is gradually weaned from the splint during this stage. Gross- and fine-pinch activities,

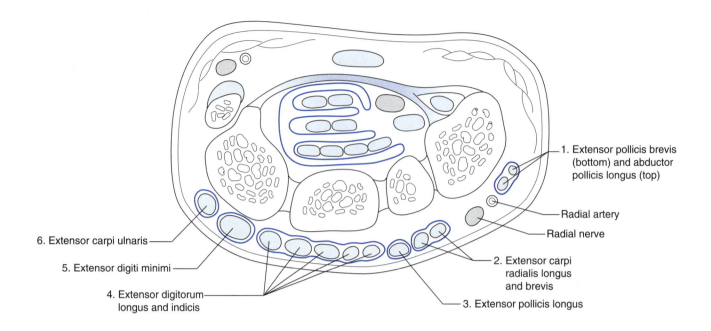

6. Extensor carpi ulnaris

5. Extensor digiti minimi

4. Extensor digitorum longus and indicis

1. Extensor pollicis brevis (bottom) and abductor pollicis longus (top)

Radial artery

Radial nerve

2. Extensor carpi radialis longus and brevis

3. Extensor pollicis longus

▶ **Figure 21.61** Cross-section showing extensor compartments in a right wrist.

■ Case Study

A 24-year-old crew team member underwent a surgical release of his right non-dominant first dorsal compartment three days ago. He has just seen the physician, who removed the surgical dressing and instructed him to begin exercising the wrist and thumb. The physician gave the patient a splint and instructed him to wear it throughout the day except during rehabilitation treatments. Some swelling and tenderness are present over the scar. The wrist has good motion, but the thumb moves 10° at the MCP joint and 30° at the IP joint. There is some tenderness to radial deviation, but the patient has full motion.

Questions for Analysis

1. What will your treatment today include?
2. What instructions will you give the patient for home treatment?
3. What precautions must be considered?
4. What kind of ROM exercises will you give him?
5. When will you start working on strength, and what will the first strengthening exercises include?
6. What functional exercises will you advance the patient to before he returns to competition?

wrist and finger exercises, strengthening activities, and endurance and coordination exercises are part of the strengthening program.

Following surgery in cases where conservative treatment failed to resolve the injury, AROM exercises begin two to three days postoperatively to promote tendon gliding and prevent loss of motion. The wrist may be in a splint for about one week, but the patient removes it frequently during the day for ROM exercises. Pain and edema are controlled with various modalities, elevation, and active motion activities. The thumb should move in all its planes through full active motion. Thumb motion exercises should also include wrist motion.

Once the sutures are removed and the scar is healed, scar-tissue desensitization and softening begins with massage. A strengthening exercise progression, which begins after 7 to 10 days, follows the same procedure as for other wrist injuries.

Long Tendon Injuries

Tendon gliding exercises have already been presented. These are important exercises to perform following any injury to the hand, because adhesions to either flexor or extensor tendons cause significant loss of motion and hand function. In addition to knowing when to apply these exercises, the rehabilitation clinician must have knowledge and understanding of the specific differences between flexor and extensor tendons so proper rehabilitation techniques to injuries affecting hand tendons occur safely and correctly.

Special Tendon Considerations

Although the biochemical structures of the hand's flexor and extensor tendons are similar, several differences govern variations in the rehabilitation of flexor and extensor tendon injuries. Some of the differences have already been mentioned and are listed in table 21.1. Among the more obvious differences is the presence of the strong pulley system for the flexor tendons versus the absence of any pulleys for the extensor tendons. The majority of the length of the flexor tendons is enclosed in sheaths, but the extensor tendons are primarily extrasynovial.

Normally, finger flexion strength is significantly greater than finger extension strength. The flexors require greater strength for activities such as grasping, propelling, and catching objects than the extensors require for opening the hand. When an injury occurs to an extensor tendon, care must be taken to prevent the stronger flexor muscles from overpowering and causing further damage to the weakened extensor tendon.

The extensor tendons are flatter and thinner than the flexor tendons; therefore overall they have less tensile strength than the larger-diameter, thicker flexor tendons. When the fingers flex into the hand, the extensor tendons undergo significant lengthening. These factors make the extensor tendon susceptible to stretch or rupture, especially when in a weakened condition following an injury.

Although the extensor tendons are not surrounded with tendon sheaths like the flexor tendons, both are at risk for adhesion formation with immobilization. Loss of extension motion can be more functionally debilitating than flexion motion loss (Stewart, 1992). Because of the intricate relationship between the extensor tendons and the intrinsic muscles, loss of mobility of the extensor tendons can have a significant impact on the function of the interossei and lumbricals and can hamper the intrinsic and extrinsic muscle balance necessary for normal hand function (von Schroeder & Botte, 2001).

Tendon ruptures and lacerations are common tendon injuries of the hand. The ruptures usually result from impact avulsions such as occur when the end of a player's finger is hit with an equipment utensil such as a baseball bat or ball like a baseball or basketball (Malanga

TABLE 21.1   Differences Between Long Flexor and Long Extensor Hand Tendons

Characteristic	Long flexor tendons	Long extensor tendons
Pulley system	Present	Absent
Sheaths	Present throughout	Not present
Strength	Greater than that of extensors	Less than for flexors
Configuration	Thick, large diameter	Thin, flatter
Tensile strength	Greater than that of extensors	Less than for flexors
Extensibility	Less than that of extensors	Greater than for extensors
Relationship with intrinsic muscles	Serve as anchor for intrinsic muscles.	Serve as distal insertion for intrinsic muscles. Long extensor tendon mobility determines the ability of the intrinsic muscles to provide their functions in hand motions.

& Chimes, 2006). Lacerations can result from cleats, contact with sharp objects hidden in the grass, and accidents in archery and many other activities. The timing of rehabilitation is crucial to a successful rehabilitation outcome. Careful application of rehabilitative techniques is important to achieving desired results. Recent advances in rehabilitation following tendon repair have improved surgical results and reduced the risk of tendon adhesions. New approaches to postoperative tendon repair include the use of early controlled motion during the first weeks after surgery rather than the more traditional three weeks or more of immobilization (Stewart, 1991). Because of the relative fragility of extensor tendons, early controlled motion was first used primarily with flexor tendon injuries in the latter half of the past century; however, more recently, early controlled motion has proven successful with extensor tendon injuries as well. At present, investigators believe that early controlled motion is advantageous for both flexor and extensor hand tendons (Buckwalter, 1996); however, there must remain a fine balance between the proper amount of motion for allowing tendon gliding, and too much motion, which causes elongation or rupture of fragile tendon tissue during the early healing phases. Careful progression and observation of treatment results is required of the rehabilitation clinician. If the clinician is in need of assistance in managing complex cases, referral to a hand specialist is an option to assure optimal patient outcomes.

Early controlled motion includes passive movement of the repaired tendon. The initial goal of early motion is to promote tendon gliding and good tendon healing simultaneously. The ultimate goal is to produce a good surgical and rehabilitative result. Areas of the hand, such as no man's land, that were previously approached with caution and misgiving because of poor surgical results can be successfully and effectively repaired using early controlled motion.

Early controlled motion is achieved using a splint that is applied approximately three days postoperatively. The splint is designed by an orthotist to limit flexion if an extensor tendon has been repaired and, likewise, to limit extension if a flexor tendon has been repaired. The angles of the splints are based on the 5 mm rule that determines the excursion of tendons during finger motion. The splints include a passive elastic force that pulls the fingers passively in the direction of the repaired tendon's pull. For example, an extensor tendon repair splint is constructed to block MCP joint flexion at 30° for the index and middle fingers, MCP joint flexion at 38° for the ring and small fingers, and extension of the IP joints with the wrist at about 40°. An elastic system, attached to the fingers, passively extends the fingers so that active motion of the tendon is not required to pull the finger into a resting position after it has flexed.

Conversely, a flexor tendon repair is placed in a dorsal splint with the wrist in about 20° of flexion, the MPs in about 40° to 50° of flexion, and the IPs in extension. An elastic system is attached to the distal finger to pull the digit passively into flexion so as not to stress the newly repaired flexor tendon.

It is necessary to take care with these splints so that the tension of the rubber band is sufficient to permit passive flexion or extension of the digits, yet not strong enough to promote a contracture with tension from the rubber band that is too much for the opposing tendon to overcome.

While the repaired flexor tendon finger is in the splint, the IP joints are passively flexed frequently throughout the day (figure 21.62). The patient performs finger extension actively to return the dorsal surface of the finger to rest on the splint's surface. Also, so that a splinted tendon-repair finger moves frequently within the splint, the patient extends the fingers against the rubber bands on the flexor surface and allows the bands to passively return the fingers to the resting position, throughout the day.

Tendon gliding and careful avoidance of adhesions are the primary concerns during the early stages of postoperative rehabilitation of tendon repairs. Extensor tendon

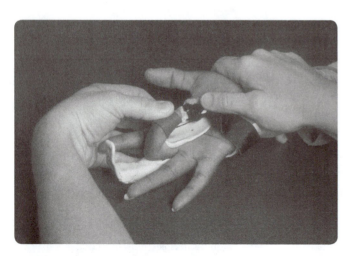

▶ **Figure 21.62** Passive range of motion in a splint.

repairs have the additional problem of possible extensor lag development. Such a condition may develop if the patient begins active extension exercises too soon or is too aggressive with them in later rehabilitation; an extensor lag occurs because the repaired sight breaks down, or dehisces, from excessive stress so the tendon elongates. The rehabilitation clinician must be aware of these potential problems and take steps to provide good care while protecting against these complications.

Observation of joint mobility is necessary for assessing the presence of these potentially debilitating conditions. You must differentiate between capsular restriction and tendon adhesions when the patient's motion is less than normal. One way to do this is to examine the digit's ROM at the individual joints and the quantity of motion with all joints involved. For example, if the patient is able to fully extend the wrist and MCP, PIP, and DIP joints of the digit one at a time when the other digit's joints are positioned in flexion, but the patient is unable to fully extend the joints all at once, the joint capsules have good mobility, but the long tendon is likely restricted.

Once sutures are removed, scar-tissue management and desensitization begins with light tapping and massage of the hypersensitive area. The patient is also instructed to perform these techniques frequently throughout the day. Since the tendons lie so close to the surface in the hand and fingers, self-massage will help reduce the risk of tendon adhesions.

When to begin strengthening exercises for repaired tendons is a point of controversy. If a tendon is adherent, strengthening exercises begin earlier than if it glides well. Strength exercises are initially light strengthening exercises, starting at four to five weeks postoperatively (Stewart, 1992). Other determining factors include the type of tendon (extensor or flexor) and the zone in which the repair is located (Evans & Burkhalter, 1986).

Long Flexor Tendons

During the initial phase of rehabilitation, goals include reducing secondary surgical inflammation signs such as swelling and pain, encouraging healing, maintaining function of unaffected joints and segments, and protecting the surgical repair site. These goals are attained, as has been presented in previous chapters, with appropriate modalities. Protection of the repair site is achieved using splints, as was discussed above. After the first two weeks, passive motion may be initiated. Passive motion places less stress on repaired tendons than active motion (Urbaniak, Cahill, & Mortenson, 1975). Passive range of motion exercises that were presented above begin in the splint. Other passive exercises for each joint with the other joints on slack reduce tendon stress. After the surgical scar is well healed, about two weeks postoperatively, gentle soft tissue mobilization to prevent adhesions may also begin. Based on surgeon approval, the patient may begin "place and hold" exercises in the first week. In these exercises, the clinician passively moves the patient's finger to end-motion flexion; the patient then attempts to hold that position actively before the fingers are passively returned to the start position. This exercise may be used as a home exercise with the patient passively positioning the finger with the uninvolved hand.

Active range of motion begins in phase II at three to six weeks for flexor tendons following surgical repair. If there is good flexion movement, in terms of quality, not necessarily quantity, gentle active motion begins. Blocking exercises that limit motion at the proximal joint while emphasizing the distal joint are used during this phase. Placing the wrist in functional extension (20° to 30°) during flexion of all the finger joints and in flexion during extension of all the finger joints, permit both tendon gliding and the desired motion at exercising joints without placing undue stress on the tendons. This wrist extension–finger flexion and wrist flexion–finger extension motion is called "wrist rocking" and is used within 1-3 weeks following a long tendon repair.

If adhesions are apparent, tendon-gliding exercises must be used in this phase. Tendon gliding must be present before the patient advances to resistive exercises. The patient's readiness is assessed based on observation skills and the techniques already described to ascertain fluidity of movement and restriction of mobility. As a rule, if the patient is unable to passively extend the wrist and MCP and IP joints simultaneously, tendon gliding is restricted and must be addressed before strengthening exercises begin.

Depending on the specific repair and the surgeon's preference, strengthening activities begin anywhere from three to six weeks after the surgery. To some extent, this timeline is determined by the zone in which the repair is performed. Zone V repairs heal quickly because of good blood supply in this zone; patients with these repairs can begin isolated AROM exercises by the third week and mild strengthening by the fifth week. Flexor digitorum superficialis tendons can withstand resistive exercises sooner than the FDP tendon.

Mild strengthening exercises include grasping exercises, prehension activities, and use of the hand in daily activities as long as the patient does not lift or hold heavy objects. Exercises that include the various power and prehensile grips are used to strengthen extrinsic and intrinsic muscles, respectively. Repetitions of the exercises begin low and increase over the next couple of weeks. Progression of resistance is slow with careful attention to the deleterious effects of too rapid a progression: pain, swelling, and stiffness. Wrist flexion-extension strength for hand stability and forearm pronation-supination strength for hand mobility are part of the program during this phase.

The therapeutic exercise program continues to progress strength, muscle endurance, and coordination through to the end of phase III, as the patient tolerates the rate of progression. The normal progression is to phase IV for functional exercises and then to the final aspect of phase IV for an activity-specific program. This entire process usually occurs within 12 weeks.

Long Extensor Tendons

The most common extensor avulsion tendon rupture is the mallet finger, in which the distal attachment of the extensor tendon is torn—usually when the digit is hit on the end and forced into sudden flexion. This rupture is frequently not surgically repaired but rather placed in a splint that maintains the DIP in 0° extension. Placing it in hyperextension risks local ischemia of the region. After six to eight weeks of continuous wear, the splint is removed and the digit is exercised with AROM, emphasizing full extension movement. Flexion exercises are active only and are gentle so that an extensor lag does not form as a result of overstretching the new connective tissue on the extensor tendon. If a lag develops, the digit must be immobilized in the splint once again for another couple of weeks before the patient resumes exercises. If the patient removes the finger splint during the initial six to eight weeks, the time count starts anew.

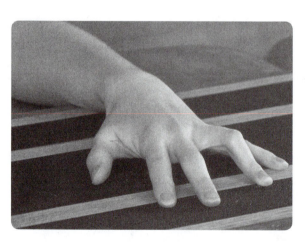

▶ **Figure 21.63** Boutonniere deformity.

Extensor tendon injuries in zones III and IV cause what is known as a boutonniere deformity (figure 21.63). The cause, a disruption of the long extensor tendon's central slip, affects other structures within the extensor mechanism. The transverse retinacular ligament and the triangular ligament stretch with repeated motion of the digit without balance of the digit's forces. This causes an extensor lag at the PIP joint. When the lag occurs, the lateral bands of the extensor tendon move anteriorly to change the angle of pull of the intrinsics and create a hyperextension force at the DIP joint.

Treatment usually includes PIP joint immobilization in extension. Surgical repair of the central slip and lateral bands is occasionally required. The splint is commonly applied for six weeks, with isometric exercises beginning at three weeks while the digit is in the splint. The finger is taken out of the splint for gentle flexion AROM exercises at three to six weeks. To prevent tendon rupture, extension should be assisted. Early protective motion using a splint similar to the early protective extension splint, mentioned previously, can be used at three weeks.

When initiated, active exercises should stress active extension, isolating joint movement by blocking the proximal joints and advancing into combined joint extension movements.

> ### ■ Case Study
>
> A 16-year-old softball catcher suffered a mallet deformity of her dominant right-hand ring finger in a game three weeks ago. It has been in a splint for the past three weeks. The doctor wants the patient to begin active exercises today and wants her to continue to wear the splint, removing it only for her treatments and to take showers. Your initial examination reveals the following ring-finger flexion/extension measurements: MCP 90°/0°, PIP 90°/0°, DIP 15°/10° from extension. When the patient simultaneously extends the wrist and finger, the DIP is lacks 20° extension. Grip strength measures 13.6 kg (30 lb) on the right and 34 kg (75 lb) on the left. Wrist extension is 4/5. Both ulnar and radial deviations have normal motion and strength. Wrist flexion is 4/5, finger flexion is 4/5, MCP extension is 4–/5, and finger abduction is 4–/5.
>
> *Questions for Analysis*
>
> **1.** What will your first treatment include?
>
> **2.** What instructions will you give the patient for home exercises?
>
> **3.** What precautions must you consider in her treatments?
>
> **4.** What determining factors will you use to decide when she should begin her strengthening exercises? Provide a rationale for your answer.
>
> **5.** List three strengthening exercises and explain why you have selected them.
>
> **6.** Identify three functional exercises and indicate your guidelines for beginning them.

Passive stretching into flexion is avoided for seven to eight weeks. Care is taken throughout the therapeutic exercise process to avoid an extensor lag and flexor contractures. The rehabilitation clinician must monitor continuously for these problems.

Mild resistive extension exercises start at 8 to 10 weeks and progress as with flexor tendon injuries.

Extensor tendon injuries in zones V, VI, and VII vary from those in the other zones because they are not impacted by the extensor mechanism. Extraneous forces and deformity are less of a problem, so motion can begin earlier.

A splint is applied for three weeks immediately after injury or repair; the wearer is then weaned from it over the next two weeks. The wrist is maintained in about 30° to 45° extension with the MCPs and IPs in 0° extension. As with other tendon injuries, extensor lag and tendon adhesions must be prevented.

Gentle active motion can begin in phase II at three weeks with blocking exercises. Wrist extension and MCP flexion-extension, with the IPs in extension, and hook exercises are good tendon-gliding exercises. At four weeks, full extension exercises for individual fingers begin, and at five or six weeks the hand exercises advance from a hook to a full fist. Resisted exercises and full stretch exercises begin in phase III after six weeks, progressing as with other hand therapeutic exercise programs.

Complex Regional Pain Syndrome

Complex regional pain syndrome (CRPS) has been known in the past as reflex sympathetic dystrophy (RSD). The name has changed to more accurately reflect the problem. This condition more commonly involves the upper extremity than the lower extremity. It can occur as the result of an injury in any part of the extremity, but the symptoms are most apparent in the hand. When it originates from a shoulder injury, it is sometimes referred to as "shoulder-hand syndrome." It can be a difficult problem to treat.

Complex regional pain syndrome is believed to occur because of a reflex sympathetic response to an injury. Characteristic complaints include pain disproportionate to the degree of injury, stiffness that is exaggerated in relation to the expected response to the injury, edema

Among the more common types of injuries to the hand are fractures, dislocations and sprains, overuse injuries including carpal tunnel syndrome, and tendon injuries. The rehabilitation clinician also infrequently encounters complex regional pain syndrome of the hand.

in the hand, cyanotic discoloration with redness around the MCP and PIP joints, coldness, and excessive sweating in the hand. The edema is initially soft and pitting, but with time, it becomes brawny and hard. X-rays can reveal bone demineralization. The skin appears tight and shiny because of immobilization and poor nutrition to the tissues. The patient tends to hold and protect the hand, moving the extremity minimally.

The most important aspect of treatment of CRPS is early intervention. It is important to stop the sympathetic reflex cycle. The physician may attempt to select from a variety of medications or try a stellate ganglion block. The rehabilitation clinician can use a variety of techniques but must keep in mind that each patient with CRPS may respond differently to these techniques.

Modalities can include a variety of methods such as various heat modalities to increase blood flow, reduce stiffness, and increase tissue extensibility for improved mobility. Heat, however, can sometimes cause increased edema. Electrical modalities, including high-voltage galvanic stimulation, transcutaneous electrical nerve stimulation, and functional electrical stimulation, can help reduce edema, decrease pain, and promote muscle activity, respectively. If tolerated, massage can be beneficial when pitting edema is present. It should be applied before exercise to maximize the effects of the exercise. Reduced edema can improve ROM and allow a greater excursion of muscle activity.

Splinting can be useful in preventing contractures. The wrist and hand are placed in a functional position with the wrist in slight extension, the MCP joints in midflexion, and the IP joints in extension. Continuous passive motion machines for the wrist and hand can also be useful in preventing contractures in the hand.

Exercises should be light and active. Exercise that is more than gentle often aggravates the patient's pain and increases stiffness. Low-repetition, active exercises are used to tolerance.

■ Case Study

An 18-year-old female gymnast is referred to you four weeks after incurring a hand injury. Your evaluation reveals pitting edema throughout the hand. The skin is red and shiny, with increased redness over the MCP and PIP joints. Active range-of-motion measurements of the fingers' extension/flexion were the following:

- Thumb MCP lacks 10° extension and can move 25° in flexion, IP lacks 15° extension and can move 20° in flexion.
- All finger MCPs lack 25° extension and can move 50° in flexion.
- Index finger PIP lacks 20° extension and can move 50° in flexion.
- Middle finger PIP lacks 30° extension and can move 50° in flexion.
- Ring finger PIP lacks 15° extension and can move 60° in flexion.
- Little finger lacks 20° extension and can move 50° in flexion.
- All DIPs are fixed at –20° extension.
- Wrist flexion is 30° and extension is 20°.

The patient reports tenderness to light touch over the entire surface of the hand. The skin is cool and clammy to the touch.

Questions for Analysis

1. What are your initial goals for this patient?
2. What will your first treatment include? Provide rationale for your treatment selections.
3. What exercises will you initiate?
4. What instructions will you give the patient?

These should include isolated joint motion and gross activities such as hook-grip, full-fist, and prehensile motions.

Passive motion and joint mobilization should not begin until the patient's pain is decreased. If pain intensifies, the exercises should return to previous levels of therapeutic activity. A gradual progression based on patient tolerance should include increased endurance exercises, strengthening, and functional activities.

SUMMARY

Just as the scapula serves to stabilize the shoulder joint, the wrist is important as a stabilizer for hand function. The hand's normal function is dependent upon a fine balance of the three elements which provide hand and finger motion: the long finger flexors, long finger extensors, and intrinsic muscle groups. If one of these is compromised from injury, the hand no longer functions as it should. The hand has various power and pinch grips that allow it to conform around and operate any object that is placed in it. Because of all the soft tissue structures and joints involved in the wrist and hand, any number of injuries may occur in this region. When injury occurs or immobilization is required, care must be taken to ensure continued gliding of tendons within the hand and fingers. Specific exercises are presented that assist in maintaining this function. Trigger point treatment, joint mobilization techniques, and progressive exercises from flexibility to functional activities were included in this chapter. Some of the more common injuries of the hand and wrist were presented along with rehabilitation programs for them.

KEY CONCEPTS AND REVIEW

1. Explain the pulley system of the fingers.

There is an elaborate pulley system on the flexor aspect of the fingers—a fibrous tunnel that extends from the metacarpal head of each digit to the insertion of the distal finger flexor tendons. These pulleys are similar to the hoops along a fishing rod, positioned to keep the fishing line in place as it travels along the pole. There are five annular pulleys and three cruciate pulleys along each finger. Disruption of the key pulleys can cause bowstringing of the flexor tendons. The key pulleys preventing bowstringing are A2 and A4. When the pulley system of any finger is disrupted, the mechanical advantage of the tendon is impaired and normal function is lost.

2. Explain why reducing edema in the hand is important.

Because the dorsal skin is loose and pliable compared to the volar skin, edema frequently accumulates in the dorsum of the hand. Pooled edema rich in proteins easily leads to contractures. Excessive swelling on the back of the hand can cause the hand arches to collapse anteriorly and adduct the thumb. Excessive swelling also requires a greater excursion of the skin for the person to flex the hand. If the skin is already stretched because of the edema, the hand's ability to move the fingers through their full motion is impaired. Fibrous tissue formation secondary to the presence of prolonged edema can cause reduced mobility and function of the hand.

3. Discuss the trimuscular system of the hand and explain why it is important to hand function.

Three muscle groups compose the trimuscular system of the hand—the extrinsic flexors, the extrinsic extensors, and the intrinsic muscles—and provide for balanced, controlled hand function. If any of these groups is unable to function normally, because of either weakness or loss of mobility, balance is lost and the hand is not able to work in its normal capacity.

4. Identify and explain the importance of the precision and power grips of the hand.

The power grips, also known as palmar grips, include the clenched fist, the cylinder grasp, the spherical grasp, and the hook. In these grasps, the thumb is positioned in opposition to the other fingers to permit a firm grasp on an object. The majority of daily hand activities involve these palmar grips. Because palmar grasping is so vital to hand function, the hand is most commonly splinted in a palmar position with the thumb in slight opposition, facing the other fingers. The precision or prehensile grips include the digital prehension grip, the lateral prehension grip, and the tip-to-tip prehension grip. These movements include fine-tuned activities such as typing, sewing, or writing. These prehensile activities occur when the thumb and finger muscles co-contract to produce an activity requiring precision.

5. Explain the difference between static and dynamic splints.

Overall, the aim of splints is either to prevent damage and maintain balance or to improve balance. Static splints restrict motion to support and protect the hand. Dynamic splints are used to increase motion of the hand. Splints are based on a three-point pressure system whereby two points of application are on one side of the hand, wrist, or forearm and the other point of application is on the opposite side.

6. Identify what motion is increased with carpal radial glide joint mobilizations.

A carpal radial glide improves ulnar flexion of the wrist.

7. Explain the force application sequence for improving long finger flexor or extensor motion.

The basic application sequence is the same for flexors and extensors. If the distal phalanx has limited flexion motion, the proximal joint is stabilized as the distal joint (DIP) is moved into flexion; then the PIP joint is moved into flexion as the MCP joint is stabilized while the DIP's flexed position is maintained. The MCP joint is then moved into flexion as the wrist is stabilized and the IP joints are kept in their flexion positions. Finally, the wrist is gradually moved into flexion. The stretch should be performed in both elbow flexion and elbow extension, and the forces applied gradually until the patient feels a stretch in the forearm.

8. Explain how the intrinsic stretches differ from the extrinsic stretches.

Because the lumbricals and interossei flex the MCP joints and extend the IP joints, the stretch is applied in the opposite direction of their function or direction of motion. The IP joints are maintained in a flexed position while a stretch is applied to increase MCP extension. The wrist should be stabilized in neutral during this activity to prevent extrinsic muscle influences on the stretch.

9. Discuss the difference in gliding exercises for the flexor profundus and superficialis tendons.

Three exercises for flexor tendon gliding include (1) keeping the MCP extended and flexing the IPs to enhance gliding between the two longer finger flexor tendons, (2) forming a fist with the IP and MCP joints in flexion to produce gliding of the profundus tendon within its sheath, and (3) positioning the MCP and PIP joints in flexion and extending the DIP joints. Flexor pollicis longus gliding exercises are performed in a similar manner by moving the IP and MCP joints through a full range of flexion and extension. These exercises are initially performed with the wrist in neutral, but as the patient progresses, the wrist should be moved into flexion with finger flexion and into extension with finger extension. A gliding exercise for the EDC is performed by moving the hand from a hook to a fist formation. The MCP joint is moved from flexion to extension while the IP joints are kept in flexion to eliminate the intrinsic muscles. If the patient has difficulty maintaining flexion of the IP joints during this activity, he or she can grasp a drinking straw or pencil in the fingers while moving the MCP joints. Wrist flexion and extension should also be added to the exercise when the patient is able to perform the exercise with the wrist in neutral.

10. Present the differences between long flexor and long extensor tendons.

Among the more obvious differences is the presence of the strong pulley system for the flexor tendons versus the absence of any pulleys for the extensor tendons. The majority of the length of the flexor tendons is enclosed in sheaths, but the extensor tendons are primarily extrasynovial. Finger flexion strength is significantly greater than finger extension strength. The extensor tendons are flatter and thinner than the flexor tendons; for this reason they have less overall tensile strength than the larger-diameter, thicker flexor tendons. When the fingers close into the hand, the extensor tendons undergo significant lengthening. The flexor tendons are surrounded with tendon sheaths and risk loss of tendon glide and formation of adhesions with immobilization. Loss of extensor motion can be more functionally debilitating than flexion motion loss.

11. Explain what procedures may used to eliminate an extensor lag of a distal phalanx.

A gliding exercise for the EDC can be used to reduce adhesions that may be causing an extensor lag and is described in the answer to question 9. If the extensor lag occurs at either IP joint, it is the result of adhesions within the extensor mechanism and can include both intrinsic and extrinsic structures, the interossei, lumbricals, and EDC. To isolate the intrinsic muscles and facilitate their movement into IP extension, the MCP is stabilized in flexion. When the patient is able to perform this exercise completely, the MCP joint is moved into extension. In the most difficult position for this exercise, the hand is flat on a table and the proximal phalanx stabilized, and the patient attempts to extend the distal phalanx off the table.

12. Identify the early signs of CRPS.

Early complaints include pain disproportionate to the degree of injury, stiffness that is exaggerated in relation to the expected response to the injury, pitting edema in the hand, cyanotic discoloration with redness around the MCP and PIP joints, coldness, and excessive sweating in the hand.

CRITICAL THINKING QUESTIONS

1. Why do you suspect that tendinopathy and overuse injuries are common in the hand and wrist? On the basis of the anatomy and the causes of overuse injuries, what sports would you suspect would have a higher-than-average incidence of overuse injuries of the hand and wrist, and why? Given this, what efforts should a clinician make to prevent these injuries in these sports?

2. If a patient suffers a scaphoid fracture, how long would you expect him or her to complain of pain? If the wrist pain continues for several weeks beyond your expectations, what would you suspect is the reason? What would you do in this situation?

3. In the opening scenario, what test did Deanna use to determine that adhesions were forming between the flexor digitorum superficialis and profundus? What specific techniques would you use to reduce these adhesions? What exercises and home program would you give Danny to help create more mobility between the tissues? How would the adhesions interfere with hand function by affecting the intrinsic muscles?

4. If a mallet finger injury begins to lose active extension after having started rehabilitation exercises, what would you suspect is the cause? How would you remedy the situation to restore active extension?

LAB ACTIVITIES

1. Locate the trigger points for the following muscles on your lab partner:
   a. Wrist extensors
   b. Wrist flexors
   c. Long finger flexors
   d. Long finger extensors
   e. Pollicis adductor

   Where were your partner's most sensitive trigger points? Perform a spray-and-stretch technique on each of them and provide your partner with a home exercise for each tender trigger point.

2. Perform the following joint mobilizations on your lab partner and identify what restrictions are best treated with each mobilization:
   a. Distal radioulnar joint
      - Distraction
      - Dorsal glide of radius
      - Ventral glide of radius
   b. Radiocarpal joint
      - Distraction
      - AP glides
      - PA glides
      - Lateral glides
   c. MCP and IP joints
      - Distraction
      - Rotation
      - AP glides
      - PA glides

3. Examine your partner's finger motion using all of the tendon-gliding exercises. Identify which structure each motion is assessing.

4. Instruct your partner in the flexor tendon gliding exercises and have him perform 10 of each. Instruct your partner in the extensor tendon gliding exercises and have him perform 10 of each. What are the differences in how each of the exercises feel as they are being performed?

5. Demonstrate how you would apply a stretch to the lumbricals. What are the key factors you need to consider in positioning for this stretch? Why?

6. List two exercises you would give a patient to strengthen the finger extensors. Identify the purpose of each exercise and when in the rehabilitation program they could be added.

7. List two strengthening exercises for the finger flexors and identify a progression for each of them. What would be your criteria for advancing a patient from one level of an exercise to another?

8. List three strengthening exercises for the intrinsic muscles of the hand and identify the substitution patterns you need to watch for during the patient's performance of each exercise.

9. List three sport-specific exercises you would have a softball left fielder perform before she returns to full participation. She is recovering from a second degree PIP sprain of the third finger. Explain why you have selected these criteria; what is your rationale?

CHAPTER 22

Foot, Ankle, and Leg

OBJECTIVES

After completing this chapter, you should be able to do the following:

1. Discuss normal foot mechanics in ambulation.
2. Identify two foot deformities and discuss their impact on injury.
3. Describe the primary structures of a shoe.
4. List the important factors in shoe considerations for a pes cavus foot.
5. Outline key factors in an orthotic examination.
6. Explain one joint mobilization technique for improving ankle dorsiflexion.
7. List three stretching exercises for the ankle and extremity, including one that is not mentioned in the text.
8. Identify three strengthening exercises for the ankle and extremity.
9. Explain three agility exercises.
10. Describe three functional exercises for the lower extremity.
11. Provide an example of a therapeutic exercise program progression for an ankle sprain.

▶ After two months of persistent heel pain, cross-country runner Hannah felt she could no longer hope the pain would go away on its own and decided to seek care for it. After Benjamin Charles performed his evaluation, he informed Hannah that the problem was plantar fasciitis.

Benjamin concluded from his examination that Hannah had a few problems that were contributing to the plantar fasciitis. Her excessive pronation would have to be corrected with orthotics; the tight hip rotators were causing altered knee alignment that contributed to increased torsional stress on the plantar fascia and would have to be stretched and corrected, as would the tightness in the iliotibial band and Achilles. The muscle imbalance between Hannah's quads and hamstrings was another possible contributing factor that would be resolved with strengthening activities. Benjamin also explained to Hannah that not only were her shoes too worn to wear running, they also did not have the proper supports her foot needs. Although there were several problems, Benjamin was optimistic that they were all correctable with proper rehabilitation and changes in footwear so that Hannah would be able to resume her normal running program.

One who walks in another's tracks leaves no footprints.

PROVERB

The foot and ankle are complex structures that impact the entire extremity, because they form the base that moves the rest of the body from one location to another. Injuries in these areas can affect the efficiency and effectiveness of body propulsion, the primary function of the lower extremities.

Injuries to the foot and ankle are common. A key responsibility of the rehabilitation clinician is to use his or her skill and knowledge of the foot and ankle to provide the patient with an appropriate and efficient recovery program that will permit a full return to full participation.

The foot, ankle, and leg, like the hand, wrist, and forearm, are complex structures composed of many bones, joints, and muscles. There are 26 bones and 33 joints in the foot, ankle, and lower leg, along with several intrinsic and extrinsic muscles. These structures are divided into segments within the foot, ankle, and leg; each segment forms integral relationships with the other segments within the area as well as with more proximal segments such as the knee, hip, and back. There is evidence to demonstrate the direct impact that foot position and mechanics have on the knee (Klingman, Liaos, & Hardin, 1997; Powers, Maffucci, & Hampton, 1995; Tiberio, 1987; Withrow, Huston, Wojtys, & Ashton-Miller, 2006) and other more distal segments (Dierks, Manal, Hamill, & Davis, 2008; Massie & Spiker, 1990). It is important, then, that you have knowledge of the structure and function of the distal lower extremity so that the rehabilitation program you establish will return the patient to full function without applying additional stresses to more proximal segments.

This chapter reviews the basic structure of the lower leg, ankle, and foot as it pertains to the normal function of those segments as well as the more proximal segments. We will pay specific attention to concepts that directly relate to rehabilitation following injury. The second half of the chapter addresses specific injuries most commonly seen in the leg, ankle, and foot, along with case studies.

GENERAL REHABILITATION CONSIDERATIONS

Before discussing the foot and ankle, we need to define some of the more common terms used to describe these body segments. These terms are often misused, so establishing definitions helps to ensure common understanding.

Terminology

One possible reason for confusion about terms relating to the foot may be that the foot is not in the same plane as the rest of the body: the foot is at roughly a 90° angle to the lower extremity. Another possible reason is that the foot seldom moves in cardinal, or straight, planes; many of the joints are multiplanar. As a point of reference, ankle and foot motions in the cardinal planes (frontal, sagittal, and transverse) and multiplanes are defined here.

Pronation is a triplanar rotational motion that occurs in the subtalar and transverse tarsal joints and is the combination of dorsiflexion, abduction, and eversion in non-weight bearing. This motion is sometimes incorrectly referred to as eversion. Dorsiflexion is the sagittal plane movement in which the ankle joint angle is decreased as the dorsal foot is moved upward toward the anterior surface of the extremity; in most other joints, this motion is flexion. Abduction is the transverse plane movement of the foot in which the lateral foot moves away from the midline. Eversion is a frontal plane movement in which the plantar foot rotates outward so that the lateral border is lifted upward.

Supination is a triplanar rotational motion that includes plantar flexion, adduction, and inversion in non-weight bearing. This combined motion is sometimes incorrectly referred to as inversion. Plantar flexion is the sagittal plane motion in which the foot moves downward and the dorsal foot moves away from the anterior surface of the extremity; in most other joints, this motion is extension. Adduction is the transverse plane movement of the foot in which the medial foot moves toward the midline. Inversion is a frontal plane movement in which the plantar foot rotates inward so that the medial border is lifted upward.

The isolated, straight-plane motions of adduction-abduction, inversion-eversion, and dorsiflexion-plantar flexion do not occur in functional ankle activities (figure 22.1). In open chain motion, pronation and supination occur as the calcaneus moves on the talus. However, in closed chain activities, the calcaneus is anchored by body weight so pronation and supination

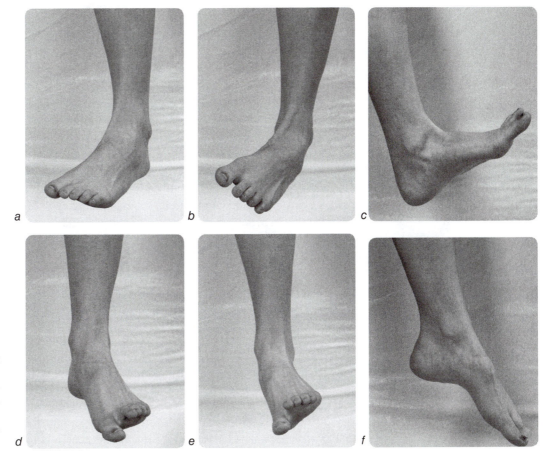

▶ **Figure 22.1** Foot planar motions: *(a)* adduction, *(b)* inversion, *(c)* dorsiflexion, *(d)* abduction, *(e)* eversion, *(f)* plantar flexion.

occur because the talus moves on the calcaneus. Therefore, in weight bearing pronation, the talus moves medially (adducts) and plantarflexes on the calcaneus, and the calcaneus everts, pulling the cuboid and navicular into abduction and eversion. The opposite occurs in weight bearing supination: the talus abducts and dorsiflexes while the calcaneus inverts to pull the cuboid and navicular into adduction and inversion. Along with pronation and supination in the closed kinetic chain, associated motions take place further up the chain. With pronation, the tibia medially rotates, the knee flexes, and the hip flexes and medially rotates. Conversely, with supination, the tibia laterally rotates; the knee extends; and the hip extends, abducts, and laterally rotates. Because supination and pronation occur in the subtalar joint, the subtalar joint is instrumental in foot motion and key in control of the other joints. For example, if the subtalar joint in the closed kinetic chain is in pronation, the tibia will medially rotate, the knee will flex, and the hip will medially rotate and flex. If the subtalar joint stays in pronation when it should be supinating during ambulation, injuries can result in either the foot or the more proximal body segments when those segments are forced to be in an abnormal position during the gait cycle because of the subtalar pronation. These injuries are discussed later in this chapter.

Extremity, Foot, and Ankle Joints

Specifics of gait analysis are discussed in chapter 12. Reviewing that chapter may help you understand some additional concepts presented here. The first foot structure to hit the ground in walking is the calcaneus. It, along with the talus, forms the subtalar joint; and the talus along with the tibia and fibula forms the talocrural joint. Normal function of these two joints permits us to land the foot on the ground and adapt to variations in ground topography while maintaining a steady gait. The talocrural joint moves primarily in dorsiflexion and plantar flexion. The subtalar joint is responsible for inversion and eversion. Pronation and its component motions loosen foot and ankle joints to allow the foot to be a mobile adapter to accommodate for uneven surfaces. Supination moves the joint into congruent positions to allow the foot to become more rigid, provide for power transfer, and permit appropriate force application needed for propulsion in ambulation. As mentioned in chapter 12, these motions must occur at specific times within the cycle for gait to be normal.

The talocrural joint is a mortise joint, with a convex talar dome in contact with a concave tibial mortise. The lateral malleolus is posterior and distal in its alignment with the medial malleolus. This arrangement allows more inversion than eversion to occur in the subtalar joint, and also causes plantar flexion to occur more in a posterolateral direction and dorsiflexion to occur more in an anteromedial direction (Hicks, 1953). As the ankle goes into plantar flexion, the talus moves anteriorly so that the posterior, narrower aspect of the talus sits in the mortise joint (Hicks, 1953). This can contribute to instability of the ankle in plantar flexion and is one reason that women wearing high-heeled shoes, and individuals landing from a jump with the foot in plantar flexion, are especially susceptible to ankle sprains. Conversely, the most stable close-packed position for the talus is with the ankle in dorsiflexion when the wider anterior talus is wedged up into the mortise joint (Lundberg et al., 1989). During dorsiflexion, the fibula glides superiorly and rotates laterally; and in plantar flexion, it moves inferiorly and rotates medially (Lundberg et al., 1989). If these fibular motions are not present, full ankle dorsiflexion and plantar flexion cannot occur. Distal to the talocrural and subtalar joints are the midtarsal joints, a combination of the talonavicular and calcaneocuboid articulations. Their position is determined by the subtalar joint position; the midtarsal joints become locked during supination and unlocked during pronation. Movements of the midtarsal joints closely follow movements of the subtalar and talocrural joints. During supination, the navicular and cuboid bones move medially and inferiorly, and they move laterally and superiorly during pronation.

The tarsometatarsal joints and their adjacent bony segments are divided into five rays. The first ray includes the first metatarsal, the medial cuneiform, and their shared joint. Although the first ray has triplanar motion, its movements are generally referred to as plantar flexion and dorsiflexion. Movement of the first ray occurs equally in plantar flexion and dorsiflexion, with each movement equivalent to about a thumb's width of motion. The second ray includes the joint and its bones, the second metatarsal, and the middle cuneiform; the third ray includes the third metatarsal and the lateral cuneiform bones and their joint; the fourth ray is the fourth metatarsal alone; and the fifth ray is the fifth metatarsal alone.

Metatarsophalangeal (MTP) joints permit active flexion-extension, abduction-adduction, and the accessory motions of rotation and dorsal-plantar glides. The interphalangeal (IP) joints, which are hinge joints, permit active flexion and extension with accessory rotation and dorsal-plantar glides. The first MTP joint must have about 65° of hyperextension for normal heel off and toe off during gait.

Muscle Function

There are 12 extrinsic muscles and 11 intrinsic muscles of the extremity and foot. The extrinsic muscles are divided into four compartments or groups: anterior, lateral, posterior superficial, and posterior deep (figure 22.2). The anterior compartment muscles cross the ankle joint anteriorly and provide for dorsiflexion, and lateral and posterior compartment muscles cross the ankle posteriorly and are plantar flexors (figure 22.3). The muscles that have the greatest mechanical advantage to produce inversion and eversion because of their positions are the anterior and posterior tibialis medially and the peroneals laterally.

The posterior leg has a superficial and a deep compartment; the two compartments are separated by deep fascia, the intermuscular septum. The superficial muscle group includes the large plantar flexors, the soleus, gastrocnemius, and plantaris. The deep posterior muscles lie closer to the tibia and include the tibialis posterior, flexor hallucis longus, and flexor digitorum longus.

The intrinsic foot muscles are completely contained within the foot itself. Their purpose is to provide stability to the toes, tarsometatarsal joints, and midfoot while extrinsic muscles move the joints. The intrinsic muscles keep the toes on the ground until toe-off during gait and convert the toes to rigid beams for propulsion in gait. These muscles weaken with ankle injuries and must be rehabilitated along with the extrinsic muscles. In a foot that is unstable or hypermobile such as one that has excessive pronation, the intrinsic muscles are required to work far beyond normal expectations. Excessive sweating of the foot and consequent foot odor are evidence of intrinsic muscle overactivity.

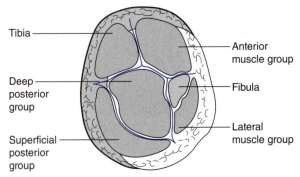

▶ **Figure 22.2** Cross section of the lower-leg muscle compartments.

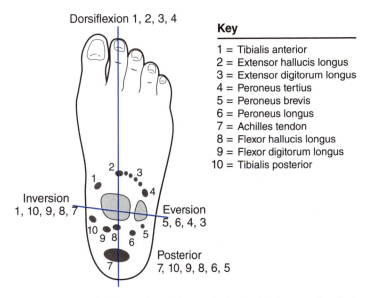

Key

1 = Tibialis anterior
2 = Extensor hallucis longus
3 = Extensor digitorum longus
4 = Peroneus tertius
5 = Peroneus brevis
6 = Peroneus longus
7 = Achilles tendon
8 = Flexor hallucis longus
9 = Flexor digitorum longus
10 = Tibialis posterior

▶ **Figure 22.3** Ankle motions. The vertical axis divides muscles that provide inversion and eversion, whereas the horizontal axis divides dorsiflexors from plantar flexors. Muscles are listed in order of their mechanical advantage for motion.

Foot Arches

There are three arches of the foot, the medial and lateral longitudinal arches and the transverse arch. These arches result from the architecture of the tarsals and their arrangement with each other, the ligaments, and the supporting muscles. The primary tensile supporting structure for the longitudinal arches is the plantar fascia; the peroneus longus supports the transverse arch. These arches protect the underlying blood vessels and nerves and provide an efficient system of support for the body's weight. If the arches are unable to maintain a normal configuration, an imbalance occurs, and these abnormal stresses applied to the foot can cause injury.

Normal foot mechanics in ambulation depends on the correct timing and coordination of the motions of many joints and the extrinsic and intrinsic muscles of the lower leg and foot. Subtalar motion and position also influence movement of the lower extremity.

The normal alignment of the longitudinal arches is determined through use of the Feiss line test. In non-weight bearing, a line is drawn from apex of the medial malleolus to the plantar aspect of the first metatarsophalangeal joint. In weight bearing, the navicular tubercle should lie on the line or near it. If the tubercle falls two-thirds the distance to the floor or more, it is pathological (Starkey, Brown, & Ryan, 2010).

Subtalar Neutral Position

Because the subtalar joint significantly influences the entire lower extremity, the rehabilitation clinician must know what normal subtalar motions and positions are to be able to assess and treat an abnormal subtalar joint.

Subtalar neutral is the position in which the talus is equally palpable from its medial or its lateral aspect within the subtalar joint. It is at this point that the talus and navicular are most congruent and the alignment of the subtalar bones is optimal (Donatelli et al., 1999). Subtalar neutral should be assessed in both weight bearing and non-weight bearing (Lattanza, Gray, & Kantner, 1988). In non-weight bearing, the patient lies prone with the opposite extremity flexed at the hip and knee and the hip in abduction and lateral rotation to stabilize the pelvis. If the patient is unable to hold this figure-4 position because of pain or inflexibility, a rolled towel secured under the proximal hip of the examined extremity may be used to stabilize the pelvis. With the patient's foot and ankle to be examined over the edge of the table, the clinician places the thumb and index finger on the medial and lateral aspects of the talus. Using his or her thumb, the clinician locates the medial aspect, in a depression slightly inferior and anterior to the medial malleolus and just proximal to the navicular. He or she locates the lateral aspect, anterior to the lateral malleolus, using the index finger (figure 22.4). As the talus is palpated with one hand, the other hand grasps the fourth and fifth metatarsal heads and rotates the forefoot in pronation and supination. When the forefoot supinates, the talus inverts so that its lateral border can be palpated; and when the forefoot pronates, the talus everts so that its medial border can be palpated. The foot is rocked back and forth in the two directions with progressively smaller arcs until the talus is centrally positioned and cannot be palpated on either the medial or the lateral aspect or is palpated equally on each side. The foot is then moved into dorsiflexion by the fingers on the fourth and fifth metatarsal heads to lock the rearfoot in place. If subtalar neutral is palpated in weight bearing, the clinician palpates the medial and lateral talus while patient elevates and lowers the longitudinal arch while keeping the toes and heel on the floor; this motion is performed until the clinician determines that the subtalar joint is in neutral.

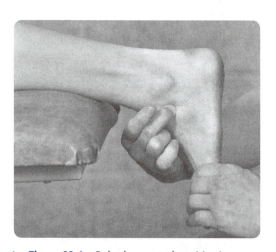

▶ **Figure 22.4** Subtalar neutral positioning.

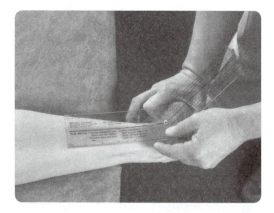

▶ **Figure 22.5** Measurement of subtalar range of motion. Lines bisecting the calcaneus and leg are used to define subtalar or rearfoot inversion and eversion range of motion.

Once subtalar neutral is identified, range of motion of the rearfoot based on calcaneal position is assessed. Normal rearfoot motion is 30° with one-third in eversion and two-thirds in inversion. A perpendicular line bisecting the posterior calcaneus and a line bisecting the posterior tibia are used as reference points. The calcaneus is passively moved into eversion and inversion, and measurements are taken at the end range of each position (figure 22.5).

COMMON STRUCTURAL DEFORMITIES

Although the deformities we will consider are not injuries but structural deviations, they can often lead to injuries. Athletic activity imposes greater-than-normal forces on the foot and thereby exaggerates the impact of a deformity. The rehabilitation clinician must be familiar with these deformities and their impact on the patient to provide appropriate treatment programs.

Pes Cavus

In pes cavus, the foot has an abnormally high longitudinal arch (figure 22.6). The navicular tubercle is above Feiss' line in both weight bearing and non-weight bearing. This is a rigid foot with limited stress-absorption abilities. The foot does not pronate as it should to absorb impact stresses, so the forces are transmitted up the extremity. Pes cavus feet can lead to fallen transverse arches, hammertoes or claw toes, corns, stress fractures, and other overuse injuries.

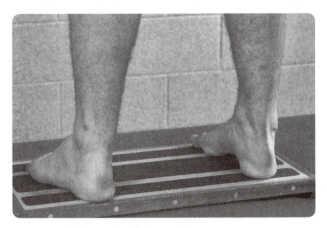

▶ **Figure 22.6** Pes cavus.

Pes Planus

In pes planus, the foot has an abnormally low longitudinal arch (figure 22.7). A rigid pes planus has the navicular tubercle below Feiss' line in both weight bearing and non-weight bearing. The more common flexible pes planus foot, however, has the navicular tubercle below Feiss' line in weight bearing but on or near Feiss' line during non-weight bearing. Either rigid or flexible pes planus can lead to injuries. During weight bearing, the foot is unable to form a rigid lever for efficiency of propulsion and remains in a pronated position when it should be supinated. This imposes additional stresses on more proximal extremity segments. During heel-off and just before toe-off, the extremity and hip are laterally rotating, a motion in conflict with pronation, so torque forces become exaggerated. This is especially true at the knee, particularly at the patellofemoral joint. The condition also places torsion on the plantar fascia and Achilles tendon, because the foot should be supinating but it is pronating. Related terms for pes planus are pronated foot, flatfoot, or pancake arch.

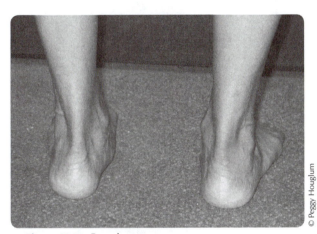

▶ **Figure 22.7** Pes planus.

Hallux Valgus

This condition is also known as a bunion. Hallux valgus is present when the first MTP joint is greater than 10° in valgus with the first toe pointed laterally toward the other toes (figure 22.8). The condition is most commonly seen in a pes planus foot. With the foot in pronation, the force at toe-off is transmitted though the medial aspect of the first ray. This increases medial joint stress at the MTP. The first ray deviates medially, and the phalanx deviates laterally.

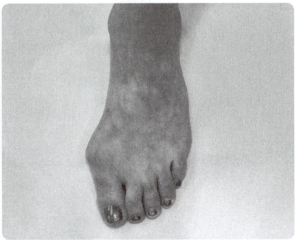

▶ **Figure 22.8** Hallux valgus.

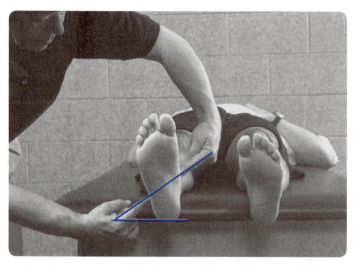

▶ **Figure 22.9** Measuring tibial torsion: Tibial torsion is the angle formed between the line through the malleoli and the plane of the tabletop when the femoral condyles on the table and the patella are facing the ceiling.

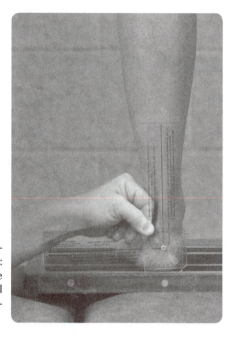

▶ **Figure 22.10** Measuring tibial varum: The line bisecting the leg should be vertical if normal tibial alignment is present.

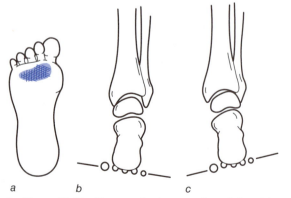

a   *b*   *c*

▶ **Figure 22.11** Varus and valgus rearfoot deformities: *(a)* callus pattern for compensated subtalar varus, *(b)* varus, *(c)* valgus.

Tibial Torsion

Tibial torsion is present when the tibia is rotated on its long axis. Normally, the midline of the patella is in line with the first- and second-toe web space. In tibial torsion, the foot is rotated laterally to the patella's midline. One can quantify this with the patient supine and the medial and lateral femoral condyles in the transverse plane and the patella facing the ceiling. The rehabilitation clinician measures the angle between the plane of the table and the line between the medial and lateral malleolus (figure 22.9). Normal value is 15°, with a normal range of 2° to 3° in either direction.

Patients with tibial torsion experience increased stress to the knee. Tibial torsion may be either excessive lateral rotation or medial rotation of the tibia on the talus, but most of the time the pathology is a lateral rotation. Because the tibia is laterally rotated relative to the patella, an increased torque is applied to the patellar tendon. Lateral rotation of the tibia may also be related to excessive pronation, lateral thigh tightness, and altered patellofemoral alignment.

Tibial Varum

Tibial varum is present when the distal tibia is closer to the midline than the proximal tibia. This is measured with the patient in standing. With the patient's feet shoulder-width apart, the rehabilitation clinician places the goniometer's stationary arm on the floor and the movable arm along a posterior line bisecting the distal tibia (figure 22.10). The movable arm should be vertical.

Tibial varum is usually accompanied by genu varum and coxa valgus. These deformities place exaggerated stresses on the knee, Achilles, and hip.

Rearfoot Varus and Valgus

The rearfoot is composed of the talus and calcaneus, and its pathological alignments are referred to as subtalar varus and subtalar valgus. Rearfoot alignment is determined by the position of the calcaneus relative to that of the leg. Rearfoot varus (figure 22.11b) is present when the calcaneus is inverted relative to the posterior bisection of the distal leg. Rearfoot valgus is present when the calcaneus is everted relative to the distal leg (figure 22.11c). The source of rearfoot varus is difficult to ascertain: it may be within the talus, the calcaneus, or both.

Rearfoot valgus is examined in both a relaxed standing position and a subtalar neutral position. Ideally, the results should be the same in the two positions. In a foot that has compensated for the deformity, the calcaneus is perpendicular to the floor in neutral and everted in resting standing. If a foot is uncompensated, the calcaneus remains in eversion in both positions, but the amount of eversion is less in subtalar neutral.

With rearfoot varus, the foot remains partially or fully pronated until heel-off during the weight-bearing phase of gait. More pronation than normal must occur to get the inverted heel to the ground. Once the foot is off the ground, the calcaneus rapidly supinates to catch up to the position it should be in at heel strike. This causes a medial heel whip immediately after toe-off, which you can see as you observe the patient posteriorly during gait.

Because the rearfoot does not supinate when it should in the gait cycle, hypermobility of the forefoot occurs, and the first ray is unable to become fully stabilized for propulsion. This causes transferal of increased shear and loading forces to the second metatarsal head, and sometimes to the third and fourth metatarsal heads. This stress transfer, in turn, causes calluses predominantly over the second metatarsal head and secondarily over the third and fourth metatarsal heads (figure 22.11a). The rearfoot position is important to recognize because it is a key determining factor for the rest of the foot and has a significant impact on knee and hip motion.

Forefoot Varus and Valgus

A forefoot varus is an inversion deformity of the midtarsal joint. It is identified through comparison of the plane of the five metatarsal heads with the perpendicular line bisecting the calcaneus. For this examination, the patient lies prone and the rearfoot is passively placed and maintained in subtalar neutral by the clinician. The forefoot is loaded on the fifth metatarsal head, and the foot is passively moved into dorsiflexion. In the normal forefoot, the line in the plane of the metatarsals and the line bisecting the calcaneus are parallel to each other (figure 22.12b). In forefoot varus, the medial forefoot is higher than the lateral side (inverted) (figure 22.12a). A related condition is first-ray dorsiflexion.

In compensated forefoot varus, the subtalar joint is pronated to allow the medial toes to touch the ground in weight bearing. This calcaneal pronation persists at a time when the joint should be starting to supinate. The rearfoot is unable to supinate in time for heel-off and toe-off because the forefoot is still in contact with the ground, forcing the rearfoot to remain pronated. A slight heel-whip may be seen at heel-off, but it usually is ineffective because the deformity in the forefoot causing the compensation is still in contact with the ground.

With the rearfoot in pronation throughout propulsion, the body's weight is distributed more medially than normal, and the midtarsal joint becomes hypermobile. This causes the first ray to become unstable and incapable of carrying its propulsive load. The weight and force are then transferred to the second and third metatarsal heads, where callus formations appear as a result of this increased shear and force stress. Because the body's weight is more medially distributed than normal, the foot abducts and a callus forms on the medial hallux from shearing stresses as the body moves over this aspect of the hallux (figure 22.12d).

If the forefoot varus is uncompensated, the individual stays on the lateral aspect of the foot and is unable to pronate as much as he or she should normally. The forefoot varus does not permit the rearfoot to pronate in relaxed standing, so the calcaneus may appear either erect or slightly inverted. Callus formation in this case occurs over the lateral aspect of the foot and over the fifth metatarsal head, because rotation occurs off the fifth metatarsal head and weight bearing is primarily over the lateral foot (figure 22.12e). The rotation is secondary to the rearfoot's failure to go through a full excursion of supination, thereby limiting extremity lateral rotation; the body attempts to abduct the foot so the tibia can tilt to evert the foot to get the propulsive forces delivered from the medial foot, as close to the first metatarsal as possible.

Forefoot valgus is the opposite condition. The metatarsal line of the heads line is higher on the lateral side than on the medial side (everted) when observed from a subtalar neutral (figure 22.12c). A related condition is first-ray plantar flexion. If the first ray is rigid with little available mobility during ambulation, the first ray will hit the ground too early and the peroneus longus will assist by moving the weight more medially in preparation to transfer weight to the other foot. In a very rigid first ray, the fifth ray's ability to get to the ground is limited because the foot supinates too early in the mid-weight-bearing phase. With the

Pes cavus and planus, hallux valgus, tibial torsion, tibial varum, and rearfoot and forefoot varus and valgus are among the common structural deformities of the foot and leg.

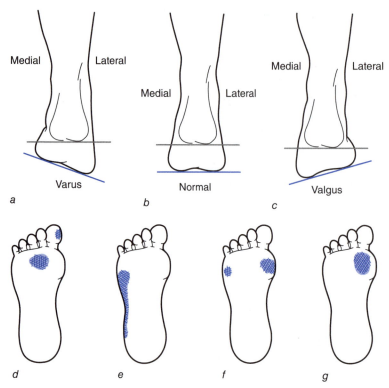

▶ **Figure 22.12** Forefoot alignment—varus and valgus deformities: *(a)* forefoot varus alignment relative to rearfoot, *(b)* normal forefoot and rearfoot alignment, *(c)* forefoot valgus, *(d)* callus pattern for compensated forefoot varus, *(e)* uncompensated forefoot varus, *(f)* callus pattern for compensated forefoot valgus with a rigid first ray, *(g)* compensated forefoot valgus and rearfoot varus with a flexible first ray.

forefoot in extreme valgus because of the rigid first ray, forefoot inversion on the rearfoot is severely limited. The rearfoot then attempts to compensate by supinating during midstance. This causes the fifth ray to hit the ground suddenly and undergo increased loading before heel-off. In turn, this causes the lateral foot to become unstable; to compensate, the rearfoot moves into pronation at heel-off. The pronation imposes increased shearing forces on the forefoot. Because of the increased shearing forces and the increased time the first ray spends on the ground, there is usually a large callus buildup over the medial first metatarsal head. There is also a callus over the fifth metatarsal head because of the increased friction (figure 22.12f).

On the other hand, if the first ray is mobile, the rearfoot will pronate normally, and no problems should become evident because motion will occur close to normal. However, a large callus forms over the first metatarsal head because of the prolonged contact of the first ray with the ground in its plantar-flexed position (figure 22.12g).

ORTHOTIC TREATMENT FOR FOOT DEFORMITIES

Normal foot mechanics during ambulation include pronation immediately after heel strike and continuing through 25% of the stance phase. During midstance, the rearfoot moves to a neutral position with the calcaneus erect and all the metatarsal heads in contact with the ground. From that point until toe-off, the rearfoot continues its progression toward supination in preparation for converting the foot from a mobile adapter to a rigid lever for propulsion. If the patient's foot does not function in this manner, increased stresses occur to segments within the foot or elsewhere in the extremity. The purpose of foot orthotics is to make the abnormal foot function in a manner closer to that of a normal foot, thereby reducing the abnormal stresses imposed on the foot and extremity. Although not all patients have correct foot alignment and function, many patients who have poor alignment do not have symptoms of pathology. For these asymptomatic patients, orthotics may not be indicated. Foot orthotics are used to correct or support symptomatic rearfoot and/or forefoot malalignments to reduce joint stresses and improve the patient's mechanical efficiency.

Premade Orthotics

Several types of orthotics are available. The type a patient uses depends on that person's specific needs. There are premade orthotics and custom-made orthotics. Premade orthotics, the off-the-shelf variety, are less expensive than custom orthotics and in some situations may meet the patient's needs adquately. These include items such as heel cushions that assist in shock absorption at heel strike and can also alter heel position if varus or valgus wedges are attached to them. A variety of pads and inserts can assist in reducing stress on specific areas of the foot. These items include metatarsal pads, arch cookies, heel pads, and other supportive devices. Premade arch supports can help support pes planus feet and feet with excessive pronation. Full-length insoles can replace the regular inner liners in shoes and further add to shock absorption.

Custom Orthotics

Custom orthotics are built to satisfy the individual's specific needs, either to absorb stress or to correct alignment. Some of the more common types of orthotics are briefly described next.

Three Types of Orthotics

Custom orthotics are either accommodating or functional and are of three basic types: rigid, semirigid, and soft. The more rigid the orthotic, the more exact the fit must be in order for the device to be effective. Soft orthotics, often made of soft polyethylene foam, are used for cavus or rigid feet to provide stress absorption. They are known as accommodative orthotics; they do not so much correct mechanics as accommodate and attempt to relieve symptoms by reducing stresses without altering the foot position.

Most athletic orthotics are of the semirigid variety. They contain a rigid shell, usually made of acrylic plastic, thermoplastic polymer, or carbon with a soft covering. These are functional orthotics but may also have accommodating aspects. Their purpose is to change the position of the rearfoot or forefoot (or both) to improve alignment, reduce shear stresses, reduce

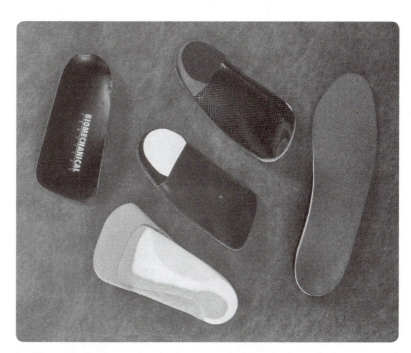

▶ **Figure 22.13** Custom orthotics are made from a variety of substances and are either corrective (rigid or semirigid) or accommodative.

shock, and stabilize and support the foot joints. The shell has either intrinsic or extrinsic posts to correct the deformities. These posts are in the rearfoot or forefoot or both, depending on the correction needed. Extrinsic posts can be made from a variety of materials with varying densities, including ethyl vinyl acetate (EVA), polyethylene, crepe rubber, and polyplastic (figure 22.13).

Specialty orthotic devices can also be constructed for specific performance needs of the patient. Special orthotics can be designed to accommodate for the stresses applied in aerobics by providing more control for loading on the anterior foot. Cycling orthotics must be lightweight and must provide control for the anterior foot, which bears the weight during cycling. A low-profile orthotic can be designed to conform to special footwear such as ski boots, soccer shoes, track racing shoes, and dress shoes.

Orthotic devices for the correction of foot deformities are either premade or custom made. The orthotist assesses a number of patient characteristics to design an orthotic device that fits that patient.

Three Impression Methods

The three most common methods of taking foot impressions are to use plaster casts, foam boxes, or wax. With the plaster cast method, the patient is prone or supine as he or she would be if you were finding subtalar neutral. A traditional plaster cast using a double layer of plaster splint material is applied to the plantar foot. While the plaster dries, the foot is passively maintained in a subtalar neutral position. This method is the most useful when the orthotic is to be functional and more accuracy is required. Although the procedure can be messy, the molds are durable after they dry and can be taken or sent through the mail to an orthotics lab without being damaged.

With the foam-box method, the patient's foot is pushed into a box of foam material much like that used by florists. The foot is actively maintained as close to subtalar neutral as possible. This is not an accurate method to use for flexible feet because it can be difficult for a patient with a flexible foot to maintain or find subtalar neutral. A foam box impression is most commonly used for an accommodative orthotic device, or devices that do not require a precision fit.

■ Orthotic Evaluation

In addition to impression molds of the feet, assessment of various patient characteristics is necessary for an orthotic to be designed to fit accurately. Information that the orthotist needs includes the following items, with the examination presented in the process often followed, moving from non-weight bearing elements to weight bearing observations:

1. The patient's gender, age, weight, and height. Some materials have limited ability to withstand stresses beyond specific weights, so the patient's size determines the material used for the orthotic.

2. The patient's shoe size and style. Different orthotics are required for different shoe styles and sizes. For example, a sprinter's practice shoe will permit insertion of a different orthotic than the sprinter's race shoe.

3. The patient's occupation and activity level. Different orthotics are designed to withstand different stresses, so the orthotist will use information about the patient's activities and sport participation to decide on the specific construction of the orthotic. For example, a soccer player will use a low-profile device that fits in the shoe and absorbs shock during quick running starts and stops.

4. Special problems. Surgery, neuromuscular deficiencies, and other medical abnormalities can alter the body's ability to tolerate changes. For example, an open reduction and internal fixation (ORIF) of the ankle may cause soft-tissue adhesions that affect the patient's ability to tolerate a great deal of change rearfoot position.

5. Chief complaints. These are what you are trying to relieve by providing the orthotic. The reason the patient is being fitted for orthotics.

6. Subtalar range of motion. Subtalar mobility is determined using the method described earlier with the subtalar joint in neutral. Normal subtalar motion is 30° with a 2 to 1 ratio of inversion to eversion. On the form, this amount of motion is indicated as "average." If the total motion is less than 15°, limited rearfoot mobility that can cause forefoot accommodation or changes is present. If eversion motion is less than 5° with the rearfoot in a neutral position, the rearfoot has restricted mobility. If the rearfoot is restricted and there is no forefoot accommodation, a rigid foot may be present. Subtalar mobility of greater than 30° indicates an unstable foot that is in pronation more than it should be. The axis measurement needs to be indicated only if there is an extreme and obvious abnormality. Normal movement of the talus and calcaneus in the subtalar joint is a 1:1 ratio. The axis is considered high if there is more movement of the talus in its transverse plane than movement of the calcaneus in the frontal plane. If, however, there is more calcaneus movement than talus movement, the axis is low.

7. Midtarsal (global) range of motion. This is a subjective assessment of gross midfoot mobility. With the rearfoot locked in subtalar neutral, the forefoot is supinated and pronated. Normal mobility should allow full but not excessive motion. This is a difficult motion to assess until you have performed the maneuver many times to obtain an impression of what is loose, what is normal, and what is restricted.

8. Midtarsal (integrity) range of motion. In the non-weight bearing position, the rearfoot is positioned with the calcaneus is supination, moving it against the cuboid to lock it in position. In this position, the clinician attempts

The wax method uses warm wax sheets that are molded to the plantar surface of the foot. The rearfoot is maintained in subtalar neutral as the wax cools and hardens. This method is not used if the impressions are to be sent elsewhere, because it is not easy to transport them and the wax melts in heat and cracks in cold weather. The method can be used if the orthotics are constructed in-house.

Regardless of the method used to obtain an impression of the feet, the form acquired is then transformed into a solid replica of the feet. The person's custom-made orthotics are created to fit the solid replica, thereby correcting the individual's foot pathology.

The firmer the orthotic, the less error is tolerated in the fit. Rigid orthotics require the most precision in creating the foot's impression. The softer accommodative orthotics tolerate a larger margin of error in the impressions from which they are made. If a semirigid orthotic is desired, an accurate impression should be used.

to move the navicular and then the cuboid. If the midtarsal is stable, there will be no motion of the cuboid and little or no motion of the navicular. If the midtarsal is unstable, there will be motion available in the navicular and may also be some in the cuboid.

9. First ray range of motion. This is the amount of flexibility of the first ray. As mentioned previously, the first ray should move about one thumb's width each in plantar flexion and in dorsiflexion. If it moves well in one direction but not the other, it is semirigid. If it is limited in both directions, it is rigid.

10. First metatarsal ray position. With the rearfoot aligned in neutral, the forefoot toes should be in the same plane. If the first ray sits above the forefoot plane, the first ray is dorsiflexed; if it sits below the plane, it is plantar flexed.

11. Hallux dorsiflexion (open chain). The hallux should have 60° to 65° of dorsiflexion for normal ambulation. In a rearfoot neutral position, the #1 MP joint should have the ability to be dorsiflexed passively to at least 65°. Patients with a lower value may have problems such as sesamoiditis, plantar fasciitis, or tendinitis. An adjustment in the orthotic may be necessary if the patient's motion is less than 60°.

12. Ankle dorsiflexion. This is measured in subtalar neutral with passive pressure applied to the ankle into dorsiflexion. Normal dorsiflexion needed for ambulation is 10¼. If the ankle does not have this motion, pronation may occur to compensate and allow the patient the mobility needed. An adjustment in the orthotic to relieve stress on the Achilles and plantar fascia may be necessary if the patient lacks full ankle dorsiflexion.

13. Toe positions (non-weight bearing). These are good indicators of rearfoot deformities. For example, hallux valgus (HAV) may be an indication of excessive pronation, and hammertoes or claw toes (contracted) are an indication

of pes cavus. A Morton's toe may necessitate a change in the orthotic to redistribute weight from the second toe onto the great toe. Normal toes should be straight.

14. Location of corns and calluses. This is important in that corns and calluses are indicators of accommodating or non-accommodating forefoot and rearfoot deformities.

15. Foot appearance: semi-weight bearing arch. The arches are examined with the patient in a sitting position. The feet are resting on the ground. The determination of high, medium, or low arch is based on Feiss' line and the relative position of the navicular.

16. Foot appearance: weight bearing arch. The same examination of arches is made with the patient in full weight bearing. Changes in arch height from resting to weight bearing may indicate accommodations in the foot.

17. Hallux dorsiflexion (closed chain). With the patient in full weight bearing, the MP joint of the great toe is passively dorsiflexed. Care must be taken to have movement occur at the MP joint and not the IP joint.

18. Tibial varum. If this value is beyond 4¼, it is abnormal. Tibial varum also adds to foot-deformity stresses and can increase pronation.

19. Knee positions. Knee positions can contribute significantly to foot deformities. For example, genu valgus can be associated with pronation.

20. Calcaneal stance position. In full weight bearing, the calcaneus position relative to the leg is observed in three different positions, subtalar neutral, relaxed standing, and in a half-squat position. These positions are useful in determining whether an accommodation is occurring.

21. Short leg. If leg length differences are greater than 0.5 inches, the differences between the two should be recorded. Differences greater than one-half inch can promote supination in the short leg and pronation in the long leg.

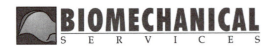

BIOMECHANICAL
S E R V I C E S

ACCOUNT NO.: _____

P.O. NO.: _____

PRACTITIONERS NAME: _____ DATE: _____

ADDRESS: _____

TELEPHONE: _ _ _ _ _ _ _ _ _ _   ALTERNATE TELEPHONE: _ _ _ _ _ _ _ _ _ _

Last Name   First Name

PATIENT NAME: _

SEX: M/F   WEIGHT: _____   HEIGHT: _____   PREVIOUS ORTHOTIC THERAPY: Y/N   DEVICE NO.: _____

SHOE SIZE: _____   SHOE STYLE: _____   SHOES ENCLOSED Y/N

OCCUPATION/ACTIVITY LEVEL: _____

SPECIAL PROBLEMS (NEUROMOTER, STRUCTURAL, SURGICAL) _____

CHIEF COMPLAINT: _____
_____
_____

OTHER COMPLAINTS: (KNEE/HIP/BACK)
_____
_____

RANGE OF MOTION:

★Subtalar:
LEFT   ❏Average   ❏<15°
        ❏<5° Eversion from Neutral
        ❏Axis_____
RIGHT   ❏Average   ❏<15°
        ❏<5° Eversion from Neutral
        ❏Axis_____

OMidtarsal (Global):
LEFT   ❏Within Normal Limits
        ❏Restricted   ❏Loose
RIGHT   ❏Within Normal Limits
        ❏Restricted   ❏Loose

OMidtarsal (Integrity):
LEFT   ❏Stable   ❏Unstable
RIGHT   ❏Stable   ❏Unstable

OFirst Ray:
LEFT   ❏Flexible   ❏Semi-Rigid
        ❏Rigid
RIGHT   ❏Flexible   ❏Semi-Rigid
        ❏Rigid

OFirst Metatarsal Ray Position:
LEFT   ❏Normal   ❏Plantarflexed
        ❏Dorsiflexed
RIGHT   ❏Normal   ❏Plantarflexed
        ❏Dorsiflexed

OHallux Dorsiflexion (Open Chain):
LEFT   ❏>65°   ❏>45°   ❏>25°
RIGHT   ❏>65°   ❏>45°   ❏>25°

OAnkle Dorsiflexion:
LEFT   ❏≥10°   ❏≤6°   ❏≤0
        ❏≤9°   ❏≤3°
RIGHT   ❏≥10°   ❏≤6°   ❏≤0
        ❏≤9°   ❏≤3°

OTOE POSITIONS Non-weight Bearing:
LEFT   ❏Contracted   ❏Straight
        ❏HAV   ❏Morton's
RIGHT   ❏Contracted   ❏Straight
        ❏HAV   ❏Morton's

OLOCATION OF CORNS/CALLUSES:

R   L

FOOT APPEARANCE:

✦ Semi-weight Bearing Arch
LEFT   ❏High   ❏Med   ❏Low
RIGHT   ❏High   ❏Med   ❏Low

✦ Weight Bearing Arch
LEFT   ❏High   ❏Med   ❏Low
RIGHT   ❏High   ❏Med   ❏Low

✦Hallux Dorsiflexion (Closed Chain):
Left   ❏>9°   ❏>4°   ❏None
Right   ❏>9°   ❏>4°   ❏None

✦TIBIAL VARUM:
Degrees Left_____   Right_____

✦KNEE POSITIONS:
Left   ❏Genu Varum   ❏Straight
        ❏Genu Valgum
Right   ❏Genu Varum   ❏Straight
        ❏Genu Valgum

CALCANEAL STANCE POSITION:

✦Neutral Subtalar
LEFT   ❏Inverted ❏Rectus ❏Everted
RIGHT   ❏Inverted ❏Rectus ❏Everted

✦Resting/Relaxed
LEFT   ❏Inverted ❏Rectus ❏Everted
RIGHT   ❏Inverted ❏Rectus ❏Everted

✦Half Squat
LEFT   ❏Inverted ❏Rectus ❏Everted
RIGHT   ❏Inverted ❏Rectus ❏Everted

SHORT LEG (If Any):
LEFT/RIGHT_____MM/INCHES

DIAGNOSIS:_____
_____
_____
_____
_____

1050 Central Ave., Suite D - Brea, CA 92821 - Phone 714.990.5932 or 800.942.2272 Fax 714.990.4060 - biomechanical.com

Patient Evaluation Form (2000) courtesy of Biomechanical Services, 1050 Central Ave., Suite D, Brea, CA 92821.

DETERMINING PROPER FOOTWEAR FOR PATIENTS

A frequently asked question regarding footwear is "What's the best shoe?" There is not a single best shoe. The best shoe is the one that meets the individual's specific needs. There are many athletic shoes to choose from and new models are released every six months; the major shoe companies produce the equivalent range of shoe models from economy to luxury cars. It is more important for the rehabilitation clinician to be aware of general functional concepts and purposes of shoe components than it is to have knowledge of specific models. Once a clinician determines the patient's shoe-construction needs, he or she can direct the patient in selecting a shoe which possesses the qualities that match the patient's needs.

Shoes have many functions, such as protecting the foot's skin and other soft-tissue structures, providing traction for improved propulsion, reducing shock impact during propulsion activities, increasing foot stability, and accommodating or correcting foot deformities. Companies emphasize style characteristics and fashion trends to increase the popularity of shoes. Ultimately, a shoe should be chosen on the basis of its structure, function, and fit, not its color, style, or name.

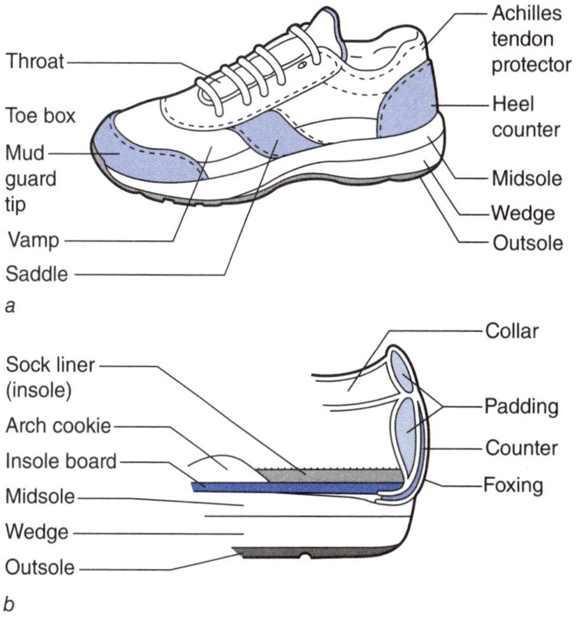

Shoe Structure

All shoes have the same basic structure consisting of an upper and a lower section. The upper section of an athletic shoe includes the vamp, toe box, saddle, collar, insole board, sock liner, and heel counter. The lower section includes the outsole, wedge, and midsole (figure 22.14). The vamp, which covers the toes and forefoot, includes the toe box. Running shoes whose vamp is made of nylon or another fabric usually have a mudguard around the rim of the toe box. The toe box can vary in width and height from one style and company to another. The toe box functions to retain the shape of the shoe's forefoot and to provide room for the toes. The saddle, the midsection of the shoe along the longitudinal arch, is usually reinforced by the company's logo or other structure to provide support to the midfoot. The heel counter is an important stabilizer for the rearfoot. A foxing, an additional piece in many athletic shoes, further reinforces the rearfoot and assists in maintaining the counter's shape. The medial aspect of the counter is sometimes extended forward to resist pronation. The collar is the top rim of the shoe's heel, often padded to reduce friction on the Achilles. Sometimes it is angled inward slightly to provide a snugger fit around the ankle. The board of the insole lies between the upper and lower segments of the shoe and serves as the attachment for these two segments. A sock liner on top of the insole board assists in shock absorption and friction reduction. The sock liner may be either glued into the shoe or inserted into it for easy removal or replacement.

The outsole is the portion of the lower segment of the shoe that is in contact with the ground. This is composed of a durable material and has a variety of designs of ripples, waves, and nubs, depending on the type of surface for which the shoe is designed. The midsole and wedge are made of a variety of substances including EVA, gas-filled or gel-filled chambers, and polyurethane. These sections provide shock attenuation, stability, and control. They can include wedges to provide stability, varying densities to reduce pronation, and special materials to reduce impact stresses.

The shoe's last is an important component of a shoe. It is the insole board, is made of a firm substance, and determines the shoe's shape, size, style, and fit. The most common types of last are the straight last and the curved last (figure 22.15). The straight last, which can be

Figure 22.14 Shoe anatomy: *(a)* upper section, *(b)* lower section.

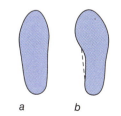

Figure 22.15 Shoe last: *(a)* straight, *(b)* curved. Last determines the shoe's shape, size, style, and fit.

bisected lengthwise into two equal parts, offers the foot the most medial support and is recommended for pronators. Curved lasts are flared inward from heel to toe to varying degrees. These lasts provide the least amount of medial support and should be avoided by persons who excessively pronate. A curve-lasted shoe is generally more flexible than a straight-lasted shoe and is used by persons with a rigid foot. Construction of the shoe around the last involves attaching the outsole and midsole to the bottom of the last and attaching the heel counter, toe box, and upper section of the shoe to the top of the last.

A last is either a board last, a slip last, or a combination last. You can easily see the last by removing the sock liner. A board last is made of a cardboard or cardboard like material that provides for a stiff sole and thus adds to the stability to the foot. A slip-lasted shoe looks similar to a moccasin inside the shoe where the last and upper section meet, with the upper section stitched along its bottom to the last. The slip-lasted shoe is appropriate for a more rigid foot and offers more flexibility than a board-lasted shoe. A combination last has a board-lasted rearfoot and a slip-lasted forefoot. This type of last is designed to offer rearfoot stability and forefoot flexibility, as well as ease of shoe bend to reduce stresses on the plantar fascia and Achilles during heel-off and toe-off.

Shoe Wear

An examination of the patient's worn shoes can give clues to foot deformities, helping the rehabilitation clinician guide the patient toward the most appropriate shoe. If the heel counter and medial heel are collapsed to the medial side of the shoe, the patient excessively pronates. A medial wedge, or increased density of the medial wedge or midsole, along with a strong heel counter will provide increased stability. This patient should use a board-lasted shoe.

If the lateral heel counter of the worn shoe is moved laterally, the patient has a rigid foot and needs a shoe with a slip last, a lot of cushion but no medial wedge, and a firm heel counter.

If the patient's hallux has a blackened toenail, the toe box may not be deep enough. If the hallux is wearing through the upper section of the shoe, the patient may have a rigid first ray and require increased shock absorption in the forefoot. The forefoot of the shoe for this type of foot needs to be rigid to protect the first ray.

Although shoe wear is a good indicator of deformities, a shoe that has noticeable wear is one that should be replaced. The life of a shoe depends on the patient, the frequency of participation, and the surfaces on which the patient plays the sport. Footwear varies greatly in longevity. It is important, however, that the shoe be replaced once a wear pattern is seen. A worn shoe changes the mechanics and stresses applied to the foot and can magnify any structural deformity.

Injury History

A profile of the patient's injury history also aids in determining the correct shoe for that person. For example, if the patient has a history of Achilles tendinopathy, the cause may be either excessive pronation or tightness in the Achilles. This patient should find a shoe that has good heel-counter stability, a straight board or combination last, good forefoot flexibility, and a higher-than-normal elevation in the wedge to relieve Achilles stress.

If the patient has a history of knee pain, excessive pronation may be the cause. A board-lasted shoe with good rearfoot control and a firm heel counter is appropriate for this patient. Plantar fasciitis is also related to excessive pronation, so a similar shoe would be appropriate for a patient with a history of plantar fasciitis.

As a general rule, a foot requires a complimentary shoe. In other words, if the foot is rigid, a flexible shoe is recommended. An individual with this type of foot will achieve a better fit with a curved last, sewn to the shoe, and cushion. On the other hand, if the foot is flexible, a more rigid shoe is more appropriate. This individual will be most comfortable in a straight, board last with good rearfoot control and a firm heel counter.

Proper Shoe Fit

Once the specific needs of the patient have been determined, the shoe must be fit properly. Shoe size is most easily determined using the Brannock measuring device found in shoe stores (figure 22.16). This devices determines the width and length of the shoe. The foot is measured in the device with the individual standing, bearing weight on the foot. A good heel fit is critical for any shoe. The shoe should fit snugly to provide adequate support for the rearfoot. There should be approximately one thumb's width between the end of the longest toe and the end of the shoe. The toe box should have adequate depth and width for the forefoot and toes. The bend in the vamp should coincide with the bend of the patient's forefoot. A good heel counter should feel firm and have little give when it is squeezed. The vamp should bend easily when you grasp the heel and try to bend the shoe by applying pressure with the index finger of your other hand. If a shoe has a board last, it should be difficult to wring the shoe and produce much motion when stabilizing the heel and rotating the vamp.

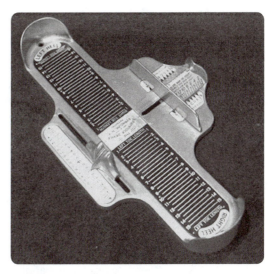

▶ **Figure 22.16** Brannock measuring device.

Shoes should be evaluated to make sure that the heel counter is perpendicular to the sole, the sole is parallel to the floor, and the last is the same on the right as on the left shoe. It is also important to ascertain that there are no abnormalities in stitching, construction, or angle from one shoe to the other. Because there is no quality control in shoe manufacturing, errors in production can occur. A construction error can cause an injury or aggravate any structural deformity.

Patients should try on shoes in the store, wearing socks of the same type and thickness as those they will use with the shoes. An individual should be able to give shoes a good trial in the store on a treadmill or track or be able to run outside before purchasing them. It is best to try on shoes in the later part of the day when foot volume is greater than in the morning. Because foot size may vary from right to left, it is advisable to try on both shoes, properly laced. It is a good idea to try on a variety of shoes and compare comfort and fit. The patient should be sure to ask about the store's return policy. The store should stand behind the product and permit exchanges if someone who has tried a shoe at home finds that it does not meet specific needs or is uncomfortable.

Sock Selection

One additional word on foot protection regards socks. The science involved in sock design and construction has improved significantly in the past several years. Athletic socks today are not the ones made several years ago, but are designed to cushion the foot, draw moisture away from the foot, and reduce friction from the foot and its skin. Some new sock materials are antibacterial, protect against odors, and cushion the foot. A variety of fibers are used in socks including common items like cotton, wool, acrylic, nylon, polyester, olefin, spandex, elastic, and some less common substances such as silk, cashmere, linen, and mohair. Proper socks are important, especially in distance events where blisters may result if the individual is not wearing a proper sock. Cotton socks do not reduce friction or moisture, but acrylic socks have the advantage of doing both. Wool absorbs moisture, but it shrinks and can be very warm. Spandex helps the socks stay up on the leg and maintain their shape. Elastic also does, but elastic fibers break down more quickly than spandex. In short, there are many different substances from which socks are made, and many socks have combinations of materials in them to provide optimal protection and support for the foot. Recommendations to patients for sock selections are important as are the recommendations clinicians make regarding shoe selections.

Shoe Types

Because different activities place different stresses on the foot, requirements for an athletic shoe differ among sports. There are as many types of shoes as there are sports. It is not advisable for a patient to wear a shoe intended for use in one sport for a second sport. The shoe is not designed to meet the demands of another sport.

There are many different compositions from which shoes are made for both the bottom and the upper portion of the shoe. Some of the newer materials have the advantage of breathability and durability for the uppers while the new lower construction materials have improved durability with reduced weight. Some shoes, however, are made to satisfy the "fashion" preference of the buyer, not the needs of the foot. It is best to obtain athletic shoes from athletic shoe stores or only after having performed adequate "homework" to know what to seek in a shoe.

Tennis Shoes

Tennis involves sudden stops and changes in direction and many lateral movements, so safe tennis participation requires good medial and lateral support to protect the lateral ligaments and peroneal muscles. Because most tennis is played on a variety of outdoor surfaces, the outsole should be durable; the material should be able to adapt to differing playing surfaces and allow some sliding on the court. A toe guard or reinforcement over the medial toes will prolong the life of the shoe and protect it against toe drag on the serve. In a shoe appropriate for tennis, the heel and toe are at about the same level, whereas a running shoe has an elevated heel to reduce stress on the Achilles. Because placing the foot in a plantar-flexed position makes the ankle susceptible to inversion sprains and because tennis involves lateral movements, a tennis shoe's sole is flat.

Running Shoes

In addition to the elevated heel, a running shoe should be flexible so that the foot does not have to work excessively to bend the shoe during heel-off. The shoe should have good cushion in the rear and forefoot yet provide stability to the heel. Many distance running shoes have used the idea from walking shoes of a rocker bottom to improve muscle efficiency during running. Race running shoes are designed for speed and not durability. They lack the support training shoes possess, and their lifespan is usually only a few races before they must be replaced. Not all competitive runners are able to use racing shoes since they do not provide necessary support some individuals require in order to run.

Aerobics Shoes

Aerobics shoes should have good forefoot cushioning, and many have additional cushioning in the sock liner. A reinforced toe box supports the forefoot primarily during forefoot-impact activities. The forefoot should have good flexibility to allow the foot to bend easily during aerobic activities; in many shoes this flexibility comes from flex bars cut into the sole. There should be good rearfoot stability with a good heel counter for adequate ankle support during medial and lateral activities. Stability is necessary for the multidirectional movements in aerobics. Stability straps in the midfoot region can provide medial-lateral stability in the midsole and the upper section. In some shoes, a mid-height upper section provides added medial-lateral support without interfering with plantar flexion-dorsiflexion. Aerobic shoes come in leather and synthetic materials; synthetic material is usually lighter and does not absorb as much moisture as the leather.

Volleyball Shoes

Volleyball shoes must meet the demands of sudden stops, starts, jumps, and lateral moves. The shoe should not have an elevation to the heel but should have a durable outsole, good medial-lateral stability, and sufficient traction; it should be lightweight and flexible enough not to contribute to jumping fatigue. Stabilizing straps and availability in mid tops and high tops add medial-lateral support as well as forefoot stability. A gum-rubber sole increases traction and durability. Additional leather guards prolong the life of the shoe by protecting the toes from excessive wear during drag.

Basketball Shoes

Basketball shoes must provide cushion during jumps, stability during quick stops and starts and changes in direction, and ease of foot-bend during running. Mid- and high-top shoes provide medial-lateral support, as do the forefoot support straps and sole design. A good heel counter also provides stability. Flex joints in the sole of the forefoot facilitate bending, and the midsole is composed of a shock-absorbing substance such as EVA. Basketball court surfaces are rough on the outsole, so a basketball shoe should have a stitched rubber outsole with a reinforced toe region.

Soccer Shoes

A soccer shoe should have a flexible sole to permit ease in dorsiflexion-plantar flexion motion of the ankle. The cleats should be placed in areas that do not promote undue pressure on or irritation of the foot; rearfoot cleat placement should be around the perimeter to avoid heel irritation. Cleats vary according to the surface the patient plays on. Short cleats are appropriate for hard turf, whereas long cleats are suitable for softer surfaces such as wet grass. Some soccer shoes are now made in mid top and high top styles for additional ankle protection.

Walking Shoes

Walking shoes have many of the same characteristics as running shoes. The heel is slightly raised, but not as much as in a running shoe, and a firm heel counter provides for rearfoot and impact stability. The forefoot is usually more flexible. The outer sole has a rocker bottom (angled rather than squared heel and curved upward at the toes) to provide efficiency and to lessen energy requirements during heel strike and rolling from heel-off to toe-off. The shank portion of the midsole is usually stiffer in a walking shoe to provide for better medial-lateral stability. Selection of a walking shoe should be based on the type of walking the individual performs. Olympic walkers require flexibility for economy of movement; off-trail walkers need stability and traction for uneven surfaces; and power and fitness walkers need stability and cushioning.

Mountaineering Shoes

Requirements for mountaineering shoes vary according to the specific activity involved. Hiking, climbing, and high-altitude climbing each place different demands on the feet and will require different shoes.

Hiking is one of the most popular mountaineering sports. A hiking shoe should provide stability and should have a good heel counter and midsole for medial-lateral support. Hiking shoes should be waterproof or water resistant and should have a very durable outsole. The outsole should have good traction for uneven and rough terrain. The upper section height should be mid to high for rough terrain and mid to low for easy terrain. A hiking shoe needs to be lightweight and comfortable; it should not have pressure points and should not need to be broken in.

Cross-Training Shoes

Cross-training shoes are designed to meet the needs of individuals involved in multiple activities. The goal is to meet all the needs of all the people all the time. The problem is that these shoes usually do not meet any specific need most of the time. There are various styles of shoes in this category. A person who wants a cross-training shoe should select the shoe that meets the demands of the activity he or she participates in most of the time.

To help a patient select a shoe, the rehabilitation clinician must understand shoe structure, identify the wear pattern on the patient's current shoes, ascertain the patient's injury history, understand how a shoe should fit, and consider the purpose for which the shoe will be used.

Lacing Patterns

Some shoes, especially running shoes, have multiple eyelets that the wearer can select from when lacing the shoe. This greater number of eyelets allows for use of a variety of lacing patterns to meet specific needs. Alternative lacing patterns can add to the support the shoe provides or accommodate for some deformities. A person who has a narrow foot should use the eyelets farthest from the tongue of the shoe, which will pull the sides of the shoe more closely together (figure 22.17a). People with wide feet should use the eyelets closest to the tongue (figure 22.17b).

Women often have the problem of a wide forefoot and a narrower heel than is accounted for in the construction of a shoe. They can accommodate for this by using two laces, one for the lower eyelets and the other for the higher eyelets, and tying the upper lace more tightly to support the heel (figure 22.17c).

Patients with high arches should avoid lacing a shoe in the traditional crisscross pattern but instead should use a straight-across pattern (figure 22.17d).

People with toe problems can obtain some relief by using the laces to lift up the forefoot of the shoe. As the shoe is tied, the lace that goes through the eyelet nearest the problem toe is brought directly to an eyelet at the top of the shoe. Pulling on this lace lifts up part of the forefoot (figure 22.17e).

Heel blisters are often caused by friction of the shoe over the heel. The wearer can decrease the friction by securing the heel more firmly in the shoe using a loop-through technique at the top of the shoe as seen in figure 22.17f. The lace should be pulled tighter at the top of the shoe than at the bottom.

A bump on the top of the foot can be painful with regular-lacing-pattern pressure. To relieve pressure on the top of the foot, don't cross the laces; instead, keep the laces on the same side of the shoe and skip the eyelet at the painful level (figure 22.17g).

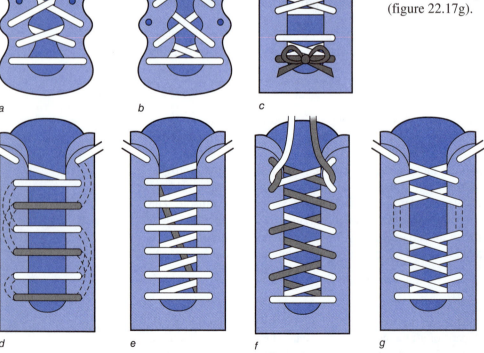

▶ **Figure 22.17** Shoe-lacing patterns for *(a)* narrow feet, *(b)* wide feet, *(c)* wide forefoot and narrow heel (using two laces), *(d)* high arches, *(e)* toe problems, *(f)* heel blisters, *(g)* dorsal foot bump.

Reprinted, by permission, from C. Frey, April 1998, "Common shoe lacing patterns." Retrieved August 28, 2000 from the World Wide Web: www.wcsportsmed.com/lacing.htm. Copyright 1998 by Carol Frey, MD.

SOFT-TISSUE MOBILIZATION

As with the upper extremity, pain and referred pain in the lower extremity can come from several sources. Sciatica is a common pain-referral source in the lower extremity, with symptoms extending anywhere from the back to the toes. Before the rehabilitation clinician treats a pain locale, he or she must identify the source. If the pain is myofascially based, soft-tissue mobilization techniques can be effective in relieving the pain. The areas discussed here are common myofascial pain-referral patterns from the muscles of the extremity and foot. These pain-referral patterns and the treatments presented are based on the work of Travell and Simons (1992). The following sections deal with identification of trigger points and pain-referral patterns for the muscles and then present trigger point release and ice/spray-and-stretch techniques. Remember that ice/spray-and-stretch or spray-and-stretch applications are repeated several times. The procedure is to apply the ice or cold spray during the passive stretch and then to perform active shortening and repeated stretches. After the ice/spray-and-stretch application, the patient should actively move the muscle through its full range of motion several times.

Superficial Intrinsic Foot Muscles

These muscles include the extensor digitorum brevis, extensor hallucis brevis, abductor hallucis, flexor digitorum brevis, and abductor digiti minimi. The muscle generally refers pain over the muscle site with a small degree of radiation that remains locally in the foot.

■ Trigger Point Releases for the Foot and Ankle Muscles

Extensor Digitorum Brevis

Referral Pattern: Over the muscle belly with less pain toward the toes (figure 22.18a).

Location of Trigger Point: Usually in the midbelly of the muscle.

Patient Position for Palpation: Supine.

Muscle Position for Palpation: Relaxed in a comfortable position.

Ischemic Treatment: Direct compression over the trigger point in the muscle belly (figure 22.18b).

Spray-and-Stretch Treatment: The foot is plantar flexed and the toes passively moved into flexion as strokes move from the anterior leg to the toes (figure 22.18c).

Notations: The intrinsic toe extensors refer to the dorsum of the foot in the area of their muscle bellies.

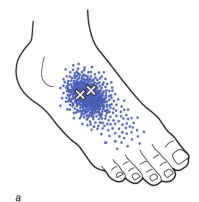

a

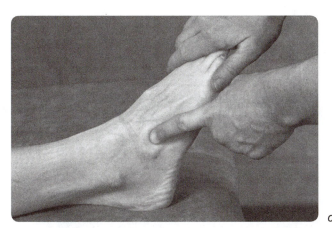

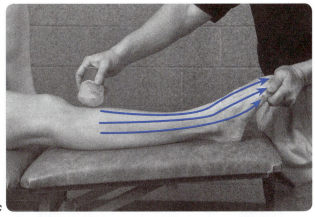

c

▶ **Figure 22.18** *(a)* Superficial intrinsic muscle pain-referral pattern of extensor digitorum brevis and extensor hallucis brevis. *(b)* Trigger point release of extensor digitorum brevis. *(c)* Ice/spray-and-stretch for toe extensors.

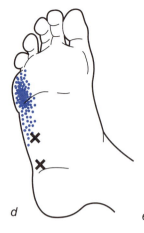

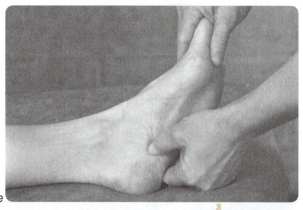

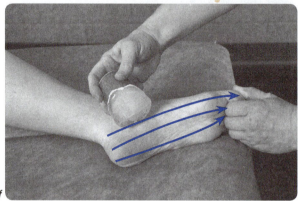

▶ **Figure 22.18** *(d)* Abductor digiti minimi pain-referral patterns of abductor hallucis. *(e)* Trigger point release of abductor hallucis. *(f)* Ice/spray-and-stretch for abductor hallucis.

Abductor Hallucis

Referral Pattern: From the heel along the medial edge of the foot near the sole (figure 22.18d).

Location of Trigger Point: In the muscle belly distal and anterior to the navicular tubercle.

Patient Position for Palpation: Supine.

Muscle Position for Palpation: Relaxed in a comfortable position.

Ischemic Treatment: Direct compression over the trigger point in the muscle belly (figure 22.18e).

Spray-and-Stretch Treatment: With the ankle in neutral, the great toe is adducted toward the others and flexed while the strokes move from plantar heel toward the toes (figure 22.18f).

Notations: The abductor hallucis brevis refers to the medial heel with some radiation into the medial arch.

Flexor Digitorum Brevis and Adductor Digiti Minimi

Referral Pattern: Flexor digitorum brevis referral is on the ball of the foot (figure 22.18h). Adductor digiti minimi referral is along the plantar surface of the fifth digit (figure 22.18g).

Location of Trigger Point: For flexor digitorum brevis over the mid-metatarsal head region; for adductor digiti minimi, between the heel and fifth metatarsal head.

Patient Position for Palpation: Supine.

Muscle Position for Palpation: Relaxed in a comfortable position.

Ischemic Treatment: Direct compression over the trigger point in the muscle belly.

Spray-and-Stretch Treatment: With the ankle in neutral, strokes move from the heel toward the toes as the toes are extended and the fifth toe is abducted (figure 22.18, i & j).

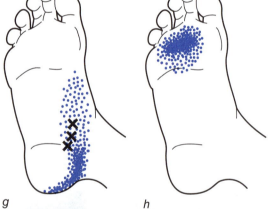

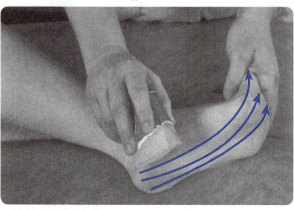

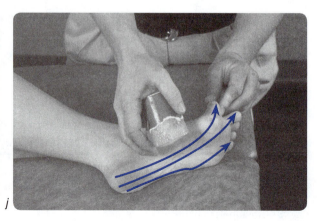

▶ **Figure 22.18** Superficial intrinsic muscle pain-referral patterns: *(g)* abductor hallucis, *(h)* flexor digitorum brevis. Ice/spray-and-stretch for *(i)* flexor digitorum brevis, *(j)* flexor hallucis brevis.

Notations: The patient can perform self-massage techniques using a tennis or golf ball, a corrugated vegetable can, or a rolling pin. In sitting, the patient places the plantar foot on top of the object being used and applies pressure downward on the knee while rolling the foot back and forth over the object (figure 22.19).

Deep Intrinsic Foot Muscles

These muscles include the quadratus plantae, lumbricals, flexor hallucis brevis, adductor hallucis, flexor digiti minimi brevis, and interossei. Like the pain-referral pattern of the superficial group, the pain-referral pattern of these muscles is primarily localized and over the region of their trigger points (figure 22.20, a-d). The pain is often described as a feeling of swelling and numbness that restricts walking.

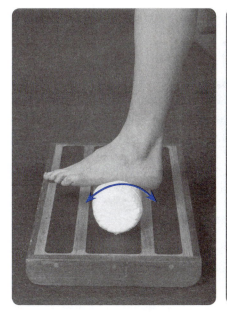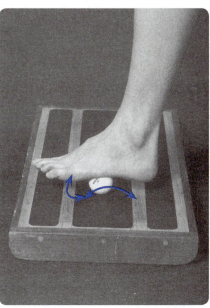

▶ **Figure 22.19** Self-application: massage to plantar foot.

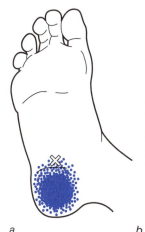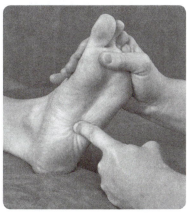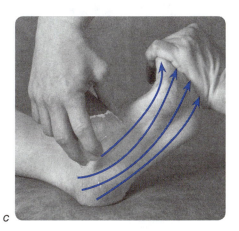

a *b* *c*

▶ **Figure 22.20** Deep intrinsic muscle pain-referral patterns: *(a)* quadratus plantae. Trigger point release of *(b)* quadratus plantae. Ice/spray-and-stretch to *(c)* intrinsic flexor muscles.

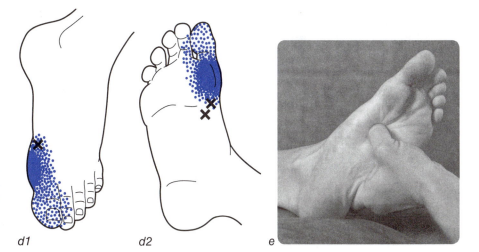

▶ **Figure 22.20** Deep intrinsic muscle pain-referral patterns: *(d)* flexor hallucis brevis. Trigger point release of *(e)* flexor hallucis brevis. See figure 22.20c for ice/spray-and-stretch to intrinsic flexor muscles.

d1 *d2* *e*

Quadratus Plantae

Referral Pattern: Pain into the plantar heel.

Location of Trigger Point: Just distal from the heel, deep in the midarch.

Patient Position for Palpation: Supine.

Muscle Position for Palpation: Relaxed in a comfortable position.

Ischemic Treatment: Deep direct compression over the trigger point.

Spray-and-Stretch Treatment: The deep flexor muscles are treated with the ankle in neutral and the hallux hyperextended as sweeps are made from the heel toward the toe.

Notations: The deep intrinsics are difficult to get to with spray-and-stretch, so one technique is used for all of them.

Flexor Hallucis Brevis

Referral Pattern: Along the lateral and posterior surface of the great toe and distal metatarsal.

Location of Trigger Point: At the base of the first metatarsal head.

Patient Position for Palpation: Supine.

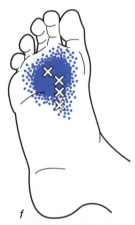
f

Muscle Position for Palpation: Relaxed in a comfortable position.

Ischemic Treatment: Deep direct compression over the trigger point.

Spray-and-Stretch Treatment: See quadratus plantae.

Notations: Because these muscles lie deep to the plantar aponeurosis, long tendons, and superficial intrinsic muscles, deep palpation is required to affect them.

Adductor Hallucis Brevis

Referral Pattern: Ball of the foot (figure 22.20f).

Location of Trigger Point: There are multiple trigger points around the muscle bellies near the proximal and lateral area of the first metatarsal head.

Patient Position for Palpation: Supine.

Muscle Position for Palpation: Relaxed in a comfortable position.

Ischemic Treatment: Deep direct compression over the trigger point (figure 22.20g).

Spray-and-Stretch Treatment: See quadratus plantae.

Notations: Because these muscles lie deep to the plantar aponeurosis, long tendons, and superficial intrinsic muscles, deep palpation is required to affect them.

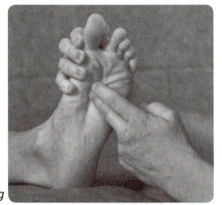
g

▶ **Figure 22.20** Deep intrinsic muscle pain-referral patterns: *(f)* adductor hallucis. Trigger point release of *(g)* adductor hallucis. See figure 22.20c for ice/spray-and-stretch to intrinsic flexor muscles.

Interossei

Referral Pattern: Ball of the foot and into the toes on the dorsal and ventral aspects (figure 22.20h1 & h2).

Location of Trigger Point: Ventral foot near where the intrinsic muscle attaches.

Patient Position for Palpation: Supine.

Muscle Position for Palpation: Relaxed in a comfortable position.

Ischemic Treatment: Deep direct compression over the trigger point (figure 22.20i).

Spray-and-Stretch Treatment: See quadratus plantae.

Notations: The pain patterns of the lumbricals and flexor digiti minimi have not been determined.

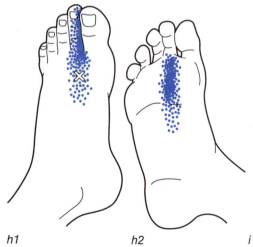
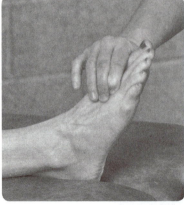

h1   h2   i

▶ **Figure 22.20** Deep intrinsic muscle pain-referral patterns: *(h)* dorsal and plantar interossei. Trigger point release of *(i)* interossei and lumbricals. See figure 22.20c for ice/spray-and-stretch to intrinsic flexor muscles.

Extrinsic Muscles

As in the upper extremity, several extrinsic muscles function in the foot and ankle. They are presented in the following sections according to the extremity compartments they lie in, moving from anterior to lateral and posterior.

Tibialis Anterior

Referral Pattern: Pain to the anteromedial ankle and over the dorsal and medial great toe (figure 22.21a). This muscle can occasionally refer pain along the anterior shin.

Location of Trigger Point: Located at the border of the proximal and middle third of the anterior extremity near the tibial ridge (figure 22.21b).

Patient Position for Palpation: Supine.

Muscle Position for Palpation: Relaxed in a comfortable position with a pillow under the knee.

Ischemic Treatment: Trigger point release is performed with flat palpation of the trigger point. If the area is tender to palpation, a taut band can be palpated. A local twitch response may be elicited with snapping palpation of the trigger point. Direct pressure to the patient's tolerance relaxes the band and relieves the pain.

Spray-and-Stretch Treatment: Applied as the foot is plantar flexed and pronated; ice sweeps are made from the knee distally toward the foot (figure 22.21c).

Notations: This trigger point usually occurs in conjunction with trigger points of other muscles.

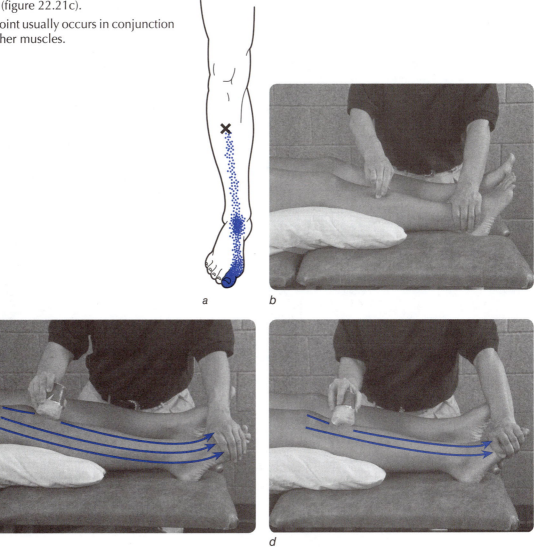

a   b

c   d

▶ **Figure 22.21** Tibialis anterior: *(a)* pain-referral pattern, *(b)* trigger point release, *(c)* ice/spray-and-stretch in plantar flexion, *(d)* ice/spray-and-stretch in plantar flexion with pronation added.

Peroneals

Referral Pattern: Peroneus longus and brevis refer pain to the lateral malleolus and proximally and distally to it (figure 22.22a). The longus pain may also spill over to the middle lateral leg. The peroneus tertius refers pain to the anterolateral ankle and into the lateral heel.

Location of Trigger Point: The peroneus longus trigger point is located about 2 to 4 cm (0.8-1.6 in.) distal to the fibular head near the shaft of the fibula (figure 22.22b). The peroneus brevis trigger point is located at the juncture of the middle and distal thirds of the extremity. The peroneus tertius trigger points are just anterior and distal to those of the peroneus brevis.

Patient Position for Palpation: Supine.

Muscle Position for Palpation: Relaxed in a comfortable position with a pillow under the knee.

Ischemic Treatment: A direct pressure is applied over the trigger point of each muscle and maintained until the pain is abated.

Spray-and-Stretch Treatment: Applied to the peroneus longus and brevis with a passive stretch of the ankle into inversion and dorsiflexion while proximal-to-distal sweeps of ice are made along the lateral extremity. To treat the peroneus tertius, the rehabilitation clinician performs a plantar-flexion and inversion stretch and applies ice more anteriorly on the distal extremity (figure 22.22c).

Notations: Individuals with a Morton's toe and excessive pronation are more prone to these complaints. Snapping palpation of the peroneus longus elicits a local twitch response that produces ankle plantar flexion and eversion.

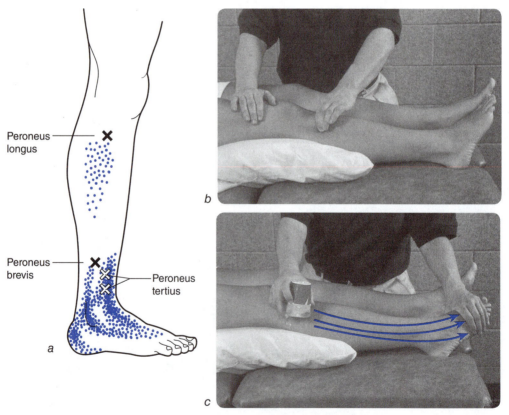

▶ **Figure 22.22** *(a)* Peroneal pain patterns, *(b)* trigger point release to peroneus longus, and *(c)* ice/spray-and-stretch for peroneus tertius.

Gastrocnemius

Referral Pattern: There are four trigger points with different referral patterns. They can refer pain to the medial arch with spillover into the medial calf (figure 22.23a1), close to the medial border of the medial gastrocnemius head (figure 22.23a2), close to the lateral border of the lateral gastrocnemius head (figure 22.23a3), and slightly more distal on the lateral head of the gastrocnemius (figure 22.23a4).

Location of Trigger Point: Trigger point causing medial arch pain is in the proximal medial belly distal to the knee (TP$_1$). The trigger point causing central posterior knee pain is located at the joint line of the knee toward the lateral edge of the medial belly (TP$_2$). The trigger point for the lateral calf is in the midbelly of the lateral calf at the fullest portion of the calf (TP$_3$). The trigger point for lateral posterior knee pain is located in the lateral calf belly distal to the knee joint (TP$_4$).

Patient Position for Palpation: Prone or kneeling.

Muscle Position for Palpation: Relaxed in a comfortable position with a pillow under the leg.

Ischemic Treatment: Either a flat thumb pressure or a pincer grasp can be used (figure 22.23b). If the muscle is taut, a flat pressure is easier and more comfortable to administer. Trigger point release is best performed with the ankle in slight plantar flexion to place the muscle on slack. A pincer grasp of the lateral head is easily used with the thumb on the lateral border and the fingers at the midline groove between the two gastrocnemius heads. Flat pressure should be used in the popliteal area.

Spray-and-Stretch Treatment: With the patient in prone and the foot over the edge of the table. While the rehabilitation clinician uses his or her knee to dorsiflex the ankle with pressure over the ball of the patient's foot, he or she applies ice from above the knee in a distal direction toward the plantar foot (figure 22.23c).

Notations: Nocturnal cramps are often associated with these trigger points.

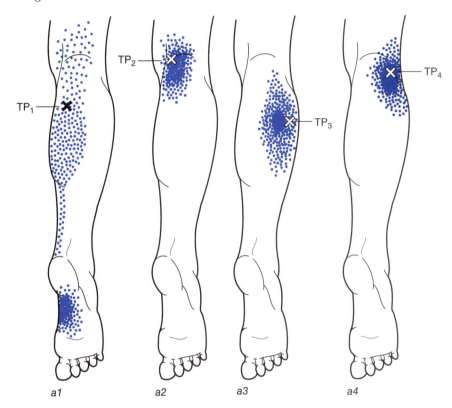

a1　　　*a2*　　　*a3*　　　*a4*

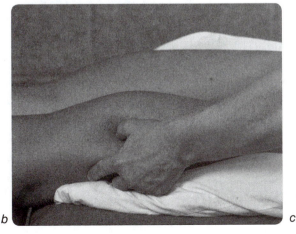

b

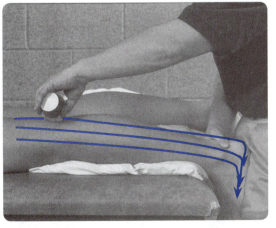

c

▶ **Figure 22.23** Gastrocnemius trigger point: *(a)* pain-referral pattern, *(b)* trigger point release of lateral head, *(c)* ice/spray-and-stretch.

Soleus

Referral Pattern: The most common site of pain referral of the soleus is into the posterior and plantar heel area and into the distal Achilles. The soleus occasionally refers pain into the upper calf and rarely into the ipsilateral sacroiliac joint (figure 22.24a).

Location of Trigger Point: The trigger point for pain referral into the calf is just distal to the knee joint between the medial and lateral gastrocnemius heads (TP_1). Trigger point for pain into the heel is located at the medial distal edge of the muscle belly, medial to the Achilles (TP_2). The trigger point for pain into the ipsilateral sacroiliac is the lateral distal edge of the muscle belly (TP_3).

Patient Position for Palpation: Prone or kneeling.

Muscle Position for Palpation: Relaxed in a comfortable position with a pillow under the leg.

Ischemic Treatment: Trigger point release uses either a pincer or flat-pressure application. The patient can be either in prone with the knee flexed to keep the gastrocnemius slack (figure 22.24b) or in a kneeling position. The distal trigger points are located just distal to the medial and lateral gastrocnemius muscle belly bulges. Direct pressure to the patient's tolerance is applied until the trigger point relaxes and the pain subsides.

Spray-and-Stretch Treatment: Performed with the knee in flexion. The patient can be kneeling or prone (figure 22.24c). As the ankle is passively dorsiflexed, the ice is swept from proximal to distal across the posterior extremity and into the plantar foot.

Notations: Heel pain during weight bearing and nocturnal deep heel pain may be primary complaints, and dorsiflexion is limited.

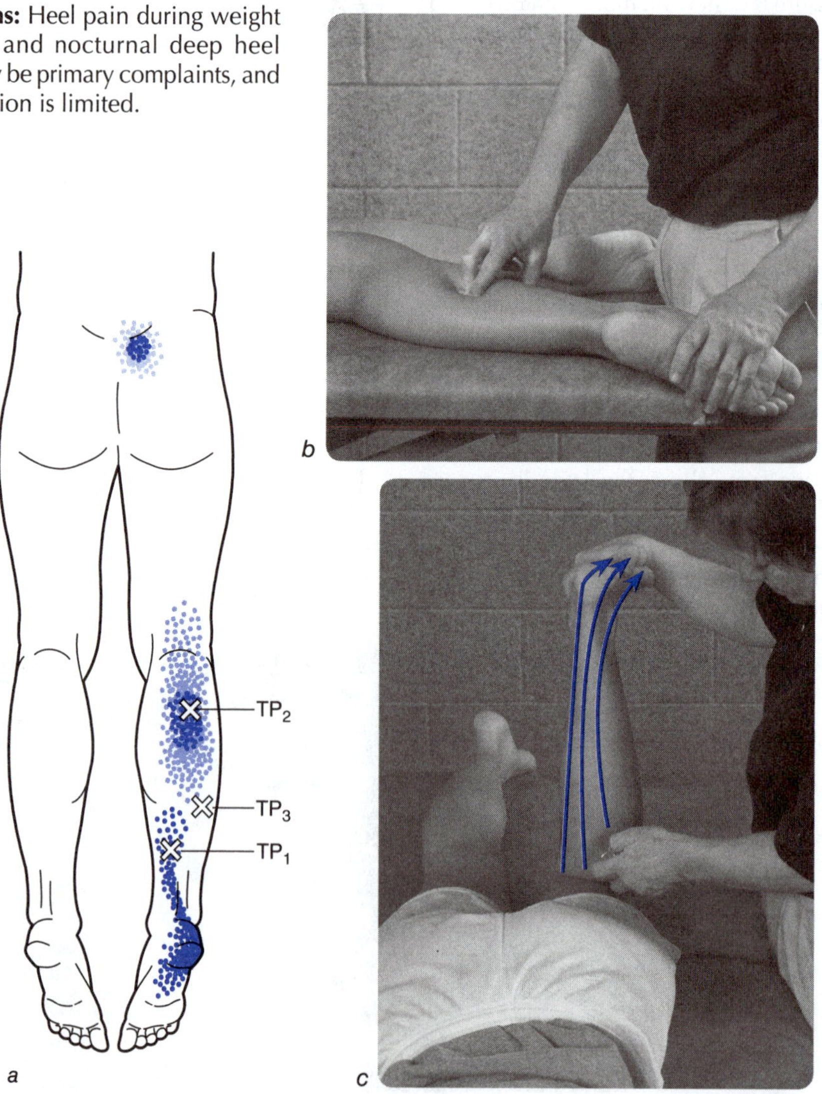

▶ **Figure 22.24** Soleus: *(a)* pain-referral pattern, *(b)* trigger point release, *(c)* ice/spray-and-stretch.

Tibialis Posterior

Referral Pattern: Pain can refer into the Achilles tendon with spillover into the midcalf proximally and the heel, instep, and plantar foot and toes distally (figure 22.25a).

Location of Trigger Point: Between the soleus and the medial border of the posterior tibia.

Patient Position for Palpation: Prone.

Muscle Position for Palpation: Relaxed in a comfortable position with a pillow under the leg.

Ischemic Treatment: Because the tibialis posterior is the deepest muscle of the extremity, it is not possible to make direct contact with it through deep pressure. Deep pressure to more superficial muscles can be used to apply indirect pressure (figure 22.25b).

Spray-and-Stretch Treatment: Applied with the patient prone and the foot over the edge of the table. The ankle is stretched into dorsiflexion and eversion as the ice sweeps begin at the posterior knee and extend distally into the plantar foot (figure 22.25c).

Notations: Trigger point activation of this muscle makes it painful for the patient to run or walk on uneven surfaces when the muscle's activity is increased to provide additional stabilization.

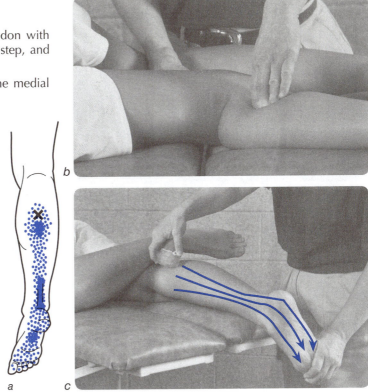

▶ **Figure 22.25** Tibialis posterior: *(a)* pain-referral pattern, *(b)* trigger point release (medial approach), *(c)* ice/spray-and-stretch.

Long Toe Extensors

Referral Pattern: The most common pain-referral pattern for these muscles is along the anterior ankle, along the dorsum of the foot over the metatarsals, and extending distally into the toes and proximally into the distal extremity (figure 22.26a).

Location of Trigger Point: The extensor digitorum longus trigger point is located about 8 cm (3 in.) distal and slightly anterior of the fibular head (figure 22.26b). The extensor hallucis longus trigger point is located at the juncture of the middle and distal thirds of the extremity (figure 22.26c).

Patient Position for Palpation: Supine.

Muscle Position for Palpation: In a comfortable, relaxed position.

Ischemic Treatment: Pressure is applied directly over the trigger points until pain is reduced and the trigger points relax.

Spray-and-Stretch Treatment: The ankle and toes are passively plantar flexed with pressure on the distal toes while ice sweeps are applied from the anterior and lateral proximal extremity distally over the ankle and foot to the toes (figure 22.26d).

Notations: These muscles include the extensor digitorum longus and the extensor hallucis longus. Trigger points can cause night cramps in the toe extensors.

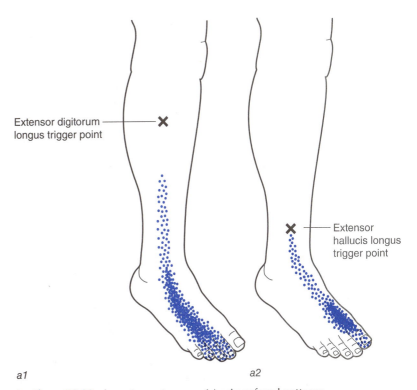

▶ **Figure 22.26** Long toe extensors: *(a)* pain-referral patterns.

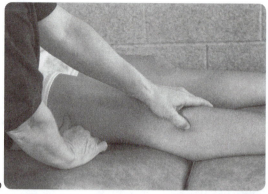

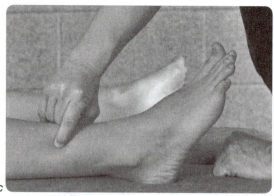

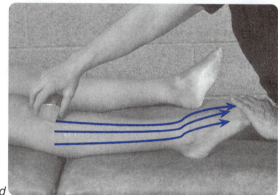

▶ **Figure 22.26** Long toe extensors: *(b)* trigger point release of extensor digitorum longus, *(c)* trigger point release of extensor hallucis longus, *(d)* ice/spray-and-stretch.

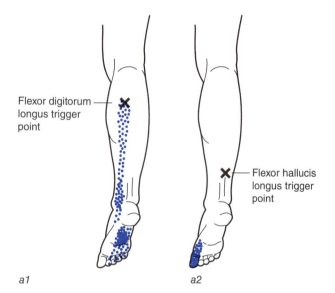

▶ **Figure 22.27** Long toe flexors: *(a1)* trigger point of flexor digitorum longus pain-referral pattern, *(a2)* trigger point of flexor hallucis longus.

Long Toe Flexors

Referral Pattern: The flexor digitorum longus refers into the sole of the forefoot with occasional spillover into the toes and medial calf (figure 22.27a1). The flexor hallucis longus refers pain to the plantar great toe and into the first metatarsal head (figure 22.27a2).

Location of Trigger Point: For the flexor digitorum longus, the trigger point is located in the medial proximal extremity between the tibia and gastrocnemius-soleus complex. The flexor hallucis longus trigger point is located with deep pressure applied to the soleus lateral to the midline at the meeting of the middle and lower third of the leg.

Patient Position for Palpation: Prone or side-lying.

Muscle Position for Palpation: Muscle is relaxed and passively positioned in a semi-shortened position.

Ischemic Treatment: For trigger point release, the patient is in side-lying on the involved side with the knee flexed and the ankle in a relaxed plantar-flexed position. Using a flat-pressure technique, the rehabilitation clinician applies pressure on the medial proximal extremity between the tibia and gastrocnemius-soleus complex (figure 22.27b). Once the gastrocnemius is pushed posteriorly, pressure is applied downward and then laterally. The flexor hallucis longus is treated with the patient in prone; deep pressure is applied through the soleus lateral to the midline and at the juncture of the middle and lower thirds of the extremity (figure 22.27c).

Spray-and-Stretch Treatment: Performed with the patient prone and the knee passively flexed. As the ankle is passively dorsiflexed and everted and the toes are extended, ice sweeps are applied from the proximal calf along the medial ankle into the plantar foot to the toes (figure 22.27d).

Notations: The most common symptom reported with active trigger points of the long toe flexors is pain in the feet during walking.

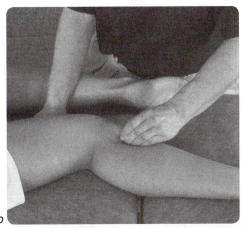

▶ **Figure 22.27** Long toe flexors: *(b)* trigger point release of flexor digitorum longus, *(c)* trigger point release of flexor hallucis longus, *(d)* ice/spray-and-stretch for flexor digitorum longus and hallucis longus.

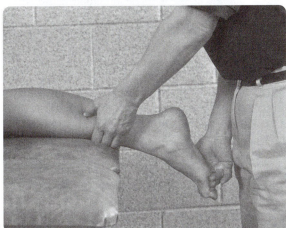

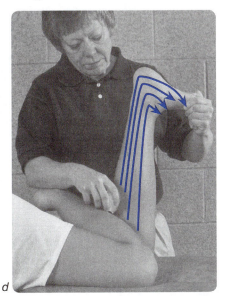

DEEP-TISSUE MASSAGE

Soft-tissue restriction often occurs after a patient has experienced excessive edema or immobilization of the ankle, foot, or extremity. Either the prolonged presence of edema or reduced tissue mobility can result in adhesions. Good tissue flexibility and restoration of normal range of motion can occur with release of adhesions. Deep-tissue massage techniques, discussed in chapter 6, can be useful in accomplishing these goals. Review the discussion of proper application of these massage techniques before using them. The patient can perform deep massage to foot intrinsic muscles that are in spasm or have myofascial tightness. Sitting in a chair, the patient places the bare foot on the side of a ribbed fruit or vegetable can positioned on the floor. Applying some downward force on the knee with the hands, the patient rolls the foot back and forth over the can to provide a self-massage (figure 22.19, p. 793).

JOINT MOBILIZATION

Joint mobilization is often necessary in the ankle, especially after periods of immobilization. The techniques can be either repeated sustained glides or oscillations. In more restricted joints, sustained glides may be more effective than oscillations. Oscillation may be more comfortable for the patient and is frequently used in distractions to aid in reduction of pain (grades I and II). More aggressive grades (III and IV) are used to improve mobility.

To determine whether joint mobilization for mobility is indicated, the rehabilitation clinician assesses the joint's capsular pattern and motion loss and also compares the involved with the uninvolved segment. The capsular pattern for the talocrural joint is more limitation of plantar flexion than of dorsiflexion; in the subtalar joint, inversion is more limited than eversion. The great toe's MTP and all the toes' IP joints have capsular patterns of more limitation of extension than flexion. Refer to chapter 6 for this information and for details on close-packed and resting positions for these joints.

As with other joints, precautions and contraindications should be respected. Body mechanics, force direction application, and amount of force should be proper in all techniques. The hands should be as close to the joint as possible, with one hand acting as the stabilizing hand and the other applying the mobilization force. The convex-concave rule determines the direction of the mobilization force. That is, when a convex surface is moved on a concave surface, the force is applied in the direction opposite than that of the bone's movement; when a concave surface is moved on a convex surface, the force is applied in the same direction as the bone's movement. Many of the mobilization techniques in this chapter are based on Maitland's (1991) work. The techniques for the foot and ankle are presented in the following sections and the images that accompany it.

Tibiofibular Joint

The tibia and fibula articulate with each other proximally in the distal knee region and distally at the ankle mortise joint. Both proximal and distal articulations must have restored mobility for ankle motion to be normal. The resting position for the proximal tibiofibular joint is 25° of knee flexion with 10° of plantar flexion, and the resting position for the distal tibiofibular joint is 10° of plantar flexion with 5° of inversion.

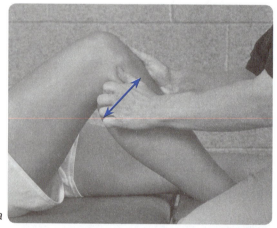

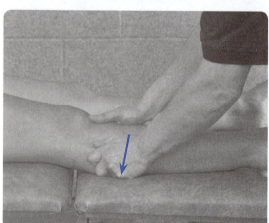

▶ **Figure 22.28** Proximal tibiofibular joint mobilization: *(a)* AP-PA mobilization, *(b)* alternative posterior glide.

■ Joint Mobilization of the Foot and Ankle Joints

Anteroposterior (AP) and Posteroanterior (PA) Glides

Joint: Proximal tibiofibular.

Resting Position: 25° knee flexion, 10° plantar flexion.

Indications: Restricted ankle dorsiflexion, plantar flexion, or both.

Patient Position: The patient is positioned to provide the clinician the best mechanical advantage and ease of force application. For an AP mobilization force, the patient is positioned supine with the knee in extension. Posteroanterior mobilization of the proximal tibiofibular joint is performed with the patient in side-lying. The weight of the extremity stabilizes the tibia while the rehabilitation clinician's distal hand stabilizes the middle extremity.

Clinician and Hand Positions: For an AP mobilization, the tibia is stabilized with the medial hand over the proximal tibia; the fleshy aspect of the thenar eminence of the lateral hand is over the fibular head and proximal fibula to provide the mobilizing force. For a PA mobilization, the mobilizing hand applies an anterior glide with the pad of the wrist against the fibular head while the stabilizing hand prevents motion of the distal leg.

Mobilization Application: For an AP mobilization, a vertical downward force is applied by the mobilizing hand on the fibular head to produce a posterior glide of the fibula (figure 22.28b). For a PA mobilization, the lateral hand glides the fibular head anteriorly and posteriorly (figure 22.28a). One direction is mobilized first and then the other direction; that is, the motion is not a full back-and-forth motion.

Notations: Mobilization of the superior tibiofibular joint should accompany any restricted movement of the distal tibiofibular joint. Normal mobility of this joint allows the fibular head to move anteriorly during knee flexion and posteriorly during knee extension.

AP and PA Glides

Joint: Distal tibiofibular.

Resting Position: 10° plantar flexion with 5° inversion.

Indications: Restricted ankle dorsiflexion, plantar flexion, or both.

Patient Position: An AP glide is performed with the patient supine. A PA glide is performed with the patient prone and the distal extremity over the edge of the table.

Clinician and Hand Positions: For an AP glide, the clinician places the medial hand over the medial malleolus to stabilize the tibia and places the thenar eminence of the lateral hand over the lateral malleolus and distal fibula. For a PA glide, the base of the lateral hand is placed over the lateral malleolus while the medial hand stabilizes the distal tibia.

Mobilization Application: For an AP mobilization, a posterior glide is performed using a downward movement of the lateral hand (figure 22.29). For a PA mobilization, the anterior force is applied perpendicular to the plane of the distal tibiofibular joint.

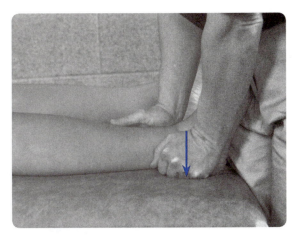

▶ **Figure 22.29** Distal tibiofibular joint mobilization, posterior glide.

Notations: During dorsiflexion, the distal fibula moves superiorly from the tibia and rotates medially. During plantar flexion, the distal fibula moves in the opposite directions. Normal ankle motion depends on good fibular mobility. Restriction of joint play between the fibula and tibia may require fibular mobilization in both AP and PA directions to restore normal motion.

Talocrural Joint

There are several joints throughout the ankle and foot. The talocrural joint is the true ankle joint, allowing flexion and extension motion. The following sections present some of the most common joint mobilization techniques for this joint.

Distraction

Joint: Talocrural.

Resting Position: 10° plantar flexion.

Indications: To increase general joint play in the ankle joint; can also be used with lower grades of mobilization to relieve pain.

Patient Position: Supine with knee and hip extended.

Clinician and Hand Positions: The rehabilitation clinician faces the foot and grasps the foot's dorsum with both hands, intertwining or overlapping the fingers of the two hands on top of the foot and placing the thumbs on the plantar aspect (figure 22.30).

Mobilization Application: Clinician leans backward to apply a distraction force.

Notations: This technique is also used to assist in relaxation prior to grade III and IV mobilization techniques.

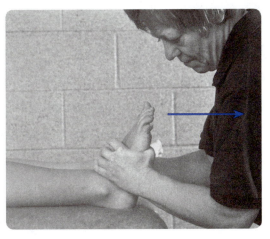

▶ **Figure 22.30** Talocrural distraction joint mobilization.

Anterior Glide

Joint: Talocrural.

Resting Position: 10° plantar flexion.

Indications: Restricted plantar flexion.

Patient Position: Supine with knee extended.

Clinician and Hand Positions: Clinician faces the foot. The stabilizing hand is placed anteriorly around the distal leg, and the mobilizing hand is placed around the proximal foot with the thumb and index finger in contact with the bottom of the malleoli.

Mobilization Application: The talus is glided posteriorly in the plane of the joint.

Notations: Also known as a ventral glide or PA movement.

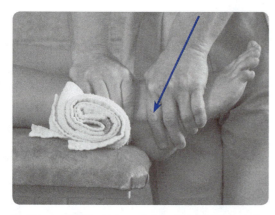

▶ **Figure 22.31** Talocrural posterior glide joint mobilization.

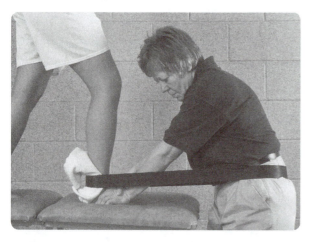

▶ **Figure 22.32** Alternative PA glide of the tibia on the talus to increase dorsiflexion.

Posterior Glide

Joint: Talocrural.

Resting Position: 10° plantar flexion.

Indications: Restricted dorsiflexion.

Patient Position: Supine with knee extended and ankle over end of table.

Clinician and Hand Positions: The clinician faces the foot. The stabilizing hand is placed anteriorly around the distal leg at the level of the malleoli, and the mobilizing hand is placed around the proximal foot with the thumb and index finger adjacent to the distal aspect of the malleoli.

Mobilization Application: The talus is glided posteriorly in the plane of the joint (figure 22.31).

Notations: Also known as a dorsal glide or AP glide.

Anterior Glide of Tibia

Joint: Talocrural.

Resting Position: 10° plantar flexion.

Indications: Restricted dorsiflexion.

Patient Position: With the patient standing in a forward-backward stride position on a table, a mobilization strap is secured around the distal tibia and fibula and the clinician's hips.

Clinician and Hand Positions: Clinician places the web of the thumb and index finger around the anterior ankle joint and also stands in a forward-backward stride position.

Mobilization Application: With the knee partially flexed, the clinician uses the hips to pull the strap forward, moving body weight from front to back leg (figure 22.32).

Notations: This is an alternative method to the one described for figure 22.31. The strap provides additional mechanical leverage.

Subtalar Joint

The subtalar joint allows inversion and eversion movements to permit ambulation on uneven surfaces without injury. Some, but not all, mobilization techniques for the subtalar joint are presented in the following sections. Hand positions for some of these techniques, such as distraction, are only subtly different from those for talocrural mobilization, but these distinctions are important.

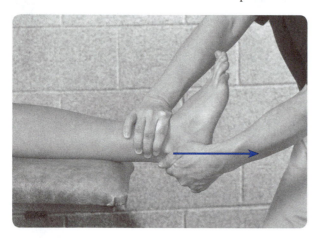

▶ **Figure 22.33** Subtalar joint distraction joint mobilization.

Distraction

Joint: Subtalar.

Resting Position: Neutral inversion-eversion.

Indications: To improve general mobility.

Patient Position: Patient is supine with the foot over the end of the table.

Clinician and Hand Positions: Clinician faces the foot. The stabilizing hand grasps the talus anteriorly, and the mobilizing hand cups the posterior calcaneus (figure 22.33).

Mobilization Application: The calcaneus is pulled distally from the long axis of the extremity.

Notations: This technique can be used to relieve pain and is good to use before and after grade III and IV techniques.

Medial Glide

Joint: Subtalar.

Resting Position: Neutral inversion-eversion.

Indications: To increase eversion.

Patient Position: Patient is side-lying on uninvolved extremity. Involved ankle is off the end of the table with a towel roll placed under the distal leg.

Clinician and Hand Positions: The distal leg is stabilized with the cephalic hand over the lateral leg; the caudal hand is positioned with its heel on the lateral calcaneus and the fingers on the plantar surface (figure 22.34).

Mobilization Application: A downward medial glide is applied to the calcaneus.

Notations: This technique may be applied with the patient in supine, but a downward force on the joint is easier to apply than a lateral-to-medial force that would be required with the patient supine.

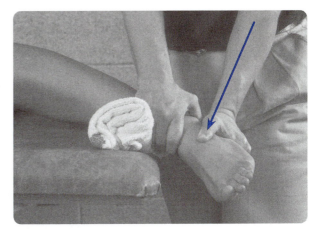

▶ **Figure 22.34** Subtalar joint mobilization, medial glide.

Lateral Glide

Joint: Subtalar.

Resting Position: Neutral inversion-eversion.

Indications: To increase subtalar inversion.

Patient Position: Patient is in side-lying on the involved side. The foot is over the end of the table and a towel is under the distal leg.

Clinician and Hand Positions: The rehabilitation clinician stabilizes the extremity with the cephalic hand over the medial distal extremity. The mobilizing hand is placed with the heel of the hand over the medial calcaneus and the fingers on the plantar aspect (figure 22.35).

Mobilization Application: The force applied occurs directly downward and parallel to the joint surface.

Notations: This technique may be applied with the patient in supine, but a downward force on the joint is easier to apply than a medial-to-lateral force that would be required with the patient supine.

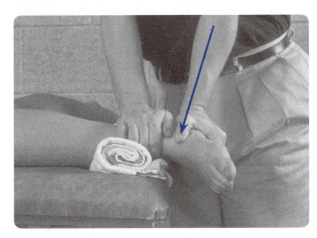

▶ **Figure 22.35** Subtalar joint mobilization, lateral glide.

Intertarsal Joints

These mobilizations can be performed on all midtarsal joints, including the talonavicular, calcaneocuboid, and naviculocuneiform. They are described in the following sections.

Anterior Glide

Joint: Intertarsal joints.

Resting Position: Neutral inversion-eversion with 10° plantar flexion.

Indications: To increase midfoot plantar flexion.

Patient Position: Prone.

Clinician and Hand Positions: Clinician grasps the midfoot with one thumb, reinforced by the other thumb over the bone to be mobilized. Forefoot is stabilized with the hands while the thumbs provide the mobilization (figure 22.36).

Mobilization Application: Thumbs perform a PA movement of the bone.

Notations: Weight of the leg helps to stabilize the ankle.

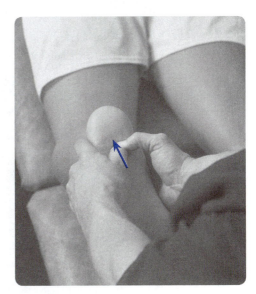

▶ **Figure 22.36** Intertarsal joint mobilization, anterior glide.

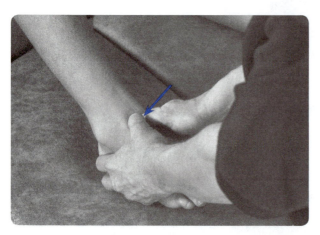

▶ **Figure 22.37** Intertarsal posterior glide joint mobilization.

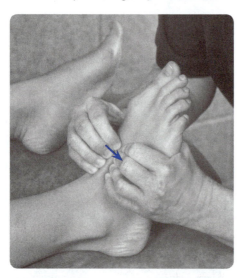

▶ **Figure 22.38** Intermetatarsal glide joint mobilization.

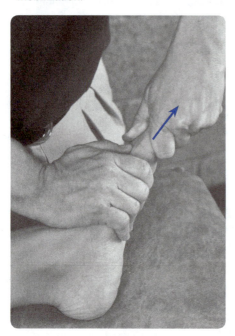

▶ **Figure 22.39** Metatarsophalangeal distraction joint mobilization.

Posterior Glide

Joint: Intertarsal joints.

Resting Position: Neutral inversion-eversion with 10° plantar flexion.

Indications: To increase midfoot dorsiflexion.

Patient Position: Supine.

Clinician and Hand Positions: Clinician stabilizes rearfoot with one hand and places the thumb of the other hand on the foot's dorsum and the fingers on the plantar aspect of the bone to be mobilized.

Mobilization Application: Mobilizing hand applies an AP movement in the plane of the joint surface (figure 22.37).

Notations: Placement of the plantar surface of the foot on the table may also be used to stabilize the rearfoot.

Anterior and Posterior Glides

Joint: Intermetatarsal joints.

Resting Position: Undefined.

Indications: To increase intermetatarsal mobility.

Patient Position: Supine on the table and extend foot.

Clinician and Hand Positions: The rehabilitation clinician stabilizes one metatarsal and grasps the adjacent one, with the thumb on the dorsum and the fingers on the plantar aspect.

Mobilization Application: Anterposterior-posteroanterior force is applied to the metatarsal (figure 22.38).

Notations: A gross AP and PA glide can also be applied to the intertarsal joints: The proximal tarsal row is stabilized, and the distal row is mobilized in either an anterior or a posterior direction.

Tarsometatarsal, Metatarsophalangeal, and Interphalangeal Joints

Many of the basic hand positions and force applications are the same for these joints, so they are grouped together in the following sections. You must realize, however, that specific finger and hand positions vary according to the particular joint being mobilized.

Distraction

Joint: Tarsometatarsal, metatarsophalangeal, and interphalangeal joints.

Resting Position: First toe: 20° dorsiflexion; toes 2 through 5: 20° plantar flexion.

Indications: To enhance general joint mobility and relaxation.

Patient Position: Patient is relaxed, supine on the table.

Clinician and Hand Positions: Phalanx is grasped with the thumb and fingers while the metatarsal is stabilized with the opposite hand (figure 22.39).

Mobilization Application: Distraction force is applied to the phalanx.

Notations: May also be used prior to and following grades II and III joint mobilization techniques.

Anterior and Posterior Glides

Joint: Tarsometatarsal, metatarsophalangeal, and interphalangeal joints.

Resting Position: First toe: 20° dorsiflexion; toes 2 through 5: 20° plantar flexion.

Indications: Anterior glides increase extension of these joints. Posterior glides increase flexion of these joints.

Patient Position: Patient is comfortable with foot over end of the table.

Clinician and Hand Positions: For the MTP and tarsometatarsal joints, the metatarsal is stabilized with one hand while the mobilizing hand grasps the proximal phalanx. For the IP joints, the proximal phalanx is stabilized by the clinician's fingers and thumb.

Mobilization Application: For MTP and tarsometatarsal joints, an AP-PA glide is applied. For IP joints, the mobilizing force is applied to the distal phalanx.

Notations: Slight traction is simultaneously applied to provide more comfort for the patient.

> Joint mobilization oscillations are used to reduce pain and swelling. Oscillations or sustained mobilizations are used to improve mobility in many joints in the ankle.

FLEXIBILITY EXERCISES

This section includes detailed information on some of the more commonly used techniques for improving ankle and foot flexibility. As with most exercises, the rehabilitation clinician must have knowledge of the body's mechanics, the muscle's function, and appropriate application of forces to design an effective flexibility exercise program.

Although there are some exceptions, the active flexibility exercises are held for 15 to 20 s and repeated four to five times. If the patient has less-than-normal flexibility, he or she should repeat the exercises frequently throughout the day.

■ Flexibility Exercises for the Foot and Ankle

Standing Stretch

Body Segment: Gastrocnemius.

Stage in Rehab: Early II.

Purpose: Increase flexibility of gastrocnemius.

Positioning: The patient is in a straddle position with the extremity to be stretched behind the opposite extremity.

Execution: The patient places his or her body weight on the arms, which are supported on the wall and on the front foot while the back extremity remains extended at the knee. The heel should remain in contact with the floor; the hip should be forward of the knee; and the foot should be in a straight line or the toes may be turned slightly inward (figure 22.40).

▶ **Figure 22.40** Gastrocnemius stretch in standing.

Possible Substitutions: Common substitutions are allowing the midfoot to collapse by rotating the foot outward, lifting the heel off the floor, bending the knee, and moving the hips posteriorly.

Notations: Because the gastrocnemius extends from above the knee to the calcaneus, both the knee and ankle joints must be placed on stretch to effectively stretch the muscle.

Seated Stretch

Body Segment: Gastrocnemius.

Stage in Rehab: Early II.

Purpose: Increase gastrocnemius flexibility.

Positioning: With the patient in a long sitting position, a stretch strap or towel is hooked around the forefoot.

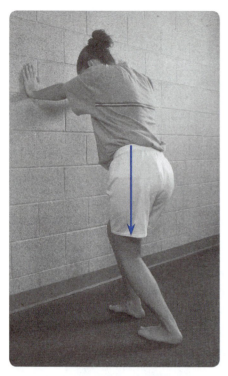

▶ **Figure 22.41** Soleus stretch in standing.

Execution: Keeping the knee straight, the patient pulls on the strap to dorsiflex the ankle. Additional stretch can be applied with active contraction of the ankle dorsiflexors.

Possible Substitutions: Hip rotation and foot pronation.

Notations: If the patient is non-weight bearing, he or she can use this gastrocnemius stretch to increase flexibility until weight bearing is permissible.

Standing Stretch

Body Segment: Soleus.

Stage in Rehab: Early II.

Purpose: Increase soleus flexibility.

Positioning: In the standing position, the patient is in a position similar to that described for the gastrocnemius. With the involved extremity behind the uninvolved extremity, he or she keeps the foot flat on the floor with the foot turned slightly inward.

Execution: Patient slowly flexes the knee until a stretch is felt in the calf (figure 22.41).

Possible Substitutions: Outward rotation of the foot, knee valgus positioning, and posterior movement of the hip as the knee is flexed.

Notations: Because the soleus does not cross the knee joint, to isolate this muscle the stretch should be applied with the knee flexed. This eliminates the stretch on the gastrocnemius and isolates the stretch to the soleus.

▶ **Figure 22.42** Soleus stretch in sitting: *(a)* with 1/2 foam roller, *(b)* with stretch strap.

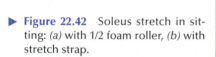

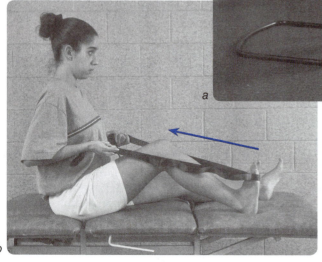

a

b

Seated Soleus Stretch

Body Segment: Soleus.

Stage in Rehab: Early II.

Purpose: Increase soleus motion.

Positioning: If partial weight bearing, patient can perform this exercise in sitting with the feet on the floor. Forefoot is on a 1/2 foam roller, and the heel is off the roller. If the patient is non-weight-bearing, a strap is placed around the forefoot with the knee in partial flexion, and the strap is pulled to apply the stretch, moving the ankle into dorsiflexion.

Execution: For the weight-bearing stretch, the patient pushes the heel to the floor until a stretch is felt in the distal calf (figure 22.42a). For the non-weight-bearing stretch, the patient pulls on the strap to move the ankle into dorsiflexion until a stretch in the lower calf is felt (figure 22.42b).

Possible Substitutions: Increasing knee flexion rather than ankle dorsiflexion and placing the strap too proximal on the foot to apply an effective stretch force.

Notations: Because the soleus does not cross the knee joint, to isolate this muscle the stretch should be applied with the knee flexed. This eliminates the stretch on the gastrocnemius and isolates the stretch to the soleus.

Prolonged Achilles Stretch

Body Segment: Achilles.

Stage in Rehab: Late II or III.

Purpose: Improve mobility of Achilles tendon.

Positioning: The patient stands with the back to a wall. The feet are positioned either on an incline (figure 22.43a) or on the edge of a book (figure 22.43b), with the heel no more than 2.5 cm (1 in.) from the wall. A towel roll is placed between the posterior knees and the wall to prevent knee hyperextension.

Execution: The patient stands in this position for a prolonged period, at least 5 min and as much as 20 min if tolerable. It is useful to place a chair next to the patient so that he or she can place the hands on the back of the chair for stabilization and support.

Possible Substitutions: Common substitutions are standing with the feet in pronation, standing too far away from the wall, and hyperextension of the knees. Some people attempt to stretch the Achilles or gastrocnemius on the edge of a step. This is ineffective because the very muscle that is being stretched is simultaneously contracting to maintain balance.

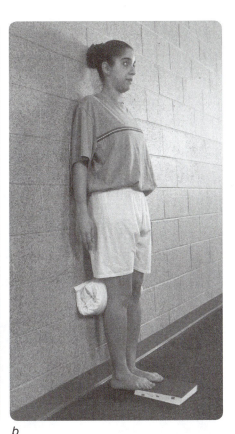

a   *b*

▶ **Figure 22.43** Achilles prolonged stretch: *(a)* using an incline, *(b)* using a book. A towel roll should be placed behind the knees to prevent knee hyperextension.

Notations: If the Achilles is the restricted structure, a prolonged stretch is most effective for increasing motion. Because of the connective tissue structure of the thick Achilles tendon, short-term stretches do not change its length. Once the stretch is released, the patient commonly feels stiffness in the posterior calf or ankle area, but this should subside quickly.

Ankle Dorsiflexor Stretch

Body Segment: Ankle dorsiflexors.

Stage in Rehab: II or III.

Purpose: Increase ankle plantar-flexion motion.

Positioning: Patient begins in a quadruped position.

Execution: Patient pushes hips back toward heels as far as tolerable. If there are no knee injuries, patient should be able to sit on the ankles. In this position, the anterior ankle should be flat on the floor (figure 22.44).

Possible Substitutions: Keeping the ankle in a flexed position, rotating the legs outward.

Notations: With very tight ankles, full weight bearing onto the ankles in this position may be too uncomfortable. A less aggressive stretch can be performed in standing, using a foam roller. The patient places the dorsum of the foot on the foam roller on the floor and pushes the ankle downward toward the floor.

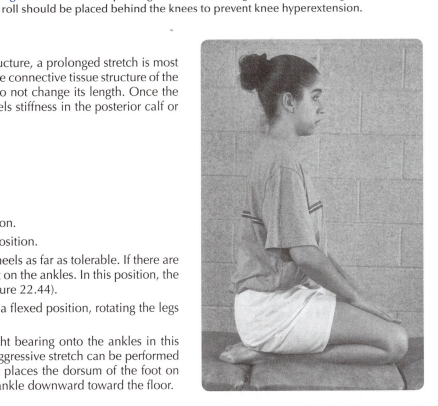

▶ **Figure 22.44** Ankle dorsiflexor stretch, sitting. If the patient has a history of knee problems, this position should be avoided.

Active Ankle Pumps, Alphabet, and Toe Exercises

Body Segment: Ankle, foot, and toes.

Stage in Rehab: II.

Purpose: Improve flexibility of ankle, foot, and toes.

Positioning: Patient is able to perform these exercises in sitting.

Execution: Leaving the heel on the floor for ankle pumps, the patient taps the foot up and down, going as high as possible each time he or she raises the foot. In another active-motion exercise, the patient spells the alphabet with the toes and foot while keeping the heel on the floor. These exercises are used as a home exercise program with instructions to perform throughout the day.

Possible Substitutions: Using the leg or hip rather than the ankle or toes to perform the motions.

Notations: These are general active exercises that the patient can perform independently throughout the day to increase ankle motion. These exercises can also be performed with the ankle elevated and can be useful in reducing edema.

BAPS Board

The BAPS board, or Biomechanical Ankle Proprioception System, is used to increase ankle flexibility and can also be used for strengthening. It consists of a board, or platform, and a variety of sizes of half-balls to which the platform is attached. The size of half-ball selected for an exercise depends on the patient's range of motion and the goal of the exercise. Patients may begin by sitting in a chair and placing the involved foot on the board to perform active range-of-motion exercises. They can advance to weight bearing on two extremities and then weight bearing on only the involved extremity to do full range-of-motion exercises for the ankle (figure 22.45). Once the patient has attained full range of motion and control on the BAPS board, you can add weights to the board to provide resistance to specific muscle groups. You can also use the board as a proprioception exercise device by having the patient stand on only the involved limb and slowly perform controlled isolated motions of inversion-eversion or plantar flexion-dorsiflexion.

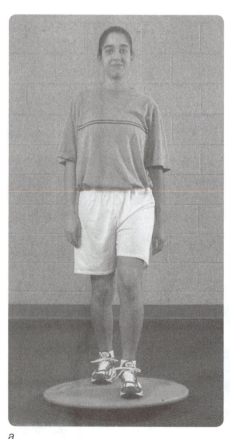 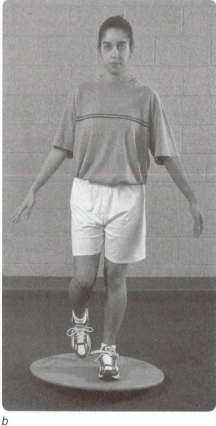

a   *b*

▶ **Figure 22.45** BAPS board: *(a)* double-leg support, *(b)* single-leg support.

Additional Active-Motion Exercises

Cardiovascular exercises that can be used to improve ankle range of motion while simultaneously contributing to cardiovascular fitness include exercises on the stationary bike and the cross-country ski machine (figure 22.46). Both machines facilitate range of motion of the ankle, especially when the patient has received careful instruction in proper exercise execution. You should teach the patient ankling on the bike: dorsiflexing the ankle on extremity lift and plantar flexing the ankle on the downstroke. On the cross-country ski machine, the patient should attempt to push off from the posterior extremity by lifting the heel, and bearing weight on the ball of the foot before pulling the extremity and ankle forward and upward.

There are many flexibility exercises for the ankle, foot, and leg. Among those often used are gastrocnemius, soleus, and Achilles stretches; ankle exercises the patient can do throughout the day; and BAPS board exercises.

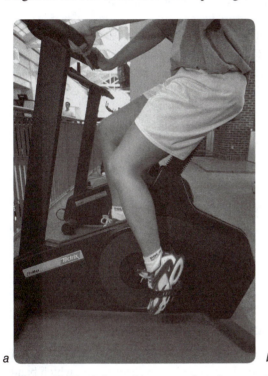
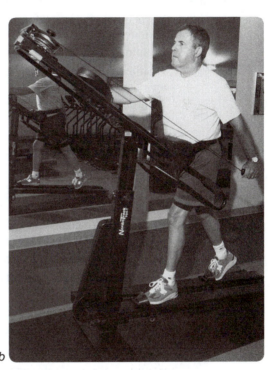

a   b

▶ **Figure 22.46** Other ankle range-of-motion exercises: *(a)* on stationary bike, *(b)* on cross-country skier.

STRENGTHENING EXERCISES

Strengthening exercises that can be used earliest in a rehabilitation program include isometrics. The patient can perform these even while the foot is in a cast or immobilizer. Normal progression is to isotonics and isokinetics. Isotonic exercises include those using resistance bands, free weights, machine weights, and body resistance. Isokinetic exercises usually do not start until the patient's foot and ankle have sufficient strength to control isotonic activities. The following sections provide examples of some of the more commonly used strengthening exercises for the ankle, foot, and toes in the early part of a rehabilitation program.

■ Early Strength Exercises for the Foot and Ankle

Isometric Inversion

Body Segment: Subtalar joint.

Stage in Rehab: Late I and early II.

Purpose: Strengthen ankle invertors.

Positioning: Patient sits with the medial aspect of the foot against a table leg.

Execution: Patient pushes the medial foot against the table leg, attempting to invert the ankle. The ankle does not move, and the patient should feel muscles working on the medial leg.

Possible Substitutions: Hip abduction, hip rotation, and tibial rotation.

Notations: Isometrics are held at the maximum contraction for 6 s, with a slow buildup and release of the force so that the total contraction is about 10 s long.

Isometric Inversion

Body Segment: Subtalar joint.

Stage in Rehab: Late I, early II.

Purpose: Strengthen peroneals.

Positioning: Patient sits with the lateral aspect of the foot against a table leg.

Execution: Patient pushes the lateral foot against the table leg, attempting to evert the ankle. The ankle does not move, and the patient should feel muscles working on the lateral leg.

Possible Substitutions: Hip abduction, hip rotation, and tibial rotation.

Notations: Isometrics are held at the maximum contraction for 6 s, with a slow buildup and release of the force so that the total contraction is about 10 s long.

Isometric Dorsiflexion

Body Segment: Talocrural joint.

Stage in Rehab: Late I, early II.

Purpose: Strengthen dorsiflexor muscles, especially tibialis anterior.

Positioning: Patient sits with uninvolved heel on top of the involved foot.

Execution: The patient pushes the involved foot upward against the top foot, attempting to dorsiflex the ankle against the opposite foot (figure 22.47).

Possible Substitutions: Hip flexion and foot eversion.

Notations: Isometrics are held at the maximum contraction for 6 s, with a slow buildup and release of the force so that the total contraction is about 10 s long.

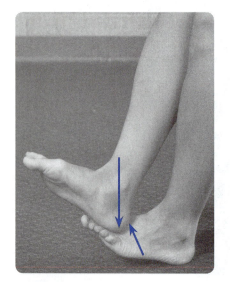

▶ **Figure 22.47** Isometric exercise for dorsiflexion.

Resistance-Band Exercises

Because the various ankle muscle groups have different strengths, you must examine the patient's strength for each exercise before determining which band's resistance is most appropriate for obtaining the desired results from the resistive exercise. Normally, ankle plantar flexors are the strongest, and ankle evertors are the weakest. Injured ankles have reduced levels of strength in all motions, but most of the time, the proportional strength remains close to normal. In other words, even though a patient's ankle has less-than-normal strength, the plantar flexors are still the strongest muscle group and the ankle evertors the weakest. Resistance-band exercises are included in the following sections.

Resistance-Band Eversion

Body Segment: Subtalar joint.

Stage in Rehab: Early II.

Purpose: Strengthen evertors.

Positioning: The patient sits in a chair, with the band around the forefoot and anchored to a table leg near the uninvolved extremity.

Execution: The ankle begins in inversion and is moved against the band into a full range of eversion (figure 22.48a).

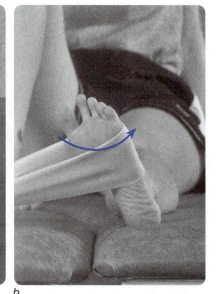

a   *b*

▶ **Figure 22.48** Band exercises: *(a)* eversion, *(b)* eversion in long sitting.

Possible Substitutions: Hip abduction and rotation. To eliminate substitutions, you should instruct the patient in the proper technique and caution against moving the knee. Placing the hands on either side of the knee to stabilize the thigh also reduces substitutions.

Notations: These exercises can be performed with either manual resistance or pulleys. The patient can also perform this exercise in a long sitting position, but it is more difficult to stabilize the thigh and avoid hip substitutions in this position (figure 22.48b).

Resistance-Band Inversion

Body Segment: Subtalar joint.

Stage in Rehab: Early II.

Purpose: Strengthen ankle inverters.

Positioning: The patient sits in a chair with the band around the forefoot and anchored to a table leg near the involved side.

Execution: Patient starts with the ankle in full eversion and moves it into a full range of motion to end-range inversion (figure 22.48c).

Possible Substitutions: Hip adduction and rotation. To eliminate substitutions, you should instruct the patient in the proper technique and caution against moving the knee. Placing the hands on either side of the knee to stabilize the thigh also reduces substitutions.

Notations: These exercises can be performed with either manual resistance or pulleys. The patient can also perform this exercise in a long sitting position, but it is more difficult to stabilize the thigh and avoid hip substitutions in this position.

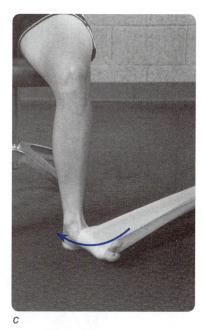

c

▶ **Figure 22.48** Band exercise: *(c)* inversion.

Resistance-Band Dorsiflexion

Body Segment: Talocrural joint.

Stage in Rehab: Early II.

Purpose: Increase strength of dorsiflexors.

Positioning: The patient sits with the band around the forefoot and anchored to a table leg, which the patient faces.

Execution: The patient pulls the foot toward the shin, dorsiflexing the ankle (figure 22.48d).

Possible Substitutions: Hip or knee flexion is the most common substitution.

Notations: These exercises can also be performed with either manual resistance or pulleys.

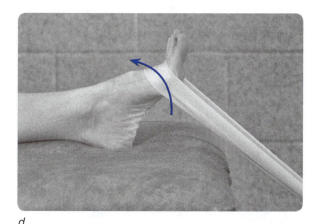

d

▶ **Figure 22.48** Band exercise: *(d)* dorsiflexion.

Resistance-Band Plantar Flexion

Body Segment: Talocrural joint.

Stage in Rehab: Early II.

Purpose: Strengthen ankle plantar flexors when patient is non-weight bearing.

Positioning: The patient is in a long sitting position with the band around the plantar foot and grasped in both hands.

Execution: Patient maintains a firm tension on the band. Starting with the foot in full dorsiflexion, the patient pushes the foot against the band to move the ankle into full plantar flexion (figure 22.48e).

Possible Substitutions: Going through an incomplete range of motion.

Notations: This exercise can also be performed with the knee in flexion and the patient sitting on a table with his or her extremity hanging off the table. In this position, plantar-flexion motion isolates and strengthens

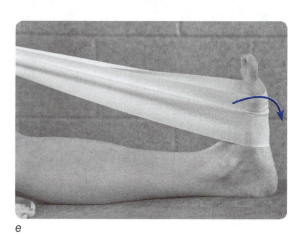

e

▶ **Figure 22.48** Band exercise: *(e)* plantar flexion.

the soleus muscle. If the patient has good strength in the early ranges of plantar flexion but is unable to stand in full plantar flexion, the band can be used to facilitate strength in the weak part of the motion. To do this, the patient places the foot in the weak range of motion and positions the band around the plantar foot. While the patient maintains the ankle position, he or she increases tension on the band by pulling on it with the arms to provide the resistance in the weak position. Maintaining good tension on the band, the patient slowly dorsiflexes the ankle to facilitate an eccentric contraction of the plantar flexors. This technique can be used to isolate weak positions in the other motions as well.

Toe Exercises

Strengthening toe muscles helps to restore optimal foot function. Both intrinsic and extrinsic toe muscles are strengthened with these exercises. The long toe muscles can also add support to the ankle. Some of these exercises are presented in the following sections.

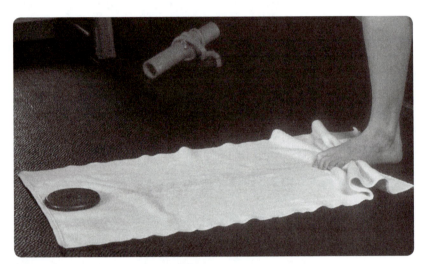

a

▶ **Figure 22.49**　Toe exercise: *(a)* towel roll.

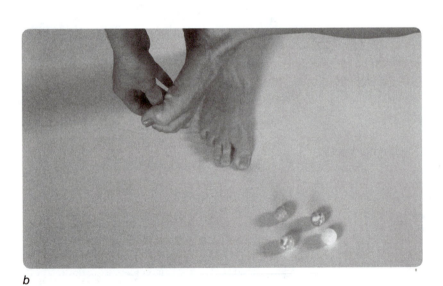

b

▶ **Figure 22.49**　Toe exercise: *(b)* marble pickup.

Towel Roll

Body Segment: Toes.

Stage in Rehab: Late I, early II.

Purpose: Strengthen intrinsic toe flexors.

Positioning: The patient sits on a chair with a towel placed on the floor in front of the chair.

Execution: Without shoes and socks on, the patient curls the toes to pull the far end of the towel toward the foot (figure 22.49). The thigh should not move during the exercise.

Possible Substitutions: Using the heel to pull the towel or flexing the knee to pull the towel.

Notations: Resistance can be added by placing a weight at the far end of the towel, using a wet towel, or using a newspaper. This exercise should be performed on a smooth surface such as a wood or vinyl floor, not on carpeting.

Marble Pickup

Body Segment: Toes.

Stage in Rehab: Late I, early II.

Purpose: Strengthen toe intrinsic and extrinsic muscles, facilitate ankle inverters and evertors.

Positioning: Patient is sitting or standing.

Execution: The patient uses the toes to pick up marbles that have been placed on the floor. The marbles are placed in the hand on the same side to facilitate eversion and in the hand on the opposite side to facilitate inversion (figure 22.49).

Possible Substitutions: Not moving the toes or ankle through full motion during the exercise.

Notations: Objects such as a pencil, pieces of paper, or a towel can be used in place of the marbles.

Body-Weight Resistance Exercises

Exercises for both the gastrocnemius and soleus are necessary for complete restoration of strength. Exercises already mentioned for the long toe extensors also help to strengthen the posterior muscles. Body weight is an excellent form of resistance that strengthens many body segments, including the ankle and foot. These exercises are introduced during phase II of the rehabilitation program once full weight bearing is permitted.

Heel Raises

This exercise strengthens the calf muscles. With feet about shoulder-width apart, the patient rises up on the toes as high as possible and then returns to feet flat on the floor. This exercise is more difficult when performed on an incline (figure 22.50) or on the edge of a stair, and also when it is performed on only the involved extremity. Common substitutions include using the hamstrings by flexing the knees during the heel raise, moving the body forward or rocking rather than moving straight upward, and placing most of the body weight on the uninvolved extremity rather than equally distributing the weight over both extremities.

Weigh-Scale Exercise

If the patient has difficulty bearing weight on the involved extremity, or is apprehensive about transferring weight onto that side, a weigh scale is an effective tool for teaching weight transfer and for helping the individual gain confidence in the involved extremity as well as improving strength.

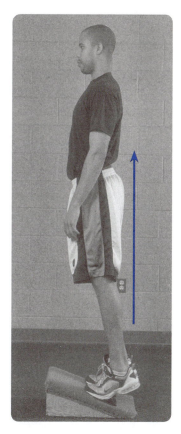

▶ **Figure 22.50** Heel raise on an incline.

This exercise uses a balance weight scale and a platform of height equal to that of the scale's foot plate. The platform is placed next to the scale. The patient stands with the uninvolved extremity on the platform and the involved extremity on the scale, and initially stands with most weight on the uninvolved extremity (figure 22.51). The scale balance is moved to a desired weight for the exercise. The patient is instructed to transfer enough weight to the involved side to move the balance arm to the top of the scale and then maintain the balance arm in the up position while performing a heel raise. As the patient's strength improves, the weight on the scale is increased until the patient is able to perform a single-extremity heel raise with full body weight. The most common substitution during this exercise is shifting the body weight to the uninvolved extremity as the patient begins to go up on the toes.

This exercise is also good for weight-transfer instruction for early gait training. The technique is similar, but the instruction is to shift body weight from the left to the right lower extremity. The scale weight is increased as the patient improves in ability to transfer weight properly. Substitutions on this activity occur commonly if a patient has been non-weight bearing for a while or is very weak in the involved extremity. The most frequently seen substitution is keeping the weight shifted to the uninvolved side but rotating the trunk toward the involved extremity. Hesitancy and reluctance to shift weight onto the involved extremity are common events as well; in these cases, it is better to start with a low percentage, such as 25%, of the individual's body weight on the scale. This way, the patient gains confidence in realizing the extremity is able to tolerate the body weight and performs the activity correctly.

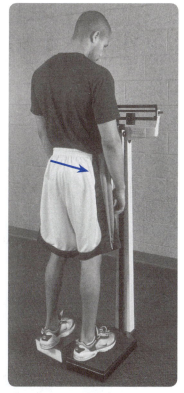

▶ **Figure 22.51** Weigh-scale exercises are used to teach weight transfer and to increase strength of the involved extremity.

Strengthening activities for the foot and ankle include isometrics, rubber-tubing activities, exercises specifically for the toes, body-weight resistance for the ankle and foot, and resistance with equipment.

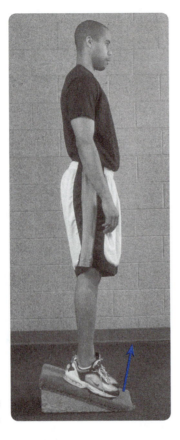

▶ **Figure 22.52** Toe raise on an incline.

Toe Raise

This exercise increases strength of the ankle dorsiflexors. The patient stands on an incline with the heel on the higher aspect of the incline. Keeping the heels in contact with the incline, he or she lifts the toes and forefoot upward and off the incline (figure 22.52). If this exercise is too difficult, the patient first performs the exercise on the floor. Using the incline requires the muscles to work through a greater range of motion and increases the difficulty of the exercise. Common substitutions include hip flexion, forward trunk flexion, and body sway. For optimal results, correct improper execution and provide verbal cueing or tactile stimulation to facilitate proper performance.

Equipment Resistance

In addition to body weight, several kinds of equipment can be used to strengthen the ankle and foot. Presented here are a few of the possibilities.

Free Weights

Cuff weights can be used in strengthening exercises for ankle inversion, eversion, and dorsiflexion. The patient, placed in an antigravity position for the muscle being exercised with the cuff weight wrapped around the midfoot, moves the ankle through a full range of motion. For dorsiflexion, the position is sitting (figure 22.53a). For inversion and eversion, the position is sidelying on the involved side and on the uninvolved side, respectively (figure 22.53b).

Machine Weights

Calf raises in the standing and seated positions using machines strengthen the gastrocnemius and soleus, respectively. Standing calf raises can be performed on machines designed specifically for that exercise, or on machines such as an upright press, bench press, or squat machine that can be modified for use as a calf-raise machine. A seated heel-raise exercise to isolate the soleus muscle can be performed on a hamstring-curl machine.

The difficulty of these exercises is increased by placing an incline under the foot in the seated heel raise or having the patient on a step in the standing heel raise. These modifications require the muscle to move through a greater range of motion, increasing the exercise difficulty.

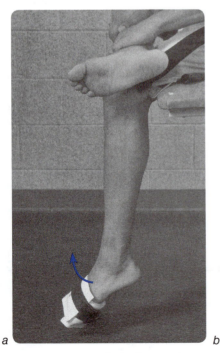

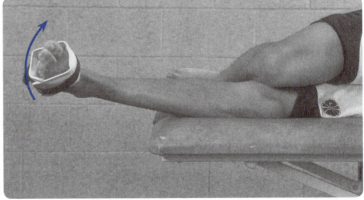

a *b*

▶ **Figure 22.53** Cuff-weight exercises: *(a)* dorsiflexion, *(b)* inversion. The weight is lifted through a full range of motion.

PROPRIOCEPTION EXERCISES

Proprioception is fundamental for kinesthesia and balance control. Research shows that deficits in these areas exist following ankle sprains, especially chronic ankle sprains (Forkin, Koczur, Battle, & Newton, 1996; Lofvenberg, Karrholm, Sundelin, & Ahlgren, 1995; Refshauge, Kilbreath, & Raymond, 2000; Willems, Witvrouw, Verstuyft, Vaes, & De Clercq, 2002). Posture and balance, important factors in controlling ankle stability, can be improved with rehabilitation (Bernier & Perrin, 1998; Hale, Hertel, & Olmsted-Kramer, 2007). It is important, then, to include proprioception exercises in an ankle rehabilitation program. If a patient is non-weight bearing, early kinesthetic exercises can include mirroring activities with the two ankles, with the patient's eyes closed. The alphabet exercise mentioned earlier can also help improve kinesthetic awareness.

Once the patient is weight bearing, additional proprioception exercises can be incorporated into the program. One of the beginning weight-bearing exercises is a tandem stance with the involved foot directly behind the uninvolved foot so the front foot's heel touches the back foot's toes. This position should be held for 30 s with no loss of balance. Another beginning exercise is the stork stand. The patient stands on the involved extremity while attempting to maintain balance for 30 s (figure 22.54). Having accomplished this, the individual performs the exercise with eyes closed to eliminate the visual component of balance. The next level is to have the patient stork stand on an unstable surface, such as a trampoline, a foam roller, or a 1/2 roller (figure 22.55).

To progress to more advanced balance activities, the patient either attempts to maintain balance while performing another activity with another body part to divert attention away from concentration on balance or performs additional activity with the lower extremity while maintaining balance. For example, a football receiver or softball or baseball player catches a medicine ball while balancing on a foam roller or trampoline. The ball is thrown at different

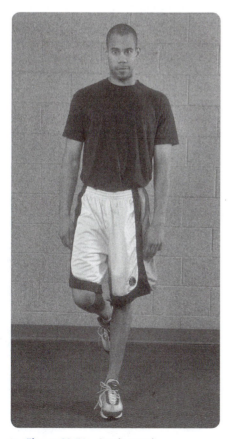

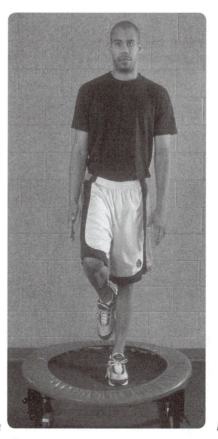

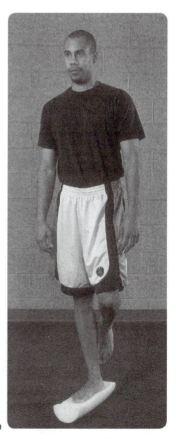

a

b

▶ **Figure 22.54** Stork stand.

▶ **Figure 22.55** Advanced stork-stand exercises: *(a)* on trampoline, *(b)* on foam roller.

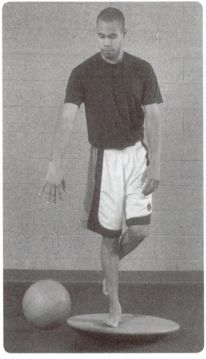

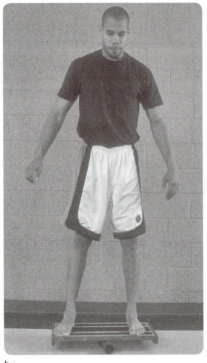

a

b

▶ **Figure 22.56** Advanced balance exercises: *(a)* sports activity on unstable surface, *(b)* balance board.

levels and to different sides of the body so the patient must move to reach for the ball and still maintain balance. If the patient is a basketball player, bouncing a ball while maintaining balance on an unstable surface is a good activity (figure 22.56a). Setting a volleyball while stork standing on an uneven surface diverts the volleyball player's conscious effort from balance to enhance autonomic responses for balance.

Various kinds of balance boards can be either made or purchased. Wobble boards, circle boards, BAPS boards, or balance boards can be used for balance activities. A board placed on top of a PVC pipe is a simple balance board. In an exercise with this type of board, the patient attempts to keep the ends of the board off the floor (figure 22.56b). This exercise becomes more difficult if the patient intentionally rolls the board side to side while keeping the ends of the board off the floor. This exercise becomes more difficult if smaller-diameter PVC pipes are used so that the ends of the board are closer to the floor.

Once the patient demonstrates good balance, he or she advances to more complex exercises that require any combination of balance, agility, control, coordination, and strength. These exercises include activities with equipment such as the Fitter, resistance band, slide board, and boxes. The Fitter and slide board develop eccentric and concentric strength and proprioception of the intrinsic and extrinsic muscles (figure 22.57a). These exercises can also assist in cardiovascular development.

Increased resistance exercises include using bands attached to the waist as the patient begins with left-to-right lateral or forward-backward jumps and progresses to single-extremity lateral and forward-backward jumps (figure 22.57b). Resistance-band exercises facilitate concentric strength, eccentric strength, power, control, coordination, and agility.

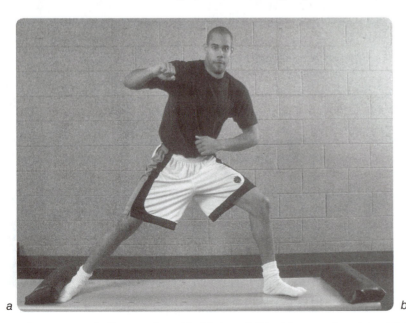

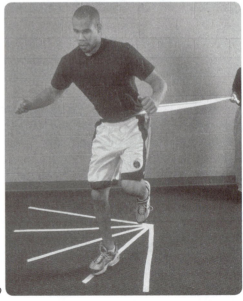

a

b

▶ **Figure 22.57** Agility exercises: *(a)* slide board, *(b)* tubing exercise—lateral, left-to-right hopping activity.

Plyometric exercises use box activities to promote power and agility. Patients can perform various plyometric exercises created and designed by the rehabilitation clinician. Generic examples of these activities include rapid lateral jumping (figure 22.58a), rapid front-to-side agility step-ups (figure 22.58b), and multidirectional-change jumps (figure 22.58, c–d). Plyometric jumps can then advance to lateral high jumps (figure 22.58e) and box drop-jumps. For additional suggestions on plyometric exercises for the lower extremities, refer to chapter 9.

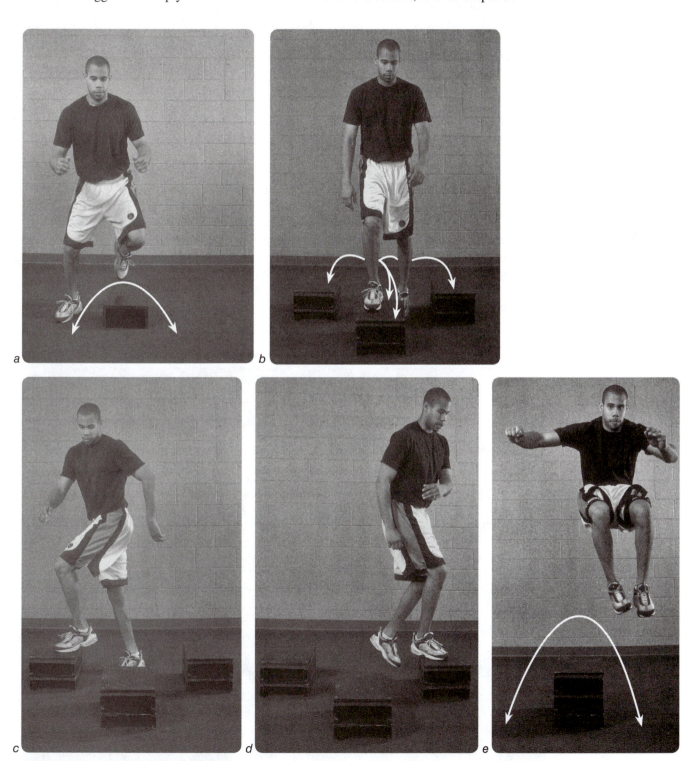

▶ **Figure 22.58** Plyometric box activities: *(a)* jump-over side-to-side, *(b)* alternate jumps side-to-front-to-side, *(c-d)* rapid sequencing from one box to another, *(e)* lateral high jumps.

Treadmill Activities

The treadmill can be used for more than gait analysis, walking, and running. It is useful in identifying subtle differences between the involved and the uninvolved extremity during running. Besides using the treadmill to visually observe walking and running mechanics, you can use it as an auditory tool for defining running abnormalities. Listening to the foot hit the treadmill surface becomes a comparative tool; if the patient's feet do not sound the same at impact, it is likely that the individual has a different pattern between the involved and uninvolved extremity. Increasing the speed of the treadmill reveals and exaggerates differences in stride, gait, and weight transfer that you may not see at slower speeds.

The treadmill may also be used for facilitation, range-of-motion, strength, agility, and coordination exercises. Walking backward on a treadmill—retro walking (figure 22.59a)—has been shown to increase range of motion and muscle activity demands on the knee and ankle (Cipriani, Armstrong, & Gaul, 1995). In retro walking, ankle dorsiflexion needs are increased, greater eccentric activity is required of the gastrocnemius, and the anterior tibialis also is more active. Many believe that these increased demands aid in facilitating the kinesthetic system and that they improve lower-extremity proprioception (Cipriani et al., 1995; Willems et al., 2002). Varying the speed of the treadmill also alters demands on the muscles.

Agility and coordination exercises on the treadmill include activities such as side shuffles and cariocas going in each left and right direction (figure 22.59b). The patient may start with sets of 30 s bouts in each direction and then increase the time on each bout or increase the number of times the bout is repeated as goals are achieved and endurance improves. Requiring the patient to make more rapid changes from left side to right side increases the agility demands of the exercise. Inclining the treadmill surface or increasing the speed also increases the difficulty.

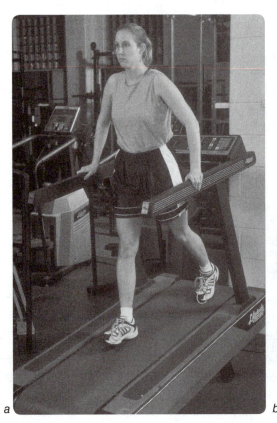
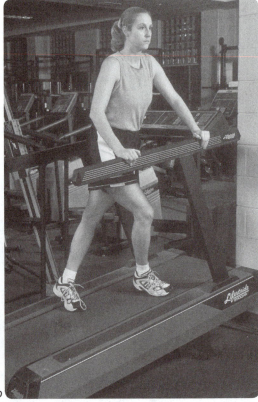

a   b

▶ **Figure 22.59** Treadmill activities: *(a)* retro walking on an incline, *(b)* carioca on an incline.

Hopping Activities

Hopping exercises are often a necessary part of an ankle rehabilitation program because many athletic events include some type of hopping or jumping. These exercises begin on a soft, force-absorbing surface such as a trampoline or mat and then advance to the patient's normal playing-field surface. Many different combinations of hopping activities are possible. Which specific patterns to select may depend on the patient's specific sport requirements, the injured ankle's deficiencies, and general conditioning demands. Some examples of patterns include box hops, side-to-side hops, forward-backward hops, cross-pattern hops, high hops, long hops, zigzag hops, and circular hops. Some of these are presented as suggestions in figure 22.60. Patients may begin with two-legged jumps and advance to one-legged hops. They may also alternate extremities or perform hops in combinations, such as two on the left and then two on the right, or two on the injured side and then one on the uninjured side.

Proprioception is an important part of any ankle rehabilitation program. Proprioceptive exercises for posture and balance help improve ankle stability.

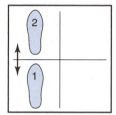

Forward-backward hop: Hop forward and backward between two quadrants.

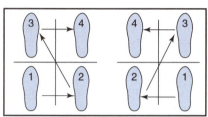

Cross-pattern hop: Hop in an X pattern.

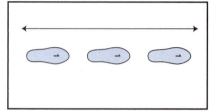

Straight-line hop: Hop forward and then backward along a 15- to 20-ft line.

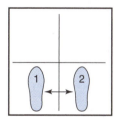

Side-to-side hop: Hop laterally between two quadrants.

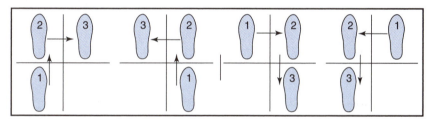

Triangular hop: Hop within three different quadrants. There are four triangles, each requiring a different diagonal hop.

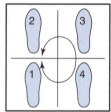

Circular hop: Hop from square to square in a circular pattern. Sets are performed clockwise and counterclockwise.

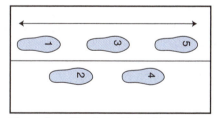

Zigzag hop: Hop from side to side across a 15- to 20-ft line while moving forward and then backward.

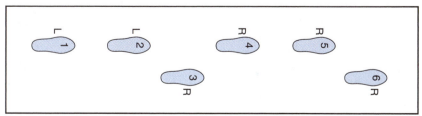

Mixed patterns: Various combination hop patterns can be used, such as two on the injured (i.e., left) side and one on the uninjured (i.e., right) side.

▶ **Figure 22.60** Suggestions for hopping patterns. You can design a number of hopping patterns, limited only by your imagination.

By the end of the rehabilitation program, a patient with a foot or ankle injury must be able to perform functional activities—for example, zigzag runs and 90° cuts to the left and right—without hesitation, smoothly, and efficiently.

FUNCTIONAL AND ACTIVITY-SPECIFIC EXERCISES

As the patient nears reentry into full participation, functional, then activity-specific exercises must become a part of the complete rehabilitation program so the patient's return to normal activity is smooth and uneventful. As mentioned throughout this book, functional activities are precursor exercises to activity-specific exercises and are designed to stress those muscles and joints used in activity-specific exercises while activity-specific exercises actually mimic the patient's activity once he or she returns to normal function. Activity-specific exercises (or drills) are also a reliable means of final examination of the patient's ability to perform accurately and safely (Bolgla & Keskula, 1997; Greenberger & Paterno, 1995).

Activity-specific exercises for individuals will vary for patients in lower-extremity sports, but many running sports include many of the same functional activities. These include activities such as single, double, or triple hops; zigzag runs with rapid changes in direction; backward running; sprinting; running circles in clockwise, counterclockwise, backward, and forward directions; 90° cuts to the left and to the right; and running figure 8s. The patient should be able to perform the functional and activity-specific exercises without hesitation, smoothly in both directions and without favoring the involved extremity, and rapidly and efficiently.

Functional exercises advance to activity-specific drills and skill activities that are unique to the demands of each patient. You must have an appreciation and understanding of each patient's activities so that you can incorporate correct drills and exercises into the final phase of the patient's rehabilitation program.

SPECIAL REHABILITATION APPLICATIONS

This section deals with specific injuries to the foot and ankle. Injuries to the extremity, especially the ankle, are among the most common orthopedic injuries. Some—certainly not all—of the more frequently seen injuries are discussed in the following sections.

Ankle Sprain or Dislocation

An ankle dislocation and ankle sprain are on the same continuum since they involve the same structures but differ in severity, so we will consider these two injuries together. As with other sprains, the severity determines the rate of rehabilitation progression and the time when various therapeutic exercises begin. The more extensive the injury and the consequent tissue damage, the less aggressive the program is, especially in the initial stages. It is important for the rehabilitation clinician to understand healing concepts and timelines and to assess the severity of the injury before proceeding with a rehabilitation program.

Discoloration is the result of bleeding in the area. It is generally a sign of the severity of the sprain as well. If no discoloration occurs, the sprain is likely to be mild, or first degree, and the patient's other symptoms should be consistent with this assessment. If discoloration occurs, at least a second-degree sprain is present. Instability indicates a possible third-degree sprain of at least one ligament. Rehabilitation for second- and third-degree sprains proceeds more slowly than for first-degree sprains. A first-degree ankle sprain may restrict the patient from normal activities for no more than one week, with return to full participation in two to three weeks or less, but a second-degree sprain may restrict the patient from participation for three weeks and full participation for four to six weeks (Glascoe, Allen, Awtry, & Yack, 1999). Third-degree ankle sprains vary widely in recovery times, which may depend, at least, on the course of treatment provided (Konradsen, Holmer, & Sondergaard, 1991). Third-degree sprains can take as little as six weeks or as much as three or more months to improve before the patient can return to full participation.

Third-degree sprains and dislocations can be treated either conservatively with rehabilitation or with surgery and rehabilitation. The choice is often made according to the patient's objective and subjective findings, age, level of sport participation, and surgeon's preference.

Ankle instabilities may be surgically repaired. Studies show that early rehabilitation with controlled weight bearing in a boot, with early active-motion and therapeutic exercise, yields better results than the more conservative approach of prolonged casting with a slower initiation of rehabilitation (Gillogly, Myers, & Reinold, 2006; Glascoe et al., 1999; Konradsen et al., 1991).

The patient's ability to recover from an ankle sprain is dependent on the history of prior injuries. Multiple episodes of ankle sprains may result in an unstable ankle, making the rehabilitation process more complex and more difficult. The clinician must obtain an accurate history from the patient before instituting a therapeutic exercise program, because a prior history of ankle sprains can alter the program progression and anticipated results if considerations are not given for this.

Chronic ankle sprains also affect other factors. One of these is additional scar tissue with probable adhesions that limits joint mobility and soft-tissue mobility. Repeated ankle sprains can result in chronic muscle weakness and reduced kinesthetic awareness, making the ankle susceptible to additional injury (Garn & Newton, 1988; Konradsen, 2002; Monaghan, Delahunt, & Caulfield, 2006; Willems et al., 2002). Chronic ankle sprains may also lead to compensatory changes with alterations in gait, strength, and flexibility, reducing the mechanical effectiveness of the ankle and foot. Because of these additional factors, chronic ankle sprains require more time to properly rehabilitate and achieve an appropriate recovery status (Seto & Brewster, 1994).

Most ankle sprains are inversion sprains. The specific ankle ligaments and structures involved and the severity of the injury depend on the mechanical forces applied and the angle of stress application. Ankle sprains may also involve other structures; for example, there may be an avulsion fracture of the malleoli, peroneal strains or dislocations, or other tendon injuries.

Of the ankle ligaments, the anterior talofibular is the most commonly injured ligament, and the calcaneofibular is the next most commonly injured ligament.

Occasionally, the tibiofibular ligament is injured. This is known as a syndesmosis ankle sprain, or a "high ankle sprain." This ligament injury deserves careful consideration. The function of the tibiofibular ligament is to hold the tibia and fibula in alignment and formation of the ankle mortise joint. When weight is borne on the extremity, the force tends to spread the two bones apart. If the tibiofibular ligament is injured, repetitive stress with weight bearing may inhibit the healing process. If this ligament is injured, the patient should be instructed in non-weight bearing or partial weight bearing on crutches to ambulate pain free until full weight bearing does not cause pain (Lin, Gross, & Weinhold, 2006). If this is not done, the ligament can develop chronic inflammation and can become difficult to treat successfully.

More typical ankle sprains permit weight bearing to tolerance. The rule of thumb is that if the patient is able to ambulate without limping, crutches are not required; however, if pain or dysfunction causes an abnormal gait, crutches with either partial or non-weight bearing are used. In most cases, weight bearing can be partial, to tolerance.

Control of edema and pain occurs in rehabilitation phase I and is the first priority, as with any injury. Common methods of reducing edema and pain include the use of ice and other modalities, such as electrical stimulation, along with strapping or bracing. Active range-of-motion exercises are instituted early, usually within the first three days, to restore ankle range of motion. Joint mobilization and soft-tissue mobilization techniques are used as indicated and on the basis of the assessment before treatment. Grades I and II are used within the first few days to relieve pain while grades III and IV are used later, in phase III or late phase II, to restore joint motion. With chronic sprains, it is common to observe scar-tissue adhesions in the joints and surrounding tissue. Sometimes intertarsal and metatarsal joints become restricted, especially if the patient used an immobilizer boot or a cast following earlier injuries.

Non-weight-bearing exercises are used early in the therapeutic exercise program for early strengthening in the initial part of phase II. These include isometric exercises, aquatic exercises, and manual resistance as tolerated. The BAPS board used in a seated position provides AROM during partial weight-bearing periods.

Ankle inversion-eversion strength is important to ankle stability. Exercises for muscles controlling these movements must certainly be included among therapeutic exercises for a sprained ankle. Isometrics, manual resistance, pulleys, rubber tubing/bands, and aquatic exercises can all provide good strengthening activities for these groups during phase II. Closed kinetic chain exercises for inversion and eversion movements during phase II make strengthening of these motions more functional and enhance proprioceptive gains.

Once full weight bearing is pain free, gait training and closed kinetic chain exercises produce additional strength and coordination. Balance activities progress from stork standing on the floor to stork standing on a 1/2 foam roller, trampoline, or other unstable surface. Initial closed chain strengthening exercises begin with low resistance, repetitions, and sets, and increase to more resistance, repetitions, and sets as the patient's ability and tolerance progresses. Early closed chain activities are performed slowly and in a controlled manner, but as the patient gains strength and control of the ankle, quicker movements requiring greater control and strength are added. This progression places demands on strength as well as the balance, coordination, and agility systems. When the patient has full, pain-free motion and approximately 90% strength, plyometrics are added to the program. The final phase includes functional activities, then activity-specific activities before return to full participation. A timeline of rehabilitation progression is outlined in figure 22.61.

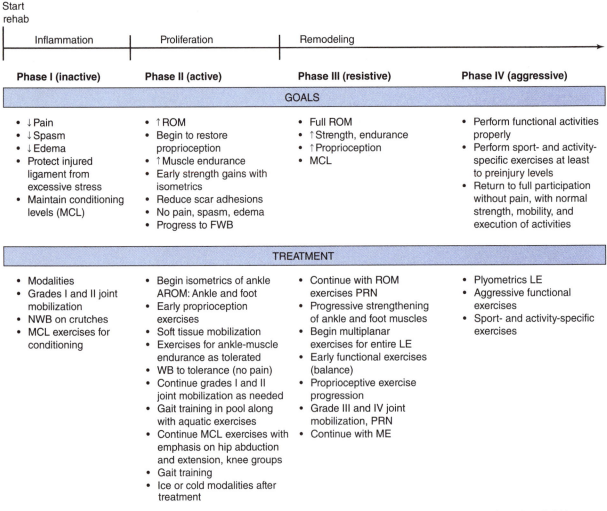

▶ **Figure 22.61** Rehabilitation progression for syndesmosis ankle sprain. AROM = active range of motion; ROM = range of motion; NWB = non-weight bearing; WB = weight bearing; FWB = full weight bearing; LE = lower extremity.

Throughout the progression, you must watch for signs of increased inflammatory response indicating that too much stress is being applied to the ankle. These signs include post-exercise swelling, and pain either during or after the treatment session. If these signs are present, you should reduce the severity of the program for one to three days, then try advancing the patient again to the next level of exercise difficulty.

It is advisable to have the patient refrain from wearing a protective brace during therapeutic exercises, but he or she may choose to use a supportive ankle device before returning to full and normal participation. During therapeutic exercises, the patient performs activities under controlled circumstances and in a restricted environment so risk of injury is reduced; but when returning to participation, he or she performs in an unpredictable environment, which creates an increased risk of injuring scar tissue that has less-than-maximum tensile strength. Because it may take a year or more for the tensile strength of injured tissue to achieve maximal levels, it is advisable for the patient to have the additional protection of ankle supports. A number of studies have demonstrated increased ankle stability of formerly injured ankles with these devices (Gross, Bradshaw, Ventry, & Weller, 1987; Karlsson & Andreasson, 1992; Kimura, Nawoczenski, Epler, & Owen, 1987; Renström, Konradsen, & Beynnon, 2000; Rovere, Clarke, Yates, & Burley, 1988; Sitler et al., 1994).

■ Case Study

A 16-year-old volleyball hitter jumped up for a hit and landed on another player's foot, causing an inversion sprain to the right ankle three days ago. She felt a pop and had immediate swelling. She was unable to bear weight on the ankle at the time. X-rays were negative, but the patient was placed on crutches, with weight bearing to tolerance. Ice, elevation, and taping have been applied periodically for the past three days, but the patient comes to you today to start her rehabilitation program. She denies any previous ankle injury. So far she has performed only alphabet exercises because it was too painful for her to do anything else. She can bear about 11 kg (25 lb) of weight on the foot in standing before she complains of pain in the lateral ankle and above the ankle joint. Her pain is located over the anterior talofibular, anterior tibiofibular, and calcaneofibular joints, with most of the pain over the first two ligaments. She has moderate swelling of the ankle, foot, and toes, with ecchymosis over the midfoot to the toes. She is able to wiggle her toes through about 50% normal motion. Her ankle range of motion is at 45° of plantar flexion, 10° of inversion with pain, 10° of eversion, and −10° dorsiflexion and is painful. Her ankle strength is restricted by pain on dorsiflexion and inversion. Since she is unable to bear weight on the foot, you cannot assess antigravity strength of the calf. You are easily able to overcome plantar flexion with manual resistance. Eversion is 4/5. Joint mobility is normal. Soft-tissue mobility is limited by the edema present, but you are unable to palpate any abnormal soft-tissue restriction.

Questions for Analysis

1. List, in order of priority, what her problems are and establish short-term and long-term goals for each of them.

2. What treatment will you provide for the patient today?

3. What home instructions will you give her?

4. What precautions will you give her?

5. What will be your guidelines for deciding when she can begin resistive weight-bearing exercises?

6. List three agility exercises that you will include in the patient's program when she is able to do them.

7. What will your functional testing include before her return to full sport participation?

Peroneal Tendon Dislocation

Peroneal tendon dislocations can often be overlooked, probably because they frequently occur in conjunction with other injuries (Alanen, Orava, Heinonen, Ikonen, & Kvist, 2001). For this reason, they are also frustrating to resolve unless discovered through the use of good evaluation techniques.

Peroneal tendon dislocation occurs most commonly through two mechanisms, ankle dorsiflexion with active peroneal contraction, and an inversion sprain (Baumhauer, Shereff, & Gould, 1997). In an inversion ankle sprain, the peroneal tendons are most susceptible to dislocation with the ankle in 15° to 25° of plantar flexion. This position places the tendons in a tenuous position along the distal fibula. If an inversion ankle sprain occurs with the ankle in less than 15° plantar flexion, the peroneal retinaculum can be stretched, leading to instability of the peroneal tendons. Skiers are commonly subjected to these injuries. If the ankle is in more than 25° of plantar flexion, the peroneal tendons move into a deep-seated position posterior to the fibular head and are stable in that position with little chance of dislocation.

Peroneal dislocations are usually self-reduced once the ankle is in a non-stressed position. The patient typically complains of a painful, snapping sensation in the posterolateral ankle with walking or ankle circumduction (Safran, O'Malley Jr, & Fu, 1999). Swelling along the tendon is sometimes observable. Treatment includes controlling the inflammation with modalities. Stabilization of the tendons with taping and pad support can sometimes help to relieve the subluxation episodes. If conservative treatment fails to prevent recurrent dislocations, surgical repair is necessary (Krause & Brodsky, 1998).

Postoperative care includes soft-tissue massage around the surgical site to reduce soft-tissue adhesions in the area once the sutures have been removed. Joint mobilization techniques should be used in areas that demonstrate restricted joint mobility. Active range of motion is permitted anywhere from 10 to 21 days postoperatively. Ankle plantar flexion and eversion are motions that cause the least disruption of the tendons and can take place passively relatively early in the program.

Once weight bearing is permitted in phase II, the exercises and progression mentioned earlier for other ankle and extremity injuries can begin. A weigh-scale weight-bearing progression can be useful in helping the patient gain confidence in the injured extremity. Balance activities once the patient is fully weight bearing begin with a stork stand and progress to more difficult exercises as strength and control are achieved during progressions of later phase II. Strengthening exercises begin with isometrics in late phase II and progress to isotonics in phase III using techniques such as manual resistance, pulleys or tubing, and progressive standing heel raises. Other lower-extremity muscle groups in the hip and knee are strengthened starting in phase I and continuing into phase II as well, because those areas have likely diminished in strength following the injury and surgery.

When the patient has achieved full range of motion and adequate strength for control, balance exercises during dynamic activities can begin while in phase III, and the patient then progresses to agility exercises in late phase III. Agility exercises on boxes, jumping with tubing resistance, and lateral movements are the final agility activities in phase III before functional and activity-specific exercises in phase IV.

Achilles Tendon Injuries

The most common injuries to the Achilles tendon are a rupture and tendinopathy. Either injury can be debilitating and can restrict the patient from a rapid return to sport participation. The rehabilitation clinician's proper management of each injury is important to a safe and prompt return.

Tendinopathy

If not treated correctly, tendinopathy can be a frustrating and prolonged condition. Causes must be addressed and the condition brought under control before therapeutic exercises can be started.

■ Case Study

A 20-year-old tennis player was downhill skiing during winter break with his family. While he was on the slopes, maneuvering to the right, he fell forward and dislocated his left peroneus longus tendon. The injury was surgically repaired. The ankle was placed in an immobilizer boot, and the patient was non-weight bearing for two weeks. He is now able to partial weight bear to about 75% on the left and is to start rehabilitation. He presents to you today still non-weight bearing on the left. He admits that he is fearful of bearing weight on the extremity. His hip and knee strength is grossly 4/5. Ankle dorsiflexion and inversion are 3/5, and ankle eversion is 2+/5. His ankle range of motion is 0° inversion, 5° eversion, 40° plantar flexion, and -5° dorsiflexion. Joint mobility is moderately restricted in the subtalar and intertarsal joints. The calcaneocuboid and cuboid-metatarsal joints are also restricted. Soft-tissue mobility around the surgical scar, along the lateral foot, and into the posterior ankle is moderately limited. There is mild to moderate swelling around the ankle.

Questions for Analysis

1. What are your patient's problems and what short-term and long-term goals will you establish to relieve these problems?
2. What will your first treatment today include?
3. What will your goals for today's treatment be?
4. What instructions will you give the patient today before he goes home?
5. What do you expect to accomplish in the next two weeks of treatment?
6. List precautions that you must respect at this point in the rehabilitation program.
7. List three strengthening exercises that you will use when the ankle is ready, and explain their progression.
8. What agility exercises will you eventually include in the therapeutic exercise program?

Achilles tendinopathy is usually a gradual-onset injury that originates secondary to overuse. Overuse of the Achilles tendon occurs when the tendon undergoes excessive stresses without sufficient time between stress applications to adjust to those stress levels. Excessive stress can be the result of cumulative forces caused by inherently poor foot mechanics, increased conditioning sessions, improper surfaces and playing fields, inadequate or improper footwear, weakness, or inflexibility. As with other tendinopathy conditions, it is necessary to correct the fundamental causative factor or factors in order for there to be complete recovery with reduced risk of reinjury.

A foot with excessive pronation increases Achilles tendon stress. The Achilles tendon's normal configuration has a medial spiral rotation from its origin in the gastrocnemius-soleus complex, where it begins as a flat, fan-shaped tendon, to its insertion on the calcaneus where it ends as a rounded cord (figure 22.62). This spiral rotation begins about 12 to 15 cm (4.7–5.9 in.) above its insertion (Stanish, Curwin, & Mandel, 2000). This twist of the tendon is an area of stress concentration, especially 2 to 5 cm (0.8–2.0 in.) above its calcaneal insertion where the rotation is at its greatest. This factor is coupled with the fact that this region is also an area of reduced circulation within the tendon. This site is the most common location for tendinopathy in the Achilles.

When the calcaneus is in eversion when it should be erect, the Achilles tendon suffers an additional torque force. If the Achilles is tight, even more pronation occurs to allow needed dorsiflexion during ambulation. If pronation is prolonged into the phase of heel-off and beyond when inversion should be occurring, a wringing of the tendon occurs, increasing stress to the Achilles at its most vulnerable site. In cases of repetitive stress and prolonged tendinopathy, a nodule of scar tissue from microscopic tears can

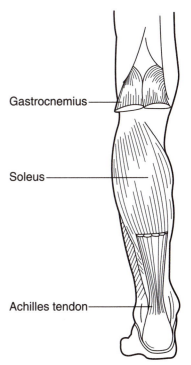

▶ **Figure 22.62** Achilles tendon.

often be palpated on the tendon 2 to 5 cm (0.8–2.0 in.) above its calcaneal insertion. The nodule is usually larger and more tender on the medial aspect, where the tendon incurs more stress.

As with other cases of tendinopathy, the patient's history typically includes a gradual progression of pain. The pain begins as tenderness during running but goes away if the individual continues running. Gradually, pain persists longer and longer into the run until it persists after running and even during simple daily activities such as walking. Stiffness can occur after periods of inactivity or prolonged sitting. Eventually, pain is present even with rest.

Common signs are reduced ankle dorsiflexion; tenderness along the Achilles, especially 2 to 5 cm (0.8–2.0 in.) above the calcaneal insertion where a nodule can be palpated; possible swelling; possible weakness; possible crepitus to palpation; and pain with unilateral hopping.

Treatment includes initially correcting the cause and reducing pain and swelling. If the cause is excessive pronation, orthotics may be necessary. A low-dye strapping technique to stabilize the calcaneus and reduce pronation can be used either alone or in combination with heel cups or medial heel wedges to assess the effectiveness of orthotics; if these devices reduce the patient's pain, it is likely that the patient will benefit from orthotics. Use of commercially available arch supports can also determine whether custom orthotics may be necessary. Inflexibility, weakness, scar-tissue adhesions and joint immobility from previous injuries, and alterations in footwear should all be assessed and corrected as necessary. A good history must include inquiries regarding recent changes in conditioning or workout sessions that may be overstressing the tendon. Changes in surfaces, for example when an individual goes from flat surfaces to hills or from soft to hard surfaces, may also be a contributing factor that must be corrected.

In extreme cases, it may be necessary to have the patient temporarily cease the aggravating activity until the injury is under control. Treatment techniques that may be beneficial include the use of various modalities, such as ultrasound, phonophoresis, iontophoresis, electrical stimulation, ice, and others presented in Denegar and colleagues (2010). Cross-friction massage over the nodule and other areas of soft-tissue restriction help to mobilize the adherent scar tissue to reduce pain and improve soft-tissue mobility.

Therapeutic exercises must include stretching and flexibility activities for restricted areas. Hamstring and hip muscle tightness can influence Achilles flexibility and should be evaluated and corrected as needed. Gastrocnemius and soleus tightness should also be addressed with the flexibility exercises presented earlier.

Once weight-bearing, the patient begins eccentric heel raises beginning with a slow heel-drop on the floor and progressing from a medium speed on the floor, to a fast speed on the floor, to a slow speed on an incline, to a medium speed on an incline, and finally to a rapid heel-drop on an incline with three sets of 15 to 25. Eccentric exercises and their benefits were provided in more detail in chapter 15.

Concentric strength exercises are initiated cautiously because it is important to avoid exacerbation of the pain. Weight-bearing strengthening exercises can begin when the patient reports pain at around 5/10. Before that, rubber band exercises for ankle inversion, eversion, and dorsiflexion strength are appropriate. The patient can perform rubber band exercises for ankle plantar flexion through a full, pain-free range of motion. Concentric weight-bearing Achilles exercises can include heel raises on a extremity press machine, standing heel raises beginning on a flat surface and progressing to an incline, and heel raises with weights. Other exercises for the lower extremity include squats, lunges, and knee flexion strengthening exercises as tolerated. When the patient's pain level is 2-3/10, agility exercises are suitable. Plyometrics start once the patient is pain free. At no time throughout the therapeutic exercise program should any exercise increase Achilles pain. If any progression results in Achilles pain, the patient should return to previous levels of activity for another one or two treatment sessions until he or she is able to progress to the next level without pain.

Once the patient is able to perform plyometric exercises well and without pain, functional and then activity-specific exercises are the last step before full return to normal activities

■ Case Study

A 24-year-old male recreational runner reports to you with complaints of pain in the right extremity just above the ankle. He reports that about two months ago while he was running, he stepped off a curb and rolled his right ankle but continued running. The ankle swelled slightly but did not require him to cut back on his running program. He did not think much about it because it did not seem to cause any problems. This patient usually runs about 8 km (5 miles) once a day but has recently increased running to twice a day in preparation for an upcoming marathon. Because the marathon course is hilly, he has recently made it a point to run at least one steep hill during his workouts. When the pain began he would continue running, and the pain would go away; but it soon lingered longer into the run until it now is present throughout the run and has forced him to reduce his mileage. He has pain after prolonged sitting, while climbing stairs, and while walking barefoot. He reports that he feels a creaking in the back of his ankle when he walks. He does a few stretches but usually does not have time after his run to do any stretch more than once, holding each stretch for 10 s.

Your examination reveals that dorsiflexion in subtalar neutral is –5°. The calcaneus inversion-eversion motion is a total of 35°, and the midfoot is loose when you lock the rearfoot and passively invert and evert the midfoot. Strength for heel raise in weight bearing is slightly less than normal, with pain occurring after about eight repetitions. There is a tender nodule about 3 cm (1.2 in.) above the base of the heel on the Achilles tendon. The nodule is significant in size, protruding about 2 mm medially and 1 mm laterally on the Achilles tendon. You can feel crepitus in the tendon as you passively dorsiflex and plantar flex the ankle.

Questions for Analysis

1. How do you think the ankle rollover incident has affected the Achilles tendon injury?
2. How will you describe for the patient the probable causes for his Achilles tendon injury?
3. What will your advice be regarding his workout program?
4. Describe what your first treatment session with the patient will include.
5. What home exercises will you give him?
6. What factors will you consider in deciding when to begin strengthening exercises?
7. What will you tell the patient when he asks you how long this will take to resolve?

and sports participation. Throughout the program, the patient must communicate to the rehabilitation clinician any changes in Achilles pain and the response to treatment. You must respect the patient's pain and realize that each person will respond differently to an exercise progression. The key to the success of the program is correcting the underlying causes of the Achilles tendinopathy and getting the signs and symptoms under control before the patient advances in the program.

Retrocalcaneal bursitis is often mistaken for Achilles tendinopathy. Bursitis occurs over the posterior aspect of the calcaneus where the bursa is located. This is an unusual location for Achilles tendinopathy to occur, so a patient presenting with complaints of pain in this area should be examined for bursitis as well as tendinopathy. A "pump bump" is frequently present because a heel-whip occurs as the calcaneus moves toward supination during late stance and heel-off after being positioned in pronation longer than it should be into midstance. The bursa becomes irritated with friction against the shoe's heel counter, especially with a heel whip. Treatment includes symptomatic relief of the bursal inflammation along with correction of the cause of the bursitis. In addition to excessive pronation, other causative factors of bursitis include tight Achilles, tight plantar fascia, and poor shoes.

Achilles Rupture

Treatment programs for Achilles ruptures have become less conservative in recent years, primarily because of better results seen with early weight bearing and rehabilitation following surgical repair (Kangas, Pajala, Siira, Hamalainen, & Leppilahti, 2003; Mortensen, Skov, & Jensen, 1999). This section presents a program of treatment and then a case study for you to solve.

An Achilles rupture most commonly occurs in individuals in the fourth and fifth decades of life. In younger athletes, a rupture occurs when the foot is anchored and the patient is thrust forward to produce a sudden stretch on the tendon. A typical history for the older patient includes an incident in which the patient was running or cutting and felt as though he or she had been shot in the extremity. A younger athlete may be in a football pileup with one player on top of his foot and then be pushed forward by another player who comes into the pileup. A pop is felt or heard. The pain is intense, and the patient is unable to walk on the extremity. Passively squeezing a normal calf muscle causes a plantar-flexion movement of the ankle, but this motion does not occur with a torn Achilles tendon (Thompson test).

Surgical repair, either open or subcutaneous, most recently has been the treatment of choice (Gigante et al., 2008). Conservative care with immobilization often lends itself to poor results, especially in the athletic population. Following repair, the leg is placed either in a series of progressively reduced plantar-flexion casts or, more commonly, in a hinged ankle walking boot with ankle immobilization. The boot is initially positioned in plantar flexion and gradually positioned to neutral. The patient may be non-weight bearing initially and progress to partial weight bearing before weight bearing as tolerated is allowed.

Initial rehabilitation treatments in phase I include cardiovascular conditioning and exercises for the uninvolved lower-extremity segments and other body segments. Isometric exercises in the immobilization boot can be encouraged, but the patient is instructed to perform a slow buildup to maximum with a maximal hold and a gradual release of muscle tension. Once the surgeon permits treatment to the involved segment, efforts to reduce edema and scar-tissue adhesions are the first priority. Soft-tissue massage and mobilization around the ankle and distal leg, along with ankle and tibiofibular joint mobilizations, often begin early in phase II to assist in restoring flexibility and range of motion. Also in phase II, active and passive range-of-motion exercises and strengthening exercises for ankle inverters, evertors, dorsiflexors, and plantar flexors begin in non-weight bearing and progress as tolerated to partial and then full weight bearing. Use of rubber bands or tubing for ankle motions once the patient's foot is out of the boot assists in promoting strength. When the patient is permitted partial weight bearing, he or she can use the BAPS board in sitting to increase active ankle range of motion. Other activities include exercise on a stationary bike, the towel-roll exercise, and marble pickups for extrinsic and intrinsic muscles. Plantar foot massage with a ribbed can, golf ball, or rolling pin is also appropriate during this time.

If the patient is partial weight bearing on crutches, it is best to encourage a correct heel-toe gait. If the patient acquires bad habits on crutches, they may extend into full weight bearing and become difficult to correct. If the patient remains on crutches after the surgical scar is healed, gait training in a pool at a depth equivalent to the patient's weight bearing restrictions may be beneficial. Gait training on land is a necessary part of the therapeutic exercise program once the patient is fully weight bearing.

Patients are typically reluctant to bear weight on the involved extremity once they are permitted full weight bearing without the boot. Weight transfer from the uninvolved to the involved extremity through the use of the weigh scale, with progressive increases in the weight placed on the scale, is a good way to help the patient develop confidence in weight bearing on the involved extremity. The scale can also be used to monitor correct technique in heel-raise exercises. Using the scale can be an especially significant exercise if the surgeon is permitting limited weight bearing on the extremity; for example, if 50% weight bearing is permitted, the scale's balance is positioned at half the patient's weight, and the patient then transfers body weight to the involved extremity until the scale's balance arm moves up, indicating that half the body weight is borne by the extremity. The scale exercise can also be used in full-weight-bearing exercise, and can be used for monitoring and recording increases in the patient's ability to bear weight on the involved extremity through a full range of motion.

When the patient is able to bear full weight on the involved extremity, stork-standing exercises are used to improve balance and proprioception. Additional strength activities in phase III should include exercises for the entire lower extremity because it is likely that with inactivity, an antalgic gait, and surgery, the entire lower extremity is weak. These exercises can include resisted open chain hip exercises and knee exercises and weight-bearing exercises such as squats and lunges. These exercises are presented in chapters 23 and 24. Other beneficial activities include step exercises, balance and agility exercises, and eventually plyometric exercises as described earlier in this chapter. Functional exercises and then activity-specific exercises are part of phase IV of the rehabilitation program and are specific to the patient's sport or occupation.

During phase I of the program, manual-resistance exercises for the hip and knee are feasible even when the extremity is immobilized. Trunk exercises can also be included in the early phase. Manual resistance to the ankle can begin once the immobilization brace or cast is off in phase II. Weight-bearing exercises are gradually increased in the program as the patient

■ Case Study

Two weeks ago, a 45-year-old male tennis player was running to return a drop shot when he suddenly felt as though he had been shot in the left calf. He had intense pain and was unable to stand or walk. He was taken to the Emergency Department, placed on crutches, given ice, and instructed to follow up with an orthopedic surgeon. He underwent surgical repair for a ruptured Achilles tendon 10 days ago. His surgeon wants him to begin his rehabilitation program today. He has a walking boot fixed at 10° plantar flexion and is permitted partial weight bearing to 50%. He is apprehensive about putting weight on the left extremity and continues to walk non-weight bearing on the left. He does not have much pain in the Achilles because he is not moving it much. Although the surgical scar is well healed, there is moderate swelling throughout the foot and distal extremity. His active ankle movement is 30° plantar flexion and −15° dorsiflexion. Inversion-eversion is stiff and has a total of 20° motion. Joint mobility of the tarsals and metatarsals is restricted overall at about 50% normal mobility. Strength of the hip and knee is 4−/5; ankle dorsiflexion, inversion, and eversion are 3/5; and plantar flexion is 2/5. Palpation reveals myofascial tenderness with soft-tissue restriction throughout the calf muscles and the presence of adhesions in the dorsum of the foot and around the ankle. The surgical site has moderate adhesions of the scar to underlying soft tissue.

Questions for Analysis

1. List this patient's problems in order of priority and identify the long-term goals for each of these problems.

2. What are your short-term goals with this patient, and when would you expect to achieve them?

3. What will your treatment include today?

4. What instructions will you give him today for a home program?

5. How aggressive will you be with your treatments during the next two weeks? Justify your answer.

6. When will you begin strengthening exercises, and what will they initially include? List your reasons.

7. List three agility exercises you will give the patient when he is able to perform them, before he progresses to functional exercises.

Start
rehab

Inflammation	Proliferation	Remodeling	
Phase I (inactive)	**Phase II (active)**	**Phase III (resistive)**	**Phase IV (aggressive)**

GOALS			
• ↓ Pain • ↓ Spasm • ↓ Edema • Protect surgical site from excessive stress • Maintain conditioning levels (MCL)	• ↑ ROM of all ankle motions; plantar flexion to neutral • ↓ Muscle endurance • Early strength gains with isometrics • Reduce scar adhesions • No pain, spasm, edema • Begin WB from toe-touch to PWB; continue with crutches	• Full ROM • ↓ Strength, endurance gradually • ↓ Proprioception • MCL • Good soft tissue mobility • Normal joint mobility	• Perform functional activities properly • Perform sport- and activity-specific exercises at least to preinjury levels • Return to full participation without pain, with normal strength, mobility, and execution of activities

TREATMENT			
• Modalities • Easy PROM; dorsiflexion and plantar flexion to 0° • Grades I and II joint mobilization • NWB on crutches • MCL exercises for conditioning with special attention to hip and knee (knee flexion with patient prone) • ROM of toes • Leg is in boot or cast	• Begin isometrics of ankle • PROM: ankle and foot • Early proprioception exercises • Soft tissue mobilization • Exercises for ankle muscle endurance to tolerance • Active dorsiflexion to 0° • Gait training in pool • Continue grades I and II joint mobilization as needed • Aquatic exercises, jogging at 6-8 weeks • Resistance-band PF:6 weeks • Stand on heels and toes alternately at 6-8 weeks • AROM at 6-8 weeks • Continue with ME with emphasis on hip abduction and extension, knee groups • Ice or cold modalities after treatment	• Continue with ROM exercises PRN • Bilateral heel raise at 9-10 weeks progressing to unilateral raise • Begin multiplanar exercises for entire LE with bands • Early functional exercises • Gastrocnemius stretches • Soleus stretches • Grade III and IV joint mobilization, PRN • CV exercise on elliptical, cycle, rowing machine, NordicTrac • Progress to jogging at 12 weeks • Continue MCL exercises	• Plyometrics for LE: stair running, jumps, eccentrics • Functional exercises • Sport- and activity-specific exercises

▶ **Figure 22.63** Rehabilitation progression for postoperative Achilles repair. PROM = passive range of motion; AROM = active range of motion; ROM = range of motion; CV = cardiovascular; NWB = non-weight bearing; WB = weight bearing; FWB = full weight bearing; LE = lower extremity; PRN = as needed; LE = lower extremity; PF = plantar flexion.

tolerates them. Initially, the resistance and repetitions are low, and emphasis should be on correct technique and proper execution. The patient may tolerate increased repetitions better than increased resistance in the early days of therapeutic exercise.

Resistance exercise beyond body weight is frequently added to the program in phase III, around 8 to 12 weeks postoperatively. Once the patient has 10° to 15° of dorsiflexion, usually toward the end of the second month or the beginning of the third, jogging activities can begin. Straight jogging on a flat surface is permitted until the patient is up to 3.2 km (2 miles). After that, agility drills are appropriate. A timeline progression of rehabilitation following an Achilles tendon repair is provided in figure 22.63.

As with any injury or surgical repair, progression of the strengthening exercises is determined by tissue healing times, the patient's flexibility and mobility, and his or her tolerance. Pain and swelling are the primary signs to avoid with any exercise. It is desirable to achieve muscle fatigue without causing pain or swelling with strengthening exercises. Exercise stress is gradually increased, and the response to any increase in exercise stress—either increased difficulty in an exercise or the addition of new exercises—must be carefully monitored. You must rely on your own observational skills, as well as on the patient's reports of the Achilles response to changes in therapeutic exercises, to gauge the effectiveness of the program. These factors dictate alterations.

Other Tendinopathy

Although several tendons in the foot, ankle, and extremity can develop tendinopathy, the most common sites are the tibialis posterior and the peroneal tendons. These tendons become inflamed most often because of overuse secondary to excessive pronation combined with increased running mileage on hard surfaces.

The tibialis posterior works eccentrically to decelerate subtalar pronation and medial rotation of the tibia at heel strike, and concentrically as a supinator and inverter of the subtalar joint and lateral rotator of the tibia during stance. The peroneus longus and brevis work as pronators of the subtalar joint and as plantar flexors and evertors of the first ray during the non-weight-bearing phase of gait. During midstance and heel-off, they evert the foot to transfer weight from the lateral to the medial foot. These lateral and medial muscles both act as stabilizers of the foot during weight bearing. The tibialis posterior stabilizes the midtarsal joint, and the peroneus longus stabilizes the first ray to accept the load as it is transferred from the lateral

■ Case Study

A 16-year-old female cross-country runner presents to you with a two-month history of medial ankle pain. She does not remember injuring the ankle. The pain was tolerable, even though it has increased in duration during her workouts, until this past week, when she increased the intensity of her workouts in preparation for the start of the cross-country competitive season. The pain now occurs throughout her workouts and does not go away when she stops running as it had in the past. She has pain if she stands too long and when she walks. She reports that she has been meaning to buy new running shoes because the ones she wears now are worn out, but she thought she would wait until she saw you to ask your advice on what to buy.

Your examination reveals ankle dorsiflexion in subtalar neutral to 0°, plantar flexion to 55°, and inversion-eversion to 30°. The midfoot is loose with the rearfoot locked. In non-weight bearing, the patient has a normal arch, but in weight bearing the navicular is close to the floor and the calcaneus is everted. In walking, the calcaneus never inverts to a vertical position. The patient's shoes are collapsed medially in the heel. Palpation reveals tenderness under the navicular and running along the tibialis posterior tendon posterior and superior to the ankle.

Questions for Analysis

1. List all of her problems, beginning with the most serious. Identify correlating long-term and short-term goals for her.

2. What will your first treatment today include, and what will you give the patient today for a home program?

3. Do you think she will need orthotics, and if so, why?

4. What will your recommendations be on shoe selection?

5. What are your short-term goals, and what is your best estimate on when to anticipate reaching them?

6. What are your criteria for when to begin strengthening exercises?

7. List three agility exercises you will include when appropriate.

8. What functional activities will you include in the patient's program?

9. What will your criteria be for her return to normal running activities?

to the medial foot at heel-off. When the foot is pronated longer than it should be in weight bearing, excessive loads are placed on these tendons. If the excessive load from changes in workouts, poor shoes, or ungiving surfaces causes breakdown that the tendon insufficiently recovers from before the next workout, tendinopathy can occur.

Tibialis posterior tendinopathy results in pain in the posteromedial ankle region and/or into the tendon's insertion site on the navicular and surrounding tarsals. Peroneal tendinopathy pain, located in the posterolateral ankle region, can run along the tendon on the lateral foot.

As with Achilles tendinopathy, it is crucial for the clinician to identify the causes if a treatment program is to have lasting effects. Once you have identified the causes, you take steps to alleviate them. If the injury is not severe, it may be possible for the patient to continue normal activities once the causes have been corrected. In severe cases it may be necessary for the patient to refrain from full participation until the symptoms are alleviated.

Initial treatment includes the use of pain-relieving modalities that have been discussed previously. The patient should be instructed in proper stretching exercises for tight areas. These may often include structures adjacent to the injured area. For example, a tight iliotibial band or piriformis may impact the tibialis posterior tendinopathy, making it necessary to include stretches for these structures in the therapeutic exercise program.

Initial strengthening activities, once pain is under control, include eccentric exercises discussed previously. The patient progresses to concentric and eccentric exercises for all ankle muscles, especially those deficient in strength or endurance, as well as the injured structures. Antigravity positioning using weights, resistance bands, or manual resistance for inverters and evertors provides additional resistance to those muscles. Marble pickups with placement of the marbles in the ipsilateral or contralateral hand, lateral towel roll, and inversion-eversion on a BAPS board or wobble board are important exercises for peroneal and tibialis posterior tendons. Balance activities provide stress to lateral ankle tendons. The Fitter and rolling balance board can also be used for lateral ankle-stressing exercises. Resistive exercises for ankle dorsiflexors and plantar flexors should also be included.

Agility exercises and functional exercises are the same as for other injuries; you should add these to the program once the patient is pain free with activity.

Shin Splints

Shin splints are also known as medial tibial stress syndrome (Batt, Ugalade, Anderson, & Shelton, 1998). More recently, it is also referred to as exercise-related leg pain (Reinking, 2007). By any name, it is a stress-reaction at the periosteal and musculotendinous fascial junctions. The pain is located in the middle and distal third of the extremity. The pain may vary in intensity, from pain that resolves after running to pain that interferes with daily activities.

This condition is usually seen in distance runners and is commonly caused by training errors coupled with improper or poor shoes and a tight Achilles (Kohn, 1997). Treatment includes correction of the causes along with reduced activity until symptoms are under control. In addition, modalities may be used to relieve pain. Stretching of the Achilles and other tight structures should be performed throughout the day. Soft-tissue release through deep-tissue massage can be useful in relieving adhesions that occur and that add to the patient's pain.

If "shin splints" complaints occur on the lateral extremity, the cause is usually an overuse reaction of the tibialis anterior and extensor digitorum communis, compounded by excessive pronation, hill running, poor shoes, or training errors. It is not technically shin splints, but it is painful, nevertheless. This condition is usually relieved with changes in shoes, training methods, and orthotics.

Athletes may experience lateral extremity pain at the outset of preseason conditioning, especially if they have not maintained an appropriate activity level up to that time. In these cases, the pain resolves with time as the patient becomes conditioned. Ice/spray-and-stretch can provide symptomatic relief in the short term. If symptoms continue beyond normal expectations, the patient should be referred to the physician to rule out anterior compartment syndrome.

Case Study

An 18-year-old male sprinter presents to you with complaints of lateral and anterior leg pain that began about one week ago. He has started training for the outdoor track season and is distance running to create a cardiovascular base. He reports that he had this pain last year but it went away after a couple of weeks, so he didn't think too much about it; however, this year, his first year as an intercollegiate athlete, the pain seems more intense. He likes the team's shoes, which he started wearing when he began training this year; he had never used the brand before.

Your examination reveals tightness in the Achilles with ankle dorsiflexion to 0°. Hamstring range of motion is 65° in a straight-extremity raise. His new shoes have a stiff sole. He is tender to palpation of the tibialis anterior.

Questions for Analysis

1. What will your first treatment today include?
2. What will you give the patient for a home program?
3. What will be your recommendations regarding his shoes?
4. What will be your recommendations regarding his workouts?
5. What are your short-term goals for him?
6. List three exercises you will include in his program.

Compartment Syndromes

There are various degrees of compartment syndromes, ranging from slight discomfort to emergency situations. This condition is also referred to as exertional compartment syndrome (Garcia-Mata, Hidalgo-Ovejero, & Martinez-Grande, 2001). There are two types of compartment syndrome, acute and chronic. The acute exertional compartment syndrome is an uncommon emergency situation that requires immediate transport of the patient to an Emergency Department. Chronic exertional compartment syndrome is more common but usually not an emergency condition.

The four compartments of the leg are divided by thick, inelastic fascial coverings. This fascia creates unyielding walls that enclose the muscles in each compartment. If volume changes occur in a compartment, there is no room for expansion, so pressure builds up within the compartment. If pressure persists, a compromise of soft tissue, blood vessels, and neural structures can result. Although any of the compartments can experience compartment syndrome, the most commonly affected one is the anterior compartment.

An increase in compartment volume is commonly the result of edema from intense activity or the result of an injury, such as a crush injury or fracture, which causes bleeding and soft-tissue swelling. Activity-induced compartment syndrome is usually chronic, whereas injury-induced compartment syndrome is acute. The acute condition results from an increase in arterial flow from the injury, with a reduction in venous return because of pressure on the vessels, and leads to ischemic pain and tissue death if it persists.

The patient complains of intense pain that is not relieved by any treatment or positioning and of pain with passive plantar flexion. Palpation of the area reveals a hardness and tension of the soft tissues. As the condition advances, the distal pulses are diminished, and neurological changes can be observed.

Because tissue life is being threatened, this is considered a medical emergency when symptoms persist or progress, and the patient must be referred to the physician immediately. A surgical fasciotomy is usually performed to release the pressure.

In chronic compartment syndrome, the symptoms are different in some ways and similar in others to the acute condition. The patient has recurrent, usually bilateral, extremity pain and tightness in the compartment during activity, but the symptoms subside with rest. Edema and tenderness can be palpated, and some patients also experience paresthesia. These symptoms occur because arterial flow secondary to increased muscle activity is greater than the capillary perfusion rate. The local blood flow is restricted—much like cars in a rush-hour traffic jam. Many fast-moving cars are suddenly forced to slow down because the number of vehicles is beyond the capacity of the road to handle them all at one time. Once the number of vehicles on the road decreases, the traffic moves smoothly again. Likewise, once pressure is reduced, blood flow is restored in the compartment.

In some chronic cases, fasciotomy for compartment release can be avoided with conservative treatment. Conservative treatment includes extremity-stretching exercises and strengthening exercises for balanced strength among all muscle groups. The patient should work out on softer surfaces and wear running shoes that absorb shock. Orthotics that reduce shock may also be helpful.

When conservative efforts do not relieve the problem, fasciotomy reduces compartment pressures and will permit the patient to return to normal activities. Patients who undergo fasciotomy may be placed on crutches, non-weight bearing, for 7 to 10 days. Isometric and active range-of-motion exercises begin within a week of surgery. Once the wound is healed, aquatic exercises are useful for gaining range of motion and strength and restoring normal gait. Myofascial release and massage for soft-tissue mobility, joint mobilization if indicated following immobilization, and gait training on land may all be necessary if the patient shows deficiencies on the initial examination. Once the patient is fully weight bearing, closed kinetic chain exercises begin in phase II with a progression of the resistive exercises discussed previ-

■ Case Study

A 16-year-old female cross-country runner fractured her right tibia in a motor-vehicle accident 5 years ago. The leg was in a cast for two months before the patient began a rehabilitation program. One month ago she was competing in a cross-country race and experienced right shin and foot numbness and burning. Since then, she has continued to experience the same symptoms during her workouts. She underwent an anterior and a posterior compartment release and removal of extensive scar tissue two weeks ago. The surgeon wants her to begin rehabilitation today.

She is partially weight bearing on the right extremity with crutches, but the surgeon has instructed her to ambulate without the crutches within the next couple of days. She admits that she doesn't have pain but lacks the confidence to get rid of the crutches. Your examination reveals well-healed surgical scars anteriorly and posteriorly on the leg. You note the presence of mild edema and stiffness to passive range of motion, but the patient has no pain. Dorsiflexion is –5°; plantar flexion is 35°. Inversion-eversion is 30°. Palpation reveals mild soft-tissue restriction around the surgical scars and moderate tissue restriction in the calf and anterior extremity.

Questions for Analysis

1. What are her problems and what are your long-term goals for her?

2. What modalities will you use today, if any, and why?

3. What exercises will you initiate today?

4. What home program and instructions will you give the patient before she leaves today?

5. What are your short-goals for her for the next two weeks, and how will you attempt to accomplish them?

6. What specific activities will you have the patient perform the first day she is on a treadmill?

7. Outline a progressive running program that you will give the patient when she is ready to begin running.

ously. Resistance-band exercises can be used before full-weight-bearing activities. At four to six weeks, the patient begins phase III with treadmill and stair-climber exercises provided the patient has shown appropriate strength and flexibility gains.

Reaching phase III and return to running activities is commonly slower in posterior compartment releases than in anterior compartment releases. Return to running activities proceeds slowly on the basis of the patient's symptoms and the healing progression. Jogging is the initial speed, which progresses to slow running, then, in phase IV, to fast running before return to normal speeds. Initial jogging distances may be no more than 0.8 km (0.5) miles with a gradual progression to 3.2 to 4.8 km (2–3 miles) before the patient is released by the surgeon to return to former running distances. Running should be on soft, flat surfaces before the patient progresses to hill running.

Foot Injuries

A number of common and some unusual foot problems can also arise. Some of the more commonly seen conditions are presented here.

Plantar Fasciitis

Of all foot injuries, plantar fasciitis is among the most common. Its cause can be any number of factors, and you must recognize and correct the cause to correct the problem and reduce the risk of reinjury.

The thick aponeurosis that covers the plantar foot from the calcaneus to the MTP joints is the plantar fascia. It is a thick connective tissue structure that protects the structures in the plantar foot, provides flexibility for shock absorption, and creates a windlass mechanism that transforms the foot into a rigid lever for transferring propulsion forces during push-off. It can become irritated when subjected to abnormal stress, usually during running activities. Patients in any sport involving these activities can be susceptible to plantar fasciitis. High arches and excessive pronation can both be culprits that increase normal stress loads and lead to plantar fasciitis. These inherent structural stresses are usually combined with other factors such as increased workout levels, poor shoes, restricted dorsiflexion from tight Achilles or calf muscles, restricted great-toe dorsiflexion, and workouts on hard surfaces.

The most classic symptom of plantar fasciitis is heel pain with weight bearing when the person arises in the morning, as well as after prolonged sitting, that decreases with continued walking. In more severe cases, pain can occur at rest and extend into the midarch region. The pain is usually unilateral. X-rays often reveal a heel spur; however, the source of pain is not the heel spur but the soft tissue that is irritated because of the stress it is experiencing. Repetitive stresses applied to the plantar fascia at its origin on the calcaneus commonly result in the development of exostosis at the location where the fascia attaches.

Treatment must include correction of the underlying causes. This frequently involves flexibility exercises for tight structures, proper shoe selection, orthotics if needed to correct abnormal foot structure, changes in conditioning, and changes in workout surfaces (De Vera Barredo, Menna, & Farris, 2007). Treatment may also include modalities such as extracorporeal shock wave to relieve the symptoms (Ogden, Alvarez, Levitt, Cross, & Marlow, 2001). Occasionally, the physician may opt for a cortisone injection into the painful area. Alternative methods that may provide relief to the tender tissues include using a heel cup with strapping techniques, applying a low-dye strapping technique to the arch to reduce the stress on the plantar fascia, putting heel lifts in the shoes to reduce the stress from a tight Achilles tendon, and providing a heel cup to increase calcaneal stability and provide a cushion to the plantar calcaneus (Hyland, Webber-Gaffney, Cohen, & Lichtman, 2006; Wilk, Fisher, & Gutierrez, 2000). Wearing a night splint that places a low-level stretch on the Achilles has been shown to reduce pain associated with plantar fasciitis (Evans, 2001). Stretching the Achilles and calf must be performed soon in the program so that the heel lift can be discarded as soon as possible; prolonged use of the heel lift can encourage tightness and prevent restoration of full motion. Calf stretching must be performed with the ankle in subtalar (Evans, 2001) neutral so that the foot does not collapse and give a false impression of stretching the calf. Stretching of the plantar fascia and great toe can be performed with the ankle in dorsiflexion and the great toe in hyperextension. Massage with golf balls, a rolling pin, or a ribbed can may provide additional relief.

If orthotics seem necessary, before they are provided the rehabilitation clinician should attempt temporary orthotic relief to assess whether an orthotic can achieve the desired result. If either a temporary orthotic or a low-dye strapping technique provides significant relief, this is a good indication that a permanent orthotic is needed.

Once pain is under control and flexibility exercises have been provided, the patient should begin strengthening exercises for the ankle inverters and the intrinsic and extrinsic toe flexors in phase II. These muscles assist in supporting the arch and plantar fascia. Marble pickups with deposit into the opposite hand and towel-roll, heel raise, and resisted inversion exercises are all appropriate for plantar fasciitis.

Only in extreme cases will the patient be compelled to refrain from normal activities. Pain is normally the limiting factor but because the fascia is weakened, it is susceptible to tears, especially during sudden acceleration or push-off movements. If a rupture of the plantar fascia occurs, acute pain and swelling will prevent the patient from ambulating normally. A stiff-soled shoe or boot or partial weight bearing on crutches for three to seven days may be necessary. Treatment for a plantar fascia rupture follows a course similar to that for plantar fasciitis. Symptom control, flexibility exercises, and the usual progression to strengthening, coordination, agility, and functional activities are normal program components for a ruptured plantar fascia.

Tarsal Tunnel Syndrome

The tarsal tunnel is formed by the medial malleolus, calcaneus, talus, and deltoid ligament's posterior aspect. Tarsal tunnel syndrome is an entrapment of the posterior tibial nerve as it passes under the flexor retinaculum posterior to the medial malleolus along with the tendons of the tibialis posterior, flexor digitorum longus, and flexor hallucis longus (figure 22.64). Excessive pronation, especially with improper shoes, can cause increased tension on the flexor retinaculum to increase compression on the nerve. Dancers, especially tap dancers who wear rigid shoes and sustain high-impact forces, are susceptible to tarsal tunnel syndrome. Swelling from trauma or tendinopathy can also cause tarsal tunnel syndrome. Symptoms during weight

---

■ Case Study

A 19-year-old basketball player has developed right plantar fasciitis over the past month. The pain is present when he gets up in the morning and when he stands after sitting in class for an hour. He is able to perform his workouts without any difficulty, but he has noticed that the pain is worse the morning after a particularly hard workout the previous day. Your examination reveals higher-than-normal arches of both feet. Ankle dorsiflexion in subtalar neutral is –5°. Great-toe hyperextension is 50°. There is tenderness to pressure over the plantar medial calcaneus where the plantar fascia inserts. Shoe wear is excessive on the lateral aspect of the shoe.

Questions for Analysis

1. What will your first treatment include?
2. What home exercises will you give the patient before he leaves today?
3. What accommodations will you place in his shoes or on his feet?
4. What strengthening exercises will you give him, and when will you give them?
5. If you decide that the patient needs orthotics, what specifications will you want in them? How will you decide that he would benefit from orthotics?

bearing include a burning pain, tingling, and numbness in the medial and plantar foot. Tinel's sign is often positive. Toe flexor and abductor hallucis weakness and decreased ability to plantar flex and invert the foot can be noted in more advanced cases.

Only severe cases require cessation of activities or surgery. Most cases can be treated conservatively. Treatment includes orthotics to reduce pronation and reduce posterior tibial nerve irritation, modalities such as phonophoresis or iontophoresis to diminish inflammation, and therapeutic exercises to resolve weakness. Properly fitted shoes and anti-inflammatory medications are also useful. Flexibility exercises and soft-tissue mobilization for release of adhesions can also be beneficial for pain relief. If shoe compression on the medial foot contributes to the problem, use of padding for nerve relief can reduce symptoms.

Cases requiring surgical release of the retinaculum may necessitate either a walking boot or a non-weight-bearing posterior splint for about 2 weeks postoperatively. A normal therapeutic exercise progression is followed by jogging at around 6 to 8 weeks and return to full participation at around 10 to 12 weeks following surgery.

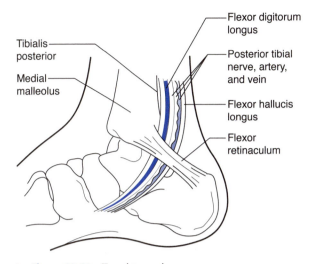

▶ **Figure 22.64** Tarsal tunnel.

Sesamoiditis

The two sesamoids under the first metatarsal head function to enhance the windlass mechanism of the foot for increased propulsion, provide improved leverage of the great toe flexor tendon, and disperse the weight-bearing forces (Jahss, 1981). A sesamoiditis does not actually involve the sesamoids but rather the soft tissue surrounding the bones. Restriction of soft tissue around the sesamoids, a tight Achilles tendon, plantar-flexed first ray, reduced great-toe hyperextension motion, and a restricted midfoot can all be underlying causes of sesamoiditis (Dietzen, 1990). Occasionally, cleat misplacement on shoes can increase pressure on the sesamoids and cause soft-tissue irritation. Hyperextension of about 65° is required for walking and running activities. Less hyperextension than that can increase forces imposed on the sesamoid region during propulsion.

The patient complains of pain with running, especially during push-off. Pain is located over the first metatarsal head. Standing heel raises with pressure over the first metatarsal head are painful, as is passive dorsiflexion of the great toe. Palpation reveals tenderness of the sesamoids.

Treatment includes relieving the symptoms and correcting the underlying cause. Flexibility exercises to correct tight structures are vital. Soft-tissue mobilization is usually necessary, because the soft tissue becomes adherent around the sesamoids and further restricts great-toe hyperextension motion. A pad or orthotic with a cutout for the first ray and with an extension pad to the second metatarsal head and toe can help to reduce stress on the sesamoids. Placing the foot in a rigid-soled shoe also limits the stress applied to the sesamoids.

This injury is self-limiting and does not usually require cessation of activity. Modification of shoe wear, correction of the causes, and modifications in activity usually will allow the patient to continue some level of participation.

Turf Toe

Turf toe is a hyperextension injury to the first MTP joint that occurs when the phalanx is jammed into the metatarsal. Improperly fitting shoes and high acceleration forces are common accompanying factors.

Symptoms include tenderness, swelling, and reduced range of motion of the great toe. Rehabilitation includes modalities to reduce the swelling and pain in phase I; scar-tissue mobilization and active range-of-motion exercises in phase II; and strength exercises in late phase II and early phase III. Ankle dorsiflexion with toe flexion-extension can be performed

---

■ **Case Study**

An 18-year-old male collegiate freshman sprinter had a plantar wart removed from the medial aspect of the ball of his left foot five years ago. Recently the ball of the foot has become progressively painful during running. He does not remember any injury to the foot recently. Your examination reveals an area of swelling with hard scar tissue around the first metatarsal head. His great-toe hyperextension is 45°. He complains of pain when you attempt to hyperextend the toe beyond that point. He is unable to stand on his toes without pain. His ankle dorsiflexion in subtalar neutral is –5°. Mobilization of the sesamoids is difficult, with mobility about 50% compared to that of the right foot. The patient reports pain when you attempt to mobilize the sesamoids with medial-lateral and superior-inferior glides.

Questions for Analysis

1. What is your determination of the cause of the patient's pain?
2. What will your treatment for him today include?
3. What modifications will you place on his foot or in his shoe that will permit him to continue his workout program?
4. What instructions will you give the patient for his workout tomorrow and for his home program?
5. How will your treatment program change as he improves over the next few weeks?

---

in a whirlpool early and then in weight bearing as tolerated. Joint mobilizations, initially in grades I and II for pain relief occur in phase I but later in phase II, grades III and IV for joint mobility, are included. Strengthening exercises including closed kinetic chain activities and progressing to jumping and plyometric exercises are added as the patient tolerates them in from late phase II into phase IV.

Shoe fit should be appropriate before the patient is allowed to return to participation. A rigid toe box and plantar-flexion positioning of the first ray with strapping or padding can be useful in reducing pain when the patient returns to the sport and unrestricted normal activities.

Fractures

The primary concern with a fracture in a young patient is that it may include the growth plates. If this occurs, further development and bone growth can be severely impaired. Stress fractures and acute fractures are more common than one might think. Each is treated differently; programs and considerations related to these fractures are outlined here.

Fractures can occur in any of the extremity, ankle, or foot bones. Stress fractures result from repetitive stress to the tibia and metatarsal bones, whereas acute fractures result from sudden application of excessive forces. In younger patients, epiphyseal plate fractures can occur, especially in the distal fibula and tibia. Acute fractures vary greatly in their presentation and according to how the forces are applied. Lateral stresses to the ankle can result in malleolar fractures; compression forces from jumping can cause talus, tibia, and metatarsal fractures; crush injuries from having the foot stepped on can cause metatarsal and phalangeal fractures; other phalangeal fractures can occur as a result of stubbing a toe; and torsional stresses can cause spiral fractures of the tibia and foot.

Phalangeal fractures are painful but seldom casted. The fractured phalanx is commonly buddy taped to an adjacent toe. Metatarsal fractures of the second, third, and fourth metatarsals are commonly placed in a controlled ankle motion (CAM) boot to restrict movement during ambulation. Crutches are sometimes needed if the patient is unable to ambulate normally. Fractures of the first metatarsal require special attention because this is a major weight-bearing bone. Fifth metatarsal fractures also deserve special attention because they can cause problems that linger, depending on the fracture's location. Tarsal fractures can be interarticular and involve interarticular ligamentous damage. If the fracture is displaced, surgery is usually indicated. Ankle fractures are often surgically repaired, because even minimal displacement of fragments has better results with surgical repair than with conservative management (Thigpen, 1983). Fractures in young patients should be referred to an orthopedic surgeon because epiphyseal fractures are serious injuries that threaten to impair normal bone growth.

Because the tibia, talus, calcaneus, and first ray are the primary weight-bearing structures of the foot and leg, fractures to these bones require immobilization and non-weight bearing. The fibula is essentially a non-weight-bearing bone, so walking boots or walking casts are usually used for fractures of this bone. Displaced fractures are surgically repaired whereas nondisplaced fractures may be immobilized with or without surgery.

Immobilization of fractures of the leg, ankle, or foot must include immobilization of the ankle. After immobilization, limited joint mobility is one of the greatest debilitating factors. The greater the damage, the more extensive the scar-tissue formation. The risk of increased scar tissue formation is greater with a greater and more prolonged presence of edema. Immobilization and soft-tissue edema with subsequent scar-tissue adhesions combine to produce restricted joint mobility of the ankle and other regional joints. Normal mobility of these joints must be restored to make full balance of function possible. If one joint is restricted, an adjacent joint suffers exaggerated stresses as it compensates for the lost mobility of the restricted joint. Over time, the increased stress can lead to tissue breakdown and injury.

In addition, the immobilization time required for fracture healing leads to capsular restriction, muscle weakness, balance and proprioception deficits, and muscle endurance deficiencies. Joint motion and soft-tissue mobility must be emphasized in early rehabilitation, because the window of opportunity for regaining these elements is narrower than for the other factors. As scar tissue matures, the opportunity to impact changes in its length diminishes. If prolonged immobilization and extensive scar-tissue formation have occurred, prolonged stretches to affect more mature scar tissue may be necessary to increase mobility of shortened tissue and adherent collagen.

The typical duration of foot, ankle, and leg fracture immobilization is three to six weeks. This time may vary for stress fractures and surgically repaired fractures. Stress fractures are not frequently casted, but activity is reduced to relieve stress on the fracture site and provide an optimal healing environment. Fractures that undergo open reduction internal fixation (ORIF) usually advance to weight bearing sooner than conservatively treated fractures. Patients with fractures that involve the primary weight-bearing bones are advanced to weight bearing with more caution, and full weight bearing is delayed.

Joint mobilization and soft-tissue mobilization techniques are initiated as soon as safely possible. Modalities, such as heat or ultrasound, applied before mobilization techniques can be useful in preparing soft tissue and achieving better treatment results. Massage is useful in relieving edema. Deep-tissue massage, friction massage, and myofascial techniques are used to improve soft-tissue mobility.

Joint mobilization techniques for pain relief occur early, in phase I, whereas grades III and IV are applied in late phase II. If a joint is very tender, grade III and IV techniques may not be possible until pain is under control. Active stretches, passive stretches, and contract-relax-stretch techniques are useful during phase II to increase motion of both joint and soft-tissue structures.

Immobilization and times of restricted weight bearing necessitate gait-training instructions once the patient is able to resume full weight bearing. Prior to weight bearing, using the pool with the patient in shoulder-high water provides only 10% of body weight on the extremity and can be used to address normal gait techniques. When the patient is partial weight bearing, it is important to instruct the patient in a normal heel-toe gait to encourage proper gait patterning in preparation for full weight bearing. Once the patient is permitted to bear full

The rehabilitation clinician sees a number of common foot and ankle injuries that call for specific approaches within the therapeutic exercise program. Some of these injuries are sprains and dislocations, Achilles tendon injuries, shin splints, compartment syndromes, a variety of foot injuries, and fractures.

weight on the extremity, pregait instruction, including weight-transfer activities and normal stride reeducation, is usually needed.

Closed kinetic chain exercises for strengthening, as well as static balance activities such as stork standing, begin when full weight bearing is permitted. Therapeutic exercises proceed in the manner discussed earlier in this chapter. Advancement follows a logical progression from light to heavier weights, few to more repetitions, static to dynamic balance and agility exercises, and simple to complex activities until the patient advances to plyometric exercises and finally to functional activities before returning to full activity.

The rate of progression is determined by the tissue-healing timeline, the tissue's response to stresses, and the individual's ability to tolerate the therapeutic exercise progression. Activity-specific testing before return to full participation must mimic demands that the patient will encounter during his or her ability to perform. Once all the parameters are improved and the patient passes all tests without any difference in performance from left to right lower extremity, he or she may resume normal participation. Depending on the extent of the injury, the time of immobilization, the age of the patient, and initial joint and soft-tissue restriction following immobilization, three to six months is a reasonable amount of time before the patient is able to resume normal participation.

■ Case Study

A 16-year-old wrestler sustained a left ankle lateral malleolar fracture during a wrestling match. He underwent an ORIF the following day and was placed on crutches, non-weight bearing for two weeks before advancing to partial weight bearing. It is now four weeks after the surgery and the patient is not yet full weight bearing, although the surgeon has instructed him to begin weight bearing to tolerance and to advance to weight bearing without the crutches. The patient admits to you that he is apprehensive about putting weight on the extremity for fear of breaking it again. The extremity had been placed in a cast following surgery until yesterday, when it was removed.

On examination, the patient's ankle moves to 10° plantar flexion for maximum dorsi-flexion. Other measures include 30° of plantar flexion, 0° of eversion, and 5° of inversion. Ankle strength in these directions is 2+/5 in the available ranges of motion. His hip and knee ranges of motion are normal, but strength is 4–/5 for all of the muscle groups. The surgical scar is well healed, but sloughing skin is present around the ankle and there are dry scabs over the wound. Palpation reveals stiffness of soft tissue around the ankle and into the foot. The foot is mildly enlarged, but there is no pitting edema. Joint mobility of the ankle joints is restricted to no more than 30% of normal, and the intertarsal and metatarsal joints are restricted to 50% normal mobility.

Questions for Analysis

1. What are your goals for today's treatment session?

2. What home program will you send with the patient today?

3. The patient wants to attend a wrestling camp in 10 weeks; what will you tell him when he asks whether he will be able to attend the camp?

4. List your long- and short-term goals for the patient for the next six weeks.

5. What will be your criteria for advancing him to closed kinetic chain exercises?

6. List three closed kinetic exercises that you will give the patient the first day these types of exercises are in his program.

7. List three non-weight-bearing exercises that you will give him in the next week.

8. List three agility exercises you will use in the patient's program and the criteria he must meet before they are used.

SUMMARY

The characteristics of a normal foot and deviations from this norm were presented in this chapter. Variations from normal can increase stresses along the closed kinetic chain. To reduce these stresses, it is important to have a foot that is well-aligned. Proper shoes, both in fit and design, will assist in optimizing foot function. The basic shoe construction and specific designs for various activities were presented. Occasionally, it may be necessary to use an orthotic to correct more profoundly misaligned feet. Either an over-the-counter or a custom made orthotic may be required to reduce stresses caused by poor foot alignment. Trigger point treatment, joint mobilization techniques, and progressive exercises from flexibility to functional activities were included in this chapter. Some of the more common injuries of the foot, ankle, and leg were presented along with rehabilitation programs for them.

KEY CONCEPTS AND REVIEW

1. Discuss normal foot mechanics in ambulation.

The first structure to hit the ground during ambulation is the calcaneus. It, along with the talus, forms the subtalar joint; and the talus, along with the tibia and fibula, forms the talocrural joint. Normal function of these two joints permits us to land the foot on the ground and adapt to variations in ground topography and stresses while maintaining a steady gait. The talocrural joint moves primarily in dorsiflexion and plantar flexion. The subtalar joint is responsible for pronation and supination. Pronation and its component motions cause the foot to convert to a mobile adapter for accommodation to uneven surfaces. Supination causes the foot articulations to become more rigid and provide for power transfer to permit appropriate force distribution needed for propulsion in ambulation. As the ankle goes into plantar flexion, the talus moves anteriorly so that the posterior, narrower aspect of the talus sits in the mortise joint. During dorsiflexion, the fibula glides superiorly and rotates laterally; and in plantar flexion, it moves inferiorly and rotates medially. In addition to the talocrural and subtalar joints, the more distal tarsal bones of the foot form the midtarsal joint. This joint's movements closely follow the subtalar and talocrural joint movements. During supination, the navicular and cuboid bones move medially and inferiorly; during pronation they move laterally and superiorly. The first-ray movement occurs in plantar flexion and dorsiflexion and is equal in each direction, with each equal to about a thumb's width of motion. The second ray includes the joint between the second metatarsal and middle cuneiform; the third ray includes the third metatarsal and the lateral cuneiform; the fourth ray is the fourth metatarsal alone; and the fifth ray is the fifth metatarsal alone. Metatarsophalangeal joints permit flexion-extension, abduction-adduction, and accessory rotation and dorsal-plantar glides. The IP joints, which are hinge joints, permit flexion and extension with accessory rotation and dorsal-plantar glides. The first MTP joint must have about 60° to 65° of hyperextension for toe roll-off during gait.

2. Identify two foot deformities and discuss their impact on athletic injury.

Pes cavus, a rigid foot, makes force absorption of the foot more limited, causing forces to be absorbed farther up the closed chain and thus risking injury to other structures. Pes planus, or flatfoot, causes the foot to move inefficiently, requiring more effort from, and subsequently applying more stress to, other structures. It also changes the mechanics of the extremity, increasing stresses applied to structures such as the Achilles, patella, and hip.

3. Describe the primary structures of a shoe.

A shoe's main components include an upper and a lower section. The upper section includes the vamp, toe box, saddle, collar, insole board, sock liner, and heel counter. The lower section includes the outsole, wedge, and midsole. The vamp covers the toes and forefoot and includes the toe box. The toe box varies in width and height and functions to retain the shape of the shoe's forefoot and provide room for the toes. The saddle is the midsection of the shoe along the longitudinal arch, which is usually reinforced to assist in supporting the midfoot. The heel counter is an important stabilizer for the rearfoot. A foxing is an additional piece often seen in athletic shoes that further reinforces the rearfoot to assist in maintaining the counter's shape. The medial aspect of the counter is sometimes extended forward to resist pronation. The collar, the top rim of the shoe, is often padded to reduce friction on the Achilles. The insole board lies between the upper and lower segments and serves as the attachment for the two segments. A sock liner on top of the insole board is used for shock absorption and friction reduction for the foot.

4. List the important factors in shoe considerations for a pes cavus foot.

Because a pes cavus foot is rigid and has limited stress-absorption capabilities, a shoe for someone with this deformity should have as much force absorption as possible. Factors such as a soft midsole, a curved last, and flexibility should be standards in a shoe for a rigid foot.

5. Outline key factors in an orthotic evaluation.

(1) The patient's height and weight; (2) type of sport and activity level of the patient; (3) medical history; (4) the patient's primary and secondary complaints; (5) the calcaneal position in relaxed standing and in subtalar neutral standing; (6) the appearance of the arches in weight bearing and non-weight bearing; (7) toe positions; (8) knee positions; (9) tibial varum; (10) first-ray positions; (11) subtalar mobility; (12) midtarsal mobility; (13) first-metatarsal mobility; (14) hallux dorsiflexion; (15) ankle dorsiflexion; and (16) location of corns and calluses. This last factor is important because corns and calluses are indicators of accommodating or nonaccommodating forefoot and rearfoot deformities.

6. Explain one joint mobilization technique for improving ankle dorsiflexion.

A dorsal glide can be used: The stabilizing hand is placed anteriorly around the distal extremity, and the mobilizing hand is placed around the proximal foot with the thumb and index finger in contact with the malleoli. The talus is glided posteriorly in the plane of the joint.

7. List three stretching exercises for the ankle and extremity, including one that is not mentioned in the text.

Some stretches for these structures are the standing gastrocnemius stretch, the seated soleus stretch with a strap, and standing sideways on an incline board with the ankle positioned in inversion.

8. Identify three strengthening exercises for the ankle and extremity.

Exercises for strengthening the ankle and extremity include calf raises, toe raises, and eversion in sidelying with a weight attached to the ankle.

9. Explain three agility exercises.

For agility the patient can do lateral jumps, zigzag runs, and rapid change-of-direction maneuvers performed on command.

10. Describe three functional exercises for the lower extremity.

Some functional exercises for the lower extremity are side-to-side sprints; run, stop and jump exercises; and running and stopping while bouncing a basketball.

11. Provide an example of a therapeutic exercise program progression for an ankle sprain.

Initial treatment in phase I includes modalities for edema and pain relief and reduction of inflammation. Joint mobilization and soft-tissue mobilization may be necessary in phase II if those structures are impaired in their normal movement. Active and passive range-of-motion exercises are accompanied by mild strengthening exercises, such as isometrics, manual resistance, and rubber band exercises in phase II. If the patient has been non-weight bearing, it may be necessary to use exercises with a weight scale to reintroduce the concept of weight bearing on the extremity as a prelude to gait training. Body-weight resistance exercises and machine-weight resistance exercises are then included as the patient progresses to phase III. Balance and proprioception exercises begin with simple stork standing and progress to standing on unstable surfaces, then moving on one extremity. Once strength, flexibility, and balance are restored, plyometric and then functional and activity-specific exercises are used in phase IV before return to participation.

CRITICAL THINKING QUESTIONS

1. Explain how Benjamin concluded that Hannah's plantar fasciitis was being caused by her pronation, hip tightness, and knee and tibial malalignments. Why would he suspect that Hannah's thigh muscle imbalance was also contributing to the plantar fasciitis? What shoe characteristics should Hannah look for when she buys her next running shoes?

2. If a patient had a leg-length discrepancy but no other major structural problems, would you expect to see an abnormal wear pattern on the bottom of his or her shoes? If so, what?

3. Using the repaired-Achilles case study presented earlier, what would you include in an aquatic exercise program for this patient for range of motion, strength, and cardio-vascular conditioning? When could you begin his aquatic program?

LAB ACTIVITIES

1. Perform a deep-tissue massage to your lab partner's leg. Are you able to locate any areas of restriction? Is that same area also tender when you apply a deep massage to it? Why would this be?

2. Instruct your partner in a home treatment to release adhesions on the plantar foot. Give precise instructions in terms of what to use, how long to apply it, how much pressure to use, and what the expected outcome should be.

3. Locate the trigger points for the following muscles on your lab partner:
   a. Peroneus longus
   b. Gastrocnemius
   c. Soleus
   d. Abductor hallucis
   e. Flexor digitorum brevis
   f. Quadratus plantae
   g. Flexor hallucis brevis

Where were your partner's most sensitive trigger points? Perform an ice/spray-and-stretch technique on each of them and provide your partner with a home exercise for each tender trigger point

4. Perform grades II and IV joint mobilizations on your lab partner and identify what restriction would be best treated with each mobilization for the following joints:

   a. Tibiofibular joints
- Superior: AP, PA glides
- Inferior: AP, PA glides

   b. Talocrural joint
- Distraction
- Anterior glide
- Posterior glide

   c. Subtalar joint
- Distraction
- Anterior glide
- Posterior glide

   d. TMT, MTP, IP joints
- Distraction
- Anterior glide
- Posterior glide

5. Have your partner perform a gastrocnemius and soleus stretch. What are the substitution patterns and where does she or he feel the stretch for each of the exercises? What verbal cues could you use to correct the errors in performance?

6. Have your partner perform a prolonged Achilles stretch for 3 minutes. How could she perform the exercise incorrectly so the stretch would not be optimally effective? When she steps out of the stretch, what does she feel?

7. Provide your partner with manual resistance to dorsiflexion, inversion, and eversion, 10 repetitions each. Be sure to provide enough resistance to make the motion smooth, accommodating your resistance to match his and still obtain a maximal output from him or her for each exercise. What position did you place him or her in to allow you to provide resistance most efficiently?

8. Now have him perform the same exercises as in question 7 with a Thera-band. First, how will you determine what color of Thera-band she should use for each exercise? Have her perform the exercise and then describe the differences in how the manual resistance and Thera-band resistance felt throughout the range of motion for each exercise. How do these results influence the factors you would use to decide what kind of exercise to include in a rehabilitation program?

9. Have your partner perform balance exercises that progress from static balance to dynamic balance to balance while performing distracting activities. Evaluate how your partner was able to perform the activities as you would for a chart note. Be sure to include the activity, repetitions, and your assessment on quality of performance.

10. Have your partner perform one agility drill that you design using tape marks on the floor. Diagram the exercise on paper. Have her perform it first without resistance then with resistance. Did your partner's ability to perform the activity change with the addition of resistance? If so, how did it change? What performance factors did you watch and correct for and what were your cues for correction? What sport athletes would benefit most from these activities as part of their rehabilitation program?

11. Design one plyometric or hopping activity. Describe it and identify why this is the one you selected. Have your partner perform it. What performance factors did you watch and correct for, and what were your cues for correction? What would be the criteria for your partner to advance to the next level of exercise? Which patients benefit most from these activities as part of their rehabilitation program?

Knee and Thigh

OBJECTIVES

After completing this chapter, you should be able to do the following:

1. Discuss the relationship and alignment between the patella and femur.
2. Identify post-injury factors that influence strength output.
3. Define quadriceps extensor lag and explain its significance.
4. Outline a general progression of rehabilitation for a knee.
5. Identify three soft-tissue mobilization techniques for the knee.
6. Identify three joint mobilization techniques for the knee, and their purpose.
7. Explain three flexibility exercises for the knee, and identify the structures they affect.
8. Explain three proprioception/balance exercises for the knee.
9. Identify three functional activities.
10. Identify three factors that influence PFD.

▶ Three mornings a week Nate Richards and his friends play a game of basketball at the university gym before going to work. It is their way of having fun and getting exercise at the same time. They have been following this routine since they were in their mid-30s, about 10 years ago. About two weeks ago their routine was suddenly disrupted. Nate jumped to retrieve a rebound and landed in severe pain. He felt as if someone had shot him in the thigh. Several hours later he underwent a quadriceps tendon repair and was placed on crutches.

Today he had his first rehabilitation appointment with Sam Joley, a clinician that has come highly recommended to Nate. After Sam Joley completed his examination, he explained to Nate what he saw as primary problems and discussed how he thought they could best resolve those problems. Nate agreed with him and realized that this was not going to be an easy or short process, but he was willing to work with Sam to get back onto the basketball court. He liked Sam's approach and appreciated the way Sam was able to explain things better than the doctor did, so he could understand them. He knew Sam would work him hard, but he also knew that if he wanted to play basketball again, he would have to work hard, and he was eager to start.

Although Sam explained to Nate that it would be a lengthy process and would require Nate to be committed and consistent in his rehabilitation, Sam also knew that the tissue's healing process had to be respected. Because it was only two weeks since Nate's surgery, stress to the newly formed tissue was important, but too much stress could be detrimental. The proper amount of stress to the patellar tendon was important, but he could also start Nate on more aggressive exercises on the hip and ankle without stressing the patellar tendon, Sam sensed that Nate was the type of person who was eager and willing to work hard but would also understand precautions if he knew about them. As he does with all his patients, Sam would keep Nate well informed throughout his program about what he should and should not be doing and why.

Never let the fear of striking out get in your way.

BABE RUTH, 1895-1948, American baseball player

Over the years, there have been many changes in rehabilitation of knee injuries. The standard of care changes as new advances in understanding and revelations of knee mechanics and healing evolve. Although current concepts may be the best at the time, sometimes advances in research demonstrate them to be erroneous. This is when we find that we have "struck out" with previous treatment and alter treatment techniques to reflect these new discoveries. In the past few years, a tremendous amount of research has provided us with a wealth of knowledge on the knee. There is still a plethora of information to be gleaned about the knee, but in the past several years, investigators have given us new insights and information regarding knee biomechanics and improved surgical procedures and optimal rehabilitation techniques.

This chapter deals with thigh and knee injuries. Thigh injuries could just as easily have been considered along with the hip in the next chapter. Indeed, I will refer you from one chapter to the other, because there is an intimate relationship between the thigh and knee and the thigh and hip. I have placed most thigh injuries in this chapter only because the knee comes before the hip in the text. Thigh injuries that impact primarily the hip are presented in chapter 24.

As with the other chapters in part IV, this one begins with general information that impacts therapeutic exercise programs for knee and thigh injuries. This information is vital if the rehabilitation clinician is to design and establish an appropriate therapeutic exercise program for the various injuries of the knee and thigh. This chapter presents specific therapeutic exercise techniques, including soft-tissue and joint mobilization and exercises for flexibility, strength, and coordination. Recommendations for functional activities before the patient's return to full sport or normal-activity participation are also included. The final section of the chapter discusses rehabilitation programs for specific injuries commonly seen in the knee and thigh.

Controversy continues on the best surgical repair technique and the most appropriate postoperative and postinjury methods of rehabilitation for the knee. Over the past several years, treatments of knee injuries and postoperative care have changed dramatically. Up until the late 1970s, postoperative knee care included cast immobilization and non-weight bearing for six weeks. Although cast immobilization is not part of postoperative care today, many surgeons choose to remain conservative while others prefer a more accelerated approach to their surgical repairs. It is important for the rehabilitation clinician to work with the physician to provide a successful rehabilitation outcome for the patient. Both the physician's and the rehabilitation clinician's protocols for rehabilitation of knee and thigh injuries should be based on the severity of the injury, the structure injured, and the tissue healing timeline. If there is to be an error, as with any rehabilitation program, it should be on the side of caution.

Specific injuries to the knee and thigh that require particular types of therapeutic exercise approaches include ligament sprains, collateral ligament sprains, meniscus injuries, patellofemoral injuries, strains and contusions, and bone injuries.

GENERAL REHABILITATION CONSIDERATIONS

The knee is one of the most frequently injured joints. The forces applied to it during running, twisting, and lifting activities are complicated by the fact that there are two long lever arms on either end of the joint, making it a joint susceptible to excessive stresses. For as shallow a joint as the knee is, complete dislocation is surprisingly rare. This rarity may be so because of the strong static and dynamic structures that surround the joint. The ligaments and muscles of the knee give the joint a sound structure so tremendous forces are required to produce an injury. The more common knee injuries are discussed later in this chapter. This section deals with unique knee structures which serve to support and protect the joint but are impacted when injury occurs.

Knee Structure

At first glance, the knee appears to be a relatively simple joint, but it is actually a complex structure. Within its anatomical structure, it possesses several elements that influence its function. When balance is lacking in structure or function, the knee becomes susceptible to injury. An understanding of the knee's structures and the ways they influence one another is basic to the ability to develop a therapeutic exercise program for any injury of the knee.

Tibiofemoral Joint

The knee joint is actually two joints, the tibiofemoral joint and the patellofemoral joint. The tibiofemoral joint has a concave tibia platform attached to a convex femur. This means that during joint mobilization, the concave tibia moves on the convex femur in the same direction as the physiological movement of the joint. In other words, a posterior glide of the tibia on the femur produces flexion and an anterior glide produces extension.

Capsule

The knee joint is the largest joint of the body and is surrounded by a capsule that aids in joint stability by merging with the collateral ligaments. The capsule also distributes the synovial fluid around the joint during movement and merges with many of the knee's bursae. If the joint capsule is restricted, a capsular pattern becomes apparent. The knee's capsular pattern is restriction of flexion more than of extension. The joint is in a resting position when it is in about 20° to 25° of flexion and in a fully close-packed position in full extension with lateral tibial rotation.

Ligaments

The collateral ligaments provide knee protection and stability against medial and lateral stresses. The medial collateral ligament (MCL) attaches to the medial meniscus. This arrangement may be one reason the medial meniscus is often injured with MCL sprains. In addition to providing protection against valgus stresses, the MCL helps to restrict lateral rotation of the tibia on the femur. The lateral collateral ligament (LCL) does not attach to the lateral meniscus and is taut during medial rotation of the tibia on the femur and when the knee incurs varus stress. Because valgus stress from lateral forces occurs more often to the knee than varus stresses, the MCL is the more frequently injured of these two ligaments.

The anterior and posterior cruciate ligaments (ACL and PCL, respectively) are structures unique to the knee. Their position within the knee joint allows them to provide distinctive anterior-posterior stability to the knee. The ligaments also provide the knee with rotational stability. Some fibers of each ligament are taut throughout the knee's range of motion. Injury to either ligament can cause instability within the knee that can be disabling.

The ACL and PCL are encased within a synovial membrane that provides the ligaments with their primary blood supply. If a partial tear of either ligament occurs, the synovial membrane may also become disrupted, compromising the ligament's vascular supply. If this happens, dehiscence, or erosion, of the ligament eventually results.

The ACL is the most researched structure of the entire musculoskeletal system within the past quarter century (Dienst, Burks, & Greis, 2002). This may be because of the frequency with which it is injured, especially in sports. The ACL protects the knee from anterior translation of the tibia on the femur. The PCL is not as frequently injured, but there is evidence indicating that injury rates to the PCL are increasing (Bosch, Kasperczyk, Oestern, & Tscherne, 1994). The PCL serves primarily to restrict knee hyperextension and posterior tibial displacement of the tibia on the femur.

All of the joint's ligaments restrain rotational stresses at the knee. The cruciate ligaments twist and become taut during medial rotation. The collateral ligaments become taut to provide stability during lateral rotation. Rotation is a primary motion of the knee in both weight bearing and non-weight bearing. In weight bearing, the femur rotates on the tibia, and in non-weight bearing, the tibia rotates on the femur. Since all ligaments restrain rotation, injury mechanisms that produce excessive rotational forces can cause damage to more than one ligament and subsequently result in joint instability.

The knee's joint capsule and intra-articular structures, including the anterior and posterior cruciate ligaments, contain various neuroreceptors that provide the neural system with position-afferent information from the knee (Safran et al., 1999). We know that the ACL contains afferent mechanoreceptors that impact the knee's stability. The joint capsule has mechanoreceptors (Ruffini endings) that are sensitive to pressure and deformation (Freeman & Wyke, 1967). Injury to the knee's ligamentous structures can damage these receptors, impairing proprioception (Lephart, Pincivero, & Rozzi, 1998). Therapeutic exercise programs must include proprioception facilitative techniques to restore the deficiencies resulting from interarticular knee injuries (Hewett, Paterno, & Myer, 2002).

Although each ligament has its own responsibility in supporting and protecting the knee, ligaments also provide assistive support to other ligaments. These protective designs are referred to as primary and secondary restraint. As an example, the ACL is the primary restraint protecting the knee against anterior tibial translation, but if it is injured, other structures such as the capsule, other ligaments, and muscles act as secondary restraints and are emphasized in non-surgical patients so joint protection continues in spite of the injury (Fitzgerald, Axe, & Snyder-Mackler, 2000). Sometimes the secondary structures are able to assume the responsibilities of providing normal stability to the joint so surgical repair is not required, but sometimes they fall short. Instability caused by ACL or PCL insufficiencies is often minimally supported by secondary structures (Butler, Noyes, & Grood, 1980).

Meniscus

The medial and lateral meniscus serve to cushion the joint, deepen the socket, increase joint congruity to better distribute weight-bearing forces, assist in joint lubrication, and provide stability. These structures are commonly referred to as cartilage, although this is a misnomer. These structures are primarily fibrocartilage (hence the name), but this is certainly not their only component. The knee joint also has articular cartilage, so the term "cartilage" is not only erroneous but sometimes confusing, especially to the patient who has injured articular cartilage, not meniscus. The medial meniscus is attached to the MCL, the ACL, and the semimembranosus. This arrangement is believed to be one cause for the greater frequency of injury to the medial meniscus (McCarty, Marx, & DeHaven, 2002). Even though the lateral meniscus is not attached to the LCL but does connect to the popliteus and PCL, it has more freedom of movement and is not impacted by collateral ligament positioning and stresses. When the knee moves in flexion and extension within the sagittal plane, the menisci follow the tibial movements. During flexion, the menisci are pulled posteriorly via the semimembranosus and popliteus, and during extension they are pulled anteriorly by the meniscopatellar ligaments. During rotation, the menisci follow the movements of the femur. During movement from extension into flexion, the femur slides posteriorly on the tibia during weight bearing so that in a squat position, the weight is borne primarily by the posterior menisci, whereas in extension, the femur is primarily on the anterior menisci. Compressive forces absorbed by the menisci are up to 50% to 60% of the knee's loads (McCarty et al., 2002). When the knee is at 90° flexion and the primary force is applied at the posterior aspect of the joint, the meniscal load increases to 85% of the total knee joint compressive forces (Ahmed & Burke, 1983). Meniscal posterior horn tears seem to be primarily degenerative tears, whereas anterior horn and lateral tears are often traumatic events. Posterior degenerative tears may be related to the increased forces absorbed by the menisci in flexion, as well as to the repetitive activity imposed on the menisci during squatting and other positional activities. On the other hand, acute tears occur most often during a running or cutting maneuver, when the knee is near extension.

The menisci are avascular except for roughly their peripheral 25%. This has a significant impact on conservative and surgical intervention following injury of the meniscus. This topic is discussed later in the chapter.

Screw Home Mechanism

The knee joint is a modified hinge joint. This means that although it is similar to a hinge joint, permitting movement in one plane, the bony segments are not entirely and purely congruent throughout. Because the medial aspect of the joint is larger and extends slightly more distally than the lateral side, when the knee moves into extension during weight bearing, the tibia rotates laterally as the medial femoral condyle rotates on the medial tibial plateau. This mechanism, called the screw home mechanism, occurs in the last 30° of extension. It affords the joint greater stability than a pure hinge-joint arrangement would because it provides a kind of locking for the joint. The popliteus is responsible for unlocking the knee during movement from full extension into flexion. It does this by laterally rotating the femoral condyles with its medial tibial insertion anchored in weight bearing. In non-weight bearing, the popliteus unlocks the knee as it medially rotates the tibia with its proximal insertion stabilized. The importance of this mechanism becomes apparent later in the chapter when discussion of full joint motion and joint mobilization are presented.

Patellofemoral Joint

The patella, the largest sesamoid bone in the body, sits within the femoral groove. Its resting position is knee extension, and its close-packed position is knee flexion. The patella serves to increase the lever-arm length of the quadriceps tendon, adds to the cosmesis of the knee joint, and protects the knee from anterior blows. It is a site of common knee pain and dysfunction.

The quadriceps tendon and its medial and lateral expansions surround the patella. The tendon attachment from the patella to the tibial tubercle is sometimes referred to as the patellar ligament because it travels from bone to bone. This structure is also called the patellar tendon.

Patellar stability is the result of static and dynamic structures. The greatest bony contributor to patellar stability is the femoral sulcus formed by the medial and higher-ridged lateral epicondyles within which the patella sits. Ligamentous stability from the patellofemoral and patellotibial joints assists in providing static restraints. Active restraints from the quadriceps provide the greatest dynamic stability. The pes anserine group and the biceps femoris with their control of tibial rotation provide indirect secondary dynamic support. Tibial rotation changes the tibial tubercle position and can alter stability provided by the patellar tendon.

Patellar alignment examination occurs in static and dynamic positions. The patella is examined in long sitting for abnormalities in resting. Position of the patella during contraction of the quadriceps in long sitting and in weight bearing is also examined, because patellar movement in open and closed kinetic chain conditions may be different. A closed kinetic chain position can change the patellar alignment because other factors, such as hip rotation and foot pronation, alter the way the patella moves when the quadriceps contract.

Superior Tibiofibular Joint

This joint is not actually a joint of the knee because it is distal to the knee joint, but it can affect the ankle and knee joints. There are no physiological movements in this joint, but it must have full accessory motion for full ankle range of motion to occur. Reduced tibiofibular joint mobility can cause lateral knee pain by restricting soft-tissue mobility in the region.

Muscles

The quadriceps and hamstrings have been the most widely addressed muscles because of their prominence in knee control. Both groups also influence the hip, and because they do, positioning of the hip must always be a consideration when one is exercising the muscles at the knee.

The quadriceps provides the most dynamic restraint for the knee. The rectus femoris is the quadriceps component that also assists in hip flexion. Hip positioning determines where in the motion the rectus femoris contributes the most at the knee. In a supine straight-leg raise, it works throughout the motion; but in sitting, the rectus femoris works only in terminal extension (Close, 1964).

Because of the angle of their pull and tendon insertions, the hamstrings also produce tibial rotation. The biceps femoris produces lateral tibial rotation, and the semimembranosus and semitendinosus produce medial tibial rotation. They provide dynamic secondary restraints to assist the ACL, and in ACL-deficient knees, they must be trained to become more prominent stabilizers.

Rehabilitation of isolated hamstring muscles should include the additional movements of tibial rotation along with hip extension and knee flexion. Eccentric and concentric activities for all their motions would most appropriately strengthen the hamstrings throughout all their functions.

Biomechanical and Physiological Concepts

An appreciation of biomechanical and physiological concepts helps the clinician understand the significance of specific therapeutic exercise applications for various knee injuries, as well as the indications and precautions.

Patellofemoral and Tibiofemoral Relationship

When the knee extends, the patella glides superiorly and during flexion it glides inferiorly for a total excursion of 5 to 7 cm (2.0-2.8 in.). The patella must glide freely for full knee motion to be possible.

In a normal resting extension, the patella's inferior pole is at the knee joint's margin and lies on the supratrochlear fat pad. A patella that lies superior to this position is called patella alta, and one that is inferior to the normal position is called patella baja. Either abnormal position restricts full range of motion of the knee. Injuries of the patellar tendon, including ACL reconstructions utilizing the quadriceps tendon, may develop patella baja. Injuries such as repaired quadriceps ruptures are susceptible to developing patella alta. Patella baja or alta requires aggressive patellar mobilization and soft-tissue-stretching techniques. These techniques are discussed in detail later.

The patella glides in the femoral groove during knee motion and makes contact with the femoral groove. When contact between the two segments is occurs, compressive forces develop between the posterior patella and anterior femur. These compressive loads can reach up to 10 times body weight during daily activities (Brownstein, Mangiene, Noyes, & Kryer, 1988). In full extension, the patella rests on the fat pad and is not in contact with the sulcus. The area of contact between the posterior patella and femoral groove migrates from the patella's inferior pole to its superior aspect as the knee moves from about 10° to 20° of flexion to 90°. The area of contact is fairly uniform across the breadth of the patella. Once the knee approaches the end of flexion, however, the contact is on the odd facet medially and the lateral-superior aspect of the patella until the patella rests on the top of the lateral condyle in full flexion (figure 23.1).

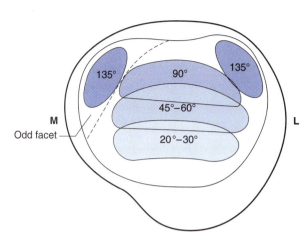

▶ **Figure 23.1** Patellofemoral contact patterns on posterior patella of a right knee.

Of significance with this change in points of contact between the patella and femur is the fact that as the knee moves into flexion, the amount of contact pressure and area of contact both increase. Contact pressure is a ratio between the patellofemoral joint reaction force and the contact area. Joint reaction force is a compressive force equivalent to the resultant vector force (of the patellofemoral quadriceps vector force and patellar tendon vector force). This vector force is perpendicular to the patella's contact surface with the femur. Stress to the patellofemoral joint is the force per area of contact. In a closed kinetic chain activity, the joint reaction forces and the area of contact both increase as the knee moves from extension to 90°, but the force applied is greater than the area of contact, so joint stress increases as the knee moves into flexion to 90°. As the knee moves from 90° toward 120°, the force decreases and the surface area of contact remains the same, so the stress decreases. The greatest compressive forces occur in the 60° to 90° positions (Grelsamer & Klein, 1998; Steinkamp, Dillingham, Markel, Hill, & Kaufman, 1993; Zwerver, Bredeweg, & Hof, 2007). If a patella is not in good alignment within the femoral groove, the congruency between the two bones is altered, so compressive forces are distributed over a smaller area. This may be one reason why malalignment of the patella results in increased pain and irritation of the patellofemoral joint.

In an open kinetic chain activity, the joint stress is lowest at 90° and greatest at 0°. Although there may be some individual variations, open kinetic chain exercises are least irritating when performed from 60° to 90°, while closed kinetic chain exercises cause the least patellofemoral joint irritation in the ranges of 0° to 30° and greater than 90° (Grelsamer & Klein, 1998; Wallace, Salem, Salinas, & Powers, 2002).

During closed kinetic chain activities such as walking, patellofemoral compressive forces of about one half of body weight are produced, while stair climbing produces about three times body weight and squatting produces compressive forces of over seven times body weight (Kaufman, An, Litchy, Morrey, & Chao, 1991; Reilly & Martens, 1972). During open kinetic chain activities the amount of compressive force changes with the type of activity and the angle at which it occurs (Wallace et al., 2002). If knee extension is performed with a weight attached to the end of the extremity, compressive forces reach their peak at 35° to 40°, but if the force is applied by a machine arm at right angles to the ankle such as in an N-K table or isokinetic machine, the peak compressive forces occur at 90° and decrease as the knee extends (Reilly & Martens, 1972; Zwerver et al., 2007). Based on mathematical formulas, it is estimated that isokinetic exercises reach a peak patellofemoral compressive force of about five times body weight (Kaufman et al., 1991).

Many functional activities are performed in the 0° to 40° range of motion. It is important when you are treating patients with patellofemoral pain to avoid painful arcs of motion. Generally, closed kinetic chain exercises from 0° to 40° of flexion provide less lateral patellar motion and less patellofemoral stress than open kinetic chain exercises, and open chain exercises in positions greater than 50° flexion are less stressful (S.A. Doucette & Child, 1996; Steinkamp et al., 1993).

These numbers may seem confusing, but you need to understand their significance when treating patients with patellofemoral stress injuries. Several points are important to remember. The most patellofemoral stress in open chain exercises occurs in the first 30° of motion, and the least amount of stress occurs in the range of 60° to 90°. The least patellofemoral stress in closed chain activities occurs in the first 30° of motion, and the greatest amount of stress occurs in the range of 60° to 90°. Because there is no contact between the femur and patella in 0° to 10°, it should be safe to strengthen in this range with any exercise (Steinkamp et al., 1993). The more inflamed the patellofemoral joint is, the more limited are the ranges of motion the patient is able to exercise within to strengthen the quadriceps without pain. Because the patella does not make contact with the femur until about 20° of flexion, very irritated patellofemoral joints may tolerate motion only in the first 20° of flexion. The exception to this generalization may be patellofemoral pain patients with hyperextended knees; these patients may experience pain in full extension. In these cases, finding a pain-free range of motion other than full extension to 20° flexion is important in order to strengthen the quadriceps.

Full squat exercises and full range-of-motion exercises with weight boots or cuff weights attached to the ankle should be avoided by patellofemoral patients until later in the treatment program when pain is reduced and strength is improved enough for the patellofemoral joint to tolerate the greater stresses of these activities. It is logical to include a slow progression in range of motion as symptoms decrease and strength increases. If you use isokinetic exercises, avoid going into the 90° range of motion where peak patellar compressive forces occur. Shortening the lever-arm length on weight machines will reduce the compressive forces, but the patient's pain is the primary guide as to whether such an adjustment is possible.

Q-Angle

Q-angle is the angle that is formed by a line from the anterior superior iliac spine to the middle patella and a line from the middle patella to the tibial tubercle (figure 23.2). Lower normal Q-angle measurement is 10°. Upper normal values may vary for men and women because of the differences in pelvic structure and range from 11° to 18° (Holmes & Clancy, 1998). The Q-angle can change from non-weight bearing to weight bearing, because tibial rotation changes the Q-angle. If the patient has pronation in weight bearing, the tibia is medially rotated and increases the Q-angle. If the leg laterally rotates, the Q-angle decreases. A weak vastus medialis oblique (VMO) can also increase the Q-angle.

In the past, many thought the Q-angle key to patellofemoral alignment and symptoms. Because it can change with functional activities, unless it is profoundly excessive its significance with patellofemoral pain is not considered as great as in the past (Livingston, 1998). The Q-angle should be assessed for gross abnormalities in non-weight bearing and for changes in standing. It may not be a primary cause of patellofemoral pain syndrome, as was once believed, but it may contribute to the syndrome when other conditions are present.

Lower-extremity Alignment

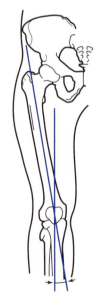

▶ **Figure 23.2** Measuring Q-angle.

As mentioned earlier, excessive rearfoot pronation influences the patella's alignment because it increases tibial rotation and changes the quadriceps tendon pull on the patella (Holmes & Clancy, 1998). You should evaluate other lower-extremity alignments during a knee examination because alterations from normal can increase stress levels of various knee structures. For example, increased hip medial rotation, squinting patellae, genu recurvatum, patella alta, tibial varum, medial tibial rotation, and compensatory pronation are malalignments that can contribute to patellofemoral pain. Because the lower extremity is a closed kinetic chain during most of its functions, malalignment in one segment results in compensatory changes in another segment. Changes at the hip or at the foot cause compensatory alterations and increased stress in the knee. Compensatory pronation and hip medial rotation with resulting medial tibial rotation are two malalignment problems that should be investigated in patients with patellofemoral pain.

■ Factors Influencing Postinjury Strength

Obviously, injury and surgery weaken the knee muscles. Other factors, however, influence knee strength and function. Some are not often considered, but all impact knee function and are important for that reason.

These factors—edema (Fahrer et al., 1988), pain (Leroux, Bélanger, & Boucher, 1995), and abnormal ambulation (Ounpuu, 1994)—lead to impaired muscle function. Reduced function leads to atrophy and weakness of the muscle. Muscle weakness leads to reduced function and control of the body segment. The rehabilitation clinician must pay attention to these factors when examining a patient before initiating a therapeutic exercise program.

EDEMA

One of the important goals of first-aid treatment of musculoskeletal injuries is minimization of edema. Once edema forms, efforts should be made to relieve it as quickly as possible. One reason this is a priority is that edema causes an inhibition of quadriceps function. Studies have demonstrated that swelling in the knee joint causes a reflex shutdown of the quadriceps (Fahrer et al., 1988; McDonough & Weir, 1996; Spencer, Hayes, & Alexander, 1984). Other researchers have injected plasma or saline in small quantities (20-30 ml) into normal knees and found a profound inhibition of quadriceps activity to levels 60% below normal (Spencer et al., 1984; Young, Stokes, & Iles, 1987). As fluid quantity increases, quadriceps activity decreases.

PAIN

It is commonly understood that pain causes a reflex inhibition of muscle activity. Pain affects both the autonomic and the conscious pathways. The reflex response in the presence of pain is to withdraw. The conscious response is to refrain from activity that produces pain. If pain persists following an injury, the patient's ability to perform active muscle contraction is impaired. Use of electrical stimulation and other modalities to control pain before therapeutic exercise may result in improved strength-output levels during exercises. This can ultimately reduce the patient's rehabilitation time by enhancing strength gains.

AMBULATION

Normal ambulation utilizes the right and left lower extremity equally, applying weight-bearing and propulsive forces equally on the two extremities. Weakness results when a patient sustains a lower-extremity injury that causes him or her to favor the extremity. An unequal gait produces less-than-normal stresses on the extremity as the patient spends less weight-bearing time on the extremity and applies less stress to it. An antalgic gait produces weakness not only in the injured segment but also throughout the entire lower extremity. Therefore, it is important to examine the total lower extremity following an injury and to correct secondary weaknesses that develop in the extremity's non-injured segments.

The quadriceps' ability to provide optimal muscle output is significantly decreased in the presence of either pain or edema.

Rehabilitation Concepts

In addition to the routine rehabilitation concepts guiding development of a therapeutic exercise program, special factors enter into knee rehabilitation. The rehabilitation clinician must address them all if a rehabilitation program is to be successful. The following sections deal with the special factors that have the most influence.

Extensor Lag

Questions that have elicited particular interest are what types of resistive knee exercises optimally strengthen the quadriceps and which quadriceps muscle works at what time within the knee's range of motion. The condition in which full passive motion is present but active extension is incomplete is an extensor lag. Two deficiencies are typically present after a knee injury: VMO atrophy and an extensor lag. Because the two problems frequently appear concurrently, a clinical presumption has been that the extensor lag is the result of VMO weakness. The VMO's oblique fiber insertion has tended to support this presumption. Research has shown, however, that the VMO does not exert any more effort than any of the other quadriceps muscles during terminal extension (Lieb & Perry, 1971). Muscle fiber atrophy is more prominent in the VMO, but the reason is unclear. This atrophy may be apparent not because it is greater in the VMO than in the other quadriceps muscles, but because the fascial covering of the muscle is thinner over the oblique fibers of the vastus medialis than in the rest of the quadriceps group. On the other hand, it may be true that VMO atrophy occurs more readily because the VMO is unable to perform its function as a patellar medial stabilizer as effectively as the other quadriceps muscles perform their task as knee extensor. Research evidence to confirm either suspicion is lacking.

Complete terminal extension is difficult for a weakened quadriceps to achieve. Some researchers maintain that because of its fiber alignment, the function of the VMO is to maintain medial patellar alignment, providing dynamic restraint for the patella (Witvrouw, Sneyers, Lysens, Victor, & Bellemans, 1996). If this is the case, an extensor lag may occur not because the VMO is deficient, but because the force required of the quadriceps to produce the last 15° of extension is twice as great as for the other ranges of knee motion (Grood, Suntay, Noyes, & Butler, 1984). The quadriceps muscles' loss of mechanical advantage (decreased lever-arm length) as the knee approaches its end range means that a much greater muscular effort is required to complete the movement.

Some of the frequently used open kinetic chain exercises for strength gains are the quad set, the straight-leg raise, and the short-arc quad. Among these, the quad set is the most effective in producing total quadriceps activity (Gough & Ladley, 1971). The rectus femoris works more during the straight-leg raise and the short-arc quad exercises. Vastus medialis activity is most apparent during a quad set. As would be expected, the quadriceps muscles work more during a knee extension exercise than during a straight-leg raise (Knight, Martin, & Londeree, 1979). Open kinetic chain exercises are an important tool in restoring isolated quadriceps strength, so these exercises are key elements in a therapeutic exercise program for a patient with isolated quadriceps weakness (Mikkelsen, Werner, & Eriksson, 2000).

Open and Closed Kinetic Chain Exercises

Open and closed kinetic chain exercises have been the subject of debate in knee rehabilitation, especially ACL rehabilitation, for the past several years. Most recently, the type of exercise most widely advocated for ACL injuries has been closed kinetic chain exercise (Beynnon, Johnson, Fleming, Stankewich, Renström, & Nichols, 1997; Bynum, Barrack, & Alexander, 1995; Mikkelsen et al., 2000). This is because research demonstrates a reduction in anterior shear stress and ACL strain in weight-bearing activities that are performed in 0° to 60°. The least amount of anterior displacement in an anterior cruciate-deficient knee during a closed chain exercise occurs at 60°, while the greatest displacement in an open chain exercise occurs at 30° (Jenkins, Munns, Jayaraman, Wertzberger, & Neely, 1997). Joint compressive forces in closed kinetic chain exercises may be responsible for reducing the shearing forces and anterior translation that occur in open kinetic chain activities (Isear, Erickson, & Worrell, 1997).

It has been assumed that closed kinetic chain exercises recruit a co-contraction of hamstrings and quadriceps to provide stability; this assumption remains controversial and inconclusive. For example, investigators have demonstrated that the lateral step-up exercise, thought to recruit co-contraction of hamstrings and quadriceps, recruits the vastus lateralis and vastus medialis components of the quadriceps significantly but does little to recruit the hamstrings (Worrell, Crisp, & LaRosa, 1998). On the other hand, it has been demonstrated that a squat exercise generated twice as much hamstring activity as a leg press (Escamilla et al., 1998). Additional investigations are needed before judgment on this topic can be determined.

In an open kinetic chain exercise as indicated in figure 23.3, less anterior shear stress is applied to the ACL in knee extension resistive exercises from 60° to 90° flexion, and more is applied in terminal-extension ranges of motion (Beynnon et al., 1995). The greatest shear stress to the ACL occurs from 0° to 40° flexion. The quandary for the clinician is that 30° is the best position for quadriceps strengthening but puts the greatest strain on the ACL. Less strain is applied to the ACL in closed kinetic chain, but increased stress is applied to the patellofemoral joint in closed kinetic chain activities beyond about 50° flexion (figure 23.4). This dichotomy creates a dilemma regarding ACL reconstruction patients with patellofemoral pain. Closed kinetic chain activities are less stressful for an ACL injury, but many patients with patellofemoral pain have difficulty performing closed kinetic chain exercises because of the pain.

Shear Stress

Aside from open kinetic chain activities, factors that also influence tibiofemoral shear stress include joint angle, location of the applied resistance, and the speed of the exercise. Peak shear stress occurs in the joint at around 28° to 14° of flexion (Wilk et al., 1996). This may be one reason open chain exercises create their greatest shear force in 15° to 30°. Additional resistance that is added to the leg increases the shear forces (Sahli, Haithem, Elleuch, Tabka, & Poumarat, 2008). Manual resistance, especially in the early phases of therapeutic exercise, should be applied immediately distal to the knee joint to reduce shear-force applications. This is also true for exercise-machine arms used in open chain exercises.

Isokinetic exercise is not used until the later phases of rehabilitation because it is open chain; its lever arm can be shortened, but it still applies significant shear stresses. When isokinetic exercise is first used, the slower speeds should be avoided because slower speeds produce a greater torque to increase anterior tibial displacement and ACL strain.

Bracing

Perhaps more than any other joint, the knee is a frequent site for braces. There are three types of braces: prophylactic, rehabilitative, and functional. The prophylactic brace is used to prevent or reduce the severity of an injury (Najibi & Albright, 2005), the rehabilitative brace restricts motion of an injured joint, and a functional brace improves stability of an unstable joint (Jenkins, Munns, & Loudon, 1998). A functional brace can also be a prophylactic brace.

There are custom-made braces and off-the-shelf braces. Custom-made braces are more expensive and can cost several hundred dollars or more. Off-the-shelf braces are similar in construction to the custom-made braces but come in generic sizes, usually ranging from extra small to extra large.

Braces are frequently used for ACL injuries. Braces provide anterior stability during low-stress loads but have not shown adequate stability during more functional athletic load applications (Moller, Forssblad, Hansson, Wange, & Weidenhielm, 2001). Subjective anecdotal reports from patients often relate a sense of security and improved performance when exercising with a brace as compared to exercising without one. Braces do seem to provide some proprioceptive feedback, and may be of value for this reason (Campbell, Yaggie, & Cipriani, 2006).

Patients who have patellofemoral pain often use knee sleeves. Once again, the proprioceptive benefit as reflected in subjective reports of decreased pain may be the primary advantage. The sleeves do not alter patellar glide or protect the knee from external stress, but there is some evidence to indicate a sleeve has some value (Garth & Flowers, 1998). Even considering the evidence, one cannot dismiss the psychological benefits of increased confidence and assurance that using a sleeve may give the patient.

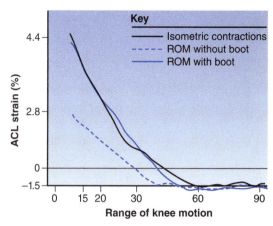

▶ **Figure 23.3** ACL strain with open kinetic chain activities.

Adapted from B.D. Beynnon et al., 1995, "Anterior cruciate ligament strain behavior during rehabilitation exercises in vivo," *American Journal of Sports Medicine* 23: 24-34.

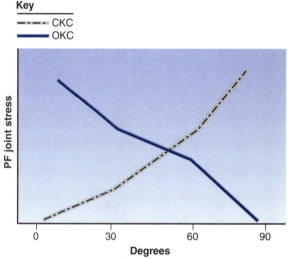

▶ **Figure 23.4** Patellofemoral joint stress at different angles.

Based on Steinkamp et al. 1993.

Program Progression

Tissue healing and the injury's response to exercise are primary factors that dictate rate of progression of a knee therapeutic exercise program. Parameters of range of motion, strength and endurance, balance and agility, and functional performance are advanced as with therapeutic exercise programs for other body segments. Careful observation by the rehabilitation clinician, as well as reliance on the patient for accurate communication regarding responses to exercise, is essential for a steady progression within a therapeutic exercise program.

As with other rehabilitation program progressions, protecting the injury, reducing pain and edema, and maintaining current levels of conditioning are all elements included in phase I of knee rehabilitation. Flexibility exercises, joint mobilization, and soft-tissue mobilization are all techniques that improve range of motion and flexibility that usually begin in phase II. Early strength and endurance exercises begin in phase III and encompass a variety of activities that advance from static to dynamic and from isometric to isotonic, and eventually in later phase III or even phase IV, to isokinetic. The method of advancing strength depends on the timing of the program, the patient's response, availability of equipment, and the rehabilitation clinician's preference. Isometric exercises are used more often in later phase II, when the knee is immobilized, when range-of-motion exercises are too painful for the patient, and when the aim is to isolate weak ranges of motion. In most cases, a combination of open and closed kinetic chain exercises is beneficial in phase III and even later phase II to improve strength.

Balance and agility exercises begin with double-support weight-bearing activities in phase III or late phase II and progress to single-limb static balancing on a stable surface. Initial double-support activities might be as simple as gait training with correct weight transfer from the right to the left extremity. From there the activities advance to single-limb stance on a stable surface then on an unstable surface in phase III. Balance activities can begin at a low level when the patient is able to bear weight on the extremity in phase II. Once the patient is able to place total body weight on the injured extremity, single-limb stance activities can begin. For these activities, the patient must be able to correctly shift weight without trunk lean onto the involved extremity. A trunk lean not only does not permit accurate body-weight transfer onto the extremity, but it also promotes bad weight-bearing habits that can become difficult to overcome.

Agility activities advance in later phase III from balance and coordination exercises used in earlier phase III rehabilitation. Prerequisites to a patient's progressing to agility exercises are an intact neuromuscular response system, and strength and motion sufficient to return the body's center of gravity to within its base of support when balance is disturbed (Wegener, Kisner, & Nichols, 1997). Agility exercises also demand appropriate coordination and muscle power, so they are the next logical step in the rehabilitation progression before functional and activity-specific exercises. Agility exercises are dynamic; they may begin with no-impact activities and progress to high-impact activities. The lower-level agility exercises are unidirectional, and more advanced agility exercises are multidirectional. Agility activities begin at reduced speeds and advance to full speed as the patient progresses in late phase III.

When adding a new agility exercise to a program, it is beneficial to include it early in the exercise session before the patient becomes fatigued. There is evidence to demonstrate that fatigue reduces the knee's proprioceptive function (Lattanzio, Petrella, Sproule, & Fowler, 1997). An agility activity requires proprioceptive feedback for proper execution (Risberg, Mork, Jenssen, & Holm, 2001). If fatigue reduces proprioceptive function, the execution will not be as good as it should be, and the application is undesirable because of the risk of engramming an incorrect execution.

Once the patient has mastered the agility exercises, the final steps—functional, and then activity-specific exercises—prepare the individual physically and psychologically for return to full participation. The program advances to this phase, phase IV, when there is no evidence of post-exercise pain or edema and when the injured knee possesses full range of motion, near-normal strength, and good balance. As with other therapeutic exercise programs, functional activities lead up to specific activity-related drills that mimic the patient's normal activities. Activity-specific exercises are designed to come as close to normal participation demands as possible. They may begin at reduced stress levels, but as the patient's skills and confidence return, the stress of the activity is akin to the stress he or she will experience on returning to full participation.

The final examination to determine the patient's readiness for return to full participation should mimic the patient's activities. The rehabilitation clinician examines the patient for accurate execution of normal activities, an ability to use both lower extremities equally and without hesitation or any inclination to favor it, and perform all motions with confidence.

SOFT-TISSUE MOBILIZATION

Pain in the soft tissue surrounding the knee can result from injury to the local tissue or to distant tissue. The foot and hip can refer pain into the knee. Sciatica can also occur as knee pain without thigh or back pain. You should examine these areas as possible sources of knee pain if there has been no frank injury. With injuries that might have involved other segments, assessment of these segments is also necessary. You must make a differential diagnosis to eliminate other sources of pain to provide appropriate rehabilitative care for the patient.

Muscles surrounding the knee have specific pain-referral patterns. They can refer pain if they suffer an injury, if they have associated soft-tissue adhesions with restrictions of normal tissue mobility or if they suffer loss of flexibility and experience increased stress during activity. Trigger points become active with abnormal or excessive stress application. These issues are discussed in chapter 6.

Soft-tissue mobilization techniques discussed in this chapter include the common pain-referral patterns and trigger point release techniques identified and advanced by Travell and Simons (Travell & Simons, 1992), deep-tissue massage for relief of scar-tissue adhesions, and cross-friction massage for tendinopathy treatment. You should review chapter 6 for information on other soft-tissue mobilization techniques, such as effleurage for edema.

Hip muscles that cross the knee joint or impact knee movement are presented in the following sections. Other hip muscles are addressed in chapter 24. For the most part, soft-tissue referral pain in the anterior aspect of the knee and thigh originates from the anterior thigh and hip muscles.

The knee encompasses two major joints, the tibiofemoral joint and the patellofemoral joint. The knee also contains a joint capsule, ligaments, menisci, and muscles. A therapeutic exercise program must take into account the knee's unique structure, as well as a number of biomechanical and physiological characteristics specific to the knee.

■ Trigger Point Releases for the Knee Muscles

Quadriceps

Referral Pattern: The pain-referral pattern for the quadriceps covers the anterior thigh and knee. The rectus femoris and vastus medialis are the only quadriceps muscles referring into the anterior knee (figure 23.5, a1 & a2). The vastus lateralis refers to the posterolateral knee. The vastus lateralis also refers pain anywhere along the lateral thigh to the knee and sometimes into the posterior knee (figure 23.5a4). The vastus intermedius refers into the midthigh and the upper thigh (figure 23.5a3).

Location of Trigger Point: The distal trigger points are at the muscle's medial distal border, whereas the proximal trigger points are in the midthigh region of the muscle's medial border. The rectus femoris trigger point is inferior to the anterior superior iliac spine (ASIS), just distal to the inguinal ligament. The vastus intermedius cannot be palpated directly but can be located lateral and deep to the rectus femoris on the proximal thigh distal and slightly lateral to the rectus femoris trigger point site. The vastus lateralis has multiple trigger points located in taut bands along the muscle and can be treated with finger-pad pressure. The distal trigger points are more often tender than the proximal trigger points.

Patient Position for Palpation: Patient is in supine.

Muscle Position for Palpation: The hip and knee are in partial flexion and hip lateral rotation, supported for comfort.

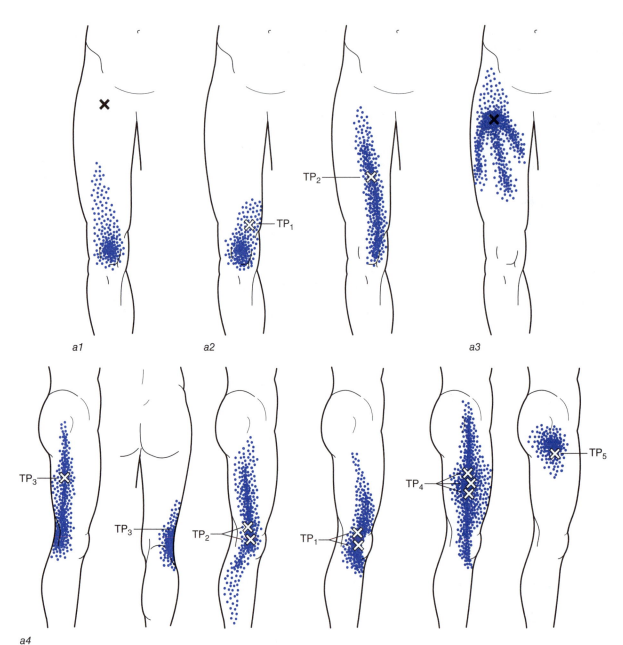

▶ **Figure 23.5** Quadriceps: pain-referral patterns for the *(a1)* rectus femoris, *(a2)* vastus medialis, *(a3)* vastus intermedius, and *(a4)* vastus lateralis.

Ischemic Treatment: You can provide trigger point release either by using finger-pad pressure or by grasping the taut band. The vastus medialis is usually treated with a finger-pad technique (figure 23.5b).

Spray-and-Stretch Treatment: Ice/spray-and-stretch treatment is performed with the patient side-lying or supine for the rectus femoris and supine for the other quadriceps muscles. The hip is extended and the knee flexed for treatment to the rectus femoris with ice sweeps from proximal to distal along the muscle. For treatment to the vastus medialis, the hip is laterally rotated and flexed and the knee is flexed as the ice is swept from the medial superior thigh to below the knee. Ice-and-stretch for the vastus intermedius and vastus lateralis is performed with a stretch moving the knee into flexion as the ice is swept from the hip to below the knee.

Notations: Proximal thigh pain caused by the vastus lateralis can make sleeping on that side uncomfortable. Rectus femoris pain is usually described as a deep thigh ache, especially at night. Referred pain from the vastus medialis can sometimes cause buckling of the knee.

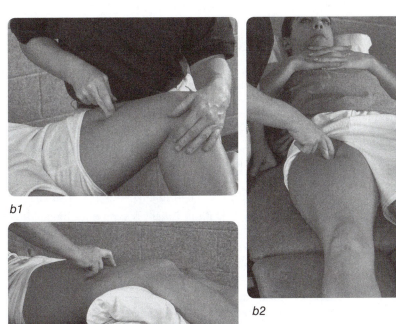

b1

b3

b2

▶ **Figure 23.5** Trigger point release for *(b1)* vastus medialis, *(b2)* vastus intermedius, and *(b3)* vastus lateralis.

Hip Adductors

Referral Pattern: The adductor longus and brevis refer pain deep into the groin, the anteromedial upper thigh, and the upper medial knee. The adductor magnus refers deep pain into the groin and distally over the anteromedial thigh. The gracilis referral pain is a superficial, hot, stinging pain along the inside of the thigh (figure 23.6a).

Location of Trigger Point: The trigger points are located along each muscle belly. The adductor magnus trigger point can be located in the proximal third of the posteromedial thigh in a triangle formed by the ischial tuberosity and pubis proximally, the medial hamstrings posteriorly, and the gracilis anteriorly. Gracilis trigger points can be found in the upper third of the muscle, but may be difficult to locate. The adductor magnus trigger points can also be located beneath the gracilis and hamstrings posteriorly, just distal to the ischial tuberosity. Adductor brevis trigger points are located under the adductor longus.

Patient Position for Palpation: Trigger point release is performed with the patient supine.

Muscle Position for Palpation: The trigger points are treated with the hip and knee flexed and the hip laterally rotated and abducted. A pillow placed beneath the thigh provides comfort.

Ischemic Treatment: A pincer grasp or flat pressure with the finger pads can be used (figure 23.6b). The adductor longus proximal trigger points are in the muscle's upper third and are best treated with a pincer grasp. Trigger points on the muscle's distal two-thirds are best treated with a flat pressure. Adductor brevis trigger points are approached with indirect flat pressure.

Spray-and-Stretch Treatment: Spray/ice-and-stretch is applied with the patient supine and the thigh abducted and laterally rotated and the knee flexed. Ice sweeps for the adductor magnus are applied from the knee proceeding proximally along the length of the muscle to the groin (figure 23.6c). The stretch is applied, moving the hip into abduction and flexion. Ice-and-stretch for the adductor magnus and brevis is performed with the patient's hip abducted and laterally rotated and the knee flexed with the foot against the opposite thigh.

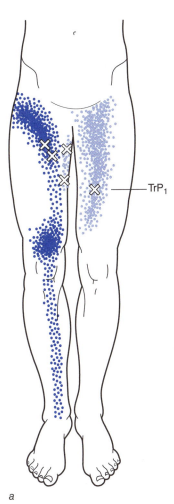

TrP$_1$

a

▶ **Figure 23.6** Hip adductors: *(a)* pain-referral patterns. Dark = adductor longus and brevis, medium = gracilis, light = adductor magnus.

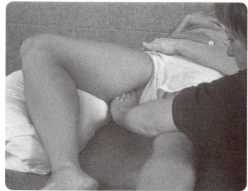

b1

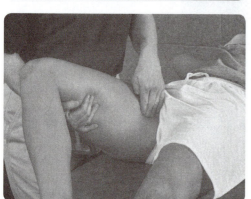

b2

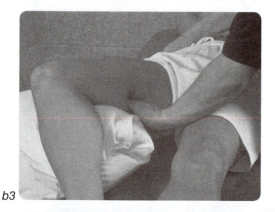

b3

As the ice sweeps are moved from the knee and along the inner thigh to the groin, the muscle is stretched, moving the hip into as much flexion and abduction as tolerated (figure 23.6c).

Notations: The gracilis muscle technique is similar to the hamstring technique with the knee straight (23.7c).

Hamstrings

Referral Pattern: In the gluteal fold and posterior knee with overflow along the muscle and into the distal medial calf (figure 23.7a).

Location of Trigger Point: Trigger points for both the medial and lateral hamstrings are located about 8 to 12 cm (3-4.5 in.) proximal to the knee.

Patient Position for Palpation: Patient is supine for medial hamstrings and prone or side-lying for lateral hamstrings.

Muscle Position for Palpation: For either the medial or lateral hamstring release, the knee is flexed. Additionally, for the medial hamstrings, the hip is abducted.

Ischemic Treatment: Either a pincer grasp or flat pressure can be used for the medial hamstrings, but the lateral hamstrings are best approached with a flat pressure (figure 23.7b).

Spray-and-Stretch Treatment: Spray/ice-and-stretch of the hamstrings is performed with the patient supine and the opposite extremity in extension. The involved extremity is supported at the ankle by the rehabilitation clinician. The initial distal-to-proximal ice sweeps are performed with the extremity abducted to passively lengthen the adductor magnus. Once the extremity is abducted as far as possible (the thigh should be almost parallel with the tabletop), the sweeps move in a proximal-to-distal direction while the hip is moved into flexion and adduction; the knee is maintained in extension throughout the motion (figure 23.7c). Once the extremity reaches a vertical position, the clinician stops the movement and dorsiflexes the ankle and extends the cold application to the calf. Passive adduction is then resumed to the end of adduction motion while in full flexion.

Notations: Semimembranosus and semitendinosus pain is often described as a sharp pain, whereas referred pain from the biceps femoris is more often a deep ache.

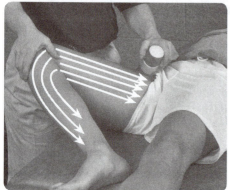

c1

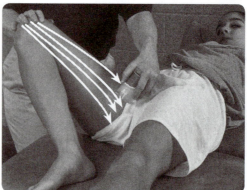

c2

▶ **Figure 23.6** Trigger point release for *(b1)* adductor magnus. Hip adductors: trigger point release for *(b2)* anterior longus and brevis, *(b3)* adductor longus. Ice-and-stretch for *(c1)* adductor longus and brevis, *(c2)* adductor magnus.

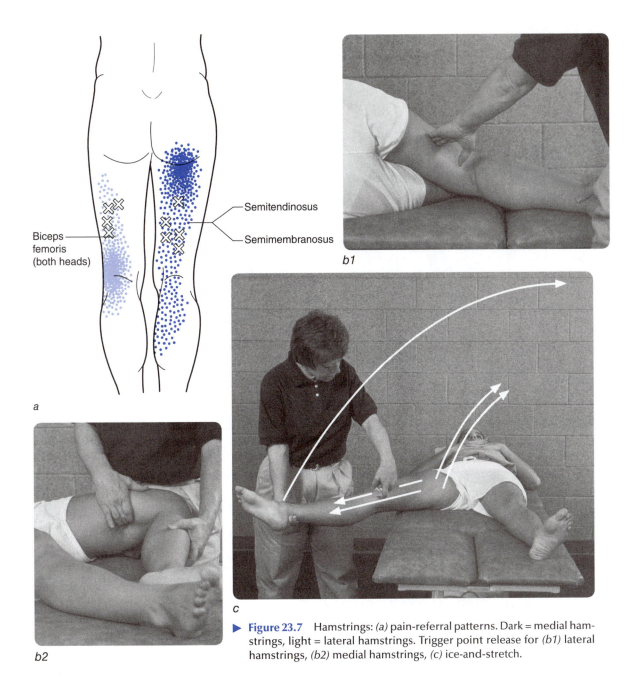

Semitendinosus

Semimembranosus

Biceps femoris (both heads)

a

b1

b2

c

▶ **Figure 23.7** Hamstrings: *(a)* pain-referral patterns. Dark = medial hamstrings, light = lateral hamstrings. Trigger point release for *(b1)* lateral hamstrings, *(b2)* medial hamstrings, *(c)* ice-and-stretch.

Popliteus

Referral Pattern: Posterior knee pain (figure 23.8a) during activities such as running, walking down stairs and hills, and squatting. The patient may complain of knee pain when fully extending the knee.

Location of Trigger Point: At the muscle's tibial insertion. Locate it by moving the soleus laterally; the popliteus is under the soleus.

Patient Position for Palpation: Side-lying on the affected side.

Muscle Position for Palpation: The knee is partially flexed, the leg laterally rotated slightly, and the ankle in moderate plantar flexion so the calf muscles are relaxed.

Ischemic Treatment: A flat pressure is applied in a downward and anterior direction medially (figure 23.8b).

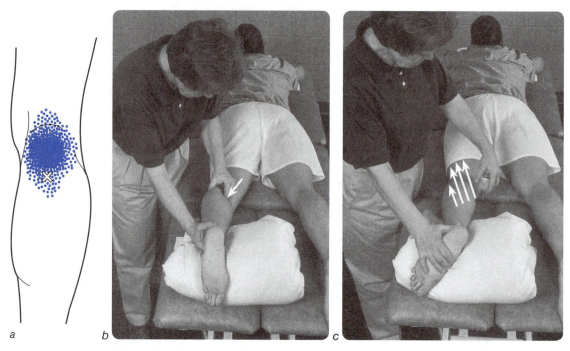

▶ **Figure 23.8** Popliteus: *(a)* pain-referral pattern, *(b)* trigger point release, *(c)* ice-and-stretch.

Spray-and-Stretch Treatment: Spray/ice-and-stretch is performed with the patient prone. Sweeps begin distally and move along the muscle's path in a proximal direction as the leg is laterally rotated and the knee extended but not locked (figure 23.8c).

Notations: Posterior knee pain is rarely caused only by this muscle's trigger point. It is usually accompanied by pain associated with trigger points from the gastrocnemius, biceps femoris, or both.

Tensor Fasciae Latae

Referral Pattern: A deep pain in the anterolateral hip is referred from the greater trochanter and can extend as far as the knee (figure 23.9a).

Location of Trigger Point: Distal to the anterior superior iliac spine and medial and proximal to the greater trochanter.

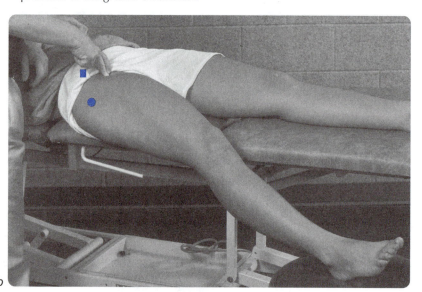

▶ **Figure 23.9** Tensor fasciae latae: *(a)* pain-referral pattern, *(b)* trigger point release. ● = greater trochanter, ■ = ASIS.

Patient Position for Palpation: Supine for ischemic compression, side-lying for spray-and-stretch.

Muscle Position for Palpation: The knee is supported in slight flexion to relax the muscle.

Ischemic Treatment: A flat palpation of the muscle is performed (figure 23.9b).

Spray-and-Stretch Treatment: Spray/ice-and-stretch is performed with the patient side-lying, the involved extremity on top. The rehabilitation clinician supports the extremity under the distal thigh and applies the ice sweeps from the anterolateral thigh distally and laterally to above the knee. The clinician applies the stretch by stabilizing the pelvis with a hand on the lateral hip and lowering the thigh with the other hand as the thigh is moved into lateral rotation (figure 23.9c).

Notations: The pain can sometimes mimic trochanteric bursitis, making it painful to lie on the side or to run.

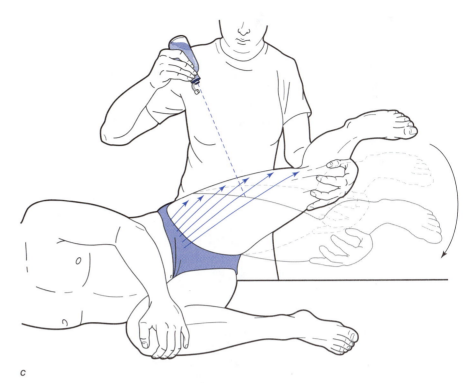

c

▶ **Figure 23.9** Tensor fasciae latae: *(c)* ice-and-stretch.

Deep-Tissue Massage

Two areas of the knee and thigh typically require deep-tissue massage: the quadriceps tendon and the iliotibial band (ITB). When the quadriceps tendon is painful because of excessive stress, irritation, or tendinopathy, cross-friction massage is frequently used to relieve scar-tissue adhesions that can occur secondarily to these conditions. The tendon fibers are cross-frictioned in the manner described in chapter 6. Because the tendon fibers run vertically from the patella to the tibial tuberosity, the cross-friction technique is applied horizontally, across the fibers.

Cross-friction massage is also used on surgical scars to prevent or reduce adhesions of skin to underlying adjacent tissues. Even the portal sites of arthroscopy should be examined and treated as needed to prevent adhesions and promote good tissue mobility following surgery.

The tensor fascia lata and its tendon are frequent sites of adhesions, especially following injury or prolonged pathomechanical stresses such as seen with genu valgus. These areas along the ITB are relieved by deep-tissue massage. The rehabilitation clinician flexes his or her hand's metacarpophalangeal and proximal interphalangeal joints and extends the distal interphalangeal joints so the finger pads rest in the palm. With the hand in this position, the clinician uses posterior surfaces of the middle and distal phalanx to apply an even pressure throughout the hand's contact on the patient's thigh while guiding the hand along the patient's lateral thigh from the knee moving toward the hip. Soft-tissue restrictions are palpated as "sticking points" as the hand moves along the lateral thigh. The clinician repeats the deep-tissue massage strokes several times, spending additional time on the more-restricted regions.

As the restrictive areas release, tissue mobility improves and the patient reports less tenderness with the massage. Range of motion of any joint affected by these soft-tissue restrictions is also improved.

In an alternative technique for a home program, the patient applies self-massage using a foam roller or massage roller. If using a foam roller, the patient lies on the involved side, with the weight on both hands and the thigh on the foam roller (figure 23.10). He or she rolls from knee to thigh on the foam roller, spending more time on the areas that are most tender and restricted. This technique should not produce tenderness in normal tissue, but tenderness

Soft-tissue mobilization for knee injuries addresses pain referred from the quadriceps, the hip adductors, the hamstrings, the popliteus, and the tensor fascia lata. Deep-tissue massage is typically used for the quadriceps tendon and the iliotibial band.

will occur in areas of soft-tissue restriction. If using a massage roller, the patient applies firm pressure with each hand on the ends of the roller as it is moved along the restricted soft tissue region.

The foam roller can also be used to massage the quadriceps muscle if it becomes restricted from immobilization or injury (figure 23.11). The patient lies prone with the body weight on both forearms and with the anterior thighs on the foam roller. He or she uses the arms to move the lower extremities from the hips to the knees on the roller, spending more time over the tender sites. Patient makes small back and forth motions on the roller until one area of pain is relieved, then moves along the muscle to the next area of tenderness and repeats the treatment at that site. This procedure is used on the entire muscle.

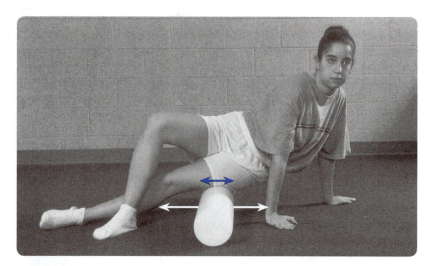

▶ **Figure 23.10** Iliotibial band foam-roller self-massage.

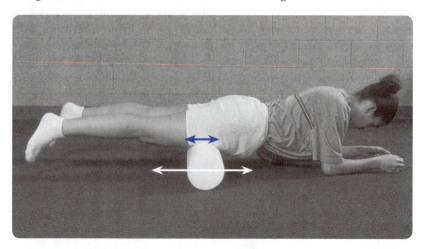

▶ **Figure 23.11** Quadriceps foam-roller massage.

JOINT MOBILIZATION

Injury, surgery, edema, and immobilization can lead to reduced joint mobility involving the patellofemoral joint, tibiofemoral joint, and proximal tibiofibular joint. Although the tibiofibular joint is not actually part of the knee, if it develops reduced mobility it can refer pain to the knee and affect ankle mobility. For this reason, you should assess the tibiofibular joint for capsular restriction during your rehabilitation examination. The following sections describe some of the most commonly used joint mobilization techniques for the knee joints.

Joint Mobilization of the Knee

Anterior and Posterior Glides

Motion: Superior tibiofibular joint.

Resting Position: Not described.

Indications: Restricted motion of the knee, ankle, or both.

Patient Position: Supine with hip and knee flexed and foot resting on the tabletop.

Clinician and Hand Positions: Clinician grasps fibular head with pads of thumb anteriorly and index and middle fingers posteriorly.

Mobilization Application: Fibular head is moved anteriorly, then posteriorly (figure 23.12).

Notations: The weight of the leg anchored with the foot on the table stabilizes the tibia.

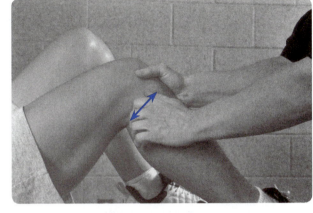

▶ **Figure 23.12** Joint mobilization: superior tibiofibular anterior and posterior glides.

Lateral Glides

Motion: Patella.

Resting Position: Knee extension.

Indications: Restricted medial motion of the patella.

Patient Position: The patient lies supine, and a rolled towel is placed under the knee for knee support.

Clinician and Hand Positions: The clinician's thumb pads are on the medial aspect of the patella.

Mobilization Application: Thumbs move the patella laterally (figure 23.13a). Care must be taken to apply a lateral force, not a downward or compressive force, on the patella.

Notations: Patellar mobility is necessary for full knee flexion-extension motion and tibial rotation.

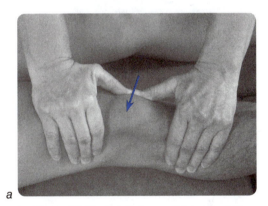

a

▶ **Figure 23.13** Patellofemoral joint mobilization: *(a)* lateral glide.

Medial Glides

Motion: Patella.

Resting Position: Knee extension.

Indications: Restricted lateral motion of the patella.

Patient Position: The patient lies supine, and a rolled towel is placed under the knee for knee support.

Clinician and Hand Positions: The clinician's index finger pads are on the lateral aspect of the patella.

Mobilization Application: Finger pads move the patella medially (figure 23.13b). Care must be taken to apply a medial force, not a downward or compressive force, on the patella.

Notations: Patellar mobility is necessary for full knee flexion-extension motion and tibial rotation.

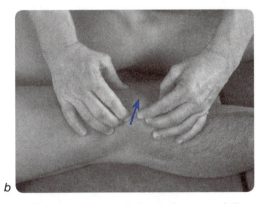

b

▶ **Figure 23.13** Patellofemoral joint mobilization: *(b)* medial glide.

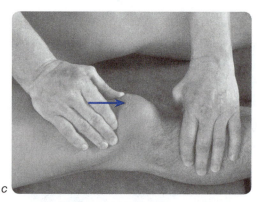

▶ **Figure 23.13** Patellofemoral joint mobilization: *(c)* inferior glide.

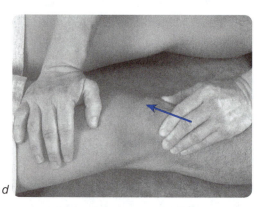

▶ **Figure 23.13** Patellofemoral joint mobilization: *(d)* superior glide.

Inferior Glides

Motion: Patella.

Resting Position: Knee extension.

Indications: Restricted inferior motion of the patella.

Patient Position: The patient lies supine, and a rolled towel is placed under the knee for knee support.

Clinician and Hand Positions: The clinician's thumb and index finger are placed around the superior rim of the patella.

Mobilization Application: The clinician glides the patella distally in an inferior direction toward the toes, being careful not to compress the patella on the femur (figure 23.13c).

Notations: Patellar mobility is necessary for full knee flexion-extension motion and tibial rotation.

Superior Glides

Motion: Patella.

Resting Position: Knee extension.

Indications: Restricted superior motion of the patella.

Patient Position: The patient lies supine, and a rolled towel is placed under the knee for knee support.

Clinician and Hand Positions: The clinician's thumb and index finger are placed around the inferior rim of the patella.

Mobilization Application: The clinician's thumb and index finger exert a cephalic force on the patella, avoiding compression of the patella on the femur (figure 23.13d).

Notations: Patellar mobility is necessary for full knee flexion-extension motion and tibial rotation.

Tibiofemoral Mobilizations

This is the joint most often mobilized to improve range of motion in the knee. Although the patellofemoral joint also can affect total range of motion, this joint has the greatest impact. For this reason, tibiofemoral mobilization techniques are included here.

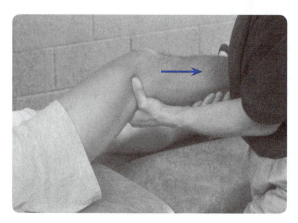

▶ **Figure 23.14** Joint mobilization: tibiofemoral distraction.

Distraction

Motion: Tibiofemoral joint.

Resting Position: 20° to 25° flexion.

Indications: General restriction or general relaxation.

Patient Position: Supine with knee supported in resting position.

Clinician and Hand Positions: The femur is stabilized with one hand proximal to the knee, and the mobilizing hand is placed above the ankle joint.

Mobilization Application: The tibia is pulled distally by the mobilizing hand while the stabilizing hand secures the thigh (figure 23.14).

Notations: This technique is often used prior to and after using grades III and IV.

Anterior Glides

Motion: Tibiofemoral joint.

Resting Position: 20° to 25° flexion.

Indications: To increase knee extension.

Patient Position: Prone. The knee is flexed with the thigh supported on the table and the patient's leg resting on the rehabilitation clinician's shoulder. A pad under the thigh will make the position more comfortable for the patient and align the thigh more appropriately for the glide.

Clinician and Hand Positions: The patient's distal leg is supported on the rehabilitation clinician's shoulder. The clinician clasps his or her hands around the proximal leg near the knee and glides the tibia anteriorly on the femur (figure 23.15).

Mobilization Application: The glide force must be parallel to the plane of the joint surface. When the knee is moved out of the resting position for mobilizations, the angle of force will change since the force must always be parallel to the joint surface.

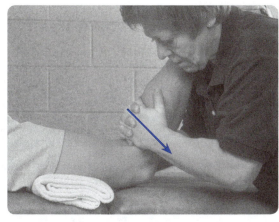

▶ **Figure 23.15** Joint mobilization: tibiofemoral anterior glide.

Notations: The hamstrings should remain relaxed to produce the most effective results. An alternative posterior-to-anterior mobilization technique is performed with the patient prone and the rehabilitation clinician supporting the tibia with the knee at 30° flexion. An anterior force is applied by the mobilizing hand just distal to the knee joint. An anterior glide can also be performed with the patient sitting with the thighs on the table and the legs freely hanging over the side. The clinician secures the patient's leg between his or her knees to place the knee in a resting position and places both hands over the posterior proximal leg just below the knee.

Posterior Glides

Motion: Tibiofemoral joint.

Resting Position: 20° to 25° flexion.

Indications: To increase knee flexion motion.

Patient Position: Patient is supine with a pad under the thigh to maintain the joint in a resting position.

Clinician and Hand Positions: The rehabilitation clinician places the heels of his or her hands on the anterior proximal tibia.

Mobilization Application: Posterior glide parallel to the joint's surface (figure 23.16).

Notations: In an alternative position, the patient is sitting with the knee over the edge of the table and the thigh supported on the table with a towel roll under the distal thigh. The clinician secures the patient's leg between his or her knees to place the knee in a resting position. The rehabilitation clinician applies a posterior glide at the tibial condyles.

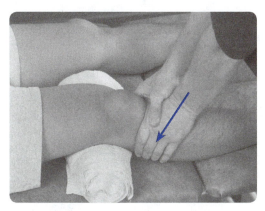

▶ **Figure 23.16** Joint mobilization: tibiofemoral posterior glide.

Joint mobilization techniques for the knee include anterior glides for extension, posterior glides for flexion, and rotational glides for terminal flexion and extension.

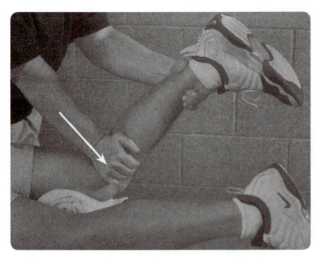

▶ **Figure 23.17** Joint mobilization: medial tibial condyle anterior glide.

Rotational Glide: Anterior Glide of the Medial Tibial Condyle

Motion: Tibiofemoral joint.

Resting Position: Resting position is 20° to 25° flexion, but this technique is usually performed in an end-range position.

Indications: Used to gain lateral tibial rotation in terminal knee extension.

Patient Position: Prone with a pad under the distal femur.

Clinician and Hand Positions: The heel of one hand is on the posterior medial tibial plateau.

Mobilization Application: An anterior-to-posterior (AP) glide of the medial tibia on the femur to produce tibial rotation (figure 23.17).

Notations: This technique is used to gain the last few degrees of extension in a knee. If the rehabilitation clinician applies the mobilizing force to the femur rather than to the tibia in AP glides or to the opposite side of the tibia in rotational glides, the opposite motions are influenced. For example, on an anterior glide of the tibia, the motion affected is knee extension. However, if the femur receives the anterior glide, knee flexion is the motion affected. So, too, if a posterior glide is applied to the lateral tibial condyle rather than to the medial tibial condyle, gains are seen in lateral rotation and extension. If the mobilizing force is applied to the femur, the tibia must be anchored.

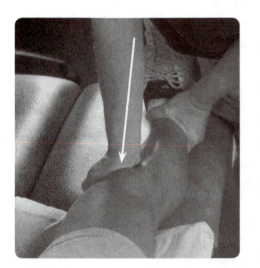

▶ **Figure 23.18** Joint mobilization: medial tibial condyle posterior glide.

Rotational Glide: Posterior Glide of the Medial Tibial Condyle

Motion: Tibiofemoral joint.

Resting Position: Resting position is 20° to 25° flexion, but this technique is usually performed in an end-range position.

Indications: Used to gain medial tibial rotation and knee flexion.

Patient Position: Patient is supine with the knee in flexion.

Clinician and Hand Positions: Clinician places the heel of the hand on the medial tibial condyle anteriorly.

Mobilization Application: An AP force is applied to the medial tibial condyle (figure 23.18).

Notations: If the rehabilitation clinician applies the mobilizing force to the femur rather than to the tibia in AP glides or to the opposite side of the tibia in rotational glides, the opposite motions are influenced. If the femur receives the anterior glide, knee flexion is the motion affected. So too, if an anterior glide is applied to the lateral rather than to the medial tibial condyle, medial rotation and knee flexion are affected. If the mobilizing force is applied to the femur, the tibia must be anchored.

FLEXIBILITY EXERCISES

Flexibility exercises for the knee can be active or passive. The specific techniques used depend on the type of tissue being stretched and how recent the injury is. Very new and developing scars in muscle tissue may not be stretched actively, but they may be able to tolerate mild passive stretches. Less immediately new scar tissue that is still in the proliferation phase and relatively-early remodeling phase may be effectively stretched with active and short-term stretches. Scar tissue that is very adherent and in the later aspects of the remodeling phase or very matured requires a combination of scar-tissue massage to loosen adhesions and long-term stretches to affect the tissue's plastic element.

Following surgical repair of the knee, orthopedic surgeons frequently have the patient's knee placed in a continuous passive motion (CPM) machine or begin early active motion. Although not used as frequently as they were a few years ago, CPMs are beneficial in reducing pain and edema and encouraging restoration of range of motion. One should not assume, however, that the CPM will restore full knee motion. You must assess the patient's knee motion at the time of the initial examination and frequently throughout the rehabilitation process.

The exercises presented in the following sections are divided into prolonged and active stretches, respectively. The active stretches include some exercises that use assistive equipment and some that require only the patient's active motion. During active stretches, it is important for the patient to contract the opposing muscle whenever possible to enhance relaxation of the stretching muscle and achieve a more effective stretch.

Prolonged Stretches

These stretches are used when scar tissue that is limiting motion is mature or is becoming mature, and short-term stretches would be ineffective.

When using prolonged stretches, the rehabilitation clinician must inform the patient that the knee will feel stiff once the stretch is released but that the stiffness sensation should resolve quickly. It may be difficult for the patient to take the first few steps after a prolonged stretch. A prolonged stretch is more effective the longer it is applied. When the force is first applied, the patient may not feel that a stretch is occurring, but as time passes he or she will feel the stretch. A patient may not be able to tolerate a prolonged stretch for more than 5 or 10 min initially. If this is the case, and a weight is being used, the stretch weight should be decreased or removed to make a longer stretch tolerable. As the patient tolerates the stretch, either the weight can be increased or the time can be lengthened, but the time should not be reduced. Keep in mind that it would be more beneficial to increase the time than the weight. These exercises may be used as clinical treatments, home exercise programs, or both. If severe restrictions are present, using prolonged stretches in both the clinic and the home may be beneficial.

■ Prolonged Flexibility Exercises for the Knee

Prolonged Knee Extension in Prone

Body Segment: Knee.

Stage in Rehab: III and beyond.

Purpose: Increase knee extension motion.

Positioning: Patient is prone with a pad under the distal thigh and the leg hanging off the table (figure 23.19).

Execution: The patient relaxes the leg and maintains this position for 10 to 15 min.

Possible Substitutions: Hip flexion or rotation. If either occurs, a strap placed across the hips and thighs and around the table will secure the extremity in position.

Notations: The prone stretch can also increase rectus femoris length if this is a factor in limited knee extension motion. A weight on the ankle will increase the stretch force, but the weight should start light and increase only as the patient tolerates.

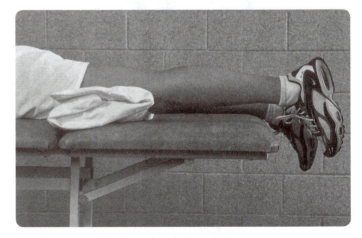

▶ **Figure 23.19** Prolonged extension stretch in prone.

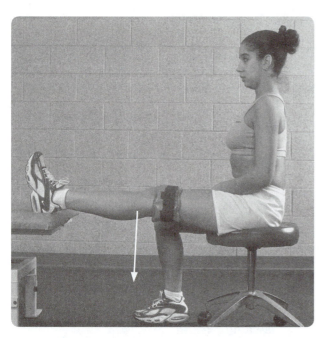

Prolonged Knee Extension in Long Sitting

Body Segment: Knee.

Stage in Rehab: III and beyond.

Purpose: Increase knee extension motion.

Positioning: The patient is sitting with the heel of the foot placed on another chair seat or table. The calf is unsupported (figure 23.20).

Execution: The patient relaxes the leg and allows gravity to pull the knee downward. A weight may be applied to the distal and proximal knee to increase gravitational forces.

Possible Substitutions: Hip lateral rotation and knee flexion.

Notations: Applying hot packs before and during the stretch may permit a greater tolerance for the stretch.

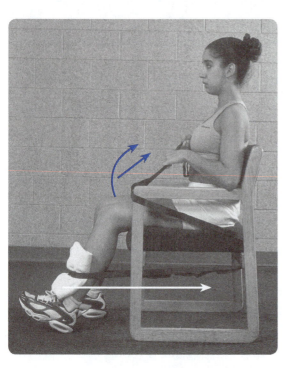

▶ **Figure 23.21** Prolonged knee flexion with rope system.

Prolonged Knee Flexion Stretch

Body Segment: Knee.

Stage in Rehab: III and beyond.

Purpose: Increase knee flexion motion.

Positioning: Patient is sitting in a chair with a pad around the distal leg and secured with a strap (figure 23.21).

Execution: The strap is anchored to the back chair leg. The strap is attached around the patient's ankle and controlled by the patient's pulling on the strap. The patient is instructed to pull the leg back to a point that feels tight but not painful. He or she holds this position for several minutes before attempting to increase flexion further.

Possible Substitutions: Rotating the leg and thigh; not holding the stretch long enough—a timer may need to be used.

Notations: An alternative method is for the patient to sit on the floor with the foot against the wall. The patient moves the buttocks toward the wall until a stretch is felt in the anterior knee. This position is maintained for 2 to 3 min before the patient moves the gluteals closer to the wall, then holds that position for several minutes. The total time for the exercise is 10 to 15 min.

Active Stretches

A number of exercises are used to gain knee flexibility. The important point to remember for each stretch is to position the muscle so it is not working during the stretch. A hamstring stretch that many athletes use, standing and bending over to touch the floor, is a good example of what not to do. The hamstrings hold the body upright in this position; therefore, stretching the muscle in this position is futile because the muscle is contracting to maintain balance.

Active stretches are repeated several times throughout the day. As discussed previously, a 20 s hold for about four repetitions is advocated. When possible, the opposing muscle should contract to produce a more effective stretch on the intended muscle. Common active stretches are presented in the following sections.

■ Active Flexibility Exercises for the Knee

Wall Slides

Body Segment: Knee (quadriceps).

Stage in Rehab: II.

Purpose: Increase knee flexion motion, especially if the patient is non-weight bearing (NWB).

Positioning: Patient is supine with buttocks about 60 cm (2 ft) or less from a wall. A towel is placed under the foot that is resting on the wall.

Execution: The patient slides the foot down the wall, bending the knee as far as possible (figure 23.22). The uninvolved extremity assists in returning the foot to the starting position. As motion improves, the buttocks are moved closer to the wall.

Possible Substitutions: Rotating the hip laterally, and hip abduction. The hip, knee, and ankle should remain in good alignment with each other throughout the exercise.

Notations: If the patient is able to tolerate more movement, he or she can encourage more flexion by using the uninvolved extremity to push on the top of the involved extremity at the ankle.

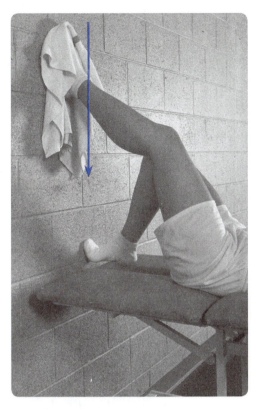

▶ **Figure 23.22** Wall slide.

Seated Knee Flexion

Body Segment: Knee (quadriceps).

Stage in Rehab: II.

Purpose: Increase knee flexion after achieving 50° of flexion.

Positioning: Patient is sitting in a chair with both feet resting on the floor. The uninvolved foot is placed on top of the involved ankle.

Execution: The uninvolved extremity pushes the involved knee into flexion as far as possible (figure 23.23).

Possible Substitutions: Laterally rotating the hip, extending the hip, abduction of the hip. The knee, hip, and ankle should all remain in the same plane.

Notations: This exercise is used throughout the day to improve knee flexion.

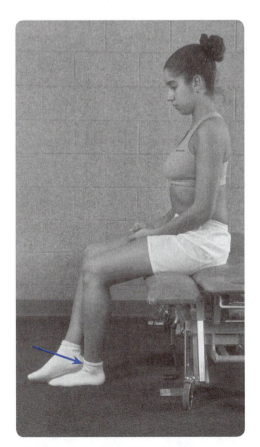

▶ **Figure 23.23** Seated knee flexion.

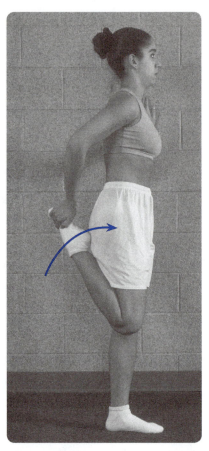

▶ **Figure 23.24** Knee flexion in standing.

Standing Knee Flexion

Body Segment: Knee (quadriceps).

Stage in Rehab: II.

Purpose: Increase knee flexion once near-normal motion is achieved.

Positioning: Patient stands near a wall or table to use as support.

Execution: The patient grasps the foot behind the back and pulls it toward the buttocks (figure 23.24).

Possible Substitutions: Forward trunk flexion, hip extension or abduction, and lateral rotation of the tibia. Provide verbal cueing to correct for improper execution.

Notations: If the patient is unable to reach the foot because of insufficient flexibility, he or she can use a stretch strap in standing. The strap is wrapped around the ankle and grasped behind the back. The strap is pulled to move the foot toward the buttock. An erect posture must be maintained for this exercise.

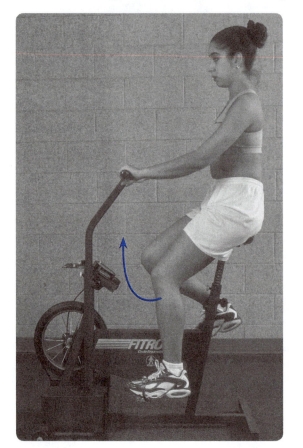

▶ **Figure 23.25** Range of motion on stationary bike.

Stationary Bike

Body Segment: Knee (quadriceps).

Stage in Rehab: II.

Purpose: Increase knee flexion motion. This exercise is especially good once the patient has 90° of flexion and is at least partial weight bearing (PWB).

Positioning: Feet are secured on foot pedals with straps. The height of the seat should be such that at the bottom of the crank position, the knee is near full extension (figure 23.25).

Execution: The patient uses the uninvolved extremity to guide and control the involved extremity during pedaling.

Possible Substitutions: Ankle plantar flexion, hip hiking, or shifting body weight to uninvolved side. Provide verbal cueing to correct technique.

Notations: It is best to begin with a backward motion, because it is easier to achieve a full circle going backward than it is forward. Once the patient is moving the pedals smoothly in reverse, he or she can do forward cycling.

Supine Hamstring Stretch

Body Segment: Knee (hamstrings).

Stage in Rehab: II.

Purpose: Increase knee extension motion.

Positioning: The patient lies supine with the uninvolved extremity extended.

Execution: The involved knee is brought toward the chest, and the hands are clasped behind the thigh. The knee is then actively extended as far as possible so that a stretch is felt behind the knee or in the thigh (figure 23.26).

Possible Substitutions: Rotating the pelvis posteriorly. To prevent this from occurring, have the patient maintain the uninvolved hip and knee in extension during the stretch.

Notations: A stretch strap can be used around the foot if it is too difficult for

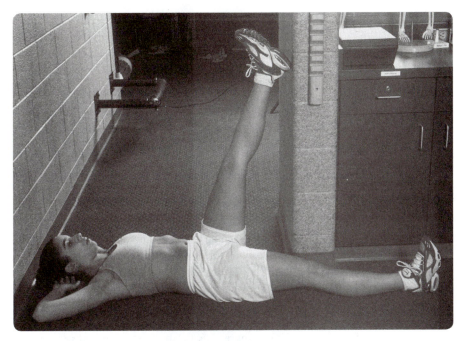

▶ **Figure 23.26** Hamstring stretch in doorway.

the patient to reach the thigh. Another alternative is to have the patient lie supine in a doorway with the uninvolved extremity extended into the doorway and the involved foot on the wall. The stretch is released by bending of the knee. As the patient's flexibility increases, the buttocks are moved closer to the doorframe.

Standing Hamstring Stretch

Body Segment: Knee (hamstrings).

Stage in Rehab: II.

Purpose: Increase knee extension motion.

Positioning: The standing leg is positioned with the foot facing forward. The involved knee is kept extended during the stretch, with the foot facing the ceiling.

Execution: The patient bends forward from the hips, not the back, and attempts to reach toward the toes with the opposite hand (figure 23.27).

Possible Substitutions: Using the same-side arm to reach forward, flexing from the back rather than the hip, rotating the standing leg, flexing the standing knee or the stretch knee. Reaching forward with the same hand allows trunk rotation. The back should remain straight during the stretch.

Notations: Standing hamstring stretches ensure stabilization of the pelvis because the supporting extremity remains in extension during the stretch. The height of the surface that the involved extremity is placed on depends on the patient's flexibility. With very tight hamstrings, it may be best to begin the stretch with the foot on a footstool or chair seat. As the patient's flexibility improves, the height of the supporting object can be raised. If flexibility is normal, an individual should be able to touch the toes of the foot elevated to hip height with the opposite hand. The patient should not bounce during this exercise. Contraction of the quadriceps improves the flexibility during the stretch.

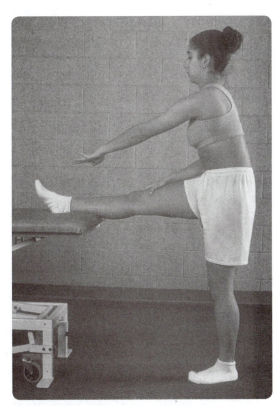

▶ **Figure 23.27** Hamstring stretch in standing.

Flexibility exercises for the knee include prolonged extension and flexion stretches, as well as active stretches for the quadriceps and hamstrings.

STRENGTHENING EXERCISES

Strengthening exercises can begin early in a therapeutic exercise program even if the knee is immobilized and the patient is non-weight bearing. Isometrics help to retard muscle atrophy. Once active motion is permitted, isotonic activities against gravity can progress to exercises against resistance in the form of free weights, manual resistance, machine resistance, body weight when weight bearing is permitted, and isokinetic exercises.

The rehabilitation clinician must bear in mind that some hip muscles and ankle muscles cross the knee joint and must be included in the rehabilitation process. The hip and lateral thigh muscles act as stabilizers for the knee and are important for knee control. Trunk muscles also are important for knee stability, so exercises for these muscles are included in knee rehabilitation. Although exercises for the trunk, hip, and ankle are not discussed here, they are part of a total therapeutic exercise program for a knee injury.

Strengthening exercises should not cause pain or swelling, either during or after the exercise. The clinician must solicit reliable feedback from the patient about how the knee responds to exercises throughout the program, especially during the initial treatment phase and whenever there are increases in the program. Increased pain and swelling indicate that the exercises are too severe. In the presence of these signs, the exercise intensity or severity must be reduced. It is important not to provide too many new exercises that stress the same tissue at one time; if the patient returns for the next treatment session with increased edema and/or pain, it cannot be determined which new exercise caused the inflammatory response. In the early phases of a therapeutic exercise program, it is better to provide a balance of exercises that include perhaps only one or two strengthening exercises for various deficient areas rather than emphasizing only the quadriceps or only the hamstrings. For example, the first treatment session's strengthening exercises may include short-arc quads; manual resistance to hip abduction, adduction, and extension; and hamstring curls. In this case, if the patient returns with increased anterior knee pain, it is likely that the short-arc quads caused the irritation. If the patient had received short-arc quad exercises along with full-arc quad and standing squat exercises, it would be difficult to determine the cause of the patient's pain. Once the cause of the knee's reaction is established, it is easier to decide what exercises are appropriate.

Isometrics

Instructions of isometric exercises should emphasize a gradual buildup of the muscle contraction to a maximum level, a hold at the maximum level for 5 to 6 s, and then a gradual decline to full relaxation before the next repetition. A sudden contraction to maximal levels can cause discomfort and yields a less-than-optimal result. You should also instruct the patient to repeat the exercise in sets of at least 10 several times throughout the day. The following sections provide some suggestions of common isometric exercises. Other exercises in these sections are a progression from non-weight bearing to weight-bearing exercises.

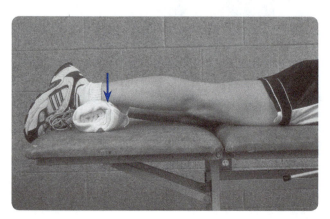

▶ **Figure 23.28** Quad set, prone.

■ Strength Exercises for the Knee

Open Kinetic Chain (OKC): Isometric Quad Set

Body Segment: Quadriceps.

Stage in Rehab: II.

Purpose: Strengthen quadriceps during early rehab when the quadriceps is very weak and the patient is NWB.

Positioning: Patient is sitting or supine with the knee extended and the uninvolved knee flexed (figure 23.28).

Execution: The patient tightens the quadriceps, attempting to push the posterior knee into the table.

Possible Substitutions: Lateral hip rotation, knee flexion, knee abduction. Verbal cueing will correct these substitutions.

Notations: Placing the hand on the quad to feel for muscle tightening helps facilitate a contraction. If the patient is unable to feel a contraction, have the individual perform the exercise with the uninvolved quadriceps to feel a normal contraction before performing the isometric with the involved knee. If the patient is still unable to facilitate a quad contraction, you can lift the heel of the involved leg off the table about 15 cm (6 in.) and instruct the patient to hold this position as you reduce hand support. You should not completely remove your hand, though, because the patient will probably not be able to hold the position independently. A patient who has difficulty producing a quad set in supine can use an alternative position. The patient lies prone with a rolled towel under the ankle, then attempts to push the ankle into the towel roll, facilitating quadriceps activation. The clinician should palpate the quadriceps to monitor active contractions. Electrical stimulation can also be useful for quadriceps facilitation if the patient is unable to produce a good quad contraction with an active exercise.

OKC: Straight-Leg Raise

Body Segment: Quadriceps.

Stage in Rehab: II.

Purpose: Strengthen the quadriceps.

Positioning: The patient is supine with the uninvolved knee flexed and the involved knee extended.

Execution: The patient first contracts the quadriceps muscle, then raises the involved extremity off the table about 20 cm (8 in.) and holds the leg at that level for about 5 s (figure 23.29). The extremity is then slowly lowered, and the quadriceps muscle is not relaxed until the extremity is on the table.

Possible Substitutions: Hip rotation, hip abduction, knee flexion.

Notations: The straight-leg raise is a hip exercise, but because it requires the quadriceps to hold the knee in extension it is essentially an isometric exercise for the quadriceps, with the exception of the rectus femoris, which also acts at the hip. The exercise becomes more difficult if the patient is in a long sitting position rather than supine. It also is more difficult if the hip is laterally rotated during the lift rather than in a neutral position. Weights can also be used to increase the difficulty of the exercise.

OKC: Hamstring Sets

Body Segment: Hamstrings.

Stage in Rehab: II.

Purpose: Increase hamstring strength during NWB and immobilization of the knee.

Positioning: Patient is either sitting or supine with the knee in some flexion.

Execution: If in sitting, the patient places the uninvolved foot behind the distal involved extremity at the ankle and pushes the involved leg against the uninvolved leg, holding the motion for 5 s. If in supine, the patient digs the heel of the involved leg into the tabletop, attempting to flex the knee but not changing the knee position.

Possible Substitutions: Hip rotation or hip extension.

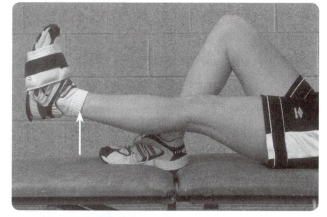

▶ **Figure 23.29** Straight-leg raise.

Notations: If the knee is not immobilized, the exercise may be performed at different points in the range of motion.

Non-Weight-Bearing Isotonic Exercises

Strengthening can begin late in phase II or in early phase III of the therapeutic exercise program even though the patient is non-weight bearing or partial weight bearing. Open kinetic chain exercises can be useful for strengthening in early strengthening activities. The following sections include some suggestions for these exercises.

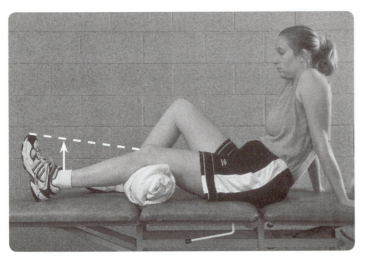

▶ **Figure 23.30** Short-arc quad exercise.

OKC: Short-Arc Quadriceps Exercise (SAQ)

Body Segment: Quadriceps.

Stage in Rehab: II.

Purpose: Strengthen the quadriceps in the terminal degrees of knee extension.

Positioning: A roll is placed under the knee to position the knee in partial flexion. The patient is supine to utilize the rectus femoris or is sitting to increase the difficulty of the exercise.

Execution: With the uninvolved knee flexed, the involved knee is straightened, held in full extension, and then returned to the starting position (figure 23.30). The patient holds the position in full extension for about 5 s.

Possible Substitutions: Hip rotation or moving the knee through incomplete extension. Also, moving through the range of motion too quickly.

Notations: This exercise applies a significant stress to the ACL; therefore, this exercise should not be used early in an ACL injury or reconstruction. A weight or manual resistance can be applied to the ankle to increase the difficulty of the exercise. The size of the towel roll can vary, depending on how much of an arc is desired.

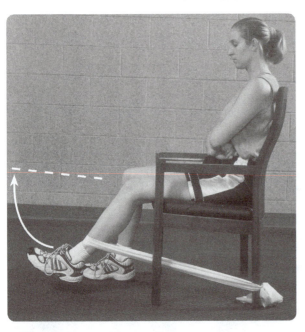

▶ **Figure 23.31** Full-arc quad exercise.

OKC: Full-Arc Quad Exercise

Body Segment: Quadriceps.

Stage in Rehab: Late II and III.

Purpose: Strengthen the quadriceps.

Positioning: The patient sits in a chair or on the edge of a table with the knees over the edge.

Execution: The foot is lifted slowly upward to straighten the knee (figure 23.31). As long as there is no pain, manual resistance, ankle weights, or rubber-band resistance can be used to increase the difficulty of the exercise.

Possible Substitutions: Using the hip to move the knee through its range of motion; moving the extremity through its motion too quickly so that momentum rather than muscle strength moves the limb.

Notations: This exercise is used with caution in early phase II or III. The patellofemoral joint may be painful during the exercise; this is especially the case during the range of motion from 0° to 60° of flexion, because this range places more joint reaction force on the patellofemoral joint. The ACL is also stressed during the 0° to 60° arc of motion, so this exercise is inappropriate for recent ACL injuries.

OKC: Hamstring Curls in Prone

Body Segment: Hamstrings.

Stage in Rehab: Late II and III.

Purpose: Strengthen hamstrings.

Positioning: The patient lies prone with the foot over the edge of the table and the knee in full extension.

Execution: The knee flexes against gravity, manual resistance, a cuff weight, or a resistance band.

Possible Substitutions: Hip flexion or moving the muscle through a partial range of motion.

Notations: Maximal resistance in this exercise occurs in the beginning of the motion, in which the muscle is strongest.

OKC: Hamstring Curls in Standing

Body Segment: Hamstrings.

Stage in Rehab: Late II and III.

Purpose: Strengthen hamstrings.

Positioning: The patient stands and is supported by the noninvolved extremity and by the hands, which grasp a stable object.

Execution: The knee is flexed against cuff weights, manual resistance, resistance bands, or pulleys, moving through a full range of motion (figure 23.32, a & b).

Possible Substitutions: Hip flexion and moving through a partial range of motion.

Notations: In this position, maximum resistance occurs at the end of the knee motion, where the hamstring is at its physiologically weakest position.

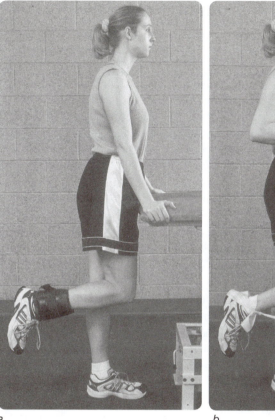
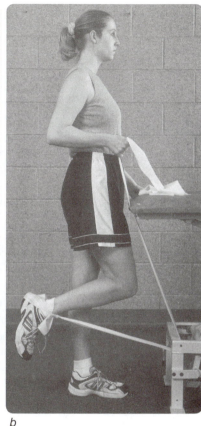

a   b

▶ **Figure 23.32** Hamstring curl: *(a)* with cuff weight, *(b)* with rubber-band resistance.

Closed Kinetic Chain (CKC): Terminal Knee Extension

Body Segment: Knee.

Stage in Rehab: Late II and III.

Purpose: Increase weight-bearing strength of the quadriceps in the final degrees of knee extension.

Positioning: A rubber band is anchored around a stable object such as an upright bar, door jamb, or table leg. It is placed around the knee. A pad or towel roll between the posterior knee and band will enhance comfort. The patient stands facing the door jamb or table with the knee slightly flexed to 30° to 45°, body weight on the involved extremity with the foot flat on the floor, and the band taut.

Execution: The quadriceps muscle is tightened to straighten but not lock the knee (figure 23.33). The position is held for up to 5 s and then slowly released. Patient repeats several times.

Possible Substitutions: Common substitutions for this exercise include lifting the heel off the floor, rotating the hips, bending the trunk, and flexing the hips.

Notations: If a four-way hip machine is available, it can be used for this exercise if the band is placed behind the distal thigh; the patient's position is otherwise the same.

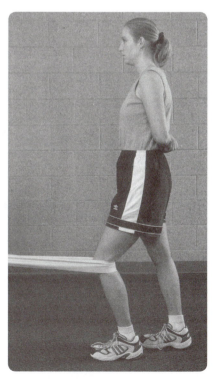

▶ **Figure 23.33** Terminal extension.

Weight-Bearing Resistive Exercises

Once the patient is able to bear weight on the injured knee, weight-transfer activities and gait training may be necessary if the individual has been on crutches, has been non-weight bearing or partial weight bearing, or demonstrates an improper gait pattern. These activities, discussed in chapter 22, include weight-transfer exercises on a scale, gait-training activities, and use of a mirror for facilitation of weight transfer and proper gait. Other weight-bearing exercise suggestions are presented in the following sections.

One note must be made of the wall squat exercise described later. Some clinicians place a ball between the knees during this exercise to facilitate an increased response from the vastus medialis (Hanten & Schulthies, 1990). Later investigations, however, discount these findings and showed evidence that hip adduction activity during a squat does not produce an isolated increase in VMO activity (Mirzabeigi, Jordan, Gronley, Rockowitz, & Perry, 1999) or any increase in quadriceps activity (Hertel, Earl, Tsang, & Miller, 2004). This discussion has become complicated by more recent research that finds there is an increase in the entire quadriceps activity when a ball is placed between the knees to facilitate hip adduction during a squat activity (Earl, Schmitz, & Arnold, 2001). The most recent evidence demonstrates that it is not possible to isolate VMO activity from other muscles within the quadriceps (Andersen et al., 2006), but if an increase in quadriceps activity is desirable, then hip adduction activity used simultaneously with squat exercises may increase quadriceps output (Earl et al., 2001; Mirzabeigi et al., 1999). Since there is disagreement among investigators of this latter point, additional research must be completed before the benefit of hip adduction activity during a squat is undisputable.

Reciprocal Training

Machines such as a stationary bike, a treadmill for gait training, a step machine, or a ski machine can be useful once weight bearing is permitted. The stationary bike produces less tibiofemoral force stress than walking; it can also be used for strengthening and cardiovascular conditioning. Step machines used with controlled degrees of knee motion, and the ski machine, facilitate strength, motion, reciprocal motion between the right and lower extremities, and cardiovascular conditioning.

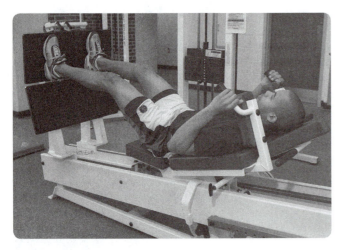

▶ **Figure 23.34** Platform leg press.

CKC: Leg Press

Body Segment: Knee and hip; possibly ankle.

Stage in Rehab: III.

Purpose: Strengthen quadriceps and gluteus maximus. May also strengthen plantar flexors if plantar-flexion motion is incorporated into the motion.

Positioning: Depending on the machine, patient is sitting, semi-reclined, or fully reclined with feet on a platform; knees and hips begin in flexed positions.

Execution: Patient pushes the platform with the legs, extending the hips and knees (figure 23.34). If also strengthening plantar flexors, the patient pushes the platform with the feet to move the ankles into plantar flexion. If the machine is to be used only for plantar flexors, the patient begins the exercises with the knees extended.

This machine can be used in a variety of ways:

1. In the supine or seated position, this exercise can provide resistive concentric and increased eccentric activity if the patient pushes off the platform and catches him- or herself as the feet return to the platform. The speed of this exercise depends on the force with which the patient pushes off the platform and the amount of resistance used.

2. If the patient is in a prone tripod position on elbows and knees with the involved foot on the platform, the foot is placed high on the platform to facilitate the quads and hip extensors. In this position, the patient performs a slow and controlled motion with special attention to gaining full knee extension.

In the prone tripod position, the patient can also perform a rapid push-off and eccentric catch; however, the faster speed is more difficult and should be used only after the patient has demonstrated proficiency with the slower exercise.

Possible Substitutions: Collapsing the knee into a valgus position, not moving through a complete range of motion, or moving the machine too quickly to utilize momentum rather than muscle force. The hip, knee, and ankle should remain in alignment with each other throughout the exercise.

Notations: The patient may use both legs or one leg to concentrate on the involved extremity. To reduce patellofemoral stress, the foot should be positioned on the platform so that the knee is flexed no more than 90° in the starting position.

CKC: Wall Squats

Body Segment: Quadriceps.

Stage in Rehab: Late II and through III.

Purpose: Strengthen quadriceps.

Positioning: The patient stands with the back to the wall and the feet out in front.

Execution: Patient squats to bend at the hips and knees, but the knees should remain over the ankles so that the leg does not go beyond a line perpendicular to the floor. The patient can hold this position in an isometric for several seconds or move up and down without pausing in the low position. A Swiss ball placed between the wall and the patient allows the patient a smoother squat motion and prevents dye in the patient's shirt from rubbing off on the wall.

Possible Substitutions: Common errors with this exercise include positioning the feet too close to the wall so that flexion goes beyond 90°, placing more weight on the uninvolved extremity, and hiking the hip so that the knee does not flex as much. If the patient is reluctant to bear weight equally on left and right extremities, a small platform placed under the uninvolved foot can facilitate increased weight bearing on the involved extremity.

Notations: If the knee is flexed more than 90°, patellofemoral stress increases and pain may result. The deeper the squat, the farther away from the wall the feet are positioned, so the knee is never flexed more than 90° in the maximum squat position. Ways to advance this exercise are to increase the repetitions or sets; to increase the depth of the squat (as long as the knee does not move in front of the ankle in the end-squat position); or to have the patient perform the exercise with only one extremity (figure 23.35), placing the uninvolved extremity on a stool or step.

CKC: Plié

Body Segment: Quadriceps.

Stage in Rehab: Late II and into III.

Purpose: Strengthen the quadriceps.

Positioning: The patient stands with the feet in a wide stance with the hips and feet turned outward about 45°.

Execution: The buttocks are squeezed as the patient slowly bends the knees, keeping the knees in line with the second toes (figure 23.36).

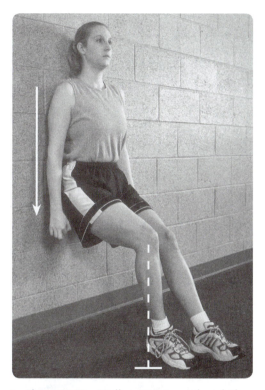

▶ **Figure 23.35** Wall squat using only right leg.

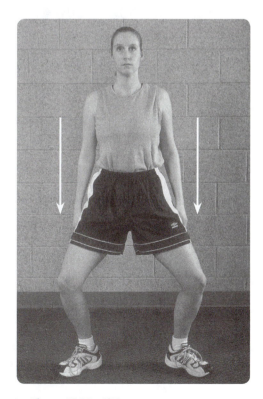

▶ **Figure 23.36** Plié.

Possible Substitutions: Not aligning the knees over the second toes; causing the knees to move into a valgus position; not keeping the weight evenly distributed over right and left legs; and not keeping the back straight.

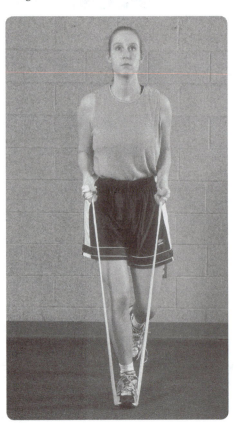

▶ **Figure 23.37**   Lunge.

Figure 23.38   Mini-squat on one leg.

Notations: The back should remain straight so that as the patient flexes the knees and hips, the trunk leans forward; the pelvis should not be allowed to move into a posterior tilt.

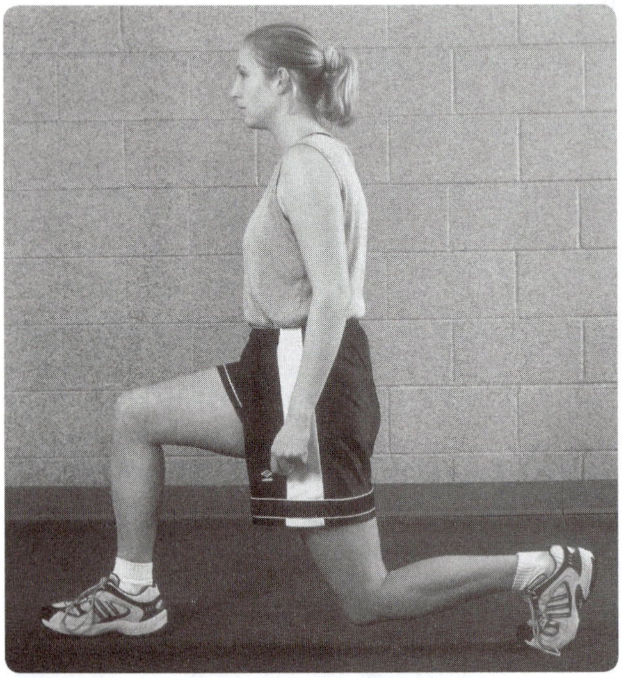

CKC: Lunge

Body Segment: Quadriceps and hip extensors.

Stage in Rehab: III.

Purpose: Strengthen quadriceps and gluteals.

Positioning: The patient stands with the feet in a forward-backward stance with the involved extremity in front.

Execution: The quadriceps and buttocks are tightened, and the weight is shifted to the front extremity as the patient bends the knee (figure 23.37). This position can be held for several seconds, or the patient can be instructed to walk across the floor in this manner. As the patient progresses forward, the body weight is lifted toward the front foot by the front leg, not pushed forward by the back leg.

Possible Substitutions: Common errors are to allow the arch to fall and the knee to move into a valgus position. The knee should not move forward ahead of the foot. The leg should remain at an angle so that it is no more than perpendicular to the floor.

Notations: Weights placed in the hands increase the resistance of this exercise. Performing the exercise on an incline also alters the resistance.

CKC: Mini-Squats

Body Segment: Quadriceps and gluteals.

Stage in Rehab: III.

Purpose: Strengthen the quadriceps and gluteals.

Positioning: The patient stands with feet shoulder-width apart and toes turned slightly outward.

Execution: Keeping the weight equally distributed, the patient squats to a comfortable position, maintaining the knees in alignment with the second toes. The back remains straight as the patient squats, so the hips flex and move posteriorly and the pelvis remains in neutral throughout the exercise.

Possible Substitutions: Common errors are valgus movement of the knees, trunk flexion, and hip hiking on the involved side to reduce knee flexion. If genu valgus is noted, the patient should be instructed to keep the knees over the second toes and to arch the foot; trunk flexion is corrected with verbal cueing for a straight back and instructions to push the hips back and to keep the chest up; hip hiking is corrected with instructions to bend the knee more and keep the hips level.

Notations: In a progression of this exercise, the patient grasps a band that is anchored under the feet to increase resistance for home exercises. Holding weights in the hands increases eccentric and concentric resistance. Performing the exercise on only one extremity increases the difficulty (figure 23.38).

CKC: Sit-to-Stand

Body Segment: Quadriceps and gluteals.

Stage in Rehab: III.

Purpose: Strengthen quadriceps in midrange and gluteals.

Positioning: The patient sits in a chair with both feet on the floor under the knees.

Execution: Without using arms for assistance, the patient moves in a slow and controlled manner from the sit position to standing and then returns to the chair. The knees should remain in line with the second toes; weight should be equally distributed over right and left extremities; and the back should remain straight with the pelvis in neutral.

Possible Substitutions: Common errors in this exercise include shifting the weight to the uninvolved side, bending the trunk, jerking up, and dropping down into the chair. Correction techniques are verbal cueing, using a mirror for visual feedback, or using a higher chair and later advancing to a lower chair as strength improves.

Notations: Once the patient performs this exercise easily, he or she can advance to a single-leg exercise.

Step Exercises

The patient should not attempt these exercises until he or she is able to bear weight on the involved extremity in a single-leg stance position. Proper weight transfer is also a prerequisite for these exercises. The step height may begin at a low level, around 10 cm (4 in.) and increase to 20 cm (8 in.) as the patient gains strength and knee control. The rehabilitation clinician observes the patient's exercise execution and correct errors as needed. The patient performs the exercise in a slow and controlled manner. As with other weight-bearing resistive exercises, the knee remains in line with the second toe throughout the motion. The knee should achieve extension at the top of the exercise, but it should not lock. During initial performance of these exercises, patients often demonstrate poor knee control, evidenced by wobbling of the knee as the individual raises and lowers body weight. With gains in strength, the knee movement becomes steady with no lateral knee motion.

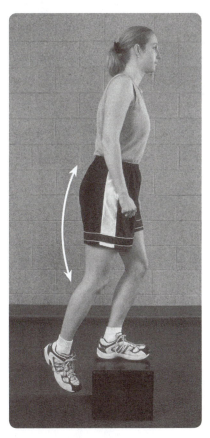

▶ **Figure 23.39** Step-up.

Common errors for these exercises include several mistakes for which the clinician observes and corrects, as indicated. These errors include flexion at the hip and trunk to reduce the amount of quadriceps activity required, locking the knee in the extension position to reduce the need for muscular control, hip hiking to reduce the amount of knee flexion motion in the lowered position, jerking up and dropping down rather than maintaining a smooth and controlled motion, moving the knee into a valgus position and flattening the foot arch, and pushing off with the uninvolved leg. Usually, corrections for these errors require verbal cueing and placing the patient in front of a mirror for visual feedback during the exercise. If pushing off with the uninvolved leg, dropping down and jerking up, and trunk and hip flexion are not corrected with these cues, the height of the step may be too great and prevent the patient from correcting the errors; in this case, it is better to use a lower step.

Advancing these exercises occurs by increasing the numbers of repetitions and sets, increasing the depth of the step, and adding weights to the hands.

Step-Up This exercise strengthens the quads. The patient stands facing a step with the involved extremity on the step. The patient shifts the weight to the involved extremity and moves the uninvolved extremity up onto the step, straightening the knee to lift the body up. The patient should not push off with the uninvolved leg (figure 23.39). He or she then returns to the starting position, stepping back and down to the floor.

Step-Down This exercise strengthens the quads and gluteal muscles. This exercise emphasizes the eccentric portion of the step activity. It stresses the knee more than the step-up exercise does because the patient is moving forward on the extremity and the knee must move in front of the foot. If the exercise causes knee pain, it is performed on a lower step, but if pain occurs on the lower step, the exercise should be deferred until knee control and strength increase. The patient stands on a step and slowly lowers the uninvolved extremity forward and downward to the floor so that the heel touches the floor first (figure 23.40). The patient then returns to the start position, lifting the body backward. The patient should not push off with the uninvolved extremity.

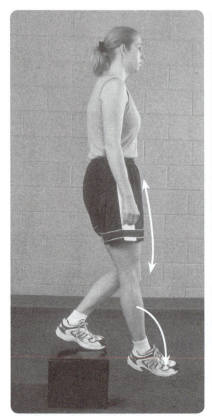

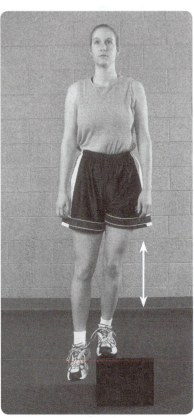

▶ **Figure 23.40** Step-down.

▶ **Figure 23.41** Lateral step-up.

Lateral Step-Up This exercise strengthens the quads and isolates the quads more than the other step exercises do. The patient stands sideways on a step, with the involved extremity on the step and the uninvolved extremity on the ground. Only the heel of the uninvolved extremity is in contact with the ground; the toes remain off the ground throughout the exercise. The patient lifts the body weight up to the step by tightening the quads and gluteals (figure 23.41). The patient then slowly lowers the heel of the uninvolved extremity to the floor. If the patient flexes at the trunk, the hamstrings are working rather than the quadriceps. If the patient feels the exercise more in the lateral hip than in the quadriceps, the patient is using the gluteus medius muscle to lift the body rather than the quadriceps; in this case, instruct the patient to flex the knee more as the uninvolved extremity is lowered to the ground.

You can provide additional overload by requiring the patient to land the heel of the uninvolved extremity away from the step to abduct the involved hip as the extremity lowers to the floor.

Machine Exercises

A number of machine and weight exercises are available for strengthening the knee. Some units vary in features or style from one brand to another but have underlying similarities and exercise the same muscles or muscle groups. Available equipment varies from one facility to another according to budget, space, and staff preferences. Whatever equipment is used, it is imperative for the rehabilitation clinician to be familiar with the machine, with the instructions for use and the indications, and with the precautions and dangers before using it with patients. The following sections describe exercises with a few of the more commonly used machines.

Knee Extension

This machine is used with caution. I do not often use it because of its potential for injury to the patellofemoral joint and ACL. It provides an open kinetic chain exercise that produces patellofemoral compression in the early portion of motion and places shear stress on the ACL in the later portion of the motion. It is essential that if this machine is used, it is used cautiously and in limited degrees of motion. Patient's pain is your primary guideline when using this machine: If pain occurs, either the motion on it is restricted or the weight is reduced. If pain still occurs with these changes, it is not used.

I mention the knee extension unit here, not because I advocate its use, but because many facilities have such a unit so it is important for the rehabilitation clinician to be aware of it and its potential hazards. It can be a beneficial exercise if used properly.

The patient sits with the ankle behind a weighted bar. To facilitate the rectus femoris, the patient inclines backward with the weight on the hands behind the hips. Some machines have the back rest positioned so the patient is naturally declined. The individual then extends the knees (figure 23.42). If pain occurs during the exercise, the machine should not be used.

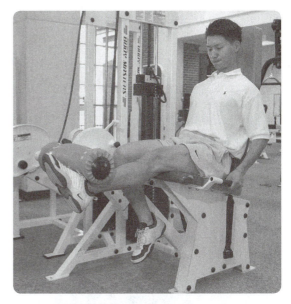

▶ **Figure 23.42** Machine knee extension.

Squat

This exercise strengthens the quads and hip extensors. It is an advanced exercise that is not performed until a patient has demonstrated good strength and knee control with the step exercises and other closed chain activities previously outlined. It is commonly placed in the latter part of phase III.

With the feet about shoulder-width apart, the weight is placed on the patient's shoulders. Keeping the back straight, the patient squats to no more than a 90° angle at the hips and knees (figure 23.43). The knees should remain in line with the second toe. The illustration demonstrates the exercise with a barbell, but the exercise can also be performed with adaptable machines such as a bench-press or heel-raise unit.

Hamstring Curl

This exercise strengthens the hamstrings. Depending on the machine, the patient may lay prone, stand, or sit on the unit with the machine secured around the posterior ankle. The knee begins in an extended position, and the patient flexes the knee (figure 23.44).

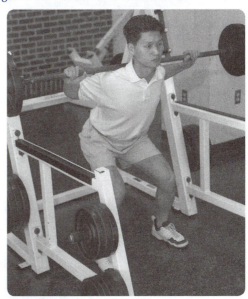

▶ **Figure 23.43** Squat.

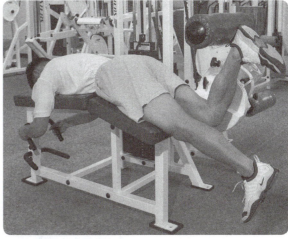

▶ **Figure 23.44** Machine hamstring curl.

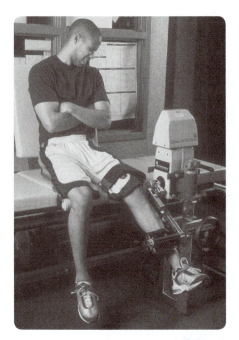

▶ **Figure 23.45** Isokinetic exercises.

Isokinetic Exercises

Isokinetic exercises for the quads and hamstrings usually begin after the patient has demonstrated control in isotonic exercises. Hamstrings and quadriceps can be exercised isokinetically, isometrically, or eccentrically on isokinetic machines. If facilitation of the rectus femoris is desired, the seat back should be reclined to extend the hip (figure 23.45). The hamstrings can be exercised in a seated position to maximize output at the knee or in prone.

PROPRIOCEPTION EXERCISES

Just as with other injured areas, balance, agility, and coordination must be restored following knee injury or surgery. Proprioception is the element basic to these parameters. Early proprioception exercises in phase II before weight bearing can include a variety of activities. For example, with eyes closed the patient can move the involved knee to mimic the uninvolved knee's position, or with eyes closed can position the knee at a designated angle. With the latter activity, the clinician measures the angle to determine the patient's ability to produce the desired angle.

Weight-bearing proprioception exercises are similar to those for the ankle as discussed in chapter 22. The patient performs stork standing on the floor with eyes open (figure 23.46a) and then eyes closed before advancing to stork standing on unstable surfaces such as the BAPS board (figure 23.46b), trampoline (figure 23.46c), or foam rollers.

The next progression is to make the balance activity more challenging and to facilitate change in the activity from a conscious to a subconscious activity. To accomplish this the patient performs a distracting activity while maintaining balance on an unstable surface. For example, the patient stands on a foam roller while using an upper-extremity device such as a B.O.I.N.G., Body Blade, or other device (figure 23.47). Another example is shown in figure 22.56a.

Patients with knee injuries perform many kinds of strengthening exercises, including isometrics, non-weight-bearing isotonics, weight-bearing resistive exercises, machine exercises, and isokinetic exercises.

▶ **Figure 23.46** Stork-standing balance progression: *(a)* on ground, *(b)* on BAPS, *(c)* on trampoline.

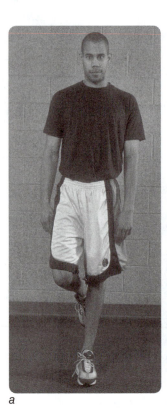

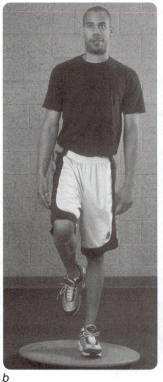

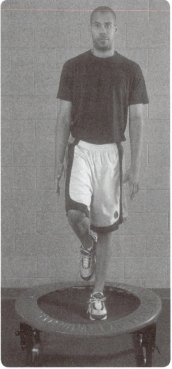

a   b   c

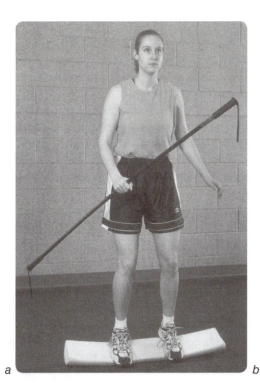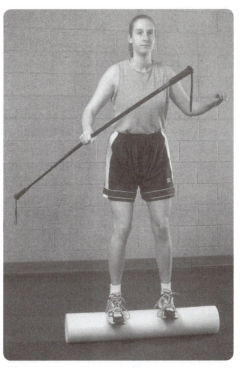

A rehabilitation program for a patient with a knee injury includes a progression of proprioception exercises aimed at restoring balance, agility, and coordination.

▶ **Figure 23.47** Advanced- and beginning-level distracting balance activities: *(a)* on 1/2 foam roller, *(b)* on foam roller.

Other balance and proprioception exercises include activities on balance boards, the Fitter, and slide boards. Activities that develop agility, coordination, and balance include jumping activities against a resistance band with both legs and then with just the involved extremity; treadmill activities such as retro walking, side shuffle, and cariocas; and bilateral and unilateral hopping and jumping activities. Plyometric exercises with boxes develop agility and power in preparation for functional exercises. These advanced proprioception exercises are discussed in chapter 22 and shown in figure 22.58.

During all of these proprioception activities, the clinician monitors and corrects the patient's performance. For example, if the patient does not maintain the body's center of gravity of the base of support, it is indicative of poor core control, so core control must be addressed before the patient progresses. If the patient is unable to perform accurate jumping activities on targets, then the targets should be spaced closer together until the patient performs the activity successfully. If the patient does not maintain balance during a single leg stance on an unstable surface, then the clinician provides the patient with verbal cues that will improve balance; for example, "tighten your quads and your glutes," or "focus on one object in front of you."

FUNCTIONAL AND ACTIVITY-SPECIFIC EXERCISES

Many of the functional and activity-specific exercises used for the knee are similar to those discussed in chapter 22 for the ankle. The exercises vary more according to the patient's activity demands than according to the lower-extremity segment injured, because a safe return to full participation depends on the entire lower extremity's ability to withstand stresses and perform properly regardless of the segment injured.

Functional activities include single, double, and triple hops; zigzag runs with sudden changes in direction; backward running with sudden changes to forward running; sprinting; running circles in clockwise and counterclockwise directions; 90° cuts to the left and to the

Functional exercises for the knee, which are similar to those for the ankle, use hopping, running, and cutting as well as sport-specific drill and skill activities.

right; and sport-specific drill and skill activities. Activity-specific drill and skill activities are dictated by the patient's specific sport or activity requirements. Because running, rapid changes of direction, and reliance on both lower extremities are vital to most sport participation, the running and hopping activities are universal and should be a part of most therapeutic exercise programs. These are discussed in detail in chapters 10 and 22.

Before returning to full participation, the patient must undergo an examination of specific activity performance. This examination uses many of the exercises and activities the patient has been performing in phase IV of the rehabilitation program. The patient should be able to perform all of these activities without psychological or physical impediment and should demonstrate equal use and performance with both lower extremities in all tests performed.

SPECIAL REHABILITATION APPLICATIONS

This section deals with specific injuries to the knee and thigh. The more common knee injuries are discussed.

Ligament Sprains

Any ligament in the knee can become injured if the stresses applied are sufficient to overstress the ligament. Depending on the magnitude and direction of the forces applied, a single ligament or multiple structures can incur injury. For the sake of simplicity, this discussion focuses primarily on injuries to individual ligaments.

Anterior Cruciate Ligament Sprain

The anterior cruciate ligament (ACL) is the knee ligament that is most frequently sprained. Considerations unique to this ligament are discussed here, and then a case study is presented.

Although daily activities apply around 454 N of stress to the ligament, it is able to tolerate up to 1,730 N before it ruptures (Dye & Cannon, 1988; Markolf, Gorek, Kabo, & Shapiro, 1990). It is in a position of maximum stress when the knee is either at full extension or at 90° flexion. The ACL is most typically injured when the knee suffers a valgus stress with lateral rotation in a foot-planted position as the athlete decelerates. The individual is often in a cutting maneuver, and the injury can occur with or without contact with another person. Sudden knee hyperextension with rotation, moving the knee into a valgus position is another mechanism of ACL injury (Krosshaug et al., 2007). Although it is likely to be a multi-factorial issue, there is evidence to demonstrate that females experience a greater frequency of ACL injuries than males because females use different landing strategies during jumping than do males (Zeller, McCrory, Kibler, & Uhl, 2003). It has been observed that women use less knee and hip flexion than men during landing and stop-jump activities, causing greater quadriceps activation than hamstrings, thereby increasing ACL stress (Chappell, Creighton, Giuliani, Yu, & Garrett, 2007). These studies provide early yet interesting if not compelling evidence for the need to alter women's conditioning programs to prevent or reduce ACL injuries.

When the ACL is injured, it is frequently only one of the structures injured. The MCL or medial meniscus, or both, can be involved along with the ACL when outside contact force is added to the internal stresses of cutting or hyperextension. When more than one structure is injured, the rehabilitation process becomes more complicated because it must address considerations other than those related to the ACL.

The individual may hear or feel a pop and then experience a giving way of the knee. Swelling occurs within the next 2 to 24 h, but is not apparent immediately.

Once an individual sustains an ACL injury, the decision about surgery must be made. Factors determining an individual's candidacy for ACL reconstructive surgery include age, activity level, desire to return to full participation, and knee instability. Long-term differences between surgically repaired and non-surgically repaired ACL ruptures indicate no differences in osteoarthritis and functional abilities, but those individuals who did not undergo surgical reconstruction developed meniscal damage and instability (Meunier, Odensten, & Good, 2007). These results seem to indicate that active persons would benefit from surgical repair of a ruptured ACL.

If a patient elects to have reconstructive surgery, motion recovery and return to participation results are best when surgery is delayed. Studies have demonstrated that surgical repair produces the best results when performed after the inflammation has subsided and full range of motion has been restored (Delay, Smolinski, Wind, & Bowman, 2001; Irrgang, Harner, Fu, Silbey, & DiGiacomo, 1997).

Over the years, many types of reconstructive surgeries for the ACL have been attempted. Surgical techniques continue to evolve, but currently the two most commonly accepted reconstructive procedures utilize the patient's patellar tendon or the medial hamstring tendons or an allograft. There are proponents of each technique, but the evidence indicates there is essentially no difference in outcomes of any of the three techniques (Marrale, Morrissey, & Haddad, 2007; Paessler & Mastrokalos, 2003; Scheffler, Sudkamp, Gockenjan, Hoffmann, & Weiler, 2002). Surgeon preference may be the primary factor determining the technique selected for a patient (Barclay, 2003). The patellar tendon graft technique, which uses the central third of the patellar tendon with bone-plug ends from the patella and tibial tuberosity, is known as the BPTB, or bone-patellar tendon-bone technique, and is considered the "gold standard" for anterior cruciate ligament reconstructions (ACLR) (Marrale et al., 2007). This technique is performed partially arthroscopically and also involves either one or two surgical incisions. The semitendinosus and gracilis are used for the hamstring tendon procedure, which is also a combined open and arthroscopic procedure. Advocates of the hamstring tendon graft procedure present the case that subjects who receive hamstring tendon grafts have fewer donor-site complications and regain quadriceps strength faster (Brown, Steiner, & Carson, 1993). However, elongation of the hamstring graft is a frequent report using these grafts (Adam et al., 2004). Allografts may be the graft of choice if the reconstruction is on a young patient or is a repeat surgery with the patient re-injuring the previously replaced ACL (Marrale et al., 2007). Allografts have been shown to heal more slowly than autografts, but one year after surgery, there is no significant difference between allografts and autografts (Gulotta & Rodeo, 2007). More than any graft selection, the choice of anchor systems for the graft appears to be most important (Scheffler et al., 2002).

Rehabilitation following ACL reconstruction follows two schools of thought, one for delay and the other for acceleration; the best course of action remains controversial (Cascio, Culp, & Cosgarea, 2004). Some clinicians advocate using the accelerated program with competitive and serious recreational athletes and the more conservative program with less serious recreational athletes (Wilk, Arrigo, Andrews, & Clancy, 1999). Of these camps, members in either commonly prefer weight bearing to tolerance following surgery (Delay et al., 2001). Those in the delayed-program camp are concerned about the vulnerability of new tissue and feel that stressing the tissue too soon will risk detachment at the graft site, compromise the graft, and render the joint unstable. Running under a conservative program is restricted until about the fifth or sixth month, with full return to activities occurring six to nine months following surgery.

Those advocating the accelerated program for ACL reconstructions believe that there are fewer complications from the surgery (Kvist, 2006). In the accelerated program, running activities begin after 12 weeks, and the patient is able to return to full participation in five to six months.

Histologically, the ACL graft undergoes necrosis and remodeling once it is transplanted. Initially it is avascular, but revascularization occurs at 6 to 8 weeks and is completed around 12 weeks postoperatively (Scheffler, Unterhauser, & Weiler, 2008). Once the graft is inserted, it goes through a process of necrosis and disintegration and then rebuilding. During this process, regardless of the graft material used, the ACL replacement is at its weakest during the first six weeks following reconstruction (Gulotta & Rodeo, 2007). New collagen is formed around the existing matrix of the graft, maturing the graft site and allowing it to manage progressively greater applied stresses. It may take at least a year for the graft to appear histologically normal, but it does not ever regain normal tensile strength (Clancy et al., 1981). Although the precise load-tolerance levels of ACL grafts are not known, it is agreed that some mechanical stress is beneficial to the healing graft (Scheffler et al., 2008). For this reason, most surgeons encourage weight bearing, either full or limited, immediately following ACL reconstruction.

If the medial meniscus is injured along with the ACL, it must be repaired to assure a successful outcome of the ACL reconstruction surgery (Meunier et al., 2007). This is important because the meniscus provides stability to the knee, so when it is injured, the knee joint's stability is compromised. An unstable knee will damage the reconstructed ACL, placing undue stress upon the structure and advance osteoarthritis within the joint (Meunier et al., 2007). Prior to performing an ACL reconstruction, the surgeon will repair the meniscus; in these cases, post-operative weight bearing may be limited or delayed in order to protect the meniscal repair (Barber & Click, 1997).

When you design a specific ACL rehabilitation program for a patient who has undergone reconstructive surgery, key considerations must include the type of graft and fixation used, the type of surgery performed, the surgeon's rehabilitation preferences, and other injuries present. Although the timing is different for exercises in delayed and accelerated programs, the exercises and the progression are essentially the same.

Two program timing progressions are provided here as examples of a delayed and an accelerated ACL program. In actuality, a patient's program may be accelerated or delayed or may be a combination of the two programs. Communication with the physician regarding the patient's progression is crucial to a safe and successful rehabilitation program.

Accelerated Postop ACL Reconstruction Program In an accelerated program, the patient ambulates with crutches, weight bearing to tolerance with full knee extension, immediately following surgery. Two days postoperatively, passive knee extension to 0°, active hip exercises including straight-leg raises, and ankle range-of-motion exercises begin. The patient may wear a knee brace, but it is set at 0° extension. Although CPM use is variable, one may be used in conjunction with electrical stimulation to the quadriceps. By the end of the first week, the patient should have 90° range of motion with full extension.

During the second week, active range-of-motion exercises for the knee begin, as do patellar mobilization and soft-tissue mobilization. By the end of the second week, the patient should be ambulating without crutches, but he or she continues to use the brace. Gait training for proper heel-toe ambulation may be necessary. Some physicians discontinue the brace during the third week, whereas others continue it for about six weeks, with removal only for showers and passive exercises. In either case, the patient is not allowed to ambulate without the brace until full active knee extension is possible; allowing the patient to ambulate with a partially flexed knee increases meniscal stress and accelerates joint degeneration. Closed kinetic activities such as mini-squats and stationary-bike exercises with minimal tension begin during the second week. Hamstring curls, toe raises, and range of motion to 105° are included at this time.

By the third week, the patient can exercise in the pool; can add other exercise equipment, such as the ski machine and the stepper with no more than a 10 cm (4 in.) step; and can leg press through a 60° range of motion. Other exercises include half squats to 40° and hamstring curls. The patient can do stork standing if weight transfer during ambulation is correct. If weight transfer is not correct, then using the weight scale for transfer activities is beneficial. By the end of the first month, the patient should have flexion motion to about 115° and full extension. Tibiofemoral joint mobilizations are used if capsular tightness is evident. The patient is now using the stepper machine and performing wall squats, heel raises, lunges, lateral step-ups, forward step-ups. None of the exercises should increase pain or edema or give the patient the sensation of increased knee laxity.

During weeks 6 to 8, if there has been no increase in swelling and the patient has full active extension and flexion to 115°-120° and good isometric quadriceps strength, he or she can begin ambulation without the brace if it has not yet been discontinued. Active knee extensions in 100° to 30° ranges of motion, and a treadmill walking program are implemented during this time. Research has demonstrated that a treadmill set at an incline slightly greater than 12% reduces ACL strain and patellofemoral strain but recruits greater quadriceps activity, and thus may be beneficial for ACL and patellofemoral rehabilitation programs (Lange, Hintermeister, Schlegel, Dillman, & Steadman, 1996).

During the weeks leading up to the third month, the exercises that the patient has done so far continue, progressing in weights, sets, and/or repetitions as tolerated provided they do not produce pain or edema. Plyometrics begin by week 12 along with jogging activities. By the third to fourth month, the patient progresses to running and sprinting. During this time the patient advances to agility drills, more aggressive plyometrics, and activity-specific drills, if full range of motion is present, strength is about 80% that of the uninvolved knee, and proprioception is good in static and dynamic balance activities.

During the fifth to sixth month, the program continues with strengthening and flexibility exercises and advances to more functional activities as the patient prepares to return to full sport participation or normal work activities. Because the physician often relies on the rehabilitation clinician for the information needed to determine readiness to return to full participation, an appropriate examination is necessary. Before returning, the patient must pass all aspects of the activity-specific examination; have full motion, strength, and normal proprioception; and be pain free without edema post-exercise. This program is condensed into a timeline in figure 23.48.

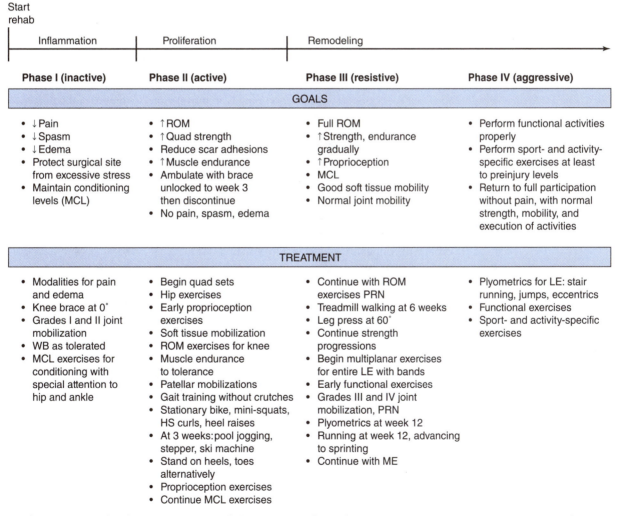

▶ **Figure 23.48** Rehabilitation progression following an accelerated ACL reconstruction program. ROM = range of motion; WB = weight bearing; LE = lower extremity; PRN = as needed; HS = hamstring.

Conservative Postop ACL Reconstruction Program A delayed program has the same progression, but at a slower rate. Weight bearing progresses from weight bearing to tolerance to full weight bearing with the brace locked in extension for one week. The brace is used to perform straight leg raises. The brace is unlocked after one week but kept on with crutches for ambulation. During the first 2 weeks, hip exercises with the brace on, heel raises, and quad sets are used for strengthening. The patient is able to remove the brace to perform wall slides to 45°, heel slides, and prone hangs with the foot over the edge of the table for range of motion. When the patient is able to perform a quad set with good quadriceps control in full extension, the crutches are removed, but the brace is used for the first 6 weeks. Patellar mobilization is started during week 2, and electrical stimulation and modalities for pain and edema

---

■ Case Study

A 16-year-old male soccer forward suffered a right ACL injury that was repaired last week. His physician instructed him in straight-leg-raise exercises and quad sets before discharging him from the hospital, but now the physician wants the patient to begin rehabilitation using an accelerated program. The patient is using crutches and bearing about 50% of his weight on the right lower extremity. He has a rehabilitative brace on the knee, with the knee joint set at 0° extension and 90° flexion. He is allowed to remove the brace for passive activities only. The knee has minor edema and some ecchymosis around the knee and into the proximal leg. The surgical repair was a patellar tendon transfer; the patient has two scars, one over the patellar tendon and one over the distal lateral thigh, in addition to portal scars from the arthroscopy. The surgical scars are healing well but still have sutures that will be removed next week. There are some soft-tissue adhesions around the knee, especially surrounding the surgical sites and the suprapatellar area. The patient reports only minor postoperative pain. Patellar mobility is about 50% normal in all planes, but the patient does not report pain with movement. Alignment of the patella is normal, without the presence of patella alta or baja. The patient is able to perform a straight-leg raise but is unable to tolerate any resistance to the motion. Hip adduction is 3+/5, hip abduction is 4–/5, and hip extension is 4–/5. He reports some pain with attempts at full weight bearing but admits that he is very apprehensive about putting full weight on the extremity.

Questions for Analysis

1. What are his problems and your long-term goals? List them in order of priority.

2. What will your first treatment for this patient include today?

3. What will your goals for this first treatment today be?

4. What pre-gait activities will you use to encourage the patient to put more weight on the right lower extremity?

5. What instructions will you give him before he leaves today?

6. What exercises will you include in his program over the next two weeks?

7. Over the next six weeks, what exercises will you assign, and what will be your criteria for advancing the exercises during that time?

8. How long do you expect the patient's program to take, assuming that he follows a program without complications or problems?

9. When will you have him start on a treadmill, and what will be your first exercise on it?

10. Outline a progression from the treadmill to a full running program.

11. List four exercises you will include in the patient's functional activities program.

12. Describe the functional tests you will use before the patient is allowed back to full sport participation.

modulation can begin during the first week. During the first week, stretching exercises for the hamstrings, gastrocnemius, ITB, and quad sets occur. Cardiovascular activities are limited to an upper-body ergometer or unilateral stationary cycling using only the uninvolved extremity.

Other exercises are not added until week 6, when the patient is able to remove the brace and good quadriceps control in knee extension become possible. The patient begins stationary-bike exercises with both legs, wall squats to 45°, leg press to 45°, lateral step-ups, forward step-ups, backward step-ups, heel raises, and static balance activities. Pool walking and jogging may begin at this time as well.

From 6-8 weeks to 5 months, the patient achieves normal gait and full range of motion of the knee. Leg press exercises advance to 60° flexion, and the patient is able to progress to the stepper and elliptical trainer. At two to three months, the patient begins fast walking.

Running is not permitted until about four to six months postoperatively. Cutting and lateral movements are permitted after the sixth month. A progression of plyometrics, agility exercises, and functional and activity-specific exercises is gradually incorporated into the program.

During the 6th through 12th month, once the patient has passed the same examination tests as in the accelerated program, return to full sport or work participation is permitted.

Recovery from ACL reconstruction can be a slow process whether the patient follows an aggressive or a conservative rehabilitation program. In a prospective study, patients who underwent ACL reconstruction took anywhere from one to two years to regain full muscle function and pain relief (Risberg, Holm, Tjomsland, Ljunggren, & Ekeland, 1999). The clinician must be careful always to consider the tissue healing timeline and to coordinate intensity levels of therapeutic exercises with the timeline. Optimal results are most likely to occur if these factors are respected.

Posterior Cruciate Ligament Sprain

Stability provided by the posterior cruciate ligament (PCL) is actually the combined result of the posterior cruciate ligament and the posterior corner structures. These posterior corner structures include an array of ligamentous and musculotendinous structures such as the popliteus complex and lateral collateral ligament that restrict external tibial rotation and varus stress (Apsingi et al., 2008). The PCL has two components, an anterolateral bundle that is the largest portion and becomes taut with knee flexion, and the posteromedial bundle that resists posterior tibial translation and becomes taut in knee extension (Margheritini, Rihn, Musahl, Mariani, & Harner, 2002). Replacement of PCL stability have included using both a double-bundle PCL to replace the original PCL elements and a combination of a double-bundle with a posterolateral corner reconstruction. Studies have shown that the latter reconstruction provides pre-injury stability but using only a double-bundle reconstruction does not (Sekiya, Haemmerle, Stabile, Vogrin, & Harner, 2005).

PCL injuries are relatively rare in sports, especially compared to ACL injuries (Margheritini et al., 2002). The common mechanisms of injury are either hyperextension of the knee or falling onto a flexed knee. Injuries to the PCL occur more often in high contact sports such as American football, soccer, and rugby and less often in sports such as basketball that require more sudden cutting and pivoting activities (Margheritini et al., 2002). Surgical repair is performed if the knee is unstable, if the posterolateral corner is injured, or if other ligaments have been injured in addition to the PCL. Surgical repair of the PCL without these other factors is controversial with many surgeons opting for a non-surgical approach (Margheritini et al., 2002)

Rehabilitation considerations for PCL reconstructions is different than ACL reconstructions since stresses to the PCL are different from those applied to the ACL. Grafts for PCL reconstructions heal more slowly than ACL grafts, so the rehabilitation progression is more prolonged. It may take the PCL graft up to 26 weeks before it has up to 62% of the stiffness of a normal PCL (Bosch et al., 1994).

During rehabilitation exercises, the PCL experiences a progressive increase in shear stress in a resisted open kinetic chain flexion exercise as the knee moves from extension to flexion.

The amount of PCL shear stress during resisted knee extension is a bit more controversial. Some investigations have found high PCL shear stresses in the 85° to 100° ranges of motion with less posterior shear as the knee reaches full extension when anterior shear stress increases (Wilk et al., 1996). In closed kinetic chain exercises, the posterior shear stress becomes progressively greater going from extension to flexion with the greatest stresses occurring in the 70° to 100° ranges of knee flexion. It is advisable, then to keep OKC extension exercises to no more than 60° of flexion, avoid OKC resisted exercises in more flexion until the PCL is adequately heeled to withstand those stresses, and keep CKC exercises in a similar range as the OKC extension exercises, 0° to 60° (Wilk et al., 1996).

PCL-deficient knees do not generally feel unstable unless the person is walking down an incline, because the PCL protects the tibia from posterior displacement on the femur (or anterior femoral displacement on the tibia). Most patients without instability are able to return to full participation following an appropriate rehabilitation program without surgical reconstruction.

The initial goals of rehabilitation are to resolve pain and edema and restore range of motion. Once signs of inflammation are managed, important goals are restoration of strength, control, and normal function. Modalities for modulation of pain and edema along with electrical stimulation for muscular facilitation are used in phase I. Range-of-motion exercises include active knee extension and passive flexion. Active and resistive hamstring exercises should be avoided because they produce posterior translation of the tibia on the femur. Strong gastrocnemius contractions should also be avoided beyond 30° of knee flexion because of the translational stress applied to the joint and stress added to the PCL (Durselen, Claes, & Kiefer, 1995).

Open kinetic chain exercises within an appropriate range of motion can provide good isolated strengthening for the quadriceps as long as patellofemoral pain is avoided. If patellofemoral pain occurs, the exercises are modified to avoid pain. Modifications can include changing the degrees of motion and angles of the exercise, reducing the resistance, reducing the lever arm of the applied resistance, and using low weights with higher repetitions. These exercises during phase II include quad sets, straight-leg raises, and quad range-of-motion exercises. Crutches are used for weight bearing to tolerance with gradual progression to weight bearing without assistive devices at six to eight weeks. A closed kinetic chain exercise in terminal extension with a resistance band can be used to strengthen the hamstrings and produce minimal posterior tibial translation. This exercise would be the reverse of the one seen in figure 23.33 and would involve having the patient facing the opposite direction and flexing the knee against a band's resistance. The hamstrings can also be strengthened in an open kinetic chain exercise for hip extension if the patient keeps the knee extended to reduce the posterior tibial shear stress.

Once the patient progresses to full weight bearing, other closed kinetic chain exercises begin in phase III. Gait training may be necessary if the patient is unable to assume a normal gait. Weight transfer activities may be indicated if the patient is reluctant to bear weight on the extremity. Proprioception exercises should emphasize recruiting the quadriceps for posterior translation control, first in static positions and advancing through dynamic activities. By the third week, exercises such as wall squats progressing to standing squats, step-ups, and other CKC exercises are added to the program.

By about the sixth to eighth week, the patient should have full knee extension without an extensor lag and knee flexion to at least 100°. Once normal gait is achieved, the patient is able to walk without assistive devices after the eighth week. At this time, the program can progress to jogging and running in the pool, the leg press, and increased weights with land exercises. Anchoring a weight behind a rolling stool and have the patient sit on the stool, using only the involved extremity to propel the stool is a good closed chain hamstring exercise.

By the end of the third month, the patient should have full knee motion. Treadmill walking begins at this time. A more advanced closed kinetic chain hamstring exercise that is performed with the patient kneeling on the table and the clinician anchoring the feet off the table may begin if the patient has sufficient hamstring strength; as the clinician secures the legs, the patient leans the trunk forward as far as possible and then returns to the upright kneeling position. The patient may have sufficient strength for this exercise by the fourth or fifth month. The stepper using small steps or the elliptical trainer is started at this time.

By the 6th month, the patient enters phase IV, jogging on a treadmill with progression to running and then moving into agility exercises, plyometrics (stressing deceleration activities, pivoting, lateral movements, and jumping), and activity-specific exercises is the next progression. Knee control for posterior tibial translation should be emphasized throughout the program.

PCL injuries that are surgically reconstructed are immobilized with a brace that is locked in 0° extension for one week and is worn for a total of six to eight weeks. The brace is removed after the first week for passive exercises only. The patient is able to ambulate with PWB on the extremity for the first three to four weeks with a progressive increase in weight bearing to full weight bearing by the end of the 3rd to 6th week. In the early phase, the knee is supported when the patient is in long sitting to prevent posterior sag of the tibia on the femur. During the first week, quad sets, straight-leg raises, ankle pumps, and short-arc quad (SAQ) exercises are started. Patellar mobilization is performed. Hip extension and knee flexion activities are avoided during the first three weeks, but hip adduction and abduction exercises can be used with resistance applied proximally on the leg. Once the patient is full weight bearing, weight transfer activities, wall squats, weight bearing proprioception and balance activities, and a stationary bike can be initiated and progressed as the patient tolerates it. Open chain exercises for the hamstrings should be avoided during the first 3 to 6 months, depending upon the physician's preference.

Although the rate is slower, the progression for a surgically reconstructed PCL is the same as for an ACL program, with advancement to agility, plyometrics, functional, and activity-specific exercises around the fifth or sixth month. The patient is able to return to full sport participation in an average of nine months, with an average range of 7 to 12 months (Harner, Fu, Irrgang, & Vogrin, 2001).

■ Case Study

Last week an 18-year-old female volleyball player injured the left posterior cruciate when landing hyperflexed after hitting a ball. The physician will not perform surgery because the knee is stable. He wants you to begin the rehabilitation process with the patient today.

Your examination reveals moderate edema around the knee. The patient has a brace and is able to bear partial weight on the left extremity. Her range of motion out of the brace is 30° to 60°. Her patellar mobility is limited by about 75%, but her knee is too flexed for you to decide whether the restriction is attributable to the knee position or to reduced patellar mobility. She has pain at 6/10. Although there is edema around the knee with some discoloration, the soft tissue feels tight from the edema pressure. Her strength is 4–/5 in hip flexors and abductors and 3+/5 in hip extensors, adductors, and quads. You have deferred hamstring testing because of the PCL injury.

Questions for Analysis

1. What will your first treatment with the patient today include?

2. What instructions will you give her to do at home?

3. What exercises will you include in today's session?

4. Outline your expected timeline for beginning hamstring exercises, walking on a treadmill, and stationary cycling. Will you use pool exercises with the patient? If you will use the pool, list three exercises.

5. List four agility exercises and functional skill activities you will include in the last phases of her therapeutic exercise program.

6. List the functional tests you will use to determine when the patient is ready to return to full sport participation.

Collateral Ligament Sprains

The medial collateral ligament (MCL) can be injured by itself or in combination with other knee structures. Collateral ligament injury treatment is different from cruciate ligament treatment.

Medial collateral ligaments are more frequently injured than lateral collateral ligaments (LCLs). An MCL injury occurs as the result of a valgus stress, and an LCL injury results from a varus stress to the knee. Medial collateral ligament injuries are rarely surgically repaired except when instability results from a combination of ACL and MCL tears. In those situations, the MCL may or may not be repaired even if the ACL is repaired.

The rehabilitation programs are similar for MCL and LCL injuries. Initial treatment includes modalities for pain and swelling modulation. The current philosophy in treating isolated collateral ligament injuries is to use a brace in conjunction with an early therapeutic exercise program (Reider, 1996). The patient's injured knee is placed in a functional or rehabilitative brace with limits set at 0° extension and 90° flexion to control ligament stress yet still allow motion. The brace is worn for three to six weeks, and crutches, with either non-weight bearing or weight bearing to tolerance, are used for two to four weeks. During this time, active range-of-motion exercises, isometric exercises to retard quad and hamstring atrophy, and hip and ankle exercises are used. Patellar mobilization may be necessary if the joint becomes stiff. Cross-friction massage to soft tissues can be helpful in promoting healing and preventing adhesions. In 7 to 10 days, pool exercises are useful for range of motion and strength. After about two weeks, the stationary bike can be used if the knee has about 105° of flexion. Before that time, the patient can use the bike as a means of increasing range of motion.

A combination of open and closed kinetic chain exercises is used to increase hamstring and quadriceps strength. These exercises follow the progression outlined for cruciate ligament injuries and must not produce patellofemoral pain or increase collateral ligament pain. Once the patient is ambulating in full weight bearing, stork standing and other balance activities

---

■ Case Study

A 17-year-old male gymnast suffered a grade II sprain of his right MCL during a rings dismount three days ago. The physician wants him started on a rehabilitation program. For the past three days he has received ice, elevation, compression, and electrical stimulation for edema control. He is on crutches with a hinged brace set at 0° and 90°. He is bearing about 75% of his body weight on the right extremity when he ambulates. There is moderate swelling with tenderness to palpation along the MCL. His hip and hamstring strength is grossly 4/5. He has an extensor lag of 15°. He reports mild pain unless he attempts to bend the knee past 60°; then the pain level becomes moderate. Patellar mobility is normal.

Questions for Analysis

1. List in order of significance, his problems and your long-term goals for each problem.
2. What will your first treatment for this patient today include? What home program will you give him before he leaves your facility today?
3. Outline the exercise program you will have the patient perform for the next week. How will you determine his progression?
4. List three open kinetic chain and three closed kinetic chain exercises you will have him perform within the next two weeks, and list them in the order that you will assign them.
5. What agility exercises will you include in his program?
6. What plyometric exercises will you use?
7. Describe the functional activities you will use in your assessment to determine when the patient is ready to return to full sport participation.

can begin. Walking on the treadmill with progression to jogging occurs once a normal walking gait has been achieved. Jogging then progresses to running and sprinting as long as pain and edema are avoided.

If full motion is not achieved by around week 5 or 6, joint mobilization techniques and prolonged stretches may be required. The patient progresses in strength and agility exercises as long as there are no deleterious signs. The program advances from agility and plyometrics to functional activities. A functional knee brace is often used before and after return to sport. The collateral ligament brace does not require the rotational stability that an ACL brace does, but it should have medial and lateral upright supports to control valgus and varus stress.

An individual's tolerance and the severity of the injury will determine the patient's rate of progression. Return to normal function can occur in as few as three to four weeks or can take as long as two to three months.

Meniscus Injuries

Among all the rehabilitation programs for knee injuries, the rehabilitation program for meniscal injuries has seen the greatest changes over the past several years. Current trends in treatment allow for a more rapid return to participation than in the past, with reduced deleterious effects.

Surgical treatment of meniscal injuries has evolved over the past several years. Arthrotomies for complete removal of damaged meniscus have been replaced by partial removal of torn segments, repair, and allograft replacements (figure 23.49), all of which are performed through arthroscopes.

Isolated injury to the medial meniscus does not result in instability to the knee, but if a meniscal tear is combined with an ACL rupture, the knee becomes unstable. Isolated meniscal tears tend to be degenerative tears, whereas meniscal tears that accompany ACL injuries are more likely to be acute (Shelbourne, Patel, Adsit, & Porter, 1996). A stable knee with a meniscal injury may not be a candidate for a meniscal repair, but an unstable knee will become more unstable if the meniscus is removed or partially removed. Knees that undergo a meniscal repair with an ACL repair do better than with an isolated meniscal repair (Tenuta & Arciero, 1994).

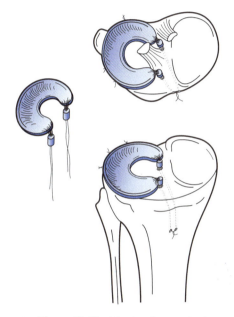

▶ **Figure 23.49** Meniscal transplant.

Meniscal repairs must have a viable blood supply to be successful. The peripheral rim of the menisci has a blood supply, but the majority of its inner substance is avascular. Meniscal blood supply can reach inward as far as 6 mm (about 0.25 in). Tears that occur over the outer third of the meniscus have the best healing capabilities. Tears that extend inward farther than the blood supply do not do well with meniscal repair procedures. Surgeon's preferences regarding the width of the meniscal tears that do well with repairs are variable, and range from 2 mm to 6 mm (Scott, Jolly, & Henning, 1986; Stone, Frewin, & Gonzales, 1990). Up to 20% of all meniscal tears are reparable. Meniscal repair is advantageous over meniscectomy because the meniscus remains, and there is consistent evidence that even partial meniscectomy leads to osteoarthritic changes in the joint (Heckmann, Barber-Westin, & Noyes, 2006). The rehabilitation process, however, is significantly longer for a meniscal repair or replacement than for a meniscectomy. Whereas a rehabilitation program for a meniscectomy generally requires four to six weeks, a patient is often restricted from sport participation after a meniscal repair for four to six months.

The patient who has a medial meniscus and ACL injury that both require surgical repair is a difficult case for the surgeon and rehabilitation clinician. Meniscal repairs do better if performed as soon after the injury as possible. Following the meniscal repair, the postoperative care is conservative, with non-weight bearing and limited motion for up to six to eight weeks. On the other hand, the ACL repair is most successful when delayed until after the inflammation is resolved and with immediate postoperative partial to full weight bearing and motion.

Traditionally, the postoperative care for meniscal repairs has been conservative, but accelerated programs have been used more recently with equal success (Barber & Click, 1997).

There is, however, much controversy about use of an accelerated program for meniscal repairs (Barber & Click, 1997). The conservative protocol guards the repair by using limited motion and weight bearing to reduce the shearing and compressive forces applied to the repair. The accelerated program limits the time on crutches and uses partial weight bearing and active motion in the early stage to apply appropriate stresses to healing tissue and prevent unwanted loss of motion and patellofemoral pain problems. The rehabilitation clinician must communicate with the physician to create a feasible rehabilitation program for the patient who has received a meniscal repair. Because of vascular supply, repaired peripheral tears will repair more quickly than complex tears that include the central portions of the meniscus. Factors that may determine whether an accelerated or conservative program is followed include not only the location of the repair but also the type and size of the repair (Heckmann et al., 2006). Conservative rehabilitation follows transplants and complex tear repairs while more aggressive rehabilitation may be possible for peripheral tear repairs.

Rehabilitation using either program involves protecting the repair or transplant from shear and excessive compression initially. Patients must be cautioned that deep squats and pivoting will risk the surgical site's integrity. Activities in a rehabilitation program should not produce increased pain or swelling at any point in the program.

Conservative Postoperative Meniscal Repair Program

A conservative postoperative meniscal repair program includes placing the patient on crutches with the knee in a brace, non-weight bearing on the involved extremity for up to six to eight weeks. Toe-touch weight bearing is sometimes allowed after two weeks, with slowly progressive increases in weight bearing to full weight bearing at six to eight weeks. A rehabilitative brace is used to keep the knee in an extended position at night for the first three weeks but allows 0° to 90° range of motion during the day for six to eight weeks after surgery. During this time, the patient performs trunk, hip and ankle exercises. Stretching exercises for the hamstrings, gastrocnemius, soleus, and hips occur during this protective phase. Manual resistance to the hip should be applied above the knee to prevent stress on the knee joint. Quad sets, straight-leg raises, and active knee extension without pain are started within the first two weeks. Once the patient demonstrates full active knee extension, the brace is unlocked for night wear. Full extension motion and active motion to 90° are the primary concerns during the first three weeks following surgery. If motion is difficult, it may be necessary to perform patellar mobilizations in all four directions.

After six to eight weeks when the brace is removed, stretching of the quadriceps along with tibiofemoral joint mobilizations can be used to gain knee flexion. Crutches are discarded when the patient is able to walk normally and has adequate quadriceps strength to control the knee. Balance and proprioception activities in weight bearing begin once the patient is full weight bearing. Strengthening the quadriceps and lower extremity with leg press, mini-squats, wall squats, and open kinetic chain knee flexion and extension exercises occurs at six to eight weeks. Initial ranges of motion are limited in open chain knee flexion to 90° and in knee extension to 30°, and in the leg press to 10° of extension. Pivoting and acceleration-deceleration activities are not allowed for four to six months after surgery. From then on, the patient progresses to functional and activity-specific exercises before returning to sport or normal activities.

Accelerated Postoperative Meniscal Repair Program

As mentioned, accelerated rehabilitation programs are usually possible following repairs of peripheral meniscal lesions. In an accelerated program, weight bearing is allowed as the patient tolerates it, but the patient uses crutches until he or she is able to walk normally. Range-of-motion exercises are used during the first postoperative week. Quad sets and straight-leg raises also begin during the first week. The goal during the first few weeks is to achieve full range of motion without increased edema in the knee. By the end of week 2 or 3, the patient who has good control of knee extension is able to ambulate normally without crutches.

In week 2 to 4, the patient can use pool exercises, closed kinetic chain exercises including a stationary bike, mini-squats, and a walking treadmill program. By week 6 to 9, isokinetic exercises are suitable. Jogging, progressing to running, is added before lateral and pivoting movements are allowed. By that time, the patient has at least 80% quad strength. The patient progresses to phase IV of rehabilitation where cutting, cariocas, and agility activities begin at month 4 to 5. These activities progress to activity-specific exercises, then to full return to normal function by month 5 to 6.

Patellofemoral Injuries

Patellofemoral injuries can be complex injuries and frustratingly slow to respond to treatment. Several factors may contribute to patellofemoral injuries, especially those that are non-traumatic. This section deals with the most frequently seen injuries.

Patellar Dislocations and Subluxation

Patellar instability is more frequently seen in women than in men. This is thought to be the result of an increased Q-angle secondary to a wider pelvis, which increases the lateral vector force on the patella. Other predisposing factors include a shallow lateral femoral condyle or posterior patella, an improper position of the patella, and a weak VMO, especially if it is combined with tight or strong lateral structures.

The mechanism for injury is lateral rotation of the thigh with knee flexion on a planted foot. If the patella is subluxed, it often relocates independently. A frank dislocation may or may not relocate on its own. First-time dislocations may not relocate, but recurrent ones often do without assistance. Pain and edema are severe.

Treatment includes use of crutches with weight bearing to tolerance. An immobilizer brace may be initially used with progression to a functional brace to stabilize the patella. Therapeutic exercise progresses to the patient's tolerance. Electrical stimulation to the quadriceps and modalities for pain and edema control are applied in phase I of a rehabilitation program,

■ Case Study

A 20-year-old male ice hockey forward experienced a left knee meniscal tear. He underwent an arthroscopic repair of the meniscus yesterday and comes to you today to begin his rehabilitation program. He is walking PWB with crutches. He reports mild pain and a sensation of tightness around the knee. Your examination reveals swelling of 2.5 cm (1 in.) around the knee's joint margin. The patient's active range of motion is –15° extension and 90° flexion. Passive range of motion is 0° extension and 100° flexion. He is able to perform a straight-leg raise but cannot tolerate resistance in the motion. Other hip motions are 4/5. Hamstring strength is 4–/5. The patella is slightly restricted in mobility.

Questions for Analysis

1. What will your first treatment with the patient include today?

2. What will you give him as home exercises and instructions before he leaves today?

3. What are your goals with him for the first week of treatment?

4. Preseason hockey practice begins in two months. What will you tell the patient when he asks you whether he will be ready by then?

5. When do you expect him to be able to begin full weight bearing? When do you expect him to begin squats with weights?

6. What will you say when the patient asks you why he cannot straighten the knee when he could before the surgery?

7. Present a progression of proprioceptive exercises that you will have in this program. Discuss the progression of agility exercises you will use. List the functional activities you will include in the final phase of the patient's program.

usually in the first two weeks. Increases in pain and edema are avoided throughout the entire program. Patellofemoral pain can be produced at any time, but especially in the early phases of rehabilitation when the tissues are still inflamed from the initial insult. All exercises should be pain free. If an exercise produces pain, it is delayed until the patient is able to perform it without pain.

It is important to work on hip stability exercises during phase I. These exercises include strengthening hip extensors and abductors especially. Additionally, core muscle strengthening should be included in any program for the patellofemoral joint, whether it is to manage a dislocation or patellofemoral stress syndrome. Both the hip and core muscles play important roles in patellofemoral joint stability. See chapters 24 and 18 for hip and core exercises, respectively.

Initial exercises in phase II include straight leg raises and pain free short-arc exercises with progression into a greater arc of motion as strength gains and pain permit. Rehabilitation exercises are a combination of open and closed kinetic chain activities. Program emphasis should be on quadriceps strength and patellar control during activities. As strength and knee control improve, exercises progress to more rapid activities until functional speeds are possible with good patellar control.

Lower-extremity alignment is examined in standing and walking, because pronation which occurs during ambulation can increase the risk of patellar instability and may require correction with orthotics.

The duration of a rehabilitation program depends on whether the dislocation or subluxation is a first-time event or a recurring injury. Recovery from an acute subluxation/dislocation can take more time than from a recurring injury. An average expected recovery period is 4 to 12 weeks; recurrent injuries are on the shorter side and first-time injuries require the longer recovery time.

Patellofemoral Pain Syndrome

Syndromes of the patellofemoral joint can be caused by many different factors, individually or in combination. The term for this frustrating injury, "syndrome," demonstrates that the medical community has been unable to identify one specific etiology.

Mechanism   Patellofemoral pain is a common complaint among athletes as well as among those who do not participate in athletics. Anterior knee pain has been classified under various headings including chondromalacia patellae, patellofemoral stress syndrome, patellofemoral pain syndrome, extensor mechanism malalignment syndrome, runner's knee, and patellofemoral malalignment syndrome. Chondromalacia is a term that was used in the past to describe anterior knee pain. Chondromalacia refers to a specific injury that involves softening and degeneration of the patella's posterior articular cartilage and it is not an accurate diagnosis for most anterior knee pain conditions. The most commonly used terms today to describe anterior knee pain include patellofemoral pain syndrome (PFPS) or patellofemoral stress syndrome (PFSS).

Signs and Symptoms   Typical signs and symptoms of PFPS include stiffness after prolonged sitting, pain with activities such as stair climbing and running, and pain after activity. Crepitus is usually present. The patient may experience a giving way of the knee because of reflex inhibition secondary to pain, especially on stairs or ramps. Swelling is usually mild, but the posterior surface of the patella is tender to palpation.

Underlying Factors   PFPS is anterior knee pain and irritation caused by abnormal stresses applied to the knee's extensor mechanism. Several underlying conditions can lead to PFPS. Patellofemoral pain syndrome can result from direct trauma to the patella, but is more often the result of cumulative stresses in the presence of additional contributing factors, both extrinsic and intrinsic to the joint itself. These factors are thought to include tightness in the ITB, hamstrings, and gastrocnemius; weakness in the VMO or imbalance of strength between the

VMO and vastus lateralis; excessive pronation; increased Q-angle; knee hyperextension; and patellar alignment (Tumia & Maffulli, 2002). More recently, it has been demonstrated that individuals with PFPS have weak hip muscles compared to persons without the condition (Bolgla, Malone, Umberger, & Uhl, 2008; Dierks, Manal, Hamill, & Davis, 2008). It is likely that a patient has more than one of these factors to develop PFPS. Each element should be evaluated when examining the patient with PFPS, because correction of or compensation for these malalignments must occur if the PFPS is to be resolved.

Normal function of all body segments relies on a balance of the surrounding structures. This balance includes adequate flexibility and proper strength so that forces are adequately and appropriately directed to produce the desired motion and force applications. If hamstring, gastrocnemius, ITB, or lateral connective tissue structures are tight, they apply an imbalance of forces on the knee. Tight hamstrings prevent full extension so the knee is in flexion during activities when it should be extended, increasing compressive forces on the patella anteriorly. If knee flexion is less than 60°, the need for increased knee flexion during ambulation is compensated by increased dorsiflexion to clear the toe. Normally 10° of dorsiflexion is necessary for ambulation, but if the gastrocnemius does not permit this motion or if the hamstrings increase the need for additional dorsiflexion but it is not available, the foot pronates in an attempt to increase flexibility. Excessive pronation necessitates tibial medial rotation, which increases the knee's valgus stress. A tight ITB pulls the patella laterally as the ITB moves posteriorly during knee flexion. In cases of severe distal tightness of the ITB, the patella is in a lateral tilt position because of the ITB's lateral pull on it.

If the hip muscles, especially the hip extensors and hip abductors, are not strong, there is no hip stability from which the knee is able to function. A weak base at the hip for the knee creates an unstable situation for knee function. An unstable condition at the knee makes it difficult to maintain the patella in proper alignment during lower extremity activities. This ultimately adds stress to the patellofemoral joint.

If either the VMO is weak or an imbalance is present between the VMO and the vastus lateralis, the patella moves laterally during quadriceps contractions. This permits the patella's lateral rim to ride more on the lateral femoral condyle than in the intercondylar groove, where it normally glides during knee motion. If the vastus lateralis is tight, the lateral pull during quadriceps contractions is exaggerated. Repetitive gliding against the condyle leads to inflammation of the patella's articular surface.

If the knee is in hyperextension, the inferior pole of the patella is frequently tilted inward. This causes the patella to push into the fat pad in full extension, and to glide with an inferior tilt during knee motion, altering the relationship between the patella and femoral groove. The patella has increased contact inferiorly as it glides in the groove, increasing stresses at the inferior pole.

Any one of these factors by themselves will create patellofemoral pain. When more than one of these factors is present, the problem becomes compounded and more difficult to resolve.

Patellar Orientation Patellar orientation and alignment are examined in a relaxed long sitting or supine position, and in closed chain positions in both static and dynamic conditions. Patellar alignment varies from one patient to another; it can also be different from left to right knee in the same individual. In a relaxed open chain position with the knee resting in slight flexion on a rolled towel and the femur in parallel alignment with the examination tabletop, the rehabilitation clinician assesses the patellar alignment in various planes. He or she examines for the presence of a lateral glide, lateral tilt, inferior tilt, and rotation. In the examination position, the patella should rest slightly lateral to the center of the knee with the inferior pole at the knee's joint margin. If the patella's position is more than a few millimeters to the lateral aspect, it has a lateral glide. A medial glide is rare. When a finger is placed on top of the medial and lateral poles of the patella, they should be in the same plane; if the lateral finger is lower than the medial finger, the patella has a lateral tilt. A medial tilt is rare. When a finger is placed on top of the mid-superior patella surface and another is placed on top of the inferior patellar pole, they should be in the same plane; if the distal finger sits deeper than the proximal finger, the patella has an inferior tilt, or posterior tilt. This tilt is also referred to as an AP tilt. Looking from directly above the patella, the superior medial and lateral poles should be in the same plane; if the lateral pole lies more superiorly on the knee and the medial pole lies more inferiorly, the patella is laterally rotated. If the medial pole lies more superiorly, the patella is medially rotated. A lateral rotation is more common than a medial rotation. These patellar positions are demonstrated in figure 23.50.

The patella's tracking pattern is examined in non-weight bearing. With the patient contracting the quadriceps in full knee extension, the clinician observes the patella for its movement. Normal patella movement occurs in a J-figure with primarily superior motion that ends some lateral motion. If lateral structures are tight or the VMO is weak, the patella will move upward in a lateral path from the start of patellar movement. During knee movement into flexion, the patella migrates medially as the Q-angle decreases and the patella becomes centered in the trochlea.

Alignment is also observed in standing, and movement of the patella is observed while the patient performs an activity such as a lunge or step-down. Changes in patellar alignment and glide during weight bearing can indicate various influential factors that should be corrected, such as pronation, weakness, incorrect firing patterns, and tightness.

Corrections Common surgical procedures to treat patellofemoral pain and patellofemoral malalignment in the past included a lateral release in which the lateral retinaculum is cut, or an advancement of the tibial tubercle medialward to allow a better patella alignment. It has been demonstrated, however, that many PFPS patients have better results with non-surgical management that consists primarily of exercise (Karlsson, Thomee, & Sward, 1996).

Determination of the underlying causes dictates what is included in the treatment program. Orthotics may be needed if pronation is present (Fulkerson, 2002); flexibility exercises and soft-tissue mobilization techniques are necessary if tightness and adhesions exist (Post, 2005); strength and control of hip muscles will reduce patellofemoral stresses (Powers, 2003); and muscle reeducation and strengthening exercises, especially for the VMO, are needed with all

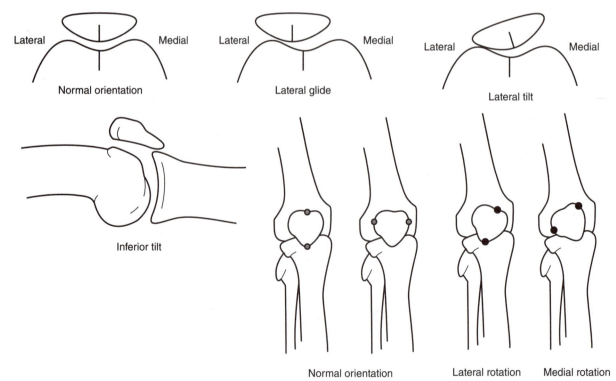

▶ **Figure 23.50** Patellar orientation.

patellofemoral pain regardless of cause (Tumia & Maffulli, 2002), because pain causes an inhibition reflex and weakens the quadriceps (Morrissey, 1989).

Patellar Taping Technique A technique developed by Jenny McConnell, an Australian physiotherapist, uses a combination of taping to the patella and exercises. Her initial theory stated that the tape corrected patellar alignment to relieve pain and allow the patient to exercise to regain strength (McConnell, 1986). More recent studies, however have shown conflicting results on the efficacy of patellar taping. Some have demonstrated that no change in patellar position occurs (Keet, Gray, Harley, & Lambert, 2007; Kowall, Kolk, Nuber, Cassisi, & Stern, 1996; Lesher et al., 2006; Wilson, Carter, & Thomas, 2003). Contrarily, others have demonstrated that a reduction in pain or minimal short-term changes in alignment do occur with the tape (Ernst, Kawaguchi, & Saliba, 1999; Somes, Worrell, Corey, & Ingersoll, 1997); these studies, however, consistently point out that the effects of taping on patellar position were limited. Patellar position changed only at 10° of knee flexion (Worrell, Ingersoll, Bockrath-Pugliese, & Minis, 1998), and no change occurred in the open chain position (Somes et al., 1997). Changes that did occur lasted less than 15 minutes after activity began. Empirical evidence persists to support the theory that McConnell taping reduces pain in spite of the now accepted fact that the tape does not change functional patellar alignment. It has been speculated that the tape may provide neural inhibition through neurosensory afferent stimulation of the large A-beta fibers (Bockrath, Wooden, Worrell, Ingersoll, & Farr, 1993).

Research has shown that patellar taping facilitates a quicker response of the VMO during step-up activities and delays the onset of vastus lateralis response while increasing the onset of VMO response during a step-down exercise (Gilleard, McConnell, & Parsons, 1998). It has yet to be determined whether this change in muscle response results from improved muscle response secondary to pain reduction or neurosensory facilitation.

Patellar Tape Application Although it has been demonstrated that patellar taping does not change the position of the patella, tape applications advocated by McConnell are presented here. The reason these techniques are presented is that the tape has been shown to consistently reduce pain in spite of the reason for this remaining elusive. When more than one malalignment is present and one of them is a posterior tilt, the posterior tilt is corrected first; otherwise, the greatest malalignment is corrected first. The tapes used for patellar taping are Cover-Roll, used as a hypoallergenic cloth undertape to protect the skin, and Leukotape, used to guide patellar alignment. The tape should reduce the patient's pain symptoms immediately. To evaluate its effectiveness, the patient performs an activity that reproduces the pain such as a step-down, and the pain level is assessed. After the tape is applied, the patient repeats the activity to reassess the pain level. Although the pain may or may not completely resolve, it will be significantly reduced with the tape application in 50% of the cases (Bockrath et al., 1993). If no change in pain is perceived, the correction tape should be reapplied in a different sequence. The tape can be worn for extended periods of time to effect a low-load, long-term stretch on soft tissues. It is worn 23 h a day with an hour off, usually after a shower, to relieve skin stress. With a reduction in pain, an increase in quadriceps strengthening can occur. The tape can get wet without any effect on its adhesion, but over time, it loses its effectiveness. The top tape strip may be readjusted if it loosens. If taping proves effective, the patient is instructed in tape application, removal, and skin care so that he or she can reapply the tape daily until symptoms subside. As quadriceps strength improves and pain decreases, the patient is weaned from the tape.

The cloth undertape is applied smoothly but without tension to the skin over the patella, medial knee area, and into the popliteal region. The correction tape is applied with force over the undertape to correct patellar position. The tape is applied with the knee in extension and a rolled towel under the knee for comfort and to prevent the knee from being locked. If pain occurs during the middle range of a squat, the tape may be applied with the knee positioned in the painful range of flexion. The quadriceps must remain relaxed during any McConnell tape application.

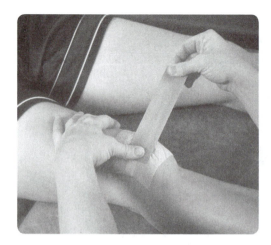

▶ **Figure 23.51** Lateral glide correction.

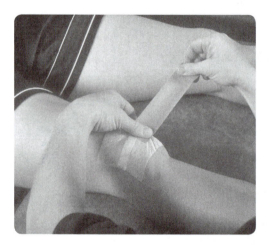

▶ **Figure 23.52** Lateral tilt correction.

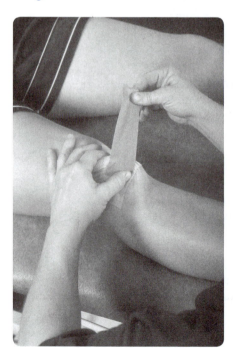

▶ **Figure 23.53** Lateral rotation correction.

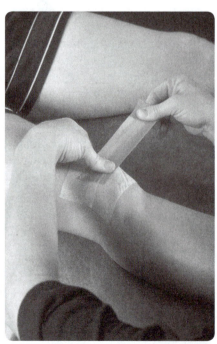

▶ **Figure 23.54** Inferior tilt correction.

For a lateral glide, the correction tape is applied from lateral to the lateral border of the patella with a medial pull on the tape over the medial femoral condyle (figure 23.51). The soft tissue over the medial femoral condyle is lifted toward the patella manually to create a fold in the skin on the medial side and ultimately provide a better pull of the tape. A couple of strips of correction tape may be necessary. Each strip should create a subsequently larger soft-tissue crease.

For a lateral tilt, a strip of tape is firmly anchored at the middle of the patella and pulled firmly toward the medial femoral condyle so that the lateral patellar border is lifted to move the patella level with the anterior femoral plane (figure 23.52). The soft tissue is lifted on the medial aspect to provide a better result.

For a lateral rotation alignment, the tape is anchored on the inferior patellar pole. The patella is manually rotated into correct alignment while the tape is pulled upward and medially (figure 23.53).

If present, a posterior or inferior tilt is taped first to reduce infrapatellar fat-pad irritation with other tape applications. A posterior tilt is usually taped in combination with a lateral tilt or lateral glide. The tape is applied over the superior half of the patella to lift the inferior pole up and away from the fat pad (figure 23.54).

Skin irritation may occur with the use of tape. To minimize this risk, the tape is removed carefully; an adhesive remover should be used after the tape has been taken off, and the skin should be carefully cleansed and conditioned with a moisturizer when the tape is not in use. If a small area of skin breakdown occurs, the area is covered with a protective dressing or, if possible, the tape should not be applied to that the area. If the skin breakdown area is too large, the tape is discontinued until the skin heals. If an allergic reaction occurs, the tape cannot be used.

Soft-Tissue Mobility Soft-tissue adhesions and tightness along the distal ITB and into the lateral retinaculum often play a role in patellar malalignment. These structures should be treated with deep-tissue massage and stretching. Deep-tissue massage can be applied by the rehabilitation clinician with the dorsal side of a flat fist (flexed MPs and PIPs, extended DIPs), with pressure delivered over the posterior middle and distal phalanges, as was discussed earlier in this chapter in the section "Deep-Tissue Massage." The patient can also use a foam roller to perform self-massage techniques (figure 23.10). The patient can perform manual massage techniques over the distal lateral thigh throughout the day while sitting (figure 23.55).

The patient is instructed to perform stretching exercises for all tight muscle groups and should perform them throughout the day. The muscle groups commonly included are the hamstrings, gastrocnemius, and tensor fascia lata.

Additional Therapeutic Exercises Therapeutic exercise is a vital part of the total rehabilitation program for patellofemoral pain. Stretching and strengthening exercises can alter patellar tracking to establish a more correct alignment (Doucette & Child, 1996; Doucette & Goble, 1992; Mascal, Landel, & Powers, 2003; Powers, 2003). Because muscle imbalance can play a role in PFPS, it is logical to assume that improvement in muscle balances can impact improvement in this condition.

As for all extremity programs, exercises for core, pelvic, and hip stabilization should be included in the therapeutic exercise program (Dierks et al., 2008; Ireland, Willson, Ballantyne, & Davis, 2003; Powers, 2003; Robinson & Nee, 2007). Deficits in strength of these areas are seen in patients with PFPS (Bolgla et al., 2008; Mascal et al., 2003). The results of these studies seem

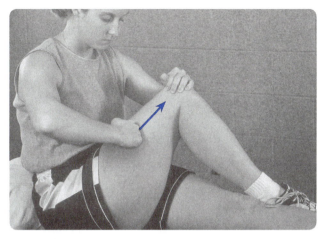

▶ **Figure 23.55** Iliotibial band massage.

to indicate that hip muscles and abdominals, especially lower abdominals, play a key role in providing adequate knee control during closed chain activities. Trunk and core exercises were presented in chapter 18 and include strengthening exercises for the abdominal obliques, lower abdominals, and spine extensors. In addition, lateral and posterior hip muscles should be strengthened to provide hip stability during knee activities. Many of these exercises are seen in chapter 24.

Lower-limb alignment and mechanics have a direct impact on the patellofemoral joint (Powers, 2003). Muscles in distal and proximal segments must be corrected for imbalances along with the knee muscles if patellofemoral pain is to be resolved. Muscles controlling foot pronation, including the posterior tibialis, anterior tibialis, and peroneals, should be strengthened and reeducated for pronation control and foot stability during closed chain activities.

Quadriceps strength is primary to a successful rehabilitation program (Mohr, Kvitne, Pink, Fideler, & Perry, 2003). Electrical stimulation and biofeedback can be used to facilitate quadriceps activation. These electrical modalities are used in open chain exercises such as straight-leg raise and SAQ and in closed chain exercises for concentric and eccentric activity such as walking, step-downs, and lunges. A combination of open and closed chain activities within a pain-free range of motion is part of a total therapeutic exercise program. Patellofemoral taping might be required, especially in the early phases of therapeutic exercise when patellofemoral pain prevents adequate quadriceps activation.

When the patient is able to perform closed chain activities in a slow and controlled manner and without pain, the speed of the activities increases to challenge muscle recruitment patterns and prepare the patient for agility, functional activities and activity-specific exercises. As the patient gains strength, control, and flexibility, he or she follows a progression of exercises similar to that for other knee injuries, advancing to increased stress and forces, more-challenging coordination and agility activities, functional activities, and finally activity-specific exercises. Return to full participation is possible once the patient is pain free; has normal flexibility, strength, agility, and power; and is able to demonstrate normal performance of activity-specific activities.

Patellar Tendinopathy

Patellar tendinopathy can be related to patellofemoral alignment, so the same factors discussed in PFPS should be assessed for patellar tendinopathy. Patellar tendinopathy is often called jumper's knee because jumping activities are the primary precipitating factor. With the energy absorption that occurs during landing from a jump, jumping on hard surfaces and excessive jump repetitions can overload the tendon beyond its stress-absorbing capabilities. Tissue breakdown then occurs. This stress becomes exaggerated with the presence of muscle imbalances such as weakness or tightness or mechanical malalignments such as foot pronation.

■ Case Study

A 16-year-old female cross-country runner has had left knee pain for the past month. The pain has progressed so that it now interferes with her workouts and occurs even during walking. The physician has diagnosed her with PFPS and wants her to begin rehabilitation. Your examination reveals genu valgus and recurvatum with foot pronation in standing. The patient's running shoes have excessive wear on the lateral posterior heel so that the midsole is showing through the outsole. The shoes have a sewn curved last. The patient's rearfoot and forefoot have excessive mobility. Straight-leg raise is to 70°; ankle dorsiflexion in rearfoot neutral is 0°. She has a positive Ober's test, and deep palpation reveals tenderness along the distal ITB. Her quadriceps strength is 4–/5, lower abdominal strength is 3/5, and hip extension strength is 4/5. Patellar alignment assessment reveals a posterior and lateral tilt. Patellar tracking in long sitting occurs primarily laterally. In standing, lateral patellar tracking is less. When the patient performs a step-down exercise, pain occurs, and the knee wobbles. Palpation of the posterior patellar surface reveals tenderness medially and laterally, especially over the inferior aspect.

Questions for Analysis

1. List in order of priority her problems. Correlate each problem with a long-term goal.
2. What will your treatment for the patient include today? What instructions will you send her home with today?
3. What will you tell her when she asks what she should do about her workouts?
4. Given her signs, what part of the range of motion would you expect the patient to have the most pain in?
5. List two elements you will use to strengthen the VMO during the first week.
6. What are your short-term for the next two weeks for the patient?

Pain occurs in the patellar tendon between the patella and tibial tuberosity. Classic activities cause patellar tendon pain: Pressure over the tendon, quadriceps tightening (especially eccentric activity), and stair climbing (especially going down). There may be slight edema in the tendon.

Initial rehabilitation goals are to reduce the painful symptoms and pain. Modalities such as phonophoresis, iontophoresis, ice, and electrical stimulation may be effective. Cross-friction massage across the tendon can be useful in promoting healing by improving mobility and reducing soft-tissue adhesions. The rehabilitation clinician applies cross-friction to one tender location on the tendon until the pain is reduced or relieved; he or she then moves to another site on the tendon and repeats the procedure until all tender sites are treated.

Therapeutic exercises include a combination of flexibility and strength. Stretching exercises for the hamstrings, quadriceps, lateral thigh, and calf muscles are taught to the patient. Strengthening exercises include primarily eccentric exercises that have been discussed in chapter 15. Eccentric exercises begin slow and through a relatively pain-free range of motion. Some pain may occur with these exercises, but the pain resolves before the next treatment. Additional exercises include open chain exercises to isolate the quadriceps and closed chain exercises for functional stresses. The rate of the program's progression is purely dependent on the patient's response to the exercises. When the patient is able to perform activity-specific exercises without pain or hesitation, return to normal activities is possible.

Tendon Rupture

Tendon ruptures occur most commonly in people 30 to 50 years old as a result of a sudden quadriceps contraction; the cause is probably a gradual degeneration, although prior complaints of tendinopathy are not usual (Sharma & Maffulli, 2005). Tendon ruptures occur more often in males than in females. As with Achilles tendon ruptures, the patient feels as though he has been shot or kicked in the knee. The patient is unable to bear weight on the extremity. The rupture can occur from either the tendon attachment between the patella and tibial tuberosity (patellar tendon rupture) or the tendon between the patella and quadriceps (quadriceps tendon rupture). Complete ruptures are surgically repaired, with the knee kept either locked in extension with a brace or on a CPM for the first few weeks. Straight-leg raises, quad sets, and hip exercises are used during the first 10 days to two weeks. Patellar mobilizations are used to maintain patellar mobility. Weight bearing is restricted initially and then advanced to weight bearing as tolerated in the brace. After about three weeks, exercises begin out of the brace and follow a progression similar to that for other surgical repair programs. The period until return to full activity is four to nine months.

Strains and Contusions

The severity of a strain determines the length of recovery. Ecchymosis indicates at least a grade II strain and necessitates a longer recovery time than a strain that does not produce bleeding. Ecchymosis is often distal to the site of muscle tear, because gravity pulls the blood caudally.

Lack of normal flexibility, fatigue, incoordination, and a sudden violent contraction or stretch of a contracting muscle can all be frequent precipitating factors for muscle strains.

Remember that rehabilitation progression must coincide with tissue healing. Initial treatment goals in phase I include relieving inflammation signs of pain, swelling, and spasm. Pulsed ultrasound is effective in promoting the absorption of ecchymosis. Electrical stimulation is useful in relieving pain and spasm. Stretches with activation of the antagonists assist in relieving muscle spasm and regaining range of motion begin in phase II.

If the patient is unable to ambulate normally, assistive devices are used with weight-bearing to tolerance. Strength exercises are incorporated into the program during late phase II or early phase III as the patient tolerates them. Active range of motion against gravity may be all that is tolerated initially, but progression to resisted open- and closed-chain exercises occurs within a few days. A variety of activities including proprioceptive neuromuscular facilitation, manual resistance, aquatic exercises and gait training, stationary-bike exercise, co-contraction exercises, and unilateral weight bearing can begin within one to three days once spasm and pain have subsided.

The program advances as tolerated to eccentric and isokinetic exercises. Eccentric exercises are important for muscle strains, because athletic activity places high eccentric demands on lower-extremity muscle groups (Stanton & Purdham, 1989). Agility activities requiring more rapid muscle responses are introduced into the program late in phase III as the patient gains strength, coordination, and balance control. After the patient moves into phase IV and is able to perform functional and activity-specific exercises, he or she is ready to be tested functionally for return to full work or sport participation.

Hamstrings

Hamstring strains most commonly occur at the musculotendinous junction, either near the ischial tuberosity or more toward the mid-lateral aspect of the muscle where the biceps femoris tendon inserts more distally. Hamstring strains often occur during high-speed activities such as sprinting or during sudden changes in muscle activity.

Stretching exercises begin within two to four days after an injury. Hamstring tightness is often a predisposing factor in strains. After an injury, additional flexibility loss occurs. Appropriately timed deep massage and cross-friction to the injury site promote healing and reduce scar-tissue adhesions that can further restrict hamstring mobility.

Strength exercises start as isometrics and progress to concentrics, and then eccentrics, before transitioning to isokinetics and faster-speed activities.

Quadriceps

The quadriceps are subject to strains, contusions, and other injuries, some severe and others not. The injuries requiring rehabilitation have unique characteristics that are outlined here, and then a case study is presented.

Strains Jumping or sudden changes in direction are activities that often produce quadriceps strains. The treatment course follows the same routine and phases as for hamstring strains. Stretching activities begin on day 2 to 4 and are accompanied initially with isometric exercises. Aquatic exercises and gait training, proprioceptive neuromuscular facilitation, passive stretching, and stationary-bike exercises are used early in the program. Isometric exercises are replaced with isotonic and open and closed chain activities and advance to eccentric activities as tolerated. Isokinetic, agility, plyometric, and functional and activity-specific exercises progress as previously mentioned for other knee rehabilitation programs.

Contusions Contusions occur more commonly in the quadriceps than strains do. Pain and spasm are the most debilitating symptoms, so initial treatment goals in phase I are to resolve these conditions and maintain flexibility. Electrical stimulation, pulsed ultrasound, and ice help to relieve spasm and pain. Mild active and passive stretches with contraction of the contralateral muscle are recommended after spasm is relaxed, usually on the second or third day postinjury when phase II begins. A stationary bike may be used to improve range of motion. Aquatic exercises can also relax the muscle. Pain reflexively inhibits the muscle, so quadriceps strengthening is necessary and can begin when muscle spasm has been relieved during later phase II. The progression into phases III and IV is the same as outlined for other injuries, with the rate of progression based on the patient's response to specific exercises. Recovery with full return to normal participation usually can occur in two to three weeks for moderate and severe contusions.

Myositis ossificans is a condition that results from either a severe direct blow or repetitive blows to the quadriceps that affects the periosteum of the femur and cause non-neoplastic bone formation in the muscle. A painful, rigid mass can be felt through deep palpation of the anterior thigh in the muscle belly. Loss of range of motion accompanies myositis ossificans.

Surgical treatment is indicated for unresolved conditions but is usually not performed until the growth has stabilized, about one year postinjury. Surgical excision before that time can exacerbate the problem. Conservative treatment involves the treatment course outlined for contusions.

■ Case Study

A 30-year-old male tennis player sprinted to return a ball at the net when he felt a tear in his right hamstring one week ago. He was unable to walk and sought medical attention. The physician has diagnosed a grade II hamstring strain and wants the patient to begin rehabilitation. The patient ambulates with a slight antalgic gait. His knee motion is 15° to 115°. Left straight-leg raise is 60°, but the patient states that he has always been tight in his hamstrings. His hamstring strength is 3/5 and painful with resistance. His quadriceps strength, ankle strength, and hip strength are each 4-/5. A large area of ecchymosis is present posteriorly from the proximal thigh below the gluteal fold to about 10 cm (3.9 in.) distal to the knee. The ecchymotic region is most tender in the darkest area of discoloration along the mid-posterolateral thigh. There is a small indentation with tenderness to palpation about 10 cm distal and 5 cm lateral to the ischial tuberosity.

Questions for Analysis

1. List in order of priority his problems and your long-term goals for him.
2. What will you include in today's treatment for the patient?
3. What home program will you give him before he leaves today?
4. What short-term goals do you expect him to achieve within the next two weeks?
5. Outline the course of exercises for this patient for the next two weeks. What functional activities will you include in his program?
6. What will your criteria be for permitting the patient to return to full sport participation?

Iliotibial Band Syndrome

Iliotibial band syndrome is an overuse syndrome that results from friction between the ITB and the lateral femoral epicondyle. It is seen most often in middle- and long-distance runners. Friction is thought to take place at 30° of knee flexion when the ITB is pulled over the lateral femoral epicondyle and occurs during running when the tensor fascia lata and gluteus maximus, the muscles attaching to the ITB, are active and are pulling on the band during the initial stance phase (Fredericson & Weir, 2006; Orchard, Fricker, Abud, & Mason, 1996). During downhill running, more time is spent in flexion, increasing ITB stress.

Predisposing factors may include leg-length discrepancy, increased Q-angle, genu valgus, and foot pronation. Running hills and increased running distances can also lead to ITB syndrome.

The patient complains of pain along the ITB (especially over the lateral femoral epicondyle), increased pain with walking or running (especially down hills), edema, and crepitus. Snapping over the lateral femoral epicondyle can sometimes be felt.

Treatment must involve correction of predisposing factors, stretching, and strengthening. Modalities to relieve the inflammation and a workout modification are useful in phase I. Running at a faster speed may reduce ITB pain, because during faster running the knee is at more than 30° flexion in the early weight-bearing phase. When pain is relieved, strengthening exercises for deficiencies should proceed in phase III with the inclusion of open and closed kinetic chain exercises, concentric and eccentric closed chain activities, and a progression as previously presented for return to full sport participation.

Osseous Injuries

Fractures of the knee bones can be traumatic or stress related. Femur fractures are not common occurrences, fortunately, but tibial fractures are seen more frequently.

Fractures

Fractures of the knee result from direct blows and impact forces, torsional stresses, or compression loads. A patellar fracture usually occurs as the result of a direct blow, but a tibial fracture occurs most often because of torsional or compression forces. Epiphyseal plate injuries of the proximal tibia or distal femur occur in adolescent patients whose growth plates have not yet matured. Damage to these sites can alter bone growth. Tibial plateau fractures require non-weight bearing for six to eight weeks because of the tibia's major role in weight bearing. Displaced fractures require open reduction and internal fixation (ORIF).

Fractures repaired with ORIF procedures become more stable more quickly and can sometimes undergo a more accelerated therapeutic exercise program.

Chondral fractures and articular cartilage defects occur as a result of trauma to the articular surface, often a direct impact. These lesions occur most often in young adults. The lesions frequently develop into localized joint degeneration. Several treatment options are available for these isolated degenerative changes in the knee. Surgical options involve either resurfacing the chondral defect or arthroscopic debridement of the chondral surface. An abrasion arthroplasty is a debridement technique while subchondral drilling, or creation of microfractures to stimulate bleeding to introduce stem cells into the area are examples of resurfacing techniques; the stem cells introduced into the area by bleeding produce hyaline-like cartilage initially. Unfortunately, the hyaline-like cartilage eventually converts to fibrocartilage. This healing process and the surgical techniques are presented in more detail in chapter 2.

Autologous-Chondrocyte Implantation As mentioned in chapter 2, one of the most recent revolutionary advances is cartilage transplantation developed by Swedish physicians (Brittberg et al., 1994). Chondral tissue is harvested from a non-weight-bearing surface of the patient's knee. The harvested cells regenerate chondrocytes in a laboratory until sufficient quantities are available to transplant into the chondral defect. Although this technique remains under investigation, it may offer patients who have a rather narrow diagnosis of focal articular defects with an opportunity to avoid osteoarthritis at the most, or delaying arthritic symptoms to prolong physical activity at the least.

Osseous/Chondral Post-op Rehabilitation   Rehabilitation following chondral-resurfacing techniques is similar to fracture rehabilitation in that weight bearing is either non-weight bearing or toe-touch weight bearing for six weeks. A brace locked in extension is used during ambulation to reduce shear stress on the lesion site. If debridement is the only procedure performed, weight bearing immediately postoperatively is to tolerance. If autologous-chondrocyte implantation is the surgical technique, the patient is initially NWB but progresses to toe-touch and full weight bearing within 4 to 6 weeks. Exercises with the knee positioned to minimize stress of the surgical site are permitted during the non-weight bearing phase: Electrical stimulation, isometric exercises, and other non-resistive open chain exercises. Biofeedback for muscle reeducation is useful for quadriceps facilitation and control. Early range of motion occurs using either CPM machine several hours a day, passive ROM activities, or a combination of both. The goal during this period is to stimulate chondral formation without applying excessive loads to the lesion site. It is appropriate to add aquatic exercises in deep water for range of motion after the operative wounds are well healed. Patellar mobilization and soft-tissue mobilization is used by the second post-op week. A stationary bike without resistance is used after the third week. Active-assistive range-of-motion exercises, progressing to active range-of-motion exercises are also used then. By week 3 or 4, the patient should be able to demonstrate good quad control without an extensor lag and should have near-normal knee range of motion. After the third week, mild resistive aquatic exercises in deep water are suitable.

After the sixth week, full weight bearing with crutches begins. Crutches are not removed until the patient is able to ambulate normally, has no extensor lag, and has full motion in knee extension. The brace can be discontinued by this time. Aquatic exercises can progress from the deep to the shallow end in chest- to waist-high water with progressive weight bearing. Progressive resistive exercises in the open- and closed-kinetic chain, using small arcs of motion initially and advancing to larger arcs of motion, start after six weeks. Exercises should remain pain free in all arcs of motion. A ski machine or stepper can also be started. Once the patient is able to ambulate without crutches, treadmill walking begins. Static balance exercises progress to dynamic balance exercises as tolerated.

A gradual progression from balance to coordination to agility exercises takes place as the patient gains strength and proprioception. Jogging, then running is allowed at 4 to 6 months postoperatively. Full return to sport participation occurs at 7 to 12 months.

Bone-fracture rehabilitation programs follow the same basic progression, but the timing for return to full sport participation is more rapid. A general range of time for return to sport following a fracture is 4 to 8 months. The time range varies according to whether the fracture is treated surgically or immobilized without surgery, the location and type of fracture, the age of the patient, and the physician's preference. See figure 23.56 for an outline of progression for rehabilitation.

Osteochondritis Dissecans

Osteochondritis dissecans (OCD) is a disease of unknown etiology without related trauma that affects the femoral epiphysis in juvenile OCD and the femoral condyle in adult OCD. A bone flake in juvenile OCD or a bone fragment in adult OCD occurs at various sites of the femoral condyle. Juvenile OCD occurs in youths under age 15 and adult OCD is seen in people over age 15. Symptoms include nonspecific knee pain, point tenderness over the site, and quadriceps atrophy. There is minimal effusion, and the patient may experience catching, locking, or giving way during ambulation.

Treatment for adult OCD includes arthroscopic debridement of loose bodies. If the lesion is small, an abrasion arthroplasty or autogenous grafting can also be performed. Treatment for juvenile OCD is more conservative, with prolonged rest, three months or more, occasionally with immobilization.

Start
rehab

Inflammation	Proliferation	Remodeling	
Phase I (inactive)	**Phase II (active)**	**Phase III (resistive)**	**Phase IV (aggressive)**

GOALS			
• ↓ Pain • ↓ Spasm • ↓ Edema • Protect surgical site from excessive stress • Maintain conditioning levels (MCL)	• ↑ ROM of knee • Protect surgical site • Reduce scar adhesions • No pain, spasm, edema • Ambulate with brace locked and TTWB • Progress in FWB • Progress to full ROM	• Full ROM • ↑ Strength, endurance gradually • ↑ Proprioception • MCL • Good soft tissue mobility • Normal joint mobility • Normal gait without assistive devices	• Perform functional activities properly • Perform sport- and activity-specific exercises at least to preinjury levels • Return to full participation without pain, with normal strength, mobility, and execution of activities

TREATMENT			
• Modalities for pain and edema • CPM 6 h/day • Grades I and II joint mobilization • NWB • MCL exercises for conditioning with special attention to hip and ankle	• Begin quad sets/ES • Active hip exercises • ROM exercises for knee • Soft tissue mobilization • Patellar mobilizations • Muscle endurance to tolerance • Aquatic exercises at 3 weeks • Gait training: TTWB • At 6 weeks: go to FWB • HS curls to 45° • Quad extension 20°-0°, 90°-120° • CKC balance when FWB • Heel raises when FWB • Continue MCL exercises	• Continue with ROM exercises PRN • Treadmill walking at 6-8 weeks • Leg press to 60° • Aquatic exercises in waist-deep water • Begin multiplanar exercises for entire LE with bands • Early functional exercises • Grades III and IV joint mobilization, PRN • Partial squats • Lateral step-up at 8-12 weeks • Jogging at 12-26 weeks • Slide board • Continue with ME	• Plyometrics for LE: stair running, jumps, eccentrics at 12-16 weeks • Functional exercises • Sport- and activity-specific exercises at 4-6 months • Return to full participation at 7-12 months

▶ **Figure 23.56** Rehabilitation progression following a chondral microfracture. AROM = active range of motion; ROM = range of motion; CPMM = continuous passive motion machine; NWB = non-weight bearing; TTWB = toe-touch weight bearing; FWB = full weight bearing; LE = lower extremity; ES = electrical stimulation; CKC = closed kinetic chain; PRN = as needed.

Rehabilitation for juvenile OCD must attempt to reverse the deleterious effects of prolonged immobilization and inactivity. Cardiovascular exercise using the upper extremities, and lower-extremity exercises for the uninvolved segments help to maintain conditioning levels. Quad sets, straight-leg raises, and electrical stimulation can assist in retarding atrophy during immobilization.

Range-of-motion exercise, joint and soft-tissue mobilization, and active exercises are used once immobilization is removed. Weight-bearing exercises include weight-transfer activities and gait training. Aquatic exercises with progressive weight bearing in progressively shallower water can be used, and activities to restore proprioception using a BAPS board and a balance board, as well as stork standing, are helpful.

Rehabilitation following surgical treatment includes immediate weight bearing unless the lesion is large; in this case, weight bearing may be restricted. A gradual progression of exercises that do not produce pain takes place as with other knee lesions. An expected recovery to full sport participation usually takes about four to six months.

SUMMARY

The knee is positioned between two long lever arms, so it is often the site of injury in any number of activities and sports. The patellofemoral joint is also a susceptible site for pain and dysfunction. Patellofemoral pain syndrome is usually a multifactorial condition, and it is important for the clinician to identify the underlying problems that lead to a specific patient's condition. Stresses for knee structures change in both open- and closed-chain activities; it is important for the clinician to understand when stresses are high and low so appropriate rehabilitation exercises are used in a patient's program. Trigger point treatment, joint mobilization techniques, and progressive exercises from flexibility to functional activities were included in this chapter. Some of the more common injuries of the knee and thigh were presented along with rehabilitation programs for them.

KEY CONCEPTS AND REVIEW

1. Discuss the relationship and alignment between the patella and femur.

Patellar stability is the result of static and dynamic structures. The bony configuration, with the patella seated within the femoral sulcus formed by the medial and higher-ridged lateral epicondyles, is the greatest bony contributor to patellar stability. Ligamentous stability from the patellofemoral and patellotibial joints assists in providing static restraints. Active restraints occur primarily from the quadriceps. The patella is in various degrees of contact within its groove in the femur during any specific point within the knee's range of motion. A combination of compressive forces and the amount of area of contact determines the patellofemoral joint stress.

2. Identify postinjury factors that influence strength output.

Edema and pain both cause automatic withdrawal of quadriceps activity. An abnormal gait, using the injured extremity less than normal, also results in reduced muscle activity. These factors in combination contribute to further reduction of strength in the injured extremity.

3. Define quadriceps extensor lag and explain its significance.

An extensor lag occurs when full passive motion of knee extension is present but the patient is unable to actively achieve full extension. It is an indication of quadriceps weakness.

4. Outline a general progression of rehabilitation for a knee.

As with other body segments, specific applications depend on specific deficiencies. Modalities are used to relieve pain and edema and to encourage the healing process in phase I. Soft-tissue and joint mobilization techniques may be necessary. Range of motion, active and passive, is used to increase motion occur in phase II. Strengthening exercises can be started late in phase II or early in phase III within a pain-free range of motion or with isometric exercises. Manual resistance can progress to machine and body-weight resistances, resistance bands, and isokinetics. Proprioception and balance activities begin with something simple like a stork stand and progress to balance activities on unstable surfaces. Once flexibility, balance, and strength have reached appropriate levels, either late in phase III or early in phase IV, plyometric exercises, such as target jumping, lateral jumps, box activities, and depth jumps, can be used. In phase IV, functional activities progress to activity-specific exercises that mimic the patient's specific sport or work demands before full participation in the patient's sport or work is permitted.

5. Identify three soft-tissue mobilization techniques for the knee.

Three such techniques include foam roller myofascial release to the ITB, trigger point release to the quadriceps, and cross-friction massage to the patellar tendon.

6. Identify three joint mobilization techniques for the knee, and the purpose of each of them.

Lateral glides of the patella are used for full flexion-extension range of motion of the knee; posterior glides of the tibia on the femur increase flexion; and rotational glides increase terminal flexion and extension of the knee.

7. Explain three flexibility exercises for the knee and identify the structure they affect.

Flexibility exercises include standing knee flexion stretch for the quadriceps with the heel behind the buttocks, standing hamstring stretch with the involved extremity on an elevated surface, and the gastrocnemius stretch with the knee straight.

8. Explain three proprioceptive/balance exercises for the knee.

Exercises for proprioception/balance include stork standing with eyes open and then closed, stork standing on a 1/2 foam roller, and standing on a foam roller while catching a ball.

9. Identify three functional activities.

Three functional activities include running and cutting while dribbling a basketball, sprinting forward and then backward with rapid changes in direction, and lateral glides with pivots to left and right.

10. Identify three factors that influence PFPS.

Three such factors are weak quadriceps, weak hip and trunk control, and tight hamstrings.

CRITICAL THINKING QUESTIONS

1. In this chapter's opening scenario, how much knee flexion motion would you expect Nate to have after two weeks of immobilization? What would be the most effective kind of motion exercise he should be able to start on his first day of rehabilitation? What strengthening exercises would you give him for his hip and ankle on his first day of rehabilitation? When you would expect him to have full knee motion? When would you start him on passive stretching exercises for his quads? Give your justification for this timetable.

2. When would you begin patellar mobilization on Nate? When would you begin soft-tissue mobilization to the quadriceps repair site? Give your rationale for these timetables.

3. If you had two patients with knee injuries, one with an ACL sprain and the other with an MCL sprain, which one (if either) would you be more cautious with and why? How would their rehabilitation programs differ?

4. If a patient complains of patellar tendinopathy, what structures would you investigate for possible causes? What key items would you include in your history questions? Would you use primarily open- or closed-chain exercises initially, and why?

5. A teenaged patient you have been rehabilitating for weakness following an anterior medial knee contusion continues to complain of pain in the knee even though his strength is improving. How would you approach the problem and what would you suspect?

LAB ACTIVITIES

1. Perform soft tissue mobilization on your lab partner's ITB. First examine the area for any restrictions, and then apply mobilization to relieve the main restrictive areas. Examine the area after your treatment. What changes do you and your partner (objectively and subjectively) observe? What do you think as occurred with the treatment? Use a foam roller to perform a soft tissue mobilization technique on the same area for the same amount of time. Compare the sensory changes between the two techniques. Based on the differences, what would be the advantages and disadvantages of each technique?

2. Locate the trigger points on your lab partner for the muscles listed. As you perform each one, indicate what the pain pattern would be if the trigger point was active.

   a. Rectus femoris
   b. Vastus lateralis
   c. Vastus medialis
   d. Popliteus
   e. Medial hamstrings

Where were your partner's most sensitive trigger points? Perform an ice-and-stretch technique on each of them, and provide your partner with a home exercise for each tender trigger point.

3. Perform grades II and IV joint mobilizations on your lab partner and identify what restriction would be best treated with each mobilization for the following joints:

    a. Patellofemoral glides
- Medial glide
- Lateral glide
- Superior glide
- Inferior glide

    b. Tibiofemoral glides
- Distraction
- Anterior
- Posterior
- Anterior glide of the medial condyle
- Posterior glide of the medial condyle

Are the medial and lateral patellofemoral glide excursions the same? Perform the tibiofemoral glides first in the resting position, and then in other open-packed positions. How does the amount of motion change with the different positions? What implications does this outcome have on treatment?

4. Have your partner perform two different prolonged stretch exercises to increase knee flexion. Is there an advantage of one over the other?

5. Identify short-term stretches you would give a patient to perform at home. Identify stretches that would be used to stretch a knee with extension limited to 15° of flexion and another stretch that could be used on a knee with extension limited to 90° of flexion. What factors do you have to consider that are unique to each condition when coming up with an exercise for each situation?

6. Have your partner perform two different exercises (same level of difficulty) to strengthen the quadriceps. How are they different? Why might you use one over the other? Explain your rationale.

7. Have your partner perform a lateral step-up exercise for 20 repetitions. What substitution patterns must you watch for and how would you correct them?

8. Have your partner perform a wall squat using three alternative ways of doing it so each exercise is a progression of the previous one. Have your partner perform 20 repetitions of each exercise. Does your partner confirm that the sequence you created is a progression, or is a later exercise easier than a previous one? What are the substitution patterns you should watch for and what verbal cues would you give to correct each substitution?

9. Have your partner perform three proprioceptive exercises, each one a progression of the previous exercise. What have you used to determine when your partner is able to progress to the next exercise (what is your criteria for progression)?

10. Evaluate your partner's patella alignment for lateral tilt, lateral shift or glide, inferior tilt, and rotation. What malalignments do you see? Is it bilateral? If there are malalignments, what might be possible reasons for them in your partner? What exercises might correct the alignment deficiencies?

11. Have your partner perform a quad set in straight leg sitting and a lunge in standing. What differences in patellar tracking do you see between the two positions? How would you correct any deficiencies you noted?

12. You are seeing a patient (basketball forward) for the first time today. She is diagnosed with an ACL reconstruction (patellar tendon graft). List in proper sequence all the exercises you would include in the rehabilitation program. You do not need to identify timing, only sequence in which you would add the exercise. Also, indicate when you might consider discontinuing an exercise in the program and your rationale for stopping the exercise.

Hip

OBJECTIVES

After completing this chapter, you should be able to do the following:

1. Discuss how anteversion and retroversion change lower-extremity mechanics.

2. Explain the mechanical factors involved in gait with hip abductor weakness and explain how a cane or single crutch assists in normal gait.

3. Identify a joint mobilization technique for the hip and explain its benefit.

4. Identify a flexibility and a strengthening exercise for the hip.

5. Identify a proprioception exercise for the hip and indicate its progression.

6. List precautions for a hip-dislocation rehabilitation program.

► Stevie Stephens has worked with dancers for several years. Having responsibility for the city ballet company's rehabilitation programs, he is quite busy. Over the years, he has come to realize that the novice dancers' injuries tend to be acute whereas the experienced dancers' injuries are more often chronic. Although he is able to resolve the acute injuries more quickly, Stevie sees the chronic injuries as a challenge—one that he is usually able to meet and resolve, much to his patients' delight.

Stevie's current patient, however, has been his greatest challenge yet. Joann Burr, the lead female dancer in the company, had been bothered with a groin strain for several months before she reported it. It occurred early in the season during rehearsal, and Joann had dismissed it as minor, not worth treating. But the problem did not go away, and now that the company is at the peak of the performance season, the injury is aggravated with each performance. Still, Joann refuses to take any time off to allow the strain to heal.

Time isn't a commodity, something you pass around like cake. Time is the substance of life. When anyone asks you to give your time, they're really asking for a chunk of your life.

ANTOINETTE BOSCO, American author, syndicated columnist

At the conclusion of this final chapter you will have acquired the information you need to work as a rehabilitation clinician, planning and providing sound therapeutic exercise programs to patients. Now it is up to you to use your time wisely and practice your skills with all the knowledge and application you have acquired to be an exceptional clinician. To ascend to new levels of knowledge is a professional goal and a responsibility shared by those who have a desire to excel within their profession; individual professional greatness is measured not by what we know but by how we share what we know. As you start to work with patients in rehabilitation, you may be hesitant for fear of failure, but fear should never be your motivation to act; rather, improving your patient's condition is the reason you have chosen this profession. If you make a mistake, you learn from it and adjust the patient's program. If you never make a mistake, you haven't done your best to make a patient better.

So, as we move through this last chapter, realize what makes the hip different from other joints, and understand how it is a lot like them as well. As with other joints we have studied, the actions of the rehabilitation clinician in hip rehabilitation must be carefully planned if you are to guide the patient to a safe return to full participation promptly and in accordance with your and your patient's mutually established goals. Primary entities that make the hip unique from other joints are its structure and importance in closed kinetic chain function.

The hip joint is secured by a deep socket and is supported by strong muscles. It is an area that experiences repetitive, microtraumatic injuries more often than acute, macrotraumatic injuries. Like other segments, this area relies on a balance of muscle flexibility and strength, along with coordination of movement, to maintain a balance for function and health. By now, you realize that if normal length, strength, or function of any element of a joint is lost or changed, other elements are impacted to make the region prone to injury; the hip is no exception.

The hip is a common site for pain referral from other sources, so pain complaints of this area warrant a look at differential diagnoses before treatment begins. Because of the various structures that can produce pain into the hip and groin, establishing the source of pain is not always easy. Hip or groin pain can be secondary to referral from pathology such as lumbar disc disruption, spondylolysis, organ disease, myofascial pain, sacroiliac dysfunction, and knee injury. The rehabilitation clinician must eliminate these possibilities as the pain source before he or she can accurately treat the patient. During the initial examination, if the patient's pain is not reproduced by stress applied to these adjacent structures but is reproduced when stress is applied to the hip, it is likely that the hip is the source of the patient's pain. If there is no change in the patient's condition after four to six sessions or two weeks of treatment, reexamination for other sources of pain is indicated.

This chapter introduces basic concepts the rehabilitation clinician must consider for hip-injury rehabilitation, focusing on topics relevant to treatment and therapeutic exercise program progression. As with the other chapters in Part IV, specific techniques for soft-tissue and joint mobilization and exercises for flexibility, strength, and proprioception are presented. Once these foundations of a hip therapeutic exercise program are provided, specific injuries commonly seen in the hip are discussed along with program progressions for these injuries. Cases are presented in connection with some injury programs to help you conceptualize how a hip program is put together and advanced for specific conditions.

> Among common hip injuries that the rehabilitation clinician encounters are muscle-imbalance syndromes, acute soft-tissue injuries, various inflammation conditions, and fractures and dislocation.

GENERAL REHABILITATION CONSIDERATIONS

The hip is a stable joint with extensive range of motion in three planes. The socket is deep and reinforced with strong ligaments for stability. Strength and motion are important for the hip because it serves as a force transmitter for both lower- and upper-limb activities and provides motion and strength for propulsion in walking and running (Ahmed & Burke, 1983).

Osseous Structures

The **acetabulum,** the hip socket, is in an inferior and anterolateral position. The femoral neck forms a 125° angle with the shaft of the femur, as shown in figure 24.1a (Kapandji, 1986). An angle greater than 125°, called coxa valga, increases pressure into the joint (figure 24.1b); an angle less than 125°, called coxa vara, increases stress on the femoral neck (figure 24.1c).

The femoral neck is rotated relative to the line of the femur's long axis. Normal alignment places the neck in a line that is 15° anterior to the line of the femur in the adult (figure 24.2). If the angle is greater than 15°, the leg is positioned in medial rotation; this condition is called **anteversion.** If it is less than 15°, **retroversion** occurs to position the leg in lateral rotation. Anteversion and retroversion alter knee alignment and change the forces acting throughout the entire lower extremity. Anteversion leads to medial hip rotation, squinting patellae, and/or foot adduction, causing the individual to ambulate with a toe-in gait. Retroversion results in lateral hip rotation, frog-eyed patellae, and/or foot abduction, and causes the person to ambulate with a toe-out gait. Anteversion and coxa valga each make the hip susceptible to dislocation.

Anteversion is measured using different methods. One measurement method is with the patient lying prone and the knee flexed to 90°. The rehabilitation clinician moves the patient's leg into medial rotation until palpation of the greater trochanter reveals that it is parallel to the tabletop (figure 24.3). A goniometer is then used to measure the difference between the tibial position and a line vertical to the tabletop. This value is the degree of anteversion.

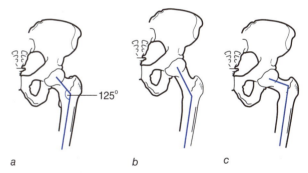

▶ **Figure 24.1** Femoral neck angles: *(a)* normal; *(b)* coxa valga—increased angle with increased joint stress; *(c)* coxa vara—decreased angle with increased femoral neck load.

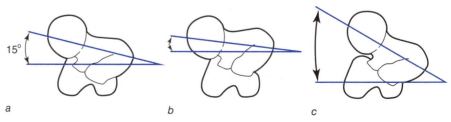

▶ **Figure 24.2** Femoral neck alignment with long axis of femur: *(a)* normal, *(b)* retroversion, *(c)* anteversion.

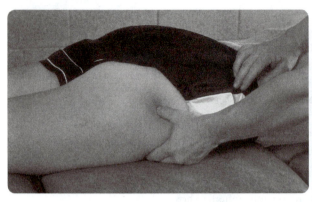

a

▶ **Figure 24.3** Craig's test for femoral anteversion: greater trochanter is positioned parallel to the tabletop *(a)*, and the angle between the tibia's position in 90° knee flexion at this point and in a vertical line is measured *(b)*.

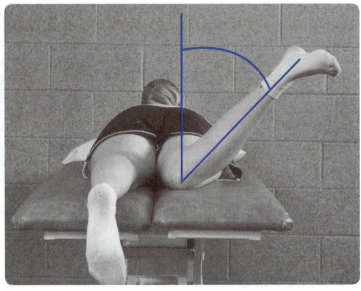

b

Neural Structures

Nerves entering the lower extremity must pass through the hip region. Nerve irritations can occur when soft tissues surrounding the hip impinge on a nerve. The sciatic nerve passes beneath, occasionally through, the piriformis muscle and through the sciatic notch before it travels along the posterior thigh. Entrapment of the nerve in the piriformis region can occur, producing neural irritation distally.

A sensory branch of the femoral nerve, the lateral femoral cutaneous nerve, travels through the psoas major muscle and then passes under the inguinal ligament near the anterior superior iliac spine (ASIS). Compression of this nerve by the inguinal ligament can cause aching and burning over the tensor fascia lata in the anterolateral thigh where the nerve provides sensory innervation.

The obturator nerve enters the pelvis from upper lumbar nerve roots and provides sensory and motor innervation to the medial thigh. Entrapment of this nerve can cause medial thigh sensory changes and adductor weakness.

Stabilization

Chapter 18 mentioned pelvic or trunk stabilization and its importance in reduced injury risk and improved upper and lower extremity performance. As you recall, a portion of trunk stabilization depends upon the hip muscles. Specifically, the hip extensors and abductors play a very important role in pelvic stability. When you think about it, this makes intuitive sense. Since athletic performance and reduced injury risk are dependent upon a stable trunk or pelvis and the gluteal muscles attach to the pelvis, then hip stability is also important for these same performance and injury-prevention elements. The hip muscles also serve as a means by which the power of the legs transfers up the chain to other body segments during upper extremity activities such as pitching, golf, and tennis. As was mentioned in chapter 19, assuming the patient performs with good sequential motion, the legs and trunk provide 51% to 55% of the total kinetic energy and total force for overhead activities (Kibler, 1995). This means that if the hips are weak, not only will there be less force applied where and when it is needed, but there will be increased stress applied to other segments within the chain that must take up the weak hip muscles' inability to provide required forces. The hips must be the platform from which the pelvis functions, just as the pelvis is the platform from which the scapula functions, and the scapula is the platform from which the shoulder joint functions. It is important, then, for the clinician to examine hip stability, especially strength of the hip extensors and abductors, for not only hip injury rehabilitation but also any extremity joint, just as the clinician examines trunk stability for upper-and-lower extremity rehabilitation programs (Leetun, Ireland, Willson, Ballantyne, & Davis, 2004; Tyler, Nicholas, Campbell, & McHugh, 2001).

Joint Mobility

The joint configuration is a convex femoral head on a concave acetabulum, so glide of the femur on the pelvis occurs in the direction opposite to movement during open chain motion. The hip's capsular pattern has its most significant restriction of motion in medial rotation. Flexion and abduction are less limited, and extension is less limited than flexion or abduction. Lateral rotation is normal (Cyriax, 1977).

The hip joint's close-packed position is full extension, abduction, and medial rotation. The resting position is 30° flexion and 30° abduction with slight lateral rotation.

Joint Mechanics

Pelvis movement has a direct influence on hip movement because the hip joint socket lies within the pelvic bones. Pelvic motion alters hip positioning, and hip abnormalities affect pelvic posture. An anterior pelvic tilt moves the anterior pelvis closer to the anterior femur, and a posterior pelvic tilt moves the posterior pelvis closer to the posterior femur. This change in position relationships alters the hip so that an anterior pelvic tilt increases hip flexion and a posterior pelvic tilt increases hip extension.

The center of gravity transfers toward the supporting leg when a person moves from a two-leg to a one-leg stance. This places rotatory stress on the weight-bearing hip because gravity's pull on the non-weight bearing leg drops the pelvis on that side. To prevent this pelvic drop and the rotatory forces accompanying it, the abductors on the weight-bearing leg work to keep the hips level with each other. The force required of the weight-bearing extremity's abductors is significantly greater than the weight of the body, because the abductors' lever-arm length is less than that of the center of gravity (figure 24.4). If the abductors are not strong enough to counter the force of gravity that is pulling the non-weight-bearing extremity downward and laterally rotating the pelvis, a normal gait is not possible. The patient either drops the non-weight-bearing hip and downwardly rotates the pelvis to the non-weight-bearing side, or the patient tilts the trunk to lean over the weak weight-bearing hip during stance on the leg so that the center of gravity is closer to the fulcrum, the femoral head. If the center of gravity is moved far enough laterally to be placed on top of or lateral to the fulcrum, the abductors do not have to work.

When a cane or one crutch is used on the side opposite the weakness, an upward force is transmitted through the appliance to counterbalance the downward gravitational force on the same side (figure 24.5). Because the lever arm from the cane to the fulcrum at the weak hip is longer than the lever arm of the

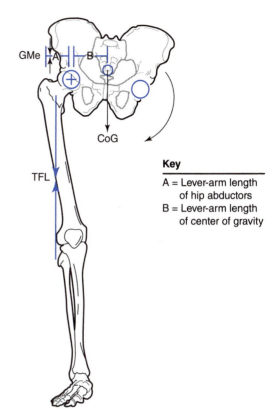

Figure 24.4 Single-leg stance mechanics.

Key

A = Lever-arm length of hip abductors
B = Lever-arm length of center of gravity

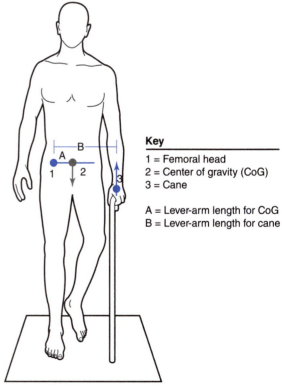

Figure 24.5 Force application with cane use in ambulation.

Key

1 = Femoral head
2 = Center of gravity (CoG)
3 = Cane

A = Lever-arm length for CoG
B = Lever-arm length for cane

body's center of gravity, the necessary counterbalance force transmitted through the cane is relatively small. Patients who use a cane or a single crutch for ambulation need only apply light pressure on the handle to offset the gravitational pull and produce adequate compensation for the weak abductors.

Leg-length discrepancies can result from actual differences in length or from other unilateral differences such as genu valgus, coxa vara, rotated sacrum, or foot pronation, as well as from soft-tissue differences such as hip flexor tightness, abductor tightness, and muscle imbalances. When one leg is shorter than the other leg, the pelvis drops on the shorter side, and the trunk bends away from the short leg when weight bearing on the short leg. The greater the discrepancy, the more notable are these compensations. If a leg-length discrepancy is suspected, shoe wear is the most obvious indication that one is present. When a leg-length discrepancy is present, the clinician should assess all possible causes; correction or adaptation of the discrepancy may be necessary to alleviate the patient's pain.

Leg-length differences can eventually lead to osteoarthritis of the hip in the longer leg. This occurs because the longer leg is in a position of adducted angulation when weight bearing. This produces increased joint incongruence in which greater weight is borne on the superior lateral aspect of the acetabulum. The weight shift to the shorter leg occurs; consequently, increased compressive forces occur to the hip joint as the abductors on the longer leg increase their exertion to keep the pelvis level.

Stress-Reduction Concepts

One rule of thumb is that if a patient is unable to ambulate normally, he or she must use assistive devices until normal ambulation is possible. An abnormal gait may result from pain, inadequate muscle control, or apprehension, and if it continues, increased stresses to the hip, back, or other lower-extremity segments resulting in additional injury will arise. When weight bearing is permitted, an assistive device is used only as much as necessary to create a normal gait. As the precipitating factor is resolved, the patient is weaned from the crutches or cane until a normal gait without assistive devices occurs.

Stress can be reduced in the hip by shortening the stride length during walking or running. A smaller stride reduces the force and motion demands on the muscles, tendons, and ligaments. Application of a hip spica wrap will assist in moderating stride length.

General Rehabilitation Procedures

Hip-pain complaints without a specific injury can sometimes be difficult to interpret because of the various possible sources. Pain in the hip joint itself commonly refers to the groin, the anterior or medial proximal thigh, or the knee. Spinal-based pain can refer to the anterior hip, buttock, or thigh. Sacral pain can refer to the buttock or posterior or lateral thigh. Internal organs and the abdomen can refer pain to the groin. When a patient complains of pain in these areas without a specific history of injury, identifying differential diagnoses is necessary to eliminate these locations as sources of hip pain. The examination tests should reproduce the patient's pain complaints for a differential diagnosis. If tests for these possibly referring segments do not reproduce the patient's pain, but the pain is reproduced with special tests to the hip joint, the clinician is safe in deducing that the pain is hip related.

Pain and inflammation control are the primary goals for initial treatment programs for hip injuries in phase I; the various means of pain control include anti-inflammatory medication, reduced activity, and modalities. Some hip injuries are self-limiting in that pain is the determining factor with respect to activity participation. The patient may wish to continue normal participation in this case, because continued activity will not make the condition worse; however, the recovery time may be longer because irritation continues to occur on a regular basis.

Therapeutic exercises include a progression of stretching or flexibility exercises, strengthening exercises, proprioception activities, and functional activities. When injuries result from predisposing factors rather than acute insult, those factors must be corrected to reduce the risk of recurrence. Since many hip muscles cross more than one joint, effective flexibility exercises require adequate stabilization of adjacent segments and proper application of the stretch force. Phase II emphasizes flexibility with early strength and proprioceptive activities while phase III includes more aggressive strength and agility exercises. Because the hip is so closely aligned with the pelvis, strengthening exercises must include pelvic and core stabilization exercises. Because the hip depends on the back, pelvis, knee, and ankle for its balance and quality of motion, exercises for deficiencies in these segments must be a part of the therapeutic exercise program for the hip. Many of these exercises for other segments besides the hip can be initiated in phase II when full strength exercises for the hip are limited yet resistive exercises to the other segments will not require hip strength. In phase IV, the patient's program concentrates on plyometrics, functional, and activity-specific exercises in preparation for a return to normal activities. Return to full sport or work participation is possible when the patient is pain free with muscle balances intact and when performance of activity-specific activities is normal.

> A rehabilitation program for the hip must be based on knowledge of the hip's osseous structures, neural structures, and joint mobility and joint mechanics. The rehabilitation clinician must also be familiar with methods of reducing stress in an injured hip.

SOFT-TISSUE MOBILIZATION

Because of the neurological, myofascial, orthopedic, and organ systems that can refer pain into the hip region, it is prudent for the rehabilitation clinician to identify any differential diagnosis that may be contributing to hip or groin pain. If myofascia is the expected source of pain, treatment can proceed. If changes in the patient's complaints do not occur with soft-tissue mobilization techniques, it is necessary to reassess for other probable causes.

Soft-tissue mobilization techniques for the hip include deep-tissue massage, scar-tissue mobilization, cross-friction massage, and myofascial release, including trigger point treatments and ice-and-stretch techniques. The myofascial release techniques and pain-referral information presented here are based on the work of Travell and Simons (Travell & Simons, 1992) and described in the following sections. The quadratus lumborum muscle is discussed in chapter 18; the rectus femoris, hamstrings, adductors, and tensor fascia lata are addressed in chapter 23.

Myofascial techniques include direct pressure with the flat finger or thumb pad or with a pincer grasp of the muscle that is held until the muscle relaxes. If soft-tissue resistance is palpated after the initial application, the technique can be repeated. Ice/spray-and-stretch techniques incorporate ice massage or cold spray applied in parallel sweeps, usually proximally to distally, with a simultaneous application of manual stretching. The rehabilitation clinician repeats this process three to five times, attempting to increase mobility with each application. He or she assists the patient in actively moving the leg to the starting position between bouts of ice-and-stretch. The patient performs several bouts of active motion following ice-and-stretch. Heat can be applied after the ice-and-stretch. Pain should not be produced during the application.

■ Trigger Point Releases for the Hip Muscles

Iliopsoas

Referral Pattern: Pain is referred either throughout the lumbar paraspinal region on the same side as the lesion or into the anterior thigh and groin (figure 24.6a).

Location of Trigger Point: The first trigger point is located on the lateral wall of the femoral triangle. The middle trigger point can be located just behind the ASIS and inside the rim of the iliac crest. The third trigger point is more difficult to access because the patient must keep the abdominal muscles relaxed, and this is sometimes difficult to do. The region is lateral and just inferior to the umbilicus on the lateral rim of the rectus abdominis.

Patient Position for Palpation: The patient is supine with the abdominal muscles relaxed.

Muscle Position for Palpation: The leg is positioned with the hip slightly flexed, abducted, and supported for relaxation.

Ischemic Treatment: The first trigger point on the lateral wall of the femoral triangle (TP$_1$) is treated with direct pressure using either the finger or the thumb pad (figure 24.6b); do not place pressure on the medial side of the muscle since the femoral nerve is located in this region. The second trigger point (TP$_2$) can be treated with finger-pad pressure pushing the muscle against the inside rim of the ilium. The third trigger point (TP$_3$) is treated with direct downward pressure exerted slowly; once past the rectus abdominis, the pressure continues downward and medially toward the spine. Depending on the patient's size, the psoas may or may not be directly palpated, but indirect pressure is effective if direct palpation is not possible.

Spray-and-Stretch Treatment: Spray/ice-and-stretch techniques are applied with the patient side-lying on the unaffected side and the top leg supported by the rehabilitation clinician in hip extension (figure 24.6c). Ice or cold spray sweeps are made from the abdomen downward past the thigh and to the knee, with stretch force applied to increase hip extension and medial rotation. Ice or cold spray sweeps are finally applied to the low back and posterior hip.

Notations: Pain from the iliopsoas trigger points is noticed particularly during weight bearing but is relieved with non-weight bearing.

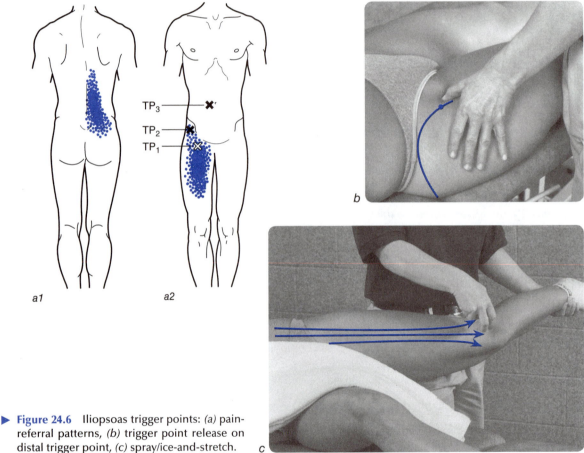

▶ **Figure 24.6** Iliopsoas trigger points: *(a)* pain-referral patterns, *(b)* trigger point release on distal trigger point, *(c)* spray/ice-and-stretch.

Gluteus Maximus

Referral Pattern: Refers pain locally in the buttock region around the sacrum and gluteal fold above the ischial tuberosity (figure 24.7a).

Location of Trigger Point: Trigger point 1 is at the superior medial gluteus maximus just distal to its insertion on the sacrum. Trigger point 2 is just proximal to the ischial tuberosity. Trigger point 3 is directly medial to trigger point 2.

Patient Position for Palpation: Patient is side-lying with the involved hip on top. A pad under the bottom hip may be placed for comfort.

Muscle Position for Palpation: Top thigh is flexed comfortably.

Ischemic Treatment: Trigger points 1 and 2 are treated with flat pressure. Trigger point 3 is best treated with a pincer grasp. A taut band is palpated in the muscle's distal medial trigger point (figure 24.7b).

Spray-and-Stretch Treatment: Ice/spray-and-stretch is applied with the patient in side-lying and the top hip flexed and adducted, with the knee resting on the table in front of the bottom extremity. The ice or cold spray sweeps start at the posterior iliac crest; they proceed along the muscle fiber direction to the mid-posterior thigh as stretch is applied, moving the hip into flexion (figure 24.7c).

Notations: Pain related to this muscle is commonly reported after prolonged sitting, walking uphill, and swimming the freestyle stroke.

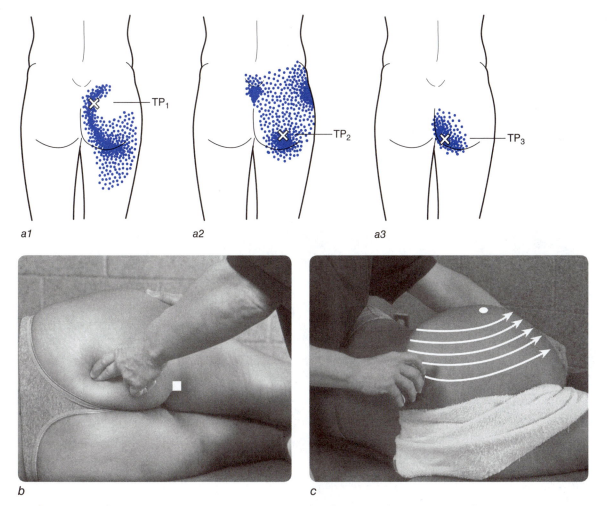

▶ **Figure 24.7** Gluteus maximus trigger points: *(a)* pain-referral patterns, *(b)* trigger point release to superior trigger point, *(c)* spray/ice-and-stretch. □ = greater trochanter, ○ = ischial tuberosity.

Gluteus Medius

Referral Pattern: Pain is along the posterior iliac crest, down the sacrum, and into the lateral posterior gluteal area (figure 24.8a).

Location of Trigger Point: The trigger points are along and inferior to the iliac crest.

Patient Position for Palpation: Side-lying with the affected hip on top.

Muscle Position for Palpation: The hip is flexed and supported with a pillow between the knees and under the bottom hip for comfort.

Ischemic Treatment: Thumb or finger-pad pressure on the trigger points against the ilium is used along the iliac crest at the tender sites until their relaxation is palpated (figure 24.8b).

Spray-and-Stretch Treatment: Spray/ice-and-stretch is applied with the patient side-lying. The hip is in adduction behind the uninvolved extremity for stretch to the anterior fibers and in front of the uninvolved extremity for stretch to the posterior fibers. Parallel ice or cold spray sweeps are made from the iliac crest, over the lateral thigh to the knee (figure 24.8c).

Notations: Pain from the gluteus medius is aggravated with walking, lying supine, side-lying on the affected side, or sitting in a slouched position. Patients with Morton's toe are more susceptible to trigger points here. Ambulating with the hip medially rotated, unilateral standing, falling on the hip, playing prolonged tennis matches, walking on soft sand, and doing aerobics are all activities that can contribute to activation of these trigger points.

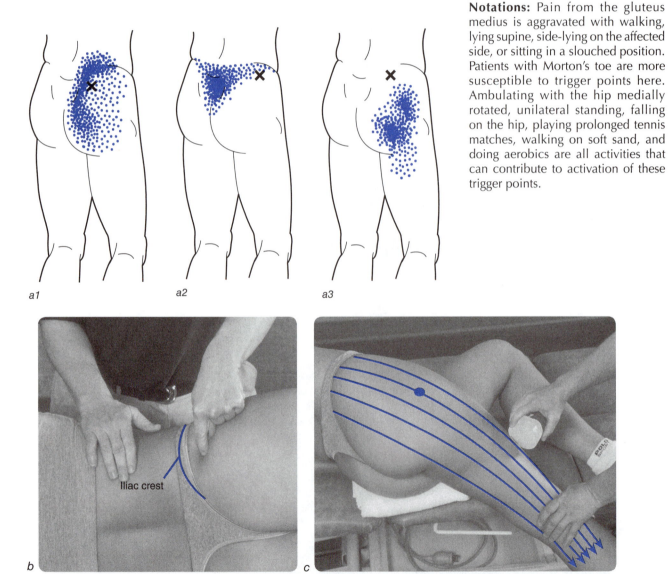

a1 *a2* *a3*

Iliac crest

b *c*

▶ **Figure 24.8** Gluteus medius trigger points: *(a)* pain-referral patterns, *(b)* trigger point release to the posterior trigger point *(a1)*, *(c)* spray/ice-and-stretch. ● = greater trochanter.

Gluteus Minimus

Referral Pattern: Pain-referral pattern is (1) over the lower lateral buttock, down the lateral thigh, and into the lateral leg to the ankle for anterior trigger points or (2) over the lower posterior buttock and posterior thigh and into the proximal posterior calf for posterior trigger points (figure 24.9a).

Location of Trigger Point: Several trigger points are located in the gluteus minimus, anteriorly and posteriorly. Anterior trigger points lie deep to the posterior border of the tensor fasciae latae muscle. The trigger point found most frequently is located in the posterior muscle cephalic to the greater trochanter about midway between the muscle's proximal and distal insertions. Other posterior trigger points are located just above the piriformis toward the middle and lateral aspects of the piriformis.

Patient Position for Palpation: Supine for anterior trigger points (figure 24.9b); side-lying with the affected leg on top for posterior trigger point treatment.

Muscle Position for Palpation: The gluteus medius and maximus should be relaxed; supportive pillows should be used for optimal effectiveness.

Ischemic Treatment: A flat palpation is used for all trigger points. The gluteus medius and maximus should be relaxed; supportive pillows should be used for optimal effectiveness. The anterior fibers are treated just distal to the ASIS and lateral and deep to the tensor fasciae latae. To locate the tensor fasciae latae, the clinician palpates for the muscle and simultaneously provides light resistance to hip medial rotation. The posterior trigger points are treated with the hip slightly flexed and adducted.

Spray-and-Stretch Treatment: Spray/ice-and-stretch is applied with the patient in side-lying with the buttock close to the end of the table (figure 24.9c). With the hip in adduction and supported by the rehabilitation clinician, ice or cold spray is applied in sweeping strokes from the iliac crest, down the lateral thigh to the lateral lower leg and ankle for the anterior trigger points and along the posterior hip, thigh, and calf for the posterior trigger points. The stretch force is applied with the hip in extension and adduction for the anterior fibers and in 30° flexion and medial rotation for the posterior fibers.

Notations: Pain from the gluteus minimus occurs with getting out of a chair and with walking.

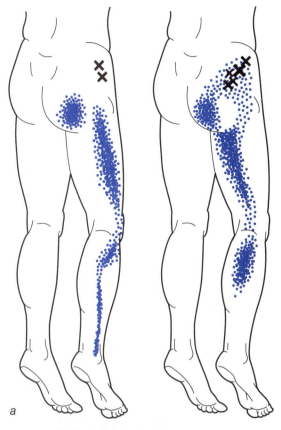

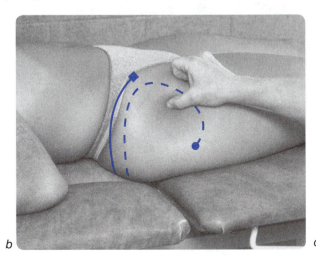

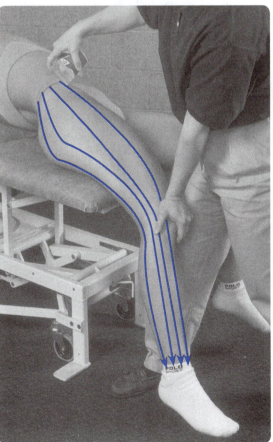

▶ **Figure 24.9** Gluteus minimus trigger points: *(a)* pain-referral patterns, *(b)* trigger point release, *(c)* spray/ice-and-stretch. ● = greater trochanter; ■ = ASIS.

Piriformis

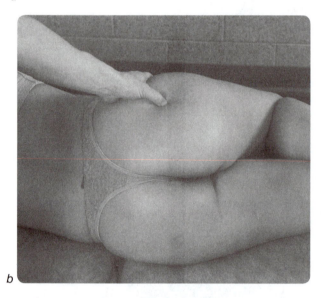

Referral Pattern: The piriformis refers pain into the sacroiliac area and the posterior hip. The pain can also extend into the upper two-thirds of the posterior thigh (figure 24.10a).

Location of Trigger Point: A line from the greater trochanter to the superior border of the sciatic foramen is the course of the muscle. Two trigger points are found on this line; one is at the junction of the medial and middle third of the line, and the other is at the junction of the middle and lateral third of the line.

Patient Position for Palpation: Prone or side-lying on the uninvolved hip (figure 24.10b).

Muscle Position for Palpation: The muscle is relaxed; if the patient is in side-lying, the leg is resting in partial hip and knee flexion, forward of the opposite extremity.

Ischemic Treatment: Flat palpation directly through the gluteus maximus.

Spray-and-Stretch Treatment: Spray/ice-and-stretch is performed with the patient side-lying and the hip in about 90° flexion and adducted in front of the bottom thigh. The side-lying patient keeps the flexed and adducted thigh anchored with his or her hand at the knee. The rehabilitation clinician then applies ice or cold spray sweeps from the sacrum to the lateral hip and down the posterior thigh (figure 24.10c). The stretch is applied at the pelvis with the clinician's hand on the patient's anterior pelvis to pull the pelvis posteriorly while the patient holds the thigh.

Notations: Activities such as sitting, standing, running, and walking aggravate myofascial pain of the piriformis. Individuals who slip but catch themselves to stop a fall may aggravate piriformis trigger points.

a

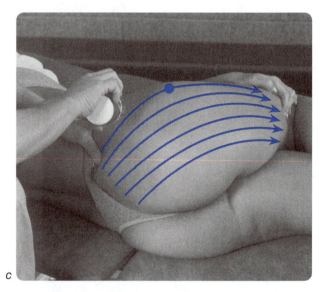

b *c*

▶ **Figure 24.10** Piriformis trigger points: *(a)* pain-referral patterns, *(b)* trigger point release to lateral trigger point, *(c)* ice-and-stretch. ● = greater trochanter.

Pectineus

Referral Pattern: Deep into the groin just below the inguinal ligament (figure 24.11a).

Location of Trigger Point: Medial to the femoral artery, lateral to the adductor longus, and inferior to the inguinal.

Patient Position for Palpation: Supine.

Muscle Position for Palpation: Hip is abducted and slightly flexed. The thigh is supported to keep muscles relaxed (figure 24.11b).

Ischemic Treatment: Finger-pad pressure directly over the trigger point.

Spray-and-Stretch Treatment: The hip is abducted and the knee and leg are over the edge of the table (figure 24.11c). The stretch force is applied so that the hip becomes progressively more abducted and moves into extension.

Notations: Trigger point activation may occur from any sudden or unexpected contraction of hip or thigh adduction with flexion. Also, gymnasts, dancers, and horseback riders may overload the muscle, especially if it is already fatigued. This trigger point may become activated after hip surgery as well.

Soft-tissue mobilization techniques for the hip, including massage, scar-tissue mobilization, and cross-friction mobilization, are directed at the iliopsoas; the gluteus maximus, medius, and minimus; the piriformis; and the pectineus.

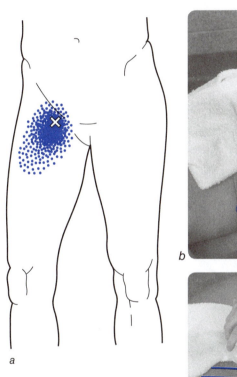

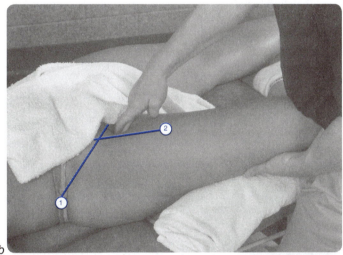

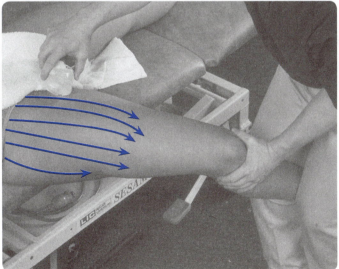

▶ **Figure 24.11** Pectineus trigger points: *(a)* pain-referral patterns, *(b)* trigger point release, *(c)* spray/ice-and-stretch. 1 = inguinal ligament, 2 = femoral artery.

JOINT MOBILIZATION

Whereas painful hip joints can benefit from grades I and II mobilization techniques, hip joints that display a capsular pattern of restricted movement can benefit from grades III and IV mobilization techniques. Although not always, oscillating techniques are often used for grades I and II and either a sustained or oscillating force is used for grades III and IV.

Because the proximal aspect of the hip joint is the pelvis, which is firmly attached to the trunk, there is little need to stabilize the hip joint of mobilization. The weight of the pelvis acts as an anchor. Some mobilizations for the hip are included in the following sections.

■ Joint Mobilization of the Hip

Inferior Glide (Also Called a Traction or Distraction Technique)

Joint: Hip.

Resting Position: 30° flexion and 30° abduction with slight lateral rotation.

Indications: To help regain joint play. In grades I and II, to relieve pain.

Patient Position: Supine.

Clinician and Hand Positions: Rehabilitation clinician grasps the distal tibia and fibula of the affected leg and places the leg in a resting position.

Mobilization Application: The clinician leans backward, using his or her body weight to supply the traction force (figure 24.12a).

Notations: If the patient has a history of knee disorders, an alternative position for an inferior glide is to have the patient's lower leg over the rehabilitation clinician's shoulder. The clinician clasps his or her hands around the proximal thigh and applies the inferior glide (figure 24.12b).

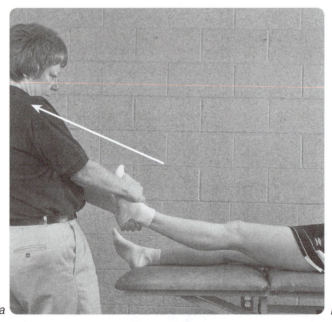
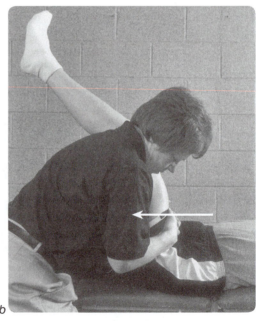

a   b

▶ **Figure 24.12** Joint mobilization—inferior glide: *(a)* with force applied in knee extension, *(b)* with force applied in knee flexion.

Lateral Glide

Joint: Hip.

Resting Position: 30° flexion and 30° abduction with slight lateral rotation.

Indications: To increase hip adduction and general mobility.

Patient Position: Patient lies supine.

Clinician and Hand Positions: Clinician stands at the patient's side by the thigh. A strap is secured around the patient's proximal thigh and the clinician's hips (figure 24.13a). The clinician places his or her cephalic hand on the lateral pelvis to stabilize it and the caudal hand on the distal thigh.

Mobilization Application: With the patient's thigh in slight flexion, the clinician transfers his or her weight from the front leg to the back leg, pushing his or her body against the strap to apply the traction force through the strap.

Notations: The patient's hip can be placed in various positions of flexion and rotation for application of superior or inferior distractions with the lateral glide (figure 24.13, b & c).

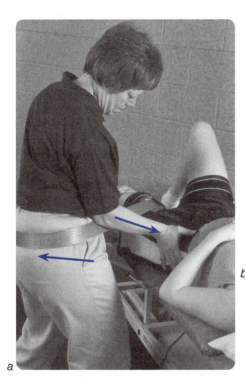
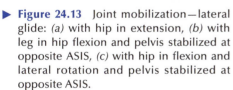
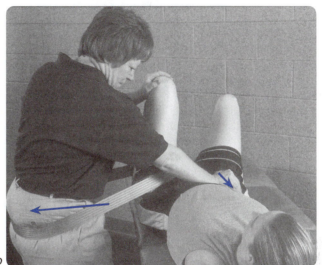
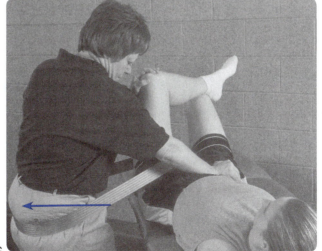

▶ **Figure 24.13** Joint mobilization—lateral glide: *(a)* with hip in extension, *(b)* with leg in hip flexion and pelvis stabilized at opposite ASIS, *(c)* with hip in flexion and lateral rotation and pelvis stabilized at opposite ASIS.

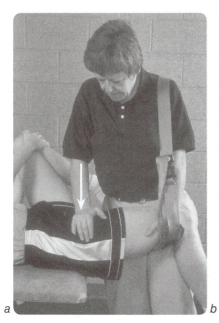 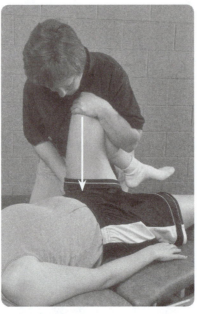

a   *b*

▶ **Figure 24.14** Joint mobilization—posterior glide: *(a)* with strap, *(b)* along the femur's long axis.

Posterior Glide (Also Known as a Dorsal Glide)

Joint: Hip.

Resting Position: 30° flexion and 30° abduction with slight lateral rotation.

Indications: To increase hip flexion and medial rotation.

Patient Position: Supine with the hip and knee flexed.

Clinician and Hand Positions: The degree of hip flexion depends on the technique used. When a belt is used, partial flexion of the joints is necessary, with the belt placed around the distal thigh and secured to the rehabilitation clinician's shoulder. The clinician places the stabilizing hand under the belt and the mobilizing hand over the anterior proximal thigh.

Mobilization Application: With the elbow kept extended, the rehabilitation clinician applies a downward force on the proximal thigh, using his or her legs, while the patient's thigh is kept stable with the belt (figure 24.14a).

Notations: An alternative position is with the hip in 90° flexion and about 10° adduction and the knee in full flexion. The rehabilitation clinician applies the posterior glide force through the long axis of the femur by leaning his or her body weight into the femur (figure 24.14b). Care must be taken not to apply the mobilizing force through the patella.

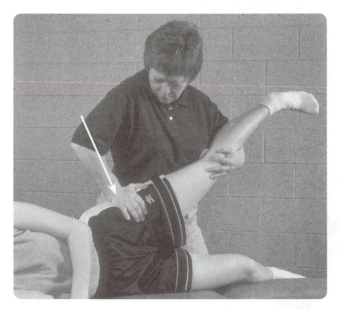

▶ **Figure 24.15** Joint mobilization: medial glide.

Medial Glide

Joint: Hip.

Resting Position: 30° flexion and 30° abduction with slight lateral rotation.

Indications: To increase hip abduction and flexion.

Patient Position: Patient is side-lying on the unaffected hip while the clinician supports the distal thigh and knee and positions the thigh in slight abduction and flexion (figure 24.15).

Clinician and Hand Positions: Mobilizing hand is placed on the proximal thigh.

Mobilization Application: The mobilizing force is applied downward, parallel to the joint's plane.

Notations: If the patient is large compared to the clinician, the assistance of another clinician to support the patient's leg may be required. This technique may also be performed with the patient in supine.

Anterior Glide

Joint: Hip.

Resting Position: 30° flexion and 30° abduction with slight lateral rotation. Also known as a postero-anterior glide or a ventral glide.

Indications: To increase hip extension and lateral rotation.

Patient Position: Prone with the knee flexed.

Clinician and Hand Positions: Clinician supports the distal thigh using the stabilizing hand or a strap.

Mobilization Application: The mobilizing hand applies a downward force through an extended elbow; body weight exerts the force (figure 24.16a). The hip can be placed in various rotation positions for additional techniques.

Notations: In an alternative position, the patient is prone, with the hips on the edge of the table and the noninvolved lower extremity supporting the body weight with the lower-extremity foot on the floor. The clinician can either support the patient's distal thigh in one hand or can have a stabilizing strap over the shoulder and wrapped around the distal thigh (figure 24.16b).

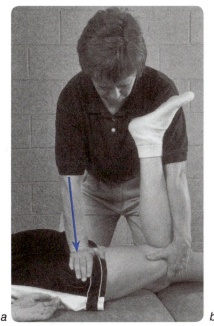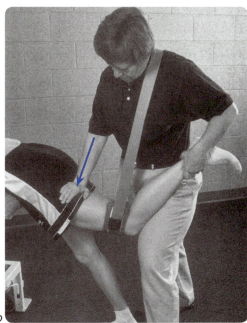

▶ **Figure 24.16** Joint mobilization—anterior glide: *(a)* prone on table, without strap; *(b)* prone off table, with strap.

Self-Mobilization

The patient can perform self-distraction using a stretch strap. The patient is supine with the strap anchored around the foot and the anterior hip; the knee and hip are placed in flexed positions, about 90° each (figure 24.17). A pad is placed on the anterior thigh for comfort. Keeping the opposite hip flexed with hands supporting the thigh, the patient pushes the involved foot against the strap, attempting to extend the hip and knee.

In an alternative position, the patient places a weight cuff around the ankle and stands with the foot off a step, allowing gravity to create a distraction force on the hip. The position is maintained for several minutes, as tolerated.

> The rehabilitation clinician used joint mobilization of the hip to improve joint play and general hip mobility, as well as hip flexion, extension, abduction, and rotation. Patients can also apply self-mobilization techniques.

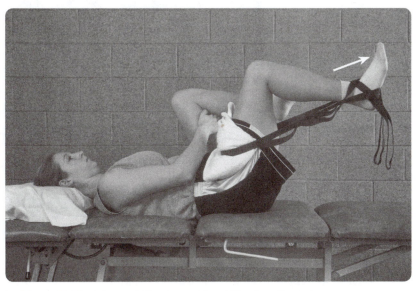

▶ **Figure 24.17** Joint mobilization: self-mobilization distraction.

FLEXIBILITY EXERCISES

Several muscles cross the hip joint, acting not only on the hip but also on the knee, back, or pelvis. For effective stretching at the hip, these segments must be positioned appropriately. Flexibility exercises for the hip muscles are presented in the following sections.

Active stretches are held for 15 to 20 s and are repeated about four times each. They should be repeated at least three to four times throughout the day. As with any stretch, active contraction of opposing muscles leads to improved results in flexibility exercises by enhancing relaxation of stretched muscle. Enough force is applied to move the muscle to a point at which the patient perceives a stretch without pain. Prolonged stretches are most effective in altering tissue length in scar tissue and connective tissue.

■ Flexibility Exercises for the Hip

Lower Lumbar Rotation

Body Segment: Lateral hip muscles.

Stage in Rehab: II.

Purpose: Increase flexibility of lower lumbar muscles.

Positioning: The patient flexes the involved hip and knee and rotates the thigh across the body, keeping the ipsilateral shoulder on the ground.

Execution: The weight of the leg provides a stretch, but additional force on the stretch can be supplied by the contralateral hand pushing on the thigh (figure 24.18).

Possible Substitutions: Rotating the body with movement of the thigh. The ipsilateral shoulder must be kept on the ground. If necessary, the arm can be placed outward, away from the side, to prevent the shoulder from rising up.

Notations: The stretch is felt in the lower back and lateral hip. The more the hip is flexed, the lower the stretch occurs.

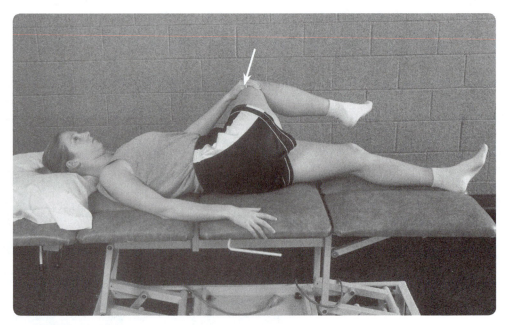

▶ **Figure 24.18** Lumbar rotation stretch.

Tensor Fasciae Latae Stretch

Body Segment: Lateral hip muscles.

Stage in Rehab: II.

Purpose: Increase flexibility of hip abductors.

Positioning: Standing with the affected side closest to a wall, about an arm's length from the wall.

Execution: Patient pushes the hips toward the wall, keeping both feet on the ground as the hand on the wall provides a push force (figure 24.19a).

Possible Substitutions: Rotating the body or flexing the elbow.

Notations: The stretch should be felt on the outside of the thigh.

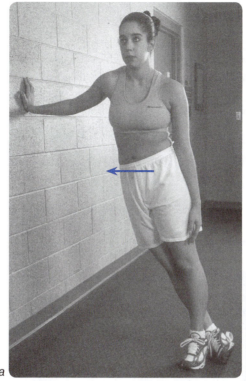

▶ **Figure 24.19** Tensor fasciae latae stretch: *(a)* standing stretch.

Tensor Fasciae Latae Stretch

Body Segment: Lateral hip muscles.

Stage in Rehab: II.

Purpose: Increase flexibility of hip abductors.

Positioning: In sitting, the patient has the uninvolved extremity out straight and the involved extremity flexed at the knee and hip; the foot of the involved extremity is flat on the ground on the outside of the uninvolved knee.

Execution: Patient uses the hands to pull the involved knee across the body toward the opposite shoulder (figure 24.19b).

Possible Substitutions: Rotating the trunk with the stretch or medially rotating the thigh.

Notations: Rotating the opposite thigh medially may stabilize the pelvis during the stretch.

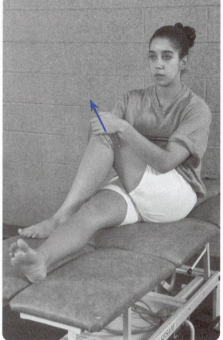

▶ **Figure 24.19** Tensor fasciae latae stretch: *(b)* seated stretch.

Tensor Fasciae Latae Stretch

Body Segment: Lateral hip muscles.

Stage in Rehab: II and III.

Purpose: Increase flexibility of hip abductors.

Positioning: Patient lies on the uninvolved extremity with the top hip extended and the knee flexed.

Execution: The top extremity drops down behind the bottom extremity (figure 24.19c).

Possible Substitutions: Rotating the trunk to place the top hip behind the bottom hip.

Notations: This position can be used as a prolonged stretch.

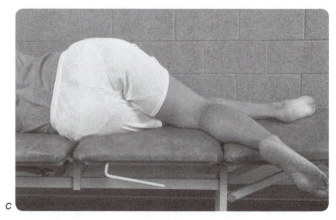

▶ **Figure 24.19** Tensor fasciae latae stretch: *(c)* side-lying position for prolonged stretch.

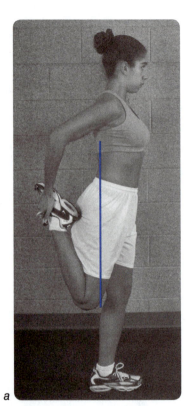

▶ **Figure 24.20** Anterior muscle stretch: *(a)* standing hip flexor stretch.

Standing Hip Flexor Stretch

Body Segment: Anterior hip muscles.

Stage in Rehab: II and III.

Purpose: Increase flexibility of the hip flexors.

Positioning: Patient is standing and grasps the foot from behind.

Execution: The foot is taken by the hand toward the buttocks while the knee remains pointing to the floor (figure 24.20).

Possible Substitutions: Trunk flexion forward or moving the knee forward of the hip.

Notations: To include the rectus femoris in the stretch, the knee is flexed. If the knee is extended, the iliopsoas will be the only hip flexor muscle stretched.

Kneeling Hip Flexor Stretch

Body Segment: Anterior hip muscles.

Stage in Rehab: II and III.

Purpose: Increase flexibility of the hip flexors.

Positioning: Patient kneels on the involved extremity, and the opposite extremity bears weight on the foot in front of the kneeling leg.

Execution: The patient transfers weight from the back knee to the front foot (figure 24.20b).

Possible Substitutions: Flexing the trunk forward.

Notations: The patient can apply additional stretch by attempting to flex the kneeling knee, although this can be a difficult maneuver. A pad can be placed under the knee for comfort.

Prone Hip Flexor Stretch

Body Segment: Anterior hip muscles.

Stage in Rehab: II and III.

Purpose: Increase flexibility of the hip flexors.

Positioning: Patient lies on the edge of a table with the uninvolved foot flat on the floor and the hip and knee slightly flexed to stabilize the pelvis.

Execution: A pillow or wedge is placed under the thigh on the table. The patient rests with weight on the elbows.

Possible Substitutions: Rotating the hip laterally or flexing the hip on the table.

Notations: Additional stretch is applied with greater pillow height or with flexing of the knee to lift the tibia off the table. This position can be used for a prolonged stretch (figure 24.20c).

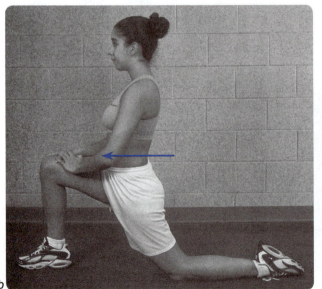

b

▶ **Figure 24.20** Anterior muscle stretch: *(b)* kneeling hip flexor stretch.

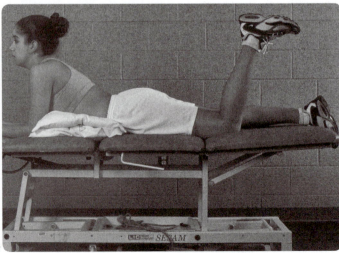

c

▶ **Figure 24.20** Anterior muscle stretch: *(c)* prone hip flexor stretch.

Thomas Hip Flexor Stretch

Body Segment: Anterior hip muscles.

Stage in Rehab: II and III.

Purpose: Increase flexibility of hip flexors.

Positioning: The patient lies with the buttocks on the end of the table. The uninvolved extremity flexes at the hip and knee, and the extremity is brought toward the chest; the position is maintained by the patient's hands.

Execution: The involved extremity hangs over the edge of the table so that the mid to upper thigh is at the edge (figure 24.20d).

Possible Substitutions: Hip abduction and hip lateral rotation.

Notations: The extremity alignment can be positioned and maintained passively by the clinician or with use of stabilization straps. This position can be used for a prolonged stretch. Weights can be applied to the ankle for additional stretch force during a prolonged stretch.

Adductor Stretch in Sitting

Body Segment: Medial hip muscles.

Stage in Rehab: II.

Purpose: Increase flexibility of hip adductors.

Positioning: In sitting, the patient flexes and abducts the hips and knees to place the bottom of the feet together. He or she pulls the feet toward the buttocks. In this position, the hands are on the ankles, and the forearms lie along the inner lower legs.

Execution: A stretch force is applied by the forearms to lower the knees (figure 24.21a).

Possible Substitutions: Flexing forward from the back. The back should be kept straight, with forward flexion occurring from hip flexion.

Notations: The long adductors pass below the knee joint, so they are stretched when the knee is extended; the shorter adductors can be stretched with the knee flexed or extended.

Adductor Stretch in Long Sitting

Body Segment: Medial hip muscles.

Stage in Rehab: II.

Purpose: Increase flexibility of hip adductors.

Positioning: Patient is in long sitting with the hips abducted and the knees extended.

Execution: The patient flexes forward from the hips, keeping the back straight, while placing the weight on the hands to keep the groin muscles relaxed (figure 24.21b).

Possible Substitutions: Flexing from the back and lifting the pelvis off the floor.

Notations: Additional stretch is provided to the long adductors by rotating to the affected extremity and reaching for the toes.

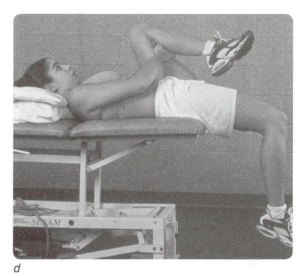

▶ **Figure 24.20** Anterior muscle stretch: *(d)* supine hip flexor stretch.

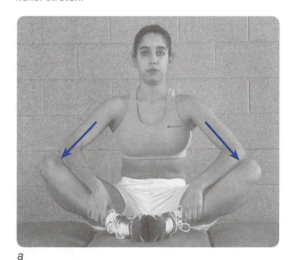

▶ **Figure 24.21** Medial hip muscle stretch: *(a)* sitting position for short adductors.

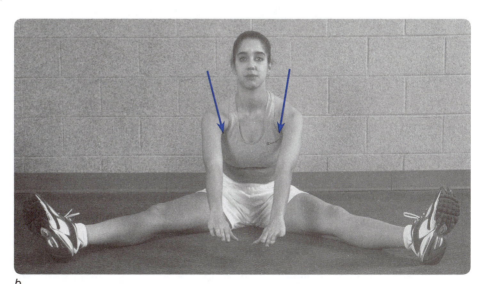

▶ **Figure 24.21** Medial hip muscle stretch: *(b)* long sitting position for long adductors.

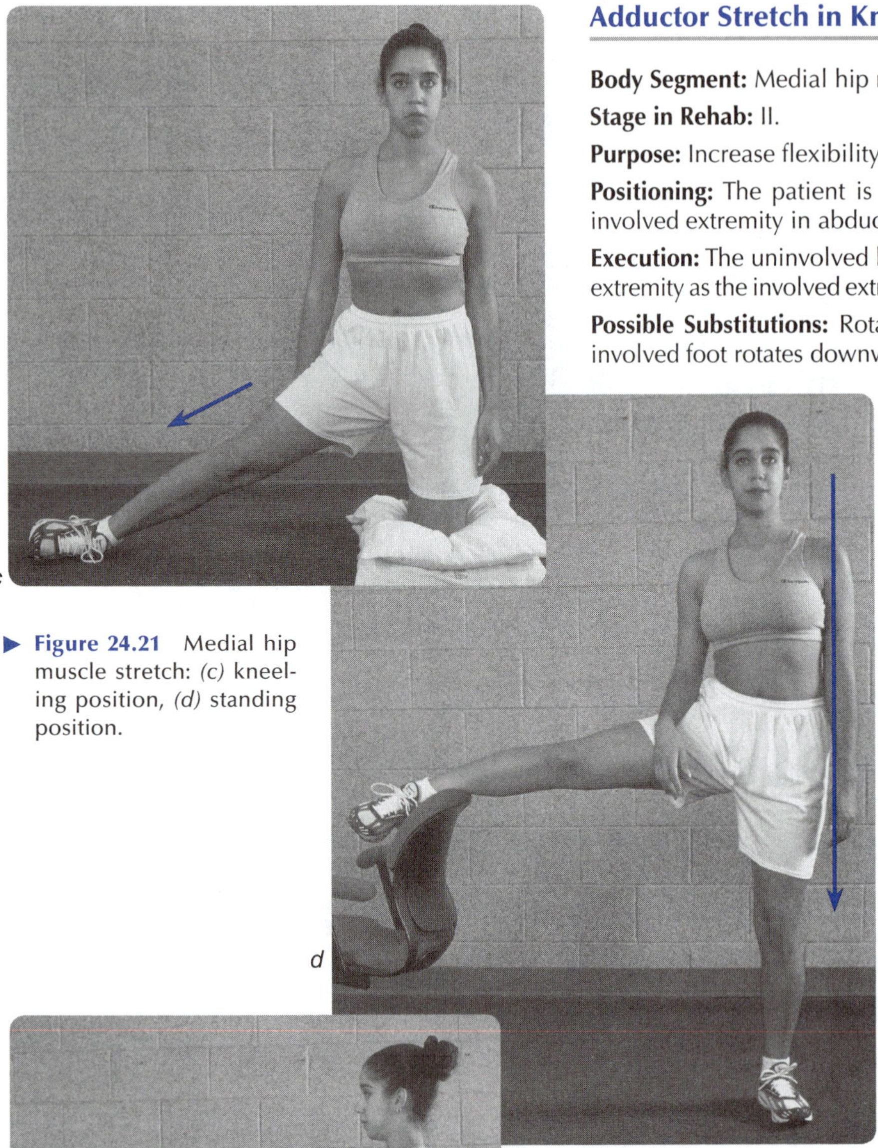

c

▶ **Figure 24.21** Medial hip muscle stretch: *(c)* kneeling position, *(d)* standing position.

d

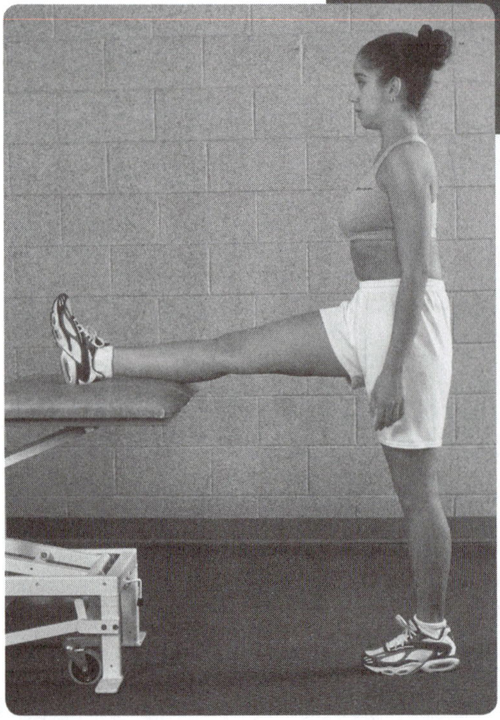

a

▶ **Figure 24.22** Hip extensor muscle stretch: *(a)* standing hamstring stretch.

Adductor Stretch in Kneeling

Body Segment: Medial hip muscles.

Stage in Rehab: II.

Purpose: Increase flexibility of hip adductors.

Positioning: The patient is on the uninvolved knee and places the involved extremity in abduction with the knee extended.

Execution: The uninvolved hip shifts laterally away from the involved extremity as the involved extremity is pushed downward (figure 24.21c).

Possible Substitutions: Rotating the hip so the inside border of the involved foot rotates downward.

Notations: A pillow can be placed under the supporting knee for comfort, and the patient can use hand support if needed.

Adductor Stretch in Standing

Body Segment: Medial hip muscles.

Stage in Rehab: II.

Purpose: Increase flexibility of hip adductors.

Positioning: The patient stands sideways to a supporting object that is about hip height and places the involved extremity's foot on top of the object (figure 24.21d).

Execution: Keeping the medial border of the foot facing downward, the patient squats on the supporting extremity while pushing on the involved lateral thigh.

Possible Substitutions: Rotation of the hip or pelvis.

Notations: A pad may be placed under the ankle for comfort.

Hamstring Stretch in Standing

Body Segment: Posterior hip muscles.

Stage in Rehab: II and III.

Purpose: Increase hamstring flexibility.

Positioning: In standing, the patient places the involved extremity on a supporting surface (figure 24.22a). The height is determined by the tightness of the hamstrings: The tighter the hamstrings, the lower the surface. The standing extremity should be positioned with the foot facing forward.

Execution: Keeping the back straight, the patient leans forward from the hips toward the elevated foot and reaches forward with the opposite hand.

Possible Substitutions: The standing extremity should not laterally rotate; the body flexes forward from the hips, not the back; and the opposite hand reaches forward to keep the pelvis from rotating.

Notations: This exercise isolates the hamstrings and prevents the pelvis from rolling posteriorly.

Hamstring Stretch in Supine

Body Segment: Posterior hip muscles.

Stage in Rehab: II.

Purpose: Increase hamstring flexibility.

Positioning: Patient is supine with uninvolved hip and knee in extension.

Execution: The patient places his or her hands around the posterior thigh and pulls the leg toward the chest to 90° of hip flexion and then extends the knee (figure 24.22b).

Possible Substitutions: Arching the back or posterior pelvic tilt.

Notations: The knee is extended until a stretch in the hamstrings is felt.

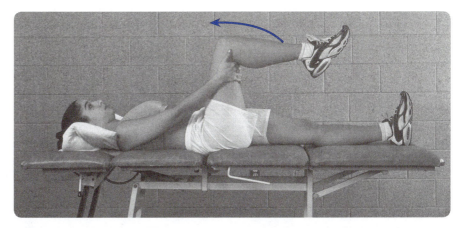

▶ **Figure 24.22** Hip extensor muscle stretch: *(b)* supine hamstring stretch.

Gluteus Maximus Stretch in Supine

Body Segment: Posterior hip muscles.

Stage in Rehab: II.

Purpose: Increase flexibility of hip extensors.

Positioning: Patient is supine as for the supine hamstring stretch.

Execution: As the patient brings the involved extremity toward the chest, the knee remains flexed (figure 24.22c).

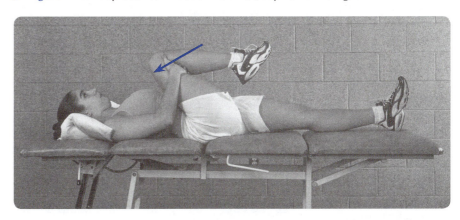

▶ **Figure 24.22** Hip extensor muscle stretch: *(c)* supine gluteal stretch.

Possible Substitutions: Posterior roll of the pelvis as indicated by the opposite leg's rise off the table.

Notations: The patient hugs the knee toward the chest until a stretch in the gluteals is felt.

Piriformis Stretch in Supine

Body Segment: Posterior hip muscles.

Stage in Rehab: II.

Purpose: Increase flexibility of lateral rotators.

Positioning: Patient is supine with knees crossed. The involved extremity is on top of the uninvolved extremity.

Execution: The knees are brought to the chest, and the patient pulls them toward the chest (figure 24.23a).

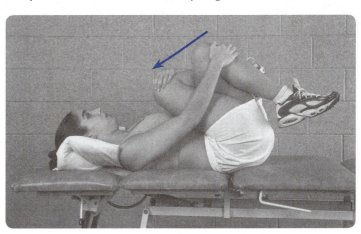

▶ **Figure 24.23** Piriformis stretch: *(a)* supine stretch.

Possible Substitutions: Rotating the pelvis.

Notations: The stretch should be felt in the posterior hip over the region of the piriformis.

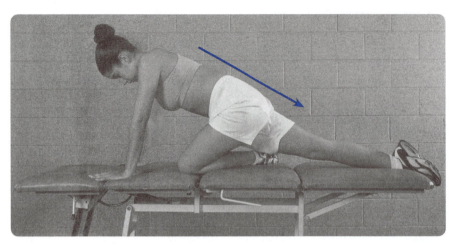

▶ **Figure 24.23** Piriformis stretch: *(b)* quadruped stretch.

Piriformis Stretch in Quadruped

Body Segment: Posterior hip muscles.

Stage in Rehab: II.

Purpose: Increase flexibility of lateral rotators.

Positioning: In a quadruped position, the patient crosses the involved extremity under the uninvolved extremity.

Execution: Patient leans the hips backward, keeping the uninvolved extremity's knee off the floor and allowing it to move back (figure 24.23b).

Possible Substitutions: Applying too much weight to the arms.

Notations: If there is a history of knee injury, this may be difficult for the patient to perform. This stretch permits the involved hip to adduct, flex, and medially rotate.

Piriformis Stretch in Standing

Body Segment: Posterior hip muscles.

Stage in Rehab: II.

Purpose: Increase flexibility of lateral rotators.

Positioning: Patient stands and rests the involved extremity's leg on a tabletop with the hip in lateral rotation and flexion.

Execution: The patient leans forward toward the tabletop.

Possible Substitutions: Rotating the body toward the stretch leg.

Notations: The patient's pelvis must remain square with the table.

Active stretches and prolonged stretches are used to improve flexibility in the hip's lateral, anterior, medial, and posterior muscles.

STRENGTHENING EXERCISES

As with other body segments, hip strengthening exercises late in phase II or early phase III may begin with isometrics that could be performed in various joint positions for optimal results. Isotonic exercises in phase III include concentric and eccentric exercises; these exercises use gravity as resistance for the least difficult exercise and advance to various other forms of resistance including manual resistance, weight cuffs, resistance bands, pulleys, and machines. Increased manual resistance and weight-cuff resistance are applied at the ankle. If less resistance is necessary, the same amount of resistance can be placed more proximally on the extremity.

The exercises are performed in a smooth, controlled motion of the hip through a full range of motion. Substitutions using other muscles occur easily in the hip, so the patient must be carefully observed and corrected as needed by the rehabilitation clinician. Low intensity, high repetition resistance is replaced with higher loads and fewer repetitions as strength and control improve.

Because the trunk, knee, and ankle are so intimately connected to the hip, strength, motion control and stabilization within each of these segments are vital to hip stability and performance quality. Exercises to satisfy deficiencies that exist within any of these parameters of any of these segments must be part of a total hip rehabilitation program. As exercises for these segments have been presented in previous chapters, they are not repeated here.

Isometric Exercises

The patient can perform isometrics independently against his or her hand or a stationary object. To perform hip adduction in long or short sitting, the patient places either the hands or a rolled towel between the knees and attempts to push the knees together (figure 24.24a).

Hip abduction isometrics are performed in sitting. The patient moves the thigh outward as he or she resists the motion at the knee on the lateral distal thigh (figure 24.24b).

Hip flexion is best performed while sitting in a chair. The patient places a hand on the distal thigh and resists attempts to lift the knee up. The patient should refrain from using the foot to push off the floor.

Hip extension is performed best in supine. The patient squeezes the buttocks to set the gluteals.

All isometric exercises are performed using a buildup to maximal tension. The tension is held for 5 or 6 s and then gradually released to full

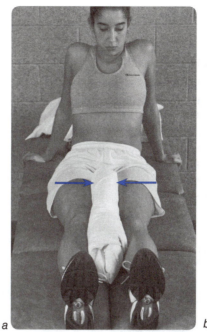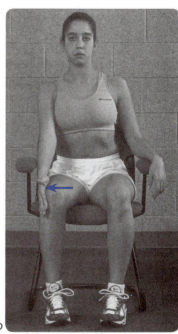

▶ **Figure 24.24**   Isometric hip exercises: *(a)* hip adduction, *(b)* hip abduction.

relaxation before the exercise is repeated. Isometrics are performed several times throughout the day in sets of at least 10 repetitions. They are used early in the rehabilitation program in either later phase I or early phase II when the muscle is very weak or when range of motion is limited either by immobilization or by restricted mobility.

Body-Weight Resistance Exercises

In a 68-kg (150-lb) patient, the lower extremity weighs about 11 kg (25 lb). This can be substantial resistance for a very weak hip muscle. Weight should not be added to the extremity until the patient is able to control movement against gravity through a full range of motion.

If the patient is unable to lift the extremity against gravity, flexing the knee to perform the exercise shortens the resistance lever-arm length. If antigravity exercises are too difficult for the patient, he or she can perform the same activity in standing; gravity affects muscle activity less in this position, but the muscle strength is still required to move the hip. Anti-gravity and other resistive strengthening exercises are presented in the following sections.

■ Strength Exercises for the Hip

Hip Abduction Against Gravity

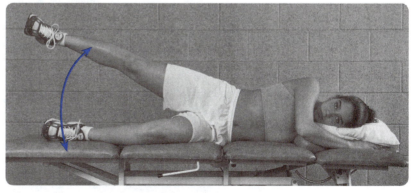

Body Segment: Hip abductors.

Stage in Rehab: Early III.

Purpose: Strengthen hip abductors.

Positioning: Patient lies on uninvolved extremity with the bottom hip and knee flexed for stability.

Execution: The patient keeps the top knee and hip extended and lifts the extremity against gravity (figure 24.25).

Possible Substitutions: Lying more on the back, moving the hip into flexion, and rotating the hip outward.

▶ **Figure 24.25**   Isotonic hip abduction exercise.

Notations: The patient may feel as though the extremity is positioned behind the body rather than in line with the trunk; this is normal.

Hip Adduction Against Gravity

Body Segment: Hip adductors.

Stage in Rehab: Early III.

Purpose: Strengthen hip adductors.

Positioning: Patient lies on the involved side with the top extremity flexed at the hip and knee and its foot placed in front of the bottom knee.

Execution: Keeping the involved extremity's knee and hip extended, the patient lifts the extremity against gravity (figure 24.26a).

Possible Substitutions: Rotating the hip, lying more on the back, and moving the hip into flexion rather than keeping it in the abduction plane.

Notations: If the patient lifts the fully extended top extremity into abduction and maintains that position while lifting the bottom extremity to meet the top extremity, the exercise is more difficult because greater trunk stabilization is required (figure 24.26b). An alternative position is with the top extremity placed on a supporting object such as the seat of a chair (figure 24.26c).

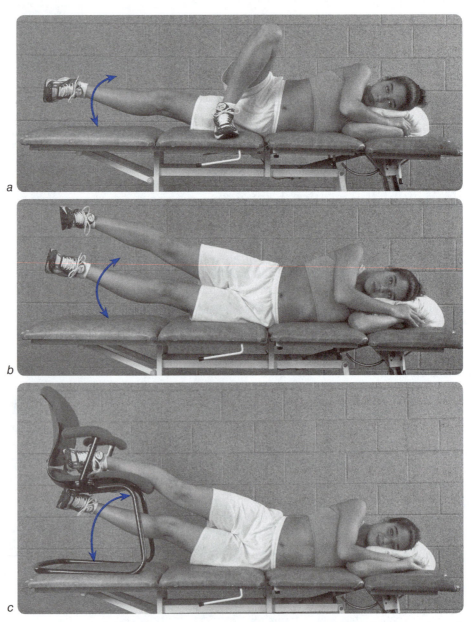

▶ **Figure 24.26** Isotonic hip adduction exercise: *(a)* without top leg support, *(b)* with additional requirements for trunk stabilization, *(c)* with top leg supported.

Hip Extension in Prone

Body Segment: Hip extensors.

Stage in Rehab: Early III.

Purpose: Strengthen gluteals and hamstrings.

Positioning: Patient is prone with the extremity either supported in extension on the table (figure 24.27a) or positioned in flexion with the leg off the table (figure 24.27b). If the patient lies prone with the extremity over the edge of a table, the hip begins in flexion and must travel through a greater range of motion.

Execution: The patient squeezes the gluteal muscles while lifting the extremity, keeping the knee extended to facilitate all hip extensor muscles. If the patient is to isolate the gluteals, the knee should be flexed; but remember that with a shorter lever-arm length, the resistance of the extremity is less.

Possible Substitutions: Hip rotation and trunk rotation.

Notations: Hip hyperextension is limited to about 15°, so when the patient begins in a fully extended position, the amount of motion the muscles produce is relatively small.

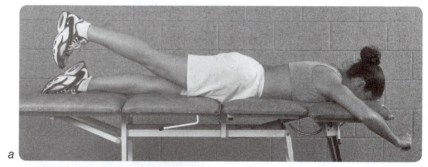

a

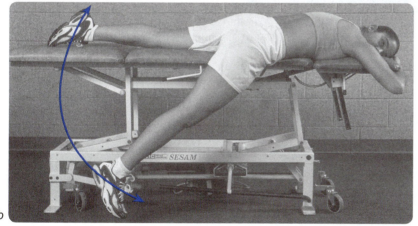

b

▶ **Figure 24.27** Isotonic hip extensor exercise: *(a)* prone on table, *(b)* over table edge.

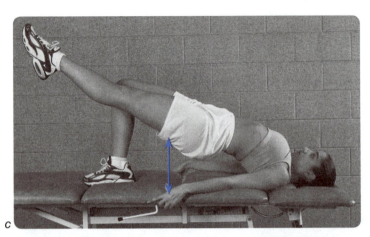

▶ **Figure 24.27** Isotonic hip extensor exercise: *(c)* supine.

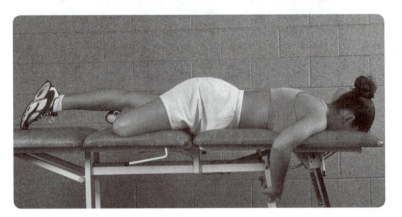

▶ **Figure 24.28** Figure-4 lift.

Bridge

Body Segment: Hip extensors.

Stage in Rehab: Early III.

Purpose: Strengthen gluteals, hamstrings, and spinal extensors.

Positioning: Patient is supine with hips and knees flexed and with the feet flat on the floor.

Execution: Patient tightens the gluteals. The hips are raised so that the hips and trunk form a straight line. The patient then holds this position for several seconds.

Possible Substitutions: Dropping the hips, moving them into flexion.

Notations: This exercise can be advanced to one-extremity support (figure 24.27c).

Figure-4 Lift

Body Segment: Hip extensors and lateral rotators.

Stage in Rehab: Early III.

Purpose: Strengthen gluteals and lateral rotators.

Positioning: The patient lies prone; the involved extremity is flexed at the hip and knee, and the ankle is under the uninvolved thigh. If the right knee is lifted, the face is turned to the left, and if the left knee is lifted, the face is turned to the right.

Execution: Patient lifts the flexed knee as high as possible (figure 24.28).

Possible Substitutions: Hip rotation or trunk rotation.

Notations: If the patient lacks enough flexibility for the position, he or she should place the involved extremity's ankle on top of the uninvolved extremity as proximal along the extremity as possible.

Straight-Leg Raise

Body Segment: Hip flexors.

Stage in Rehab: Early III.

Purpose: Strengthen iliopsoas and rectus femoris.

Positioning: Patient is supine; the uninvolved extremity is flexed at the hip and knee with the foot flat on the floor.

Execution: Patient tightens the abdominal muscles and quadriceps, then lifts the leg about 18 in. (about 0.5 m) off the floor, keeping the knee extended.

Possible Substitutions: Arching the back (prevented with abdominal tensing), hip rotation, and hip abduction.

Notations: The patient may be asked to raise the leg as high as possible, but as the leg is raised more, the resistance becomes less because the angle of the force of gravity changes.

Resistance-Band Exercises

Resistance bands or weighted pulleys can be used progressively once the patient is able to perform antigravity exercises through a full range of motion. In the descriptions of the exercises in the following sections, the involved extremity is used as the exercising extremity, so it is advisable to use upper-body support devices for balance to allow better exercise execution.

Resistance band exercises can also be performed with the resistance attached to the uninvolved extremity so that the involved extremity must work to support and stabilize the body during activities for the uninvolved extremity. When exercises are used with that goal, upper-extremity support is limited or eliminated to facilitate a greater effort from the weight-bearing hip. When the exercises are used for balance and proprioception, they can be executed as explained here or in the more challenging diagonal proprioceptive neuromuscular facilitation planes.

If the patient performs the exercise using a substitution pattern, correct the execution by providing verbal or tactile cueing (or both) or visual feedback with a mirror. If substitution continues with these corrections, the resistance may be too much for the patient to control properly; in this case, he or she should use the next-lightest resistance band instead. The motion should be full and should be controlled by the patient throughout the entire exercise.

Resistance-Band Hip Abduction

Body Segment: Hip abductors.

Stage in Rehab: III.

Purpose: Strengthen hip abductors against resistance.

Positioning: With the band attached to a doorway or table leg, the patient places the band around the involved extremity's ankle. The patient stands sideways with the uninvolved side closest to the anchor site and takes the slack out of the band.

Execution: Patient tightens the quadriceps and gluteals and abducts the extremity out to the side (figure 24.29).

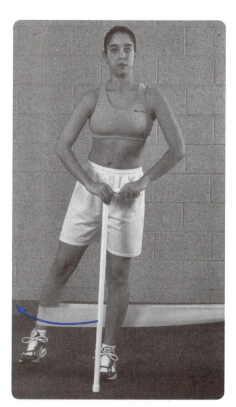

▶ **Figure 24.29** Resistance-band hip abduction.

Possible Substitutions: Moving the hip into flexion, using a forward lean of the trunk, side bending to the opposite side, and hiking the hip.

Notations: Once the patient performs this exercise correctly, it may be transferred to a part of the home exercise program.

Walking Abduction

Body Segment: Hip abductors.

Stage in Rehab: III.

Purpose: Strengthen hip abductors.

Positioning: A short-length band is wrapped around both ankles. The patient stands in a partial squat position with the back straight.

Execution: Patient takes a large step laterally and controls the opposite leg as weight is transferred to the front leg. This motion occurs to the left and to the right (figure 24.30a).

Possible Substitutions: Standing too erect, flexing the back rather than the hips, taking small steps, moving body weight over the weight-bearing leg rather than keeping it between the two feet, flexing the trunk too far forward.

Notations: If the patient is partial weight bearing or does not have the balance to walk during this exercise, he or she may perform it facing a wall with the hands on the wall for balance. In this position, the patient tightens the quadriceps and gluteals and extends the involved hip backward and outward to about a 45° angle.

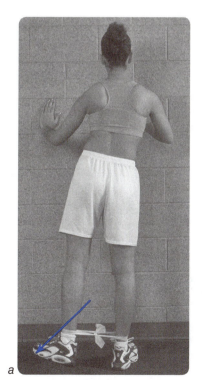

a

▶ **Figure 24.30** Gluteus medius strengthening: *(a)* with short-length Thera-Band.

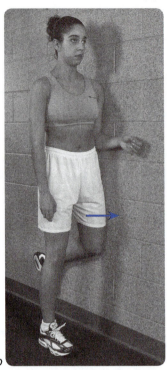

▶ **Figure 24.30** Gluteus medius strengthening: *(b)* The standing leg is the involved leg.

Standing Rotation

Body Segment: Hip abductors and lateral rotators.

Stage in Rehab: III.

Purpose: Strengthen hip rotator abductors.

Positioning: The patient is standing sideways with the uninvolved side about 5 to 10 cm (2-4 in.) from the wall. The uninvolved extremity's knee is flexed to 90° and the lateral pelvis, knee, and leg are pressed into the wall. The involved extremity is flexed slightly at the knee and should be in line with the ipsilateral shoulder and the second toe (figure 24.30b).

Execution: The standing knee rotates laterally while the foot stays flat on the floor and the pelvis remains stable.

Possible Substitutions: Rotating the weight to the outside foot, rotating the pelvis away from the wall.

Notations: The motion is very small, so the patient must be cautioned that the foot should remain entirely on the floor and the pelvis should stay in contact with the wall.

Hip Adduction With Resistance Band

Body Segment: Hip adductors.

Stage in Rehab: III.

Purpose: Strengthen hip adductors.

Positioning: With the band anchored around a table leg or secured low in a closed doorway, the patient places the band around the involved extremity's ankle and stands sideways from the anchor site, with the involved side closest to the anchor site, and takes the slack out of the band.

Execution: Patient moves the extremity across and in front of the uninvolved extremity.

Possible Substitutions: Trunk rotation as the extremity moves across the body, flexing the hip too far forward, hip flexion, knee flexion, and trunk lean toward the band anchor site.

Notations: Once the patient performs this exercise correctly, it may be transferred to a part of the home exercise program.

Hip Extension With Resistance Band

Body Segment: Hip extensors.

Stage in Rehab: III.

Purpose: Strengthen gluteus maximus and hamstrings.

Positioning: With the band anchored around a table leg or low in a closed doorway, the patient places the band around the involved extremity's ankle and faces the anchor site, taking the slack out of the band.

Execution: The patient tightens the quadriceps and gluteals and extends the hip (figure 24.31).

Possible Substitutions: Backward trunk lean and knee flexion.

Notations: Once the patient performs this exercise correctly, it may be included in the home exercise program. These muscles are usually stronger than other hip muscles and will require a more resistive band.

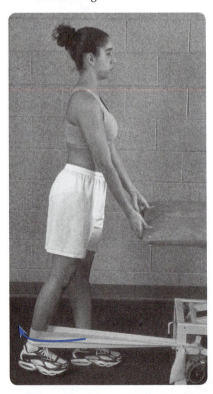

▶ **Figure 24.31** Resistance-band hip extension.

Hip Flexion Resistance With Resistance Band

Body Segment: Hip flexors.

Stage in Rehab: III.

Purpose: Strengthen iliopsoas and rectus femoris.

Positioning: With the band anchored around a table leg or low in a closed doorway, the patient stands with the band around the involved ankle and his or her back to the anchor site, removing the slack from the band.

Execution: Patient tightens the quadriceps, then flexes the hip.

Possible Substitutions: Backward trunk lean and knee flexion during the exercise.

Notations: Once the patient performs this exercise correctly, it may be included in the home exercise program.

Medial Rotation Against Resistance Band

Body Segment: Hip medial rotators.

Stage in Rehab: III.

Purpose: Strengthen hip medial rotators.

Positioning: The band is anchored between a closed door and doorframe about 30 to 45 cm (12-18 in.) from the floor. With the uninvolved side closest to the band anchor, the patient lies prone on the floor with the band around the involved ankle. The involved extremity's knee is flexed to 90°, and the slack is taken out of the band.

Execution: Patient rotates the hip, moving the band away from the anchor site (figure 24.32).

Possible Substitutions: Pelvis rotation rather than hip rotation; extending the hip during the exercise.

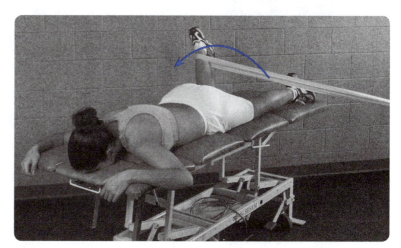

▶ **Figure 24.32** Resistance-band medial rotation.

Notations: This exercise may also be performed with the patient sitting in a chair.

Hip Lateral Rotation Against Resistance Band

Body Segment: Hip lateral rotators.

Stage in Rehab: III.

Purpose: Strengthen hip lateral rotators.

Positioning: With the band anchored as for hip medial rotation, the patient lies prone on the floor with the involved extremity closest to the anchor site and the band around the extremity's involved ankle. With the knee flexed to 90°, the patient takes the slack out of the band.

Execution: Patient pulls the involved extremity's foot toward the uninvolved extremity, keeping the knee at 90°.

Possible Substitutions: Rotating the pelvis or extending the knee.

Notations: This exercise may also be performed with the patient sitting in a chair.

Machine and Equipment Exercises

Many resistive exercises for the hip are the same as those used for the knee as discussed in chapter 23. Some additional exercises are mentioned here, but you should revisit chapter 23 for additional hip exercises. Some of these include step exercises, wall squats, mini-squats, the plié, lunges, sit-to-stand, and leg press machine exercises.

Reciprocal-Exercise Equipment

Reciprocal-exercise equipment can be useful for range-of-motion gains, strengthening, and coordination. These can be used early in strengthening work when the patient may not have antigravity strength but is able to tolerate resistance in an upright posture that does not require full antigravity strength. These exercises include activities on machines such as the step machine, ski machine, or stationary bike (figure 24.33).

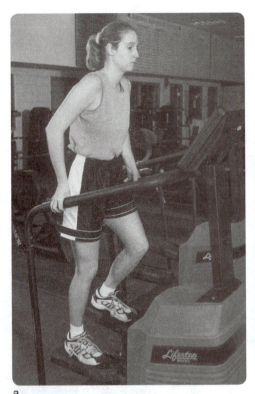

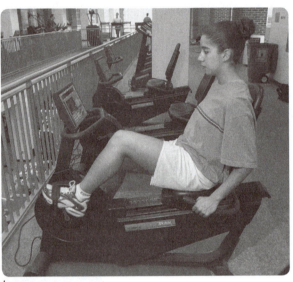

a   b

▶ **Figure 24.33** Reciprocal machines, such as the step machine *(a)* or stationary bike *(b)*, can be used to increase strength, ROM, and coordination.

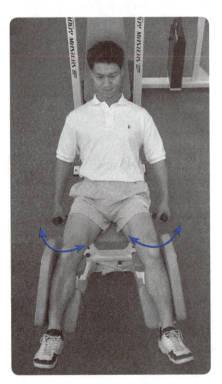

▶ **Figure 24.34** Isolated hip-motion exercises.

Resistance Machines

Machines are used primarily during phase III of the rehabilitation program. Machines have a variety of resistance mechanisms, including weights pans, hydraulics, rubber, and asymmetrical cam systems. They all provide progressive resistance for a variety of exercises. Resistive increments vary from one type machine to another. Although there are many machines on the market, only a few are mentioned here.

Hip Abduction, Adduction, Extension, and Flexion Some machines provide exercise for the hip only in one plane of motion while others provide resistance exercises in several planes of hip motion. In each case, the machine isolates one hip motion at a time and does not allow motion from other joints or other hip motions (figure 24.34). It is essential to provide instruction in the proper use of these machines prior to a patient's use. These instructions include correct alignment, proper weight selection that the patient can control throughout the motion, and precise execution without improper substitution.

Recliner Leg Press There are different models of leg presses on the market. The machines are closed-kinetic chain devices that utilize hip, knee, and ankle motions. The hip can be exercised in supine with the involved extremity placed on the platform so the knee and hip start the exercise at 90°. The patient pushes the extremity into extension so that the body moves away from the platform (figure 24.35).

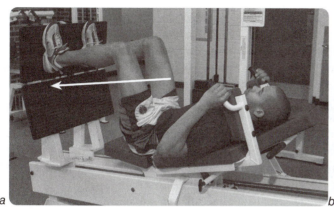
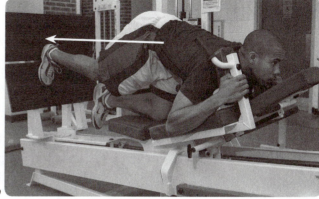

▶ **Figure 24.35** Recliner leg press exercises: *(a)* supine position, *(b)* prone position.

The patient can take an alternative position to further increase hip-extension activity. With the patient in a quadruped position on the machine, the involved extremity is placed high on the platform and the patient bears weight on the elbows and the uninvolved extremity's knee. The patient pushes on the platform to extend the involved extremity.

Free-Weight Squats and Split Squats

Barbells and dumbbells can provide resistance to squat and split-squat exercises. The patient is cautioned to keep good alignment of the knee and back in executing these exercises (figure 24.36). Weights should begin light and progress as the patient demonstrates control and adequate strength. These exercises are advanced with the patient standing with the involved extremity in the regular squat position and the uninvolved extremity on a box or step to place more resistance on the involved limb.

Swiss-Ball Exercises

Swiss-ball exercises can involve activities such as bridging with leg curls, first with both legs and then with the involved extremity only. This exercise facilitates the hip extensors. Hip flexor exercises on the Swiss ball are performed with the patient prone with hands on the floor and tibias on the ball. The patient pulls the knees toward the chest while maintaining balance on the ball (figure 24.37). Both of these exercises become more difficult when manual resistance is applied to the movement of the ball: The clinician's hands provide friction against ball motion during the exercise.

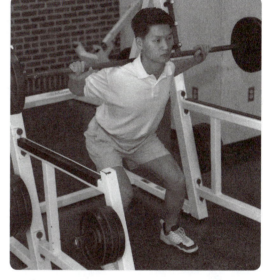

▶ **Figure 24.36** Squat exercise with free weights. Correct body alignment should be maintained.

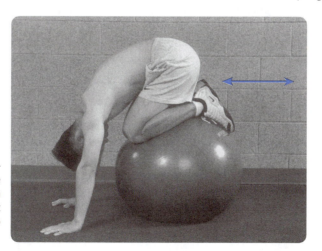

▶ **Figure 24.37** Swiss-ball hip-flexion exercise: With legs on the ball, the knees and hips begin in an extended position. The patient pulls the knees toward the chest to end in the position shown.

Strengthening exercises for the hip, which are analogous in their progression to those for other body segments, include isometric, body-weight resistance, resistance bands, machine, free-weight, and Swiss-ball activities.

Proprioception exercises for the hip progress from static balance activities to distracting balance activities, then to agility exercises such as rapid box exercises, and finally to plyometrics.

PROPRIOCEPTION EXERCISES

Balance exercises begin early in the therapeutic exercise program when the patient is able to bear weight on the extremity. As with other lower-extremity injuries, progression during phase II is from weight-transfer activities and gait training to stork standing with eyes open and then eyes closed. Balance begins with static activities and advances to distracting activities in which static balance is challenged while the patient performs other functions and dynamic activities. These can include the resistance-band exercises performed with the uninvolved extremity while the patient balances on the involved extremity on the ground or on a 1/2 foam roller; stork standing on a trampoline or BAPS board while catching or bouncing a ball; and using a balance board or other machine such as a Fitter or slide board.

As balance, proprioception, strength, and coordination improve, the patient progresses to agility exercises in later phase III that demand higher proprioceptive responses and control. These include resistive weight-transfer activities, exercises using increased speed of movement, and finally explosive exercises using jumping and plyometrics.

Agility exercises were introduced in chapters 22 and 23. Some of these include rapid box exercises such as rapid step-up-and-step-down activities, changes in direction from left to center to right box steps, and hopping over boxes.

Resistance bands can be used to increase resistance of rapid-direction-change exercises. With the band attached to the waist, the patient can be required to jump to different targets on the floor, change directions of movement, and alternate patterns of jumps. Some of these exercises are detailed in chapter 22.

Plyometric exercises maximize use of the patient's agility, strength, power, and coordination; these begin when the patient has demonstrated good control in rapid agility exercises and has good strength and adequate flexibility to perform the exercises safely.

Plyometric exercises such as drop-and-jump activities, lateral jumps, and cone jumps can all be used for all lower-extremity injuries, including hip injuries. These activities are discussed in chapters 9 and 22.

FUNCTIONAL AND ACTIVITY-SPECIFIC EXERCISES

A wide variety of functional exercises can be included in hip rehabilitation. Some suggestions for functional exercises include squats, step exercises, lunges, lateral lunges, cariocas, and stair running. The primary factor in determining which activity-specific exercises to use in a hip program is the patient's sport and position within the sport or the patient's work demands. If the sport includes primarily running activities, then those types of activities are included in the functional and sport-specific program. If the patient's activity includes rapid changes of direction, acceleration, and deceleration, then the sport-specific portion of the program includes those activities. If the patient's activity demands include squatting and lifting heavy objects up ladders, then those are added to the activity-specific program.

Speed, distance, repetitions, and difficulty of the exercises are at a low level at first and are increased progressively as the patient is able to tolerate the added stress. A continuous progression to activities that precisely mimic the demands of the patient's activity is provided, as long as pain and other deleterious signs or symptoms are avoided.

The patient may return to normal activity participation once he or she is pain free; has normal strength, flexibility, and agility; can perform equally on the left and right lower extremities without hesitating or favoring the involved extremity; and uses both lower extremities normally.

The rehabilitation clinician selects functional and activity-specific exercises for the hip, when the patient is ready for them, according to the patient's specific sport and position or work demands.

SPECIAL REHABILITATION APPLICATIONS

Although hip injuries do not occur as often as injuries of the ankle and knee, they can be just as disabling and need proper rehabilitation if the patient is to have a successful return to normal activities. Younger patients whose bones have not matured sustain more growth plate injuries in the hip than ligamentous or musculotendinous injuries (Mellman, McPherson, Dorr, & Kwong, 1996). Some of the more common injuries and dysfunctions of the hip and their rehabilitation programs are discussed next.

Muscle-Imbalance Syndromes

Many of the soft-tissue injuries around the pelvis, hip, and thigh result from muscle imbalances (Geraci, 1994). These syndromes are characterized by tightness of a muscle group and weakness of its antagonist and compensatory muscle firing patterns in adjacent areas (Sahrmann, 2002). The resulting symptoms typically include pain and reduced function and can cause structural changes. Changes in myofascial tissue are also commonly seen.

Hip Flexor Tightness Syndrome

This problem is common in gymnasts and dancers. Hip flexors are tight, and their antagonists, the hip and lumbar extensors, are weak and inhibited. This imbalance is characterized by an exaggerated anterior pelvic tilt and lumbar lordosis in standing. Lower lumbar spine dysfunctions including disc degeneration, spondylosis, spondylolysis, or spondylolisthesis can develop. Myofascial restriction is common in the lumbar paraspinals, quadratus lumborum, and latissimus dorsi.

Objective assessment findings demonstrate a positive Thomas test for hip tightness. In prone, assessment of muscle firing in hip extension reveals an asynchronous pattern. Normal firing sequence in prone hip extension is initiated by the hamstrings; next, the gluteus maximus fires; the firing sequential order is then the contralateral lumbosacral paraspinals, followed by the ipsilateral lumbosacral paraspinals, followed by the contralateral thoracolumbar paraspinals, and finally the ipsilateral thoracolumbar paraspinals fire (Geraci, 1994). Excessive scapular muscle firing is seen as a compensation for weak, inhibited extensor muscles (Geraci & Brown, 2005).

Treatment of this syndrome requires correction of shortened muscles, myofascial release of restricted soft tissue, correction of posture, strengthening of the weak muscles, and muscle reeducation to facilitate correct muscle firing patterns. When the antagonistic muscles are weak secondary to tightening of agonists, lengthening of the tight muscles often has a significant impact on positive strength changes in the antagonists. Pelvic stabilization activities and strengthening lower abdominals for pelvic support provide a base for posture correction. The use of electrical stimulation and instruction in muscle firing sequence patterns, beginning with slow sequences and progressing to more rapid firing sequences and finally to functional activities, can be helpful in muscle reeducation.

The patient can usually continue with some activities during the rehabilitation process, but he or she should be cautioned that performance may change as muscle firing patterns change. This can be frustrating for a patient who has adapted specific sport skills to compensate for imbalances.

Piriformis Syndrome

Buttock and leg pain are the most distinguishing symptoms of piriformis syndrome (Benzon, Katz, Benzon, & Iqbal, 2003). The leg pain can radiate distally into the thigh and lower leg, mimicking an S1 nerve root syndrome. Running, standing, or prolonged sitting can aggravate the piriformis. Clinical examination reveals tightness of the piriformis that is often accompanied by weakness. When the patient is relaxed in supine, the involved extremity is more laterally rotated than the contralateral leg. Palpation reveals tenderness, tightness, and soft-tissue restriction in the piriformis muscle. Active trigger points are often the source of pain referral into the lower extremity. Sciatic nerve irritation that occurs as the tight piriformis presses on the nerve can also refer pain into the lower extremity. The 15% of the population whose sciatic nerves pass through the piriformis muscle are more susceptible to this condition as the source of referred leg pain from the piriformis.

Common causes of piriformis syndrome include sacroiliac dysfunction; leg-length discrepancies; running on canted surfaces, creating a false leg-length difference; and muscle imbalances including tightness of the piriformis, hamstrings, and lateral thigh muscles.

Treatment includes correction of underlying causes, myofascial release and trigger point release techniques, stretching exercises, and strengthening exercises. The patient can usually continue sport participation during treatment. It is a self-limiting condition in that pain dictates the patient's ability to perform.

Acute Soft-Tissue Injuries

Injuries in this category include sprains, strains, and contusions. Traumatic bursitis can also come under this heading, but bursitis will be discussed in connection with repetitive stress injuries.

Contusions

Hip contusions are very common, especially in athletics. When they occur along the crest of the ilium, they are called a hip pointer. A hip pointer usually does not require rehabilitation unless it is severe and disabling. In these cases, the patient experiences a rapid progressive onset of pain within 24 h following the injury; this pain increase is the result of edema and spasm of the muscles that attach to the iliac crest. These injuries involve hip and abdominal muscles that attach or cross the contusion site, so activities that elicit complaints of pain include hip motions of flexion and abduction and trunk motions, especially resisted motions. Ambulation is painful, especially long striding and faster speeds. Ecchymosis becomes evident within a day or two.

Treatment includes anti-inflammatory medication and modalities during phase I of rehabilitation to absorb the ecchymosis, relieve muscle spasm, and encourage healing. The injury is self-limiting, primarily because of the muscle spasm and tenderness from the ecchymosis.

■ Case Study

A 25-year-old distance runner presents with complaints of right buttock and posterior thigh pain that has become progressively worse over the past three weeks. He has recently increased his distance from 6.4 to 9.7 km (4-6 miles). The pain occurs about 4.8 km (3 miles) into his run and remains. The patient reports that when he gets up from his desk after sitting for about 45 min, his right buttock is painful until he walks around for a few minutes. He had a back injury about five years ago that was treated, and he has not had any back problems since then. Standing trunk motions do not elicit pain in any direction. When he lies supine on the treatment table, his right leg is laterally rotated about 20° more than his left. Placing the hip in 60° flexion, adduction, and medial rotation elicits pain in the right buttock. Straight-leg raise is to 70° and negative for sciatic pain. Palpation of the right buttock reveals tenderness in the mid-buttock region to deep pressure. You can feel tightness in the piriformis. Resisted hip lateral rotation in this position is painful. Hip rotation is weak.

Questions for Analysis

1. What other tests should you perform to eliminate any other possible cause of the patient's problem?
2. What do you suspect is his problem?
3. What will be your first treatment for him today?
4. What instructions for home treatments will you give him before he leaves today?
5. What will your goals for the first week of treatment include?
6. What will you tell the patient when he asks you if he can continue running?

Range of motion with the aid of electrical stimulation can be useful in phase II in restoring early active mobility and should be encouraged within the first or second day of the injury. Ultrasound is helpful for ecchymotic absorption. Light resistive strengthening exercises should be possible by day 2 or 3 at the end of phase II and start of phase III, depending on the severity of the injury and pain level. Resistive exercises progress in phase III with increasing repetitions and resistance as the patient tolerates them.

Recovery depends on the severity of the injury; the quality of initial treatment in controlling the swelling, bleeding, and muscle spasm; and the timing of rehabilitation. With a moderate injury and appropriate care, the patient may return to full participation in less than one week, but more severe injuries with delayed care can disable the patient for at least a couple of weeks.

Groin Strain

Groin strains are defined as strains not only to the hip adductors but also to the hip flexors. The iliopsoas, rectus femoris, adductor longus, brevis, magnus, or sartorius may be involved. Most often, an adductor or the iliopsoas is the muscle injured. The muscle is injured when it is either brought beyond its normal limits of motion or produces a rapid forceful contraction. Pre-morbid contributing factors include muscle tightness, weakness, or imbalances. The injury is usually at the site of the musculotendinous junction and can be disabling in moderate or severe cases.

Since other injuries may mimic groin strains, differential diagnoses must be eliminated. Other possible conditions include osteitis pubis, stress fractures, avulsion fractures, and sports hernias (Lynch & Renstrom, 1999).

The patient has an antalgic gait favoring the injured leg, with an uneven stride cadence, shortened stride length, and reduced knee and hip motion. Muscle spasm, swelling, and tenderness to palpation of the injury site can also be present. Ecchymosis occurs in second- and third-degree strains.

Examination of the injured muscle includes resisted muscle activity tests to determine which motion produces the greatest pain response. Hip flexion with knee extension tests the iliopsoas; hip flexion with knee flexion tests the rectus femoris; hip flexion, lateral rotation, and abduction with resisted knee flexion tests the sartorius; and hip adduction tests the adductors.

Treatment in phase I includes modalities for pain control and spasm reduction. Electrical stimulation for muscle spasm reduction, along with assistive active range of motion and active range of motion, is used to regain lost range of motion as soon as possible. If the patient displays an antalgic gait, crutches are necessary until he or she demonstrates a normal gait. A hip spica wrap supports the muscle and reduces range of motion during ambulation to make walking more comfortable. Aquatic exercises and reciprocal-motion machines can be helpful in phase II after day 2 or 3. The patient begins with isometric exercises on day 2 or 3, and a gradual transition to phase III for a progressive resistive exercise program starts when the patient is able to move the limb in antigravity positions. Once the patient is able to transfer weight from one extremity to the other correctly, stork standing and progressive proprioception exercises are used to develop balance and, later, agility. Treadmill activities can begin when the patient walks normally without crutches; the treadmill progression starts first with walking, then jogging, and finally running. Agility activities on the treadmill can be used when the patient demonstrates good muscle control and range of motion with closed kinetic chain exercises towards the end of phase III. Soft-tissue massage is helpful in reducing scar-tissue adhesions and stimulating blood flow to encourage healing after day 5 to 10, depending on the injury's severity and the extent of tissue damage.

Resistance-band jumping, box drills, and lateral movements begin when good dynamic balance and muscle control are present in early phase IV. The patient advances to plyometrics, then functional, and finally activity-specific exercises prior to his or her return to full activity.

Depending on the severity of the injury, the patient's program may span from less than a week to several weeks.

Sprains

Ligament sprains in the hip are relatively rare. The joint is stable because of its deep socket and strong ligamentous support and does not succumb easily to outside forces. Hip ligaments can incur sprains when a violent injury involving severe forces occurs. The hip is placed in a position of combined extreme flexion, abduction, and lateral rotation or combined extreme flexion, adduction, and medial rotation during these events.

Grades I and II joint mobilizations can relieve joint pain following a sprain. The patient can do aquatic exercises in small arcs of motion initially, with progression in the size of the arc of motion as the joint responds. Therapeutic exercises for flexibility and strength progress as in other hip rehabilitation programs.

Other Conditions

These injuries are primarily overuse based and are the result of repetitive stresses applied at a rate greater than the body's ability to recover. Among the number of conditions that fall into this category are bursitis, tendinopathy, and osteitis.

Bursitis

The most common bursitis in the hip is greater trochanteric bursitis, but other hip bursae, including the ischiogluteal and iliopectineal bursae, are also subject to irritation.

If the patient's symptoms persist in spite of treatment efforts, other diagnoses must be considered. Additional diagnoses that should be ruled out include lumbar disc injury, facet syndrome, fracture, nerve entrapment, inguinal hernia, abdominal visceral diseases, hip joint disease, and bone tumor. Additional diagnoses for males are testicular torsion and chronic prostatitis.

Greater Trochanteric Bursitis The greater trochanteric bursa is susceptible to bursitis when the patient's running mechanics increases stress to the bursa because the person has a greater-than-normal adduction angle or is running on a canted surface. Muscle imbalance between adductors and abductors, an increased Q-angle, leg-length discrepancy, and a wider pelvis are also precipitating causes for trochanteric bursitis. Falling on the lateral hip can cause a traumatic bursitis. Pain in the lateral hip can radiate distally down the thigh or proximally into the lateral buttock. There is pain with lying on the involved side and crossing the legs, as well as during running or walking (Hammer, 1993).

■ Case Study

A 16-year-old sprinter injured her left hip when she was practicing three days ago. She has continued pain in the proximal inner thigh with some discoloration along the middle aspect of the inner thigh. She is unable to walk normally because of the pain. Your examination reveals hip abduction to 20°, limited by pain. The patient is unable to adduct the leg against gravity. Hip flexion is 4/5 but is not as tender as adduction. The inner thigh area feels tight and is tender to palpation from the middle thigh to the groin.

Questions for Analysis

1. What do you suspect is the patient's injury?
2. What other differential diagnoses tests will you do?
3. What will her treatment today include?
4. What instructions for home care will you give her today?
5. Outline the progression of therapeutic exercises you will provide for this patient. What modalities will you use with her and why?

The examination reveals tenderness to palpation over the greater trochanter, pain with hip rotation, and tightness of the ITB as demonstrated with a positive Ober's test. Resisted abduction is tender because of the pressure placed on the bursa by the contracting muscles. Passive hip flexion with adduction and medial rotation press the bursa against the greater trochanter and cause irritation. The patient may stand with the involved extremity more abducted or may place more weight on the contralateral leg.

Iliopectineal Bursitis   Dancers and skaters are the athletes who most commonly experience iliopectineal bursitis, although it can occur in most sports. The iliopectineal bursa lies superficially to the anterior acetabulum and deep to the iliopsoas tendon. Sudden flexion-extension activities, especially resisted motions, can aggravate the bursa. The bursa lies adjacent to the femoral nerve and can often irritate the nerve if it becomes painful and swollen. Pain occurs with either stretch or contraction of the iliopsoas muscle. The pain is located at the site of the bursa in the inguinal area, but it can also radiate into the hip, anterior thigh, or knee if the femoral nerve is also affected.

Ischiogluteal Bursitis   The ischiogluteal bursa lies between the ischial tuberosity and gluteus maximus. A traumatic bursitis can develop if the patient falls and lands on the buttocks, or it can develop over time consequent to prolonged sitting on hard surfaces or sitting with the legs crossed. Pain is present with hip or trunk flexion, stair climbing, walking or running, and sitting, especially on a hard chair. Palpation of the ischial tuberosity with the patient in sidelying reveals localized tenderness with occasional radiation into the hamstrings or hip.

Treatment   Ultrasound and thermal techniques are the modalities most commonly employed for hip bursitis (Gerber & Herrin, 1994). Anti-inflammatory medications are medically prescribed and provided either orally or by injection. Cross-friction massage reduces adhesions and pain (DeDomenico, 2007). Therapeutic exercises should include stretching exercises to increase flexibility of tight muscles and strengthening to correct muscle imbalances. Correction of underlying causes such as running mechanics and running surfaces is necessary and probably the most important treatment step in reducing the risk of recurrence. The bursitis injury is self-limiting, and although a modification of activity level may be advantageous, total cessation of sport participation is left to the discretion of the rehabilitation clinician and/or physician. The amount of activity restriction depends on factors such as severity of the injury, type of sport, intensity of participation, and correction of mechanics.

Tendinopathy

The adductor longus, iliopsoas, and rectus femoris tendons are the most common sites of tendinopathy at the hip (Micheli & Coady, 1997). Mechanisms of injury relate to overuse and can involve additional factors such as tightness, muscle imbalances, leg-length discrepancy, running on canted surfaces, increasing workloads too quickly, and incorrect mechanics. A gradual onset of pain in the groin (adductor longus) or inguinal area (rectus femoris or iliopsoas) is the primary complaint. The course of tendinopathy in the hip follows that of tendinopathy in other body segments, with a progression of pain into the patient's workout until daily activities such as walking and stair climbing are painful.

Examination reveals tenderness to palpation of the tendon. Crepitus may be felt. Stretching or resisted contraction can be painful. Flexibility is often reduced. Reduced stride length and diminished hip motion may be present in an antalgic gait.

Treatment follows the same course as for other tendinopathy conditions. Pain-relieving medications and modalities for pain control accompany therapeutic exercises. Stretching exercises and a graduated program of primarily eccentric strengthening exercises are used as exercises initially. Later, other types of exercises are added. Correction of the underlying causes is necessary to minimize tendinopathy recurrence. Cross-friction massage on the tendon reduces adhesion formation and pain. The patient's sport participation may require reduction during treatment, depending on the severity of the injury.

Osteitis Pubis

Athletes who are susceptible to osteitis pubis include distance runners, race walkers, dancers, fencers, soccer players and other athletes who place excessive shearing forces on the pubic symphysis by requiring multi-directional motion during single-limb weight bearing of deceleration activities. This is an inflammatory condition of shear stresses caused by either repeated trauma or strain on the symphysis pubis joint. Pain onset is gradual and localized, with occasional radiation to the abdomen or groin. Aggravating activities include pivoting, jumping, sprinting, kicking, and sudden direction changes. Daily activities such as stair climbing can be painful. Stretching the hips into full abduction is painful, as is resisted hip adduction.

Treatment includes anti-inflammatory medication, modalities for pain relief, and a gradual progression of therapeutic exercises for flexibility and strength as tolerated. The treatment progression follows that of a tendinopathy program. This injury is self-limiting, but an initial reduction in normal activity helps to improve the response to treatment efforts and reduce recovery time.

Rice Krispie Syndromes

Snap, crackle, and pop sounds in the hip, resulting from a variety of factors, occur most commonly in dancers and gymnasts, but they can also occur in athletes in other sports such as skating and running.

The ITB can be the source of snapping in the hip. The snapping occurs when a tight ITB moves across the trochanteric bursa during hip flexion-extension (Sammarco, 1983). The condition becomes more noticeable with medial rotation when the band is moved across the bursa. It can cause pain and result in irritation of the trochanteric bursa or the proximal ITB.

Another snapping malady found in dancers is the iliopsoas snap syndrome, which occurs when the hip is in about 45° flexion and moving into extension (Mellman et al., 1996). In this position, the iliopsoas snaps against the iliopectineal bursa and anterior ridge of the acetabulum (Schaberg, Harper, & Allen, 1984). Tightness of the iliopsoas or an anterior pelvic tilt can be the source of this syndrome, which can cause either bursitis or tendinopathy in the area if it persists.

■ Case Study

A 16-year-old male competitive figure skater has been diagnosed with right iliopectineal bursitis. His physician has referred him to you for treatment. The patient presents with tenderness in the inguinal area for the past four weeks. Over that time, the pain has increased to the point that it interferes with his practices. He is unable to lift his partner during their practices without intense pain. He also experiences pain throughout the practice, especially when he pivots, jumps, or lands on the right leg. During the past week, he has noticed pain extending down the front of the thigh. Your examination reveals pain with resisted hip flexion and stretch into hip extension. The patient has pain and weakness to resisted hip flexion. He has a moderate lumbar lordosis and weakness in the lumbar extensors, and his hip-extension firing-pattern test reveals increased scapular activity with mild to moderate gluteal firing last in the sequence.

Questions for Analysis

1. List other tests for all differential diagnoses that you should perform today.
2. What is your goal for treatment today and what treatment will you give the patient today?
3. What home instructions will you discuss with him?
4. What will you tell the patient when he asks if he can continue his workouts?
5. Outline your program for the patient for the next two weeks. What functional activities will you include in his program before full return to sport participation?

A clicking sound that accompanies pivoting movements may result from a torn acetabular labrum (Yamamoto, Hamada, Ide, & Usui, 2005). The pivoting motion of the femur catches the labrum when the hip is in extension. A torn acetabular labrum presents with a sharp pain into the groin or anterior thigh (Martin, Trapuzzano, Enseki, Draovitch, & Philippon, 2006).

Patients with the acetabular click syndrome should be referred to the physician for orthopedic examination and for diagnostic tests to rule out other diagnoses. Patients with either iliopsoas or ITB syndrome should learn proper stretching exercises to lengthen shortened structures, use stabilization techniques for proper pelvic and hip alignment, and strengthen muscles if imbalances exist. Deep-tissue massage can reduce adhesions, stimulate circulation, and reduce pain.

Fractures and Dislocation

Fractures fall into three main categories: traumatic, stress, and growth plate fractures. Traumatic fractures are not commonly seen in athletics because of the great forces required. Stress fractures, however, are more common. Growth plate fractures occur in younger athletes whose epiphyseal plates remain immature.

Traumatic Fractures

The traumatic fractures include avulsion fractures involving an apophysis to which a muscle is attached and non-apophyseal fractures that can include the pelvis or femur. Both types occur as the result of a high-energy violent trauma—the apophyseal fractures because of an internal force and the non-apophyseal fractures because of an external force.

Avulsion Fractures   Avulsion fractures occur because of a sudden, forceful contraction of a muscle that pulls the apophysis away from the bone; these injuries occur primarily in males from pre-teens to early 20s (Miller, 1982). The sites of avulsion fractures are at the origins of the hip's strong muscles. These locations include the ischium, ASIS, anterior inferior iliac spine, lesser trochanter, inferior pubic ramus, and iliac crest—the origin sites for the hamstrings, sartorius, rectus femoris, iliopsoas, adductors, and abdominals, respectively. The greater trochanter rarely is a site of avulsion fractures.

The patient has pain with active movement and attempts to shorten the muscle's motion during ambulation. For example, if the ischium is fractured, the patient ambulates with a shortened stride length and keeps the leg from moving very far in front of the body to reduce pull on the ischium by the hamstrings. Resistance against the muscle is more painful than stretching the muscle, but both elicit significant pain responses. The site is very tender to palpation, and edema and discoloration are present.

Treatment depends on the size of avulsion and its location. An open reduction and internal fixation may be necessary but often is not. Crutches with partial weight bearing to tolerance are used for the first three to six weeks until the patient is able to walk normally. Pain-free isometric exercises and active range-of-motion exercises are used early in the therapeutic exercise program in phase II. Modalities for modulation of pain, edema, and muscle spasm are used initially. Strength exercises progress from isometric to isotonic in phase III. Aquatic exercises can be used after the first or second week. Isotonic exercises progress as the patient tolerates them pain free, moving to antigravity resistance and weight-resistance activities as tolerated. When the patient is able to bear total body weight on the extremity during phase III, he or she can perform stork standing and other static balance activities and then advance to dynamic balance activities and agility exercises. From this point, the typical progression into phase IV includes plyometrics and then functional exercises before activity-specific exercises that precede a return to full sport participation.

Rehabilitation may take up to three months following an avulsion fracture. The time required for full recovery depends on the site of the fracture, type of treatment (surgical or non-surgical), and the individual patient's ability to progress.

Non-Avulsion Fractures Common sites of these fractures include the pelvis, acetabulum, femoral neck, and intertrochanteric femur. Fractures of this type, which are rare in athletics, cause significant pain. Most often, they require hospitalization and surgical treatment, especially if the fracture is displaced. The rehabilitation process is prolonged, a minimum of three months. During immobilization or after surgery, isometric exercises are used to reduce muscle atrophy. Other exercises and weight bearing may be delayed in comparison to the timing for avulsion fractures, but the program progression is similar.

Stress Fractures

Stress fractures occur most commonly in patients who suddenly increase their training intensity. This type of fracture is most often seen in distance runners and soccer players. The common sites of stress fractures are the pubic ramus, femoral neck, and subtrochanteric region of the femur. In patients with coxa vara, stress loads placed on the femoral neck may be increased, predisposing these individuals to femoral neck stress fractures.

The patient reports a sharp, deep, localized pain that is aggravated with jumping and running. In the early stages, rest relieves the pain, but as the injury progresses, the pain continues during rest. Nocturnal pain may also be present.

Treatment includes, most importantly, correction of the causative factors. Non-weight bearing or partial weight bearing on crutches is used for up to three weeks. Exercises on reciprocal machines such as the stationary bike or upper-body ergometer, pain-free open kinetic chain exercises, and aquatic exercises including deep-water running can take place early in the program during restricted weight bearing. Hip, knee, ankle, and trunk exercises should be included in the program. As the patient progresses to full weight bearing with a normal gait and without pain, he or she performs progressive closed kinetic chain and proprioception exercises to make additional strength, balance, coordination, and agility gains.

Growth Plate Fractures

Slipped capital femoral epiphysis is a displacement of the femoral head from the femoral neck because of a weakness in the epiphyseal plate. The approximate age range this condition occurs is ages 13 to 16 in boys and ages 11 to 14 in girls (Loder et al., 1993). It is seen in youths who have predisposing factors such as a recent growth spurt, an imbalance of sex hormones and growth hormones, and who are overweight or have a lanky build. The patient reports an insidious, gradual onset of pain in the groin that can refer to the thigh and knee in chronic slips. Less often, the patient experiences an acute slipped capital femoral epiphysis that presents with a sudden onset of pain and disability following a traumatic event. Pain produces an antalgic gait.

Examination reveals restriction of hip medial rotation, abduction, and flexion, with the greatest restriction in medial rotation. During active hip flexion, the hip also moves into lateral rotation. In a relaxed position, the leg is in greater lateral rotation than the contralateral limb. Hip abductors are weak.

Possible differential diagnoses with groin, anterior thigh, and knee pain must be investigated. Other possible diagnoses are fracture, tumor, hernias, strains, and contusions. An evaluation of the patient's history, hip motion, motion patterns, pain level, and strength helps the clinician determine other possible sources of the patient's pain.

Treatment includes open reduction and internal fixation followed by partial weight bearing for two to six weeks. Isometric exercises immediately postoperatively, followed by open kinetic chain exercises, are used early in the rehabilitation process. Aquatic exercises after the surgical incision has healed and the patient is still partial weight bearing are used to achieve range-of-motion and strength gains. Once full weight bearing is permitted, the patient continues to use the crutches until normal gait and hip control are evident. Stork standing and other proprioception exercises progress as tolerated when unilateral weight-bearing activities are permissible. The therapeutic exercise progression follows that for other fractures once the patient is full weight bearing.

Dislocation

Because the hip socket is deep and the ligaments surrounding it are strong, the hip is rarely dislocated in sports: a large, violent force is required to disrupt the joint. One may see dislocations in high-energy sports with large external force applications such as downhill skiing, soccer, football, and rugby. Rarely are orthopedic injuries considered medical emergencies, but hip dislocations are emergencies because of the risk of arterial damage.

Rehabilitation of hip dislocations follows up to three weeks of bed immobilization. During this time, isometric hip exercises and isotonic exercises for the knee and ankle are used to retard atrophy. Thera-band exercises for the ankle and knee are performed in bed several times throughout the day. Manual resistance exercises can also be used. Activities that put the hip at risk for redislocation include hip adduction, hip flexion, and trunk forward bending. For this reason, the patient must not cross the legs, sit in a chair with the hip at 90° to the trunk, or bend over from the waist for 12 to 16 weeks postinjury.

Once the patient is permitted crutch ambulation, usually partial weight bearing to tolerance, active range-of-motion exercises can begin. All exercises should be pain free and should not include motion beyond active abilities. The patient uses crutches for about 6 to 8 weeks postinjury, until he or she is able to ambulate normally and demonstrates good hip control. Closed kinetic chain exercises begin when the patient begins weight bearing, but hip flexion beyond 90° is avoided for up to 12 to 16 weeks post-injury. Machine squats, leg press, and other resistive machines for the hip are appropriate after week 12. Aquatic exercises can be started around week 8; however, swimming should be avoided until week 12 when the hip strength is sufficient to provide hip stability against the water's resistance; the breaststroke should be avoided until week 16. The stationary bike can begin at week 12 to 16; treadmill walking begins during week 10 and is performed without an incline until week 12. When the patient demonstrates good hip control, walking can progress to jogging after week 14 to 16. The patient transitions to running, then to agility and sport-specific activities as he or she makes further gains in strength, control, and coordination, usually anywhere from week 20 to week 30.

Acetabular Labral Tears

An athlete with complaints of hip pain that has not responded to treatment may have a labral tear. This sharp anterior hip, thigh, or groin pain may be accompanied by popping, clicking, or catching. The most common location of acetabular labral tear is seen in the anterior labrum (Farjo, Glick, & Sampson, 1999). If the anterior labrum is torn, pain will increase with hip extension. Whether or not the patient reports a previous hip injury, if the complaints include persistent vague, recurrent groin or thigh pain that is either sharp or dull and occurs primarily with activity along with reports of joint locking, the clinician should rule out a labrum tear (Binningsley, 2003; Burrnett, Prather, et al., 2006). The previously preferred method of treatment of labral tears was arthroscopic debridement (O'Kane, 1999). However, it is now realized how crucial the acetabular labrum is to hip stability, so now more physicians find it advantageous to preserve the labrum (Philippon, 2001; Robertson, Kadrmas, & Kelly, 2007).

Acetabular labral repairs are surgically managed using arthroscopy today. Either the labral tear is debrided or repaired. The most frequently repaired acetabular labral tears are the anterior and anterosuperior aspects of the labrum. If the tear is macerated rather than acute, debridement is the surgery of choice (Newman et al., 2007).

Labral repair patients remain either NWB or TTWB for up to six weeks. Immediately post-operative, rehabilitation treatments during phase I include the use of modalities to reduce swelling and pain. Ankle pumping exercises and knee motion activities occur within the first week. After two weeks, the patient moves on to phase II where PROM of the hip begins, moving to no more than 90° of flexion, 25° of abduction, and 0° of extension. PROM for internal and external pain-free ranges of motion with the hip in neutral flexion-extension can also be used during this time. Grades I and II joint mobilization may be provided for pain relief. Once the surgical wounds are healed, the patient is able to perform gait training in shoulder-deep water. Core exercises as long as the hip does go beyond the restrictive motions can also be performed at this time. After the third week, active motion exercises begin for the hip. Flexion is remains restricted to 90° and abduction to 25°.

At five to six weeks, the patient is in phase III and begins partial weight bearing and is full weight bearing by week 6 to 7. At that time, the patient transitions off the crutches and is able to ambulate without crutches when there is no extensor lag at the knee and the patient is able to ambulate normally. Stretching exercises become more aggressive but should not cause hip pain; the patient should feel the stretch in the muscles being stretched, not the joint. These stretches include flexibility exercises for the piriformis, iliopsoas and rectus femoris, and hip adductors. If necessary, joint mobilizations for additional motion are used. Proprioception static exercises also begin once the patient is full weight bearing. Strength exercises also become more progressive as tolerated by the patient. Resistance-band exercises for all hip motions, squats, lunges, side-walking with a resistance band, step ups, and bridging can be used to increase hip strength. The patient begins with high repetitions and low resistance and progresses as tolerated to increased resistance. At the end of phase III, more aggressive exercises include the leg press, open chain knee extensions with weight machines, slide board, treadmill walking.

Phase III begins post-operative week 9-12. By this time the patient should have full hip motion without pain. If not, aggressive grade IV joint mobilizations are required along with aggressive active stretching exercises. The patient now begins agility exercises such as Sport-Cord resisted walking exercises, jogging on the treadmill, and low-level jumps on a padded surface.

Phase IV, the final phase, begins at week 12-15. A this time, rotational movements are added to agility exercises. Agility then moves from rotational to rotational with jumping activities. Activity-specific exercises are then provided once the patient has completed all the agility and plyometric exercises. The patient returns to full and normal activities once he or she passes the specific criteria that have been established as part of the activity-specific pre-participation tests. This rehabilitation progression is summarized in figure 24.38.

■ Case Study

A 17-year-old female forward soccer player reports that she has had progressive anterior hip pain for the past four weeks. The pain has increased to the point that it bothers her on stairs and during walking and standing. She ambulates with an antalgic gait, using a shortened stride length and keeping the hip flexed and in a forward trunk lean. Your examination reveals tenderness to resisted hip flexion that increases with resisted knee extension applied simultaneously. Hip flexion is weak. Passive stretch of prone hip extension with knee flexion is more uncomfortable than hip extension with the knee extended. There is tenderness to palpation of the anterior inferior iliac spine, and pressure on this area reproduces the patient's pain.

Questions for Analysis

1. What do you suspect is the patient's problem?
2. What other differential diagnoses should you eliminate, and how would you accomplish this?
3. Explain what your treatment for her today will include.
4. What home instructions will you give the patient before she leaves today?
5. Outline the rehabilitation program you will place the patient on over the next two weeks. How will you decide when she is ready to resume full sport participation?

Start
rehab

Inflammation	Proliferation	Remodeling	
Phase I (inactive)	**Phase II (active)**	**Phase III (resistive)**	**Phase IV (aggressive)**

GOALS			
• ↓Pain • ↓Spasm • ↓Edema • Protect surgical site from excessive stress • Maintain conditioning levels (MCL)	• ↑ROM of hip to restricted limits • Reduce scar adhesions • Relieve pain/edema • NWB on crutches • No pain, spasm, edema • Protect repaired labrum	• Full ROM • ↑Strength, endurance gradually • ↑Proprioception • MCL • Good soft tissue mobility • Normal joint mobility	• Perform functional activities properly • Perform sport- and activity-specific exercises at least to preinjury levels • Return to full participation without pain, with normal strength, mobility, and execution of activities

TREATMENT			
• Modalities for pain and edema • Grades I and II joint mobilization • NWB 6 weeks • MCL exercises for conditioning with special attention to knee and ankle	• Begin PROM to: flexion 90˚, abduction 25˚, extension 0˚ • Soft tissue mobilization PRN • Strength exercises • Joint mobilization for pain • Aquatic gait training • ROM for hip MR/LR • Hip AROM after week 3 • Continue MCL exercises • Core exercises	• ↑ROM exercises PRN • Tranfer to FWB without assistive devices • Treadmill walking at 6 weeks • Grades II and IV joint mobilization if not full ROM • Add resistance-band exercises, lunges, leg press, side-walking, step ups, bridging at high reps, low resistance; progress PRN • At week 9-12 begin rubber band resistance, jogging, low-level jumps on padded surface • Continue with ME	• Add rotational motions to agility • Move to combined or more complex rotational and jumping exercises • Plyometric exercises after agility • Functional activities • Sport- and activity-specific exercises

▶ **Figure 24.38** Rehabilitation progression following an arthroscopic repair of acetabular labrum. ROM = range of motion; AROM = active range of motion; NWB = non-weight bearing; FWB = full weight bearing; PROM = passive range of motion; PRN = as needed; MR = medial rotation; LR = lateral rotation.

SUMMARY

Since lower-extremity stresses occur primarily during closed-chain activities, the hip's alignment, or misalignment, has an impact on other joints up and down the closed chain. A common problem in the hip is hip abductor weakness. Such a problem can occur as a primary factor that has been caused by an injury to the abductors or as a secondary factor caused by an injury to another segment. Regardless of the cause, the clinician must recognize the problem and correct it to reduce abnormal stresses being applied to other elements of the closed chain. Injuries to the hip do not occur as frequently as in other joints, but they can be disabling and require accurate assessment and treatment for sustained correction. Trigger point treatment, joint mobilization techniques, and progressive exercises from flexibility to functional activities were included in this chapter. Some of the more common injuries of the hip were presented along with rehabilitation programs for them.

KEY CONCEPTS AND REVIEW

1. Discuss how anteversion and retroversion change lower-extremity mechanics.

Normal alignment places the neck in a line that is 15° anterior to the line of the femur in the adult. If the angle is greater than 15°, the hip is in anteversion. If it is less than 15°, the hip is in retroversion. Retroversion and anteversion alter knee alignment and change the forces acting throughout the entire lower extremity. Retroversion results in frog-eyed patellae, or calcaneal inversion, and causes the individual to ambulate with a toe-out gait. Anteversion causes squinting patellae, or foot pronation, and causes the individual to ambulate with a toe-in gait. Anteversion makes the hip susceptible to dislocation.

2. Explain the mechanical factors involved in gait with hip abductor weakness and explain how a cane assists in normal gait.

When the person stands on the involved extremity, the abductors are not strong enough to counter the force of gravity pulling the non-weight-bearing hip downward and laterally rotating the pelvis, so a normal gait is not possible. The patient either drops the non-weight-bearing hip and downwardly rotates the pelvis to that side, or tilts the trunk to lurch over the weak hip during stance on the leg so that the center of gravity is closer to the fulcrum, the femoral head. If the center of gravity is moved far enough laterally to put it lateral to the fulcrum, the abductors do not have to work and the pelvis does not drop. If a cane is used on the side opposite the weakness, an upward force is transmitted through the cane to counterbalance the downward gravitational force on the same side. Because the lever-arm from the cane to the fulcrum is longer than the center of gravity's lever arm, the force that must be transmitted through the cane is relatively small.

3. Identify a joint mobilization technique for the hip and explain its benefit.

Medial glide increases hip extension and lateral rotation.

4. Identify a flexibility and a strengthening exercise for the hip.

Thomas stretch is used to gain hip extension. A resistance-band exercise moving into extension is used to increase hip extensor strength.

5. Identify a proprioceptive exercise for the hip and indicate its progression.

In a proprioceptive exercise progression for the hip, the patient stork-stands with eyes open, then with eyes closed, then on an unstable surface, then on an unstable surface while performing a distracting activity, and finally on the involved extremity while performing a resisted exercise with the uninvolved extremity.

6. List precautions for a hip-dislocation rehabilitation program.

Activities that put the hip at risk for redislocation include hip adduction, hip flexion, and trunk forward bending. Therefore, the patient should not cross the legs, sit in a chair with the leg at 90° to the trunk, or bend over from the waist for 12 to 16 weeks postinjury.

CRITICAL THINKING QUESTIONS

1. If you were Stevie in the opening scenario, how would you manage Joann's injury? Would you insist that she take time off from her performances; would you rehabilitate the injury as if Joann were not performing daily; would you treat the injury to keep it from getting worse until the season was over and fully rehabilitate it then; would you refuse to treat her unless she complied with your recommendations; or would you use some other approach? Give justifications for your decisions and explain your treatment program.

2. If a patient complains of anterior hip pain, what possible diagnoses will you need to differentiate before beginning a rehabilitation program? (Hint: Do a mental review of all the structures from superficial to deep.) What differences would there be in the rehabilitation programs for those diagnoses?

3. If a gymnast sustained an anterior hip contusion on the bars, what possible secondary problems would cause her to require rehabilitation? What would be your rehabilitation approach to these problems?

LAB ACTIVITIES

1. Locate the trigger points on your lab partner for the muscles listed below. As you perform each one, indicate what the pain pattern would be if the trigger point was active.
   a. Piriformis
   b. Iliopsoas
   c. Gluteus medius
   d. Gluteus minimus

   Where were your partner's most sensitive trigger points? Perform an ice-and-stretch technique on each of them and provide your partner with a home exercise for each tender trigger point.

2. Perform grades I, II, III, and IV of joint mobilizations on your lab partner's hip joint for any motion. Examine the joint's total range of capsular mobility in a posterior glide. Where does the joint's resistance occur relative to the entire joint's mobility? Is it the same for the other hip joint? How does your partner's joint excursion and point of resistance compare with two other people in your class? Of what relevance is this to your thoughts on hip joint mobilization?

3. Perform grades II and IV joint mobilizations on your lab partner's hip and identify what motion restriction would be best treated with each mobilization:
   a. Anterior glide
   b. Posterior glide
   c. Inferior glide
   d. Medial glide

   Which one was the easiest to perform? Which one allowed you to feel the greatest motion within the joint? Given the size of the leg, what accommodations did you have to make in order to manage the leg during joint mobilization treatment?

4. Check your partner's sequential firing pattern during prone hip extension. Looking at when these muscles fire, what is his sequence? What is the normal sequence? Compare your partner's sequential firing pattern with the opposite leg. Are they the same? What would you do to correct the sequence-firing pattern if it was abnormal? Why should an abnormal sequence-firing pattern be corrected?

5. Examine your partner's hip ROM for flexion, extension, abduction, lateral rotation, and medial rotation. What are the ranges of motion for each movement? What is normal for each motion? Measure medial and lateral rotation with your partner in seated and prone positions. Do you get differences between the two positions? Why?

6. Have your partner perform the TFL stretch in standing, sitting, and sidelying as demonstrated earlier in the chapter. Hold each stretch for 30 to 60 seconds. Observe and correct for substitutions. Which one did she feel the greatest stretch? What do you think is the reason for this?

7. Have your partner perform the hip flexor stretches demonstrated earlier in this chapter. Hold each stretch for 30 to 60 seconds. Observe and correct for substitutions. Which position created the greatest stretch for him? What do you think is the reason for this?

8. Instruct your partner in a piriformis stretch. Notice if she performs it correctly and give verbal cueing to correct for any errors. Reverse positions so you are now the patient and have your partner instruct you in a different piriformis stretch, correcting with verbal cues any errors in your performance. What kind of substitutions could each of you use in these exercises?

9. Have your partner perform each of the hip extension exercises in figures 24.27 and 24.28 for 20 repetitions. Which exercise was the most difficult? Why?

10. Using rubber tubing or bands that provide sufficient resistance, have your partner perform resisted hip extension and abduction, each for 15 repetitions. What are the substitutions he could use for each exercise? What verbal cues should you use to correct these errors?

11. Have your partner perform two different exercises for proprioception. Which one was the easier one and which one was more difficult? How could you make them each more difficult?

12. Have your partner perform two plyometric exercises and identify how you would determine when she has progressed in one to go to the next. What substitutions would you be looking for and how would you correct them with verbal cues?

13. A cross-country runner strained his piriformis three weeks ago when he slipped on wet grass running up a hill. He has noticed that he is limping and does not have the stride length he usually has when he runs. He reports that he has pain with sitting, walking, and running. Why do you think he continues to have pain three weeks after the injury? What do you think will need to be resolved before he is able to resume racing without pain? Describe a progressive rehabilitation program, including all types of exercises you would incorporate into the program. What would be your guidelines for progression throughout the program?

GLOSSARY

A band—The portion of the sarcomere where the thick filaments inter-digitate with the thin filaments.

ABCs of proprioception—Agility, balance, and coordination.

abduction—Lateral movement of a limb or segment away from the midline of the body or part.

absolute refractory period—The time immediately following a stimulus when depolarization prevents another response of the muscle cell from occurring.

acceleration—Rate at which velocity increases.

acceleration phase—That portion of swing in which momentum is increased and the non-weight-bearing limb has propulsion forward. Also known as *early swing*.

accessory joint motion—Necessary mobility for normal joint motion that cannot be voluntarily performed or controlled.

accommodating resistance—An activity where the resistance provided a muscle changes as the muscle moves through its range of motion. Isokinetic activity.

acetabulum—The socket portion of the hip joint.

acetylcholine—A neurotransmitter at the myoneural junction of striated muscles. Causes vasodilation.

actin—One of two primary proteins of the thin filament of the sarcomere.

action peak—The second ground reaction force peak. The peak occurs during the last half of support and is usually less than impact peak.

action potential—A brief nerve impulse created from a rapid change in the membrane potential to cause a muscle contraction.

active assistive range of motion (AAROM)—Range of motion that is performed with a combination of voluntary activity of the muscles and passive assistance from an outside source.

active range of motion (AROM)—The amount of movement produced at a joint by the patient without assistance.

active stretch—A stretch that uses the patient's active muscle force to control and provide the force for the stretch.

active trigger point—A trigger point that is always tender and that can produce referred pain whether the muscle is active or inactive.

activity-specific exercises—Exercises that include drills or mimic tasks found within a specific sport or job.

adduction—Lateral movement of a limb or segment toward the midline of the body or part.

adenosine diphosphate (ADP)—A phosphate compound that, when combined with a phosphate, forms adenosine triphosphate (ATP) for energy production. It is also the product of the breakdown of ATP during energy production.

adenosine triphosphate (ATP)—A phosphate compound that provides energy for muscle activity.

adrenaline—See *epinephrine*.

afferent muscle nerve fiber—A sensory nerve fiber from the muscle spindle and Golgi tendon organ. There are two primary types, A and C fibers. C fibers are pain receptors; A fibers are tension and length receptors. Group III delta are A receptors that responds to pressure pain. Group I are A receptors: Group Ia form muscle spindle primary endings and Group Ib form Golgi tendon organs. Group II are A receptors and form muscle spindle secondary endings.

afferent receptors—Sensory receptors that transmit information from the periphery to the central nervous system.

agility—The ability to control the direction of a body or its parts during rapid movement.

agonist(ic)—A muscle acting as a prime mover to produce a motion.

allogenic graft—a graft taken from one individual and transplanted into another.

all-or-none principle—A motor unit does not respond until the stimulus is sufficient to produce an action potential. The action potential produces a reaction from the entire motor unit.

alpha motor neuron—An efferent nerve from the ventral horn of the spinal cord to the muscle.

AMBRI—**A**traumatic, **m**ultidirectional, **b**ilateral, **r**ehabilitation effective, **i**nferior capsular shift required. A condition of non-traumatic shoulder instability that is multi-directional but usually responds well to the conservative treatment of rehabilitation.

amortization phase—The second phase of a plyometric activity that is the rapid transition from eccentric to concentric motion.

angiogenesis—Formation of new blood vessels.

angle of pull of a muscle—Angle formed by the muscle's line of pull and the line of the bone. Maximal isometric force occurs at a 90° angle of pull.

angular motion—Rotational movement on an axis through an arc.

antagonist(ic)—A muscle that opposes the motion of another muscle.

anteversion—Excessive anterior angulation of the femoral head, resulting in a toe-in gait.

apophysis—An outgrowth of bone where a tendon attaches, not fully formed in immature bones.

arachidonic acid—An unsaturated essential fatty acid. Works as a precursor in the production of substances, including leukotrienes, prostaglandins, and thromboxanes.

Archimedes' principle of buoyancy—Principle stating that a body partially or fully immersed in a fluid will experience an upward thrust of that fluid that is equal to the weight of the fluid the body displaces.

areolar connective tissue—Loose connective tissue with unorganized structure and relatively long distances between cross-links.

arthrokinematics—The motions between the bones that make up a joint, including roll, slide, spin, compression, and distraction.

arthroplasty—Joint replacement surgery.

arthroscopy—Use of an endoscope to examine or surgically treat the interior aspect of a joint.

assessment—A conclusion based on the gathering of information through an evaluation.

ATPase (adenosine triphosphatase)—Myosin enzyme that is a catalyst the body uses to break down ATP into ADP and phosphate for energy production.

atrophy—Wasting away of tissue with a decrease in size and strength, especially from lack of use.

autogenic inhibition—A protective mechanism provided by the Golgi tendon organ, in which a Golgi tendon organ stimulus facilitated by a sudden stretch causes a reflex activation of the antagonist and relaxation of the agonist.

autologous graft—a graft of articular cartilage and bone plug that is taken from the individual's same joint as the damaged cartilage, but it is removed from a part of the joint that does not bear weight.

balance—The body's ability to maintain an equilibrium by controlling the body's center of gravity over its base of support.

ballistic stretching—A rapid stretch or bouncing technique used primarily in sport activities but seldom used in rehabilitation because of the increased risk of injury.

Bankart lesion—Tear of the capsulolabral complex from the glenoid rim.

barrier—A resistance that is felt when a part is moved through its passive range of motion in muscle energy techniques.

Barton's fracture—A fracture of the wrist that occurs with a sudden, violent wrist extension and pronation.

base of support—Two-dimensional area that lies within the points of contact between an object and the supporting surface.

basophil—See *granular leukocyte*.

Bennett's fracture—A fracture of the first metacarpal.

body mechanics—The way the body is positioned and used during activity; correct body mechanics makes efficient use of the body's forces and lever systems.

boutonniere deformity—Deformity characterized by flexion of the PIP joint and hyperextension of the DIP joint.

boxer's fracture—Fracture of the metacarpals secondary to a compressive force.

bradykinin—A local tissue hormone that is activated by the interaction of proteases upon the Hageman factor. A very potent local vasodilator. It increases vascular permeability and stimulates local pain receptors.

brain stem—Includes the midbrain, pons, medulla oblongata, and diencephalon to form the stem of the brain between the spinal cord and cerebrum.

Brannock measuring device—Used to determine shoe size (length and width).

bursa—Synovial-filled membrane that lies between adjacent structures to limit friction and ease movement.

bursitis—Inflammation or swelling of a bursa.

callus—Fibrous matrix formed at a bone's fractured sites. Immobilizes the bone fragments and serves as the foundation for eventual bone replacement.

capsular pattern—A characteristic pattern of motion unique to each joint when a loss of motion is caused by capsular tightness.

carpal tunnel syndrome—A condition of the wrist and hand characterized by compression of the median nerve as it passes through the carpal tunnel.

center of buoyancy—The center of gravity of the fluid displaced by a body in water and the point at which the buoyant force acts on the body.

center of gravity—The point on an object around which its weight is balanced.

central nervous system (CNS)—The brain and spinal cord comprise the central nervous system.

cerebellum—That section of the brain that lies below the posterior cerebrum and behind the brain stem and is connected to the brain stem by paired peduncles.

cerebral cortex—The surface of the brain that contains primarily gray matter and nerve cell bodies.

cerebrum—The largest portion of the brain encompassing most of the skull.

chemoattractant—See *chemotactic factor*.

chemotactic factor—A chemical gradient. Also referred to as a *chemotactin* or *chemoattractant*. Occurs after an injury. Cells either become oriented along a chemical concentration gradient or move in the direction of that gradient. Example: Chemicals attract platelets, red blood cells, and polymorphonuclear leukocytes into an injured area.

chemotactin—See *chemotactic factor*.

chemotaxis—Movement of cells or chemicals in response to a chemical stimulus. Vital activities in wound healing that occur through complex and not totally understood processes.

claw toes—Toes that are extended at the metatarsophalangeal joints and flexed at the proximal and distal interphalangeal joints.

closed kinetic chain—Characterizing a motion in which the distal segment of an extremity is weight bearing and the body moves over the hand or foot.

close-packed position—The joint position in which the joint surfaces are most congruent with each other.

Codman's exercises—Low-level passive flexibility exercises for the shoulder that are performed by the patient. Also known as *pendulum exercises*.

cogwheel resistance—An abnormal response during muscle testing that is observed as a series of catch-and-release tensions rather than a smooth resistance, indicative of the individual's providing a less than maximal effort.

collagen—Major structure of the body's protein. There are five types in the body: Type I, the most abundant type, is high in tensile strength and is found in dermis, fascia, and bone; Type II is found in cartilage; Type III is found in embryonic connective tissue; Types IV and V are found in basement membranes. Forms inelastic bundles to provide structure, integrity, and tensile strength to tissues.

collagenase—An enzyme produced by newly formed epithelial cells and fibroblasts. Involved in the degradation of collagen during tissue repair. It is important in controlling the collagen content in a wound.

collar—The top rim of the shoe that is often padded to reduce friction on the Achilles.

Colles fracture—A fracture in which the distal radius proximal to the wrist is fractured and is displaced dorsally.

comparable sign—A sign produced by an active or passive movement or test that reproduces a patient's symptom, such as pain or protective muscle spasm.

compartment syndrome—A significant rise in intracompartmental pressure caused by severe bleeding within a muscular compartment that can compromise neurovascular structures.

complement cascade—Specific proteins interacting with one another in a specific sequence.

complement system—Various proteins found in serum. Act as chemotactic factors for neutrophils and phagocytosis.

concave-convex rule—Roll and slide occur in the same direction when a concave surface moves on a convex surface.

concentric motion—Dynamic activity in which the muscle shortens.

concentric phase—The third phase of a plyometric activity, resulting from the combined eccentric and amortization phases. The concentric phase is the outcome phase. If the eccentric activity has been quickly performed and the amortization has occurred rapidly, the concentric phase will produce the desired powerful outcome.

contact pressure—Pressure that occurs between two objects in contact with each other.

contractile components—Myofibrils, the portion of a muscle that actively shortens to produce movement.

contractility—The ability of a muscle fiber to contract.

contraction phase—That part of the mechanical response of a muscle twitch that follows the latency period during which the sarcomere's actin and myosin cross-bridge activity occurs.

contracture—Failure of a muscle to relax. Can occur after fatigue.

convex-concave rule—Roll and slide occur in opposite directions when a convex surface moves on a concave surface.

coordination—The ability of muscles and muscle groups to perform complicated movements.

coxa valga—Femoral neck angulation greater than 135°.

coxa vara—Femoral neck angulation less than 120°.

creep—Permanent tissue elongation caused by low-level stress applied over an extended period.

crepitus—A cracking or grating sound or sensation caused by inflammation or degenerative changes.

cross-bridges—The "head" projections from the myosin filaments that link the thick filaments to the thin filaments through a complex process.

cross-training—A process in which exercising the contralateral body part results in strength gains in the opposite extremity.

cross-training shoes—These are shoes designed to meet the needs of individuals involved in multiple activities. However, these shoes usually do not meet any specific need most of the time.

cycle time—In running, the time it takes to perform one step length. Also known as *stride time*.

De Quervain's disease—Tenosynovitis of the abductor pollicis longus and extensor pollicis brevis tendons and their sheaths on the radial side of the thumb.

deceleration—Negative acceleration.

deceleration phase—That portion of swing in which the limb slows down in preparation for making initial contact with the ground. Also known as *late swing*.

dense irregular connective tissue—Connective tissue consisting of collagen fibers arranged in a haphazard or disarrayed alignment.

dense regular connective tissue—Connective tissue with highly organized, parallel collagen fibers and more cross-links than loose connective tissue.

depression—A downward movement of the scapula.

direct techniques—Manual therapy techniques that load or bind tissue and structures, moving toward the point of limitation of mobility.

dislocation—Complete disassociation or displacement of one joint surface on another.

dorsiflexion—The sagittal plane movement in which the ankle joint angle is decreased as the dorsal foot is moved upward toward the anterior surface of the lower leg.

double-crush syndrome—A condition in which an injury at one site produces signs and symptoms at another site.

double float—The nonsupport phase in a running stride.

double-limb support—The point of the gait cycle that occurs at the beginning of the stance phase during heel strike for one leg and the end of the stance phase just before toe-off for the other.

downward rotation—A movement of the scapula that causes the glenoid to face downward and backward. The inferior angle of the scapula moves medially, and the scapula slides backward.

drag—The water's resistance to a body moving through it. There are three types of drag: form drag, wave drag, and frictional drag.

drug interaction—A reaction in which one drug either enhances or reduces the effectiveness of other drugs that are also being taken.

duration of drug action—Amount of time the blood level of a drug is at or above the level needed to obtain a minimum therapeutic effect. Determined by the drug's half-life.

dynamic activity—Activity in which movement occurs.

dynamic restraint—One of two systems a joint has for its stability. Dynamic restraints are the neuromuscular components that provide movement.

dynamic splint—Splint used to increase motion or limit unwanted activity. It incorporates springs, rubber bands, or other elastic elements to provide a continual low-grade passive stretch, passive assistive motion, or active assistive motion to an area.

dynamometer—A device used to measure strength.

eccentric motion—A dynamic activity in which the muscle lengthens.

eccentric phase—The first phase of a plyometric activity during which the muscle is pre-stretched as it actively lengthens in preparation for performing the activity. The slack is taken out of the muscle, and its elastic components are put on stretch.

early swing—The first part of the swing phase of gait.

eddy—Circular motion of water layers pulling against a moving object.

elasticity—An object's ability to return to normal shape or size after a deforming force is applied.

elastin—An essential protein of connective-tissue elastic structures. Arranged in a wavy orientation. The wavy arrangement allows tissue to change with stress and to resume normal conditions after stress removal. It plays an as yet unknown role in the remodeling phase.

electrothermally assisted capsular shift—A relatively recently developed arthroscopic procedure used in the shoulder to reduce joint laxity.

elevation—An upward movement of the scapula.

end-feel—The nature of resistance that is felt at the end of joint movement.

endomysium—Connective-tissue layer covering a muscle fiber and continuous with the muscle fiber's membrane.

endotenon—Tissue, continuous with the epitenon, that extends itself between the collagen bundles in a tendon.

endothelial cells—Large flat cells that line blood and lymphatic vessels.

endothelial leukocyte—A large white blood cell that circulates in the bloodstream and tissues. Acts as a phagocyte to remove debris from an injured area.

endurance limit—See *fatigue failure.*

energy—The capacity to do work.

engram—A memory trace of an activity accomplished through repetitive application of stimuli.

eosinophil—See *granular leukocyte.*

epicondylitis—An overuse injury to the tendinous attachments of the flexor/pronator group at the medial epicondyle or the extensor/supinator group at the lateral epicondyle. Also referred to as *tennis elbow.*

epimysium—Connective-tissue layer covering an entire muscle.

epinephrine—A hormone. Also called *adrenaline.* A potent stimulator of the sympathetic nervous system. It is also a powerful vasopressor, increasing blood pressure, stimulating the heart muscle, accelerating the heart rate, and increasing cardiac output. It also increases such metabolic activities as glycogenolysis and glucose release.

epitenon—The loose areolar tissue that surrounds a tendon and contains the tendon's blood vessels and nerves.

erythrocyte—An element of blood. Also known as a *red blood cell* or *corpuscle.* Used by the body for oxygen transport.

eversion—Outward-turning motion of the foot that causes the bottom of the foot to face laterally.

examination—Includes subjective and objective components by which a clinician determines the severity, irritability, nature, and stage of a patient's injury. It serves as the basis upon which a rehabilitation program is based.

excursion—Amount of movement from one point to another.

extensible—Able to lengthen. When muscle temperature increases, the muscle fibers and its connective tissue become more easily stretched.

extension—Straightening of a joint so that the two body segments move apart and increase the joint angle.

extensor lag—Inability to fully extend the knee during active motion, but full passive motion is present.

extracellular matrix—The basic material from which tissue develops. Produced by fibroblasts in wounds. Composed of fibers and ground substance. Serves as a foundation on which anything is cast.

extrafusal fiber—A regular muscle fiber. Also known as a *myofibril.*

extrinsic foot muscles—Muscles that provide function of the toes, foot, and ankle but originate in the lower leg and terminate in the foot.

extrinsic muscles—Muscles that originate proximally from the hand or foot and terminate within the hand or foot.

exudate—Material that escapes from blood vessels following an injury. It contains high concentrations of protein, cells, and other materials from injured cells. As polymorphonuclear leukocytes die and decompose, the exudate may resemble pus although no infection is present.

factor XII—See *Hageman factor.*

fast-twitch fiber—A muscle fiber, also called a *type II fiber* or *fast oxidative fiber,* that is lighter in color than a slow-twitch fiber and that reaches its maximum tension approximately 50 ms after being stimulated.

fatigue—An inability to continue an activity.

fatigue failure—The point at which the cumulative stress of a repetitive submaximal load results in tissue failure. Also called *endurance limit.*

Feiss line—A line from the tip of the medial malleolus to the first metatarsal head. It is used as a point of reference to determine relative position of the navicular tubercle.

fibrin—Insoluble fibrous protein. Formed by fibrinogen. Important in clotting.

fibrinogen—A globulin present in plasma. Converts to fibrin to form a fibrin plug at the injury site.

fibrinolysin—An enzyme in plasma that is released in later healing. Converts fibrin into a soluble substance to unplug lymphatics.

fibroblast—A connective-tissue cell. Fibroblasts differentiate into chondroblasts, osteoblasts, and collagenoblasts. They form the fibrous tissues to support and bind a variety of the body's tissues.

fibrocyte—An inactive fibroblast. See *fibroblast.*

fibronectin—An adhesive glycoprotein found in most body tissues and serum. Fibronectin is plentiful in early granulation tissue formation but gradually disappears during the remodeling phase. Fibronectins cross-link to collagen in connective tissue, thereby playing a role in the adhesion of fibroblasts to fibrin. They are also involved in the collection of platelets in an injured area and enhance myofibroblast activity.

first-class lever—A lever in which the fulcrum is between the resistance and the force.

first ray—The joint between the first metatarsal and the medial cuneiform. This is the primary weight-bearing ray of the foot and has triplanar motion.

fixation—A state of stabilization in which motion is restricted or prevented.

flexibility—Mobility of a body segment, dependent on soft-tissue tolerance to movement and the ability of soft tissue to move with forces applied to it. Flexibility can involve soft-tissue mobility alone or in combination with joint motion. Used interchangeably with *range of motion.*

flexion—Bending of a joint so that the two body segments approach each other and decrease the joint angle.

foam roller—Cylindrical therapeutic tool made of Ethafoam or polyurethane and used in rehabilitation in neurological, orthopedic, and sports medicine facilities.

foot abduction—The transverse plane movement of the foot in which the lateral foot is moved away from the midline.

foot adduction—The transverse plane movement of the foot in which the medial foot is moved toward the midline.

foot eversion—The frontal-plane movement in which the plantar foot rotates inward so that the medial border is lifted upward.

foot flat—That portion of the stance phase of the gait cycle in which the foot is flat on the floor. Also known as *loading response*.

foot inversion—The frontal-plane movement in which the plantar foot rotates outward so that the lateral border is lifted upward.

foot strike—Initial foot contact with the ground in running. The term replaces *initial contact* or *heel strike*.

force—A strength or energy that causes movement and has direction and magnitude.

force couple—Two equal forces acting in opposite but parallel directions to create a rotatory motion.

force deformation—The amount of force applied to maintain a change of length or deformation of tissue.

forefoot valgus—An eversion deformity of the midtarsal joint causing the medial forefoot to be lower than the lateral forefoot in non-weight bearing when viewed in the same plane as a perpendicular line bisecting the calcaneus.

forefoot varus—An inversion deformity of the midtarsal joint causing the medial forefoot to be higher than the lateral forefoot in non-weight bearing when viewed in the same plane as a perpendicular line bisecting the calcaneus.

form drag—The resistance an object encounters in a fluid, as determined by the object's size and shape.

foxing—An additional piece of the heel counter that is often seen in athletic shoes to further reinforce the rearfoot in order to help maintain the heel counter's shape.

free nerve endings—Small-diameter, unmyelinated afferent nerve endings located throughout soft-tissue and articular structures that perceive pain and temperature. They are nociceptors that are stimulated by pain and inflammation. Although they do not play a role in proprioception, they respond to any extreme joint position.

friction—Resistance to movement between two surfaces.

frictional drag—The result of water's surface tension. This is not a factor in therapeutic exercise.

frog's eye—Condition in which the patellae face outward in relation to each other rather than forward.

frontal (coronal) plane—Any vertical plane that divides the body into front and back parts.

functional evaluation—An assessment of the patient's ability to perform accurately and safely an exercise or skill drill before that patient is allowed to advance to the next level.

functional exercise—Activities that mimic the stresses, demands, and skills of the sport and advance a patient toward a safe and prompt return to sport participation.

gait cycle—The time from the point at which the heel of one foot touches the ground to the point at which it touches the ground again.

genu recurvatum—Excessive knee hyperextension.

genu valgus—Knee alignment in which the knees are angled toward each other. Also called *genu valgum*.

genu varum—Knee alignment in which the knees are bowed outward. Also called *genu varus*.

glycoprotein—One of a number of protein–carbohydrate compounds that are elements of ground substance. Includes fibronectin. Probably cross-links with collagen so that tissue is able to withstand pressure without harming tissue integrity.

glycosaminoglycan (GAG)—One of a number of compounds occurring mostly in proteoglycans. Glycosaminoglycans are non-fibrous elements of ground substance in the extracellular matrix. Examples: hyaluronic acid, proteoglycans. Different glycosaminoglycans have different functions—for example, stimulating fibroblast proliferation, promoting collagen synthesis and maturation, contributing to tissue resilience, and regulating cell function.

Golgi-Mazzoni corpuscles—These afferent receptors are located in joint capsules. They are stimulated by joint compression but not by joint motion. Any weight-bearing activity stimulates these slowly adapting receptors. They are not believed to play a role in proprioception except in identification of joint compression.

Golgi tendon organ (GTO)—A stretch receptor found in series within the musculotendinous structure. It responds to muscle contraction more than to muscle stretch to signal force.

goniometer—A tool used to measure joint range of motion. The device uses either a 180° or a 360° system.

goniometric terms—See *abduction, adduction, depression, dorsiflexion, downward rotation, elevation, eversion, extension, external rotation, flexion, frontal (coronal) plane, horizontal extension, horizontal flexion, internal rotation, inversion, opposition, plantar flexion, pronation, protraction, radial deviation, retraction, sagittal plane, supination, transverse (horizontal) plane, ulnar deviation, upward rotation*.

granular leukocyte—White blood cells, divided into three groups: neutrophils, eosinophils, and basophils. Among their functions are chemotaxis and phagocytosis, as well as release of histamine and serotonin to produce vasoactive reactions following injury.

granulation tissue—Newly formed vascular tissue that is produced during wound healing. Consists of fibroblasts, macrophages, and neovascular structure within a base of connective-tissue matrix of collagen, hyaluronic acid, and fibronectin. It has the velvety appearance of small, red, nodular masses seen in new tissue. It eventually forms the cicatrix of the wound.

granuloma—Hard mass of fibrous tissue. Occurs in chronic inflammatory conditions when the body produces collagen around a foreign substance to protect itself from that substance.

grasshopper eye—See *frog's eye*.

ground substance—Gel-like material in which connective-tissue cells and fibers are embedded. Part of the connective tissue or extracellular matrix. Reduces friction between the connective-tissue fibers when forces are applied to the structure. Adds to the area's density.

growth factor—A factor released by platelets and macrophages. Growth factors perform complex and numerous roles, including the stimulation of re-epithelialization, and are chemotactic for macrophages, monocytes, and neutrophils. The role of growth factors is not thoroughly understood but is believed to be important throughout tissue repair. Also referred to as *growth hormone factor*.

H band—That portion of the sarcomere that contains only thick filaments.

Hageman factor—An enzyme present in the blood. It initiates the blood coagulation process by converting prothrombin to thrombin following trauma to an area.

half-life—Amount of time it takes for the level of a drug in the bloodstream to diminish by one half. Determines the frequency with which a medication is taken.

hallux valgus—A condition also known as a *bunion*. Present when the first metatarsophalangeal joint is greater than 10° in valgus, so that the first toe points laterally toward the other toes.

hammertoe—Condition in which the toe is extended at the metatarso-phalangeal joint, flexed at the proximal interphalangeal joint, and extended at the distal interphalangeal joint.

heel counter—The portion of a shoe that circles the calcaneus and serves as an important rearfoot stabilizer.

heel-off—The portion of the stance phase of the gait cycle in which the weight begins to transfer to the front of the foot and the heel is lifted off the floor. Also known as *terminal stance*.

heel strike—The portion of the stance phase of the gait cycle in which the heel first comes in contact with the floor. Also known as *initial contact*.

hemiarthroplasty—A joint replacement surgery in which only half of the joint is replaced.

hip pointer—a contusion along the iliac crest.

histamine—A local tissue hormone released by mast cells and granulo-cytes. Increases vascular permeability to proteins and fibronectin.

Hooke's law—Law stating that the stress applied to a body to deform it is proportional to the strain as long as the body's elasticity limit is not exceeded.

horizontal extension—A motion of the upper extremity in a transverse plane away from the midline of the body. Also called *horizontal abduction*.

horizontal flexion—A motion of the upper extremity in a transverse plane toward the midline of the body. Also called *horizontal adduction*.

hyaluronic acid—See *glycosaminoglycan*. A major component of early granulation tissue. Greatest amounts are seen in a wound during the first four to five days. Promotes cell movement and migration during repair. Stimulates fibroblast proliferation. Produces edema by absorbing large amounts of water to increase fibroblast migration.

hypertrophy—An increase in muscle bulk from an increase in size of the muscle fibers, not the number of muscle fibers. Hypertrophy occurs with strength gains.

hysteresis—The process of tissue lengthening that results when the tissue is unable to withstand forces that are progressively applied to it.

I band—The portion of the sarcomere that contains only thin filaments.

impact peak—The ground reaction force that is a rapid peak occurring very quickly with impact at the foot's initial contact with the ground.

indirect techniques—Manual therapy techniques that move tissue away from the direction of limitation.

inertia—The tendency of an object at rest or in uniform motion to remain in that state until an external force is applied. See also *Newton's first law of motion*.

inflare—A pelvic girdle dysfunction in which the iliosacral joint is medially rotated.

inhibition—Transmission of an impulse that results in the cessation or decrease of an activity.

initial contact—See *heel strike*.

initial swing—The portion of the swing phase that includes early swing and acceleration.

insole board—The part of a shoe that lies between the upper and lower segments and that serves as the attachment for the two segments. Also called *last*.

internuncial neuron—A neuron that is interposed between two other neurons. The transmission rate for messages that use this type of neuron is slower than that for monosynaptic transmission.

intrafusal muscle fiber—Modified muscle fiber that lies within a muscle spindle. The two types of muscle fibers are nuclear bag fibers and nuclear-chain fibers.

intrinsic foot muscles—Muscles that control the foot and toes and originate and terminate within the foot.

intrinsic muscles—Muscles that originate and terminate within the hand or foot.

inversion—An inward-turning motion of the foot that causes the bottom of the foot to face medially.

irritability—The amount of stimulation that is required to initiate a response, such as pain.

isokinetic—Characterizing a dynamic activity in which the velocity of movement remains the same and the resistance varies.

isometric—Characterizing an activity produced when muscle tension is created without a change in the muscle's length. An isometric activity is a static activity.

isotonic—Characterizing an activity during which a muscle's length changes.

joint reaction force—Forces that are transmitted from one segment to another through the connecting joint.

jump sign—A reflex response to a trigger point palpation that includes a wincing or withdrawal reaction by the patient.

juncturae tendinum—A fibrous band that limits independent motion of the extensor tendons of the hand.

kallikrein—A proteolytic enzyme found in blood plasma, lymph, and other exocrine secretions. Activated by the Hageman factor. Forms kinins and activates plasminogen, a precursor of plasmin. Increases vascular permeability and vasodilation.

kinetic energy—Energy that a body has because of its motion.

kinin—A generic term for polypeptides related to bradykinin. Kinins are potent local tissue hormones and are found in injured-tissue, released from plasma proteins. Examples: bradykinin, kallidin. Kinins mediate the classic signs of inflammation. Their action in the microvascular system is similar to that of histamine and serotonin in the early inflammation phase to cause increased microvascular permeability.

lactic acid—A by-product of muscle activity that leads to fatigue by reducing the muscle's calcium-binding capacity and impairing glycogen breakdown.

last—An important component of a shoe that determines the shoe's shape, size, style, and fit. It can be straight or curved. A shoe is constructed around a last that can be formed as a board last, slip last, or combination last.

latent trigger point—A trigger point that is painful only when it is palpated.

lateral rotation (LR)—Rotation of a joint around its axis away from the body's midline. Also inaccurately referred to as external rotation.

leukocyte—White blood cell or corpuscle. Types include polymorphonuclear leukocytes and mononuclear cells. These cells have notable phagocytic properties for removal of debris from an injury site.

leukotriene—A compound formed from arachidonic acid. Leukotrienes regulate inflammatory reactions. Some stimulate the movement of leukocytes into the area.

lever—A simple machine with a rigid bar and a fulcrum.

lever arm—The length of the distance from where a force is applied to the axis of motion.

linear motion—Movement in a straight line.

line of gravity—Imaginary line through an object's center of gravity to the center of the earth.

line of pull of a muscle—The long axis of the muscle along which it exerts force.

lipid—A heterogeneous group of fats and fatlike substances, including fatty acids and steroids. Lipids serve as a source of fuel and are important to the structure and makeup of cells.

Little League elbow—A valgus traction force injury of the medial elbow that may start out as an inflammatory response or apophysitis and progress to an avulsion of the apophysis if the repetitive stress continues.

loading response—See *foot flat*.

local twitch response—An involuntary contraction of the muscle fibers in response to the snapping palpation.

loose-packed position—A joint position in which there is not complete congruency of joint surfaces with each other. Also called *open-packed position*. A joint demonstrates its greatest laxity in a loose-packed position.

lordosis—Excessive anterior convexity of the cervical and lumbar spine.

lymphocyte—A non-phagocytic leukocyte found in blood and lymph. These cells serve as important structures in the body's immune system by producing antibodies.

M band—The center of the A band where the thick filaments are attached.

macrophages—Mononuclear phagocytes that arise from stem cells in bone marrow. Considered one of the regulators of the repair process. They serve to phagocytize injury areas of debris, kill microorganisms, and secrete substances into an injury site, including enzymes, fibronectin, and coagulation factors. They play a role in keeping the inflammatory process localized and enhance collagen deposition and fibroblast proliferation.

mallet deformity—Avulsion of the extensor digitorum longus from the distal phalanx. Also known as *baseball finger*.

manipulation—Passive joint movement used to increase joint mobility. It incorporates a sudden, forceful thrust that is beyond the patient's control.

manual muscle test—An evaluation technique that uses manual resistance against a muscle or muscle group to provide a grade for that muscle or muscle group. Muscle grades range from 0 (zero) to 5 (normal).

manual therapy—The use of hands-on techniques for evaluating, treating, and improving the status of neuromusculoskeletal conditions.

massage—Manual manipulation of soft tissue to effect changes in the neuromuscular, lymph, cardiovascular, and connective-tissue systems.

mast cells—Connective-tissue cells. Also referred to as *mastocytes* and *labrocytes*. Store and produce various mediators of inflammation. Through their release of histamine, enzymes, and other mediators, mast cells cause increased local blood flow, attract immune cells, stimulate cell production of fibroblasts and endothelial cells, and promote and control remodeling of extracellular matrix.

matrix—Substance of a tissue. Can refer to intracellular or extra-cellular structure. Forms the basis from which a structure develops.

medial rotation (MR)—Rotation of a joint around its axis toward the midline of the body. Also incorrectly referred to as internal rotation.

Meissner's corpuscles—Sensory nerve endings that transmit light-touch sensation.

midsole—The middle portion of a shoe's outer sole that can be composed of a variety of substances. It can also include a wedge. The midsole provides shock attenuation, stability, and control.

midstance—The portion of the stance phase of the gait cycle in which the foot is directly under the body's weight and the entire foot is in contact with the floor. Also known as *single-leg support*.

mitochondria—Organelles of a cell that are the primary energy source for the cell and that contain the enzyme used to metabolize lactic acid for energy to form adenosine triphosphate.

mobilization—Passive joint movement for increasing joint mobility or reducing pain. The applied force is light enough that the patient can stop the movement at any time.

modality—A physical agent used to relieve pain, improve circulation, reduce spasm, and promote healing.

moment arm—A length measure equivalent to lever arm. Moment arm rather than lever arm is used when discussing torque and rotational forces. Moment arm length is the perpendicular distance from the rotational axis of motion to the line of force application.

momentum—Amount of motion that a moving object has.

monocyte—Mononuclear phagocytic leukocyte. Monocytes are formed in the bone marrow and transported to tissues to become macrophages. They debride an injury site.

mononuclear phagocyte—Any cell capable of ingesting particulate matter. The term usually refers to macrophages (polymorphonuclear leukocytes) and monocytes (mononuclear phagocytes). These ingest microorganisms and debride an injury site.

monosynaptic response—A reflex response involving only one synapse that is between the afferent and efferent nerves.

monosynaptic transmission—The direct connection between a sensory nerve and a motor neuron. Also called a *monosynaptic reflex*.

motor unit—A neuromuscular unit composed of the nerve, or motor neuron, and the muscle fibers that it innervates.

mucopolysaccharide—Polysaccharide. Also called *GAG*. See *glycosaminoglycan*.

muscle endurance—Ability of a muscle or muscle group to perform repeated contractions against a less-than-maximal load.

muscle energy—A manual therapy technique using precisely applied active muscle contraction against a counterforce to correct alignment and improve function.

muscle energy technique—The use of muscle contraction to precipitate a correction of a joint's malalignment.

muscle spasm—Prolonged reflex muscle contraction.

muscle spindle—A neuromuscular spindle, composed of intrafusal muscle fibers, that lies between regular muscle fibers. With its complex afferent and efferent supply, it provides the body with sensory stimulation and motor responses. The muscle spindle is sensitive to stretch and signals muscle length and rate of change in the muscle's length.

muscle stiffness—The change in a muscle's tension that occurs as the muscle's length changes; related to the strength of the muscle's cross-bridge connections and the amount of muscle hypertrophy. The more stiffness a muscle has, the more resistant it is to stretching. Muscle stiffness is related to muscle tone.

muscular endurance—A muscle or muscle group's ability to sustain a submaximal force during either static or dynamic activity over time.

muscular strength—The amount of force a muscle or muscle group exerts. The ability to resist or produce a force.

myoblast—A cell formed from myogenic cells in muscle. Myoblasts form myotubes that eventually evolve into muscle fiber.

myofibroblasts—Fibroblasts that have the ultrastructural features of a fibroblast as well as the qualities of a smooth muscle cell. They are responsible for wound contraction.

myogenic cells—Cells that arise from muscle and later become myoblasts. See *myoblast*.

myosin—The chief protein structure of the thick filament of the sarcomere.

myotatic reflex—See *stretch reflex*.

neural mobilization—A manual therapy technique that stretches neural and connective tissue structures to affect neural symptoms, restore tissue balance, and improve function.

neurotransmitters—Hormones such as norepinephrine, epinephrine, and acetylcholine that are found in capillary, arteriole, and artery walls. They are released at the injury site to enhance platelet and leukocyte adherence to the vessel surface.

neutral spine—See *pelvic neutral*.

neutrophil—See *polymorphonuclear leukocyte*.

Newton's first law of motion—Law stating that a body remains at rest or in uniform motion until an outside force acts on it.

Newton's second law of motion—Law stating that acceleration of an object is directly proportional to the force causing the motion and inversely proportional to the mass of the object being moved.

Newton's third law of motion—Law stating that for every action there is an equal and opposite reaction.

nociceptors—Afferent nerve endings that transmit pain stimuli.

norepinephrine—A hormone that acts as a powerful vasoconstrictor at the immediate onset of injury. It may last from a few seconds to a few minutes.

nuclear bag fiber—One of two intrafusal muscle fibers within a muscle spindle, named for its nuclei arrangement. The nuclei are bunched together in the middle of the fiber's central region.

nuclear chain fiber—One of two intrafusal muscle fibers within a muscle spindle. Its nuclei are arranged in a chain or row. It is the smaller of the intrafusal muscle fibers.

nystagmus—A reflexive attempt to keep the eyes steady during body motion.

objective examination—The portion of an examination by which the clinician discovers the observable signs and effects of an injury: The portion of observation, testing for quality and quantity of movement, strength, neurological and other special testing, and palpation.

oculomotor system—An afferent system for balance that uses the eyes to provide the central nervous system with information regarding the body's relative position in space.

open kinetic chain—Characterizing a motion in which the distal segment of an extremity moves freely in space.

open reduction internal fixation (ORIF)—Surgical reduction of a fracture with application of a fixation device, such as a pin or screw, to stabilize the fracture site.

opposition—A diagonal movement of the thumb across the palm of the hand to permit the thumb to make contact with one of the other fingers.

orthotic—In reference to the foot, an appliance designed to correct body-segment or foot alignment or function, absorb stress, or reduce pressure or symptoms. Orthotics can be custom made or preformed and can vary in composition, degree of control, and type of correction.

Osgood-Schlatter disease—An inflammation or avulsion of the tibial apophysis, occurring in active, prepubescent children.

osteitis pubis—An inflammatory condition of shear stresses caused by either repeated trauma or strain on the symphysis pubis joint.

osteoarthritis—A condition caused by wearing and thinning of articular cartilage in a joint, eventually producing degeneration of the joint's articular surface. Also known as *degenerative joint disease (DJD)*.

osteoblasts—Osteogenic cells from periosteum. Lay down the callus of fractured bone. Convert later to chondrocytes.

osteochondritis dissecans—Avascular necrosis of a joint's articular surface.

osteoclasts—Large multinuclear cells. Resorb dead, necrotic bone tissue.

osteocyte—A cell characteristic of adult bone. Maintains new bone mineralization.

osteopenia—A mild to moderate bone density loss that places the individual at risk for developing osteoporosis.

osteophytes—Bone spurs, or bony outgrowths, within a joint.

osteoporosis—A marked decrease in bone density causing bone porosity and brittleness.

outsole—The portion of a shoe that includes the lower segment and is in contact with the ground.

overflow—Also known as *irradiation*. With increased voluntary effort or prolonged effort, motor activity spreads to additional motor units of the same muscle and to motor units of other muscles.

overload principle—To gain strength, a muscle must be overloaded beyond its accustomed level.

overpressure—Movement of a joint beyond its normal mobility to assess and feel or produce a comparable sign.

pacinian corpuscles—Afferent nerve endings that lie throughout the joint capsule and periarticular structures. They are rapidly adapting receptors thought to be compression sensitive, especially during high-velocity changes when the joint accelerates or decelerates as it moves into its limits of motion.

parallel elastic component (PEC)—One of the non-contractile elements of muscle, composed of the muscle's connective tissue.

paratendinitis—An inflammation and thickening of the paratenon sheath of tendons that do not have synovial sheaths.

Pascal's law—Law stating that pressure from a fluid is exerted equally on all surfaces of an immersed object at any given depth (i.e., the deeper the object is immersed, the greater the pressure it encounters).

passive physiological range of motion—The amount of range of motion achieved without the assistance of the patient.

passive range of motion (PROM)—See *passive physiological range of motion.*

passive stretch—A stretch for which application relies on an outside force. The patient remains relaxed throughout the stretch.

patella alta—Position of the patella higher than normal in the patellofemoral groove.

patella baja—Position of the patella lower than normal in the patellofemoral groove.

pathoneurodynamics—A term coined by David Butler to describe pathological conditions that produce referral patterns proximally and distally from the site of pathology.

pelvic neutral—The position in which the spine and sacrolumbar junction incur the least stress. This is usually a midposition between the extremes of anterior and posterior pelvic tilt. Because of its impact on spine position, the position is also referred to as *neutral spine* or *straight spine.*

pelvic stabilization—Activities or exercises that are used to position and maintain the body in a pelvic neutral position. Also referred to as *core stabilization* or *spinal stabilization* activities.

performance evaluation—An assessment of the patient's ability to perform and complete an exercise or skill drill safely and accurately before he or she is allowed to advance to the next level.

periarticular connective tissue—Soft tissue surrounding a joint, such as ligaments, the joint capsule, fascia, tendons, and synovial membranes.

perimysium—Connective-tissue layer covering a group of muscle fibers (fascicle).

pes cavus—An abnormal condition in which the foot has an abnormally high longitudinal arch. Associated with a rigid foot.

pes planus—An abnormal condition in which the foot has a low longitudinal arch. Associated with a hypomobile foot. Also known as a *pancake arch, flatfoot,* or *excessive pronation.* Associated with a flexible foot.

phagocyte—Any cell that ingests particulate matter. Commonly referred to as *polymorphonuclear leukocyte* and *mononuclear phagocyte,* otherwise known as *macrophage* and *monocyte.* These cells ingest microorganisms and other particulate antigens to debride an area.

phospholipids—Lipids that contain phosphoric acid. Found in all cells and in layers of plasma membranes. Stimulate the clotting mechanism.

physically active—Characterizing an individual who engages in occupational, recreational, or athletic activities that require physical skills and utilize strength, power, endurance, speed, flexibility, range of motion, or agility. (Based on the National Athletic Trainers' Association definition.)

physiological advantage—A muscle's ability to shorten. A muscle has its greatest physiological advantage when at its resting length.

physiological joint motion—Joint motion that can be performed voluntarily, such as shoulder flexion and ankle inversion.

physis—A complex cartilaginous matrix that lies near the end of the longitudinal bone and forms new bone, providing growth of the long bone. Also called a *growth plate.*

plan of treatment program—The components, frequency, and duration of a treatment program. Includes the establishment of short-term and long-term goals.

plantar flexion—An extension of the ankle that causes the dorsum (top) of the foot to move away from the lower leg so that the angle of the ankle increases.

plasmin—An enzyme that occurs in plasma as plasminogen. It is activated by kallikrein and other activators. It converts fibrin to soluble substances.

plasminogen activator—An enzyme. See *fibrinolysin.* Converts fibrin to a soluble substance.

plasticity—In muscle physiology, a permanent change in length that occurs after an elongation force is applied.

platelet-derived growth factor (PDGF)—Substance found in platelets. It is essential for the growth of connective-tissue cells and stimulates the migration of polymorphonuclear leukocytes.

platelets—Irregular cell fragments found in blood. The first cells seen at an injury site, platelets are classified as regulatory cells of healing. Release growth factors. Form a plug at the injury to stop bleeding.

plica—A redundant fold in the knee's synovial lining, palpated as a band extending medially from the patella.

plumb line—A string with a weight (formerly a lead weight, but any weight object will do) at the end. When suspended, the string forms a vertical line.

plyometric exercise—A lengthening of a muscle followed by a sudden shortening to produce increased power. Also called *stretch-shortening exercise.*

polymorphonuclear leukocytes—One of the granular leukocytes. Also referred to as *PMNs* or *neutrophils.* These cells are chemotactic and phagocytic in the healing process.

posture—The relative alignment of the various body segments with one another.

potential energy—Energy that is stored in a body.

power—Work produced over time.

preswing—See *toe-off.*

primary intention—Healing that occurs with minor or surgical wounds. Reepithelialization closes the wound within 48 h. Scarring is minimal when healing by primary intention occurs.

procedure (vs. modality)—A treatment technique that involves the clinician's active participation or supervision.

pronation—Movement of the palm backward or downward so that the palm faces in a posterior direction, opposite the anatomical position. Also, a multiplanar rotation of the subtalar and transverse tarsal joints that is the combination of dorsiflexion, abduction, and eversion.

proprioception—The body's ability to transmit afferent information regarding position sense, to interpret the information, and to respond consciously or unconsciously to stimulation through appropriate execution of posture and movement.

proprioceptive neuromuscular facilitation (PNF)—A combined movement pattern that uses neural stimulation to facilitate a proper muscle response.

prostaglandins (PGs)—Components stemming primarily from arachidonic acid. Release of these substances requires the presence of the complement system and follows kinin formation. Specific PG compound compositions are designated by adding a letter, "A" through "I," and a subscript number, 1 through 3, to designate the number of hydrocarbon bonds. Examples: PGE_1 and PGE_2. Prostaglandins mediate cell migration during inflammation and modulate serotonin and histamine. Some PGs increase pain sensitivity, induce fever, and suppress lymphocyte transformation, thereby inhibiting the inflammatory reaction. Mediate myofibroblasts. Prostaglandins initiate early phases of injury repair as well as playing a role in the later stages of inflammation.

protease—An enzyme that acts as a catalyst to split interior peptide bonds in protein. Activates kallikrein to release bradykinin, ultimately causing increased vascular permeability to result in an increase in concentration of proteins and cells in the wound spaces.

proteoglycan—Substances found in tissues, including synovial fluid and connective-tissue matrix. Proteoglycan solutions are very viscous lubricants and are sulfated glycosaminoglycans. See *glycosaminoglycan.* A proteoglycan provides a resilient matrix for inhibiting cell migration. Regulates cell function and proliferation and regulates collagen fibrillogenesis.

protraction—A forward movement of the scapula. Also called *scapular abduction.*

pump bump—Increased prominence of the posterior calcaneal tuberosity. Also know as a *calcaneal exostosis.*

Q-angle—The angle formed by a line from the anterior superior iliac spine to the middle patella and a line from the middle patella to the tibial tubercle.

radial deviation—A movement of the wrist toward the thumb side of the forearm. Also called *radial flexion.*

range of motion—Amount of movement within a joint. Range of motion is affected by soft-tissue mobility and can be influenced by strength when performed actively. Used interchangeably with *flexibility.*

rearfoot valgus—An abnormal condition in which the calcaneus is everted relative to the tibia.

rearfoot varus—An abnormal condition in which the calcaneus is inverted relative to the posterior bisection of the lower leg.

refraction—When a light ray moves from air through water, it bends as it moves from the air, which has a lower density than the water does, into the water with its higher density. This makes the pool bottom appear closer than it actually is and makes objects within the water appear distorted.

refractory period—The time immediately following a stimulation, when the muscle fiber is unable to respond to additional stimuli. It is divided into an absolute refractory period and a relative refractory period.

rehabilitation clinician—The medical professional responsible for the design, progression, supervision, and administration of a rehabilitation program for individuals involved in physical activity. Medical professionals who most often assume these responsibilities include certified athletic trainers and physical therapists.

relative density—See *specific gravity.*

relative refractory period—A period that follows depolarization after a membrane has become partially repolarized. During this period the membrane is able to respond again if the stimulus is stronger than the normal threshold level.

resisted range of motion (RROM)—Motion that occurs with resistance applied to the movement. Also referred to as *strengthening exercises* or *progressive resistive exercises.*

resting membrane potential—The electrical potential difference across an inactive cell's membrane.

resting position—The position of a joint that allows the joint capsule the greatest amount of play and where the volume within the joint is at its greatest.

reticulin—A collagen-like fiber. Some consider reticulin a Type III collagen fiber. Forms the early framework for collagen deposition in a wound.

retraction—A backward movement of the scapula. Also called *scapular adduction.*

retroversion—Decreased anterior angulation of the femoral neck, resulting in a toe-out gait.

Romberg test—A test for balance in which a patient stands with feet together and eyes closed. Increased postural sway compared to when eyes are open is a positive sign.

Ruffini nerve endings—These afferent receptors are in the joint capsule on the flexion side of the joint. They are slowly adapting and respond more to loads on the connective tissue in which they are contained than to displacement of that connective tissue. These receptors are stimulated by extreme joint motion when the capsule is stressed in extension with rotation.

running cycle—A cycle that includes two running strides; a running stride is from toe-off of one foot to toe-off of the opposite foot.

saddle—The portion of a shoe that includes the midsection along the longitudinal arch, usually reinforced to assist in supporting the midfoot.

sagittal plane—The anterior-posterior vertical plane through which the longitudinal axis passes and which divides the body into right and left halves.

SAID principle—Specific adaptation to imposed demands. Tissue will adapt to the specific stresses applied to it. This is a principle upon which a therapeutic exercise program is designed.

sarcolemma—The outer membrane of a muscle fiber.

sarcomere—The smallest contractile element of a muscle fiber.

sarcopenia—A decrease in muscle mass secondary to aging.

sarcoplasmic reticulum—A highly specialized intracellular membrane system that stores and transports calcium.

satellite cells—Cells present in muscle that regenerate new muscle tissue.

scaption—Elevation of the shoulder in the scapular plane 30° forward of the frontal plane. This alignment of the glenohumeral joint with the scapula on the rib cage places the rotator cuff in the least stressful position for exercise.

scoliosis—A lateral or S curvature of the spinal column.

secondary intention—Healing that occurs in large wounds associated with soft-tissue loss. The wound heals with granulation tissue from the bottom and sides of the wound. Epithelial tissue does not form until granulation tissue has filled the wound. Larger scar formation occurs with healing by secondary intention. Wound contraction is evident with this healing.

second-class lever—A lever in which the resistance is between the fulcrum and the force.

series elastic component (SEC)—One of the non-contractile elements of muscle, composed primarily of the tendons, sheath, and sarcolemma.

serotonin—A hormone released by mast cells and platelets. Produces vasoconstriction in small vessels after norepinephrine activity is completed; occurs only when blood vessel endothelial walls are damaged. In later phases, it is responsible for initiating reactions leading to collagen cross-linking. It also is involved in granuloma formation.

shin splints—A general term used to describe pain and inflammation of the musculotendinous unit and/or periosteum along the anteromedial border of the tibia. Also know as *medial tibial stress syndrome.*

single-leg support—The portion of the gait cycle in which the body weight is transferred entirely to the one supporting leg and the other leg is in the middle of its swing phase. Also known as *midstance.*

sinusoidal curve—A curve that takes the shape of a sine wave.

SLAP lesion—Superior labrum tear anterior and posterior in location. A tear in the labrum appearing superiorly either on the posterior or anterior glenoid.

slow-twitch fiber—A muscle fiber that is a type I fiber or slow oxidative fiber, is darker in color than the fast-twitch fiber, and takes about 110 ms to reach its peak tension when stimulated.

Smith's fracture—A type of fracture in which the distal radius is fractured and the fragment is displaced palmarly.

sock liner—The portion of a shoe that lies on top of the insole board, used for shock absorption and friction reduction for the foot.

somatosensory system—Another term for the body's proprioceptive system.

specific gravity—The ratio of an object's weight to the weight of an equal volume of water. The term refers to the density of an object relative to that of water. This ratio is also called *relative density.* The specific gravity of water is 1.

spinal cord—Part of the central nervous system that extends from the brain to the second lumbar vertebra and contains a cervical and a lumbar enlargement where the dorsal and ventral roots leading to the extremities are contained.

spinal reflex—When an impulse goes from a dorsal root afferent nerve either to an internuncial connecting nerve or directly to an efferent nerve in the spinal cord, and then immediately out the ventral root to the muscle.

sprain—Stretching or tearing of a ligament or capsular structure.

squinting patellae—Patellae that are angled toward each other rather than facing forward.

stable—A condition where the body is secure, usually occurs when the center of mass remains within its base of support and is not in danger of losing balance.

stance phase—The portion of the gait cycle during which the foot is in contact with the floor and the extremity is bearing partial or total body weight. In running, sometimes called the *support phase.*

static activity—An isometric activity in which no movement occurs.

static progressive splint—Change of static splints as motion of a segment changes so the desired goals, usually including increased motion, are achieved.

static restraint—One of two systems a joint has for its stability. Static restraints include ligaments, capsule, and other inert structures such as the glenoid labrum in the shoulder and the meniscus in the knee.

static splint—Splint used to support, protect, or restrict motion. It does not have any moving parts.

steady state of a drug—The state in which the average level of a drug remains constant in the blood: The amount of drug leaving the body is equal to the amount being absorbed. On average, a steady state occurs after five doses equal to the drug's half-life are administered.

step length—The distance from heel strike of one foot to heel strike of the other foot in one gait cycle.

stiffness—The ability of an object to resist deformation when a stress is applied to it. The stiffer an object, the less elastic it is.

stretch-shortening exercise—An exercise that makes use of the elastic properties of muscle, using a lengthening of a muscle followed by a sudden shortening to produce increased power. Also called *plyometric exercise.*

strain—Amount of change in size or shape of an object caused by stress.

strength—A muscle's relative ability to resist or produce a force.

stress—Force required to change the shape or form of a body.

stretch reflex—The most basic sensorimotor response. Does not involve an internuncial neuron, but instead goes directly from the afferent sensory nerve (muscle spindle) to the spinal cord, where it makes contact with the motor nerve to permit a rapid muscle response.

stride length—The distance from heel strike of one foot to heel strike of the same foot in one gait cycle.

stride rate—In running, the inverse of cycle time or stride time: the number of step lengths over a given period.

stride width—The body's side-to-side movement as weight is shifted from one lower extremity to the other.

structural fatigue—The point at which stress exceeds the tissue's ability to resist it and breakdown occurs.

subjective evaluation—The portion of an examination that includes the history of an injury, including the mechanism of injury, the patient's experience of pain and other symptoms, prior injuries, medical conditions, medications, and other pertinent social and medical factors. This information is provided by the patient or other individual.

subtalar joint—The joint formed by the talus and calcaneus. This joint allows inversion and eversion motion of the rearfoot.

subtalar neutral—The position in which the talus is palpable from its medial or its lateral aspect within the subtalar joint. The point at which the talus and navicular are most congruent and the alignment of the subtalar bones is optimal.

summation of forces—Sequential movement of body segments to increase force production for a desired motion.

supination—Movement of the palm forward or upward into the anatomical position. Also, the multiplanar rotation of the subtalar and transverse tarsal joints that includes plantar flexion, adduction, and inversion.

swan-neck deformity—A deformity caused by hyperextension at the PIP joint and hyperflexion at the DIP joint due to disruption of the volar plate and tensioning of the flexor tendons.

swing phase—The time during which the foot is not in contact with the floor and no weight is borne on the extremity.

swing-through—The middle of the swing phase. Also called *mid-swing*.

swing-through gait—A three-point gait pattern with crutches in which the weight-bearing leg is advanced far enough to land in front of the crutches.

swing-to gait—A three-point gait pattern with crutches in which the individual swings the weight-bearing leg to the crutches.

Swiss ball—A large, vinyl ball developed by an Italian toy manufacturer that is used in physical therapy and therapeutic exercise programs.

synergist(ic)—A muscle that assists an agonist muscle.

synovial fluid—A lubricating fluid secreted by membranes in joints and tendon sheaths.

synovial sheaths—Sheaths that surround tendons subjected to greater than normal friction stresses, such as the Achilles and biceps tendons.

talocrural joint—The true ankle joint that is formed by the talus and tibia with the fibula. The joint allows dorsiflexion and plantar flexion motions.

tarsal tunnel—Formed by the medial malleolus, calcaneus, talus, and deltoid ligament's posterior aspect.

tendinitis—The global term used to identify an inflammation of a tendon. Also spelled *tendonitis*.

tendinopathy—Condition of a tendon that demonstrates signs and symptoms of pain, swelling, and reduced function.

tendinosis—A condition that involves microscopic tears of the tendon caused by repeated trauma.

tenocyte—Tendon cell. Converts to fibroblasts during healing of tendons.

tenosynovitis—An inflammation of the synovial sheath that surrounds a tendon.

tensile strength—Maximal amount of stress or force that a structure is able to withstand before tissue failure occurs. Tensile strength varies as tissue healing proceeds. One must take tensile strength of an injured structure into account when determining appropriate stress application in rehabilitation.

terminal stance—See *heel-off*.

terminal swing—The portion of the swing phase that includes late swing, or deceleration.

tetanus—An intermittent contraction of a muscle that is demonstrated as a fibrillation of the muscle.

tetany—A sustained maximal contraction of a muscle.

third-class lever—A lever in which the force is between the fulcrum and the resistance.

thoracic kyphosis—Excess posterior convexity of the thoracic spine.

thoracic outlet syndrome (TOS)—A clinical term that describes compression of the neurovascular structures as they exit through the thoracic outlet at the base of the neck.

threshold stimulation—The minimal stimulation required to initiate a muscular response.

thrombin—An enzyme that converts fibrinogen to fibrin to form a fibrin plug early in the inflammation phase. In later inflammation, it stimulates fibronectin production and fibroblast proliferation.

thromboxane—A compound that is produced by platelets and is unstable. Its half-life is 30 s. Related to prostaglandins. Acts as a vasoconstrictor and is a potent inducer of platelet aggregation.

tibial torsion—An abnormal structural condition in which the tibia is rotated along its longitudinal axis so that the foot is rotated laterally beyond the normal 15° in relation to the patella's midline.

tibial varum—An abnormal condition in which the distal tibia is closer to the midline than the proximal tibia.

toe box—The upper portion of the shoe that covers the toes. It varies in width and height, and functions to retain the shape of the shoe's forefoot and provide room for the toes.

toe-off—The portion of the gait cycle during which the foot comes off the floor and the swing phase begins. Also called *push-off* or *preswing*.

torque—The ability of a force to produce rotational movement.

transverse (horizontal) plane—A plane that divides the body or a body part into upper and lower parts. It is parallel to the horizon.

Trendelenburg gait—An abnormal gait secondary to gluteus medius weakness. The gait is also known as a *gluteus medius gait* and is seen as a drop of the pelvis on the uninvolved side during weight bearing on the involved side.

trigger point—According to Travell and Simons (1983, p. 3), a "focus of hyperirritability in a tissue that, when compressed, is locally tender and, if sufficiently hypersensitive, gives rise to referred pain and tenderness, and sometimes to referred autonomic phenomena and distortion of proprioception." A myofascial trigger point includes a taut band of muscle with its surrounding fascia.

tropomyosin—One of two primary proteins of the thin filament of the sarcomere.

troponin—A protein on the actin filament to which calcium ions bind during a sarcomere's cross-bridging process.

TUBS—**T**raumatic, **u**nilateral, **b**ankart lesion, **s**urgery required. A traumatic shoulder injury involving a tear of the anterior capsulolabral complex and requiring surgical repair.

ulnar deviation—A movement of the wrist toward the little-finger side of the forearm. Also called *ulnar flexion*.

ultimate strength—The greatest load a tissue can tolerate before it reaches failure.

upward rotation—A movement of the scapula that causes the glenoid to face forward and upward. The inferior angle of the scapula moves laterally away from the spine, and the scapula slides forward.

Valsalva maneuver—When the breath is held, intrathoracic pressure is increased. This can lead to impeded venous return to the right atrium, causing increased peripheral venous pressure, increasing blood pressure and reducing cardiac output because of diminished cardiac volume.

vamp—The upper portion of a shoe that covers the toes and forefoot and includes the toe box.

velocity—Rate of change of position.

vestibular system—An afferent system within the inner ear that is responsible for sending messages to the central nervous system regarding vertical and horizontal position and motion.

viscoelasticity—The property of being both viscous and elastic.

viscosity—The resistance to movement within a fluid or fluid-like substance that is caused by the friction of the fluid's molecules. Viscosity limits the rate of muscle contraction: The faster the contraction, the greater the internal resistance and the less the force that can be generated.

volitional—The conscious performance or an activity.

wave drag—The water's resistance as a result of turbulence.

weight—The force of gravity. Commonly measured in kilograms (grams) or pounds (ounces).

work—Product of a force and the distance through which it is applied.

Z-disc—The end of the sarcomere element where the thin filaments attach. Also known as the Z-line or Z-band.

REFERENCES

Chapter 1

Appell, H. J. (1990). Muscular atrophy following immobilization: A review. *Sports Medicine, 10*, 42-58.

Binkley, J. M., Stratford, P. W., Lott, S. A., & Riddle, D. L. (1999). The lower extremity functional scale (LEFS): scale development, measurement properties, and clinical application. *Physical Therapy, 79*, 371-383.

Denegar, C. R., Saliba, E., & Saliba, S. (2010). *Therapeutic Modalities for Musculoskeletal Injuries*. Champaign, IL: Human Kinetics.

Fisher, A. C., Mullins, S. A., & Frye, P. A. (1993). Athletic trainers' attitudes and judgmetns of injured athletes' rehabilitation adherence. *Journal of Athletic Training, 28*, 43-47.

Keith, R. H., Granter, C. V., Hamilton, B. B., & Sherwin, F. S. (1987). The functional independence measure: a new tool for rehabilitation. In M. G. Eisenberg & R. C. GRzesink (Eds.), *Advances in Clinical Rehabilitation*. New York: Springer.

Kubler-Ross, E. (1969). *On Death and Dying*. New York: Macmillan.

Peterson, P. (1986). The grief response and injury. *Athletic Training, 21*, 312-314.

Quealy, J., & Langan-Fox, J. (1998). Attributes of delivery media in computer-assisted instruction. *Ergonomics, 41*(3), 257-279.

Rastall, M., Brooks, B., Klarneta, M., Moylan, N., McCloud, W., & Tracey, S. (1999). An investigation into younger and older adults' memory for physiotherapy exercises. *Physiotherapy, 85*(3), 122-128.

Ray, R. (2010). *Management Strategies in Athletic Training* (4th ed.). Champaign, IL: Human Kinetics.

Rotella, R. J. (1985). The psychological care of the patient. In R. J. Rotella (Ed.), *Psychological Consideration in Maximizing Sport Performance*. Ann Arbor, MI: McNaughton and Gun.

Staron, R. S., Leonardi, M. J., Karapondo, D. L., Malicky, E. S., Falkel, J. E., Hagerman, F. C., et al. (1991). Strength and skeletal muscle adaptations in heavy-resistance-trained women after detraining and retraining. *Journal of Applied Physiology 70*, 631-640.

Stratford, P. W., Binkley, J. M., Riddle, D. L., & Guyatt, G. H. (1998). Sensitivity to change on the Roland-Morris Pain Questionnaire: Part 1. *Physical Therapy, 78*, 1186-1196.

Ware, J. E., Jr., Kosinski, M., Bayliss, M. S., McHorney, C. A., Rogers, W. H., & Raczek, A. (1995). Comparisons of methods for the scoring and statistical analysis of the SF-36 health profile and summary measures: Summary of results from the Medical Outcomes Study. *Medical Care, 33*, AS264-279.

Ware, J. E., Jr., & Sherbourne, C. D. (1992). The MOS 36-Item Short Form Health Survey (SF-36), I: Conceptual framework and item selection. *Medical Care, 30*, 473-483.

Wingfield, A., & Byrnes, D. L. (1981). *The Psychology of Human Memory*. New York: Academic Press.

Chapter 2

Almekinders, L. C., & Gilbert, J. A. (1986). Almekinders, L.C., and J.A. Gilbert. 1986. Healing of experimental muscle strains and the effects of non-steroidal antiinflammatory medication. American Journal of Sports Medicine 14:303–308. *American Journal of Sports Medicine, 14*, 303-308.

Andriacchi, T. P., Sabiston, K., DeHaven, K., Dahners, L., Woo, S., Frank, C., et al. (1988). Ligament: Injury and repair. In S. L.-Y. Woo & J. A. Buckwalter (Eds.), *Injury and Repair of the Musculoskeletal Soft Tissues*. Park Ridge, IL: American Academy of Orthopaedic Surgeons.

Angel, M. J., Sgaglione, N. A., & Grande, D. A. (2006). Clinical applications of bioactive factors in sports medicine. Current concepts and future trends. *Sports Medicine and Arthroscopy Review, 14*, 138-148.

Bartha, L., Vajda, A., Duska, Z., Rahmeh, H., & Hangody, L. (2006). Autologous osteochondral mosaicplasty grafting. *Journal of Orthopaedic & Sports Physical Therapy, 36*, 739-750.

Beredjiklian, P. K. (2003). Biologic aspects of flexor tendon laceration and repair. *Journal of Bone and Joint Surgery (Am), 85-A*(3), 539-550.

Best, T. M., & Hunter, K. D. (2000). Muscle injury and repair. *Physical Medicine and Rehabilitation Clinics of North America, 11*(2), 251-266.

Betz, P., Norlich, A., Wilske, J., Tubel, J., Penning, R., & Eisenmenger, W. (1992). Time-dependent appearance of myofibroblasts in granulation tissue of human skin wounds. *International Journal of Legal Medicine, 150*, 99-103.

Breuing, K., Andree, C., Helo, G., Slama, J., Liu, P. Y., & Eriksson, E. (1997). Growth factors in the repair of partial thickness porcine skin wounds. *Plast reconstr surg, 100*(3), 657-664.

Brittberg, M., Lindahl, A., Nilsson, A., Ohlsson, C., Isaksson, O., & Peterson, L. (1994). Treatment of deep cartilage defects in the knee with autologous chondrocyte transplantation. *N Engl J Med, 331*, 889-895.

Browne, J. E., & Branch, T. P. (2000). Surgical alternatives for treatment of articular cartilage lesions. *Journal of the American Academy of Orthopaedic Surgeons, 8*(3), 180-189.

Buckwalter, J. A., Rosenberg, L., Coutts, R., Hunziker, E., Reddi, A. H., & Mow, V. (1988). Articular cartilage: Injury and repair. In S. Woo & J. A. Buckwalter (Eds.), *Injury and Repair of Musculoskeletal Soft Tissues*. Park Ridge, IL: American Academy of Orthopaedic Surgeons.

Butterfield, T. A., Best, T.M., & Merrick, M. A. (2006). The dual roles of neutrophils and macrophages in inflammation: A critical balance between tissue damage and repair. *Journal of Athletic Training, 41*(4), 457-465.

Caplan, A. B., Carlson, J., Faulkner, J., Fischman, D., & Garrett, W., Jr. . (1988). Skeletal muscle. In S. Woo & J. A. Buckwalter (Eds.), *Injury and Repair of the Musculoskeletal Soft Tissues*. Park Ridge, IL: American Academy of Orthopaedic Surgeons.

Connolly, J. F. (1988). *Fracture complications, recognition, prevention, and management*. Chicago: Year Book Medical.

Cromack, D. T., Porras-Reyes, B., & Mustoe, T. A. (1990). Current concepts in wound healing: growth factor and macrophage interaction. *Journal of Trauma, 30*(12), S129-S133.

Denegar, C. R., Saliba, E., & Saliba, S. (2010). *Therapeutic Modalities for Athletic Injuries* (3rd ed.). Champaign, IL: Human Kinetics.

Detterline, A. J., Goldberg, S., Bach, B. R. J., & Cole, B. J. (2005). Treatment options for articular cartilage defects of the knee. *Orthopedic Nursing, 24*(5), 361-368.

Diegelmann, R. F., & Evans, M. C. (2004). Wound healing: An overview of acute, fibrotic and delayed healing. *Frontiers in Bioscience, 9*, 283-289.

Folland, J. P., & Williams, A. G. (2007). The Adaptations to Strength Training: Morphological and Neurological Contributions to Increased Strength. *Sports Medicine, 37*(2), 145-168.

Gelberman, R., An, K.-A., Banes, A., & Goldberg, V. (1988). Tendon. In S. Woo & J. A. Buckwalter (Eds.), *Injury and Repair of the Musculoskeletal Soft Tissues*. Park Ridge, IL: American Academy of Orthopaedic Surgeons.

Gelberman, R. H., Woo, S. L.-Y., Lothringer, K., Akeson, W. H., & Amiel, D. (1982). Effects of early intermittent passive mobilization on healing canine flexor tendons. *Journal of Hand Surgery (Am), 7*, 170-175.

Gill, T. J., Asnis, P. D., & Berkson, E. M. (2006). The treatment of articular cartilage defects using the microfracture technique. *Journal of Orthopaedic & Sports Physical Therapy, 36*(10), 728-738.

Grundnes, O., & Reikeras, O. (1992). Grundnes, O., and O. Reikeras. 1992. Blood flow and mechanical properties of healing bone. Acta Orthopaedica Scandinavica 63:487–491. *Acta Orthopaedica Scandinavica, 63*, 487-491.

Heppenstall, R. B. (1980). Fracture healing. In R. B. Heppenstall (Ed.), *Fracture Treatment and Healing*. Philadelphia: Saunders.

Hildebrand, K. A., Gallant-Behm, C. L., Kydd, A. S., & Hart, D. A. (2005). The basics of soft tissue healing and general factors that influence such healing. *Sports Medicine and Arthroscopy Review, 11*(3), 136-144.

Hillman, S. (2010). *Introduction to Athletic Training*. Champaign, IL: Human Kinetics.

Hom, D. B. (1995). Growth factors in wound healing. *Otolaryngologic Clinics of North America, 28*, 933-953.

Houglum, J. E. (1998). Pharmacologic considerations in the treatment of injured athletes with nonsteroidal anti-inflammatory drugs. *Journal of Athletic Training, 33*, 259-263.

Houglum, J. E., Harrelson, G. L., & Leaver-Dunn, D. (2005). *Principles of Pharmacology for Athletic Trainers*. Thorofare, N.J.: Slack, Inc.

Jones, G., Ding, C., Glisson, M., Hynes, K., Deqiong, M. A., & Cicuttini, F. (2003). Knee articular cartilage development in children: A longitudinal study of the effect of sex, growth, body composition, and physical activity. *Pediatric Research, 54*, 230-236.

Khan, K. M., Cook, J. L., Bonar, F., Harcourt, P., & Astrom, M. (1999). Histopathology of common tendinopathies. Update and implications for clinical management. *Sports Medicine, 27*(6), 393-408.

LaStayo, P. C., Winters, K. M., & Hardy, M. (2003). Fracture healing: Bone healing, fracture management, and current concepts related to the hand. *Journal of Hand Therapy, 16*(2), 81-93.

Leadbetter, W. B. (1994). Soft tissue athletic injury. In F. H. Fu & D. A. Stone (Eds.), *Sports injuries: Mechanisms, prevention, treatment,* . Baltimore: Williams & Wilkins.

Lewis, P. B., McCarty, L. P., 3rd, Kang, R. W., & Cole, B. J. (2006). Basic science and treatment options for articular cartilage injuries. *J Orthop Sports Phys Ther, 36*(10), 717-727.

Martinez-Hernandez, A., & Amenta, P. S. (1990). Basic concepts in wound healing. In W. B. Leadbetter, J. A. Buckwalter & S. L. Gordon (Eds.), *Sports-induced Inflammation*. Park Ridge, IL: American Academy of Orthopaedic Surgeons.

Mehallo, C. J., Drezner, J. A., & Bytomski, J. R. (2006). Practical management: Nonsteroidal antiinflammatory drug (NSAID) use in athletic injuries. *Clinics in Sports Medicine, 16*, 170-174.

Miura, K., Ishibashi, Y., Tsuda, E., Sato, H., & Toh, S. (2007). Results of arthroscopic fixation of osteochondritis dissecans lesion of the knee with cylindrical autogenous osteochondral plugs. *American Journal of Sports Medicine, 35*(2), 216-222.

Mosher, T. J., & Dardzinksi, B. J. (2004). Cartilage MRI T2 relaxation time mapping: overview and applications. *Seminars in Musculoskeletal Radiology, 8*, 355-368.

Nordin, M., & Frankel, V. H. (1980). Biomechanics of collagenous tissues. In V. H. Frankel & N. Nordin (Eds.), *Basic Biomechanics of the Skeletal System*. Philadelphia: Lea & Febiger.

Pandit, A., Ashar, R., & Feldman, D. (1999). The effect of TGF-beta delivered through a collagen scaffold on wound healing. *Journal of Investigative Surgery, 12*(2), 89-100.

Peacock, E. E. (1984). *Wound Repair* (3rd ed.). Philadelphia: Saunders.

Scott, A., Cook, J. L., Hart, D. A., Walker, D. C., Duronio, V., & Khan, K. M. (2007). Tenocyte responses to mechanical loading in vivo: a role for local insulin-like growth factor 1 signaling in early tendinosis in rats. *Arthritis rheum, 56*(3), 871-881.

Silver, F. H., & Glasgold, A. I. (1995). Cartilage wound healing. *Otolaryngologic Clinics of North America, 28*, 847-864.

Steadman, J. R., Forster, R. S., & Silferskiold, J. P. (1989). Steadman, J.R., Forster, R.S., and J.P. Silferskiold. 1989. Rehabilitation of the knee. Clinics in Sports Medicine 8:605–627. *Clinics in Sports Medicine, 8*, 605-627.

Steadman, J. R., Rodkey, W. G., & Briggs, K. K. (2003). Microfracture chondroplasty: indications, techniques, and outcomes. *Sports Medicine and Arthroscopy Review, 11*, 236-244.

Tohyama, H., & Yasuda, K. (2005). Anterior cruciate ligament (ACL) healing. ACL graft biology. *Sports Medicine and Arthroscopy Review, 13*, 156-160.

Urban, M. K. (2000). COX-2 Specific inhibitors offer improved advantages over traditional NSAIDs. *Orthoapedics, 23*, 761s-764s.

Wang, J. H.-C., Iosifidis, M. L., & Fu, F. H. (2006). Biomechanical basis for tendinopathy. *Clinical Orthopaedics and Related Research, 443*, 320-332.

Chapter 3

Nimni, M. E. (1983). Collagen: Structure, function, and metabolism in normal and fibrotic tissues. *Seminars in Arthritis and Rheumatism 13*, 1-86.

Smith, L. K., Weiss, E. L., & Lehmkuh, L. D. (1996). *Brunnstrom's Clinical Kinesiology* (5th ed.). Philadelphia: FA Davis.

Chapter 4

Borcherding, S. (2000). *Documentation Manual for Writing SOAP Notes in Occupational Therapy*. Thorofare, NJ: Slack.

Corrigan, B., & Maitland, G. D. (1989). *Practical Orthopedic Medicine*. Boston: Butterworth.

Cyriax, J. H. (1982). *Textbook of Orthopaedic Medicine. Vol. 1. Diagnosis of Soft Tissue Lesions* (8th ed.). London, England: Bailliere Tindall.

Kaltenborn, F. M. (2002). *Manual Mobilization of the Joints. The Kaltenborn Method of Joint Examination and Treatment* (6th ed.). Oslo, Norway: Olaf NOrlis Bokhandel.

Maitland, G. D. (1991). *Peripheral Manipulation* (3rd ed.). Boston: Butterworth-Heinemann.

Paris, S. V., & Patla, C. (1988). *E1 course notes: Extremity dysfunction and manipulation*. St. Augustine, FL: Patris.

Ray, R. (2010). *Management Strategies in Athletic Training* (4th ed.). Champaign, IL: Human Kinetics.

Shultz, S. J., Houglum, P. A., & Perrin, D. H. (2010). *Examination of Musculoskeletal Injuries* (3rd ed.). Champaign, IL: Human Kinetics.

Chapter 5

AAOS. (1965). *Joint motion: Method of measuring and recording*. Chicago: American Academy of Orthopaedic Surgeons.

Bandy, W., Irion, J., & Briggler, M. (1997). The effect of time and frequency on static stretching on flexibility of the hamstring muscles. *Phys ther, 77*(10), 1090-1096.

Bradley, P. S., Olsen, P. D., & Portas, M. D. (2007). The effect of static, ballistic, and proprioceptive neuromuscular facilitation stretching on vertical jump performance. *J Strength Cond Res, 21*(1), 223-236.

Brander, V., & Stulberg, S. D. (2006). Rehabilitation after hip- and knee-joint replacement. An experience- and evidence-based approach to care. *Am J Phys Med Rehabil, 85*, S98-118.

Buckwalter, J. A. (1996). Effects of early motion on healing of musculoskeletal tissues. *Hand Clinics, 12*, 13-24.

Butler, D. L., Grood, E. S., Noyes, F. R., & Zernicke, R. F. (1978). Biomechanics of ligaments and tendons. *Exercise and Sport Sciences Review, 6*, 125-281.

Church, J. B., Wiggins, M. S., Moode, F. M., & Crist, R. (2001). Effect of warm-up and flexibility treatments on vertical jump performance. *ournal of Strength & Conditioning Research, 15*, 332-336.

Cook, J. R., Baker, N. A., Cham, R., Hale, E., & Redfern, M. S. (2007). Measurements of wrist and finger postures: a comparison of goniometric and motion capture techniques. *Journal of Applied Biomechanics, 23*(1), 70-78.

Daniels, L., & Worthingham, C. (1986). *Muscle Testing: Techniques of Manual Examination* (ed 5 ed.). Philadelphia: WB Saunders.

Davis, D. S., Ashby, P. E., McCale, K. L., McQuain, J. A., & Wine, J. M. (2005). The effectiveness of 3 stretching techniques on hamstring flexibility using consistent stretching parameters. *J Strength Cond Res, 19*(1), 27-32.

Donatelli, R., & Owens-Burkhart, A. (1981). Effects of immobilization on the extensibility of periarticular connective tissue. *Journal of Orthopaedic and Sports Physical Therapy, 9*, 67-72.

Eldred, E. (1967). Peripheral receptors: Their excitation and relation to reflex patterns. *American Journal of Physical Medicine, 46*(1), 69-87.

Esch, D., & Lepley, M. (1974). *Evaluation of joint motion: Methods of measurement and recording*. Minneapolis: University of Minnesota Press.

Evans, E. B., Eggers, G. W. N., Butler, J. K., & Blumel, J. (1960). Experimental immobilization and remobilization of rat knee joints. *Journal of Bone and Joint Surgery, 42A*, 737-758.

Finsterbush, A., & Friedman, B. (1975). Reversibility of joint changes produced by immobilization of rabbits. *Clinical Orthopaedics and Related Research, 111*, 290-298.

Flowers, K. R., & LaStayo, P. (1994). Effect of total end range time on improving passive range of motion. *J hand ther, 2*, 150-157.

Friemert, B., Bach, C., Schwarz, W., Gerngross, H., & Schmidt, R. (2006). Benefits of active motion for joint position sense. *Knee surg sports traumatol arthroscopy, 14*(6), 564-570.

Garrett, W. E., Jr. . (1990). Muscle strain injuries: Clinical and basic aspects. *Medicine & Science in Sports & Exercise, 22*, 436-443.

Garrett, W. E. J. (1996). Muscle strain injuries. *American Journal of Sports Medicine, 24*(6), S2-S8.

Gerhardt, J. J., & Russe, O. A. (1975). *International SFTR Method of Measuring and Recording Joint Motion*. Hans Huber, Bern, Switzerland: Year Book Medical Publishers.

Gomez, M. A., Woo, S. L.-Y., Amiel, D., Hardwood, F., Kitabayashi, L., & Matyas, J. R. (1991). The effects of increased tension on healing medial collateral ligaments. *American Journal of Sports Medicine, 19*, 347-354.

Heckmann, T. P., Barber-Westin, S. D., & Noyes, F. R. (2006). Meniscal repair and transplantation: indications, techniques, rehabilitation, and clinical outcome. *J orthop sport phys ther, 36*(10), 795-814.

Hewett, T., Paterno, M., & Myer, G. (2002). Strategies for enhancing proprioception and neuromuscular control of the knee. *Clin orthop, 402*, 76-94.

Hoppenfeld, S. (1676). *Physical examination of the spine and extremities*. New York: Appleton-Century-Crofts.

Kapandji, I. A. (1982). *The Physiology of the Joints, Vol 1, Upper Limb* (5 ed.). Edinburgh: Churchill Livingstone.

Kapandji, I. A. (1987). *The Physiology of the Joints, Vol 2, Lower Limb* (5 ed.). Edinburgh: Churchill Livingstone.

Karpovich, P. V., Herden, E. L., Jr., Asa, M. M., & Karpovich, G. P. (1959). Electrogoniometer: A new device for study of joints in action. *Federation Proceedings, 18*, 79.

Kendall, F. P., McCreary, E. K., & Provance, P. G. (1993). *Muscles: Testing and function* (4th ed.). Baltimore: Williams & Wilkins.

Klein, L., Heiple, K. G., Torzilli, P. A., Goldberg, V. M., & Burstein, A. H. (1989). Prevention of ligament and meniscus atrophy by active joint motion in a non-weight-bearing model. *Journal of Orthopaedic Research, 7*, 80-85.

Kottke, F. J., & Lehmann, J. F. (1990). *Krusen's handbook of physical medicine and rehabilitation* (4th ed.). Philadelphia: Saunders.

Kottke, F. J., Pauley, D. L., & Ptak, R. A. (1966). The rationale for prolonged stretching for correction of shortening of connective tissue. *Arch phys med rehabil, 47*(6), 345-352.

Kovacs, M. S. (2006). The argument against static stretching before sport and physical activity. *Athletic Therapy Today, 11*(3), 6-8, 30-31, 60.

Light, K. E., Nuzik, S., Personius, W., & Barstrom, A. (1984). Low-load prolonged stretch vs. high-load brief stretch in treating knee contractures. *Physical Therapy, 64*, 330-333.

Lundberg, A., Malmgren, K., & Schomburg, E. D. (1977). Cutaneous facilitation of transmission in reflex pathways from Ib afferents to motorneurones. *J Physiol, 265*, 763-780.

Lundberg, A., Malmgren, K., & Schomburg, E. D. (1987). Reflex pathways from group II muscle afferents. 2. Functional characteristics of reflex pathways to alpha motorneurons. *Exp Brain Res, 65*, 282-293.

Malliaropoulos, N., Papalexandris, S., Papalada, A., & Papacostas, E. (2004). The role of stretching in rehabilitation of hamstring injuries: 80 athletes follow-up. *Med Sci Sports Exerc, 36*(5), 756-759.

McNair, P. J., Stanley, S. N., & Strauss, G. R. (1996). Knee bracing: effects on proprioception. *Arch phys med rehabil, 77*, 287-289.

Moll, J., & Wright, V. (1971). Normal range of spinal mobility: A clinical study. *Annals of the Rheumatic Diseases, 30*, 381-386.

Montgomery, J. B., & Steadman, J. R. (1985). Rehabilitation of the injured knee. *Clinics in Sports Medicine, 4*, 333-343.

O'Driscoll, S. W., & Nicholas, J. G. (2000). Continuous passive motion (CPM): Theory and principles of clinical application. *Journal of Rehabilitation Research and Development, 37*, 178.

Ono, T., Tsuboi, M., Oki, S., Shimizu, M. E., Otsuka, A., Shiraiwa, K., et al. (2007). Preliminary report: Another perspective on the effect of prolonged stretching for joint contracture. *Journal of Physical Therapy Science, 19*, 97-101.

Pratt, K., & Bohannon, R. (2003). Effects of a 3-minutes standing stretch on ankle-dorsiflexion range of motion. *Journal of Sport Rehabilitation, 12*, 162-173.

Prentice, W. E. (1983). Comparison of static stretching and PNF stretching for improving hip joint flexibility. *Athl Train, 18*, 556-559.

Provenzano, P. P., Martinez, D. A., Grindeland, R. E., Dwyer, K. W., Vailas, A. C., & Vanderby, R. J. (2003). Hindlimb loading alters ligament healing. *Journal of Applied Physiology, 94*, 314-324.

Saal, J. S. (Ed.). (1987). *Flexibility training. In rehabilitation of sports injuries*. Philadelphia: Hanley & Belfus.

Sady, S. P., Wortman, M., & Blanke, D. (1982). Flexibility training: ballistic, static or proprioceptive neuromuscular facilitation. *Archives of Physical Medicine & Rehabilitation, 63*, 261-263.

Sahrmann, S. (2002). *Diagnosis and treatment of movement impairment syndromes*. St. Louis: Mosby.

Sexton, P., & Chambers, J. (2006). The importance of flexibility for functional range of motion. *Athletic Therapy Today, 11*(3), 13-15.

Sharman, M. J., Cresswell, A. G., & Riek, S. (2006). Proprioceptive neuromuscular facilitation stretching: mechanisms and clinical implications. *Sports Medicine, 36*(11), 929-939.

Shellock, F. G., & Prentice, W. E. (1985). Warming-up and stretching for improved physical performance and prevention of sports-related injuries. *Sports Medicine, 2*, 267-278.

Shrier, I., & Gossal, K. (2000). Myths and truths of stretching: individualized recommendations for healthy muscles. *Physician Sportsmed, 28*(8), 57-63.

Smith, L. K., Weiss, E. L., & Lehmkuh, L. D. (1996). *Brunnstrom's Clinical Kinesiology* (5th ed.). Philadelphia: FA Davis.

Sullivan, M. K., Dejulia, J. J., & Worrell, T. W. (1992). Effect of pelvic position and stretching method on hamstring muscle flexibility. *Med Sci Sports Exerc, 24*, 1383-1389.

Swenson, C., Swärd, L., & Karlsson, J. (1996). Cryotherapy in sports medicine. *Scandinavian Journal of Medicine and Science in Sports, 6*, 193-200.

Taylor, D. C., Dalton, J. D., Jr., Seaber, A. V., & Garrett, W. E., Jr. (1990). Viscoelastic properties of muscle-tendon units: The biomechanical effects of stretching. *American Journal of Sports Medicine, 18*, 300-309.

Thacker, S. B., Gilchrist, J., Stroup, D. F., & Kimsey, C. D., Jr. (2005). The impact of stretching on sports injury risk: a systematic review of the literature. *Med Sci Sports Exerc, 36*(3), 371-378.

Warren, C. G., Lehmann, J. K., & Koblanski, J. N. (1971). Elongation of rat tail tendon: Effect of load and temperature. *Archives of Physical Medicine and Rehabilitation, 52*, 465-474.

Warren, C. G., Lehmann, J. K., & Koblanski, J. N. (1976). Heat and stretch procedures: An evaluation using rat tail tendon. *Archives of Physical Medicine and Rehabilitation, 57*, 122-126.

Chapter 6

Bengtsson, A., Henrikkson, K. G., & Larsson, J. (1986). Reduced high-energy phosphate levels in the painful muscles of patients with primary fibromyalgia. *Arthritis & Rheumatism, 29*(7), 817-821.

Bernau-Eigen, M. (1998). Rolfing: a somatic approach to the integration of human structures. *Nurse Practitioner Forum, 9*(4), 235-242.

Brander, V., & Stulberg, S. D. (2006). Rehabilitation after hip- and knee-joint replacement. An experience- and evidence-based approach to care. *American Journal of Physical Medicine and Rehabilitation, 85,* S98-118.

Butler, D. S. (1991). *Mobilization of the nervous system.* New York: Churchill Livingstone.

Butler, D. S. (1994). *Mobilization of the nervous system. Level II. course handbook.* Marina Del Rey, CA: Neuro Orthopedic Institute.

Castel, J. C. (1979). *Pain management: Acupuncture and transcutaneous electrical nerve stimulation techniques.* Lake Bluff, IL: Pain Control Services.

Corrigan, B., & Maitland, G. D. (1989). *Practical Orthopedic Medicine.* Boston: Butterworth.

Cyriax, J. H. (1977). *Textbook of orthopedic medicine. Vol. 2, Treatment by manipulation, massage and injection.* Baltimore: Williams & Wilkins.

Cyriax, J. H. (1982). *Textbook of Orthopaedic Medicine. Vol. 1. Diagnosis of Soft Tissue Lesions* (8th ed.). London, England: Bailliere Tindall.

D'Ambrogio, K. J., & Roth, G. B. (1997). *Positional Release Therapy. Assessment & treatment of musculoskeletal dysfunction.* St. Louis: Mosby.

DeDomenico, G. (2007). *Beard's massage principles and practice of soft tissue manipulation.* Philadelphia: Saunders.

Dommisse, G. F. (1975). Morphological aspects of the lumbar spine and lumbosacral region. *Orthopedic Clinics of North America, 6,* 163-175.

Flynn, T. W., Wainner, R. S., & Fritz, J. M. (2006). Spinal manipulation in physical therapist professional degree education: A model for teaching and integration into clinical practice. *Journal of Orthopaedic & Sports Physical Therapy, 36*(8), 577-587.

Gerwin, R. D. (1994). Neurobiology of the myofascial trigger point. *Baillieres Clinical Rheumatology, 8*(4), 747-762.

Giammatteo, S. W., & Kain, J. B. (2005). *Integrative Manual Therapy. For the Connective Tissue System. Myofascial Release: The 3-Planar Fascial Fulcrum Approach* (Vol. IV). Berkeley, CA: North Atlantic Books.

Godges, J. J., Mattson-Bell, M., Thorpe, D., & Shah, D. (2003). The immediate effects of soft tissue mobilization with proprioceptive neuromuscular facilitation on glenohumeral external rotation and overhead reach. *Journal of Orthopaedic & Sports Physical Therapy, 33*(12), 713-718.

Greenman, P. E. (1996). *Principles of manual medicine.* Baltimore: Williams & Wilkins.

Gunn, C. (1997). Radiculopathic pain: diagnosis and treatment of segmental irritation or sensitisation. *Journal of Musculoskeletal Pain, 5,* 119-134.

Hanten, W. P., Olsen, S. L., Butts, N. L., & Nowicki, A. L. (2000). Effectiveness of a home program of ischaemic pressure followed by sustained stretch for treatment of myofascial trigger points. *Physical Therapy, 80*(10), 997-1003.

Huguenin, L. K. (2004). Myofascial trigger points: the current evidence. *Physical Therapy in Sport, 5*(1), 2-12.

Hunter, G. (1998). Specific soft tissue mobilization in the management of soft tissue dysfunction. *Manual Therapy, 3*(1), 2-11.

Johnson, A. J., Godges, J. J., Zimmerman, G. J., & Ounanian, L. L. (2007). The effect of anterior versus posterior glide joint mobilization on external rotation range of motion in patients with shoulder adhesive capsulitis. *Journal of Orthopaedic & Sports Physical Therapy, 37*(3), 88-99.

Jones, J. H., Kusunose, R. S., & Goering, E. K. (1995). *Strain-counterstrain.* Boise, ID: Jones Strain-CounterStrain, Inc.

Kaltenborn, F. M. (2002). *Manual Mobilization of the Joints. The Kaltenborn Method of Joint Examination and Treatment* (6th ed.). Oslo, Norway: Olaf NOrlis Bokhandel.

Konradsen, L., Holmer, P., & Sondergaard, L. (1991). Early mobilizing treatment for grade III ankle ligament injuries. *Foot Ankle, 12,* 69-73.

Lewis, C., & Flynn, T. W. (2001). The use of strain-counterstrain in the treatment of patients with low back pain. *Journal of Manual & Manipulative Therapy, 9*(2), 92-98.

Maitland, G. D. (1991). *Peripheral Manipulation* (3rd ed.). Boston: Butterworth-Heinemann.

Manheim, C. J. (1994). *The myofascial release manual* (2nd ed.). Thorofare, NJ: Slack.

McPartland, J. M., & Goodridge, J. P. (1997). Counterstrain and traditional osteopathic examination of the cervical spine compared. *Journal of Bodywork & Movement Therapies, 1*(3), 173-178.

Melzack, R. (1973). *The Puzzle of Pain.* New York: Basic Books.

Mennell, J. M. (1964). *Joint Pain: Diagnosis and Treatment Using Manipulative Techniques.* Boston: Little, Brown & Co.

Mesequer, A. A., Fernández-de-las-Peñas, C., Navarro-Poza, J. L., Rodríguez-Blanco, C., & Gandia, J. J. B. (2006). Immediate effects of the strain/counterstrain technique in local pain evoked by tender points in the upper trapezius muscle. *Clinical Chiropractic, 9*(3), 112-118.

Michlovitz, S. L., Harris, B. A., & Watkins, M. P. (2004). Therapy interventions for improving joint range of motion: A systematic review. *J hand ther, 17*(2), 118-131.

Mitchell, F. L. (1958). Structural pelvic function. In *Yearbook of the American Academy of Ostepathy.* Carmel, CA: American Academy of Osteopathy.

Molinary, R. (2006). A new word for relief. *Health, 20*(7), 88, 92.

Paris, S. V., & Patla, C. (1988). *E1 course notes: Extremity dysfunction and manipulation.* St. Augustine, FL: Patris.

Quintner, J. L., & Cohen, M. L. (1994). Referred pain of peripheral nerve origin: an alternative to the "myofascial pain" construct. *Clinical Journal of Pain, 10*(3), 243-251.

Simons, D. G. (1981). Myofascial trigger points: A need for understanding. *Archives of Physical Medicine & Rehabilitation, 62,* 97-99.

Smith, J. (2005). *Structural Bodywork.* Philadelphia: Elsevier.

Stone, J. A. (2000). Prevention and rehabilitation. Strain -- counterstrain. *Athletic Therapy Today, 5*(6), 30-31.

Sutton, G. S., & Bartel, M. R. (1994). Soft-tissue mobilization techniques for the hand therapist. *Journal of Hand Therapy, 7,* 185-192.

Travell, J. (1976). Myofascial trigger points: Clinical view. In J. J. Bonica & D. Albe-Fessard (Eds.), *Advances in pain research and therapy, vol. 1.* New York: Raven Press.

Travell, J. G., & Simons, D. G. (1983). *Myofascial pain and dysfunction. The trigger point manual. Vol. 1.* Baltimore: Williams and Wilkins.

Travell, J. G., & Simons, D. G. (1992). *Myofascial pain and dysfunction. The trigger point manual. Vol. 2.* Baltimore: Williams and Wilkins.

Unsworth, A., Dowson, D., & Wright, V. (1971). "Cracking joints". A bioengineering study of cavitation in the metacarpophalangeal joint. *Annals of the Rheumatic Diseases, 30*(4), 348-358.

Upton, A. R. M., & McComas, A. J. (1973). The double crush in nerve entrapment syndromes. *Lancet, 2,* 359-362.

van der Wees, P. J., Lenssen, A. F., Hendriks, E. J., Stomp, D. J., Dekker, J., & de Bie, R. A. (2006). Effectiveness of exercise therapy and manual mobilisation in acute ankle sprain and functional instability: a systematic review. *Australian Journal of Physiotherapy, 52*(1), 27-37.

Vicenzino, B., Collins, D., Benson, H., & Wright, A. (1998). An investigation of the interrelationship between manipulative therapy-induced hypoalgesia and sympathoexcitation. *Journal of Manipulative and Physiological Therapeutics, 21*(7), 448-453.

Wong, C. K., & Schauer, C. (2004). Reliability, validity and effectiveness of strain counterstrain techniques. *Journal of Manual & Manipulative Therapy, 12*(2), 107-112.

Yoder, E. (1990). Physical therapy management of nonsurgical hip problems in adults. In J. L. Echternach (Ed.), *Physical Therapy of the Hip.* New York, N.Y.: Churchill Livingstone.

Chapter 7

AAP., & fitness, C. o. s. m. a. (2001). Strength training by children and adolescents. *Pediatrics, 107*(6), 1470-1472.

ACSM. (1998). Position Stand. The recommended quantity and quality of exercise for developing and maintaining cardiorespiratory and muscular fitness, and flexibility in healthy adults. *Medicine & Science in Sports & Exercise, 30,* 975-991.

Akihiko, S. E. O., & Shinichi, U. D. A. (1997). Trunk rotation monitor using angular velocity sensors. *Industrial Health, 35,* 222-228.

Baechle, T. R., Earle, R. W., & Wathen, D. (2000). Resistance training. In T. R. Baechle & R. W. Earle (Eds.), *Essentials of Strength Training and Conditioning.* Champaign, IL: Human Kinetics.

Berger, R. A. (1962). Optimal repetitions for the development of strength. *Res Q, 33,* 334-338.

Billeter, H., & Hoppeler, H. (1992). Muscular basis of strength. In P. V. Komi (Ed.), *Strength and power in sport.* Boston: Blackwell Scientific.

Braatz, J. H., & Gogia, P. P. (1987). The mechanics of pitching. *J Orthop Sports Phys Ther, 9,* 56-69.

Brown, D. R. (1980). *Neurosciences for allied health therapies.* St. Louis: Mosby.

Clark, R. G. (1975). *Manter and Gatz's Essentials of Clinical Neuroanatomy and Neurophysiology* (5th ed.). Philadelphia: F.A.Davis.

Clarke, D. H. (1971). The influence on muscular fatigue patterns of the intercontraction rest interval. *Medicine and Science in Sports, 3,* 83-88.

Conley, M. (2000). Bioenergetics of exercise and training. In T. R. Baechle & R. W. Earle (Eds.), *Essentials of Strength Training and Conditioning.* Champaign, IL: Human Kinetics.

Conroy, B., & Earle, R. W. (2000). Bone, muscle, and connective tissue adaptations to physical activity. In T. R. Baechle & R. W. Earle (Eds.), *Essentials of Strength Training and Conditioning* (2nd ed.). Champaign, IL: Human Kinetics.

de Ruiter, C. J., Van Leeuwen, D., Heijblom, A., Bobbert, M. F., & de Haan, A. (2006). Fast unilateral isometric knee extension torque development and bilateral jump height. *Med sci sports exerc, 38*(10), 1843-1852.

DeLorme, T. L., & Watkins, A. L. (1948). Technics of progressive resistance exercise. *Arch Phys Med, 29,* 263-273.

Denegar, C. R., Saliba, E., & Saliba, S. (2010). *Therapeutic Modalities for Athletic Injuries* (3rd ed.). Champaign, IL: Human Kinetics.

Enoka, R. M. (1995). Morphological features and activation patterns of motor units. *Journal of Clinical Neurophysiology, 12,* 538-559.

Enoka, R. M., Christou, E., Hunter, S., Kornatz, K., Semmler, J., Taylor, M., et al. (2003). Mechanisms that contribute to differences in motor performance between young and old adults. *J Electromyogr Kinesiol, 13,* 1-12.

Feigenbaurm, M. S., & Pollock, M. L. (1999). Prescription of resistance training for health and disease. *Med Sci Sports Exerc, 31*(1), 38-45.

Folland, J. P., & Williams, A. G. (2007). The Adaptations to Strength Training: Morphological and Neurological Contributions to Increased Strength. *Sport med, 37*(2), 145-168.

Gabriel, D. A., Kamen, G., & Frost, G. (2006). Neural adaptations to resistive exercise: mechanisms and recommendations for training practices. *Sport med, 36*(2), 133-149.

Hale, S. A., Hertel, J., & Olmsted-Kramer, L. C. (2007). The effect of a 4-week comprehensive rehabilitation program on postural control and lower extremity function in individuals with chronic ankle instability. *J orthop sports phys ther, 37*(6), 303-311.

Hettinger, T., & Müller, E. (1953). Muscle strength and muscle training. *Arbeits Physiology, 15,* 111-126.

Hislop, H. J., & Montgomery, J. (2002). *Daniels and Worthingham's muscle testing. Techniques of manual examination* (7th ed ed.). Philadelphia: WB Saunders.

Hortobágyi, T., & Katch, F. I. (1990). Eccentric and concentric torque-velocity relationships during arm flexion and extension. *European Journal of Applied Physiology, 60,* 395-401.

Houglum, P. (1977). The modality of therapeutic exercise: Objectives and principles. *Athletic Training, 12,* 42-45.

Hunter, G. R. (2000). Muscle physiology. In T. R. Baechle & R. W. Earle (Eds.), *Essentials of Strength Training and Conditioning* (2nd ed.). Champaign, IL: Human Kinetics.

Johnson, E. W., & Wiechers, D. (1982). Electrodiagnosis. In F. J. Kottke, G. K. Stillwell & J. F. Lehmann (Eds.), *Krusen's Handbook of Physical Medicine and Rehabilitation* (3rd ed.). Philadelphia: WB Saunders.

Kendall, F. P., McCreary, E. K., & Provance, P. G. (1993). *Muscles: Testing and Function* (4th ed.). Baltimore: Williams & Wilkins.

Knight, K. L. (1985). Guidelines for rehabilitation of sports injuries. *Clinics in Sports Medicine, 4,* 405-416.

Knott, M., & Voss, D. E. (1968). *Proprioceptive Neuromuscular Facilitation*. New York: Harper & Row.

Kottke, F. J. (1982). Therapeutic exercise to maintain mobility. In F. J. Kottke, G. K. Stillwell & J. F. Lehmann (Eds.), *Krusen's Handbook of Physical Medicine and Rehabilitation*. Philadelphia: Saunders.

Kotzamanidis, C., Chatzopoulos, D., Michailidis, C., Papaiakovou, G., & Patikas, D. (2005). The effect of a combined high-intensity strength and speed training program on the running and jumping ability of soccer players. *J Strength Cond Res, 19*(2), 369-375.

Kraemer, W. J. (2000). Physiological adaptations to anaerobic and aerobic endurance training programs. In T. R. Baechle & R. W. Earle (Eds.), *Essentials of Strength Training and Conditioning*. Champaign, IL: Human Kinetics.

Lieber, R. L. (1992). *Skeletal Muscle Structure and Function. Implications for Rehabilitation and Sports Medicine*. Baltimore: Williams & Wilkins.

Lind, A. R. (1959). Muscle fatigue and recovery from fatigue induced by sustained contractions. *Journal of Physiology (London), 147*, 162-171.

MacDougall, J. D., Elder, G. C. B., Sale, D. G., Moroz, J. R., & Sutton, J. R. (1980). Effect of training and immobilization on human muscle fibers. *European Journal of Applied Physiology, 43*, 25-34.

Moritani, T., & DeVries, H. A. (1979). Neural factors versus hypertrophy in the time course of muscle strength gain. *Am j phys med, 58*(3), 115-130.

Müller, E. A. (1970). Influence of training and of inactivity on muscle strength. *Archives in Physical Medicine and Rehabilitation, 51*, 449-492.

Page, P. (2003). More than meets the eye. *Advance phys ther PT assist, 14*, 47-48.

Page, P. A., Labbe, A., & Tropp, R. V. (2000). Clinical force production of Thera-band elastic bands. *J Orthop Sports Phys Ther, 30*(1), A-47-48.

Sinacore, D. R., Bander, B. L., & Delitto, A. (1994). Recovery from a 1-minute bout of fatiguing exercise: Characteristics, reliability, and responsiveness. *Physical Therapy, 74*, 234-244.

Stamford, B. (1985). The difference between strength and power. *Physician and Sportsmedicine, 13*, 155.

Threlkeld, A. J. (1992). The effects of manual therapy on connective tissue. *Physical Therapy, 72*, 893-902.

van der Hoeven, J. H., van Weerden, T. W., & Zwarts, M. J. (1993). Long-lasting supernormal conduction velocity after sustained maximal isometric contraction in human muscle. *Muscle Nerve, 16*(3), 312-320.

Wallis, E. L., & Logan, G. A. (1964). *Figure Improvement and Body Conditioning Through Exercise*. Englewood Cliffs, NJ: Prentice-Hall.

Wilmore, J. H., & Costill, D. C. (2004). *Physiology of Sport and Exercise* (3rd ed.). Champaign, IL: Human Kinetics.

Zinovieff, A. N. (1951). Heavy-resistance exercises. The "Oxford Technique". *British Journal of Physical Medicine, 14*, 129-132.

Chapter 8

Barrack, R. L., Lund, P. J., & Skinner, H. B. (1994). Knee joint proprioception revisited. *J Sport Rehabil, 3*, 18-42.

Beynnon, B. D., Good, L., & Risberg, M. A. (2002). The effect of bracing on proprioception of knees with anterior cruciate ligament injury. *J orthop sports phys ther, 32*(1), 11-15.

Blackburn, T., Guskiewicz, K. M., Petschauer, M. A., & Prentice, W. E. (2000). Balance and joint stability: the relative contributions of proprioception and muscular strength. *J sport rehabil, 9*(4), 315-328.

Callaghan, M. J., Selfe, J., Bagley, P. J., & Oldham, J. A. (2002). The effects of patellar taping on knee joint proprioception. *Journal of Athletic Training, 37*, 19-24.

Ellaway, P. H. (1995). Fusimotor reflexes from joint and cutaneous afferents. In W. R. Ferrell & U. Proske (Eds.), *Neural Control of Movement* (pp. 89-96). New York: Plenum Press.

Gabriel, D. A., Kamen, G., & Frost, G. (2006). Neural adaptations to resistive exercise: mechanisms and recommendations for training practices. *Sport med, 36*(2), 133-149.

Grigg, P. (1994). Peripheral neural mechanisms in proprioception. *J Sport Rehabil, 3*, 2-17.

Hewett, T., Paterno, M., & Myer, G. (2002). Strategies for enhancing proprioception and neuromuscular control of the knee. *Clin orthop, 402*, 76-94.

Kottke, F. J. (1982). Therapeutic exercise to develop neuromuscular coordination. In F. Kottke, G. Stillwell & J. Lehmann (Eds.), *Krusen's handbook of physical medicine and rehabilitation*. Philadelphia: Saunders.

Lephart, S. M., Kocher, M. S., Fu, F. H., Borsa, P. A., & Harner, C. D. (1992). Proprioception following ACL reconstruction. *J Sport Rehabil, 1*, 188-196.

Leroux, A., Bélanger, M., & Boucher, J. P. (1995). Pain effect on monosynaptic and polysynaptic reflex inhibition. *arch phys med rehabil, 76*, 576-582.

Perlau, R., Frank, C., & Fick, G. (1995). The effect of elastic bandages on human knee proprioception in the uninjured population. *Am J Sports Med, 23*, 251-255.

Risberg, M. A., Beynnon, B. D., Peura, G. D., & Uh, B. S. (1999). Proprioception after anterior cruciate ligament reconstruction with and without bracing. *Knee Surgery, Sports Traumatology, Arthroscopy, 7*(5), 303-309.

Strasmann, T., van der Wal, J. C., Halata, Z., & Drukker, J. (1990). Functional topography and ultrastructure of periarticular mechanoreceptors in the lateral elbow region of the rat. *Acta Anat, 138*, 1-14.

Verhagen, E., van der Beek, A., Twisk, J., Bouter, L., Bahr, R., & van Mechelen, W. (2004). The effect of a proprioceptive balance board training program for the prevention of ankle sprains. A prospective controlled trial. *American Journal of Sports Medicine, 32*, 1385-1393.

Willems, T., Witvrouw, E., Verstuyft, J., Vaes, P., & De Clercq, D. (2002). Proprioception and muscle strength in subjects with a history of ankle sprains and chronic instability. *J Athletic Train, 37*(4), 487-493.

Chapter 9

Allerheiligen, B., & Rogers, R. (1995). Plyometrics program design. *Strength Condit, 17*, 26-31.

Bosco, C., Komi, P. V., & Ito, A. (1981). Prestretch potentiation of human skeletal muscle during ballistic movement`. *Acta Physiol Scand, 111*, 135-140.

Chmielewski, T., Kauffman, D., Myer, G. D., & Tillman, S. M. (2006). Plyometric Exercise in the Rehabilitation of

Athletes: Physiological Responses and Clinical Application. *Journal of Orthopaedic & Sports Physical Therapy, 36*(5), 308-319.

Chu, D. (1989). *Plyometric exercises with medicine balls.* Livermore, CA: Bittersweet.

Chu, D. (1998). *Jumping into plyometrics* (2nd ed ed.). Champaign, IL: Human Kinetics.

Dean, E. (1988). Physiology and therapeutic implications of negative work. A review. *Phys Ther 68,* 233-237.

Gambetta, V. (1986). In Roundtable discussion: Practical considerations for utilizing plyometrics. Part 1. *Nat Strength Coach Assoc J, 8,* 14-22.

Koutedakis, Y. (1989). Muscle elasticity - plyometrics : some physiological and practical considerations. *Journal of Applied Research in Coaching Athletics, 4,* 35-49.

Lundin, P. (1985). A review of plyometric training. *Strength Condit, 7,* 69-74.

Rassier, D. E., & Herzog, W. (2005). Force enhancement and relaxation rates after stretch of activated muscle fibers. *Procedures in Biological Science, 272,* 475-480.

Rimmer, J. H. (2005). Exercise and physical activity in persons aging with a physical disability. *Physical Medicine and Rehabilitation Clinics of North America, 16*(1), 41-56.

Roberts, T. J. (2002). The integrated function of muscles and tendons during locomotion. *Molecular Integrated Physiology, 133,* 1087-1099.

Sexton, P., & Chambers, J. (2006). The importance of flexibility for functional range of motion. *Athletic Therapy Today, 11*(3), 13-15.

Siff, M. C. (2004). *Supertraining* (6th ed.). Denver: Supertraining Institute.

Toumi, H., Thiery, C., Maitre, S., Martin, A., Vanneuville, G., & Poumarat, G. (2001). Training effects of amortization phase with eccentric/concentric variations - the vertical jump. *International Journal of Sports Medicine, 22,* 605-610.

Wilk, K. E., Voight, M. L., Keirns, M. A., Gambetta, V., Andrews, J. R., & Dillman, C. J. (1993). Stretch-shortening drills for the upper extremities: theory and clinical application. *Journal of Orthopaedic & Sports Physical Therapy, 17,* 223-239.

Wilt, F. (1975). Plyometrics. What it is-how it works. *Athletic Journal, 55,* 76-79.

Chapter 10

Kottke, F. J. (1980). From reflex to skill: The training of coordination. *Archives in Physical Medicine and Rehabilitation, 61*(12), 551-561.

Monfils, M.-H., Plautz, E. J., & Kleim, J. A. (2005). In search of the motor engram: Motor map plasticity as a mechanism for encoding motor experience. *Neuroscientist, 11*(5), 471-483.

Chapter 11

Alon, R. (1990). *Mindful spontaneity: Moving in tune with nature: Lessons in the Feldenkrais Method.* New York: Harper & Row.

Barlow, W. (1977). *The Alexander Technique.* New York: Knopf.

Kendall, F. P., McCreary, E. K., & Provance, P. G. (1993). *Muscles: Testing and Function* (4th ed.). Baltimore: Williams & Wilkins.

Sahrmann, S. A. (2002). *Diagnosis and treatment of movement impairment syndromes.* St. Louis: Mosby.

Siler, B. (2000). *The Pilates Body.* New York: Broadway Books.

Chapter 12

Chambers, H. G., & Sutherland, D. H. (2002). A practical guide to gait analysis. *Journal of the American Academy of Orthopaedic Surgeons, 10,* 222-273.

Childress, D. S., & Gard, S. A. (1997). Investigation of vertical motion of the human body during normal walking. *Gait and Posture, 5,* 161.

Dillman, C. J. (1975). Kinematic analyses of running. *Exercise and Sport Sciences Review, 3,* 193-218.

Gard, S. A., & Childress, D. S. (1999). The influence of stance-phase knee flexion on the vertical displacement of the trunk during normal walking. *Arch Phys Med Rehabil, 90,* 26.

Klopsteg, P. E., & Wilson, P. D. (1968). *Human Limbs and Their Substitutes.* New York: McGraw Hill.

Kumar, R., Roe, M. C., & Scremin, O. U. (1995). Methods for estimating the proper length of a cane. *Archives of Physical Medicine and Rehabilitation, 76*(12), 1173-1175.

Lehmann, J. F. (1990). Gait analysis: Diagnosis and management. In F. J. Kottke & J. F. Lehmann (Eds.), *Krusen's handbook of physical medicine and rehabilitation* (4th ed.). Philadelphia: Saunders.

Mann, R., & Inman, V. T. (1964). Phasic activity of intrinsic muscles of the foot. *J Bone Joint Surg, 46,* 469.

Mann, R. A., & Hagy, J. (1980). Biomechanics of walking, running, and sprinting. *American Journal of Sports Medicine, 8*(3), 345-350.

Murray, M. P., Drought, A. B., & Kory, R. C. (1964). Walking patterns of normal men. *J Bone Joint Surg Am, 46A,* 335-360.

Ounpuu, S. (1994). The biomechanics of walking and running. *Clin Sport Med, 13,* 843-863.

Perry, J. (1990). Gait analysis in sports medicine. *Instr Course Lect, 39,* 319-324.

Perry, J. (1992). *Gait Analysis: Normal and Pathological Function.* Thorofare, NJ: Slack.

Rodgers, M. M. (1988). Dynamic biomechanics of the normal foot and ankle during walking and running. *Phys Ther, 68,* 1822-1830.

Saunders, J. B. d. M., Inman, V. T., & Eberhart, H. D. (1953). The major determinants in normal and pathological gait. *Journal of Bone and Joint Surgery (Am), 35-A,* 543-558.

Williams, K. R. (1985). The biomechanics of running. *Exerc Sport Sci Rev, 13,* 389-441.

Winter, D. A. (1987). *The biomechanics and motor control of human gait.* Waterloo, ON, Canada: University of Waterloo Press.

Chapter 13

Davis, B. C., & Harrison, R. A. (1988). *Hydrotherapy in practice.* New York: Churchill Livingstone.

Denegar, C. R., Saliba, E., & Saliba, S. (2010). *Therapeutic Modalities for Athletic Injuries* (3rd ed.). Champaign, IL: Human Kinetics.

Edlich, R. F., Towler, M. A., Goitz, R. J., Wilder, R. P., Buschbacher, L. P., Morgan, R. F., et al. (1987). Bioengineering principles of hydrotherapy. *J Burn Care Rehabil, 8,* 580-584.

Harrison, R. A., Hillman, M., & Bulstrode, S. (1992). Loading of the lower limb when walking partially immersed: implications for clinical practice. *Physiother, 78*(3), 164-166.

Hay, J. (1993). *The biomechanics of sports techniques* (4th ed.). Englewood Cliffs, NJ: Prentice-Hall.

Koury, J. M. (1996). *Aquatic Therapy Programming*. Champaign, IL: Human KInetics.

McWaters, J. G. (1988). *Deep water exercise for health and fitness*. Laguna Beach, CA: Publitec Editions.

Thein, J. M., & Brody, L. T. (1998). Aquatic-based rehabilitation and training for the elite athlete. *Journal of Orthopaedic & Sports Physical Therapy, 27*, 32-41.

Chapter 14

Drake, J. D. M., S. L. Fischer, et al. (2006). "Do Exercise Balls Provide a Training Advantage for Trunk Extensor Exercises? A Biomechanical Evaluation." *Journal of Manipulative and Physiological Therapeutics* 29: 354-362.

Naughton, J., R. Adams, et al. (2005). "Upper-body wobble-board training effects on the post-dislocation shoulder." *Physical Therapy in Sport* 6(1): 31-37.

Posner-Mayer, J. (1995). *Swiss ball applications for orthopedic and sports medicine*. Denver, Ball Dynamics International.

Chapter 15

Alfredson, H. (2005). The chronic painful Achilles and patellar tendon: research on basic biology and treatment. *Scandinavian Journal of Medicine and Science in Sports, 15*(4), 252-259.

Alfredson, H. (2006). Strategies in treatment of tendon overuse injury. The chronic painful tendon. *European Journal of Sport Science, 6*(2), 81-85.

Alfredson, H., & Cook, J. (2007). A treatment algorithm for managing Achilles tendinopathy: new treatment options. *British Journal of Sports Medicine, 41*(4), 211-216.

Alfredson, H., Pietila, T., Jonsson, P., & Lorentzon, R. (1998). Heavy-load eccentric calf muscle training for the treatment of chronic Achilles tendinosis. *American Journal of Sports Medicine, 26*(3), 360-366.

Elliot, D. H. (1965). Structure and function of mammalian tendon. *Biological Reviews, 40*, 392-421.

Eriksson, E. (2006). Eccentric training of painful supraspinatus tendinosis. *Knee Surgery, Sports Traumatology, Arthroscopy, 14*(1), 1.

Fenwick, S. A., Hazleman, B. L., & Riley, G. P. (2002). The vasculature and its role in the damaged and healing tendon. *Arthritis Research, 4*(4), 252-260.

Gross, M. T. (1992). Chronic tendinopathy: Pathomechanics of injury, factors affecting the healing response, and treatment. *Journal of Orthopaedic & Sports Physical Therapy, 16*, 248-261.

Jonsson, P., & Alfredson, H. (2007). Superior results with eccentric compared to concentric quadriceps training in patients with jumper's knee: a prospective randomised study. *British Journal of Sports Medicine, 39*(11), 847-890.

Jonsson, P., Wahlstrom, P., & Ohberg, L. (2006). Eccentric training in chronic painful impingement syndrome of the shoulder. *Knee Surgery, Sports Traumatology, Arthroscopy, 14*, 76-81.

LaStayo, P. C., Woolf, J. M., Lewek, M. D., Snyder-Mackler, L., Reich, T., & Lindstedt, S. L. (2003). Eccentric muscle contractions: their contribution to injury, prevention, rehabilitation, and sport. *Journal of Orthopaedic & Sports Physical Therapy, 33*(10), 557-571.

Maffulli, N., Khan, K. M., & Puddu, G. (1998). Overuse tendon conditions: time to change a confusing terminology. *Arthroscopy, 14*(8), 840-843.

Ohberg, L., Lorentzon, R., & Alfredson, H. (2004). Eccentric training in patients with chronic Achilles tendinosis: normalised tendon structure and decreased thickness at follow up. *British Journal of Sports Medicine, 38*(1), 8-11.

Rees, J. D., Wilson, A. M., & Wolman, R. L. (2006). Current concepts in the management of tendon disorders. *Rheumatology, 45*(5), 508-521.

Stanish, W. D., Curwin, S., & Mandel, S. (2000). *Tendinitis: its etiology and treatment*. New York: Oxford University Press.

Tasto, J. P., Cummings, J., Medlock, V., Harwood, F., Hardesty, R., & Amiel, D. (2004). Tendon treatment center. *Sports Medicine and Arthroscopy Review, 12*(4), 210-219.

Wang, J. H.-C., Iosifidis, M. I., & Fu, F. H. (2006). Biomechanical basis for tendinopathy. *Clinical Orthopaedics and Related Research, 443*, 320-332.

Woodley, B. L., Newsham-West, R. J., & Baxter, G. D. (2007). Chronic tendinopathy: effectiveness of eccentric exercise. *British Journal of Sports Medicine, 41*(4), 188-198.

Young, M. A., Cook, J. L., Purdam, C. R., Kiss, Z. S., & Alfredson, H. (2005). Eccentric decline squat protocol offers superior results at 12 months compared with traditional eccentric protocol for patellar tendinopathy in volleyball players. *British Journal of Sports Medicine, 39*, 102-105.

Chapter 16

Bauman, S., Williams, D., Petruccelli, D., Elliott, W., and J. de Beer. 2007. Physical activity after total joint replacement: A cross-sectional survey. *Clinical Journal of Sports Medicine* 17(2):104–108.

Berry, D.J., Berger, R.A., Callaghan, J.J., Dorr, L.D., Duwelius, P.J., Hartzband, M.A., et al. 2003. The orthopaedic forum. Minimally invasive total hip arthroplasty. Development, early results, and a critical analysis. *Journal of Bone and Joint Surgery Am* 85(11):2235–2246.

Bourdeau, S., Bourdeau, E., Higgins, L.D., and I.R.B. Wilcox. 2007. Rehabilitation following reverse total shoulder arthroplasty. *Journal of Orthopaedic and Sports Physical Therapy* 27(12):734–743.

Brady, O.H., Masri, B.A., Garbuz, D.S., and C.P. Duncan. 2000. Joint replacement of the hip and knee—when to refer and what to expect. *Canadian Medical Association Journal* 163(10):1285–1291.

Brander, V., and S.D. Stulberg. 2006. Rehabilitation after hip- and knee-joint replacement. An experience- and evidence-based approach to care. *American Journal of Physical Medicine and Rehabilitation* 85:S98–118.

Brief, A.A., Maurer, S.G., and P.E. DiCesare. 2001. Use of glucosamine and chondroitin sulfate in the management of osteoarthritis. *Journal of the American Academy of Orthopaedic Surgeons* 9:71–78.

Centers for Disease Control and Prevention. 2008. National Center for Health Statistics. Web site home page. Retrieved December 30, 2008, from www.cdc.gov/nchs/index.htm.

Dines, D.M., and M. Levinson. 1995. The conservative management of the unstable shoulder including rehabilitation. *Clinics in Sports Medicine* 14(4):797–816.

Dines, J.S., Fealy, S., Strauss, E.J., Allen, A., Craig, E.V., Warren, R.F., et al. 2006. Outcomes analysis of revision total shoulder replacement. *Journal of Bone and Joint Surgery Am* 88(7):1494–1500.

Fahrer, H., Rentsch, H.U., Gerber, N.J., Beyeler, C., Hess, C.W., and B. Grunig. 1988. Knee effusion and reflex inhibition of the quadriceps. A bar to effective retraining. *Journal of Bone and Joint Surgery Am* 70:635–638.

Guery, J., Favard, L., Sirveaux, F., Oudet, D., and D. Mole. 2006. Reverse total shoulder arthroplasty: Survivorship analysis of eighty replacements followed for five to ten years. *Journal of Bone and Joint Surgery Am* 88(8):1742–1747.

Hartzband, M.A. 2006. Posterolateral mini-incision total hip arthroplasty. *Operative Techniques in Orthopaedics* 16(2):93–101.

Hawker, G.A. 2006. Who, when, and why total joint replacement surgery? The patient's perspective. *Current Opinion in Rheumatology* 18(5):526–560.

Liem, D., van Fabeck, K., Poetzl, W., Winkelmann, W., and G. Gosheger. 2006. Golf after total hip arthroplasty: A retrospective review of 46 patients. *Journal of Sport Rehabilitation* 15(3):206–215.

McMullen, J., and T. Uhl. 2000. A kinetic chain approach for shoulder rehabilitation. *Journal of Athletic Training* 35(3):329–337.

Nicholson, G.P. 2006. Current concepts in reverse shoulder replacement. *Current Opinion in Orthopaedics* 17(4):306–309.

O'Driscoll, S.W., and J.G. Nicholas. 2000. Continuous passive motion (CPM): Theory and principles of clinical application. *Journal of Rehabilitation Research and Development* 37:178.

Pagnano, M.W., Trousdale, R.T., Meneghini, M., and A.D. Hanssen. 2006. Patients preferred a mini-posterior THA to a contralateral two-incision THA. *Clinical Orthopaedics & Related Research* 453:156–159.

Ulrich, S.D., Bonutti, P.M., Thorsten, M.S., Marker, D.R., Jones, L.C., and M.A. Mont. 2007. Outcomes-based evaluations supporting computer-assisted surgery and minimally invasive surgery for total hip arthroplasty. *Experimental Reviews of Medical Devices* 4(6):873–883.

Weng, H.H., and J. Fitzgerald. 2006. Current issues in joint replacement surgery. *Current Opinion in Rheumatology* 18(2):163–169.

Wilcox, R.B. III, Arslanian, L.E., and P.J. Millett. 2005. Rehabilitation following total shoulder arthroplasty. *Journal of Orthopaedic and Sports Physical Therapy* 35(12):821–836.

Chapter 17

Abbassi, V. 1998. Growth and normal puberty. *Pediatrics* 102(2):507–511.

Ahmed, M.S., Matsumura, B., and A. Cristian. 2005. Age-related changes in muscles and joints. *Physical Medicine and Rehabilitation Clinics of North America* 16(1):19–39.

American Academy of Pediatrics. 2001. Strength training by children and adolescents. *Pediatrics* 107(6):1470–1472.

Andrish, J.T. 1984. Overuse syndromes of the lower extremity in youth sports. In *Advances in Pediatric Sport Sciences,* ed. R.A. Boileau. Champaign, IL: Human Kinetics.

Ausubel, J.H., and A. Grübler. 1995. Working less and living longer: Long-term trends in working time and time budgets. *Technological Forecasting and Social Change* 50:113–131.

Backx, F.J.G., Erich, W.B.M., Kemper, A.B.A., and A.L.M. Verbeek. 1989. Sports injuries in school-aged children: An epidemiologic study. *American Journal of Sports Medicine* 17(2):234–240.

Baezner, H., Blahak, C., Poggesi, A., Pantoni, L., Inzitari, D., Chabriat, H., et al. 2008. Association of gait and balance disorders with age-related white matter changes: The LADIS study. *Neurology* 70(12):935–942.

Bar-Or, O., and T.W. Rowland. 2004. *Pediatric exercise medicine. From physiologic principles to health care application.* Champaign, IL: Human Kinetics.

Bijur, P.E., Thrumble, A., Harel, Y., Overpeck, M.D., Jones, D., and P.C. Scheidt. 1995. Sports and recreation injuries in US children and adolescents. *Archives of Pediatric and Adolescent Medicine* 149:1009–1016.

Cronin, A., and M.B. Mandich. 2005. *Human development and performance throughout the lifespan.* Clifton Park, NY: Thomson Delmar Learning.

Draper, D.O., and A.J. Dustman. 1992. Avulsion fracture of the anterior superior iliac spine in a collegiate distance runner. *Archives of Physical Medicine and Rehabilitation* 73:881–882.

Faigenbaum, A.D., Kraemer, W.J., Cahill, B., Chandler, J., Dziados, J., Elfrink, L.D., et al. 1996. Youth resistance training: Position statement paper and literature review. *Strength and Conditioning Journal* 18(6):62–75.

Feigenbaum, M.S., and M.L. Pollock. 1999. Prescription of resistance training for health and disease. *Medicine and Science in Sports and Exercise* 31(1):38–45.

Fernhall, B., and V.B. Unnithan. 2002. Physical activity, metabolic issues, and assessment. *Physical Medicine and Rehabilitation Clinics of North America* 13(4):925–947.

Frontera, W. 2006. Aging muscle. *Critical Reviews of Physical Rehabilitation Medicine* 18(1):63–93.

Hara, T., and T. Shimada. 2007. Effects of exercise on the improvement of the physical functions of the elderly. *Journal of Physical Therapy Science* 19(1):15–26.

Hellebrandt, F.A., and J.C. Waterland. 1962. Indirect learning: The influence of unimanual exercise on related muscle groups of the same and the opposite side. *American Journal of Physical Medicine* 41(4):45–55.

Hutchinson, M.R., and S. Wynn. 2004. Biomechanics and development of the elbow in the young throwing athlete. *Clinics in Sports Medicine* 23:531–544.

Jones, G., Ding, C., Glisson, M., Hynes, K., Ma, D., and F. Cicuttini. 2003. Knee articular cartilage development in children: A longitudinal study of the effect of sex, growth, body composition, and physical activity. *Pediatric Research* 54(2):230–236.

Kallinen, M., and A. Markku. 1995. Aging, physical activity and sports injuries. An overview of common sports injuries in the elderly. *Sports Medicine* 20(1):41–52.

Kemp, B.J. 2005. What the rehabilitation professional and the consumer need to know. *Physical Medicine and Rehabilitation Clinics of North America* 16(1):1–18.

Kocher, M.S. 2006. Anterior cruciate ligament reconstruction in the skeletally immature patient. *Operative Techniques in Sports Medicine* 14(3):124–134.

Koester, M.C. 2002. Adolescent and youth sports medicine: A "growing" concern. *Athletic Therapy Today* 7(6):6–12.

Kottke, F.J. 1982. Therapeutic exercise to develop neuromuscular coordination. In *Krusen's handbook of physical medicine and rehabilitation,* ed. F. Kottke, G. Stillwell, and J. Lehman. Philadelphia: Saunders.

Lane, L.B., and P.G. Bullough. 1980. Age-related changes in the thickness of the calcified zone and the number of tidemarks in adult human articular cartilage. *Journal of Bone and Joint Surgery Br* 62(3):372–375.

Mase, K., Kamimura, H., Imura, S., and K. Kitagawa. 2006. Effect of age and gender on muscle function-analysis by muscle fiber conduction velocity. *Journal of Physical Therapy Science* 18(1):81–87.

Mazzeo, R.S., Cavanagh, P., Evans, W.J., Fiatarone, M., Hagberg, J., McAuley, E., et al. 1998. Position stand. Exercises and physical activity for older adults. *Medicine and Science in Sports and Exercise* 30(6): 992-1008.

McDermott, A.Y., and H. Mernitz. 2006. Exercise and older patients: Prescribing guidelines. *American Family Physician* 74(3):437–444.

Micheli, L.J., Moseley, J.B., Anderson, A.F., Browne, J.E., Erggelet, C., Arciero, R.A., et al. 2006. Articular cartilage defects of the distal femur in children and adolescents: Treatment with autologous chondrocyte implantation. *Journal of Pediatric Orthopaedics* 26(4):455–460.

Milgrom, C., Miligram, M., Simkin, A., Burr, D., Ekenman, I., and A. Finestone. 2001. A home exercise program for tibial bone strengthening based on in vivo strain measurements. *American Journal of Physical Medicine and Rehabilitation* 80(6):433–438.

Narici, M.V., and C.N. Maganaris. 2006. Adaptability of elderly human muscles and tendons to increased loading. *Journal of Anatomy* 208(4):433–443.

Narici, M., and C. Maganaris. 2007. Plasticity of the muscle-tendon complex with disuse and aging. *Exercise and Sport Sciences Reviews* 35(3):126–134.

Natri, A., Jarvinen, M., Latvala, K., and P. Kannus. 1996. Isokinetic muscle performance after anterior cruciate ligament surgery. Long-term results and outcome predicting factors after primary surgery and late-phase reconstruction. *International Journal of Sports Medicine* 17(3):223–238.

Omey, M.L., and L.J. Micheli. 1999. Foot and ankle problems in the young athlete. *Medicine and Science in Sports and Exercise* 31(7):S470–S486.

Poluri, A., Mores, J., Cook, D.B., Findley, T.W., and A. Cristian. 2005. Fatigue in the elderly population. *Physical Medicine and Rehabilitation Clinics of North America* 16(1):91–108.

Reeves, N.D., Narici, M.V., and C.N. Maganaris. 2006. Musculoskeletal adaptations to resistance training in old age. *Manual Therapy* 11(1):192–196.

Riegger-Krugh, C.L., McCarty, E.C., Robinson, M.S., and D.A. Wegzyn. 2008. Autologous chondrocyte implantation: Current surgery and rehabilitation. *Medicine and Science in Sports and Exercise* 40(2):206–214.

Runnels, E.D., Bemben, D.A., Anderson, M.A., and M.G. Bemben. 2005. Influence of age on isometric, isotonic, and isokinetic force production characteristics in men. *Journal of Geriatric Physical Therapy* 28(3):74–84.

Salter, R.B., and W.R. Harris. 1963. Injuries involving the epiphyseal plate. *Journal of Bone and Joint Surgery Am* 45(3):587–622.

Shigematsu, R., and T. Okura. 2006. A novel exercise for improving lower-extremity functional fitness in the elderly. *Aging Clinical and Experimental Research* 18(3):242–248.

Steadman, T.L. 1990. *Steadman's medical dictionary.* 25th ed. Baltimore: Williams & Wilkins.

Tanigawa, M. 1972. Comparison of the hold-relax procedure and passive mobilization on increasing muscle length. *Physical Therapy* 52:725–735.

Tanner, J.M., and J.M. Buckler. 1997. Revision and update of Tanner-Whitehouse clinical longitudinal charts for height and weight. *European Journal of Pediatrics* 156(3):248–249.

Tanner, J.M., and P.S.W. Davies. 1985. Clinical longitudinal standards for height and height velocity for North American children. *Journal of Pediatrics* 107:317–329.

Tanner, J.M., and R.H. Whitehouse. 1976. Clinical longitudinal standards for height, weight, height velocity, weight velocity, and stages of puberty. *Archives of Disease in Childhood* 51(3):170–179.

Thompson, L.V. 2002. Skeletal muscle adaptations with age, inactivity, and therapeutic exercise. *Journal of Orthopaedic & Sports Physical Therapy* 32(2):44–57.

Warren, C.G., Lehmann, J.K., and J.N. Koblanski. 1976. Heat and stretch procedures: An evaluation using rat tail tendon. *Archives of Physical Medicine and Rehabilitation* 57:122–126.

Wasserlauf, B.L., and G.A. Paletta Jr. 2003. Shoulder disorders in the skeletally immature throwing athlete. *Orthopedic Clinics of North America* 34:427–437.

Williams, C.A. 2007. Exercise and environmental conditions. In *Paediatric exercise physiology,* ed. N. Spurway and D. MacLaren. Philadelphia: Churchill Livingstone Elsevier.

Youdas, J.W., Krause, D.A., Hollman, J.H., Harmsen, W.S., and E. Laskowski. 2005. The influence of gender and age on hamstring muscle length in healthy adults. *Journal of Orthopaedic & Sports Physical Therapy* 35(4):246–252.

Part IV

Fahrer, H., Rentsch, H. U., Gerber, N. J., Beyeler, C., Hess, C. W., & Grunig, B. (1988). Knee effusion and reflex inhibition of the quadriceps. A bar to effective retraining. *Journal of Bone and Joint Surgery, 70,* 635-638.

Leroux, A., Bélanger, M., & Boucher, J. P. (1995). Pain effect on monosynaptic and polysynaptic reflex inhibition. *Archives of Physical Medicine & Rehabilitation, 76,* 576-582.

Maitland, G. D. (1991). *Peripheral Manipulation* (3rd ed.). Boston: Butterworth-Heinemann.

Chapter 18

Beattie, P. (1992). The use of an eclectic approach for the treatment of low back pain: A case study. *Physical Therapy, 72*(12), 923-928.

Bergmark, A. (1989). Stability of the lumbar spine. A study in mechanical engineering. *Acta Orthopaedica Scandinavica, 60*(230 (suppl)), 1-54.

Cappaert, T. A. (2000). The sacroiliac joint as a factor in low back pain: A review. *Journal of Sport Rehabilitation, 9*(2), 169-183.

Childs, J. D., Flynn, T. F., Fritz, J. M., Piva, S. R., Wainner, R. S., & Whitman, J. M. (2005). Screening for Vertebrobasilar Insufficiency in Patients With Neck Pain: Manual Therapy Decision Making in the Presence of Uncertainty. *Journal of Orthopaedic & Sports Physical Therapy, 35*(5), 300-306.

Cholewicki, J., Panjabi, M. M., & Khachatryan, A. (1997). Stabilizing function of trunk flexor-extensor muscles around a neutral spine posture. *Spine, 22,* 2207-2212.

Cibulka, M. T. (1992). The treatment of the sacroiliac joint component to low back pain: A case report. *Physical Therapy, 72*(12), 917-922.

Clark, M. A., Fater, D., & Reuterman, P. (2000). Core (trunk) stabilization and its importance for closed kinetic chain rehabilitation. *Orthopaedic physical therapy clinics of north america, 9*(2), 119-135.

Cook, C., Hegedus, E., Showalter, C., & Sizer, P. S., Jr. (2006). Coupling behavior of the cervical spine: A systematic review of the literature. *Journal of Manipulative and Physiological Therapeutics, 29*(7), 570-575.

Ebenbichler, G. R., Oddsson, L. I. E., Kollmitzer, J., & Erim, Z. (2001). Sensory-motor control of the lower back: implications for rehabilitation. *Medicine & Science in Sports & Exercise, 33*(11), 1889-1198.

Ekstrom, R. A., Donatelli, R. A., & Carp, K. C. (2007). Electromyographic Analysis of Core Trunk, Hip, and Thigh Muscles During 9 Rehabilitation Exercises. *Journal of Orthopaedic & Sports Physical Therapy, 37*(12), 754-762.

Fryette, H. H. (1980). *Principles of Osteopathic Technique.* Carmel, CA: Academy of Applied Osteopathy.

Grenier, S., & McGill, S. M. (2007). Quantification of Lumbar Stability by Using 2 Different Abdominal Activation Strategies. *Archives of Physical Medicine & Rehabilitation, 88*(1), 54-62.

Hubley-Kozey, C. L. (2005). Training the abdominal musculature. *Physiotherapy of Canada, 57*(1), 5-17.

Jull, G. A., & Richardson, C. A. (2000). Motor control problems in patients with spinal pain: a new direction for therapeutic exercise. *Journal of Manipulative and Physiological Therapeutics, 23,* 115-117.

Kasai, R. (2006). Current trends in exercise management for chronic low back pain: comparison between strengthening exercise and spinal segmental stabilization exercise. *Journal of Physical Therapy Science, 18*(1), 97-105.

Kennedy, B. A. (1967). A muscle-bracing technique utilizing intra-abdominal pressure to stabilize the lumbar spine. *Australian Journal of Physiotherapy, 11,* 102-106.

Kofotolis, N., & Kellis, E. (2006). Effects of two 4-week proprioceptive neuromuscular facilitation programs on muscle endurance, flexibility, and functional performance in women with chronic low back pain. *Physical Therapy, 86*(7), 1001-1012.

Leetun, D. T., Ireland, M. L., Willson, J. D., Ballantyne, B. T., & Davis, I. M. (2004). Core stability measures as risk factors for lower extremity injury in athletes. *Medicine & Science in Sports & Exercise, 36*(6), 926-934.

Legaspi, O., & Edmond, S. L. (2007). Does the evidence support the existence of lumbar spine coupled motion? A critical review of the literature. *Journal of Orthopaedic & Sports Physical Therapy, 37*(4), 169-178.

Liebenson, C. (2006). Functional training for performance enhancement—Part 1: The basics. *Journal of Bodywork and Movement Therapies, 10,* 154-158.

Mannion, A. F., Taimela, S., Müntener, M., & Dvorak, J. (2001). Active therapy for chronic low back pain part 1. Effects on back muscle activation, fatigability, and strength. *Spine, 26*(8), 897-908.

McConnell, J. (2002). Recalcitrant chronic low back and leg pain – a new theory and different approach to management. *Manual Therapy, 7*(4), 183-192.

McGill, S. M. (2001). Low back stability: from formal description to issues for performance and rehabilitation. *Exercise and Sport Sciences Review, 29*(1), 26-31.

McGill, S. M., Grenier, S., Kavcic, N., & Cholewicki, J. (2003). Coordination of muscle activity to assure stability of the lumbar spine. *Journal of Electromyography & Kinesiology, 13*(4), 353-359.

McKenzie, R. A. (1981). *The Lumbar Spine: Mechanical Diagnosis and Therapy.* Lower Hutt, New Zealand: Spinal Publications.

McKenzie, R. A. (1989). *The Lumbar Spine: Mechanical Diagnosis and Therapy.* Raumati Beach, New Zealand: Spinal Publications.

Norris, C. (1995). Stabilisation Mechanisms of the Lumbar Spine. *Physiotherapy, 81*(2), 72-79.

Norris, C. (2001). Functional load abdominal training: part 2. *Physical Therapy in Sport, 2*(3), 149-156.

Nourbakhsh, M. R., & Arab, A. M. (2002). Relationship between mechanical factors and incidence of low back pain. *Journal of Orthopaedic & Sports Physical Therapy, 32,* 447-460.

O'Sullivan, P. B., Beales, D. J., Beetham, J. A., Cripps, J., Graf, F., Lin, I. B., et al. (2002). Altered motor control strategies in subjects with sacroiliac joint pain during the active straight-leg-raise test. *Spine, 27*(1), E1-8.

O'Sullivan, P. B., Burnett, A. F., Floyd, A. N., & al., e. (2003). Lumbar repositioning deficit in a specific low back pain population. *Spine, 28*(10), 1074-1079.

Panjabi, M. M., Abumi, K., Duranceau, J., & Oxland, T. (1989). Spinal stability and intersegmental muscle forces. A biomechanical model. *Spine, 14*(2), 194-200.

Radebold, A., Cholewicki, J., Panjabi, M. M., & Patel, T. C. (2000). Muscle response pattern to sudden trunk loading in healthy individuals and in patients with chronic low back pain. *Spine, 25*(8), 947-954.

Richardson, C. A., Jull, G., Hodges, P. W., & Hides, J. A. (1999). *Therapeutic exercise for spinal segmental stabilization in low back pain: Scientific basis and clinical approach.* Edinburgh, UK: Churchill Livingstone.

Rosatelli, A. L., Agur, A. M., & Chhaya, S. (2006). Anatomy of the interosseous region of the sacroiliac joint. *Journal of Orthopaedic & Sports Physical Therapy, 36*(4), 200-208.

Rydeard, R., Leger, A., & Smith, D. (2006). Pilates-based therapeutic exercise: Effect on subjects with nonspecific chronic low back pain and functional disability: A randomized controlled trial. *Journal of Orthopaedic & Sports Physical Therapy, 36*(7), 472-484.

Sahrmann, S. (2002). *Diagnosis and treatment of movement impairment syndromes*. St. Louis: Mosby.

Thorstensson, A., & Carlson, H. (1987). Fiber types in human lumbar back muscles. *Acta Physiologica Scandinavia, 131*, 195-202.

Travell, J. G., & Simons, D. G. (1983). *Myofascial pain and dysfunction. The trigger point manual. Vol. 1*. Baltimore: Williams and Wilkins.

Wilke, H. J., Wolf, S., Claes, L. E., Arand, M., & Wiesend, A. (1995). Stability increases of the lumbar spine with different muscles groups. A biomechanical in vitro study. *Spine, 20*(2), 192-198.

Williams, P. C. (1955). Examination and conservative treatment for disk lesions of the lower spine. *Clinical Orthopaedics 5*, 28-40.

Zazulak, B. T., Hewett, T. E., Reeves, N. P., Goldberg, B., & Cholewicki, J. (2007). Deficits in neuromuscular control of the trunk predict knee injury risk: a prospective biomechanical-epidemiologic study. *American Journal of Sports Medicine, 35*(7), 1123-1130.

Chapter 19

Akeson, W. H., Woo, S. L.-Y., Amiel, D., Coutts, R. D., & Daniel, D. (1973). The connective tissue response to immobility: Biochemical changes in periarticular connective tissue of the immobilized rabbit knee. *Clinical Orthopaedics, 93*, 356-362.

Andrews, J. R., Carson, W. G. J., & McLeod, W. D. (1985). Glenoid labrum tears related to the long head of the biceps. *American Journal of Sports Medicine, 13*(5), 337-341.

Bagg, S. D., & Forrest, W. J. (1988). A biomechanical analysis of scapular rotation during arm abduction in the scapular plane. *American Journal of Physical Medicine, 67*, 238-245.

Bishop, J. Y., & Kaeding, C. (2006). Treatment of the acute traumatic acromioclavicular separation. *Sports Medicine and Arthroscopy Review, 14*, 237-245.

Blackburn, T. A., McLeod, W. D., White, B., & Wofford, L. (1990). EMG analysis of posterior rotator cuff exercises. *Athletic Training, 25*(1), 40,42-45.

Borich, M. R., Bright, J. M., Lorello, D. J., Cieminski, C. J., Buisman, T., & Ludewig, P. M. (2006). Scapular angular positioning at end range internal rotation in cases of glenohumeral internal rotation deficit. *Journal of Orthopaedic & Sports Physical Therapy, 36*(12), 926-934.

Borsa, P. A., Lephart, S. M., Kocker, M. S., & Lephart, S. P. (1994). Functional assessment and rehabilitation of shoulder proprioception for glenohumeral instability. *Journal of Sport Rehabilitation, 3*(1), 84-104.

Braatz, J. H., & Gogia, P. P. (1987). The mechanics of pitching. *Journal of Orthopaedic & Sports Physical Therapy, 9*, 56-69.

Bradley, J. P., & Tibone, J. E. (1991). Electromyographic analysis of muscle action about the shoulder. *Clinics in Sports Medicine, 10*, 789-805.

Burkhart, S. S., Morgan, C. D., & Kibler, W. B. (2003a). The disabled throwing shoulder: Spectrum of pathology Part I: Pathoanatomy and biomechanics. *Arthroscopy, 19*(4), 404-420.

Burkhart, S. S., Morgan, C. D., & Kibler, W. B. (2003b). The disabled throwing shoulder: Spectrum of pathology part III: The SICK scapula, scapular dyskinesis, the kinetic chain, and rehabilitation. *Journal of Arthroscopic and Related Surgery, 19*(6), 641-661.

Chan, R. H., & Lam, J. J. (2006). Glenoid Labrum Lesion in an Elite Tennis Player: A Clinical Challenge in Diagnosis. *Journal of Sport Rehabilitation, 15*, 168-177.

Cools, A., Witvrouw, E., Declercq, G., Danneels, L., & Cambier, D. (2003). Scapular muscle recruitment patterns: trapezius muscle latency with and without impingement symptoms. *American Journal of Sports Medicine, 31*(4), 542-549.

Cyriax, J. H. (1982). *Textbook of Orthopaedic Medicine. Vol. 1. Diagnosis of Soft Tissue Lesions* (8th ed.). London, England: Bailliere Tindall.

Decker, M. J., Hintermeister, R. A., Faber, K. J., & Hawkins, R. J. (1999). Serratus Anterior Muscle Activity During

Denegar, C. R., Saliba, E., & Saliba, S. (2010). *Therapeutic Modalities for Athletic Injuries* (3rd ed.). Champaign, IL: Human Kinetics.

Dietz, A., & Dreese, J. C. (2007). Anterior shoulder instability in the overhead athlete: current concepts. *Current Opinions in Orthopaedics, 18*(2), 172-176.

Dillman, C. J., Fleisig, G. S., & Andrews, J. R. (1993). Biomechanics of pitching with emphasis upon shoulder kinematics. *Journal of Orthopaedic & Sports Physical Therapy, 18*(2), 402-408.

Ebaugh, D. D., Karduna, A. R., & McClure, P. W. (2006). Scapulothoracic and Glenohumeral Kinematics Following an External Rotation Fatigue Protocol. *Journal of Orthopaedic & Sports Physical Therapy, 36*(8), 557-571.

Ekstrom, R. A., Bifulco, K. M., Lopau, C. J., Andersen, C. F., & Gough, J. R. (2004). Comparing the function of the upper and lower parts of the serratus anterior muscle using surface electromyography. *Journal of Orthopaedic & Sports Physical Therapy, 34*, 235-243.

Ellenbecker, T. S., & Mattalino, A. J. (1999). Glenohumeral joint range of motion and rotator cuff strength following arthroscopic anterior stabilization with thermal capsulorraphy. *Journal of Orthopaedic & Sports Physical Therapy, 29*, 160-167.

Gerber, A., & Warner, J. J. (2002). Thermal capsulorrhaphy to treat shoulder instability. *Clinical Orthopaedics, 400*, 105-116.

Goldstein, B. (2004). Shoulder anatomy and biomechanics. *Phys med rehabil clin North Am, 15*(2), 313-349.

Hardwick, D. H., Beebe, J. A., McDonnell, M. K., & Lang, C. E. (2006). A comparison of serratus anterior muscle activation during a wall slide exercise and other traditional exercises. *Journal of Orthopaedic & Sports Physical Therapy, 36*(12), 903-910.

Hayashi, K., & Markel, M. D. (2001). Thermal Capsulorrhaphy Treatment of Shoulder Instability. *Clinical Orthopaedics and Related Research, 390*, 59-72.

Hayashi, K., Thabit, G., III, Massa, K. L., Bogdanske, J. J., Cooley, A. J., Orwin, J. F., et al. (1997). The effect of thermal heating on the length and histologic properties of the glenohumeral joint capsule. *American Journal of Sports Medicine, 25*, 107-112.

Hintermeister, R. A., Lange, G., Schultheis, J. M., Bey, M. J., & Hawkins, R. J. (1998). Electromyographic activity and applied load during shoulder rehabilitation exercises using elastic resistance. *American Journal of Sports Medicine, 26*(2), 210-220.

Host, H. H. (1995). Scapular taping in the treatment of anterior shoulder impingement. *Physical Therapy, 75*, 803-812.

Hume, P. A., Keogh, J., & Reid, D. (2005). The role of biomechanics in maximising distance and accuracy of golf shots. *Sports Medicine, 35*(5), 429-449.

Jobe, F. W., Moynes, D. R., & Antonelli, D. J. (1985). Rotator cuff function during a golf swing. *American Journal of Sports Medicine, 14*, 388-392.

Jobe, F. W., Moynes, D. R., Tibone, J. E., & Perry, J. (1984). An EMG analysis of the shoulder in pitching. A second report. *American Journal of Sports Medicine, 12*(3), 218-220.

Jobe, F. W., Tibone, J. E., Perry, J., & Moynes, D. R. (1983). An EMG analysis of the shoulder in throwing and pitching. A preliminary report. *American Journal of Sports Medicine, 11*(1), 3-5.

Kamkar, A., Irrgang, J. J., & Whitney, S. L. (1993). Nonoperative management of secondary shoulder impingement syndrome. *Journal of Orthopaedic & Sports Physical Therapy, 17*, 212-224.

Kelly, B., Kadrmas, W., & Speer, K. (1996). The manual muscle examination for rotator cuff strength. An electromyographic investigation. *American Journal of Sports Medicine, 24*(5), 581-588.

Kibler, W. B. (1995). Biomechanical analysis of the shoulder during tennis activities. *Clinics in Sports Medicine, 14*, 79-85.

Kuechle, D. K., Newman, S. R., Itoi, E., Niebur, G. L., Morrey, B. F., & An, K. N. (2000). The relevance of the moment arm of shoulder muscles with respect to axial rotation of the glenohumeral joint in four positions. *Clinical Biomechanics, 15*(5), 322-329.

Kuhn, J. E., Lindholm, S. R., Huston, L. J., Soslowsky, L. J., & Blasier, R. B. (2003). Failure of the biceps superior labral complex: A cadaveric biomechanical investigation comparing the late cocking and early deceleration positions of throwing. *Journal of Arthroscopy & Related Research, 19*(4), 373-379.

Lear, L.J. & Gross, M.T. (1998). An electromyographical analysis of the scapular stabilizing synergists during a push-up progression. *Journal of Orthopaedic & Sports Physical Therapy, 28*, 146-157.

Lephart, S. M., & Henry, T. J. (1996). The physiological basis for open and closed kinetic chain rehabilitation for the upper extremity. *Journal of Sport Rehabilitation, 5*, 71-87.

Lewis, L. S., Wright, C., & Green, A. (2005). Subacromial impingement syndrome: The effect of changing posture on shoulder range of movement. *Journal of Orthopaedic & Sports Physical Therapy, 35*, 72-87.

Lukasiewicz, A. C., McClure, P., Michener, L., Praff, N., & Senneff, B. (1999). Comparison of 3-dimensional scapular position and orientation between –subjects with and without shoulder impingement *Journal of Orthopaedic & Sports Physical Therapy, 29*, 574-586.

Mazzocca, A. D., Arciero, R. A., & Bicos, J. (2007). Evaluation and treatment of acromioclavicular joint injuries. *American Journal of Sports Medicine, 35*(2), 316-329.

McCabe, R., Orishimo, K., McHugh, M., & Nicholas, S. (2007). Surface electromyographic analysis of the lower trapezius muscle during exercises performed below ninety degrees of shoulder elevation in healthy subjects. *North American Journal of Sports Physical Therapy, 2*(1), 34-43.

McCann, P.D,, Wootten, M.E., Kadaba, M.P., & Bigliani, L.U. (1993). A kinematic and electromyographic study of shoulder rehabilitation exercises. *Clinical Orthopaedics and Related Research*, 288, 178-188.

McQuade, K. J., Dawson, J., & Smidt, G. L. (1998). Scapulothoracic muscle fatigue associated with alterations in scapulohumeral rhythm kinematics during maximum resistive shoulder elevation. *Journal of Orthopaedic & Sports Physical Therapy, 28*(2), 74-80.

Mileski, R. A., & Synder, S. J. (1998). Superior labral lesions in the shoulder: Pathoanatomy and surgical management. *Journal of American Academic of Orthopaedic Surgeons, 6*, 121-131.

Miniaci, A., & Codsi, M. J. (2006). Thermal Capsulorrhaphy for the Treatment of Shoulder Instability. *American Journal of Sports Medicine, 34*(8), 1356-1363.

Moseley, J. B., Jr. , Jobe, F. W., Pink, M., Perry, J., & Tibone, J. (1992). EMG analysis of the scapular muscles during a shoulder rehabilitation program. *American Journal of Sports Medicine, 20*(2), 128-134.

Moynes, D. R., Perry, J., Antonelli, D. J., & Jobe, J. W. (1986). Electromyography and motion analysis of the upper extremity in sports. *Physical Therapy, 66*, 1905-1911.

Myers, J. B., Wassinger, C. A., & Lephart, S. M. (2006). Sensorimotor contribution to shoulder stability: Effect of injury and rehabilitation. *Manual Therapy, 11*, 197-201.

Nuber, G. W., Jobe, F. W., Perry, J., Moynes, D. R., & Antonelli, D. (1986). Fine wire electromyography analysis of muscles of the shoulder during swimming. *American Journal of Sports Medicine, 14*(7-11).

Pappas, A. M., Zawacki, R. M., & Sullivan, T. J. (1985). Biomechanics of baseball pitching, a preliminary report. *American Journal of Sports Medicine, 13*(216-222).

Park, H. B., Lin, S. K., Yokota, A., & McFarland, E. G. (2004). Return to play for rotator cuff injuries and superior labrum anterior posterior (SLAP) lesions. *Clinics in Sports Medicine, 23*(3), 321-334.

Park, S. S., Loebenberg, M. L., Rokito, A. S., & Zuckerman, J. D. (2002/2003a). The shoulder in baseball pitching. Biomechanics and related injuries. Part 1. *Bulletin (Hospital for Joint Diseases (New York, N.Y.)), 61*(1/2), 68-79.

Park, S., Loebenberg, M., Rokito, A., & Zuckerman, J. (2002/2003b). The shoulder in baseball pitching. Biomechanics and related injuries. Part 2. *Bulletin (Hospital for Joint Diseases (New York, N.Y.)), 61*(1/2), 80-88.

Perry, J. (1978). Normal upper extremity kinesiology. *Phys Ther, 58*, 265-278.

Perry, J. (1983). Anatomy and biomechanics of the shoulder in throwing, swimming, gymnastics, and tennis. *Clinics in Sports Medicine, 2*(2), 247-270.

Perry, J. (1993a). The Shoulder and Elbow. In M. W. Chapman (Ed.), *Operative Orthopaedics* (2nd ed., Vol. 2, Part VI, pp. 1642-1649). Philadelphia: J.P. Lippincott.

Perry, J. (1993b). Shoulder Function for the Activities of Daily Living. In F. A. Matsen, F. H. Fu & R. J. Hawkins (Eds.), *The Shoulder: A Balance of Mobility and Stability* (pp. 185-191). Rosemont, IL: AAOS.

Pink, M., Perry, J., Browne, A., Scovazzo, M. L., & Kerrigan, J. (1991). The normal shoulder during freestyle swimming. *American Journal of Sports Medicine, 19*, 569-576.

Reinold, M. M., Macrina, L. C., Wilk, K. E., Fleisig, G. S., Dun, S., Barrentine, S. W., et al. (2007). Electromyographic analysis of the supraspinatus and deltoid muscles during 3 common rehabilitation exercises. *Journal of Athletic Training, 42*(4), 464-469.

Reinold, M. M., Wilk, K. E., Fleisig, G. S., Zheng, N., Barrentine, S. W., Chmielewski, T., et al. (2004). Electromyographic analysis of the rotator cuff and deltoid musculature during common shoulder external rotation exercises. *Journal of Orthopaedic & Sports Physical Therapy, 34*, 385-394.

Richardson, A. B., Jobe, F. W., & Collins, H. R. (1980). The shoulder in competitive swimming. *Am J Sports Med, 8*, 159-163.

Ryu, R. K. N., McCormick, J., Jobe, F. W., Moynes, D. R., & Antonelli, D. J. (1988). An electromyographic analysis of shoulder function in tennis players. *American Journal of Sports Medicine, 16*, 481-485.

Sagano, J., Magee, D., & Katayose, M. (2006). The effect of glenohumeral rotation on scapular upward rotation in different positions of scapular-plane elevation. *Journal of Sport Rehabilitation, 15*, 144-155.

Sauers, E. L. (2005). Effectiveness of rehabilitation for patients with subacromial impingement syndrome. *Journal of Athletic Training, 40*(3), 221-223.

Selected Rehabilitation Exercises. *American Journal of Sports Medicine, 27*(6), 784-791.

Selkowitz, D. M., Chaney, C., Stuckey, S. J., & Vlad, G. (2007). The effects of scapular taping on the surface electromyographic signal amplitude of shoulder girdle muscles during upper extremity elevation in individuals with suspected shoulder impingement syndrome. *Journal of Orthopaedic & Sports Physical Therapy, 37*(11), 694-702.

Sheridan, M. A., & Hannafin, J. A. (2006). Upper extremity: emphasis on frozen shoulder. *Orthopedic Clinics of North America, 37*(4), 531-539.

Synder, S. J., Karzel, R. P., Del Pizzo, W., Ferkel, R. D., & Friedman, M. J. (1990). SLAP lesions of the shoulder. *Arthroscopy, 6*, 274-279.

Townsend, H., Jobe, F. W., Pink, M., & Perry, J. (1991). Electromyographic analysis of the glenohumeral muscles during a baseball rehabilitation program. *American Journal of Sports Medicine, 19*(3), 264-271.

Travell, J. G., & Simons, D. G. (1983). *Myofascial pain and dysfunction. The trigger point manual. Vol. 1.* Baltimore: Williams and Wilkins.

Uhl, T. L., Carver, T. J., Mattacola, C. G., Mair, S. D., & Nitz, A. J. (2003). Shoulder musculature activation during upper extremity weight bearing exercise. *Journal of Orthopaedic & Sports Physical Therapy, 33*, 109-117.

Wilk, K., Reinold, M., Dugas, J., Arrigo, C., & Andrews, J. (2005). Current concepts in the recognition and treatment of superior labral (SLAP) lesions. *Journal of Orthopaedic & Sports Physical Therapy, 35*(5), 273-291.

Zhang, Q. (2007). Influence of knee joint position on co-contractions of agonist and antagonist muscles during maximal voluntary isometric contractions: Electromyography and Cybex movement. *Journal of Physical Therapy Science, 19*, 125-130.

Chapter 20

Alcid, J. G., Ahmad, C. S., & Lee, T. Q. (2004). Elbow anatomy and structural biomechanics. *Clinics in Sports Medicine, 23*(4), 503-517.

Ciccotti, M. C., Schwartz, M. A., & Ciccotti, M. G. (2004). Diagnosis and treatment of medial epicondylitis of the elbow *Clinics in Sports Medicine, 23*(4), 693-705.

Croisier, J., Foidart-Dessalle, M., Tinant, F., Crielaard, J., & Forthomme, B. (2007). An isokinetic eccentric programme for the management of chronic lateral epicondylar tendinopathy. *British Journal of Sports Medicine, 41*(4), 269-275.

Denegar, C. R., Saliba, E., & Saliba, S. (2010). *Therapeutic Modalities for Athletic Injuries* (3rd ed.). Champaign, IL: Human Kinetics.

Donkers, M. J., An, K. N., Chao, E. Y., & Morrey, B. F. (1993). Hand position affects elbow joint load during push-up exercise. *Journal of Biomechanics, 26*, 625-632.

Ellenbecker, T. S., & Mattalino, E. G. (1997). *The Elbow in Sport*. Champaign, IL: Human Kinetics.

Feltner, M., & Dapena, J. (1986). Dynamics of the shoulder and elbow joints of the throwing arm during a baseball pitch. *International Journal of Sport Biomechanics, 2*, 235-259.

Groppel, J. L., & Nirschl, R. P. (1986). A mechanical and electromyographical analysis of the effects of various joint counterforce braces on the tennis player. *American Journal of Sports Medicine, 14*, 195-200.

Hume, P., Reid, D., & Edwards, T. (2006). Epicondylar injury in sport. Epidemiology, type, mechanisms, assessment, management and prevention. *Sports Medicine, 36*(2), 151-170.

Jobe, F. W., Stark, H., & Lombardo, S. J. (1986). Reconstruction of the ulnar collateral ligament in athletes. *Journal of Bone and Joint Surgery, 68A*, 1158-1163.

Keefe, D. T., & Lintner, D. M. (2004). Nerve injuries in the throwing elbow. *Clinics in Sports Medicine, 23*, 723-742.

Kibler, W. B. (1995). Pathophysiology of overload injuries around the elbow. *Clinics in Sports Medicine, 14*.

Kibler, W. B., & Sciascia, A. (2004). Kinetic chain contributions to elbow function and dysfunction in sports. *Clinics in Sports Medicine, 23*(4), 545-552.

Kohia, M., Brackle, J., Byrd, K., Jennings, A., Murray, W., & Wilfong, E. (2008). Effectiveness of physical therapy treatments on lateral epicondylitis. *Journal of Sport Rehabilitation, 17*(1), 113-136.

Kottke, F. J., Pauley, D. L., & Ptak, R. A. (1966). The rationale for prolonged stretching for correction of shortening of connective tissue. *Archives of Physical Medicine & Rehabilitation, 47*(6), 345-352.

Light, K. J. (2008). Golf injuries take a swing at rehab and prevention. *Biomechanics, 15*(6), 22-31.

Loftice, J., Fleisig, G. S., Zheng, N., & Andrews, J. R. (2004). Biomechanics of the elbow in sports. *Clinics in Sports Medicine, 23*(4), 519-530.

Mero, A., Komi, P. V., Korjus, T., Navarro, E., & Gregor, R. J. (1994). Body segment contributions to javelin throwing during final thrust phases. *Journal of Applied Biomechanics, 10*.

Nassab, P. F., Mark, S., & Schickendantz, M. (2006). Evaluation and treatment of medial ulnar collateral ligament injuries in the throwing athlete. *Sports Medicine and Arthroscopy Review, 14*, 221-231.

Nirschl, R. P. (1977). Tennis elbow. *Primary care, 4*, 367-382.

Rees, J. D., Wilson, A. M., & Wolman, R. L. (2006). Current concepts in the management of tendon disorders. *Rheumatology, 45*(5), 508-521.

Sabick, M. B., Kim, Y.-K., Torry, M. R., Keirns, M. A., & Hawkins, R. J. (2005). Biomechanics of the shoulder in youth baseball pitchers. *American Journal of Sports Medicine, 33*(11), 1716-1722.

Travell, J. G., & Simons, D. G. (1983). *Myofascial pain and dysfunction. The trigger point manual. Vol. 1.* Baltimore: Williams and Wilkins.

Chapter 21

Bowers, W. H., & Tribuzi, S. M. (1992). Functional anatomy. In B. G. Stanley & S. M. Tribuzi (Eds.), *Concepts in Hand Rehabilitation*. Philadelphia: F.A. Davis.

Boyes, J. R. (1970). *Bunnell's Surgery of the Hand* (ed 5 ed.). Philadelphia: JB Lippincott.

Buckwalter, J. A. (1996). Effects of early motion on healing of musculoskeletal tissues. *Hand Clinics, 12*, 13-24.

Buterbaugh, G. A., Brown, T. R., & Horn, P. C. (1998). Ulnar-sided wrist pain in athletes. *Clinics in Sports Medicine, 17*(3), 567-583.

Doyle, J. R., & Blythe, W.F., (1975). The finger flexor tendon sheaths and pulleys. Anatomy and reconstruction. In *A.A.O.S.: Symposium on tendon surgery of the hand*. St. Louis: Mosby.

Duran, R. J., & Houser, R. G. (1975). Controlled passive motion following flexor tendon repair in zones 2 and 3. In *A.A.O.S. Symposium on tendon surgery of the hand*. St. Louis: Mosby.

Evans, R. B., & Burkhalter, W. E. (1986). A study of the dynamic anatomy of extensor tendons and implications for treatment. *Journal of Hand Surgery (Am), 11*, 774-779.

Malanga, G. A., & Chimes, G. P. (2006). Rehabilitation of basketball Injuries. *Physical Medicine and Rehabilitation Clinics of North America, 17*(3), 565-587.

McFee, S. D. (1987). Functional hand evaluations: A review. *American Journal of Occupational Therapy, 41*, 158-163.

Moore, J. S. (1997). De Quervain's tenosynovitis: Stenosing tenosynovitis of the first dorsal compartment. *Journal of Occupational and Environmental Medicine, 39*, 990-1002.

Stewart, K. M. (1991). Review and comparison of current trends in the postoperative management of tendon repair. *Hand Clinics, 7*, 447-460.

Stewart, K. M. (1992). Tendon injuries. In B. G. Stanley & S. M. Tribuzi (Eds.), *Concepts in Hand Rehabilitation*. Philadelphia: F.A. Davis.

Travell, J. G., & Simons, D. G. (1983). *Myofascial pain and dysfunction. The trigger point manual. Vol. 1.* Baltimore: Williams and Wilkins.

Urbaniak, J. R., Cahill, J. D., & Mortenson, R. (Eds.). (1975). *Tendon suturing methods: Anaylsis of tensile strength*. St. Louis, MO: CV Mosby.

von Schroeder, H. P., & Botte, M. J. (2001). Anatomy and functional significance of the long extensors to the fingers and thumb. *Clinical Orthopaedics, 383*, 74-83.

Chapter 22

Alanen, J., Orava, S., Heinonen, O. J., Ikonen, J., & Kvist, M. (2001). Peroneal tendon injuries. Report of thirty-eight operated cases. *Annales Chirurgiae et Gynaecologiae, 90*, 43-46.

Batt, M. E., Ugalade, V., Anderson, M. W., & Shelton, D. K. (1998). A prospective controlled study of diagnostic imaging for acute shin splints. *Medicine and Science in Sports and Exercise, 30*(11), 1564-1571.

Baumhauer, J., Shereff, M., & Gould, J. (1997). Ankle pain in runners. In G. N. Guten (Ed.), *Running injuries*. Philadelphia: Saunders.

Bernier, J. N., & Perrin, D. H. (1998). Effect of coordination training on proprioception of the functionally unstable ankle. *Journal of Orthopaedic & Sports Physical Therapy, 27*, 264-275.

Bolgla, L. A., & Keskula, D. R. (1997). Reliability of lower extremity functional performance tests. *Journal of Orthopaedic & Sports Physical Therapy, 26*, 138-142.

Cipriani, D. J., Armstrong, C. W., & Gaul, S. (1995). Backward walking at three levels of treadmill inclination: An electromyographic and kinematic analysis. *Journal of Orthopaedic & Sports Physical Therapy, 22*, 95-102.

De Vera Barredo, R., Menna, D., & Farris, J. W. (2007). An evaluation of research evidence for selected physical therapy interventions for plantar fasciitis. *Journal of Physical Therapy Science, 19*(1), 41-56.

Dierks, T. A., Manal, K. T., Hamill, J., & Davis, I. S. (2008). Proximal and distal influences on hip and knee kinematics in runners with patellofemoral pain during a prolonged run. *Journal of Orthopaedic & Sports Physical Therapy, 38*(8), 448-456.

Dietzen, C. J. (1990). great toe sesamoid injuries in the athlete. *Orthopaedic Review, 19*(11), 966-972.

Donatelli, R., Wooden, M., Ekedahl, S. R., Wilke, J. S., Cooper, J., & Bush, A. J. (1999). Relationship between static and dynamic foot postures in professional baseball players. *Journal of Orthopaedic & Sports Physical Therapy, 29*, 316-325.

Evans, A. (2001). Podiatric medical applications of posterior night stretch splinting. *Journal of the American Podiatric Medical Association, 91*(7), 356-360.

Forkin, D. M., Koczur, C., Battle, R., & Newton, R. A. (1996). Evaluation of kinesthetic deficits indicative of balance control in gymnasts with unilateral chronic ankle sprains. *Journal of Orthopaedic & Sports Physical Therapy, 23*, 245-250.

Garcia-Mata, S., Hidalgo-Ovejero, A., & Martinez-Grande, M. (2001). Chronic exertional compartment syndrome of the legs in adolescents. *Journal of Pediatric Orthopaedics, 21*(3), 328-334.

Garn, S. N., & Newton, R. A. (1988). Kinesthetic awareness in subjects with multiple ankle sprains. *Physical Therapy, 68*, 1667-1671.

Gigante, A., Moschini, A., Verdenelli, A., Torto, M., Ulisse, S., & Palma, L. (2008). Open versus percutaneous repair in the treatment of acute Achilles tendon rupture: a randomized prospective study. *Knee Surgery, Sports Traumatology, Arthroscopy, 16*(2), 204-209.

Gillogly, S. D., Myers, T. H., & Reinold, M. M. (2006). Treatment of full-thickness chondral defects in the knee with autologous chondrocyte implantation. *Journal of Orthopaedic & Sports Physical Therapy, 36*(10), 751-764.

Glascoe, W. M., Allen, M. K., Awtry, B. F., & Yack, H. J. (1999). Weight-bearing immobilization and early exercise treatment following a grade II lateral ankle sprain. *Journal of Orthopaedic & Sports Physical Therapy, 29*, 394-399.

Greenberger, H. B., & Paterno, M. V. (1995). Relationship of knee extensor strength and hopping test performance in the assessment of lower extremity function. *Journal of Orthopaedic & Sports Physical Therapy, 22*, 202-206.

Gross, M. T., Bradshaw, M. K., Ventry, L. C., & Weller, K. H. (1987). Comparison of support provided by ankle taping and semirigid orthosis. *Journal of Orthopaedic & Sports Physical Therapy, 9*, 33-39.

Hale, S. A., Hertel, J., & Olmsted-Kramer, L. C. (2007). The effect of a 4-week comprehensive rehabilitation program on postural control and lower extremity function in individuals with chronic ankle instability. *Journal of Orthopaedic & Sports Physical Therapy, 37*(6), 303-311.

Hicks, J. H. (1953). The mechanics of the foot: I. The joints. *Journal of Anatomy, 87*, 345.

Hyland, M. R., Webber-Gaffney, A., Cohen, L., & Lichtman, S. W. (2006). Randomized controlled trial of calcaneal taping, sham taping, and plantar fascia stretching for the short-term management of plantar heel pain. *Journal of Orthopaedic & Sports Physical Therapy, 36*(6), 364-371.

Jahss, M. H. (1981). The sesamoids of the hallux. *Clinical Orthopaedics, 157*, 88-97.

Kangas, J., Pajala, A., Siira, P., Hamalainen, M., & Leppilahti, J. (2003). Early functional treatment versus early immobilization in tension of the musculotendinous unit after Achilles rupture repair: a prospective, randomized, clinical study. *Journal of Trauma, 54*(6), 1171-1180.

Karlsson, J., & Andreasson, G. O. (1992). The effect of external ankle support in chronic lateral ankle joint instability. *American Journal of Sports Medicine, 20*, 257-261.

Kimura, I. F., Nawoczenski, D. A., Epler, M., & Owen, M. G. (1987). Effect of the AirStirrup in controlling ankle inversion stress. *Journal of Orthopaedic & Sports Physical Therapy, 9*, 190-193.

Klingman, R. E., Liaos, S. M., & Hardin, K. M. (1997). The effect of subtalar joint posting on patellar glide position in subjects with excessive rearfoot pronation. *Journal of Orthopaedic & Sports Physical Therapy, 25*, 185-191.

Kohn, H. S. (1997). Shin pain and compartment syndromes in running. In G. N. Guten (Ed.), *Running injuries*. Philadelphia: Saunders.

Konradsen, L. (2002). Factors contributing to chronic ankle instability: kinesthesia and joint position sense. *Journal of Athletic Training, 37*(4), 381-385.

Konradsen, L., Holmer, P., & Sondergaard, L. (1991). Early mobilizing treatment for grade III ankle ligament injuries. *Foot Ankle, 12*, 69-73.

Krause, J. O., & Brodsky, J. W. (1998). Peroneus brevis tendon tears: pathophysiology, surgical reconstruction, and clincial results. *Foot and Ankle International, 19*(5), 271-279.

Lattanza, L., Gray, G. W., & Kantner, R. M. (1988). Closed versus open kinematic chain measurements of subtalar joint eversion: implications for clinical practice. *Journal of Orthopaedic & Sports Physical Therapy, 9*, 310-314.

Lin, C.-F., Gross, M. T., & Weinhold, P. (2006). Ankle syndesmosis injuries: Anatomy, biomechanics, mechanism of injury, and clinical guidelines for diagnosis and intervention. *Journal of Orthopaedic & Sports Physical Therapy, 36*(6), 372-384.

Lofvenberg, R., Karrholm, J., Sundelin, G., & Ahlgren, O. (1995). Prolonged reaction time in patients with chronic lateral instability of the ankle. *American Journal of Sports Medicine, 23*, 414-417.

Lundberg, A., Goldien, I., Kalin, B., & Selvik, G. (1989). Kinematics of the foot/ankle complex: plantar flexion and dorsiflexion. *Foot & Ankle, 9*, 194-200.

Massie, D. L., & Spiker, J. C. (1990). *Foot biomechanics and the relationship to rehabilitation of lower extremity injuries*. Berryville, VA: Forum Medicum.

Monaghan, K., Delahunt, E., & Caulfield, B. (2006). This ankle function during gait in patients with chronic ankle instability compared to controls. *Clinical Biomechanics, 221*(2), 168-174.

Mortensen, N. H. M., Skov, O., & Jensen, P. E. (1999). Early motion of the ankle after operative treatment of a rupture of the Achilles tendon: A prospective randomized clinical trial and radiographic study. *Journal of Bone and Joint Surgery, 81A*, 983-990.

Ogden, J. A., Alvarez, R., Levitt, R., Cross, G. L., & Marlow, M. (2001). Shock wave therapy for chronic proximal plantar fasciitis. *Clinical Orthopaedics, 387*, 47-59.

Powers, C. M., Maffucci, R., & Hampton, S. (1995). Rearfoot posture in subjects with patellofemoral pain. *Journal of Orthopaedic & Sports Physical Therapy, 22*, 155-160.

Refshauge, K. M., Kilbreath, S. L., & Raymond, J. (2000). The effect of recurrent ankle inversion sprain and taping on proprioception at the ankle. *Medicine & Science in Sports & Exercise, 32*, 10-15.

Reinking, M. F. (2007). Exercise related leg pain (ERLP): a review of the literature. *North American Journal of Sports Physical Therapy, 2*(3), 170-180.

Renström, P. A., Konradsen, L., & Beynnon, B. D. (2000). Influence of knee and ankle support on proprioception and neuromuscular control. In S. M. Lephart & F. H. Fu (Eds.), *Proprioception and Neuromuscular Control in Joint Stability* (pp. 301-309). Champaign, IL: Human Kinetics.

Rovere, G. D., Clarke, T. J., Yates, C. S., & Burley, K. (1988). Retrospective comparison of taping and ankle stabilizers in preventing ankle injuries. *American Journal of Sports Medicine, 16,* 228-233.

Safran, M. R., O'Malley Jr, D., & Fu, F. H. (1999). Peroneal subluxation in athletes: new exam technique, case reports, and review. *Medicine & Science in Sports & Exercise, 31*(7), S487-S492.

Seto, J. L., & Brewster, C. E. (1994). Treatment approaches following foot and ankle injury. *Clinics in Sports Medicine, 13,* 695-718.

Sitler, M., Ryan, J., Wheeler, B., McBride, J., Arciero, R., Anderson, J., et al. (1994). The efficacy of a semirigid ankle stabilizer to reduce acute ankle injuries in basketball. *American Journal of Sports Medicine, 22,* 454-461.

Stanish, W. D., Curwin, S., & Mandel, S. (2000). *Tendinitis: its etiology and treatment.* New York: Oxford University Press.

Starkey, C., Brown, S., & Ryan, J. (2010). *Orthopedic & Athletic Injury Evaluation Handbook.* Philadelphia: F.A. Davis.

Thigpen, C. M. (1983). Early management of fractures of the foot and ankle. *Current Issue Trauma Care, 6,* 4-8.

Tiberio, D. (1987). The effect of excessive subtalar joint pronation on patellofemoral mechanics: A theoretical model. *Journal of Orthopaedic & Sports Physical Therapy, 9,* 160-165.

Travell, J. G., & Simons, D. G. (1992). *Myofascial pain and dysfunction. The trigger point manual. Vol. 2.* Baltimore: Williams and Wilkins.

Wilk, B. R., Fisher, K., & Gutierrez, W. (2000). Defective running shoes as a contributing factor in plantar fasciitis in a triathlete. *Journal of Orthopaedic & Sports Physical Therapy, 30,* 21-31.

Willems, T., Witvrouw, E., Verstuyft, J., Vaes, P., & De Clercq, D. (2002). Proprioception and muscle strength in subjects with a history of ankle sprains and chronic instability. *Journal of Athletic Training, 37*(4), 487-493.

Withrow, T. J., Huston, L. J., Wojtys, E. M., & Ashton-Miller, J. A. (2006). The relationship between quadriceps muscle force, knee flexion, and anterior cruciate ligament strain in an in vitro simulated jump landing. *American Journal of Sports Medicine, 34*(2), 299-311.

Chapter 23

Adam, F., Pape, D., Schiel, K., Steimer, O., Kohn, D., & Stefan Rupp, S. (2004). Biomechanical properties of patellar and hamstring graft tibial fixation techniques in anterior cruciate ligament reconstruction. *American Journal of Sports Medicine, 32*(1), 71-78.

Ahmed, A. M., & Burke, D. L. (1983). In vitro measurement of static pressure distribution in synovial joints: I. Tibial surface of the knee. *Journal of Biomedical Engineering, 105,* 216-225.

Andersen, L. L., Magnusson, S. P., Nielsen, M., Haleem, J., Poulsen, K., & Aagaard, P. (2006). Neuromuscular activation in conventional therapeutic exercises and heavy resistance exercises: Implications for rehabilitation. *Physical Therapy, 86*(5), 683-697.

Apsingi, S., Nguyen, T., Bull, A., Unwin, A., Deehan, D., & Amis, A. (2008). The role of PCL reconstruction in knees with combined PCL and posterolateral corner deficiency. *Knee Surgery, Sports Traumatology, Arthroscopy, 16*(2), 104-111.

Barber, F. A., & Click, S. D. (1997). Meniscus repair rehabilitation with concurrent anterior cruciate reconstruction. *Arthroscopy, 13*(4), 433-437.

Barclay, L. (2003). Outcomes similar for patellar or hamstring tendon ACL repair. *American Journal of Sports Medicine, 31,* 564-573.

Beynnon, B. D., Fleming, B. C., Johnson, R. J., Nichols, C. E., Renström, P. A., & Pope, M. H. (1995). Anterior cruciate ligament strain behavior during rehabilitation exercises in vivo. *American Journal of Sports Medicine, 23,* 24-34.

Beynnon, B., Johnson, R., Fleming, B., Stankewich, C. R., Renström, P. A., & Nichols, C. (1997). The strain behavior of the anterior cruciate ligament during squatting and active flexion-extension. A comparison of an open and a closed kinetic chain exercise. *American Journal of Sports Medicine, 25*(6), 823-829.

Bockrath, K., Wooden, C., Worrell, T., Ingersoll, C. D., & Farr, J. (1993). Effects of patella taping on patella position and perceived pain. *Medicine & Science in Sports & Exercise, 25,* 989-992.

Bolgla, L. A., Malone, T. R., Umberger, B. R., & Uhl, T. L. (2008). Hip strength and hip and knee kinematics during stair descent in females with and without patellofemoral pain syndrome. *Journal of Orthopaedic & Sports Physical Therapy, 38*(1), 12-18.

Bosch, U., Kasperczyk, W. J., Oestern, H. J., & Tscherne, H. (1994). Biology of posterior cruciate ligament healing. *Sports Medicine and Arthroscopy Review, 2,* 288-299.

Brown, C. H., Steiner, M. E., & Carson, E. W. (1993). The use of hamstring tendons for anterior cruciate ligament reconstruction. Technique and results. *Clinics in Sports Medicine, 12,* 723-756.

Brownstein, B., Mangiene, R. E., Noyes, F. R., & Kryer, S. (1988). Anatomy and biomechanics. In R. E. Mangiene (Ed.), *Physical therapy of the knee.* New York: Churchill Livingstone.

Butler, D. L., Noyes, F. R., & Grood, E. S. (1980). Ligamentous restraints to anterior-posterior drawer in the human knee. A biomechanical study. *Journal of Bone and Joint Surgery, 62-A,* 259-270.

Bynum, E. B., Barrack, R. L., & Alexander, A. H. (1995). Open versus closed chain kinetic exercises after anterior cruciate ligament reconstruction. A prospective randomized study. *American Journal of Sports Medicine, 23*(4), 401-406.

Campbell, B., Yaggie, J., & Cipriani, D. (2006). Temporal influences of functional knee bracing on torque production of the lower extremity. *Journal of Sport Rehabilitation, 15,* 216-227.

Cascio, B. M., Culp, L., & Cosgarea, A. J. (2004). Return to play after anterior cruciate ligament reconstruction. *Clinics in Sports Medicine, 23*(3), 395-408.

Chappell, J. D., Creighton, R. A., Giuliani, C., Yu, B., & Garrett, W. E. (2007). Kinematics and Electromyography of Landing Preparation in Vertical Stop-Jump Risks for Noncontact Anterior Cruciate Ligament Injury. *American Journal of Sports Medicine, 35*(2), 235-241.

Clancy, W. G., Jr., Narechania, R. G., Rosenberg, T. D., Gmeiner, J. G., Wisnefske, D. D., & Lange, T. A. (1981). Anterior and posterior cruciate ligament reconstruction in rhesus monkeys. *Journal of Bone and Joint Surgery, 63A,* 1270-1284.

Close, J. R. (1964). *Motor Function in the Lower Extremity: Analyses of Electronic Instrumentation.* Springfield, IL: Charles C Thomas.

Delay, B. S., Smolinski, R. J., Wind, W. M., & Bowman, D. S. (2001). Current practices and opinions in ACL reconstruction and rehabilitation: results of a survey of the American Orthopaedic Society for Sports Medicine. *American Journal of Knee Surgery, 14*(2), 85-91.

Dienst, M., Burks, R. T., & Greis, P. E. (2002). Anatomy and biomechanics of the anterior cruciate ligament. *Orthopedic Clinics of North America, 33*(4), 605-620.

Dierks, T. A., Manal, K. T., Hamill, J., & Davis, I. S. (2008). Proximal and distal influences on hip and knee kinematics in runners with patellofemoral pain during a prolonged run. *Journal of Orthopaedic & Sports Physical Therapy, 38*(8), 448-456.

Doucette, S. A., & Child, D. D. (1996). The effect of open and closed chain exercise and knee joint position on patellar tracking in lateral patellar compression syndrome. *Journal of Orthopaedic & Sports Physical Therapy, 23,* 104-110.

Doucette, S. A., & Goble, E. M. (1992). The effect of exercise on patellar tracking in lateral patellar compression syndrome. *American Journal of Sports Medicine, 20,* 434-440.

Durselen, L., Claes, L., & Kiefer, H. (1995). The influence of muscle forces and external loads on cruciate ligament strain. *American Journal of Sports Medicine, 23,* 129-136.

Dye, S. F., & Cannon, W. D., Jr. (1988). Anatomy and biomechanics of the anterior cruciate ligament. *Clinics in Sports Medicine, 7,* 715-725.

Earl, J. E., Schmitz, R. J., & Arnold, B. L. (2001). Activation of the VMO and VL during dynamic mini-squat exercises with and without isometric hip adduction. *Journal of Electromyography & Kinesiology, 11*(6), 381-386.

Ernst, G. P., Kawaguchi, J., & Saliba, E. (1999). Effect of patellar taping on knee kinetics of patients with patellofemoral pain syndrome. *Journal of Orthopaedic & Sports Physical Therapy, 29*(11), 661-667.

Escamilla, R., Fleisig, G., Zheng, N., Barrentine, S., Wilk, K., & Andrews, J. (1998). Biomechanics of the knee during closed kinetic chain and open kinetic chain exercises. *Medicine & Science in Sports & Exercise, 30*(4), 556-569.

Fahrer, H., Rentsch, H. U., Gerber, N. J., Beyeler, C., Hess, C. W., & Grunig, B. (1988). Knee effusion and reflex inhibition of the quadriceps. A bar to effective retraining. *Journal of Bone and Joint Surgery, 70,* 635-638.

Fitzgerald, G. K., Axe, M. J., & Snyder-Mackler, L. (2000). The efficacy of perturbation training in nonoperative anterior cruciate ligament rehabilitation programs for physically active individuals. *Physical Therapy, 80*(2), 128-151.

Fredericson, M., & Weir, A. (2006). Practical management of iliotibial band friction syndrome in runners. *Clinical Journal of Sport Medicine, 16*(3), 261-268.

Freeman, M. A., & Wyke, B. (1967). The innervation of the knee joint. An anatomical and histological study in the cat. *J Anat, 101,* 505-532.

Fulkerson, J. P. (2002). Current concepts. Diagnosis and treatment of patients with patellofemoral pain. *American Journal of Sports Medicine, 30*(3), 447-456.

Garth, W. P., Jr., & Flowers, K. (1998). Efficacy of knee sleeves in the management of patellofemoral dysfunction. *Athletic Therapy Today, 3,* 23-27.

Gilleard, W., McConnell, J., & Parsons, D. (1998). The effect of patellar taping on the onset of vastus medialis obliquus and vastus lateralis muscle activity in persons with patellofemoral pain. *Physical Therapy, 78,* 25-32.

Gough, J. V., & Ladley, G. (1971). An investigation into the effectiveness of various forms of quadriceps exercises. *Physiotherapy, 57,* 356-361.

Grelsamer, R. P., & Klein, J. R. (1998). The biomechanics of the patellofemoral joint. *Journal of Orthpaedic & Sports Physical Therapy, 28,* 286-298.

Grood, E. S., Suntay, W. J., Noyes, F. R., & Butler, D. L. (1984). Biomechanics of the knee-extension exercise. Effect of cutting the anterior cruciate ligament. *Journal of Bone and Joint Surgery, 66-A,* 725-734.

Gulotta, L. V., & Rodeo, S. A. (2007). Biology of autograft and allograft healing in anterior cruciate ligament reconstruction. *Clinics in Sports Medicine, 26,* 509-524.

Hanten, W. P., & Schulthies, S. S. (1990). Exercise effect on electromyographic activity of the vastus medialis oblique and vastus lateralis muscles. *Physical Therapy, 70,* 561-565.

Harner, C. D., Fu, F. H., Irrgang, J. J., & Vogrin, T. M. (2001). Anterior and posterior cruciate ligament reconstruction in the new Millennium: a global perspective. *Knee Surgery, Sports Traumatology, Arthroscopy, 9*(6), 330-336.

Heckmann, T. P., Barber-Westin, S. D., & Noyes, F. R. (2006). Meniscal repair and transplantation: indications, techniques, rehabilitation, and clinical outcomes. *Journal of Orthopaedic & Sports Physical Therapy, 36*(10), 795-814.

Hertel, J., Earl, J. E., Tsang, K. K. W., & Miller, S. J. (2004). Combining isometric knee extension exercises with hip adduction or abduction does not increase quadriceps EMG activity. *British Journal of Sports Medicine, 38*(2), 210-213.

Hewett, T., Paterno, M., & Myer, G. (2002). Strategies for enhancing proprioception and neuromuscular control of the knee. *Clinical Orthopaedics, 402,* 76-94.

Holmes, S. W., Jr., & Clancy, W. G., Jr. (1998). Clinical classification of patellofemoral pain and dysfunction. *Journal of Orthopaedic & Sports Physical Therapy, 28*(5), 299-306.

Ireland, M. L., Willson, J. D., Ballantyne, B. T., & Davis, I. M. (2003). Strength in females with and without patellofemoral pain. *Journal of Orthopaedic & Sports Physical Therapy, 33,* 671-676.

Irrgang, J. J., Harner, C. D., Fu, F. H., Silbey, M. B., & DiGiacomo, R. (1997). Loss of motion following ACL reconstruction: A second look. *Journal of Sport Rehabilitation, 6,* 213-225.

Isear, J. A., Erickson, J. R., & Worrell, T. W. (1997). EMG analysis of lower extremity muscle recruitment patterns during an unloaded squat. *Medicine & Science in Sports & Exercise, 29*(4), 532-539.

Jenkins, W. L., Munns, S. W., Jayaraman, G., Wertzberger, K. L., & Neely, K. (1997). A measurement of anterior tibial displacement in the closed and open kinetic chain. *Journal of Orthopaedic & Sports Physical Therapy, 25*, 49-56.

Jenkins, W. L., Munns, S. W., & Loudon, J. (1998). Knee joint accessory motion following anterior cruciate ligament allograft reconstruction: a preliminary report. *Journal of Orthopaedic & Sports Physical Therapy, 28*(1), 32-39.

Karlsson, J., Thomee, R., & Sward, L. (1996). Eleven year follow-up of patello-femoral pain syndrome. *Clinical Journal of Sport Medicine, 6*, 22-26.

Kaufman, K. R., An, K.-N., Litchy, W. J., Morrey, B. F., & Chao, E. Y. S. (1991). Dynamic joint forces during knee isokinetic exercise. *American Journal of Sports Medicine, 19*, 305-316.

Keet, J. H. L., Gray, J., Harley, Y., & Lambert, M. I. (2007). The effect of medial patellar taping on pain, strength, and neuromuscular recruitment in subjects with and without patellofemoral pain. *Physiotherapy, 93*, 45-52.

Knight, K. L., Martin, J. A., & Londeree, B. R. (1979). EMG comparison of quadriceps femoris activity during knee extension and straight leg raises. *American Journal of Sports Medicine, 58*, 57-67.

Kowall, M. G., Kolk, G., Nuber, G. W., Cassisi, J. E., & Stern, S. H. (1996). Patellar taping in the treatment of patellofemoral pain. A prospective randomized study. *American Journal of Sports Medicine, 24*, 61-66.

Krosshaug, T., Nakamae, A., Boden, B. P., Engebretsen, L., Smith, G., Slauterbeck, J. R., ll , et al. (2007). Mechanisms of anterior cruciate ligament injury in basketball. *American Journal of Sports Medicine, 35*(3), 359-367.

Kvist, J. (2006). Tibial translation in exercises used early in rehabilitation after anterior cruciate ligament reconstruction exercises to achieve weight-bearing. *Knee, 13*(6), 460-463.

Lange, G. W., Hintermeister, R. A., Schlegel, T., Dillman, C. J., & Steadman, J. R. (1996). Electromyographic and kinematic analysis of graded treadmill walking and the implications for knee rehabilitation. *Journal of Orthopaedic & Sports Physical Therapy, 23*(5), 294-301.

Lattanzio, P. J., Petrella, R. J., Sproule, J. R., & Fowler, P. J. (1997). Effects of fatigue on knee proprioception. *Clinical Journal of Sport Medicine, 7*, 22-27.

Lephart, S. M., Pincivero, D. M., & Rozzi, S. L. (1998). Proprioception of the ankle and knee. *Sports Medicine, 25*(3), 149-155.

Leroux, A., Bélanger, M., & Boucher, J. P. (1995). Pain effect on monosynaptic and polysynaptic reflex inhibition. *Archives of Physical Medicine & Rehabilitation, 76*, 576-582.

Lesher, J. D., Sutlive, T. G., Miller, G. A., Chine, N. J., Garber, M. B., & Wainner, R. S. (2006). Development of a clinical prediction rule for classifying patients with patellofemoral pain syndrome who respond to patellar taping. *Journal of Orthopaedic & Sports Physical Therapy, 36*(11), 854-866.

Lieb, F. J., & Perry, J. (1971). Quadriceps function. An electromyographic study under isometric conditions. *Journal of Bone and Joint Surgery, 53A*, 749-758.

Livingston, L. A. (1998). The quadriceps angle: a review of the literature. *Journal of Orthopaedic & Sports Physical Therapy, 28*, 105-109.

Margheritini, F., Rihn, J., Musahl, V., Mariani, P. P., & Harner, C. (2002). Posterior cruciate ligament injuries in the athlete: An anatomical, biomechanical and clinical review. *Sports Medicine, 32*(6), 393-408.

Markolf, K. L., Gorek, J. F., Kabo, J. M., & Shapiro, M. S. (1990). Direct measurement of resultant forces in the anterior cruciate ligament. An in vitro study performed with a new experimental technique. *Journal of Bone and Joint Surgery, 72A*, 557-567.

Marrale, J., Morrissey, M. C., & Haddad, F. S. (2007). A literature review of autograft and allograft anterior cruciate ligament reconstruction. *Knee Surgery, Sports Traumatology, Arthroscopy, 15*, 690-704.

Mascal, C. L., Landel, R., & Powers, C. (2003). Management of patellofemoral pain targeting hip, pelvis, and trunk muscle function: 2 case reports. *Journal of Orthopaedic & Sports Physical Therapy, 33*(11), 647-660.

McCarty, E. C., Marx, R. G., & DeHaven, K. E. (2002). Meniscus Repair: Considerations in Treatment and Update of Clinical Results. *Clinical Orthopaedics, 402*, 122-134.

McConnell, J. (1986). The management of chondromalacia patellae: a long term solution. *Australian Journal of Physiotherapy, 32*, 215-223.

McDonough, A. L., & Weir, J. P. (1996). The effect of post-surgical edema of the knee joint on reflex inhibition of the quadriceps femoris. *Journal of Sport Rehabilitation, 5*, 172-182.

Meunier, A., Odensten, M., & Good, L. (2007). Long-term results after primary repair or non-surgical treatment of anterior cruciate ligament rupture: a randomized study with a 15-year follow-up. *Scandinavian Journal of Medicine and Science in Sports, 17*(3), 230-237.

Mikkelsen, C., Werner, S., & Eriksson, E. (2000). Closed kinetic chain alone compared to combined open and closed kinetic chain exercises for quadriceps strengthening after anterior cruciate ligament reconstruction with respect to return to sports: a prospective matched follow-up study. *Knee Surgery, Sports Traumatology, Arthroscopy, 8*(6), 337-342.

Mirzabeigi, E., Jordan, C., Gronley, J. K., Rockowitz, N. L., & Perry, J. (1999). Isolation of the vastus medialis oblique muscle during exercise. *American Journal of Sports Medicine, 27*, 50-53.

Mohr, K. J., Kvitne, R. S., Pink, M. M., Fideler, B., & Perry, J. (2003). Electromyography of the quadriceps in patellofemoral pain with patellar subluxation. *Clinical Orthopaedics and Related Research, 415*, 261-271.

Moller, E., Forssblad, M., Hansson, L., Wange, P., & Weidenhielm, L. (2001). Bracing versus nonbracing in rehabilitation after anterior cruciate ligament reconstruction: a randomized prospective study with 2-year follow-up. *Knee Surgery, Sports Traumatology, Arthroscopy, 9*(2), 102-108.

Morrissey, M. C. (1989). Reflex inhibition of thigh muscles in knee injury. Causes and treatment. *Sports Medicine, 7*, 263-276.

Najibi, S., & Albright, J. P. (2005). The use of knee braces, part 1. Prophylactic knee braces in contact sports. *American Journal of Sports Medicine, 33*(4), 602-611.

Orchard, J. W., Fricker, P. A., Abud, A. T., & Mason, B. R. (1996). Biomechanics of iliotibial band friction syndrome in runners. *American Journal of Sports Medicine, 24*(3), 375-379.

Ounpuu, S. (1994). The biomechanics of walking and running. *Clin Sport Med, 13*, 843-863.

Paessler, H. H., & Mastrokalos, D. S. (2003). Anterior cruciate ligament reconstruction using semitendinosus and gracilis tendons, bone patellar tendon, or quadriceps tendon-graft with press-fit fixation without hardware. A new and innovative procedure. *Orthopedic Clinics of North America, 34*(1), 49-64.

Post, W. R. (2005). Patellofemoral pain results of nonoperative treatment. *Clinical Orthopaedics and Related Research, 436*, 55-59.

Powers, C. M. (2003). The influence of altered lower-extremity kinematics on patellofemoral joint dysfunction: A theoretical perspective. *Journal of Orthopaedic & Sports Physical Therapy, 33*, 639-646.

Reider, B. (1996). Medial collateral ligament injuries in athletes. *Sports Med, 21*, 147-156.

Reilly, D. T., & Martens, M. (1972). Experimental analysis of the quadriceps muscle force and patellofemoral joint reaction force for various activities. *Acta Orthop Scand, 43*, 126.

Risberg, M., Mork, M., Jenssen, H., & Holm, I. (2001). Design and implementation of a neuromuscular training program following anterior cruciate ligament reconstruction. *Journal of Orthopaedic & Sports Physical Therapy, 31*(11), 620-631.

Risberg, M. A., Holm, I., Tjomsland, O., Ljunggren, E., & Ekeland, A. (1999). Prospective study of changes in impairments and disabilities after anterior cruciate ligament reconstruction. *J Orthop Sports Phys Ther, 29*, 400-412.

Robinson, R. L., & Nee, R. J. (2007). Analysis of hip strength in females seeking physical therapy treatment for unilateral patellofemoral pain syndrome. *J orthop sports phys ther, 37*(5), 232-238.

Safran, M. R., Harner, C. D., Giraldo, J. L., Lephart, S. M., Borsa, P. A., & Fu, F. H. (1999). Effects of injury and reconstruction of the posterior cruciate ligament on proprioception and neuromuscular control. *Journal of Sport Rehabilitation, 8*(4), 304-321.

Sahli, S., Haithem, R., Elleuch, M. H., Tabka, Z., & Poumarat, G. (2008). Tibiofemoral joint kinetics during squatting with increasing external load. *Journal of Sport Rehabilitation, 17*(3), 300-315.

Scheffler, S. U., Sudkamp, N. P., Gockenjan, A., Hoffmann, R. F., & Weiler, A. (2002). Biomechanical comparison of hamstring and patellar tendon graft anterior cruciate ligament reconstruction techniques: The impact of fixation level and fixation method under cyclic loading. *Arthroscopy, 18*(3), 304-315.

Scheffler, S. U., Unterhauser, F., & Weiler, A. (2008). Graft remodeling and ligamentization after cruciate ligament reconstruction. *Knee Surgery, Sports Traumatology, Arthroscopy, 16*(9), 834-842.

Scott, G. A., Jolly, B. L., & Henning, C. E. (1986). Combined posterior incision and arthroscopic intra-articular repair of the meniscus. *J Bone Joint Surg Am, 68A*, 847-861.

Sekiya, J. K., Haemmerle, M. J., Stabile, K. J., Vogrin, T. M., & Harner, C. D. (2005). Biomechanical analysis of a combined double-bundle posterior cruciate ligament and posterolateral corner reconstruction. *American Journal of Sports Medicine, 33*(3), 360-369.

Sharma, P., & Maffulli, N. (2005). Tendon injury and tendinopathy: healing and repair. *Journal of Bone and Joint Surgery (Am), 87-A*(1), 187-202.

Shelbourne, K. D., Patel, D. V., Adsit, W. S., & Porter, D. A. (1996). Rehabilitation after meniscal repair. *Clinics in Sports Medicine, 15*, 595-612.

Somes, S., Worrell, T. W., Corey, B., & Ingersoll, C. D. (1997). Effects of patellar taping on patellar position in the open and closed kinetic chain: a preliminary study. *Journal of Sport Rehabilitation, 6*, 299-308.

Spencer, J. D., Hayes, K. C., & Alexander, I. J. (1984). Knee joint effusion and quadriceps reflex inhibition in man. *Archives of Physical Medicine & Rehabilitation, 64*, 171-177.

Stanton, P., & Purdham, C. (1989). Hamstring injuries in sprinting: The role of eccentric exercise. *Journal of Orthopaedic & Sports Physical Therapy, 10*(9), 343-349.

Steinkamp, L. A., Dillingham, M. F., Markel, M. D., Hill, J. A., & Kaufman, K. R. (1993). Biomechanical considerations in patellofemoral joint rehabilitation. *Am J Sports Med, 21*, 438-444.

Stone, R. G., Frewin, P. R., & Gonzales, S. (1990). Long-term assessment of arthroscopic meniscus repair: A two- to six-year follow-up study. *Arthroscopy, 6*, 73-78.

Tenuta, J. J., & Arciero, R. A. (1994). Arthroscopic evaluation of meniscal repairs. Factors that effect healing. *American Journal of Sports Medicine, 22*, 797-802.

Travell, J. G., & Simons, D. G. (1992). *Myofascial pain and dysfunction. The trigger point manual. Vol. 2*. Baltimore: Williams and Wilkins.

Tumia, N., & Maffulli, N. (2002). Patellofemoral pain in female athletes. *Sports Medicine and Arthroscopy Review, 10*, 69-75.

Wallace, D. A., Salem, G. J., Salinas, R., & Powers, C. M. (2002). Patellofemoral joint kinetics while squatting with and without an external load. *Journal of Orthopaedic & Sports Physical Therapy, 32*, 141-148.

Wegener, L., Kisner, C., & Nichols, D. (1997). Static and dynamic balance responses in persons with bilateral knee osteoarthritis. *J Orthop Sports Phys Ther, 25*, 13-18.

Wilk, K., Escamilla, R., Fleisig, G., Barrentine, S., Andrews, J., & Boyd, M. (1996). A comparison of tibiofemoral joint forces and electromyographic activity during open and closed kinetic chain exercises. *American Journal of Sports Medicine, 24*(4), 518-527.

Wilk, K. E., Arrigo, C., Andrews, J. R., & Clancy, W. G. (1999). Rehabilitation after anterior cruciate ligament reconstruction in the female athlete. *Journal of Athletic Training, 34*, 177-193.

Wilson, T., Carter, N., & Thomas, G. (2003). A multicenter, single-masked study of medial, neutral, and lateral patellar taping in individuals with patellofemoral pain syndrome. *Journal of Orthopaedic & Sports Physical Therapy, 33*, 437-448.

Witvrouw, E., Sneyers, C., Lysens, L., Victor, J., & Bellemans, J. (1996). Reflex response times of vastus medialis oblique and vastus lateralis in normal subjects and in subjects with patellofemoral pain syndrome. *Journal of Orthopaedic & Sports Physical Therapy, 24*, 160-165.

Worrell, T., Ingersoll, C. D., Bockrath-Pugliese, K., & Minis, P. (1998). Effect of patellar taping and bracing on patellar position as determined by MRI in patients with patellofemoral pain. *Journal of Athletic Training, 33*, 16-20.

Worrell, T. W., Crisp, E., & LaRosa, C. (1998). Electromyographic reliability and analysis of selected lower extremity muscles during lateral step-up conditions. *J Athl Train 33*, 156-162.

Young, A., Stokes, M., & Iles, J. F. (1987). Effects of joint pathology on muscle. *Clin Orthop, 219*, 21-27.

Zeller, B. L., McCrory, J. L., Kibler, W. B., & Uhl, T. L. (2003). Differences in kinematics and electromyographic activity between men and women during the single-legged squat. *Am J sports med, 31*(3), 449-456.

Zwerver, J., Bredeweg, S. W., & Hof, A. L. (2007). Biomechanical analysis of the single-leg decline squat. *Br J Sport Med, 41*(4), 264-268.

Chapter 24

Ahmed, A. M., & Burke, D. L. (1983). In vitro measurement of static pressure distribution in synovial joints: I. Tibial surface of the knee. *Journal of Biomedical Engineering, 105*, 216-225.

Benzon, H. T., Katz, J. A., Benzon, H. A., & Iqbal, M. S. (2003). Piriformis Syndrome: Anatomic Considerations, a New Injection Technique, and a Review of the Literature. *Anesthesiology, 98*(6), 1442-1448.

Binningsley, D. (2003). Tear of the acetabular labrum in an elite athlete. *British Journal of Sports Medicine, 37*(1), 84-88.

Burrnett, R. S., Rocca, G. J., Prather, H., Curry, M., Maloney, W. J., & Clohisy, J. C. (2006). Clinical presentation of patients with tearws of the acetabular labrum. *Journal of Bone and Joint Surgery, 88-A*, 61-66.

Cyriax, J. H. (1977). *Textbook of orthopedic medicine. Vol. 2, Treatment by manipulation, massage and injection.* Baltimore: Williams & Wilkins.

DeDomenico, G. (2007). *Beard's massage principles and practice of soft tissue manipulation.* Philadelphia: Saunders.

Farjo, L. A., Glick, J. M., & Sampson, T. G. (1999). Hip arthroscopy for acetabular labral tears. *Arthroscopy, 15*, 132-137.

Geraci, M. C., Jr. (1994). Rehabilitation of pelvis, hip, and thigh injuries in sports. *Physical Medicine and Rehabilitation Clinics of North America, 5*(1), 157-173.

Geraci, M. C., Jr, & Brown, W. (2005). Evidence-based treatment of hip and pelvic injuries in runners. *Physical Medicine and Rehabilitation Clinics of North America, 16*(3), 711-747.

Gerber, J. M., & Herrin, S. O. (1994). Conservative treatment of calcific trochanteric bursitis. *Journal of Manipulative Physiological Therapeutics, 17*(4), 250-252.

Hammer, W. I. (1993). The use of transverse friction massage in the management of chronic bursitis of the hip or shoulder. *Journal of Manipulative and Physiological Therapeutics, 16*(2), 107-111.

Kibler, W. B. (1995). Biomechanical analysis of the shoulder during tennis activities. *Clinics in Sports Medicine, 14*, 79-85.

Leetun, D. T., Ireland, M. L., Willson, J. D., Ballantyne, B. T., & Davis, I. M. (2004). Core stability measures as risk factors for lower extremity injury in athletes. *Medicine & Science in Sports & Exercise, 36*(6), 926-934.

Loder, R. T., Farley, F., Herzenberg, J., Hensinger, R. N., & Kuhn, J. (1993). Narrow window of bone age in children with slipped capital femoral epiphysis. *Journal of Pediatric Orthopaedics, 13*, 290-293.

Lynch, S. A., & Renstrom, P. A. (1999). Groin injuries in sport. Treatment strategies. *Sports Medicine, 28*(2), 137-144.

Martin, R. L., Trapuzzano, T., Enseki, K. R., Draovitch, P., & Philippon, M. J. (2006). Acetabular Labral Tears of the Hip: Examination and Diagnostic Challenges. *Journal of Orthopaedic & Sports Physical Therapy, 36*(7), 503-515.

Mellman, M. F., McPherson, E. J., Dorr, L. D., & Kwong, K. (1996). Differential diagnosis of back and lower extremity problems. In R. G. Watkins (Ed.), *The spine in sports.* St. Louis: Mosby.

Micheli, L. J., & Coady, C. M. (1997). Approaching hip, pelvis, and groin injuries in athletes. *Biomechanics, 4*, 22-26.

Miller, M. L. (1982). Avulsion fractures of the anterior superior iliac spine in high school track. *Athletic Training, 17*(1), 57-59.

Newman, G., Menducuti, A. D., Zou, K. H., Minas, T., Coblyn, J., Winalski, C. S., et al. (2007). Prevalence of labral tears and cartilage loss in patients with mechanical symptoms of the hip: evaluation using MR arthrography. *Osteoarthritis and Cartilage, 15*(8), 909-917.

O'Kane, J. W. (1999). Anterior hip pain. *American Family Physician, 60*, 1687-1696.

Philippon, M. J. (2001). The role of arthroscopic thermal capsulorrhaphy in the hip. *Clinics in Sports Medicine, 20*(4), 817-829.

Robertson, W. J., Kadrmas, W. R., & Kelly, B. T. (2007). Arthroscopic management of labral tears in the hip: A systematic review. *Clinical Orthopaedics, 455*, 88-92.

Sahrmann, S. (2002). *Diagnosis and treatment of movement impairment syndromes.* St. Louis: Mosby.

Sammarco, G. J. (1983). The dancer's hip. *Clinics in Sports Medicine, 2*(3), 485-498.

Schaberg, J. E., Harper, M. C., & Allen, W. C. (1984). The snapping hip syndrome. *American Journal of Sports Medicine, 12*(5), 361-365.

Travell, J. G., & Simons, D. G. (1992). *Myofascial pain and dysfunction. The trigger point manual. Vol. 2.* Baltimore: Williams and Wilkins.

Tyler, T. F., Nicholas, S. J., Campbell, R. J., & McHugh, M. P. (2001). The association of hip strength and flexibility with the incidence of adductor muscle strains in professional ice hockey players. *American Journal of Sports Medicine, 29*(2), 124-128.

Yamamoto, Y., Hamada, Y., Ide, T., & Usui, I. (2005). Arthroscopic surgery to treat intra-articular type snapping hip. *Arthroscopy, 21*(9), 1120-1125.

INDEX

Note: The italicized *f* and *t* following page numbers refer to figures and tables, respectively.

ABOUT THE AUTHOR

Peggy A. Houglum, **PhD, ATC, PT,** is an associate professor at the Rangos School of Health Sciences at Duquesne University in Pittsburgh. She has nearly 40 years of experience providing patient and athlete care in a variety of settings, including university athletic training facilities, sports medicine clinics, rehabilitation hospitals, acute care hospitals, burn care, workers' compensation clinics, and extended care facilities. She has also served as an athletic trainer with the United States Olympic Sports Festivals, Olympic Games, and World University Games.

Houglum's extensive background as a certified athletic trainer, physical therapist, clinical and classroom educator, and program director provides her with a unique perspective on the appropriate use of therapeutic exercise techniques in rehabilitation programs for treatment of athletic injury.

In 1991, Houglum created the National Athletic Trainers' Association's (NATA) first formal continuing education program. Since that time, Houglum has served as chair of the NATA Continuing Education Committee and as a member of the organization's Education Council and the Council on Employment. In 2002, she was named to the NATA Hall of Fame, the association's highest award, and received NATA's Most Distinguished Athletic Trainer Award in 1996.

Houglum is a member of the American Physical Therapy Association and its Sports Medicine Section. She is also a member of NATA and serves on the NATA's CEPAT committee and the BOC's Role Delineation #6 Committee. Houglum is an associate

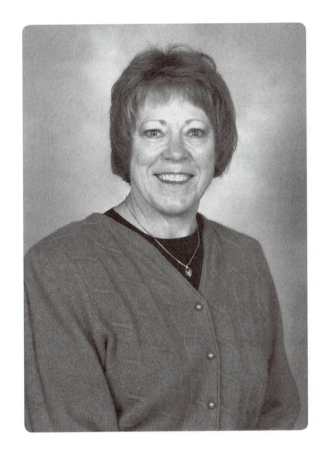

editor for *Sports Rehabilitation* and clinical applications editor of the *Journal of Athletic Training*.

In her free time, Houglum enjoys spending time with family, reading, and painting. She resides in Gibsonia, Pennsylvania.

Athletic Training Education Series

Human Kinetics' Athletic Training Education Series contains six textbooks, each with its own supporting instructional resources. Featuring the work of respected athletic training authorities, the series parallels and expounds on the content areas established by the NATA Executive Committee for Education. To learn more about the books in this series, visit the Athletic Training Education Series website at **www.HumanKinetics.com/AthleticTrainingEducationSeries**.

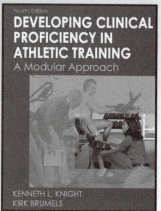

DEVELOPING CLINICAL PROFICIENCY IN ATHLETIC TRAINING
A Modular Approach

KENNETH L. KNIGHT
KIRK BRUMELS

Kenneth L. Knight, PhD, and Kirk Brumels, PhD
©2010 • Spiral-bound
352 pp
ISBN 978-0-7360-8361-4

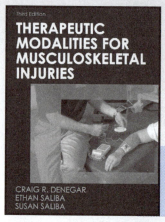

THERAPEUTIC MODALITIES FOR MUSCULOSKELETAL INJURIES

CRAIG R. DENEGAR
ETHAN SALIBA
SUSAN SALIBA

Craig R. Denegar, PhD, ATC, PT, Ethan Saliba, PhD, ATC, PT, and Susan Saliba, PhD, ATC, PT
©2010 • Hardback • 304 pp
Print: ISBN 978-0-7360-7891-7
E-book: ISBN 978-0-7360-8558-8

Ancillaries: instructor guide, test package, image bank
www.HumanKinetics.com/
TherapeuticModalitiesFor
MusculoskeletalInjuries

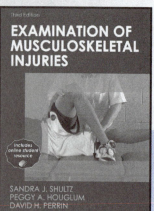

EXAMINATION OF MUSCULOSKELETAL INJURIES

Includes online student resource

SANDRA J. SHULTZ
PEGGY A. HOUGLUM
DAVID H. PERRIN

Sandy J. Shultz, PhD, ATC, CSCS, Peggy A. Houglum, PhD, ATC, PT, and David H. Perrin, PhD, ATC
©2010 • Hardback • 720 pp
Print: ISBN 978-0-7360-7622-7
E-book: ISBN 978-0-7360-8694-3

Ancillaries: instructor guide, test package, image bank
Online Student Resource: examination checklists, tables, full-color photos
www.HumanKinetics.com/
ExaminationOfMusculoskeletalInjuries

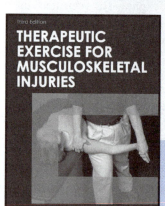

THERAPEUTIC EXERCISE FOR MUSCULOSKELETAL INJURIES

PEGGY A. HOUGLUM

Peggy A. Houglum, PhD, ATC, PT
©2010 • Hardback • 1040 pp
Print: ISBN 978-0-7360-7595-4
E-book: ISBN 978-0-7360-8560-1

Ancillaries: instructor guide, test package, presentation package plus image bank
www.HumanKinetics.com/
TherapeuticExerciseFor
MusculoskeletalInjuries

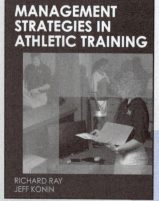

MANAGEMENT STRATEGIES IN ATHLETIC TRAINING

RICHARD RAY
JEFF KONIN

Richard Ray, EdD, ATC, and Jeff Konin, PhD, ATC, PT, FACSM, FNATA
©2011 • Hardback • 360 pp
Print: ISBN 978-0-7360-7738-5
E-book: ISBN 978-1-4504-1623-8

Ancillaries: instructor guide, test package, image bank
www.HumanKinetics.com/
ManagementStrategiesIn
AthleticTraining

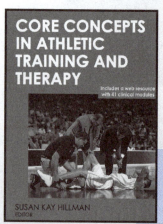

CORE CONCEPTS IN ATHLETIC TRAINING AND THERAPY

Includes a web resource with 41 clinical modules

SUSAN KAY HILLMAN
EDITOR

Susan Kay Hillman, ATC, PT
©2012 • Hardback • 640 pp
Print: ISBN 978-0-7360-8285-3
E-book: ISBN 978-1-4504-2355-7

Ancillaries: instructor guide, test package, image bank, web resource
www.HumanKinetics.com/
CoreConceptsInAthleticTraining
AndTherapy

HUMAN KINETICS
The Information Leader in Physical Activity & Health

For more information:
(800) 747-4457 US • (800) 465-7301 CDN • 44 (0) 113-255-5665 UK
(08) 8372-0999 AUS • 0800 222 062 NZ • (217) 351-5076 International
Or visit **www.HumanKinetics.com**